MOSBY'S

Manual of Diagnostic and Laboratory Tests

Fifth Edition

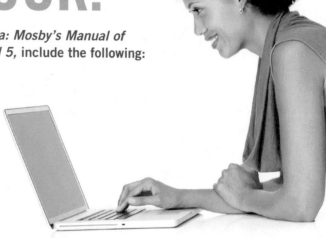

FIFTH EDITION

MOSBY'S
Manual of Diagnostic and Laboratory Tests

Kathleen Deska Pagana, PhD, RN
Professor Emeritus
Department of Nursing
Lycoming College
President, Pagana Keynotes & Presentations
http://www.KathleenPagana.com
Williamsport, Pennsylvania

Timothy J. Pagana, MD, FACS
Medical Director, Emeritus
The Kathryn Candor Lundy Breast Health
    Center and The SurgiCenter
Susquehanna Health System
Williamsport, Pennsylvania

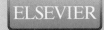

ELSEVIER
MOSBY

3251 Riverport Lane
St. Louis, Missouri 63043

Notices

Knowledge and best practice in this field are constantly changing. As new research and experience broaden our understanding, changes in research methods, professional practices, or medical treatment may become necessary.

Practitioners and researchers must always rely on their own experience and knowledge in evaluating and using any information, methods, compounds, or experiments described herein. In using such information or methods they should be mindful of their own safety and the safety of others, including parties for whom they have a professional responsibility.

With respect to any drug or pharmaceutical products identified, readers are advised to check the most current information provided (i) on procedures featured or (ii) by the manufacturer of each product to be administered, to verify the recommended dose or formula, the method and duration of administration, and contraindications. It is the responsibility of practitioners, relying on their own experience and knowledge of their patients, to make diagnoses, to determine dosages and the best treatment for each individual patient, and to take all appropriate safety precautions.

To the fullest extent of the law, neither the Publisher nor the authors, contributors, or editors, assume any liability for any injury and/or damage to persons or property as a matter of products liability, negligence or otherwise, or from any use or operation of any methods, products, instructions, or ideas contained in the material herein.

International Standard Book Number 978-0-323-08949-4

Senior Content Strategist: Tamara Myers
Content Manager: Jean Sims Fornango
Publishing Services Manager: Deborah L. Vogel
Senior Project Manager: Jodi M. Willard
Design Direction: Margaret Reid

Printed in Canada

Last digit is the print number: 9 8 7 6 5 4 3 2 1

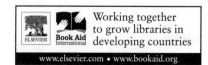

We lovingly dedicate this book to our delightful grandchildren:

Ella Marie Gaul

Jocelyn Elizabeth Gaul

Timothy William Gaul

Justin Aquinas Gaul

Juliana Kathleen Pericci

Luke Michael Pericci

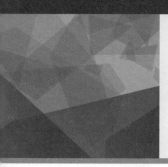

Reviewers

Michael Andary, MD, MS
Professor
College of Osteopathic Medicine
Michigan State University
East Lansing, Michigan

Valerie Bush, PhD, FACB
Clinical Laboratory Director
Bassett Medical Center
Cooperstown, New York

Karmen A. Grant, MS, RN, CNDR
Nursing Instructor
Rogers State University
Claremore, Oklahoma

Joseph Hawkins, MS Ed., CNMT
Associate Professor and Program Director
Nuclear Medicine Technology
Florida Hospital College of Health Sciences
Orlando, Florida

Michael Horner, DO
Department of Michigan State University
Lansing, Michigan

Mary Anne Jessee, MSN, RN
Assistant Professor
School of Nursing
Vanderbilt University
Nashville, Tennessee

Stephen Krau, PhD, RN, CNE
Associate Professor
School of Nursing
Vanderbilt University
Nashville, Tennessee

Geralyn López-de-Victoria, PhD, MS
Science Department Chair
Midlands Technical College
West Columbia, South Carolina

Carla R. Lynch, MS, RN
Nursing Instructor
Rogers State University
Claremore, Oklahoma

Naser Nejadi, BS, MSc
Tehran University of Medical Sciences
Tehran, Iran

Sandra Rome, RN, MN, AOCN
Clinical Nurse Specialist
Cedars-Sinai Medical Center
Los Angeles, California

Bonnie L. Welniak, MSN, RN
Assistant Professor of Nursing
Monroe County Community College
Monroe, Michigan

Preface

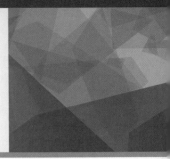

This book provides the user with an up-to-date, extensive manual that allows rapid access to clinically relevant laboratory and diagnostic tests. A unique feature of this manual is its consistent format, which provides a comprehensive approach to laboratory and diagnostic tests. Tests are categorized according to either the method of testing (e.g., x-ray, ultrasound, nuclear scan) or the type of specimen (e.g., blood, urine, stool) used for testing. Every chapter of this book is based on this categorization. Each chapter begins with an alphabetical listing of all tests in the chapter to aid the user in locating discussions quickly. An overview follows the list and contains general information concerning test methods and related patient care.

Chapter 1 includes a discussion of guidelines for proper test preparation and performance. New coding requirements for ordering tests have been added along with a description of common laboratory methods. Standard Precautions and other clinically important information for the health care provider are included to ensure accurate diagnostic and laboratory testing. This information is essential for health care economics so that tests are performed in a timely fashion and do not need to be repeated because of problems in patient preparation, test procedure, or specimen handling. Communication and collaboration with other health care providers are emphasized. The privacy rules resulting from the Health Insurance Portability and Accountability Act (HIPAA) are explained in relationship to diagnostic and laboratory test results.

Throughout the book, information is explained in a comprehensive manner to enhance full understanding of each particular test. Every feature of test discussion is geared to provide complete information in a sequence that best simulates priorities in clinical practice. The following information is provided, whenever possible, for a thorough understanding of each diagnostic test:

- *Name of test.* Tests are listed by their complete name. A complete list of abbreviations and alternative test names follows each main entry.
- *Normal findings.* Normal values are listed, when applicable, for the infant, child, adult, and elderly person. Also, where appropriate, values are separated into categories of male and female. We realize that normal ranges for laboratory tests vary significantly depending on the method of testing and the particular laboratory. For this reason, we strongly encourage the user to check the normal values at the institution where the test is performed. This should be relatively easy because most laboratory reports indicate normal values.
- *Critical values.* These values give an indication of results that are well outside the usual range for normal. These results generally require immediate intervention.
- *Indications.* This section describes the main uses for each test. Emphasis is placed on the type of patient signs and symptoms that lead to the indications for each test.
- *Test explanation.* This section provides a comprehensive description of each test. The explanation includes fundamental information about basic pathophysiology related to the test methods, what diseases the test results may indicate, and the location where the test is generally performed. Also, in this section, patient sensation, test duration, and the type of health care professional involved in the testing are described.

- *Contraindications.* This information alerts the user to patients who should not have the test performed. As in other segments of the book, each contraindication is fully explained with an in-depth rationale. Patients frequently highlighted in this section include those who are pregnant, who are allergic to iodinated or contrast dye, or who have bleeding disorders.
- *Potential complications.* This section alerts the user to potential problems that will necessitate astute posttesting assessments and interventions. Not only is each complication fully explained in detail, but also patient symptoms and appropriate interventions are described. For example, a potential complication of an intravenous pyelogram is renal failure, especially in the elderly patient. An appropriate intervention may be to hydrate the patient before the test and force fluids afterward.
- *Interfering factors.* This section includes a thorough discussion of factors that can invalidate or alter the test results. An important feature of this section is the inclusion of drugs that can interfere with test results. Drugs that increase or decrease test values are indicated by a drug icon (▤) for quick access.
- *Procedure and patient care.* This section emphasizes the role of nurses and other health care providers in diagnostic and laboratory testing by addressing psychosocial and physiologic interventions. Patient teaching priorities are noted with a special icon (▨) to highlight information to be communicated to patients. For quick location of essential information concerning the testing procedure, this section is divided into before, during, and after time sequences.
    - *Before.* This section addresses the need to explain the procedure and to allay patient concerns or anxieties. Dietary restrictions, bowel preparations, baseline pretest assessment, and the need for informed consent are discussed.
    - *During.* This section provides a complete and thorough description of the testing procedure, alternative procedures, and methods of testing. In most instances, a step-by-step description of testing procedures is provided. This information is important because all health care providers involved in the particular test should have a good understanding of what the procedure entails so they can assist more completely in the testing process.
    - *After.* This section includes vital information that the nurse or other health care provider should know concerning postprocedure care of the patient. This includes information on specific posttest assessment, medication administration, recognition of posttest complications (with suggestions for interventions), home care, and follow-up.
- *Test results and clinical significance.* As the name implies, this section describes the significance of the test findings. A unique feature of this manual, compared with other books on diagnostic and laboratory tests, is an extensive discussion of the pathophysiology of the disease process and how it relates to the test result. This provides enhanced understanding of the diagnostic test and better understanding of many disease processes.
- *Related tests.* This section, another unique feature of the text, includes a list of tests that are related to the main test under discussion. This includes tests that provide similar information, tests that provide confirmatory information, and other tests used to evaluate the same organ, disease process, or symptom complex. A short description and page numbers for all related tests are included for ease in cross-referencing. This aids the reader to develop a broader understanding of diagnostic testing and indicates where the reader may go to obtain more information on the topic of interest.

This logical format emphasizes clinically relevant information. The clarity of the format facilitates a full understanding of content essential to both students and health care providers, and its uniformity allows the user to quickly recognize where information of interest may be found.

Multiple colors have been used to help locate tests, highlight critical information, and generally improve the readability of the text. Another key feature is the use of color photographs and illustrations throughout the book. Many tables are also included to simplify or summarize complex material regarding clinical care, test categories, or disease processes.

Feature boxes are used throughout the book to highlight and summarize important clinical data. They allow the reader to assimilate important information at a glance. There are three types of feature boxes: Clinical Priorities, Age-Related Concerns, and Home Care Responsibilities. *Clinical Priorities* boxes emphasize pertinent information specific to understanding and performing a particular test. For example, coagulation studies must be assessed before invasive studies (e.g., liver biopsy) that may cause bleeding. Chest x-ray examinations should be performed after procedures (e.g., pleural biopsy) that may cause a pneumothorax. *Age-Related Concerns* boxes primarily address pediatric and geriatric priorities. For example, the risk for dye-induced renal failure is emphasized in the dehydrated elderly patient scheduled for an intravenous pyelogram. The bowel preparation for children of different ages is described in the barium enema study. *Home Care Responsibilities* boxes focus on factors that need to be addressed after a test is performed. With an increasing number of procedures being performed on an outpatient basis, the patient has the responsibility for detecting problems and knowing what to do when they occur. Often, the patient returns home with instructions or guidelines for recognizing problems such as infection, bleeding, or urinary retention.

New to this edition is a comprehensive listing of diagnostic and laboratory tests used when evaluating a patient with a common disease or condition. These are based on the International Classification of Disease (ICD) codes (see p. xi). This alphabetical list should be invaluable to readers who want to know the testing possibilities for common problems such as adrenal abnormalities, AIDS, Alzheimer's disease, bowel obstruction, breast cancer, and others. For emphasis, this material is placed before Chapter 1.

Also new is a description of commonly performed laboratory methods, which is placed in Chapter 1. This section explains methods used to evaluate blood, urine, spinal fluid, and other specimens. Methods such as latex agglutination, agglutination inhibition, hemagglutination, electrophoresis, immunoassay, polymerase chain reaction, and FISH techniques are examples.

Appendix A, Alphabetical List of Tests, helps the user locate specific tests at a glance. *Appendix B, List of Tests by Body System,* familiarizes the user with other related studies the patient or client may need or the user may want to review. This information should be especially useful for students and health care providers working in specialized areas. For example, all tests related to infertility are listed in the Reproductive System section. *Appendix C* provides a list of *Panel Tests* such as cardiac enzymes, lipid profile, liver profile, and thyroid studies. *Appendix D* contains a list of *Abbreviations for Diagnostic and Laboratory Tests.* Finally, a comprehensive Index includes the names of all tests and their synonyms and other relevant terms found within the tests. Typical Abbreviations and Units of Measurement are located on the inside cover.

Many new studies such as anti-glycan antibodies, laboratory genetics, neuron-specific enolase, galectin-3, and ProstaScint scan have been added. All other studies have been revised and updated. Outdated tests have been eliminated. Illustrations and photographs have been extensively updated, and many new ones have been added.

We sincerely thank Mosby/Elsevier for invaluable assistance and dedication to our books over 30 years. We also thank our editors—Jean Sims Fornango, Brandi Flagg, and Jodi Willard—for their enthusiasm and support. We invite comments from users of this book so that we may improve our goal of providing useful and relevant diagnostic and laboratory test information to users of future editions.

Kathleen D. Pagana

Timothy J. Pagana

Contents

Testing for Common Diseases and Conditions

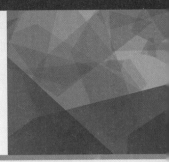

This listing is designed to help the health care provider focus on possible tests ordered with certain common diseases or conditions. The numbers and letters reflect ICD-10 codes, which are described on pp. 1 and 2.

Adrenal Functional Abnormalities: E 24-27, E 35, C 74

- 17-Hydroxycorticosteroids
- 17-Ketosteroids
- 21 Hydroxylase antibodies
- Adrenal steroid precursors
- Adrenocorticotropic hormone (ACTH)
- Adrenocorticotropic hormone stimulation test
- Adrenocorticotropic hormone stimulation with metyrapone
- Aldosterone
- Cortisol, blood
- Cortisol, urine
- Dexamethasone suppression
- Glucose

AIDS/Immunologic Deficiency: B 20-24

- Bone marrow aspiration
- Cell surface immunophenotyping
- Complement assay
- Complete blood count (CBC)
- Immunoglobulin quantification
- Cytokines
- Fungal testing
- Hepatitis virus studies
- HIV drug resistance testing
- HIV serology
- HIV RNA quantification
- Human lymphocyte phenotyping
- Immunoglobulin quantification
- Protein quantification
- Tuberculosis testing
- Viral Testing: cytomegalovirus, toxoplasmosis, herpes simplex, Epstein-Barr

Allergy: T 78

- Allergy blood testing
- Allergy skin testing
- Cutaneous immunofluorescence antibodies
- HLA-B27
- Immunoglobulin quantification

Alzheimer's Disease/Dementia: G 30, F 00-03

- Amyloid beta protein
- Cerebrospinal fluid analysis
- CT scan of the brain
- Electroencephalography
- Electrolytes
- MRI of the brain
- Nuclear brain scan
- PET scan
- Tau protein
- Thyroid function studies

Anemia: D 50, D 51, D 55, D 60-61, D 65

- Anti-parietal cell antibody
- Blood smear
- Bone marrow biopsy
- Complete blood count (CBC)
- 2,3-Diphosphoglycerate
- Erythropoietin
- Ferritin
- Folic acid
- Heinz body
- Hematocrit (Hct)
- Hemoglobin (Hgb)
- Hemoglobin electrophoresis
- Intrinsic factor
- Iron testing

- Alkaline phosphatase
- Alpha$_1$-antitrypsin
- Alpha-fetoprotein
- Ammonia
- Antimitochondrial antibody
- Anti-liver/kidney microsomal antibody
- Anti-nuclear antibody
- Anti-smooth muscle antibody
- Antithrombin III
- Aspartate aminotransferase
- Bilirubin
- Ceruloplasmin
- Cold agglutinins
- Complete blood count (CBC)
- Copper
- Electrolytes
- Endoscopic retrograde cholangiopancreatography (ERCP)
- Ethyl alcohol
- Febrile agglutinins
- Gamma glutamyl transpeptidase
- Hepatitis virus studies
- Immunoglobulin quantification
- Iron
- Lactic dehydrogenase
- Leucine aminopeptidase
- Liver biopsy
- Liver/spleen scan
- 5′-Nucleotidase
- Paracentesis
- Prothrombin time
- Urine for bilirubin and urobilinogen
- Zinc

Coagulation Abnormalities: D 68, P 61

- Activated clotting time
- Antithrombin III
- Bilirubin
- Coagulating factor concentration
- Complete blood count (CBC)
- D-Dimer
- DIC screening
- Fibrinogen
- Partial thromboplastin time (PTT)
- Plasminogen
- Plasminogen activator inhibitor-1 (PAI-1) antigen
- Platelet aggregation
- Platelet antibody

- Platelet count
- Platelet function assay
- Protein C, protein S
- Prothrombin time (PT)
- Thromboelastography
- Thrombosis indicators

Colitis: A 00-09, K 50-52

- Anti-glycan antibody
- *Clostridium difficile* testing
- Lactoferrin
- Stool culture
- Stool for ova and parasites

Colorectal Cancer: C 17-21

- Barium enema
- Carcinoembryonic antigen (CEA)
- Colon cancer tumor analysis
- Colonoscopy
- CT scan of the abdomen
- Genetic testing
- Septin 9 DNA methylation assay
- Sigmoidoscopy
- Stool for occult blood
- Ultrasound of the rectum

Coma: R 40

- Alcohol
- Ammonia
- Anion gap
- Arterial blood gases (ABG)
- Carboxyhemoglobin
- Electrolytes
- Ethyl alcohol
- Glucose
- Ketones
- Lactic acid
- Osmolality, blood
- Osmolality, urine
- Salicylate
- Substance abuse testing

Congestive Heart Failure: I 50

- Anti-myocardial antibody
- Cardiac catheterization
- Cardiac enzymes
- Cardiac nuclear scanning
- Chest x-ray
- Complete blood count (CBC)

- Creatine kinase
- Drug monitoring
- Echocardiography
- Electrocardiography (EKG)
- Electrolytes
- Erythropoietin
- Lipoproteins
- MRI of the heart
- Natriuretic peptides
- Pericardiocentesis
- PET scan
- Thyroid function studies
- Total blood volume
- Transesophageal echocardiography
- Triglycerides
- Viral studies

Coronary Occlusive Disease: I 20-25

- Aldolase
- Anti-myocardial antibody
- Apolipoproteins
- Aspartate aminotransferase
- Cardiac nuclear scanning
- Creatinine kinase
- D-Dimer
- Echocardiography
- Electrocardiography
- Homocysteine
- Ischemia-modified albumin
- Lactic dehydrogenase
- Lipoprotein-associated phospholipase
- Lipoproteins
- Magnesium
- Microalbumin
- MRI of the heart
- Myoglobin
- PET scan
- Triglycerides
- Troponins

Diabetes: E10-14

- Anion gap
- C-peptide
- Diabetes mellitus autoantibody panel
- Electrolytes
- Glucagon
- Glucose tolerance
- Glucose, blood
- Glucose, postprandial

- Glucose, urine
- Glycosylated hemoglobin
- Insulin assay
- Lactic acid
- Lipid profile
- Ketones
- Lactic acid
- Microalbumin
- Osmolality, blood
- Osmolality, urine
- Urinalysis

Diarrhea: A02-09

- Anti-glycan antibodies
- Colonoscopy
- Carcinoid studies
- *Clostridium difficile* testing
- D-xylose absorption
- Febrile antibodies
- Electrolytes
- Fecal fat
- Gastrin
- Lactose tolerance
- Pancreatic enzymes
- Prealbumin
- Stool for occult blood
- Stool for ova and parasites

Dysfunctional Uterine Bleeding: N 85, N 92-93

- Activated thromboplastin time (aPTT)
- Complete blood count
- CT scan of the abdomen and pelvis
- Endometrial biopsy
- Estrogen fractions
- Follicular stimulating hormone (FSH)
- HCG/pregnancy test
- Hysteroscopy
- Laparoscopy
- Luteinizing hormone (LH)
- Papanicolaou test/ThinPrep
- Platelet count
- Prothrombin time (PT)
- STD testing
- Ultrasound of the pelvis

Gallbladder/Biliary Disease: C 22-24, K 80/K 87

- Abdomen ultrasound
- Alanine aminotransferase (ALT)

- Alkaline phosphatase (ALP)
- Amylase
- Bilirubin, blood and urine
- Cholangiography
- Electrolytes
- Endoscopic retrograde cholangiopancreatography (ERCP)
- Gallbladder nuclear scanning
- Laparoscopy
- Leucine aminopeptidase (LAP)
- Lipase
- Magnetic resonance cholangiopancreatography

Gastrointestinal Bleeding: K 92

- Blood typing
- BUN
- Coagulation panel (see Appendix C)
- Complete blood count (CBC)
- Esophagogastroduodenoscopy
- Gastrointestinal bleeding scan
- Sigmoidoscopy/colonoscopy
- Stool for occult blood

Hematuria: R 31

- Antiglomerular basement membrane antibody
- Complete blood count (CBC)
- Creatinine/BUN
- Electrolytes
- Kidney biopsy
- Myoglobin
- Pyelography
- Streptococcus
- Urinalysis
- Urine culture and sensitivity

Hemolysis: T 80, P 55

- Alanine aminotransferase (ALT)
- Blood smear
- Complete blood count (CBC)
- Coombs test, direct
- Creatinine/BUN
- Electrolytes
- Erythrocyte fragility
- Haptoglobin
- Myoglobin
- Reticulocyte count

Hypertension: I 13-15

- Aldosterone
- Arteriography, kidney
- Catecholamines
- Cortisol
- Creatinine/BUN
- Creatinine clearance
- Electrolytes
- Metanephrines
- Magnetic resonance angiography, kidney
- Renin
- Thyroxine, triiodothyronine, TSH
- Tilt table testing
- Total blood volume
- Urinalysis
- Vanillylmandelic acid (VMA)

Infertility: N 97, N 46

- Anti-spermatozoal antibody
- Estrogen fractionation
- Follicle-stimulating hormone (FSH)
- Human chorionic gonadotropin (pregnancy tests)
- Hysterosalpingogram
- Luteinizing hormone
- Papanicolaou smear/thin prep
- Progesterone
- Semen analysis
- Sims-Huhner test
- Testosterone
- Thyroid function studies
- Ultrasound of the pelvis

Leukemia/Lymphoma: C 81-96

- Bence Jones protein
- 11-Beta prostaglandin
- Blood smear
- Bone marrow biopsy
- Cell surface immunophenotyping
- Complete blood count (CBC)
- Cryoglobulins
- Cytokines
- Human T-cell lymphotrophic virus
- Microglobulin
- Proteins
- White blood cell count

Liver Diseases/Cirrhosis: K 70-77

- Alanine aminotransferase (ALT)
- Aldolase
- Alkaline phosphatase (ALP)
- Alpha-fetoprotein
- Ammonia
- Anti-liver/kidney microsomal antibody
- Antimitochondrial antibody
- Aspartate aminotransferase (AST)
- Bilirubin
- CT scan of the liver
- Gamma glutamyl transpeptidase (GGTP)
- Hepatitis virus studies
- Lactic dehydrogenase (LDH)
- Leucine aminopeptidase (LAP)
- Liver biopsy
- Liver/spleen scan
- MRI of the liver
- 5′-Nucleotidase
- Paracentesis
- Prealbumin
- Ultrasound of the liver

Lung Cancer: C 34, C 38, C 39

- Alpha$_1$-antitrypsin
- Bone scan
- Bronchoscopy
- Chest x-ray
- CT scan of the chest
- Lung biopsy
- Mediastinoscopy
- Neuron-specific enolase
- PET scan
- Pleural biopsy
- Pulmonary function tests
- Sputum cytology
- Thoracentesis and fluid analysis
- Thoracoscopy

Lupus Erythematosus: L 93, M 32

- Antichromatin antibody
- Anticardiolipin antibody
- Anti-DNA antibody
- Anti-extractable nuclear antigen
- Antinuclear antibody
- Complement assay
- Cryoglobulins
- Cutaneous immunofluorescence antibodies
- Erythrocyte sedimentation rate (ESR)
- Immunoglobulin quantification
- Ribosome P antibodies

Maternal/Fetal Evaluation: O 00-99

- Abdominal ultrasound
- Alpha-fetoprotein
- Amino acid profiles
- Amniocentesis
- Apt test
- Blood typing
- Chorionic villus sampling (CVS)
- Chromosome karyotype
- Cytomegalovirus testing
- Fetal biophysical profile
- Fetal contraction stress test (CST)
- Fetal fibronectin
- Fetal hemoglobin testing
- Fetal nonstress test (NST)
- Fetal nuchal translucency
- Fetal oximetry
- Fetal scalp blood pH
- Fetoscopy
- Genetic testing
- Glucose tolerance test (GTT)
- Hepatitis virus studies
- Herpes simplex testing
- Hexosaminidase
- Human chorionic gonadotropin (pregnancy tests)
- Human placental lactogen
- Immunoglobulin quantification
- Laboratory genetics
- Maternal screen testing
- Newborn metabolic screening
- Papanicolaou test/ThinPrep
- Pelvic ultrasonography
- Pregnancy-associated plasma protein
- Pregnanediol
- Progesterone assay
- Rubella/rubeola titer
- Sexually transmitted disease culture
- Thyroid testing
- Thyroxine
- TORCH
- Toxoplasmosis antibody
- Urinalysis

Menopause: N 95

- Bone mineral density scan
- Estrogen fractionation
- Follicular stimulating hormone (FSH)
- Luteinizing hormone (LH)
- Mammogram
- Papanicolaou test/ThinPrep

Osteoporosis: M 80

- Alkaline phosphatase (ALP)
- Bone densitometry
- Bone turnover markers
- Spinal x-rays
- Vertebral fracture analysis
- Vitamin D

Ovarian Cancer: C 57

- CA-125
- Chest x-ray
- Complete blood count (CBC)
- CT scan of the abdomen and pelvis
- Laparoscopy
- Metabolic assay (see Appendix C)
- Paracentesis
- Pelvic ultrasound
- Pyelography
- Sigmoidoscopy

Pancreatitis: K 85-86

- Amylase, blood
- Amylase, urine
- Bilirubin
- CA 19-9
- Cholesterol
- CT scan of the abdomen
- Endoscopic retrograde cholangiopancreatography (ERCP)
- Gallbladder ultrasound
- Lipase
- Lipoproteins
- Magnetic resonance cholangiopancreatography (MRCP)
- MRI of the pancreas and biliary tract
- Pancreatobiliary FISH testing
- Triglycerides
- Ultrasound of the pancreas

Parathyroid Functional Abnormalities: E 20-E 21, C 75

- Alkaline phosphatase (ALP)
- Bone densitometry
- Bone turnover markers
- BUN
- Creatinine
- Creatinine clearance
- Calcium, blood
- Calcium, urine
- Magnesium
- Parathyroid hormone (PTH)
- Parathyroid scan
- Phosphate

Peptic Ulcer: K 25-30

- Barium swallow
- Complete blood count (CBC)
- Esophageal function studies
- Esophagogastroduodenoscopy (EGD)
- Gastrin
- Gastroesophageal reflux scan
- *Helicobacter pylori* testing
- Upper gastrointestinal tract x-ray
- Urea breath test

Pheochromocytoma: C 74

- Abdominal ultrasound
- Catecholamines
- CT scan of the adrenal glands
- Homovanillic acid (HVA)
- Metanephrine, plasma free
- MRI
- Pheochromocytoma suppression and provocative testing
- Vanillylmandelic acid (VMA)

Pituitary Functional Abnormalities: E 22-23, C 75

- Adrenocorticotropic hormone (ACTH)
- Adrenocorticotropic hormone stimulation with metyrapone
- Antidiuretic hormone (ADH)
- Cortisol, blood
- CT scan of the brain
- Dexamethasone suppression test
- Electrolytes
- Growth hormone

- Growth hormone stimulation test
- Insulin-like growth factor
- MRI of the brain
- Prolactin level
- Thyroid releasing hormone
- Thyroid stimulating hormone (TSH)
- Thyroid stimulating hormone stimulation test
- Thyroxine (T_4)
- Triiodothyronine (T_3)

Pneumonia: J 09-18

- Alpha$_1$-antitrypsin
- Arterial blood gases (ABG)
- Blood culture and sensitivity
- Chest x-ray
- Cold agglutinins
- Complete blood count (CBC)
- CT scan of the lung
- Fungal testing
- Legionnaires disease antibody
- *Mycoplasma pneumoniae* antibodies
- Pulmonary function studies
- SARS virus testing
- Sputum culture and sensitivity
- Virus testing

Prostate Cancer: C 61

- Acid phosphatase
- Bone scan
- CT scan of the pelvis
- Cystoscopy
- MRI of the prostate
- PET scan
- ProstaScint scan
- Prostate and rectal ultrasound
- Prostate specific antigen (PSA)
- Ultrasound of the abdomen
- Ultrasound of the prostate and rectum
- Urine flow studies

Pulmonary Disease Acute/Chronic: J 00-99

- Alpha$_1$-antitrypsin
- Arterial blood gases (ABG)
- Bronchoscopy
- Chest x-ray
- CO_2 content

- CT scan of the chest
- Drug monitoring
- Oximetry
- Pulmonary function tests
- Sputum for culture and sensitivity
- Sputum cytology

Renal Disease: N 00-19

- BUN/creatinine
- Creatinine clearance
- CT scan of the abdomen
- Electrolytes
- Microalbumin
- Microglobulin
- Neutrophil gelatinase–associated lipocalin
- Osmolality, blood/urine
- PET scan
- Pyelography
- Renal biopsy
- Renal scan
- Ultrasound of the kidney
- Urinalysis
- Urine culture and sensitivity

Renal Failure: N 17-19

- Aluminum/chromium
- Anion gap
- Arterial blood gases (ABG)
- BUN/creatinine
- CO_2 content
- Complete blood count (CBC)
- Creatinine clearance
- Electrolytes, blood/urine
- Homocysteine
- Immunoglobulin quantification
- Magnesium
- Microglobulin
- Myoglobin
- Osmolality, blood/urine
- Phosphate
- Protein quantification
- Pyelography
- Renal biopsy
- Renal scan
- Uric acid
- Urinalysis

Sexually Transmitted Diseases: A 50-64

- Chlamydia
- Herpes simplex
- Human papillomavirus (HPV)
- Papanicolaou smear
- Sexually transmitted disease culture
- Syphilis detection
- Ultrasound of the pelvis

Shortness of Breath J 44, J 45

- Arterial blood gases
- Chest x-ray
- CO_2 content
- Complete blood count (CBC)
- CT scan of the chest
- D-Dimer
- Electrocardiography (EKG)
- Lung scan
- Oximetry

Sleep Apnea: P 28, G 47

- Chest x-ray
- Oximetry
- Sleep studies

Streptococcus Infection: A38, A 40

- Antiglomerular basement membrane
- Complement assay
- Streptococcus serology
- Throat and nose culture

Stroke Syndrome: I 60-69

- Activated partial thromboplastin time (aPTT)
- Brain scan
- Carotid artery duplex scan
- CT scan of the brain
- D-Dimer
- Echocardiography
- Electrolytes
- Homocysteine
- Lipoprotein-associated phospholipase
- Lumbar puncture and cerebral spinal fluid analysis
- MRI of the brain
- Platelet count

- Prothrombin time (PT)
- Transesophageal echocardiography (TEE)

Thrombocytopenia: D 69

- Bone marrow biopsy
- Capillary fragility test
- Complete blood count (CBC)
- Platelet antibody
- Platelet count
- Platelet mean volume
- Tourniquet test

Thromboembolism: D 68, I 74

- Anticardiolipin antibody
- Antithrombin activity and antigen assay
- Arterial blood gases (ABG)
- CT pulmonary angiography
- D-Dimer
- Factor V-Leiden
- Lung scan
- Oximetry
- Partial thromboplastin time (PTT)
- Plasminogen
- Plasminogen activator inhibitor-1 (PAI-1)
- Platelet count
- Prothrombin time
- Pulmonary angiography
- Thrombosis indicators
- Thromboelastography
- Venography, lower extremity
- Venous duplex scan

Thyroid Functional Abnormalities: E 00-07, C 73

- Antithyroglobulin antibody
- Antithyroid peroxidase antibody
- CT scan of the thyroid
- Thyroglobulin
- Thyroid scan
- Thyroid stimulating hormone (TSH)
- Thyroid stimulating hormone stimulation
- Thyroid stimulating immunoglobulins
- Thyroid ultrasonography
- Thyrotropin releasing hormone
- Thyroxine (T_4), total and free
- Thyroxine binding globulin
- Triiodothyronine (T_3)

Transfusion Reaction: T 80

- Blood culture
- Blood typing
- Complete blood count (CBC)
- Coombs test, direct
- Coombs test, indirect
- Haptoglobin
- HLA-B27
- Neutrophil antibody screen
- Urinalysis

Tuberculosis: A 15-19

- Acid-fast bacilli (AFB)
- Chest x-ray
- CT scan of the chest
- Tuberculin skin testing
- Tuberculosis culture
- Tuberculosis testing

Urinary Stones: N 20-23

- BUN
- Calcium
- Creatinine
- CT scan the abdomen

- Electrolytes
- KUB
- MRI
- Pyelography
- Renal ultrasound
- Uric acid, urine/serum
- Urinalysis
- Urinary stone analysis
- Urine culture and sensitivity

Vascular Disease: I 65-70, I 77

- Apolipoprotein
- Arteriography
- Fluorescein angiography
- Glucose
- Homocysteine
- Intravascular ultrasound
- Lactic acid
- Lipoprotein associated phospholipase
- Lipoproteins
- Plethysmography, arterial
- Triglycerides
- Vascular ultrasound studies

Guidelines for Proper Test Preparation and Performance

 Overview

A complete evaluation of patients with signs or symptoms of disease usually requires a thorough history and physical examination, as well as efficient diagnostic testing. The correct use of diagnostic testing can confirm or eliminate the presence of disease and improve the cost efficiency of screening tests in a community of people without signs or symptoms of disease. Finally, appropriate and thoughtfully timed use of diagnostic testing allows monitoring of disease and treatment.

Furthermore, health care economics demands that laboratory and diagnostic testing be performed accurately and in a timely fashion. Tests should not have to be repeated because of improper patient preparation, test procedures, or specimen collection technique. The following guidelines will describe the responsibilities of health care providers to ensure safety and accuracy in diagnostic testing.

Patient education is the single most important factor in ensuring accuracy and success of test results. All phases (before, during, and after) of the testing process must be thoroughly explained to the patient. A complete understanding of these factors is essential to the development of nursing processes and standards of care for diagnostic testing.

The interpretation of diagnostic testing is no longer left to the physician alone. In today's complex environment of high-tech testing and economic restrictions, individuals representing many health care professions must be able to interpret diagnostic tests to develop a timely and effective treatment plan.

CODING FOR DIAGNOSTIC AND LABORATORY TESTS

The International Classification of Diseases, Clinical Modification (ICD-CM) is used to code and classify disease (morbidity data). The ICD-Procedure Coding System (PCS) is used to code inpatient procedures. "ICD-10" is the abbreviated way to refer to 10th revision of these codes. In October

2014, use of ICD-10 will be mandated as a HIPAA requirement. These codes provide an alphanumeric designation for diagnoses and inpatient procedures. These codes are developed, monitored, and copyrighted by the World Health Organization. In the United States, the NCHS (National Center for Health Statistics) which is part of CMS (Centers for Medicare and Medicaid Services) oversees the ICD codes. Using these codes, government health authorities can track diseases and causes of death, and compare mortality. All of the patient's diseases and conditions are converted to an ICD code.

This information is required for use by third-party health care payers and providers and all points of service. Each diagnostic test must reflect the ICD code that most accurately identifies the patient's medical condition. Accurate coding is necessary so that data can be accurately collected, testing accurately interpreted, and medical care properly reimbursed. Complying with this coding requirement is no small task because there are there are about 140,000 codes in the ICD-10 catalogs. See p. xi for a listing of common codes. For additional information about this coding requirement, see http://www.cdc.gov/nchs/icd/icd10.htm; http://www.cms.gov/Medicare/Coding/ICD10/downloads/ICD10FAQs.pdf.

LABORATORY METHODS

To understand laboratory diagnostic testing, it is helpful to have a basic understanding of commonly performed laboratory methods that can be used on blood, urine, spinal fluid, and other bodily specimens. Most laboratory diagnostic tests use serologic and immunologic reactions between an antibody and an antigen. *Precipitation* is a visible expression of the aggregation of soluble antigens. *Agglutination* is a visible expression of the aggregation of particulate antigens or antibodies. As the specimen is progressively diluted, persistent precipitation or agglutination indicates greater concentrations of the antigen or antibody. Dilution techniques are therefore used to quantify the pathologic antigen or antibody in the specimen. Commonly used laboratory methods and their variations are described in the following.

Latex Agglutination

Latex agglutination is a common laboratory method in which latex beads (that become visibly obvious when agglutination occurs) are coated with antibody molecules. When mixed with the patient's specimen containing a particular antigen, agglutination will be visibly obvious. C-reactive proteins are identified by this method. In an alternative latex agglutination method (for example, as needed for pregnancy testing or rubella testing), latex beads are coated with a specific antigen. In the presence of antibodies in the patient's specimen to that specific antigen on the latex particles, visible agglutination occurs.

Agglutination Inhibition

Agglutination inhibition is another laboratory method based on the agglutination process. In this process, if one is trying to identify a particular molecule, for example hCG, the patient's specimen is incubated with anti-hCG. Latex particles coated with hCG are then added to the mixture. If the patient's specimen contains hCG, those molecules will attach to the anti-hCG during incubation leaving no anti-hCG molecules to attach to the hCG coated latex beads. Therefore, agglutination would not occur because the patient's endogenous hCG "inhibited" the agglutination.

Hemagglutination

Hemagglutination laboratory methods are used to identify antibodies to antigens on the cell surface of red blood cells (RBCs). Like latex, RBC agglutination is visible. Blood typing for transfusions uses this laboratory method. In an alternate method of hemagglutination, different antigens can be bound to the RBC surface. When added to the patient's specimen, specific antibodies can be identified by RBC agglutination.

Electrophoresis

Electrophoresis is an analytic laboratory method where an electrical charge is applied to a medium on which the patient's specimen has been placed. Migration of charged molecules (particularly proteins) in the specimen can be separated in an electrical field. Proteins can then be identified based on their rate of migration. Serum protein electrophoresis utilizes this method.

Immunoelectrophoresis. Immunoelectrophoresis is a laboratory method that allows the previously electrophoresed proteins to act as antigens to which known specific antibodies are added. This provides specific protein identification. With dilution techniques as described, these particular proteins can be quantified. This method is used to identify gammopathies, hemoglobinopathies, and Bence Jones proteins.

Immunofixation Electrophoresis. Immunofixation electrophoresis (IFE) is particularly helpful in the identification of certain diseases. In this method, a specific known antibody is added to a previously electrophoresed specimen. The antigen/antibody complexes become fixed (that is attached) to the electrophoretic gel medium. When the non-fixed proteins are washed away, the protein immune complexes that remain fixed to the gel are stained with a protein-sensitive stain and can be identified and quantified. IFE is particularly helpful in identifying proteins that exist in very small quantities in the serum, urine, or CSF.

Immunoassay

Immunoassay is an important laboratory method of diagnosing disease. In the past, *radioimmunoassay (RIA)* was performed using a radioactive label that could identify an antibody/antigen complex at very low concentrations. Unfortunately, there are significant drawbacks of using radioactive isotopes as labels. Radioactive labels have a short half-life and are hard to keep on the shelf. These labels require considerable care to avoid environmental exposure. And finally, the costs associated with disposal of radioactive waste are high.

Enzyme-Linked Immunosorbent Assay. *Enzyme linked immunosorbent assay (ELISA)* techniques are able to detect immunocomplexes more easily when compared to RIA. This ELISA technique (also known as *enzyme immunoassay [EIA]*) is able to detect antigens or antibodies by producing an enzyme-triggered color change. In this method, an enzyme-labeled antibody or antigen is used in the immunologic assay to detect either suspected abnormal antibodies or antigens in the patient's specimen. In this method, a plastic bead (or a plastic test plate) is coated with an antigen (e.g., virus). The antigen is incubated with the patient's serum. If the patient's serum contains antibodies to the pathologic viral antigen, an immunocomplex forms on the bead (or plate). When a chromogenic chemical is then added, a color change is noted and can be spectrophotometrically compared with a control (or reference) serum identification. Then, quantification of abnormal antibodies in the patient's serum instigated by the viral infection can be performed. Similarly EIA can also be used for detection of pathologic antigens in the patient's serum. Testing for HIV, hepatitis, or cytomegalovirus commonly uses these methods.

Autoimmune Enzyme Immunoassay. *Autoimmune enzyme immunoassay* screening tests are commonly used for the detection of antinuclear antibodies. EIA techniques (similar to what have been described in the preceding) are used as the purified nuclear antigens are bound to a series of microwells to which the patient's serum is serially diluted and added. After adding up peroxidase conjugated antihuman IgG, a complex antibody/antigen "sandwich" is identified by color changes.

Chemiluminescent Immunoassays. ***Chemiluminescent immunoassays*** are extensively used in automated immunoassays. In this technique, chemiluminescent labels can be attached to an antibody or antigen. After appropriate immunoassays are obtained (as described), light emission produced by the immunologic reaction can be measured and quantified. This technique is commonly used to detect proteins, viruses, and nucleic acid sequences associated with disease.

Fluorescent Immunoassays. ***Fluorescent immunoassays*** consist of labeling antibody with fluorescein. This fluorescein-labeled antibody is able to bind either directly with a particular antigen or indirectly with antiimmunoglobulins. Under a fluorescent microscope, the fluorescein becomes obvious as yellow-green light. Testing for *Neisseria gonorrhea* or antinuclear antibodies may use these laboratory methods.

With the increasing use of automated analyzers, the use of chemiluminescence and *nephelometry* has become extremely important to allow analyzers to quantify results in great numbers of specimens tested in a short period of time. *Nephelometry* (in auto analyzers) depends on the light-scattering properties of antigen/antibody complexes as light is passed through the test medium. The quantity of the cloudiness or turbidity in a solution then can be measured photometrically. Automated C-reactive protein, alpha antitrypsin, haptoglobins, and immunoglobulins are often measured using nephelometry.

Polymerase Chain Reaction

Since the complete human genome sequence became available in 2003, laboratory molecular genetics has become an integral part of diagnostic testing. Molecular genetics depends on an in vitro method of amplifying low levels of specific DNA sequences in a patient specimen to raise quantities of a potentially present specific DNA sequence to levels that can be quantitated by further analysis. This process is called Polymerase Chain Reaction (PCR). This is particularly helpful in the identification of diseases caused by gene mutations (e.g., BRCA mutations), in the identification and quantitation of infectious agents such as HPV or HIV, and in the identification of acquired genetic changes that may be present in hematologic malignancies or colon cancer.

In PCR procedures, a known particular target short DNA sequence (ranging from 100 to 1000 nucleotide pairs) is used. This known DNA sequence "primer" is then placed in a series of reactions with the patient's specimen. These reactions are designed to markedly increase the number of comparable abnormal DNA sequences that potentially exist in the patient's specimen. The increased number of abnormal DNA sequences then can be identified and quantified. In many instances, the nucleic acid of interest is ribonucleic acid (RNA) rather than DNA. In these circumstances, the PCR procedure is modified by reverse transcription (*reverse transcriptase PCR [RT PCR]*). With RT PCR, abnormal RNA can be amplified (increased in number), detected, and quantified.

Real-time PCR uses the same reaction sequence as described. In real-time PCR, fluorescence resonance energy transfer is used to quantitate the DNA sequences of interest and identify points of mutation. Real-time PCR provides a product that can be more accurately quantified.

Quantification of PCR derived DNA/RNA products can be performed in many ways. This can be performed by simple gel electrophoresis, *DNA sequencing*, or using *DNA probes*. DNA probes are presynthesized DNA primers that are used to identify and quantify the amplified DNA produced by the PCR process. Hybridization techniques such as *liquid phase hybridization* interact with a defined DNA probe and the potential targeted DNA in solution. DNA probes have become a very important part of commercial laboratory molecular genetics. Microarray DNA chip technology (*Microarray analysis*) places thousands of major DNA probes on one glass chip. After interaction with the patient's specimen, the microarray chip can then be scanned with high speed fluorescent detectors that can quantify each DNA micro sequence. This process is used to identify gene expression of malignancies and has led to a new understanding of the classification, pathophysiology, and treatment of cancer.

Fluorescence in Situ Hybridization (FISH)

Fluorescence in situ hybridization (FISH) uses nucleic probes (short sequences of single-stranded DNA) that are complementary to the DNA sequence to be identified. These nucleic probes are labeled with fluorescent tags that can identify the exact location of the complementary DNA sequence that is being targeted. This method is particularly helpful in the detection of inherited and acquired chromosomal abnormalities common in hematologic and other oncologic conditions, such as lymphomas and breast cancer. Laboratory genetics are also discussed on p. 1104.

STANDARD PRECAUTIONS

The risk of spread of diseases such as hepatitis B virus (HBV) and human immunodeficiency virus (HIV) has made all health care organizations aware of the need to protect health care providers. These threats prompted the Centers for Disease Control and Prevention (CDC) to release its guidelines for universal precautions, now called Standard Precautions (Box 1-1). This policy recommends that blood and body fluid precautions be used for all patients regardless of their infection status. All patients should be considered potentially infectious. The Standard Precautions apply to all blood, body fluids, and tissues. Serous fluids such as pleural, peritoneal, amniotic, cerebrospinal, and synovial fluids are included. Semen and vaginal secretions should also be considered hazardous. Other clinical specimens (e.g., sputum, stool, urine) are of less concern, and the Standard Precautions apply only if these specimens contain visible amounts of blood.

These precautions require the use of protective barriers (gloves, gowns, masks, protective eyewear) to avoid skin and mucous membrane exposure to blood and body fluids. A fundamental principle of Standard Precautions is frequent handwashing between patients and when gloves are changed. All specimens should be collected and transported in containers that prevent leakage. Blood or body fluid spills must be decontaminated immediately. All needles and other sharp items must be handled carefully and discarded in puncture-resistant containers. Needles should not be recapped, broken, bent, or removed from a syringe to avoid the risk of puncturing the finger or hand. All needle sticks need to be reported and followed up with appropriate testing for infectious disease. Special reusable needles are placed in metal containers for transport to a designated area for sterilization or disinfection.

Vaccination against HBV is another safety precaution recommended by the CDC.

PROPER SEQUENCING AND SCHEDULING OF TESTS

Because of the cost and complexity of laboratory and diagnostic testing, it is important that tests be scheduled in the most efficient sequential manner. Because one type of test can interfere with another, certain guidelines apply when multiple tests must be performed in a limited amount of time. X-ray examinations that do not require contrast material should precede examinations that do require contrast media. X-ray studies using barium should be scheduled after ultrasonography studies. For example, x-ray studies using barium should follow x-rays using iodine contrast dye (such as intravenous pyelography [IVP]), which should follow x-ray studies using no contrast because contrast agents can obscure visualization of other body areas on subsequent x-ray tests. Also, stool specimens should be collected before x-ray studies using barium.

BOX 1-1	Standard Precautions

These precautions have been mandated by the Occupational Safety and Health Administration (OSHA). Their purpose is to protect health care workers from contracting illnesses from the specimens they handle, the patients they care for, and the environment in which they work. The precautions are as follows:

- Wear gowns, gloves, protective eyewear, face masks, and protective clothing (including laboratory coat) whenever exposed to blood or other body fluids.
- If the health care worker's skin is opened, gloves should be worn whenever direct patient care is performed.
- Mouth-to-mouth emergency resuscitation equipment should be available in strategic locations. The mouthpieces should be individualized for each health care worker. Ambu bags are preferable. Saliva is considered an infectious fluid.
- Dispose of all sharp items in puncture-resistant containers.
- Do not "recap," bend, break, or remove needles from syringes.
- Immediately remove gloves that have a hole or tear in them.
- All disposed patient-related wastes must be labeled as a "biohazard."
- All specimens must be transported in leak-proof containers.
- Eating, drinking, applying cosmetics, or handling contact lenses is prohibited in patient care areas.
- Assume that every person is potentially infected or colonized with an organism that could be transmitted in the health care setting.
- Implement respiratory hygiene/cough etiquette instructions to contain respiratory secretions in patients and accompanying individuals who have signs and symptoms of a respiratory infection. These include posting signs with instructions about covering mouths/noses, using and disposing of tissues, and hand hygiene. Offer masks to coughing patients and encourage them to keep a distance of at least three feet from others.
- If a health care worker has experienced an exposure incident to blood or other body fluids (e.g., needle stick), testing of the health care worker and the patient for HBV and HIV is necessary.

Data from Centers for Disease Control and Prevention, 2007.

Test sequencing affects the ability to efficiently perform tests in a limited time period. An essential component of this process is communication and collaboration with other health care workers in numerous departments.

PROCEDURE AND PATIENT CARE

Before the Test

Patient preparation is vital to the success of any diagnostic test. Patient education is essential and is discussed later in this chapter. Development of and adherence to patient care guidelines in regard to patient preparation for the test require an understanding of the procedure. A thorough history to identify contraindications to the specific test is vital. Recognizing patients at risk for potential complications and counseling them about those complications is important. The fears and concerns of the patient should be elicited and addressed prior to testing. Documentation and a thorough understanding of ongoing factors (e.g., medications, previous tests, other variables as discussed later in this chapter) that could interfere with the test results are essential to avoid misinterpretation of diagnostic testing.

Pretest preparation procedures must be followed closely. Dietary restriction is often an important factor in preparing the patient for tests. Studies requiring fasting should be performed as early in the morning as possible to diminish patient discomfort. Adherence to dietary restriction is important for test accuracy. Many blood tests and procedures require fasting. Studies such as a barium enema, colonoscopy, upper gastrointestinal (GI) series, and IVP are more accurate if the patient has been on NPO (nothing by mouth) status for several hours before the test. Sometimes dietary restrictions are important for safety, especially if a sedative is to be administered during testing. For example, upper GI endoscopy requires that the patient remain NPO for 8 to 12 hours before the test to prevent gagging, vomiting, and aspiration. Bowel preparation is necessary for many procedures designed to evaluate the mucosa of the GI tract.

Equally important to total patient care is the coordination of ongoing therapy (e.g., physical therapy, administration of medications, other diagnostic testing). Finally, correct timing of testing is key to accurate interpretation of results. For example, blood samples for cortisol, parathormone, and fasting glucose levels (among others) must be obtained in the early morning hours.

Patient Identification. Proper identification of the patient is a critical safety factor. The conscious patient should be asked to state his or her full name. The name should be verified by checking the identification band and requisition slip. The identity of an unconscious patient should be verified by family or friends. No specimens should be collected or procedure performed without properly identifying the patient. Costly tests on the wrong patient are useless and may instigate legal action. Confusion can occur when patients with the same name are on the same nursing unit. Most units have some type of warning or "name alert" to address this concern.

Patient Education. Once the patient is properly identified and the proper test or procedure is scheduled, patient education begins. Patients want to know what tests they are having and why they are needed. An informed patient is less apprehensive and more cooperative. Patient education helps ensure that the test will not need to be repeated because of improper preparation. Fasting requirements and bowel preparations must be clearly explained to the patient. Written instructions are essential. If used, the patient's literacy and understanding of the material should be validated. Sometimes medications need to be discontinued for a period of time before certain tests. This information should be determined in consultation with the physician. Medications that are not discontinued may be listed on the requisition to aid in interpretation of test results. Finally it is extremely important to inform the patient regarding the need to discontinue medications or foods that may interfere with testing results.

Variables Affecting Test Results. Many laboratory tests are affected by individual variables that must be considered in test result interpretation. Several of these key variables are discussed in the following paragraphs.

Age. Pediatric reference values differ from adult values. For some tests, values vary according to the week of life of the infant. For example, in the first week of life, newborns have elevated levels of serum bilirubin, growth hormone, blood urea nitrogen (BUN), and fetal hemoglobin. They have decreased levels of cholesterol and haptoglobin. Healthy newborns also have an increase in total white blood cells and decreases in immunoglobulin (Ig) M and IgA. For some tests, children have different reference values based on their developmental stage. For example, alkaline phosphatase levels in children are much higher than adult values because of rapid bone growth.

Age-related changes are also apparent in the middle adult and older adult years. For example, albumin and total protein levels begin to decline in the mid-adult years. Reference values for cholesterol and triglyceride levels begin to increase in the mid-adult years. Creatinine clearance levels decrease with age relative to changes in glomerular filtration rate.

Gender. Gender is another variable that affects values in men and women. Differences are usually related to increased muscle mass in men and differences in hormonal secretion. For example, men usually have higher reference values for hemoglobin, BUN, serum creatinine, and uric acid. Men also have higher serum levels of cholesterol and triglycerides as compared with premenopausal women. Sex-specific hormones will also differ, with men having higher testosterone levels and women having higher levels of estrogens, follicle-stimulating hormone, and luteinizing hormones.

Race. Generally race has little effect on laboratory values. It has a greater effect on genetic diseases, such as sickle cell anemia in blacks and thalassemia in individuals with origins near the Mediterranean Sea.

Pregnancy. Many endocrine, hematologic, and biochemical changes occur during pregnancy. Pregnant women have increased levels of cholesterol, triglycerides, lactic dehydrogenase, alkaline phosphatase, and aspartate aminotransferase. They may have lower values of hemoglobin, hematocrit, serum creatinine, urea, glucose, albumin, and total protein.

Food Ingestion. Several serum values are markedly affected by food. For example, levels of glucose and triglycerides rise after a meal. To avoid the effects of diet on laboratory tests, many tests are obtained when the patient is in the fasting state.

Posture. Changes in body position affect the concentration of several components in the peripheral blood. Therefore it is sometimes important to note whether the patient was in the supine, sitting, or standing position when blood was drawn. Examples of laboratory values affected by posture include norepinephrine, epinephrine, renin, aldosterone, protein, and potassium.

During Testing

Often many different health care professionals are needed to successfully perform a diagnostic procedure. The health care provider's knowledge of the procedure will be a major determinant of the success of the procedure. Furthermore, the presence of a knowledgeable and supportive health care provider during any procedure is invaluable to the patient and to the accuracy of the test.

Specimen Collection. Protocols and guidelines are available for each type of specimen collection. These are essential for appropriate preparation and collection. For example, the selection of the color-coded tube varies with the type of blood test needed. Guidelines for the collection of a 24-hour urine collection must be followed to obtain a representative urine sample. These and other examples are described in detail in the following chapter overviews.

Transport and Processing of the Specimen. Preparing the patient and collecting the specimen are essential. Getting the specimen to the laboratory in an acceptable state for examination is just as important. In general, the specimen should be transported to the laboratory as soon as possible after collection. Delays may result in rejection of the specimen. Specimens are usually refrigerated if transportation is delayed.

A Note About SI Units. The International System of Units (SI units) is a system for reporting laboratory values in terms of standardized international measures. This system is currently used in many countries, and it is expected to be adopted worldwide. Throughout this book results are given in conventional units and SI units when possible.

After the Test

Posttest care is an important aspect of total patient care. Attention should be directed to the patient's concerns about possible results or the difficulties of the procedure. Appropriate treatment subsequent to testing must be provided. For example, after a barium test, a cathartic is indicated. However, if a bowel obstruction has been identified, catharsis is contraindicated.

Recognition and rapid institution of treatment of complications (e.g., bleeding, shock, bowel perforation) is essential in caring for the patient who has just had a diagnostic procedure. More invasive tests often require heavy sedation or a surgical procedure. In these situations, aftercare is similar to routine postoperative care.

Reporting Test Results. Although proper patient preparation and skill and accuracy in performing test procedures are vital, timeliness in reporting test results is no less essential. To be clinically useful, results must be reported promptly. Delays in reporting test results can make the data useless. The data must be included in the appropriate medical record and presented in a manner that is clear and easily interpreted. As in all phases of testing, communication among health care professionals is important. Health care providers need to understand the significance of test results. For example, nurses on the evening shift may be the first to see the results of a culture and sensitivity report on a patient with a urinary tract infection. If the results indicate that the infecting organism is not sensitive to the prescribed antibiotic, the doctor should be informed and an appropriate antibiotic order obtained.

Ethical standards for disclosure of test results must be strictly followed. In 1996, the Health Insurance Portability and Accountability Act (HIPAA) became law. Its purpose was to improve the health care of each individual by insuring the ability for each person to obtain reasonable health care, and to allow each individual access to and protection of his or her health care information. In response to the HIPAA mandate, Health and Human Services published the *Standards for Privacy of Individually Identifiable Health Information (the Privacy Rule)* in December 2000, which became effective on April 14, 2001. The Privacy Rule set national standards for the protection of an individual's health information. Compliance with this rule is particularly important when providing diagnostic test results. The Privacy Rule generally gives patients the right to examine and obtain a copy of their own health records and to request corrections. It limits who can have access to results of diagnostic tests. Information regarding test results can only be provided to the patient and to persons the patient indicates (by signature). Only health care workers who have a provider relationship with a patient may obtain access to a patient's test results. The federal government has responsibility for enforcing these laws and violators are subject to civil and criminal prosecution. Fines can be levied against both the individual and the health organization. The penalties for violation of these laws are fines up to $250,000 and up to 10 years in jail.

As a result of the Privacy Rule, test results are not given over the phone to patients. Results, no matter if normal or not, are never left on "answering machines." Results cannot be given to family or friends unless written consent is provided. These restrictions include providing test results to spouses, parents of adult children, siblings, or children. If the patient presents in the laboratory or a clinical area, the patient is usually required to show a photo identification to confirm his or her identity and to verify his or her signature on a Release of Information Authorization form. The Privacy Rule does not negate state regulations that affect test result reporting. For example, in most states, HIV results are released only to the ordering physician/provider and are not provided by the laboratory to the patient. Compliance with the Privacy Rule is an extremely important part of diagnostic testing and patient education. The impact of an abnormal test result on the patient must always be appreciated, and support must be provided.

Knowledge of the implications of various test results and an understanding of the disease process are as important as the communicative skills required to inform the patient and the family. Succinct documentation of test results may be required before the "official" result is included in the patient's chart. Again, a thorough understanding of the test is essential. Adequate follow-up is as important as all previously mentioned factors for successful diagnostic testing. The patient must be educated about home care, the next doctor's visit, and treatment options.

• • •

Knowledgeable interpretation of diagnostic tests is key for effective collaboration among health care providers if the most efficient patient care is to be provided. The safety and success of diagnostic testing often depend on the nurse and other health care professionals. The safety of the patient and health care professionals depends on the creation of practice guidelines and standards of care. These can be effectively developed only with a thorough understanding of laboratory and diagnostic testing.

Blood Studies

Continued

TESTS—cont'd

TESTS—cont'd

Continued

Overview

REASONS FOR OBTAINING BLOOD STUDIES

Blood is the body fluid most frequently used for analytic purposes. Blood studies are used to assess a multitude of body processes and disorders. Common studies assess the quantity of red and white blood cells, and the levels of enzymes, lipids, clotting factors, and hormones. Most blood studies are performed for one of the following reasons:

1. To establish a diagnosis (e.g., high blood urea nitrogen [BUN] and creatinine levels are indicative of renal failure).
2. To rule out a clinical problem (e.g., hypokalemia is ruled out with a normal potassium level).
3. To monitor therapy (e.g., glucose levels are used to monitor treatment of diabetic patients, and partial thromboplastin time [PTT] values are used to regulate heparin therapy).
4. To establish a prognosis (e.g., declining CD4 counts reflect a poor clinical prognosis for the acquired immunodeficiency syndrome [AIDS] patient).
5. To screen for disease (e.g., prostate-specific antigen levels are used to detect prostate cancer).
6. To determine effective drug dosage and to prevent toxicity. (Peak and trough levels are drawn at designated time periods; see p. 21.)

METHODS OF BLOOD COLLECTION

There are three general methods for obtaining blood: venous, arterial, and skin puncture. Blood collected from these sites differs in several important aspects. For example, arterial blood is oxygenated by the lungs and pumped from the heart to body organs and tissues. It is essentially uniform in its composition throughout the body. Venous blood composition varies depending on the metabolic activity of the organ or tissue being perfused. Venous blood is oxygen-deficient in comparison to arterial blood. Variations between arterial and venous blood are often seen in measurements of pH, CO_2 concentration, and glucose, lactic acid, and ammonia levels. On the other hand, blood obtained by skin puncture is a mixture of arterial and venous blood. Skin puncture blood also includes intracellular and interstitial fluid. By far the most common access for blood withdrawal is venous puncture.

Venous Puncture

Background Information. The ease of obtaining venous blood makes this the primary source of blood collection. It is relatively free of any complications. Venipuncture is usually obtained by drawing a specimen of blood from a superficial vein (Figure 2-1). The site most often used is the antecubital fossa of the arm because there are several large superficial veins at that location. The basilic, cephalic, and median cubital veins are the most commonly used sites. Veins of the wrist or hand can also be used.

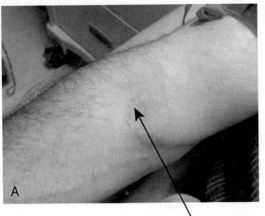
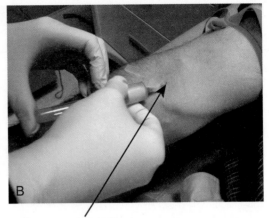

Right arm antecubital vein used for venipuncture

Figure 2-1 Venipuncture.

When venous puncture cannot be performed on the upper extremities, the femoral vein is the most easily accessible for puncture.

Collection Tubes. Venipuncture is usually accomplished using needles attached to glass tubes under specified vacuum. A needle and a syringe can also be used to collect the blood sample and then to inject it into the appropriate tube. Tubes come in various sizes (2, 3, 5, 7, 10, and 15 mL). The rubber stoppers are color-coded to distinguish whether the tube is a plain tube (e.g., no preservatives or anticoagulants added), whether the tube contains a specific anticoagulant (such as heparin, oxalate, citrate, or ethylenediamine tetraacetic acid salts [EDTA]), or whether the tube is chemically clean (e.g., iron determination). Depending on the tests needed, the analysis is performed on whole blood, serum, or plasma. A centrifuge is used to separate the blood components and to obtain either serum or plasma. Whole blood collected without anticoagulant clots, and *serum* can be separated out for testing. Whole blood collected with an anticoagulant prevents clotting, and *plasma* can be tested. Plasma contains fibrinogen, which is missing from serum.

The selection of the color-coded tube is based on the requirements of the test. Charts are available from the laboratory that indicate the type of tube needed for a particular blood test. Colors and amount of blood required may vary according to the laboratory. A representative chart is shown in Table 2-1.

The recommended order of draw must be followed when collecting multiple tubes of blood. Specimens should be drawn into nonadditive tubes (e.g., red top) before tubes are drawn that contain additives. The tubes should be filled in the following order:

1. Blood culture tubes first (to maintain sterility)
2. Nonadditive tubes (e.g., red top)
3. Coagulation tubes (e.g., blue top)
4. Heparin tubes (e.g., green top)
5. EDTA-K3 tubes (e.g., lavender top)
6. Oxalate-fluoride tubes (e.g., gray top)

Technique
Before
- Identify the patient. Assemble all equipment and supplies and put on gloves (Figure 2-2).
- Explain the procedure to the patient. Explain that mild, brief discomfort may result from the needlestick.
- If fasting is required, verify that this requirement has been followed.

TABLE 2-1	Blood Studies		
Color of Top	**Additive**	**Purpose**	**Examples**
Red	None	To allow blood sample to clot. This permits separation of serum when the serum needs to be tested	Chemistry, Bilirubin, Blood urea nitrogen (BUN), Calcium
Red/black	None	Serum separator tube for serum determinations in chemistry and serology	Chemistry, Serology
Purple or lavender	Ethylenediamine tetraacetic acid (EDTA)	To prevent blood from clotting	Hematology, Complete blood cell count, Platelet count
Gray	Sodium fluoride oxalate	To prevent glycolysis	Chemistry, Glucose, Lactose tolerance
Green	Heparin	To prevent blood from clotting when plasma needs to be tested	Chemistry, Ammonia, Carboxyhemoglobin
Blue	Sodium citrate	To prevent blood from clotting when plasma needs to be tested	Hematology Prothrombin time (PT), Partial thromboplastin time (PTT)
Black	Sodium citrate	Binds calcium to prevent blood clotting	Westergren erthrocyte sedimentation rate (ESR)
Yellow	Citrate dextrose	Preserves red cells	Blood cultures
Gold serum separator tube (SST)	None	Collects serum	Chemistry

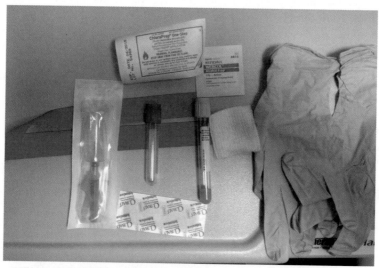

Figure 2-2 Supplies for venipuncture: tourniquet, Vacutainer and needle, specimen tubes, skin preparation antiseptics, protective gloves, gauze, Band-Aid.

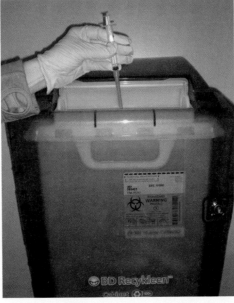

Figure 2-3 Proper disposal of needles and other sharp disposable instruments.

During
- Position the patient properly for easy access to the antecubital fossa.
- Ask the patient to make a fist to distend the veins.
- Select a vein for venipuncture.
- Apply a tourniquet several inches above the puncture site.
- Cleanse the venipuncture site with an antiseptic solution (such as chlorhexidine, 70% isopropyl alcohol, or Betadine). Allow the area to dry.
- Perform the venipuncture by entering the skin with the needle bevel up and the needle at approximately a 15-degree angle to the skin.
- If using a *Vacutainer,* ease the tube forward in the holder as soon as the needle is in the vein. When the tube is filled, remove it. Another tube can then be inserted into the holder. If using a *syringe,* pull back on the barrel with slow, even tension as blood fills the syringe. Transfer the blood to the appropriate color tubes. Butterfly needles can also be used for collection.
- Release the tourniquet when the blood begins to flow.

After
- After the blood is drawn, place a cotton ball over the site. Withdraw the needle and apply pressure to the site. A Band-Aid applied over the cotton ball usually stops the bleeding.
- Discard the needle in an appropriate receptacle to prevent inadvertent needle sticks (Figure 2-3).
- Mix tubes with the additives by gently rolling the tubes. Do not vigorously shake the tubes. Specimens collected in the syringe should be transferred to appropriate test tube containers.
- Properly dispose of contaminated materials, syringes, and cotton balls.
- Initial the label and record the date and time of blood collection. Attach a label to each vial of blood.
- Arrange for prompt delivery of the blood specimen to the laboratory.
- If the patient fasted before the test, remove diet restrictions as per physician recommendations.

Potential Complications

- *Bleeding.* After the specimen is drawn, apply pressure or a pressure dressing to the venipuncture site. Assess the venipuncture site for bleeding.
- *Hematoma.* Hematomas can form under the skin when the vein continues to leak blood. This results in a large, bruised area. This can usually be prevented by applying pressure to the venipuncture site until clotting occurs. If a hematoma does occur, reabsorption of the blood can be enhanced by the application of warm compresses.
- *Infection.* Instruct the patient to assess the venipuncture site for redness, pain, swelling, or tenderness. This is more common in immunocompromised patients or patients who have had lymph node dissection above the venipuncture site.
- *Dizziness and fainting.* If this occurs, prevent injury by helping the patient to a sitting or reclining position. Lowering the head between the knees or using smelling salts can also help.

Preventing Interfering Factors

- Hemolysis may result from vigorous shaking of a blood specimen. This may invalidate test results.
- Collect the blood specimen from the arm without an intravenous (IV) device if possible. IV infusion can influence test results. If it is necessary to draw blood from the arm with an IV device, never draw blood above the IV needle site. Satisfactory samples may be obtained by drawing the blood below the IV needle after turning the IV infusion off for 2 minutes before the venipuncture. Select a vein other than the one with the IV device and draw 5 mL of blood. Discard this sample before drawing blood for analysis.
- Do not use the arm with the dialysis arteriovenous fistula for a venipuncture unless the physician specifically authorizes it.
- Because of the risk for cellulitis, specimens should not be taken from the side on which an axillary lymph node dissection has been performed.
- To obtain valid results, do not fasten the tourniquet for longer than 1 minute. Prolonged tourniquet application can cause stasis, localized acidemia, and hemoconcentration.

Drawing Blood from an Indwelling Venous Catheter. Follow the institutional guidelines for drawing blood from an indwelling venous catheter, such as a central venous catheter or a peripherally inserted central catheter. Guidelines will specify the amount of blood to be drawn from the catheter and discarded before blood is collected for laboratory studies. The guidelines also indicate the amount and type of solution needed to flush the catheter to prevent it from being clogged by blood.

Drawing a Panel of Blood Studies. Blood tests are often part of a panel or group of specified tests. This is because patterns of abnormalities may be more useful than single test changes. See Appendix C for blood tests included in disease and organ panels.

Arterial Puncture

Background Information. Arterial blood is used to measure oxygen, CO_2, and pH. These are often referred to as arterial blood gases (ABGs) and are described on p. 109. If a patient will require frequent sampling, an indwelling arterial catheter is usually placed. Arterial puncture is used for single or infrequent sampling.

Arterial punctures are more difficult to perform than venipuncture. They also cause a significant amount of patient discomfort. The brachial and radial arteries are the arteries most often used for arterial puncture. The femoral artery is usually avoided because bleeding occurs more often after the procedure and may not be noted because it is hidden by bed covers. Large amounts of blood could be lost before the problem is detected.

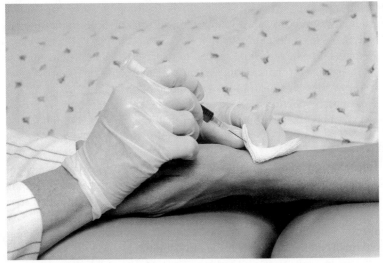

Figure 2-4 Drawing arterial blood. Note that the needle is at a 45-degree angle.

Technique

Before

- Explain the procedure to the patient. Inform the patient why this blood test is necessary. Tell the patient that the test causes more discomfort than a venipuncture.
- Notify the laboratory before drawing arterial blood samples so the necessary equipment can be calibrated before the blood sample arrives.
- Perform the *Allen test* to assess collateral circulation before performing the arterial puncture on the radial artery. To perform the Allen test, make the patient's hand blanch by obliterating both the radial and ulnar pulses. Then release the pressure over the ulnar artery only. If flow through the ulnar artery is good, flushing will be observed immediately. The Allen test is then positive and the radial artery can be used for venipuncture. If the Allen test is negative (no flushing), repeat it on the other arm. If the results are negative in both arms, choose another artery for puncture. The Allen test is important because it ensures collateral circulation to the hand if thrombosis of the radial artery occurs after the puncture.
- Assemble appropriate equipment and specimen container for the specimen. Put on protective gloves.

During

- Cleanse the arterial site with 70% isopropyl alcohol. Allow the site to dry.
- Attach a 20-gauge needle to a syringe containing approximately 0.2 mL of heparin. Insert the needle at a 45- to 60-degree angle into the skin over the palpable artery (Figure 2-4).
- After drawing approximately 3 to 5 mL of blood, remove the needle and apply pressure to the arterial site for 3 to 5 minutes. Expel any air bubbles in the syringe and activate the protective cover.
- Cap the syringe and gently rotate to mix the blood and the heparin.

After

- Indicate on the laboratory slip if the patient is receiving any oxygen therapy or is attached to a ventilator.
- Place the arterial blood on ice and immediately take it to the chemistry laboratory for analysis.
- If the patient has an abnormal clotting time or is taking anticoagulants, apply pressure for approximately 15 minutes. A pressure dressing is usually applied.

Potential Complications

- *Arterial thrombosis.* Thrombosis can result and impair arterial circulation. This can result in ischemia or necrosis of tissue on the extremity.
- *Hematoma formation.* Pressure must be applied to the arterial puncture site for at least 3 to 5 minutes to prevent hematoma formation (longer if the patient is anticoagulated). If a hematoma results, warm compresses will enhance absorption of the blood.
- *Bleeding.* The site must be carefully assessed for bleeding. An arterial puncture can cause rapid bleeding. This is especially important if the patient has an abnormal clotting time or is taking anticoagulants.

Skin Puncture

Background Information. Skin puncture (sometimes called capillary puncture) is the method of choice for obtaining blood from pediatric patients, especially infants, because large amounts of blood required for repeated venipuncture could result in anemia. However, skin punctures are also used in adult patients.

Common puncture sites include the fingertips, earlobes, and heel surfaces. The fingertips are often used in adults and small children. The heel is the most commonly used site for infants. The earlobe can be used to obtain blood in adults and older pediatric patients. The earlobe can also be used to obtain arterialized capillary blood as a possible substitute for arterial blood in determining the pH, Pco_2, and Po_2.

With changes in health care economics and delivery, the use of skin punctures will probably increase. Blood monitoring will be increasingly performed in outpatient settings. Clinical laboratory tests will be performed more frequently at the bedside using a skin puncture.

Technique

Before

Identify the patient using two separate identifiers. Explain the procedure to the patient and/or family. Assemble all supplies. Put on gloves.

- Select an appropriate puncture site. For *infants,* the lateral or medial heel surface is commonly used. For *older* infants, children, or adults, the lateral aspect of the second, third, or fourth fingertip may be used to avoid the central tip of the fingers where the nerve supply is more dense.

During

- Warm the puncture site with a warm, moist towel to increase blood flow.
- Cleanse the puncture site with 70% isopropyl alcohol. Allow the site to dry.
- Make the puncture with a sterile lancet or skin puncture device.
- Discard the first drop of blood by wiping it away with a sterile pad.
- Do not milk the site, as this may hemolyze the specimen and introduce excess tissue fluid. Also avoid using excess pressure on the fingers during blood collection. This may cause hemolysis of the sample.
- Collect the specimen in capillary tubes or on special filter papers.
- If using capillary tubes, seal the capillary tubes by inserting clay into the end of the micropipette.

After

- Initial the blood label and record the time and date of blood collection. Indicate that the blood was collected by skin puncture.
- Arrange for prompt transportation of the blood specimen to the laboratory.

Potential Complications

- *Infection.* Assess the skin puncture site for redness, swelling, pain, or tenderness. Although this is a serious complication, the incidence is very low.

- *Hematoma and bruising.* Check the skin puncture site for discoloration, bruising, or swelling. Look for bleeding onto the skin. Avoid frequent skin punctures or excessive squeezing of the tissue during blood collection to prevent this problem.

TIMING OF BLOOD COLLECTION

Although many blood specimens can be obtained randomly, some must be drawn at specific times. For example, lipoproteins (see p. 342) should be drawn after a 12- to 14-hour fast (except for water), because food can alter lipoprotein values. Because glucose levels are related to food intake, fasting blood glucose specimens require an 8-hour fast. Glucose tolerance tests (see p. 261) require a fasting blood glucose level and a glucose level drawn at 30 minutes, 1 hour, 2 hours, 3 hours, and sometimes 4 hours after glucose administration.

Specimens for therapeutic drug monitoring (see p. 211) must be obtained at specific times determined by the method of drug delivery (e.g., IV or oral), dosage interval, absorption characteristics of the drug, and half-life of the drug. Drug monitoring is especially important in patients taking medications (such as antiarrhythmics, bronchodilators, antibiotics, anticonvulsants, and cardiotonics), because the margin of safety between therapeutic and toxic levels may be narrow. Blood levels can be taken at the drug's *peak level* (highest concentration) or at the drug's *trough level* (lowest concentration). Peak levels are useful when testing for toxicity, and trough levels are useful for demonstrating a satisfactory therapeutic level.

TRANSPORT AND PROCESSING OF BLOOD SPECIMENS

Once blood specimens are obtained, they should be promptly transported to the laboratory. Because the blood cells continue to live in the collection tubes, they will metabolize some of the components in the blood. This can result in alterations in the concentration of some blood components before analysis in the laboratory. Therefore blood specimens should be delivered to the laboratory for processing within 1 hour, depending on the test. Stat specimens should be delivered immediately after being drawn. Laboratories have written criteria for rejecting a specimen as unsuitable for testing. Box 2-1 lists common reasons for rejecting a blood specimen.

In general, specimens should be tested within 1 hour of collection. If this is not possible, the sample may need to be refrigerated or frozen depending on the compound for testing. Some blood specimens must be sent by mail or special courier from physicians' offices or small hospitals to large reference laboratories. As a result, delays of 24 hours may occur before specimen analysis.

After testing, the remainder of the blood sample should be saved by the laboratory along with the original sample for 24 hours to be retested if needed to verify discrepant results. These samples can also be used for additional ("add-on") tests ordered by the physician while avoiding additional

---

| **BOX 2-1** | **Criteria for Rejection of Blood Sample** |

- Improper sample identification
- Wrong collection tube used
- Insufficient blood quantity
- Hemolyzed blood sample
- Improper transport of sample
- Insufficient filling of anticoagulated tube

venipunctures. With retesting or "add-on" requests, the stability of the requested serum constituent becomes an important consideration.

Multiphasic screening machines can perform many blood tests quickly and simultaneously using a very small blood sample. An example is the *Astra-7* or *Chem-7,* which usually includes the following seven studies: sodium, potassium, chloride, CO_2 content, BUN, creatinine, and glucose. See Appendix C for a listing of common panels. The basic metabolic panel and comprehensive metabolic panel have replaced the Chem-7 and Astra panels. These changes are the result of the recent federal guidelines to standardize the nomenclature for chemistry panels. The advantage of these machines is that results are available quickly and the cost is cheaper when compared to performing each test individually.

REPORTING OF RESULTS

Although accuracy and processing are the prerequisites of good laboratory practice, timeliness in reporting results is essential. To be clinically useful, a test result must be reported promptly. Delays in reporting a result can make the data useless and potentially could be life-threatening to the patient. Verbal reporting of result to the clinician should be provided by a licensed health care provider after using two patient identifiers (e.g., patient's name and medical record number/date of birth). A "read-back" of the information from the clinician should also occur.

BOX 2-2	Adult Critical Laboratory Values*
Bicarbonate (Total CO_2)	<10 or >40 mmol/L
Bilirubin, total	>15 mg/dL
Blood culture	Positive
Calcium	<6 or >13 mg/dL
Digoxin	>2.4 ng/mL
Direct Coombs	Positive
Glucose	<40 or >450 mg/dL
Glucose, point of care (Chemstrip)	≤60 or ≥450 mg/dL
Hematocrit	≤21% or ≥65%
Hemoglobin	≤7 or ≥21g/dL
Magnesium	≤1 or ≥9 mg/dL
Partial thromboplastin time	≥85 seconds
P_{CO_2}	≤20 or ≥60 mm Hg
pH	≤7.25 or ≥7.6
Platelet count	<20,000 or >1,000,000 /mcL
PO_2	≤40 mm Hg
Potassium	<3 or >6.1 mmol/L
Prothrombin time/International Normalized Ratio (INR)	≥5
Sodium	<120 or >160 mmol/L
Theophylline, trough	>25 mcg/mL
Tobramycin, peak	>12 mcg/mL
Tobramycin, trough	>2 mcg/mL
White blood cell count	≤2,000 or ≥40,000/mcL

*Critical values should be reported to the treating health care provider immediately so therapeutic action can be instigated.

The report must also be entered in the appropriate medical record and must be presented in a manner that is clear and easily interpreted. A listing of the patient's medications will help with test result interpretation.

The results should include the test results, reporting units, and reference ranges. It is important to note that normal ranges for laboratory tests vary from institution to institution. Often serial listing of results is useful for tests in which trends and values make interpretation easier. Comments may be added to help interpret test results; for example, the technologist would indicate if the sample was hemolyzed.

Because acronyms are used to shorten test names, these code names must be understood for proper interpretation. For example, the acronym LAP could stand for leucine amino peptidase or for leukocyte alkaline phosphatase.

Proper reporting of a "critical" or "panic" value is essential. These values are results well outside the usual range of normal and generally require immediate intervention. Common examples are shown in Box 2-2. If these results were phoned to a physician or nurse, verification of this notification must be properly documented.

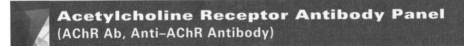

Acetylcholine Receptor Antibody Panel
(AChR Ab, Anti–AChR Antibody)

NORMAL FINDINGS

ACh receptor (muscle) binding antibodies: ≤0.02 nmol/L
ACh receptor (muscle) modulating antibodies: 0-20% (reported as % loss of AChR)
Striational (striated muscle) antibodies: <1:60

INDICATIONS

Antibodies to AChR are used to diagnose acquired myasthenia gravis (MG) and also to monitor patient response to immunosuppressive therapy.

TEST EXPLANATION

These antibodies may cause blocks in neuromuscular transmission by interfering with the binding of acetylcholine (ACh) to ACh receptor (AChR) sites on the muscle membrane, thereby preventing muscle contraction. It is this phenomenon that characterizes myasthenia gravis (MG). Myasthenia gravis (MG) is an autoimmune disease usually caused by antibodies that block or destroy receptors for the neurotransmitter acetylcholine, leading to muscle weakness and fatigue. Antibodies to AChR occur in more than 85% to 90% of patients with acquired MG, and 63% of patients with only ocular MG have elevated levels. The presence of these antibodies is virtually diagnostic of MG, but a negative test does not exclude the disease. The measured titers do not correspond well with the severity of MG. In an individual patient with MG, however, antibody levels are particularly useful in monitoring response to immunosuppressive or plasmapheresis therapy. As the patient improves, antibody titer decreases.

In adults with MG, there is at least a 20% occurrence of thymoma or other neoplasm. Neoplasms are an endogenous source of the antigens driving production of AChR autoantibodies. Among patients who have a thymoma, 59% have MG. Because congenital MG is not an autoimmune disease, this antibody test is not helpful in the diagnosis of congenital MG.

There are several AChR antibodies that can be associated with MG binding, blocking, and modulating antibodies. The *AChR-binding antibody* can activate complement and lead to loss of AChR. The

AChR-binding antibody is most commonly used. The *AChR-modulating antibody* causes receptor endocytosis resulting in loss of AChR expression, which correlates most closely with clinical severity of disease. It is most sensitive. A positive modulating antibody test may indicate subclinical MG, contraindicating the use of curare-like drugs during surgery. Approximately 10% to 15% of individuals with confirmed myasthenia gravis have no measurable binding, blocking, or modulating antibodies. The *AChR-blocking antibody* may impair binding of acetylcholine to the receptor, leading to poor muscle contraction. It is the least sensitive test (positive in only 61% of patients with MG), but it can be quantified more accurately. The blocking and modulating antibodies are not often positive for about 1 year after onset of MG symptoms.

The most commonly used method for the detection of these AChR antibodies is the Quantitative Radioimmunoassay/Semi-Quantitative Radioreceptor Assay.

Anti-Striated Muscle Antibody (Striated Muscle Antibody, IgG) titers greater than or equal to 1:80 are suggestive of myasthenia. This antibody is detectable in 30% to 40% of anti-AChR-negative patients (particularly those with bulbar symptoms only). However, striated muscle antibody can be found in rheumatic fever, myocardial infarction, and a variety of post-cardiotomy states.

INTERFERING FACTORS

- False-positive results may occur in patients with amyotrophic lateral sclerosis who have been treated with cobra venom.
- False-positive results may be seen in patients with penicillamine-induced or Lambert-Eaton myasthenic syndromes.
- Patients with autoimmune liver disease may have elevated results.
- The use of muscle relaxant drugs (metocurine and succinylcholine) or penicillamine may cause false-positive results.
- Immunosuppressive drugs may suppress the formation of these antibodies in patients with subclinical MG.

PROCEDURE AND PATIENT CARE

Before

- Explain the procedure to the patient.
- Tell the patient that no fasting is required.
- Inform the patient that the blood sample is usually sent to a reference laboratory. It will take several days before the results are available.

During

- Collect a venous blood sample in a red-top tube.

After

- Apply pressure or a pressure dressing to the venipuncture site.
- Assess the venipuncture site for bleeding.

TEST RESULTS AND CLINICAL SIGNIFICANCE

▲   Increased Levels

MG,
Ocular MG,

Thymoma:
Fifty-nine percent of patients with thymoma have MG and 10% of MG patients have a thymoma.

RELATED TESTS

Cholinesterase (p. 159). Patients with an acquired or congenital deficiency of this enzyme will experi
ence acute MG-like muscle paralysis when a depolarizing agent, such as succinylcholine, is used for
anesthesia induction.
Electromyography (p. 554). Repetitive stimulation or single-fiber electromyogram is positive in 90% of
MG patients.
Chest x-ray (p. 1014) or chest CT (p. 1029). These tests are used to identify thymoma.

Acid Phosphatase (Prostatic Acid Phosphatase [PAP],
Tartrate-Resistant Acid Phosphatase [TRAP])

NORMAL FINDINGS

Adult/elderly: 0.13-0.63 units/L (Roy, Brower, Hayden, 37° C) or 2.2-10.5 units/L (SI units)
Child: 8.6-12.6 units/mL (30° C)
Newborn: 10.4-16.4 units/mL (30° C)

INDICATIONS

Total acid phosphatase and specifically the PAP isoenzyme is primarily used to document rape cases. It
was used in the diagnosis of prostate cancer, but has been replaced by the use of prostate specific antigen
(PSA, p. 420). Otherwise this test has very little clinical usefulness.

TEST EXPLANATION

Acid phosphatase is found in many tissues, including liver, red blood cells, bone marrow, and platelets. The highest levels are found in the prostate gland—the PAP isoenzyme. Usually (but not always)
elevated levels are seen in patients with prostatic cancer, especially if it has metastasized beyond the
capsule to other parts of the body.

Because acid phosphatase is also found at high concentrations in seminal fluid, this test can be
performed on vaginal secretions to investigate alleged rape. This is now the primary use of PAP
testing. High levels of acid phosphatase also exist in white blood cells (mostly monocytes and lymphocytes). They are helpful in determining the clinical course of patients with lymphoproliferative
diseases and hairy cell leukemia. Acid phosphatase is a lysosomal enzyme; therefore lysosomal
storage diseases (such as Gaucher disease and Niemann-Pick disease) are associated with elevated
levels.

INTERFERING FACTORS

- Falsely high levels of acid phosphatase (and specifically PAP) may occur in males after a digital rectal
  examination or after instrumentation of the prostate (e.g., cystoscopy) because of prostatic stimulation. Elevated levels of 25% to 50% may occur for up to 48 hours after prostate manipulation. The test
  should be repeated if elevated levels occur after a rectal or prostate examination.

- Alkaline and acid phosphatase are very similar enzymes that function at different pH levels. Any condition associated with very high levels of alkaline phosphatase may falsely indicate high acid phosphatase levels.
- Drugs that may cause *increased* levels of acid phosphatase include alglucerase, androgens (in females), and clofibrate (Atromid-S).
- Drugs that may cause *decreased* levels include alcohol, fluorides, heparin, oxalates, and phosphates.

PROCEDURE AND PATIENT CARE

Before
- Explain the procedure to the patient.
- Tell the patient that no food or drink restrictions are necessary.
- Note that some laboratories request notification before the blood sample is drawn so that immediate attention (<1 hour) can be given to the sample.

During
- Collect a venous blood sample in a red-top tube.
- Avoid hemolysis. RBCs contain acid phosphatase.
- Note on the laboratory slip if the patient has had a prostatic or rectal examination or instrumentation of the prostate within the past 24 to 48 hours.

After
- Apply pressure or a pressure dressing to the venipuncture site.
- Assess the venipuncture site for bleeding.
- Promptly deliver the specimen to the laboratory.
- Do not leave the specimen at room temperature for 1 hour or longer; the enzyme is heat and pH sensitive, and acid phosphatase activity will decrease. Once the specimen is received by the laboratory, the use of a preservative and prompt refrigeration are important.

TEST RESULTS AND CLINICAL SIGNIFICANCE

▲ Increased Levels

Prostatic carcinoma,
Benign prostatic hypertrophy,
Prostatitis:

Acid phosphatase and specifically PAP exist in the lysosomes of prostate cells. Diseases affecting prostate tissue will destroy those cells, and the lysosomal contents will spill into the bloodstream, where they will be detected.

Multiple myeloma,
Paget disease,
Hyperparathyroidism,
Metastasis to the bone:

Because acid phosphatase exists in the lysosomes of the bone marrow, diseases affecting the bone will be associated with elevated blood levels.

Multiple myeloma,
Sickle cell crisis,
Thrombocytosis:

Because acid phosphatase exists in the lysosomes of blood cells, diseases affecting blood cells will be associated with elevated blood levels.

Lysosomal disorders (e.g., Gaucher disease): *Because acid phosphatase exists in the lysosomes of many tissues affected by these diseases, elevated blood levels can be expected.*

Renal diseases,

Liver diseases, such as cirrhosis:

Because acid phosphatase is present in these organs, diseases affecting these organs will be associated with elevated blood levels.

Rape:

PAP will be elevated in vaginal secretions of a woman having been recently raped. The PAP assay is a well-documented presumptive assay for the presence of semen.

Related Tests

Prostate Specific Antigen (PSA) (p. 420). This is a more specific test for prostatic cancer.

Alkaline Phosphatase (p. 47). This is a similar enzyme that is more easily identified in an alkaline environment. It is useful in the evaluation of diseases of the liver and bone.

Activated Clotting Time (ACT, Activated Coagulation Time)

NORMAL FINDINGS

70-120 seconds

Therapeutic range for anticoagulation: 150-600 seconds

(Normal ranges and anticoagulation ranges vary according to particular therapy.)

INDICATIONS

The ACT is primarily used to measure the anticoagulant effect of heparin or other direct thrombin inhibitors during cardiac angioplasty, hemodialysis, and cardiopulmonary bypass (CPB) surgery.

TEST EXPLANATION

This test measures the time for whole blood to clot after the addition of particulate activators. Like the activated partial thromboplastin time (aPTT, p. 383), it measures the ability of the *intrinsic pathway* (reaction 1) to begin clot formation by activating factor XII (see Figure 2-12, p. 167). By checking the blood clotting status with ACT, the response to unfractionated heparin therapy can be easily and rapidly monitored. Equally important is the use of the ACT in determining the appropriate dose of protamine sulfate required to reverse the effect of heparin on completion of surgical procedures and hemodialysis.

Both the aPTT and the ACT can be used to monitor heparin therapy in patients on CPB. However, the ACT has several advantages over the aPTT. First, the ACT is more accurate than the aPTT when high doses of heparin are used for anticoagulation. This makes it especially useful during clinical situations requiring high-dose heparin, such as during CPB when high-dose anticoagulation is necessary at levels 10 times those used for venous thrombosis. The aPTT is not measurable at these high doses. The accepted goal for the ACT is 400-480 seconds during CPB.

Second, the ACT is not only less expensive, but it is also more easily and rapidly performed than the aPTT, which is time consuming and requires full laboratory facilities. The ACT can be performed at the bedside. This provides immediate information on which further therapeutic anticoagulation decisions can be based. The capability to perform the ACT at the "point of care" makes the ACT particularly useful for patients requiring angioplasty, hemodialysis, and CPB.

A nomogram adjusted to the patient's baseline ACT is often used as a guide to reach the desired level of anticoagulation during these procedures. This same nomogram is used in determining the dose of protamine to be administered to neutralize the heparin when a return to normal coagulation is desired on completion of these procedures. The ACT is used in determining when it is safe to remove the vascular access after these procedures. The *modified ACT test* requires a smaller-volume blood specimen, automated blood sampling, standardized blood/reagent mixing, and faster clotting time results than the conventional ACT. The modified ACT is now being used more frequently.

INTERFERING FACTORS

- The ACT is affected by several biologic variables, including hypothermia, hemodilution, and platelet number and function.
- Factors affecting the pharmacokinetics of heparin (e.g., kidney or liver disease) and heparin resistance due to antithrombin deficiency and contact factor deficiencies can affect ACT measurements.
- A partially or completely occluded specimen can increase ACT measurements.

PROCEDURE AND PATIENT CARE

Before

🖉 Explain the procedure to the patient.

During

- Less than 1 mL of blood is collected into a commercial container. This container is then placed into a whole blood microcoagulation analyzer at the bedside. When a clot is formed, the ACT value is displayed on the machine's panel.
- If the patient is receiving a continuous heparin drip, the blood sample is obtained from the arm without the intravenous catheter.

After

- Apply pressure to the venipuncture site. Remember that the bleeding time will be prolonged because of anticoagulation therapy.
- Assess the patient to detect possible bleeding. Check for blood in the urine and all other excretions and assess the patient for bruises, petechiae, and low back pain.
- For clinical significance, the test results must be correlated with the time of heparin administration. A clinical flow sheet is used to list the test results with the time and route of heparin administration.

TEST RESULTS AND CLINICAL SIGNIFICANCE

▲ Increased Levels

Heparin administration: *Heparin, along with antithrombin III, interrupts in the action of several coagulation proteins (except factor VII). As a result, the intrinsic pathway of coagulation is inhibited. This pathway is measured by the ACT and is therefore prolonged.*

Clotting factor deficiencies: *Deficiencies in any clotting factor associated with the intrinsic pathway will be associated with prolonged ACT.*

Cirrhosis of the liver: *Coagulation factors are proteins that are synthesized in the liver. Liver pathology therefore is associated with a reduction in coagulation factors; this prolongs the time required for the reactions of the intrinsic pathway and prolongs the ACT.*

Coumadin administration: *Deficiencies in the vitamin K clotting factors associated with the intrinsic pathway will cause a prolonged ACT.*

Lupus inhibitor: *Lupus inhibitors are autoantibodies against components involved in the activation of the coagulation cascade and thus prolong the ACT.*

▼ Decreased Levels

Thrombosis: *In thrombotic syndromes in which secondary hemostasis is inappropriately stimulated, the ACT may be shortened.*

RELATED TESTS

Partial Thromboplastin Time (PTT) (p. 383). The PTT is another test used to evaluate the intrinsic pathway of secondary hemostasis. It, too, is commonly used to monitor heparin therapy.

Prothrombin Time (p. 434). The PT is used to evaluate the extrinsic and common pathways of secondary hemostasis.

Coagulating Factor Concentration (p. 163). This is a quantitative measurement of specific coagulation factors.

Adrenal Steroid Precursors (Androstenediones [AD], Dehydroepiandrosterone [DHEA], Dehydroepiandrosterone Sulfate [DHEA S], 11-Deoxycortisol, 17-Hydroxyprogesterone, 17-Hydroxypregnenolone, Pregnenolone)

NORMAL FINDINGS

		Female	Male
AD	Tanner Stage I	0.05-0.51 ng/mL	0.04-0.32 ng/mL
	Tanner Stage II	0.15-1.37 ng/mL	0.08-0.48 ng/mL
	Tanner Stage III	0.37-2.24 ng/mL	0.14-0.87 ng/mL
	Tanner Stage IV-V	0.35-2.05 ng/mL	0.27-1.07 ng/mL
DHEA	Tanner Stage I	0.14-2.76 ng/mL	0.11-2.37 ng/mL
	Tanner Stage II	0.83-4.87 ng/mL	0.37-3.66 ng/mL
	Tanner Stage III	1.08-7.56 ng/mL	0.75-5.24 ng/mL
	Tanner Stage IV-V	1.24-7.88 ng/mL	1.22-6.73 ng/mL
DHEA S	Tanner Stage I	7-209 mcg/dL	7-126 mcg/dL
	Tanner Stage II	28-260 mcg/dL	13-241 mcg/dL
	Tanner Stage III	39-390 mcg/dL	32-446 mcg/dL
	Tanner Stage IV and V	81-488 mcg/dL	65-371 mcg/dL

INDICATIONS

This test is used for evaluating virilizing syndromes and amenorrhea.

TEST EXPLANATION

Androstenediones (ADs, DHEA, and the sulfuric ester, DHEA S) are precursors of testosterone and estrone, and are made in the gonads and the adrenal gland. 11-Deoxycortisol, 17-hydroxyprogesterone,

17-hydroxypregnenolone, and pregnenolone are precursors of cortisol. ACTH stimulates their adrenal secretion. Children with congenital adrenal hyperplasia (CAH) have genetic mutations that cause deficiencies in the enzymes involved in the synthesis of cortisol, testosterone, aldosterone, and estrone. When defects in enzyme synthesis occur along the path of hormone synthesis, the listed precursors exists in levels that exceed normal through the increased stimulation of ACTH. In most cases, CAH is a genetic autosomal recessive disorder.

The symptoms of this disorder depend on which steroids are overproduced and which are deficient. As a result, CAH may present with various symptoms, including virilization of the affected female infant, signs of androgen excess in males and females, signs of sex hormone deficiency in males and females, salt-wasting crisis secondary to cortisol and aldosterone deficiency, or hormonal hypertension caused by increased mineralocorticoids. A milder, nonclassic form of CAH is characterized by premature puberty, acne, hirsutism, menstrual irregularity, and infertility.

These same precursors can occur in adults because of adrenal or gonadal tumors that produce one of these precursors. Patients with polycystic ovary (Stein-Leventhal) syndrome have particularly elevated levels of ADs. Levels of DHEA S are particularly high in patients with adrenal carcinoma.

In patients suspected of CAH, testing for a panel of steroids involved in the cortisol biosynthesis pathway may be performed to establish the specific enzyme deficiency. In most cases, basal concentrations within the normal reference interval rule out CAH. The ratio of the precursor to the final pathway product (with and without ACTH stimulation) may be used to diagnose which enzyme is deficient.

Testing is performed by Quantitative High Performance Liquid Chromatography-Tandem Mass Spectrometry. Results vary considerably based on testing method.

INTERFERING FACTORS

- A radioactive scan performed 1 week before the test may invalidate the test results, if it is performed by radioimmunoassay.
- Drugs that may *increase* levels of androstenedione are clomiphene, corticotropin, and metyrapone.
- Steroids may *decrease* levels of androstenedione.

PROCEDURE AND PATIENT CARE

Before

- Explain the procedure to the patient.
- Tell the patient that the specimen should be collected 1 week before or after the menstrual period.
- Note that fasting is preferable.
- Because peak production of androstenedione is around 7 AM, blood should be drawn around that time.

During

- Collect a venous blood sample in a red-top or gold-top tube.
- Indicate the date of the last menstrual period on the laboratory form.

After

- Apply pressure or a pressure dressing to the venipuncture site.
- Assess the venipuncture site for bleeding.

TEST RESULTS AND CLINICAL SIGNIFICANCE

▲ Increased Levels

Adrenal tumor: *Some tumors make large amounts of androstenediones, which is then converted by the ovaries and fatty tissue to testosterone and estrogen. The relatively high level of testosterone causes the virilizing signs.*

Congenital adrenal hyperplasia: *This disease is characterized by enzyme defects that prevent conversion of androstenediones to cortisol. Androstenediones levels are increased.*

Ectopic ACTH-producing tumors,

Cushing disease:
 ACTH stimulates the adrenal gland to make large amounts of hormones, including androstenediones.

Cushing syndrome: *Large amounts of hormones, including androstenediones, are made in the adrenal gland.*

Stein-Leventhal syndrome

Ovarian sex cord tumor

▼ Decreased Levels

Primary or secondary adrenal insufficiency,

Ovarian failure,

Oophorectomy:
 There is a decreased production and conversion of androstenediones.

RELATED TESTS

Testosterone (p. 476). This is a direct measurement of testosterone.

Estradiol (p. 226). This is a direct measurement of one of the conjugated estrogens.

Cortisol, Blood (p. 179). This is a direct measurement of cortisol, the major adrenal glucocorticosteroid.

Adrenocorticotropic Hormone (ACTH, Corticotropin)

NORMAL FINDINGS

Adult/elderly:
 Female: 19 years and older: 6-58 pg/mL
 Male: 19 years and older: 7-69 pg/mL
Children:
 Male and female: 10-18 years: 6-55 pg/mL
 Male and female: 1 week-9 years: 5-46 pg/mL

INDICATIONS

The serum ACTH study is a test of anterior pituitary gland function that affords the greatest insight into the causes of either Cushing syndrome (overproduction of cortisol) or Addison disease (underproduction of cortisol).

TEST EXPLANATION

An elaborate feedback mechanism for cortisol coordinates the function of the hypothalamus, pituitary gland, and adrenal glands. ACTH is an important aspect of this mechanism.

TABLE 2-2	Cortisol/ACTH Levels in Diagnosis of Adrenal Dysfunction	
Disease	**Cortisol Level**	**ACTH Level**

Cushing syndrome
    Adrenal micronodular hyperplasia
    Adrenal tumor (adenoma, cancer)
	High	Low

Cushing syndrome
    Cushing disease (ACTH-producing pituitary tumor)
    Ectopic ACTH-producing tumor (e.g., lung cancer)
	High	High

Addison disease
    Adrenal gland failure (e.g., infarction, hemorrhage,
        congenital adrenal hyperplasia)
	Low	High

Hypopituitarism	Low	Low

Corticotropin-releasing hormone (CRH) is made in the hypothalamus. This stimulates ACTH production in the anterior pituitary gland, which in turn stimulates the adrenal cortex to produce cortisol. The rising levels of cortisol act as negative feedback and curtail further production of CRH and ACTH.

In the patient with Cushing syndrome, an elevated ACTH level can be caused by a pituitary ACTH-producing tumor or a nonpituitary (ectopic) ACTH-producing tumor, usually in the lung, pancreas, thymus, or ovary. ACTH levels greater than 200 pg/mL usually indicate ectopic ACTH production. If the ACTH level is below normal in a patient with Cushing syndrome, an adrenal adenoma or carcinoma is probably the cause of the hyperfunction (Table 2-2).

In patients with Addison disease, an elevated ACTH level indicates primary adrenal gland failure, as in adrenal gland destruction caused by infarction, hemorrhage, or autoimmunity; surgical removal of the adrenal gland; congenital enzyme deficiency; or adrenal suppression after prolonged ingestion of exogenous steroids. If the ACTH level is below normal in a patient with adrenal insufficiency, hypopituitarism is most probably the cause of the hypofunction (see Table 2-2).

ACTH can be directly measured by Quantitative Chemiluminescent Immunoassay. ACTH levels exhibit diurnal variations that correspond to cortisol levels. Levels in evening (8 PM to 10 PM) samples are usually one half to two thirds those of morning (4 AM to 8 AM) specimens. This diurnal variation is lost when disease (especially neoplasm) affects the pituitary or adrenal glands. Likewise stress can blunt or eliminate this normal diurnal variation.

ACTH is measured in amniotic fluid when anencephaly is suspected. Decreased levels are noted in anencephalic fetuses (see discussion of amniocentesis on p. 632).

INTERFERING FACTORS

- Stress (trauma, pyrogen, hypoglycemia), menses, and pregnancy cause increased levels of cortisol. This is accomplished through elevation of ACTH.
- Recently administered radioisotope scans can affect levels measured by radioimmunoassay or immunoradiometry.
- Drugs that may cause *increased* levels include aminoglutethimide, amphetamines, estrogens, ethanol, insulin, levodopa, metyrapone, spironolactone, and vasopressin.
- Exogenously administered corticosteroids decrease ACTH levels.

| **Clinical Priorities** |

- Evaluate the patient for stress factors that could invalidate test results.
- Remember that there is a diurnal variation in ACTH levels that corresponds to cortisol levels. With a normal sleep pattern, levels are highest in the morning and lowest in the evening.

PROCEDURE AND PATIENT CARE

Before

✗ Explain the procedure to the patient. Allow plenty of time to answer questions so the patient's stress is diminished as much as possible.

✗ Keep the patient on nothing by mouth (NPO) status after midnight the day of the test.

- Evaluate the patient for stress factors that could invalidate the test results.
- Evaluate the patient for sleep pattern abnormalities. With a normal sleep pattern, the ACTH level is highest between 4 AM and 8 AM and lowest around 9 PM.
- Assess the patient for self-administration of drugs that could affect test results.

During

- Collect a venous blood sample in a lavender (EDTA) or pink-top (K_2 EDTA) tube or as required by your reference laboratory.
- Chill the blood tube to prevent enzymatic degradation of ACTH.

After

- Place the specimen in ice water and send it to the chemistry laboratory immediately. ACTH is a very unstable peptide in plasma and should be stored at −20° C to prevent artificially low values.
- Apply pressure or a pressure dressing to the venipuncture site.
- Assess the venipuncture site for bleeding.

TEST RESULTS AND CLINICAL SIGNIFICANCE

▲ Increased Levels

Addison disease (primary adrenal insufficiency),
Adrenogenital syndrome (congenital adrenal hyperplasia):
   The adrenal glands are not making enough cortisol for the body's needs. The reduced serum cortisol level is a strong stimulus to pituitary production of ACTH.
Cushing disease (pituitary-dependent adrenal hyperplasia),
Ectopic ACTH syndrome,
Stress:
   ACTH is overproduced as a result of neoplastic overproduction of ACTH in the pituitary or elsewhere in the body by an ACTH-producing cancer. Stress is a potent stimulus to ACTH production.

▼ Decreased Levels

Secondary adrenal insufficiency (pituitary insufficiency),
Hypopituitarism:
   The pituitary gland is incapable of producing adequate ACTH.
Adrenal adenoma or carcinoma,
Cushing syndrome,

Exogenous steroid administration:
Overproduction or availability of cortisol is a strong inhibitor to pituitary production of ACTH.

RELATED TESTS

Cortisol, Blood, and Urine (pp. 179 and 920). Cortisol is a hormone produced by the adrenal gland and is the main determinant of Cushing syndrome (overproduction) or Addison disease (underproduction).
Adrenocorticotropic Hormone (ACTH) Stimulation (p. 34). This test is used to determine the cause of adrenal insufficiency.
Dexamethasone Suppression (p. 204). This test is used to determine the cause of Cushing syndrome.
Adrenocortotropic Hormone Stimulation With Metyrapone (p. 36). This test is used to determine the cause of Cushing syndrome.

Adrenocorticotropic Hormone Stimulation (ACTH Stimulation With Cosyntropin, Cortisol Stimulation)

NORMAL FINDINGS

Rapid test: cortisol levels increase >7 mg/dL above baseline
24-hour test: cortisol levels >40 mcg/dL
3-day test: cortisol levels >40 mcg/dL

INDICATIONS

This test evaluates the ability of the adrenal gland to respond to ACTH administration. It is useful in evaluating the cause of adrenal insufficiency and also in evaluating patients with cushingoid symptoms.

TEST EXPLANATION

This test is performed on patients found to have adrenal insufficiency. An increase in plasma cortisol levels after the infusion of an ACTH-like drug indicates that the adrenal gland is normal and capable of functioning if stimulated. In that case the cause of adrenal insufficiency would lie within the pituitary gland (hypopituitarism, which is called secondary adrenal insufficiency). If little or no rise in cortisol levels occurs after the administration of the ACTH-like drug, the adrenal gland is the source of the problem and cannot secrete cortisol. This is called primary adrenal insufficiency (Addison disease), which may be caused by adrenal hemorrhage, infarction, autoimmunity, metastatic tumor, surgical removal of the adrenal glands, or congenital adrenal enzyme deficiency.

This test can also be used to evaluate patients with Cushing syndrome. Patients with Cushing syndrome caused by bilateral adrenal hyperplasia have an exaggerated cortisol elevation in response to the administration of the ACTH-like drug. Those experiencing Cushing syndrome as a result of hyperfunctioning adrenal tumors (which are usually autonomous and relatively insensitive to ACTH) have little or no increase in cortisol levels over baseline values.

Cosyntropin (Cortrosyn) is a synthetic subunit of ACTH that has the same corticosteroid-stimulating effect as endogenous ACTH in healthy persons. During this test, cosyntropin is administered to the patient, and the ability of the adrenal gland to respond is measured by plasma cortisol levels.

The *rapid stimulation test* is only a screening test. A normal response excludes adrenal insufficiency. An abnormal response, however, requires a 1- to 3-day prolonged ACTH stimulation test to differentiate primary insufficiency from secondary insufficiency. It should be noted that the adrenal gland can also be stimulated by insulin-induced hypoglycemia as a stressing agent. When insulin is the stimulant, cortisol and glucose levels are measured.

INTERFERING FACTORS

🍴 Drugs that may cause artificially *increased* cortisol levels include prolonged corticosteroid administration, estrogens, and spironolactone.

PROCEDURE AND PATIENT CARE

Before

✂ Have the patient remain on nothing by mouth (NPO) status after midnight the day of the test.

During

Rapid Test

- Obtain a baseline plasma cortisol level less than 30 minutes before cosyntropin administration.
- Administer an intravenous (IV) injection of cosyntropin over a 2-minute period. An intramuscular (IM) injection may also be used.
- Measure plasma cortisol levels 30 and 60 minutes after drug administration. Serum or heparinized blood is acceptable.

24-Hour Test

- Obtain a baseline plasma cortisol level.
- Start an IV infusion of synthetic cosyntropin for administration over 24 hours.
- After 24 hours, obtain another plasma cortisol level.

3-Day Test

- Obtain a baseline plasma cortisol level.
- Administer cosyntropin intravenously over an 8-hour period on 2 to 3 consecutive days.
- Plasma cortisol is then measured at 12, 24, 36, 48, 60, and 72 hours after the start of the test.

After

- Apply pressure or a pressure dressing to the venipuncture site.
- Check the venipuncture site for bleeding.

TEST RESULTS AND CLINICAL SIGNIFICANCE

▲ Exaggerated Response

Cushing syndrome: *Bilateral adrenal hyperplasia.*

Adrenal insufficiency: *Secondary adrenal insufficiency caused by hypopituitarism, exogenous steroid ingestion, or endogenous steroid production from nonendocrine tumor.*

▼ Normal or Below-Normal Response

Cushing syndrome: *Adrenal adenoma, adrenal carcinoma, ACTH-producing tumor, chronic steroid ingestion.*

Adrenal insufficiency: *Primary adrenal insufficiency (Addison disease) caused by adrenal infarction, hemorrhage, infection, or metastatic tumor to adrenal gland.*

Congenital enzyme adrenal insufficiency, surgical removal of adrenal gland, and ingestion of drugs, such as mitotane, metyrapone, or aminoglutethimide.

RELATED TESTS

Cortisol (p. 179). Cortisol is a hormone produced by the adrenal gland and is the main determinant of Cushing syndrome (overproduction) or Addison disease (underproduction).

Adrenocorticotropic Hormone (ACTH) (p. 31). This test is used to determine the cause of Cushing syndrome or Addison disease.

Dexamethasone Suppression (p. 204). This test is used to determine the cause of Cushing syndrome.

Adrenocortotropic Hormone Stimulation With Metyrapone (see following test). This test is used to determine the cause of Cushing syndrome.

Adrenocorticotropic Hormone Stimulation With Metyrapone (Metyrapone, ACTH Stimulation With Metyrapone)

NORMAL FINDINGS

24-Hour Urine

Baseline excretion of urinary 17-hydroxycorticosteroid (OCHS) more than doubled

Blood

11-Deoxycortisol increased to >7 mcg/dL and cortisol <10 mcg/dL

INDICATIONS

This test is useful in differentiating adrenal hyperplasia from a primary adrenal tumor by determining whether the pituitary-adrenal feedback mechanism is intact.

TEST EXPLANATION

Metyrapone (Metopirone) is a potent blocker of an enzyme involved in cortisol production. Cortisol production is therefore reduced. When this drug is given, the resulting decrease in cortisol production should stimulate pituitary secretion of adrenocorticotropic hormone (ACTH) by way of a negative-feedback mechanism. Cortisol itself cannot be synthesized because of the metyrapone inhibition at the 11-beta-hydroxylation step, but an abundance of cortisol precursors (11-deoxycortisol and OCHS) will be formed. These cortisol precursors can be detected in the urine or in the blood. This test is similar to the ACTH stimulation test.

In patients with adrenal hyperplasia caused by pituitary overproduction of ACTH, the cortisol precursors are greatly increased. This is because the normal adrenal-pituitary feedback response mechanism is still intact. No response to metyrapone occurs in patients with Cushing syndrome resulting from adrenal adenoma or carcinoma, because the tumors are autonomous and therefore insensitive to changes in ACTH secretion. This test has no significant advantage over the ACTH stimulation test in the differential diagnosis of Cushing disease.

This test is also used to evaluate the pituitary reserve capacity to produce ACTH. It can document that adrenal insufficiency exists as a result of pituitary disease (secondary adrenal insufficiency) rather than primary adrenal pathology. This test should not be performed if primary adrenal insufficiency is likely. A severe, life-threatening adrenal crisis could be precipitated. A normal response to ACTH should be demonstrated before metyrapone is given.

CONTRAINDICATIONS

- Patients with possible primary adrenal insufficiency, because metyrapone could reduce the production of what little cortisol is produced and precipitate an adrenal crisis.
- Patients taking glucocorticoids.

POTENTIAL COMPLICATIONS

- Addison disease and addisonian crisis, because metyrapone inhibits cortisol production

INTERFERING FACTORS

- Recent administration of radioisotopes can interfere with test results performed by radioimmunoassay (RIA).
- Chlorpromazine (Thorazine) interferes with the response to metyrapone and should not be administered during the testing.

Clinical Priorities

- This test evaluates the intactness of the pituitary-adrenal feedback mechanism.
- This test should not be performed on patients with adrenal insufficiency. A severe, life-threatening adrenal or addisonian crisis could result.
- Patients should be carefully assessed for impending signs of addisonian crisis, which include glucocorticoid deficiency, drop in extracellular fluid volume, and hyperkalemia. This is a medical emergency and must be treated vigorously.

PROCEDURE AND PATIENT CARE

Before

 Explain the procedure to the patient.
- Obtain a baseline 24-hour urine specimen for 17-OCHS level for the urine test.
- Obtain a baseline cortisol level (see p. 179) for the blood test.

During

Blood

- Administer a prescribed dose of metyrapone at 11 PM the night before the blood specimen is to be collected. Collect a blood specimen in the morning.

Urine

- Obtain a 24-hour urine specimen for a 17-OCHS baseline level. Then collect a 24-hour urine specimen for the 17-OCHS level during and again 1 day after the oral administration of a dose of metyrapone, which may be given every 4 hours for 24 hours.

After

- Assess the patient for impending signs of addisonian crisis (muscle weakness, mental and emotional changes, anorexia, nausea, vomiting, hypotension, hyperkalemia, vascular collapse).
- Note that addisonian crisis is a medical emergency that must be treated vigorously. Basically, the immediate treatment includes replenishing steroids, reversing shock, and restoring blood circulation.

TEST RESULTS AND CLINICAL SIGNIFICANCE

▲   Increased Levels

Adrenal hyperplasia: *Cortisol precursors will be significantly increased as a result of accentuating the ACTH effect.*

Adrenal tumor: *Tumors are autonomous and are not affected by inhibitory or stimulatory feedback. There is no apparent change in cortisol precursors.*

Ectopic ACTH syndrome: *This syndrome occurs when neoplasms (usually lung cancer) produce ACTH without regard to regulatory mechanisms. There is no apparent change in cortisol precursors.*

Secondary adrenal insufficiency: *There will be no significant change in cortisol precursors, because there is no pituitary function to stimulate the production of ACTH.*

RELATED TESTS

Adrenocorticotropic Hormone (ACTH) (p. 31). This is a direct measurement of ACTH, which is used in the evaluation of Cushing syndrome and Addison disease.

Adrenocorticotropic Hormone (ACTH) Stimulation (p. 34). This test is used similarly to the metyrapone test for evaluation of Addison disease and Cushing syndrome.

Age-Related Macular Degeneration Risk Analysis (Y402H and A69S)

NORMAL FINDINGS

No mutation noted.

INDICATIONS

This test is used for risk assessment and as supportive documentation of macular degeneration.

TEST EXPLANATION

Age-related macular degeneration (ARMD) is recognized as a leading cause of blindness in the United States. Blurred or distorted vision and difficulty adjusting to dim light are common symptoms. ARMD, both wet and dry types, is considered a multifactorial disorder, as it is thought to develop because of the interplay among environmental (smoking), genetic (gender, ethnicity) risk, and protective (antioxidants) factors. At least two genetic variants (Y402H and A69S) have been found to be associated with an increased risk for ARMD. The Y402H and A69S variant genetic variants are common polymorphisms in ARMD. An individual with two copies of the Y402H variant in the gene *CFH* and two copies of the A69S variant in the gene *LOC387715* has an approximate 60-fold increased risk for ARMD. This is significant given how common ARMD is in the general population.

This information can be clinically useful when making medical management decisions (e.g., the use of inflammatory markers) and emphasizing to patients the benefits of smoking cessation and dietary modification. In some cases, genotype information may also assist with clinical diagnosis.

PROCEDURE AND PATIENT CARE

Before

Explain the procedure to the patient.

During

- Collect a venous sample of blood in a lavender- (EDTA) or a yellow-top (ACD) tube.

After

- Apply pressure to the venipuncture site.
- Tell the patient that results may not be available for a few weeks.

ABNORMAL FINDINGS

▲ **Increased**

ARMD—*Patients with abnormal genetics as described are at a marked increased risk for developing macular degeneration.*

Alanine Aminotransferase (ALT, formerly Serum Glutamic-Pyruvic Transaminase [SGPT])

NORMAL FINDINGS

Elderly: may be slightly higher than adult values
Adult/child: 4-36 international units/L at 37° C or 4-36 units/L (SI units)
Values may be higher in men and in African Americans.
Infant: may be twice as high as adult values

INDICATIONS

This test is used to identify hepatocellular diseases of the liver. It is also an accurate monitor of improvement or worsening of these diseases. In jaundiced patients an abnormal alanine aminotransferase (ALT) will incriminate the liver rather than red blood cell (RBC) hemolysis as a source of the jaundice.

TEST EXPLANATION

ALT is found predominantly in the liver; lesser quantities are found in the kidneys, heart, and skeletal muscle. Injury or disease affecting the liver parenchyma will cause a release of this hepatocellular enzyme into the bloodstream, thus elevating serum ALT levels. Most ALT elevations are caused by liver dysfunction. Therefore this enzyme is not only sensitive but also quite specific for hepatocellular disease. In hepatocellular disease other than viral hepatitis the ALT/AST (aspartate aminotransferase) ratio (DeRitis ratio) is less than 1. In viral hepatitis the ratio is greater than 1. This is helpful in the diagnosis of viral hepatitis.

INTERFERING FACTORS

- Previous intramuscular (IM) injections may cause elevated levels.
- Drugs that may cause *increased* ALT levels include acetaminophen, allopurinol, aminosalicylic acid, ampicillin, azathioprine, carbamazepine, cephalosporins, chlordiazepoxide, chlorpropamide, clofibrate, cloxacillin, codeine, dicumarol, indomethacin, isoniazid (INH), methotrexate, methyldopa, nafcillin, nalidixic acid, nitrofurantoin, oral contraceptives, oxacillin, phenothiazines, phenylbutazone, phenytoin, procainamide, propoxyphene, propranolol, quinidine, salicylates, tetracyclines, and verapamil.

PROCEDURE AND PATIENT CARE

Before

- Explain the procedure to the patient.
- Tell the patient that no fasting is required.

During

- Collect a venous blood sample in a red-top tube and send it to the laboratory for analysis.

After

- Apply pressure or a pressure dressing to the venipuncture site.
- Assess the venipuncture site for bleeding. Patients with liver dysfunction often have prolonged clotting times.

TEST RESULTS AND CLINICAL SIGNIFICANCE

▲ Significantly Increased Levels

Hepatitis
Hepatic necrosis
Hepatic ischemia

▲ Moderately Increased Levels

Cirrhosis
Cholestasis
Hepatic tumor
Hepatotoxic drugs
Obstructive jaundice
Severe burns
Trauma to striated muscle

▲ Mildly Increased Levels

Myositis,
Pancreatitis,
Myocardial infarction,
Infectious mononucleosis,
Shock:
  Injury or disease affecting the liver, heart, or skeletal muscles will cause a release of this enzyme into the bloodstream, thus elevating serum ALT levels.

RELATED TESTS

Aspartate Aminotransferase (AST) (p. 119). This is another enzyme existing predominantly in the liver.

Gamma-Glutamyl Transpeptidase (GGTP) (p. 246). This is another enzyme predominantly existing in the liver.

Alkaline Phosphatase (p. 47). This is another enzyme existing predominantly in the liver.

5′-Nucleotidase (p. 376). This is another enzyme existing predominantly in the liver.

Creatine Kinase (CK) (p. 186). This enzyme is used similarly to AST and exists predominantly in heart and skeletal muscle.

Lactic Dehydrogenase (LDH) (p. 329). This is an intracellular enzyme used to support the diagnosis of injury or disease involving the heart, liver, RBCs, kidneys, skeletal muscle, brain, and lungs.

Leucine Aminopeptidase (p. 337). This enzyme is specific to the hepatobiliary system. Diseases affecting that system will cause elevation of this enzyme.

Aldolase

NORMAL FINDINGS

Adult: 3.0-8.2 Sibley-Lehninger units/dL or 22-59 mU/L at 37° C (SI units)
Child: approximately two times adult
Newborn: approximately four times adult

INDICATIONS

This test is used to aid in the diagnosis and surveillance of skeletal muscle diseases.

TEST EXPLANATION

Serum aldolase is very similar to the enzymes aspartate aminotransferase (AST) (see p. 119) and creatine kinase (CK) (see p. 186). Aldolase is an enzyme used in the glycolytic breakdown of glucose. As with AST and CPK, aldolase is present in most tissues of the body. This test is most useful for identifying muscular or hepatic cellular injury or destruction. The serum aldolase level is very high in patients with muscular dystrophies, dermatomyositis, and polymyositis. Levels also are increased in patients with gangrenous processes, muscular trauma, and muscular infectious diseases (e.g., trichinosis). Elevated levels are also noted in chronic hepatitis, obstructive jaundice, and cirrhosis.

Neurologic diseases causing weakness can be differentiated from muscular causes of weakness with this test. Normal values are seen in patients with such neurologic diseases as poliomyelitis, myasthenia gravis, and multiple sclerosis. Elevated aldolase levels are seen in patients with primary muscular disorders.

INTERFERING FACTORS

- Previous intramuscular (IM) injections may cause elevated levels.
- Strenuous exercise can cause a transient spike in aldolase.
- Drugs that may cause *increased* aldolase levels include hepatotoxic agents.
- Drugs that may cause *decreased* levels include phenothiazine.

PROCEDURE AND PATIENT CARE

Before

🖎 Explain the procedure to the patient.
🖎 Note that a short period of fasting usually will provide more accurate results.

During

- Collect a venous blood sample in a red-top tube.

After

- Apply pressure or a pressure dressing to the venipuncture site.
- Observe the venipuncture site for bleeding.

TEST RESULTS AND CLINICAL SIGNIFICANCE

▲ Increased Levels

Muscular Diseases

Muscular dystrophy (highest aldolase levels associated with Duchenne muscular dystrophy)
Dermatomyositis
Polymyositis

Muscle Injury

Muscular trauma (examples include severe crush injuries, muscular infections [such as trichinosis], delirium tremens, severe burns),
Gangrenous/ischemic processes (such as prolonged shock):
Disease of or injury to muscle causes lysis of the muscle cells. Intracellular enzymes such as aldolase spill out into the bloodstream and are detected at elevated levels.

Hepatocellular Diseases

Hepatitis,
Cirrhosis:
Diseases of the liver cause lysis of the liver cells. Intracellular enzymes such as aldolase spill out into the bloodstream and are detected at elevated levels.

Myocardial Infarction

Infarction of heart muscle causes lysis of the muscle cells. Intracellular enzymes such as aldolase spill out into the bloodstream and are detected at elevated levels.

▼ Decreased Levels

Muscle wasting diseases,
Late muscular dystrophy:
As muscle mass decreases, aldolase values decrease.
Hereditary fructose intolerance: *Without an adequate source of glycogen (i.e., fructose), normal levels of aldolase are not needed.*

RELATED TEST

Creatine Kinase (CK) (p. 186). CK is another muscular enzyme and is more frequently used for identifying cardiac and skeletal injury.

Aldosterone

NORMAL FINDINGS

Blood

Supine: 3-10 ng/dL or 0.08-0.30 nmol/L (SI units)
Upright (sitting for at least 2 hours)
    Female: 5-30 ng/dL or 0.14-0.80 nmol/L (SI units)
    Male: 6-22 ng/dL or 0.17-0.61 nmol/L (SI units)
    Child/adolescent
    Newborn: 5-60 ng/dL
    1 week-1 year: 1-160 ng/dL
    1-3 years: 5-60 ng/dL
    3-5 years: 5-80 ng/dL
    5-7 years: 5-50 ng/dL
    7-11 years: 5-70 ng/dL
    11-15 years: 5-50 ng/dL

Urine

2-26 mcg/24 hour or 6-72 nmol/24 hour (SI units)

INDICATIONS

This test is used to diagnose hyperaldosteronism. To differentiate primary aldosteronism (adrenal pathology) from secondary aldosteronism (extraadrenal pathology), a plasma renin assay must be performed simultaneously.

TEST EXPLANATION

Aldosterone, a hormone produced by the adrenal cortex, is a potent mineralocorticoid. Production of aldosterone is regulated primarily by the renin-angiotensin system. This system works as follows: a decreased effective renal blood flow triggers pressure-sensitive renal glomerular elements to release renin. The renin then stimulates the liver to secrete angiotensin I, which is converted to angiotensin II in the lung and kidney. Angiotensin II is a potent stimulator of aldosterone (see Figure 2-26, p. 448).

    Secondarily, aldosterone is stimulated by adrenocorticotropic hormone (ACTH), low serum sodium levels, and high serum potassium levels. Aldosterone in turn stimulates the renal tubules to absorb sodium (water follows) and to secrete potassium in the urine. In this way, aldosterone regulates serum sodium and potassium levels. Because water follows sodium transport, aldosterone also partially regulates water absorption (and plasma volume).

    Increased aldosterone levels are associated with primary aldosteronism in which a tumor (usually an adenoma) of the adrenal cortex (Conn syndrome) or bilateral adrenal nodular hyperplasia causes increased production of aldosterone. The typical pattern for primary aldosteronism is an increased aldosterone level and a decreased renin level. The renin level is low because the increased aldosterone level "turns off" the renin-angiotensin system. Patients with primary aldosteronism characteristically have hypertension, weakness, polyuria, and hypokalemia.

Increased aldosterone levels also occur with secondary aldosteronism caused by nonadrenal conditions. These include the following:

- Renal vascular stenosis or occlusion
- Hyponatremia (from diuretic or laxative abuse) or low salt intake
- Hypovolemia
- Pregnancy or use of estrogens
- Malignant hypertension
- Potassium loading
- Poor perfusion states (e.g., congestive heart failure)
- Decreased intravascular volume (e.g., cirrhosis, nephrotic syndrome).

In secondary aldosteronism, aldosterone levels and renin levels are high.

The aldosterone assay can be performed on a 24-hour urine specimen or a plasma blood sample. The advantage of the 24-hour urine sample is that short-term fluctuations are eliminated. Plasma values are more convenient to sample, but they are affected by short-term fluctuations. Factors that can rapidly cause fluctuation in aldosterone levels include the following:

- *Diurnal variation:* Peak aldosterone levels occur in early morning. In late afternoon the levels are cut in half.
- *Body position:* In the upright position, plasma aldosterone levels are greatly increased.
- *Diet:* Levels of both urine and plasma aldosterone are increased by low-sodium diets and are decreased by high-sodium diets. (Diets high and low in potassium have the opposite effect.)

A 24-hour urine collection is therefore much more reliable because the effect of these interfering factors is dampened.

Primary aldosteronism can be diagnosed by demonstrating little or no increase in renin levels after aldosterone stimulation (using salt restriction as the stimulant). This is because aldosterone is already maximally secreted by the pathologic adrenal gland. Also, patients with primary aldosteronism fail to suppress aldosterone after saline infusion (1.5 to 2 L of normal saline solution infused between 8 AM and 10 AM). Aldosterone can be measured in blood obtained from adrenal venous sampling. In this situation, high levels from the right and left adrenal veins are diagnostic of bilateral adrenal hyperplasia. Unilateral high aldosterone levels are found in patients with aldosterone-producing tumors of the adrenal gland or renal artery stenosis. Renin levels are usually obtained at the same time. High unilateral renin levels with unilateral high aldosterone levels indicate renal artery stenosis. Aldosterone-producing tumors of the adrenal gland are characterized by unilateral high adrenal vein aldosterone and low renin levels.

INTERFERING FACTORS

- Strenuous exercise and stress can stimulate adrenocortical secretions and increase aldosterone levels.
- Excessive licorice ingestion can cause decreased levels, because it produces an aldosterone-like effect.
- Values are influenced by posture, diet, pregnancy, and diurnal variations.
- Patient position can significantly affect aldosterone levels.
- If the test is performed by radioimmunoassay, recently administered radioactive medications will affect test results.
- Drugs that may cause *increased* levels include diazoxide (Hyperstat), hydralazine (Apresoline), nitroprusside (Nipride), diuretics, laxatives, potassium, and spironolactone.
- Drugs that may cause *decreased* levels include angiotensin-converting enzyme inhibitors (e.g., captopril), fludrocortisone (Florinef), licorice, and propranolol (Inderal).

✔ **Clinical Priorities**

- Aldosterone levels exhibit a diurnal variation, with peak levels occurring early in the morning and lower levels in the late afternoon.
- Body position affects aldosterone levels. Levels are greatly increased in the upright position. Usually patients should be sitting up for at least 2 hours before blood is drawn.
- Levels of both urine and plasma aldosterone are increased by low-sodium diets and are decreased by high-sodium diets. Patients should maintain a normal-sodium diet (approximately 3 g/day) for at least 2 weeks before blood or urine collection.

PROCEDURE AND PATIENT CARE

Before

✗ Explain the procedure for blood collection to the patient. Usually the patient is asked to be in the upright position (at least sitting) for a minimum of 2 hours before blood is drawn. Occasionally blood will be drawn again before the patient gets out of bed. Inform nonhospitalized patients when to arrive at the laboratory and to maintain the upright position for at least 2 hours.

✗ Tell the patient that no fasting is necessary.

✗ Explain the procedure for collecting a 24-hour urine sample.

✗ Give the patient verbal and written instructions regarding dietary and medication restrictions.

✗ Instruct the patient to maintain a normal-sodium diet (approximately 3 g/day) for at least 2 weeks before blood or urine collection.

✗ Have the patient ask the physician whether drugs that alter sodium, potassium, and fluid balance (e.g., diuretics, antihypertensives, steroids, oral contraceptives) should be withheld. Test results will be more accurate if these are suspended at least 2 weeks before either the blood or urine test.

✗ Inform the patient that renin inhibitors (e.g., propranolol) should not be taken 1 week before the test if confirmed by the physician.

✗ Tell the patient to avoid licorice for at least 2 weeks before the test because of its aldosterone-like effect.

During

Blood Collection

- Collect a venous blood sample in a gold-top (serum separator) tube. For hospitalized patients, the sample is occasionally drawn first with the patient in the supine position. A second specimen (upright sample) is collected 4 hours later after the patient has been up and moving.
- Obtain the specimen in the morning.
- Indicate on the laboratory slip if the patient was supine or standing during the venipuncture.
- Handle the blood specimen gently. Rough handling may cause hemolysis and alter the test results.
- Transport the specimen on ice to the laboratory.
- Indicate the source of the specimen (i.e., peripheral or adrenal vein).

Urine Collection

✗ Instruct the patient to begin the 24-hour urine collection after discarding the first morning specimen. This is the start time of the 24-hour collection.

- Collect all urine passed over the next 24 hours into a container containing a boric acid preservative.

✗ Instruct the patient to void before defecating so that the urine is not contaminated by feces.

✗ Remind the patient not to put toilet paper in the collection container.

- Keep the urine specimen on ice or keep it refrigerated during the 24 hours.
- Collect the last specimen as close as possible to the end of the 24 hours.

After
Blood Collection
- Apply pressure or a pressure dressing to the venipuncture site.
- Assess the venipuncture site for bleeding.

Urine Collection
- Transport the urine specimen promptly to the laboratory.

TEST RESULTS AND CLINICAL SIGNIFICANCE
▲   Increased Levels
Primary Aldosteronism
Aldosterone-producing adrenal adenoma (Conn disease),
Adrenal cortical nodular hyperplasia,
Bartter syndrome (renal wasting of potassium associated with poor sodium tubule absorption):
> *Aldosterone is produced in abnormally high quantities by the pathologic adrenal gland. This is reflected in serum and urine levels.*

Secondary Aldosteronism
Hyponatremia,
Hyperkalemia,
Diuretic ingestion resulting in hypovolemia and hyponatremia,
Laxative abuse:
> *These are all direct stimulants of aldosterone.*

Stress,
Malignant hypertension,
Poor perfusion states (e.g., congestive heart failure),
Decreased intravascular volume (e.g., cirrhosis, nephrotic syndrome),
Renal arterial stenosis,
Pregnancy and oral contraceptives,
Hypovolemia or hemorrhage:
> *The renin-angiotensin system is stimulated in these conditions. Renin levels are high, and aldosterone secretion is stimulated.*

Cushing disease: *Abnormally high ACTH levels secreted by a pituitary adenoma act as a direct stimulant to aldosterone.*

▼   Decreased Levels
Aldosterone deficiency
Renin deficiency: *This is very rare and results in aldosterone deficiency.*
Steroid therapy: *ACTH is suppressed and therefore aldosterone is suppressed.*
Addison disease: *The adrenal cortex is not functional and therefore aldosterone cannot be secreted.*
Patients on a high-sodium diet,
Hypernatremia:
> *The above act as potent inhibitors to aldosterone secretion.*

Toxemia of pregnancy
Antihypertensive therapy: *Some antihypertensive medications inhibit aldosterone secretion.*

RELATED TESTS

Sodium, Blood (p. 466), Urine (p. 946), and Potassium, Blood (p. 409), Urine (p. 942). These are direct measurements of these electrolytes.

Adrenocorticotropic Hormone (ACTH) (p. 31). This is a test of anterior pituitary gland function.

Renin Assay (p. 447). This test is helpful in the differential diagnosis of primary versus secondary aldosteronism.

 Alkaline Phosphatase (ALP)

NORMAL FINDINGS

Elderly: slightly higher than adult
Adult: 30-120 units/L or 0.5-2.0 μkat/L (SI units)
Child/adolescent
      <2 years: 85-235 units/L
      2-8 years: 65-210 units/L
      9-15 years: 60-300 units/L
      16-21 years: 30-200 units/L

INDICATIONS

ALP is used to detect and monitor diseases of the liver or bone.

TEST EXPLANATION

Although ALP is found in many tissues, the highest concentrations are found in the liver, biliary tract epithelium, and bone. The intestinal mucosa and placenta also contain ALP. This phosphatase enzyme is called alkaline because its function is increased in an alkaline (pH of 9 to 10) environment. This enzyme test is important for detecting liver and bone disorders. Within the liver, ALP is present in Kupffer cells. These cells line the biliary collecting system. This enzyme is excreted into the bile. Enzyme levels of ALP are greatly increased in both extrahepatic and intrahepatic obstructive biliary disease and cirrhosis. Other liver abnormalities, such as hepatic tumors, hepatotoxic drugs, and hepatitis, cause smaller elevations in ALP levels. Reports have indicated that the most sensitive test to indicate tumor metastasis to the liver is the ALP.

Bone is the most frequent extrahepatic source of ALP; new bone growth is associated with elevated ALP levels. Pathologic new bone growth occurs with osteoblastic metastatic (e.g., breast, prostate) tumors. Paget disease, healing fractures, rheumatoid arthritis, hyperparathyroidism, and normal-growing bones are sources of elevated ALP levels as well.

Isoenzymes of ALP are also used to distinguish between liver and bone diseases. These isoenzymes are most easily differentiated by the heat stability test and electrophoresis. The isoenzyme of liver origin (ALP1) is heat stable; the isoenzyme of bone origin (ALP2) is inactivated by heat. The detection of isoenzymes can help differentiate the source of the pathologic condition associated with the elevated total ALP. ALP1 would be expected to be high when liver disease is the source of the elevated total ALP. ALP2 would be expected to be high when bone disease is the source of the elevated total ALP. Another way to separate the source of elevated ALP is to simultaneously test for 5′-nucleotidase. This later enzyme is made predominantly in the liver. If total ALP and 5′-nucleotidase are concomitantly elevated, the disease is in the liver. If 5′-nucleotidase is normal, the bone is the most probable source.

Age-Related Concerns

- Young children have increased ALP levels because their bones are growing. This increase is magnified during the "growth spurt," which occurs at different ages in males and females.

INTERFERING FACTORS

- Recent ingestion of a meal can increase the ALP level.
- Age: Young children with rapid bone growth have increased ALP levels. This is most magnified during the growth spurt. Females and males differ in age of growth spurt.
- Drugs that may cause *increased* ALP levels include albumin made from placental tissue, allopurinol, antibiotics, azathioprine, colchicine, fluorides, indomethacin, isoniazid (INH), methotrexate, methyldopa, nicotinic acid, phenothiazine, probenecid, tetracycline, and verapamil.
- Drugs that may cause *decreased* levels include arsenicals, cyanides, fluorides, nitrofurantoin, oxalates, and zinc salts.

PROCEDURE AND PATIENT CARE

Before

- Explain the procedure to the patient.
- Tell the patient that fasting is preferred but not required. Overnight fasting may be required for isoenzymes. The ALP level is generally higher after eating.

During

- Collect a venous blood sample in a red-top tube.

After

- Apply pressure or a pressure dressing to the venipuncture site.
- Assess the venipuncture site for bleeding. Patients with liver dysfunction often have prolonged clotting times.

TEST RESULTS AND CLINICAL SIGNIFICANCE

▲   Increased Levels

Primary cirrhosis,
Intrahepatic or extrahepatic biliary obstruction,
Primary or metastatic liver tumor:
  ALP is found in the liver and biliary epithelium. It is normally excreted into the bile. Obstruction, no matter how mild, will cause elevations in ALP.
Metastatic tumor to the bone,
Healing fracture,
Hyperparathyroidism,
Osteomalacia,
Paget disease,
Rheumatoid arthritis,
Rickets:
  The ALP comes from the bone in the above-noted diseases.

Intestinal ischemia or infarction
Myocardial infarction
Sarcoidosis

▼ **Decreased Levels**

Hypophosphatemia: *There is insufficient phosphate to make ALP.*
Hypophosphatasia
Malnutrition
Milk-alkali syndrome
Pernicious anemia
Scurvy (vitamin C deficiency)

RELATED TESTS

Alanine Aminotransferase (ALT) (p. 39). This liver enzyme can aid in the differential diagnosis of causes of ALP elevation. If the ALT is elevated along with the ALP, hepatocellular disease is suspected.

Aspartate Aminotransferase (AST) (p. 119). This liver enzyme can aid in the differential diagnosis of causes of ALP elevation. If the AST is elevated along with the ALP, hepatocellular disease is suspected.

Gamma-Glutamyl Transpeptidase (GGT) (p. 246). This liver enzyme can aid in the differential diagnosis of causes of ALP elevation. If the GGT is elevated along with the ALP, diseases affecting the biliary tree are suspected.

5′-Nucleotidase (p. 376). This liver enzyme can aid in the differential diagnosis of causes of ALP elevation. If the 5′-nucleotidase is elevated along with the ALP, diseases affecting the biliary tree are suspected.

Acid Phosphatase (p. 25). This bone enzyme can aid in the differential diagnosis of causes of ALP elevation. If the acid phosphatase is elevated along with the ALP, bone disease is suspected.

Creatine Kinase (CK) (p. 186). This enzyme exists predominantly in heart and skeletal muscle.

Lactic Dehydrogenase (LDH) (p. 329). This intracellular enzyme is used to support the diagnosis of injury or disease involving the heart, liver, red blood cells, kidneys, skeletal muscle, brain, and lungs.

Leucine Aminopeptidase (p. 337). This enzyme is specific to the hepatobiliary system. Diseases affecting that system will cause elevation of this enzyme.

Allergy Blood Testing (IgE Antibody Test, Radioallergosorbent test [RAST])

NORMAL FINDINGS

Total immunoglobulin (IgE) serum
Adult: 0-100 international units/ml
Child
    0-23 months: 0-13 international units/mL
    2-5 years: 0-56 international units/mL
    6-10 years: 0-85 international units/mL

RAST Rating	IgE Level (KU/L)	Comment
0	<0.35	Absent or undetectable allergen specific IgE
1	0.35-0.69	Low level of allergen specific IgE
2	0.70-3.49	Moderate level of allergen specific IgE
3	3.50-17.49	High level of allergen specific IgE
4	17.50-49.99	Very high level of allergen specific IgE
5	50-100	Very high level of allergen specific IgE
6	>100	Extremely high level of allergen specific IgE

INDICATIONS

Allergy blood testing is an alternative to allergy skin testing in diagnosing allergy as a cause of a particular symptom complex. It is also useful in identifying the specific allergen affecting a patient. It is particularly helpful when allergy skin testing is contraindicated.

TEST EXPLANATION

Measurement of serum IgE is an effective method to diagnose allergy and specifically identify the allergen (the substance to which the person is allergic). Serum IgE levels increase when allergic individuals are exposed to the allergen. Various classes of allergens can initiate the allergic response. They include animal dandruff, foods, pollens, dusts, molds, insect venoms, drugs, and agents in the occupational environment.

Although skin testing (see p. 1079) can also identify a specific allergen, measurement of serum levels of IgE is helpful when a skin test result is questionable, when the allergen is not available in a form for dermal injection, or when the allergen may incite an anaphylactic reaction if injected. IgE is particularly helpful in cases in which skin testing is difficult (e.g., in infants or in patients with dermatographism or widespread dermatitis), and it is not always necessary to remove the patient from antihistamines. The decision concerning which method to use to diagnose an allergy and to identify the allergen depends on the elapsed time between exposure to an allergen and testing, class of allergen, age of patient, the possibility of anaphylaxis, and the affected target organ (such as skin, lungs, or intestine). In general, allergy skin testing is the preferred method in comparison with various in vitro tests for assessing the presence of specific IgE antibodies because it is more sensitive and specific, simpler to use, and less expensive.

IgE levels, like provocative skin testing, are used not only to diagnose allergy, but also to identify the allergen so that an immunotherapeutic regimen can be developed. Increased levels of total IgE can be diagnostic of allergic disease in general. Specific IgE blood allergy testing, however, is an in vitro test for specific IgE directed to a specific allergen. Since the development of liquid allergen preparations, the use of in vitro blood allergy testing has increased considerably. It is more accurate and safer than skin testing.

Once the allergen has been identified, for most patients, the treatment would include avoidance of the allergen and use of bronchodilators, antihistamines, and possibly steroids. If aggressive antiallergy treatment is provided before testing, IgE levels may not rise despite the existence of an allergy.

Allergy to latex-containing products is an increasingly common allergy for which certain industrial and most medical personnel are at risk. It is an allergy that may develop in otherwise nonallergic patients because of overexposure. Furthermore, patients with latex exposure are at risk for allergic reaction if they undergo operative procedures or any procedure for which the health care personnel wear latex gloves. In these patients a latex-specific IgE can be easily identified with the use of an enzyme-labeled immunometric assay. This test is 94% accurate.

There are many methods of measuring IgE. One of the most commonly used methods is the radioallergosorbent test (RAST). In this method, the serum of a patient suspected of having a specific allergy is mixed with a specific allergen. The antibody-allergen complex is then incubated with one or more radiolabeled monoclonal anti-IgE antibodies. The total amount of IgE can be measured. Enzyme-conjugated, radioimmunometric, colorimetric, fluorometric, or chemiluminometric methods are used for allergen-specific IgE quantification. Accuracy varies between 45% and 95% depending on the allergen.

Allergy testing of IgG antibodies can also be performed and may provide a more accurate correlation between allergen and allergic symptoms. Like IgE antibody testing, IgG antibody testing is often performed in "panels." For example, there are meat panels that might include IgE or IgG testing for chicken, duck, goose, and turkey. Testing a fruit panel might include IgE or IgG antibody testing for apples, bananas, peaches, and pears. Testing in panels diminishes the cost of testing. Specific allergen antibody testing can follow panel testing. Testing methods vary by laboratory. They may include ELISA/EIA or Quantitative Immunofluorescence Enzyme Assay.

CONTRAINDICATIONS

- Patients with multiple allergies because no information will be obtained regarding identification of the specific allergen.

INTERFERING FACTORS

- Concurrent diseases associated with elevated IgG levels will cause false-negative results.
- Drugs that may cause *increased* IgE levels include corticosteroids.

PROCEDURE

Before

- Explain the procedure to the patient.
- Remind the patient that the suspected allergen will be mixed with the patient's blood specimen in the laboratory. The patient will not experience any allergic reaction by this method of testing.
- Determine if the patient has recently been treated with a corticosteroid for allergies.

During

- Collect a venous blood sample in a gold-top serum tube.

After

- Apply pressure or a pressure bandage to the venipuncture site.

TEST RESULTS AND CLINICAL SIGNIFICANCE

Allergy-Related Diseases

Asthma,
Dermatitis,
Food allergy,
Drug allergy,
Latex allergy,
Occupational allergy,
Allergic rhinitis,

Angioedema:
> *All of the above diseases are immunoreactive conditions in their pathophysiology. IgE is the mediator of the "allergic response" and can be expected to be elevated in these diseases.*

RELATED TESTS

Allergy Skin Testing (p. 1079). Skin testing is the easiest and cheapest manner of determining specific allergic reactions. However, skin testing is not available for many allergens and may instigate an anaphylactic response.

Immunoglobulin Quantification (p. 312). This test is used to assist in the diagnosis of several different disease states. Elevated levels of IgE are occasionally detected, indicating that the disease is associated with an allergic response.

Alpha₁-Antitrypsin (AAT, A₁AT, AAT phenotyping)

NORMAL FINDINGS

85-213 mg/dL or 0.85-2.13 g/L (SI Units)

INDICATIONS

Serum alpha₁-antitrypsin (AAT) determinations are obtained in patients with a family history of emphysema, because there is a familial tendency for a deficiency of this anti-enzyme. Deficient or absent serum levels of this enzyme can cause the early onset of disabling emphysema. A similar deficiency in AAT is seen in children with cirrhosis and other liver diseases.

AAT is also an acute-phase reactant protein that is elevated in the presence of inflammation, infection, or malignancy. It is not specific regarding the source of the inflammatory process.

TEST EXPLANATION

AAT inactivates endoproteases (protein catabolic enzymes that are released in the body by degenerating and dying cells), such as trypsin and neutrophil elastase, that can break down elastic fibers and collagen, especially in the lung. Deficiencies of AAT can be genetic or acquired. Acquired deficiencies in AAT can occur in patients with protein-deficiency syndromes (e.g., malnutrition, liver disease, nephrotic syndrome, neonatal respiratory distress syndrome). People with AAT deficiency develop severe panacinar (although usually more severe in the lower third of the lungs) emphysema in the third or fourth decade of life. Their major clinical symptoms usually include progressive dyspnea with minimal coughing. Chronic bronchitis is prominent in those patients with deficient AAT levels who smoke. Bronchiectasis can also occur in these patients.

Inherited AAT deficiency is associated with symptoms earlier in life than acquired AAT disease. Inherited AAT is also commonly associated with liver and biliary disease. *AAT Genetic Phenotyping (AAT phenotyping)* has shown that most persons have two AAT "M" genes (designated as MM) and AAT levels over 250 mg/dL. "Z" and "S" gene mutations are typically associated with alterations in serum levels of AAT. Individuals who are ZZ or SS homozygous have serum levels below 50 mg/dL and often near zero.

Individuals who are MZ or MS heterozygous have diminished or low-normal serum levels of AAT. Approximately 5% to 14% of the adult population have this heterozygous state, which is considered to be a risk factor for emphysema. Homozygous individuals have severe pulmonary and liver disease very early in life. AAT Phenotyping is particularly helpful when blood AAT levels are suggestive but not definitive.

AAT is qualitatively measured using immunochemical methods. Quantification is possible but rarely useful with phenotyping. Routine serum protein electrophoresis (p. 424) is a good screening test for AAT deficiency, because AAT accounts for about 90% of the protein in the alpha$_1$-globulin region on electrophoresis.

INTERFERING FACTORS

- Serum levels of AAT can double during pregnancy.
- Drugs that may cause *increased* levels include oral contraceptives.

PROCEDURE AND PATIENT CARE

Before

- Explain the procedure to the patient.
- Note that no fasting is usually required. Verify this with the laboratory performing the study.

During

- Collect a venous blood sample in a red-top tube.

After

- Apply pressure or a pressure dressing to the venipuncture site.
- Observe the venipuncture site for bleeding.
- If the results show the patient is at risk for emphysema, begin patient teaching. Include such factors as avoidance of smoking, infection, and inhaled irritants; proper nutrition; adequate hydration; and education about the disease process of emphysema.
- If the test is positive, genetic counseling is indicated. Other family members should be tested to determine their and their children's risks.

TEST RESULTS AND CLINICAL SIGNIFICANCE

▲ Increased Levels

Acute and chronic inflammatory disorders,

Stress,

Infection,

Thyroid infections:

    Because AAT is an acute-phase reactant protein, elevated levels can be expected when the body is subjected to any inflammatory reaction or stress.

▼ Decreased Levels

Early onset of emphysema (adults),

Neonatal respiratory distress syndrome,

Cirrhosis (children):

    These diseases are a result of endoproteases working uninhibited (no AAT available) within the body. Collagen is broken down, setting up the destruction of lung and liver structures.

Low serum proteins: *Diseases such as malnutrition, end-stage cancer, nephrotic syndrome, protein-losing enteropathy, and hepatic failure are associated with lack of protein synthesis. AAT is a protein and therefore will not be produced in adequate quantities in these diseases.*

RELATED TESTS

C-Reactive Protein (p. 184). This also is an acute-phase reactant protein.
Erythrocyte Sedimentation Rate (p. 221). This also is an acute-phase reactant protein.

Alpha-Fetoprotein (AFP, Alpha1-Fetoprotein)

NORMAL FINDINGS

Adult: <40 ng/mL or <40 mcg/L (SI units)
Child younger than 1 year: <30 ng/mL
Ranges are stratified by weeks of gestation and vary among laboratories.

INDICATIONS

This test is used as a screening marker indicating increased risk for birth defects, such as fetal body wall defects, neural tube defects, and chromosomal abnormalities. It can also be used as a tumor marker to identify cancers.

TEST EXPLANATION

AFP is an oncofetal protein normally produced by the fetal liver and yolk sac. It is the dominant fetal serum protein in the first trimester of life and diminishes to very low levels by the age of 1 year. Normally it is found in very low levels in the adult.

AFP is an effective screening serum marker for fetal body wall defects. The most notable of these is neural tube defects, which can vary from a small myelomeningocele to anencephaly. If a fetus has an open body wall defect, fetal serum AFP leaks out into the amniotic fluid and is picked up by the maternal serum. Normally AFP from fetal sources can be detected in the amniotic fluid or the mother's blood after 10 weeks' gestation. Peak levels occur between 16 and 18 weeks. Maternal serum reflects that change in amniotic AFP levels. When elevated maternal serum AFP levels are identified, further evaluation with repeat serum AFP levels, amniotic fluid AFP levels, and ultrasound is warranted. Other examples of fetal body wall defects would include omphalocele and gastroschisis.

Elevated serum AFP levels in pregnancy may also indicate multiple pregnancy, fetal distress, fetal congenital abnormalities, or intrauterine death. Low AFP levels after correction for age of gestation, maternal weight, race, and presence of diabetes are found in mothers carrying a fetus with trisomy 21 (Down syndrome). There are other indicators of trisomy that are often performed simultaneously. See Maternal Screen Testing (p. 354) and Fetal Nuchal Translucency (p. 888).

AFP is also used as a tumor marker. Increased serum levels of AFP are found in as many as 90% of patients with hepatomas. The higher the AFP level, the greater the tumor burden. A decrease in AFP is seen if the patient is responding to antineoplastic therapy. AFP is not specific for hepatomas, although extremely high levels (above 500 ng/mL) are diagnostic for hepatoma. Other neoplastic conditions, such as nonseminomatous germ cell tumors and teratomas of the testes, yolk sac and germ cell tumors of the ovaries, and to a lesser extent Hodgkin disease, lymphoma, and renal cell carcinoma, are also associated with elevated AFP levels. Testing methods for AFP quantification include radioimmunoassay or enzyme-linked immunosorbent assay (ELISA) with a commercially available kit. Noncancerous causes of elevated AFP levels occur in patients with cirrhosis or chronic active hepatitis.

INTERFERING FACTORS

- Fetal blood contamination, which may occur during amniocentesis, can cause increased AFP levels.
- Multiple pregnancies can cause increased levels.
- Recent administration of radioisotopes can affect values because results are determined by radioimmunoassay.

PROCEDURE AND PATIENT CARE

If an AFP test is to be performed on amniotic fluid, follow "Procedure and Patient Care" for amniocentesis, p. 632.

Before

- Explain the procedure to the patient.
- Tell the patient that no food or fluid restriction is required.

During

- Collect a venous blood sample in a red-top tube.

After

- Apply pressure or a pressure dressing to the venipuncture site.
- Assess the venipuncture site for bleeding.
- Include the gestational age on the laboratory slip.

TEST RESULTS AND CLINICAL SIGNIFICANCE

▲ Increased Maternal Serum Levels

Neural tube defects (e.g., anencephaly, encephalocele, spina bifida, myelomeningocele),
Abdominal wall defects (e.g., gastroschisis, omphalocele):

If a fetus has an open body wall defect, fetal serum AFP leaks out into the amniotic fluid and is picked up by the maternal serum.

Multiple-fetus pregnancy: *The multiple fetuses make large quantities.*
Threatened abortion
Fetal distress or congenital anomalies
Fetal death

▲ Increased Nonmaternal Serum Levels

Primary hepatocellular cancer (hepatoma),
Germ cell or yolk sac cancer of the ovary,
Embryonal cell or germ cell tumor of the testes,
Other cancers (e.g., stomach, colon, lung, breast, lymphoma),
Liver cell necrosis (e.g., cirrhosis, hepatitis):

Cancers contain undifferentiated cells that may carry the surface markers of their fetal predecessors.

▼ Decreased Maternal Levels

Trisomy 21 (Down syndrome)
Fetal wastage

RELATED TESTS

Maternal Screen Testing (p. 354). This testing includes AFP and other serum markers that are accurate indicators of increased risk for birth defects.

Amniocentesis (p. 632). This is a procedure to obtain amniotic fluid for evaluation of fetal health.

Pelvic Ultrasonography (p. 887). Nuchal Translucency is an accurate indicator of trisomy chromosomal abnormalities.

 Aluminum (Chromium and Other Heavy Metals)

NORMAL FINDINGS

0-6 ng/mL (all ages)
<60 ng/mL (dialysis patients all ages)

INDICATIONS

This test is used to evaluate aluminum levels in patients with renal failure. Elevated concentrations of aluminum in a patient with an aluminum-based joint implant suggest significant prosthesis wear.

TEST EXPLANATION

Under normal physiologic conditions, the usual daily dietary intake of aluminum (5-10 mg) is completely excreted by the kidneys. Patients in renal failure (RF) lose the ability to clear aluminum and are at risk for aluminum toxicity. Aluminum-laden dialysis water and aluminum-based phosphate binder gels designed to decrease phosphate accumulation increase the incidence of aluminum toxicity in RF patients. Furthermore, the dialysis process is not highly effective at eliminating aluminum. If a significant load exceeds the body's excretory capacity, the excess is deposited in various tissues, including bone, brain, liver, heart, spleen, and muscle. This accumulation causes morbidity and mortality through various mechanisms. Brain deposition has been implicated as a cause of dialysis dementia. In bone, aluminum replaces calcium and disrupts normal osteoid formation.

Aluminum is absorbed from the GI tract in the form of oral phosphate-binding agents (aluminum hydroxide), parenterally via immunizations, via dialysate on patients on dialysis, via total parenteral nutrition (TPN) contamination, via the urinary mucosa through bladder irrigation, and transdermally in antiperspirants. Lactate, citrate, and ascorbate all facilitate GI absorption.

Serum aluminum concentrations are likely to be increased above the reference range in patients with metallic joint prosthesis. Serum concentrations >10 ng/mL in a patient with an aluminum-based implant suggest significant prosthesis wear. *Chromium* and other metals can be determined using similar laboratory techniques.

INTERFERING FACTORS

- Most of the common evacuated blood collection devices have rubber stoppers that are comprised of aluminum-silicate. Simple puncture of the rubber stopper for blood collection is sufficient to contaminate the specimen with aluminum; therefore special evacuated blood collection tubes are required for aluminum testing.
- Gadolinium- or iodine-containing contrast media that has been administered within 96 hours can alter test for heavy metals including aluminum.

PROCEDURE AND PATIENT CARE

Before

 Explain the procedure to the patient.

Tell the patient that no fasting is required.

During

• Collect a venous blood in a royal blue-top tube. A tan-top (lead only) Becton-Dickinson tube can be used.

• Have the blood sample sent to a central diagnostic laboratory. The results will be available to the local hospital in 7 to 10 days.

After

• Apply pressure to the venipuncture site.

ABNORMAL FINDINGS

▲ Increased Levels

Aluminum toxicity—Approximately 95% of aluminum load is eliminated renally. If the load exceeds the ability of the kidney to excrete it, aluminum toxicity may occur.

Amino Acid Profiles (Amino Acid Screen)

NORMAL FINDINGS

Normal values vary for different amino acids

INDICATIONS

Measurement of certain amino acids is performed to identify diseases associated with specific essential amino acid deficiencies.

TEST EXPLANATION

Amino acids are "building blocks" of proteins, hormones, nucleic acids, and pigments. They can act as neurotransmitters, enzymes, and coenzymes. There are eight essential amino acids that must be provided to the body by the diet. The body can make the others. The essential amino acids must be transported across the gut and renal tubular lining cells. The metabolism of the essential amino acids is critical to the production of other amino acids, proteins, carbohydrates, and lipids. Amino acid levels can thereby be affected by defects in renal tubule or gastrointestinal (GI) transport of amino acids.

When there is a defect in the metabolism or transport of any one of these amino acids, excesses of their precursors or deficiencies of their "end product" amino acid are evident in the blood and/or urine. There are more than 90 diseases described that are associated with abnormal amino acid function.

Clinical manifestations of these diseases may be precluded if diagnosis is early, and appropriate dietary replacement of missing amino acids is provided. Usually urine testing (see phenylketonuria [PKU] testing, p. 374) for specific amino acids is used to screen for some of these errors in amino acid metabolism and transport. Blood testing is very accurate. Federal law now requires hospitals to test all newborns for inborn errors in metabolism, including amino acids. Testing is required for errors in amino acid metabolism such as phenylketonuria (PKU), maple syrup urine disease (MSUD), and homocystinuria. Testing for more rare disorders may include testing for tyrosinemia and argininosuccinic aciduria.

A few drops of blood are obtained from the heel of a newborn baby to fill a few circles on filter paper (Guthrie card) labeled with names of infant, parent, hospital, and primary physician. The sample is usually obtained on the second or third day of life, after protein-containing feedings (i.e., breast milk or formula) have started,

Once a presumptive diagnosis is made, amino acid levels can be determined by chromatographic methods on blood or amniotic fluid. The genetic defects for many of these diseases are becoming more defined, allowing for even earlier diagnosis to be made in utero. Common examples of amino acid diseases include PKU, cystinosis, and cystic fibrosis.

INTERFERING FACTORS

- Amino acid levels are affected by the circadian rhythm. Levels are usually lowest in the morning and highest by mid-day.
- Levels of amino acids are generally higher in infants and children compared to adults.
- Pregnancy is associated with reduced levels of some amino acids.
- Normal values vary widely and only extremely abnormal results are diagnostic without genetic corroboratory evidence.
- Drugs that may *increase* amino acid levels include bismuth, heparin, steroids, and sulfonamides.
- Drugs that may *decrease* some amino acid levels include estrogens and oral contraceptives.

PROCEDURE AND PATIENT CARE

Before

- Obtain a history of the patient symptoms.
- Obtain a pedigree highlighting family members with amino acid disorders.
- Inform the patient that a 12-hour fast is generally required before blood collection. Occasionally, a particular protein or carbohydrate load is ordered to stimulate production of a particular amino acid metabolite.

During

- Collect a venous blood sample in a red-top tube.
- Usually a 24-hour random urine specimen is required. Screening is done on a spot urine using the first voided specimen in the morning.

After

- Generally, genetic counseling is provided before testing. However, acute anxiety by the patient or parents often requires emotional support immediately after obtaining a specimen.

TEST RESULTS AND CLINICAL SIGNIFICANCE

▲ Increased Blood Levels

Specific aminoacidopathies (e.g., PKU, maple syrup disease): *The parent amino acid is present at increased quantities because of a genetic defect that impairs catabolism of that particular amino acid. It is the excessive build up of that amino acid that causes disease.*

Specific aminoacidemias (e.g., glutaric aciduria): *Products in the catabolic pathway of a particular amino acid accumulate. Which particular product accumulates depends on which enzyme is deficient (usually as a result of a genetic defect).*

▼ Decreased Blood Levels

Hartnup disease,
Nephritis,
Nephrotic syndromes:
   These diseases result in amino acid deficiencies secondary to increased renal excretion.

▲ Increased Urine Levels

Specific aminoacidurias (e.g., cystinuria, homocystinuria): *Genetic defects in amino acid metabolism cause buildup of precursor amino acids that are then excreted by the kidney. Several other mechanisms affect the pathophysiology of these diseases.*

RELATED TEST

Phenylketonuria (PKU) (p. 374). This test is routinely performed on infants to exclude the diagnosis of PKU. It is part of the newborn screening panel.

 Ammonia

NORMAL FINDINGS

Adult: 10-80 mcg/dL or 6-47 μmol/L (SI units)
Child: 40-80 mcg/dL
Newborn: 90-150 mcg/dL

INDICATIONS

Ammonia is used to support the diagnosis of severe liver diseases (fulminant hepatitis or cirrhosis), and for surveillance of these diseases. Ammonia levels are also used in the diagnosis and follow-up of hepatic encephalopathy.

TEST EXPLANATION

Ammonia is a by-product of protein catabolism. Most of it is made by bacteria acting on proteins present in the gut. By way of the portal vein, it goes to the liver, where it is normally converted into urea and then secreted by the kidneys. Ammonia cannot be catabolized in the presence of severe hepatocellular dysfunction. Furthermore, when portal blood flow to the liver is altered (e.g., in portal hypertension), ammonia cannot reach the liver to be catabolized. Ammonia blood levels rise. Plasma ammonia levels do not correlate well with the degree of hepatic encephalopathy. Inherited deficiencies of urea cycle enzymes, inherited metabolic disorders of organic acids, and the dibasic amino acids lysine and ornithine are a major cause of high ammonia levels in infants and adults. Finally, impaired renal function diminishes excretion of ammonia, and the blood levels rise. High levels of ammonia result in encephalopathy and coma. Arterial ammonia levels are more reliable than venous levels but more difficult to obtain and are therefore not routinely used.

INTERFERING FACTORS

- Hemolysis increases ammonia levels because the red blood cells (RBCs) have about three times the ammonia level content of plasma.
- Muscular exertion can increase ammonia levels.
- Cigarette smoking can produce significant increases in ammonia levels within 1 hour of inhalation.
- Ammonia levels may be factitiously increased if the tourniquet is too tight for a long period.
- Drugs that may cause *increased* ammonia levels include acetazolamide, alcohol, ammonium chloride, barbiturates, diuretics (loop, thiazide), narcotics, and parenteral nutrition.
- Drugs that may cause *decreased* levels include broad-spectrum antibiotics (e.g., neomycin), lactobacillus, lactulose, levodopa, and potassium salts.

PROCEDURE AND PATIENT CARE

Before

- Explain the procedure to the patient.
- Note that no fasting is usually required.

During

- Collect a venous blood sample in a green-top tube. Note that some institutions require the specimen be sent to the laboratory in an iced container.
- Avoid hemolysis and send the specimen promptly to the laboratory.

After

- Apply pressure or a pressure dressing to the venipuncture site.
- Assess the venipuncture site for bleeding. Many patients with liver disease have prolonged clotting times.

TEST RESULTS AND CLINICAL SIGNIFICANCE

▲ Increased Levels

Primary hepatocellular disease,
Reye syndrome,
Asparagine intoxication:
    There are not enough functioning liver cells to metabolize the ammonia.
Portal hypertension,
Severe heart failure with congestive hepatomegaly:
    The portal blood flow from the gut to the liver is altered. The ammonia cannot get to the liver to be metabolized for excretion. Furthermore, the ammonia from the gut is rapidly shunted around the liver (by way of gastroesophageal varices) and into the systemic circulation.
Hemolytic disease of newborn (erythroblastosis fetalis): *RBCs contain high amounts of ammonia. The newborn liver is not mature enough to metabolize all the ammonia presented to it by the hemolysis that occurs in this disease.*
GI bleeding with mild liver disease,
GI obstruction with mild liver disease:
    Ammonia production is increased because the bacteria have more protein (blood) to catabolize. An impaired liver may not be able to keep up with the increased load of ammonia presented to it.

Hepatic encephalopathy and hepatic coma: *These neurologic states are a result of ammonia acting as false neurotransmitters. The brain cannot function properly.*

Genetic metabolic disorder of urea cycle: *Ammonia is catabolized by the urea cycle. Disruption of that cycle will inhibit excretion of ammonia and levels can be expected to rise.*

▼ Decreased Levels

Essential or malignant hypertension
Hyperornithinemia

RELATED TESTS

Alanine Aminotransferase (ALT) (p. 39), Aspartate Aminotransferase (AST) (p. 119), and Alkaline Phosphatase (ALP) (p. 47). These tests are all used to evaluate liver function.

Amylase, Blood

NORMAL FINDINGS

Adult: 60-120 Somogyi units/dL or 30-220 units/L (SI units)
Newborn: 6-65 units/L
Values may be slightly increased during normal pregnancy and in older adults.

🛑 Critical Values

More than three times the upper limit of normal (depending on the method)

INDICATIONS

This test is used to detect and monitor the clinical course of pancreatitis. It is frequently ordered when a patient presents with acute abdominal pain.

TEST EXPLANATION

The serum amylase test, which is easy and rapidly performed, is most specific for pancreatitis. Amylase is normally secreted from pancreatic acinar cells into the pancreatic duct and then into the duodenum. Once in the intestine it aids in the catabolism of carbohydrates to their component simple sugars. Damage to pancreatic acinar cells (as in pancreatitis) or obstruction of the pancreatic duct flow (as in pancreatic carcinoma or common bile duct gallstones) causes an outpouring of this enzyme into the intrapancreatic lymph system and the free peritoneum. Blood vessels draining the free peritoneum and absorbing the lymph pick up the excess amylase. An abnormal rise in the serum level of amylase occurs within 12 hours of the onset of disease. Because amylase is rapidly cleared (2 hours) by the kidney, serum levels return to normal 48 to 72 hours after the initial insult. Persistent pancreatitis, duct obstruction, or pancreatic duct leak will cause persistent elevated amylase levels.

Although serum amylase is a sensitive test for pancreatic disorders, it is not specific. Other nonpancreatic diseases can cause elevated amylase levels in the serum. For example, during bowel perforation, intraluminal amylase leaks into the free peritoneum and is picked up by the peritoneal blood vessels. This results in an elevated serum amylase level. A penetrating peptic ulcer into the pancreas will also cause elevated amylase levels. Duodenal obstruction can be associated with less significant elevations in amylase. Because salivary glands contain amylase, elevations can be expected in patients with parotiditis (mumps). Amylase isoenzyme testing can differentiate pancreatic from salivary hyperamylasemia. Amylase is also found in low levels in the ovaries and skeletal muscles. Ectopic pregnancy and severe diabetic ketoacidosis are also associated with hyperamylasemia.

Patients with chronic pancreatic disorders that have resulted in pancreatic cell destruction or patients with massive hemorrhagic pancreatic necrosis often do not have high amylase levels, because there may be so few pancreatic cells left to make amylase.

INTERFERING FACTORS

- Serum lipemia may factitiously decrease amylase levels.
- Intravenous dextrose solutions can lower amylase levels and cause a false-negative result.
- Drugs that may cause *increased* serum amylase levels include aminosalicylic acid, aspirin, azathioprine, corticosteroids, dexamethasone, ethyl alcohol, glucocorticoids, iodine-containing contrast media, loop diuretics (e.g., furosemide), methyldopa, narcotic analgesics, oral contraceptives, and prednisone.
- Drugs that may cause *decreased* levels include citrates, glucose, and oxalates.

PROCEDURE AND PATIENT CARE

Before

- Explain the procedure to the patient.
- Tell the patient that no fasting is required.

During

- Collect a venous blood sample in a red-top tube.

After

- Apply pressure or a pressure dressing to the venipuncture site.
- Check the venipuncture site for bleeding.

TEST RESULTS AND CLINICAL SIGNIFICANCE

▲ Increased Levels

Acute pancreatitis,
Chronic relapsing pancreatitis:
   Damage to pancreatic acinar cells, as in pancreatitis, causes an outpouring of amylase into the intrapancreatic lymph system and the free peritoneum. Blood vessels draining the free peritoneum and absorbing the lymph pick up the excess amylase.
Penetrating peptic ulcer into the pancreas: *The peptic ulcer penetrates the posterior wall of the duodenum into the pancreas. This causes a localized pancreatitis with elevated amylase levels.*
Gastrointestinal disease: *In patients with perforated peptic ulcer, necrotic bowel, perforated bowel, or duodenal obstruction, amylase leaks out of the gut and into the free peritoneal cavity. The amylase is picked up by the blood and lymphatics of the peritoneum, where levels are demonstrated in excess.*
Acute cholecystitis,
Parotiditis (mumps),
Ruptured ectopic pregnancy:

Amylase is also present in the salivary glands, gallbladder, and fallopian tubes. Diseases affecting these organs will be associated with elevated levels of amylase.

Renal failure: *Amylase is cleared by the kidney. Renal diseases will reduce excretion of amylase.*

Diabetic ketoacidosis

Pulmonary infarction

After endoscopic retrograde pancreatography

RELATED TESTS

Urine Amylase (p. 909). Amylase can be detected in the urine long after serum amylase has cleared. If serum amylase levels are normal and pancreatitis is suspected, the period of peak amylase levels may have passed. Elevated amylase levels may still be found in the urine.

Lipase (p. 339). Lipase is similar to amylase except that it is more specific for the pancreas.

Angiotensin

NORMAL FINDINGS

Angiotensin I: ≤25 pg/mL

Angiotensin II: 10-60 pg/mL

INDICATIONS

This test is performed to identify renovascular hypertension.

TEST EXPLANATION

Renin (p. 447) is an enzyme that is released by the juxtaglomerular apparatus of the kidney. Its release is stimulated by hypokalemia, hyponatremia, decreased renal blood perfusion, or hypovolemia. Renin stimulates the release of angiotensinogen. Angiotensin-converting enzyme (ACE) (p. 64) metabolizes angiotensinogen to angiotensin I and subsequently to angiotensin II and III. Angiotensin then stimulates the release of catecholamines, antidiuretic hormone, ACTH, oxytocin, and aldosterone. Angiotensin is also a vasoconstrictor. Angiotensin is used to identify renovascular sources of hypertension. It can be measured as angiotensin I or angiotensin II. The test is performed by direct radioimmunoassay.

INTERFERING FACTORS

See Plasma Renin Assay, p. 447.

PROCEDURE AND PATIENT CARE

Before

 Explain the procedure to the patient.

Instruct the patient to maintain a normal diet with a restricted amount of sodium (approximately 3 g/day) for 3 days before the test.

Instruct the patient to check with a health care provider about discontinuing any medications that may interrupt in renin activity.

During

- Collect a venous blood sample and place it in a chilled lavender-top tube with ethylene diamine tetraacetic acid (EDTA) as an anticoagulant. Heparin can falsely decrease results.
- Gently invert the blood tube to allow adequate mixing of the blood sample and the anticoagulant.
- Record the patient's position, dietary status, and time of day on the laboratory slip.
- Place the tube of blood on ice, and immediately send it to the laboratory.
- In the laboratory, the blood will be centrifuged and the serum frozen.

After

- Apply pressure or a pressure dressing to the venipuncture site.
- Observe the venipuncture site for bleeding.
- Tell the patient that usually a normal diet and medications may be resumed.

TEST RESULTS AND CLINICAL SIGNIFICANCE

▲ Increased Levels

Essential hypertension: *A small percentage of these patients have renin hypertension and elevated angiotensin levels.*

Malignant hypertension: *A large percentage of these patients with aggressive hypertensive episodes have elevated angiotensin levels.*

Renovascular hypertension: *Renal artery stenosis or occlusion decreases the renal blood flow, which is a strong stimulant to angiotensin production.*

▼ Decreased Levels

Primary hyperaldosteronism: *This is usually caused by an adrenal adenoma. Aldosterone levels are high and angiotensin levels are low.*

Steroid therapy: *Glucocorticosteroids also have an aldosterone effect, which acts to increase serum sodium levels, decrease potassium levels, and increase blood volume. These responses all tend to diminish angiotensin levels.*

Congenital adrenal hyperplasia: *An enzyme defect in cortisol synthesis causes an accumulation of cortisol precursors, some of which have strong aldosterone-like activity. These act to increase serum sodium levels, decrease potassium levels, and increase blood volume, all of which tend to diminish angiotensin levels.*

RELATED TEST

Aldosterone (p. 43). This is a direct measurement of aldosterone level. It is used to evaluate hypertension and aldosteronism.

Plasma Renin Assay (p. 447). Plasma renin and angiotensin levels are parallel for each cause of hypertension.

Angiotensin-Converting Enzyme (ACE, Serum
Angiotensin-Converting Enzyme [SACE])

NORMAL FINDINGS

8-53 U/L

INDICATIONS

ACE is used to detect and monitor the clinical course of sarcoidosis (a granulomatous disease that affects many organs, especially the lungs). Furthermore, it is used to differentiate between sarcoidosis and other granulomatous diseases. It is also used to differentiate active and dormant sarcoid disease.

TEST EXPLANATION

ACE is found in pulmonary epithelial cells and converts angiotensin I to angiotensin II (a potent vasoconstrictor). Angiotensin II is a significant stimulator of aldosterone. ACE is vital in the renin/aldosterone mechanism and therefore important in controlling blood pressure. Despite this, ACE is not very helpful in the evaluation of hypertension. Its value is in the detection of sarcoidosis.

Elevated ACE levels are found in a high percentage of patients with sarcoidosis. This test is primarily used in patients with sarcoidosis to evaluate the severity of disease and the response to therapy. Levels are especially high with active pulmonary sarcoidosis and can be normal with inactive (dormant) sarcoidosis. Elevated ACE levels also occur in conditions other than sarcoidosis, including Gaucher disease (a rare familial lysosomal disorder of fat metabolism), leprosy, alcoholic cirrhosis, active histoplasmosis, tuberculosis, Hodgkin disease, myeloma, scleroderma, pulmonary embolism, and idiopathic pulmonary fibrosis. ACE is elevated in the CSF of patients with neurosarcoidosis. An ACE assay can be performed using spectrophotometry or radioimmunoassay.

INTERFERING FACTORS

- Patients under 20 years of age normally have very high ACE levels.
- Hemolysis or hyperlipidemia may factitiously decrease ACE levels.
- Drugs that may cause *decreased* ACE levels include ACE inhibitor antihypertensives and steroids.

PROCEDURE AND PATIENT CARE

Before
- Explain the procedure to the patient.
- Tell the patient that no fasting is required.

During
- Collect a venous blood sample in a red-top tube.

After
- Apply pressure or a pressure dressing to the venipuncture site.
- Assess the venipuncture site for bleeding.

TEST RESULTS AND CLINICAL SIGNIFICANCE

▲ Increased Levels

Sarcoidosis: *This is the disease for which this test is primarily performed. The more severe the sarcoidosis, the greater the likelihood that ACE will be increased.*

Other rare diseases that have been found to be associated with ACE elevations include Gaucher disease, tuberculosis, leprosy, alcoholic cirrhosis, active histoplasmosis, Hodgkin disease, myeloma, idiopathic pulmonary fibrosis, diabetes mellitus, primary biliary cirrhosis, amyloidosis, hyperthyroidism, scleroderma, and pulmonary embolism.

 Anion Gap (AG, R factor)

NORMAL FINDINGS

16 ± 4 mEq/L (if potassium is used in the calculation)
12 ± 4 mEq/L (if potassium is not used in the calculation)

INDICATIONS

Calculation of the anion gap (AG) assists in the evaluation of patients with acid-base disorders. It is used to attempt to identify the potential cause of the disorder and can also be used to monitor therapy for acid-base abnormalities.

TEST EXPLANATION

The anion gap (AG) is the difference between the cations and the anions in the extra-cellular space that are routinely calculated in the laboratory (i.e., AG = [sodium + potassium] − [chloride + bicarbonate]). In some laboratories, the potassium is not measured because the level of potassium in acid-base abnormalities varies. The normal value of the anion gap is adjusted downward if potassium is eliminated from the equation. The anion gap, although not real physiologically, is created by the small amounts of anions in the blood (such as lactate, phosphates, sulfates, organic anions, and proteins) that are not measured. Further, it is important to realize that the HCO_3^- that is measured is actually the venous CO_2, not the arterial HCO_3^-.

This calculation is most often helpful in identifying the cause of metabolic acidosis. As acids such as lactic acid or ketoacids accumulate in the bloodstream, bicarbonate neutralizes them to maintain a normal pH within the blood. Mathematically, when bicarbonate decreases, the AG increases. In general, most metabolic acidotic states (excluding some types of renal tubular acidosis) are associated with an increased anion gap. The higher the gap above normal, the more likely this will be the case. Proteins can have a significant effect on AG. As albumin (usually negatively charged) increases, AG will increase. In the face of normal albumin, a high AG is usually a result of an increase in non–chloride-containing acids or organic acids (such as lactic acid or ketoacids).

A decreased AG is very rare but can occur when there is an increase in unmeasured (calcium or magnesium) cations. A reduction in anionic proteins (nephrotic syndrome) will also decrease AG. For example, a 1 g/dL drop in serum protein is associated with a 2.5 mEq/L drop in AG. Because the anion proteins are lost, the HCO_3^- increases to maintain electrical neutrality. Increase in cationic proteins (some immunoglobulins) will also decrease AG. Except for hypoproteinemia, conditions that cause a reduced or negative anion gap are relatively rare compared to those associated with an elevated anion gap.

AG measurement is also helpful in identifying the presence of a mixed acid-base situation. The arterial blood gases do not always tell the whole story, especially if there is a mixed metabolic acidosis and a concomitantly occurring alkalosis. An increased AG, despite a normal pH will indicate an acidotic component to the metabolic picture. When AG measurement is combined with the ABGs and electrolytes, complex metabolic clinical pictures can be more clearly elucidated. The AG calculation is indicated whenever an acid-base problem exists.

INTERFERING FACTORS

- Hyperlipidemia may cause under measurement of sodium and falsely decrease AG.
- Normal values of AG vary according to different normal values for electrolytes, depending on laboratory methods of measurement.
- Drugs that *increase* AG are many. Examples include carbenicillin, carbonic anhydrase inhibitors (e.g., acetazolamide), diuretics, ethanol, methanol, penicillin, and salicylate.
- Drugs that *decrease* AG are also many. Examples include acetazolamide, lithium, polymyxin B, spironolactone, and sulindac.

PROCEDURE AND PATIENT CARE

Before
- Explain the procedure to the patient.
- Tell the patient that no food or fluid is restricted.

During
- Collect a venous blood sample in a red-top or green-top tube.
- If the patient is receiving an intravenous infusion, obtain the blood from the opposite arm.

After
- The sodium, potassium, chloride, and bicarbonate levels are determined by an automated multi-channel analyzer. The AG is then calculated as indicated in the test explanation section.
- Apply pressure to the venipuncture site.

TEST RESULTS AND CLINICAL SIGNIFICANCE

▲ Increased Levels

Lactic acidosis,
Diabetic ketoacidosis,
Alcoholic ketoacidosis,
Alcohol intoxication,
Starvation:
  These diseases are associated with increased acid ions such as lactate, hydroxybutyrate, or acetoacetate. HCO_3^- neutralizes these acids, HCO_3^- levels fall and AG mathematically increases.
Renal failure: *Uremic organic acid anions (phosphate, sulfates, etc.) accumulate in the blood as a result of poor excretion of these acids. The hydrogen combines with the bicarbonate to maintain a homeostatic pH. Bicarbonate levels diminish and AG mathematically rises.*
Increased gastrointestinal (GI) losses of bicarbonate (e.g., diarrhea or fistulae): *HCO_3^- and other base losses can occur, thereby mathematically increasing AG. Not all GI losses result in AG differences, if mixed electrolyte imbalances occur.*
Hypoaldosteronism: *Aldosterone stimulates acid secretion in the distal renal tubule in exchange for sodium. With deficient quantities of aldosterone, acid builds up and is combined with bicarbonate. Bicarbonate levels diminish and AG rises.*

▼ Decreased Levels

Excess alkali ingestion: *Increase in alkali products (antacids, boiled milk), especially in children, causes increased HCO_3^- products and mathematically decreases AG.*

Multiple myeloma: *The M-chain component of the proteins produced by the neoplastic plasma cells are cationic, causing a compensatory decrease in measured cations and an increase in measured anions to maintain electrical neutrality.*

Chronic vomiting or gastric suction: *The loss of HCl causes a decrease in chloride and an increase in HCO_3^- that mathematically decreases AG.*

Hyperaldosteronism: *These patients lose great amounts of potassium and hydrogen ions causing a metabolic alkalosis associated with a decreased AG.*

Hypoproteinemia: *Loss of anionic proteins directly causes a decrease in the AG.*

Lithium toxicity: *An increase in inorganic cations decreases the measured cations and thereby decreases AG.*

RELATED TESTS

Electrolytes (Sodium [p. 466], Potassium [p. 409], Chloride [p. 152], Bicarbonate [p. 141]). Measurement of these electrolytes is necessary to calculate the AG.

Arterial Blood Gases (ABGs) (p. 109). This is the method by which acid-base balance is identified and evaluated.

Anticardiolipin Antibodies (aCL Antibodies, ACA, Antiphospholipid Antibodies, Lupus Anticoagulant)

NORMAL FINDINGS

<23 GPL (IgG phospholipid units)
<11 MPL (IgM phospholipid units)

INDICATIONS

This test is positive in some patients with systemic lupus erythematosus (SLE). The presence of this antibody places the patient at higher risk for "antiphospholipid syndrome" (i.e., venous or arterial thrombosis, thrombocytopenia, recurrent spontaneous abortions). This test is performed on patients with SLE to determine if the patient is at risk for developing the above-noted complications.

TEST EXPLANATION

Anticardiolipin antibodies (immunoglobulins G and M to cardiolipin) are antiphospholipid autoantibodies that attach to phospholipids of cell membranes and can interfere with the coagulation system. Antiphospholipid autoantibodies include *anticardiolipin antibodies* and the "lupus anticoagulant antibody." Phospholipid antibodies occur in patients with a variety of clinical signs and symptoms, notably thrombosis (arterial or venous), pregnancy morbidity (unexplained fetal death, premature birth, severe preeclampsia, or placental insufficiency), unexplained cutaneous circulation disturbances (livido reticularis or pyoderma gangrenosum), thrombocytopenia or hemolytic anemia, and nonbacterial thrombotic endocarditis. Phospholipid antibodies and lupus anticoagulants are found with increased frequency in patients with systemic rheumatic diseases, especially lupus erythematosus. The term "antiphospholipid syndrome" (APS) or "Hughes syndrome" is used to describe the triad of thrombosis, recurrent fetal loss, and thrombocytopenia accompanied by phospholipid antibodies or a lupus anticoagulant. Both antibodies may be found in other autoimmune diseases, drug-induced lupus, and infection. These antibodies may be considered normal in the elderly person.

Antiphospholipid IgG and IgM antibodies are directed against a mixture of phosphatidylserine, phosphatidic acid, and beta-2 glycoprotein I antigens and are more specific than cardiolipin IgG and IgM antibodies in the diagnosis of antiphospholipid syndrome (APS). Testing is commonly performed by Semi-Quantitative Enzyme-Linked Immunosorbent Assay.

INTERFERING FACTORS

- Patients who have or had syphilis infections can have a cross reaction to the radiolabeled antibody used for radioimmune assay or the antibody used for enzyme-linked immunosorbent assay. These patients therefore will have a false-positive result.
- These transient antibodies can occur in patients with infections, acquired immunodeficiency syndrome (AIDS), inflammation, autoimmune diseases, or cancer.
- *False-positive results* have been seen in patients who take medications such as chlorpromazine, hydralazine, penicillin, phenytoin, procainamide, and quinidine.

PROCEDURE AND PATIENT CARE

Before

 Explain the procedure to the patient.

Tell the patient that no fasting is required.

During

- Collect a venous blood sample according to the laboratory protocol.

After

- Apply pressure or a pressure dressing to the venipuncture site.
- Assess the venipuncture site for bleeding.

TEST RESULTS AND CLINICAL SIGNIFICANCE

▲ Increased Levels

Systemic lupus erythematosus: *A patient's results are considered positive, and therefore the patient is at risk for antiphospholipid syndrome if either anticardiolipin antibodies or the lupus anticoagulant is present.*

Antiphospholipid syndrome

RELATED TESTS

Anti-DNA Antibody (p. 78). This test is used to diagnose SLE.
Antinuclear Antibody (p. 88). This test is used to diagnose SLE.

Anticentromere Antibody (Centromere Antibody)

NORMAL FINDINGS

Negative (If positive, serum will be titrated.)
Weak positive: positive screening titer (1:40 for human epithelial type 2 cells [HEp-2 cells], 1:20 for kidney cells)

Moderately positive: one dilution above screening titer
Strong positive: two dilutions above screening titer

INDICATIONS

This test is used to support the diagnosis of CREST syndrome.

TEST EXPLANATION

A centromere is the region of the chromosome referred to as the primary constriction that divides the chromosome into arms. During cell division the centromere exists in the pole of the mitotic spindle.

Anticentromere antibodies are a form of antinuclear antibodies. They are found in a very high percentage of patients with CREST syndrome, a variant of scleroderma. CREST is characterized by calcinosis, Raynaud phenomenon, esophageal dysfunction, sclerodactyly (a hand deformity), and telangiectasia (permanent dilation of superficial capillaries and venules). Anticentromere antibodies, on the contrary, are present in only a small minority of patients with scleroderma, a disease that is difficult to differentiate from CREST. No correlation exists between antibody titer and severity of CREST disease.

PROCEDURE AND PATIENT CARE

Before

🖉 Explain the procedure to the patient.
🖉 Tell the patient that no fasting is usually required.

During

• Collect one red-top tube of venous blood.

After

• Apply pressure or a pressure dressing to the venipuncture site.
• Assess the venipuncture site for bleeding.

TEST RESULTS AND CLINICAL SIGNIFICANCE

Positive

CREST syndrome

RELATED TESTS

Antinuclear Antibody (p. 88). This test is used to diagnose autoimmune-related diseases.

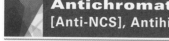

Antichromatin Antibody (Antinucleosome Antibodies
[Anti-NCS], Antihistone Antibody [Anti-HST, AHA])

NORMAL FINDINGS

Antinucleosome antibodies
    No antibodies present in <1:20 dilution

Antihistone antibody
    None detected: <1.0 units
    Inconclusive: 1.0-1.5 units
    Positive: 1.6-2.5 units
    Strong positive: >2.5 units

INDICATIONS

This test is used to diagnose systemic lupus erythematosus (SLE).

TEST EXPLANATION

There are several chromatin antinuclear antibodies associated with autoimmune diseases. Nucleosome (NCS) represents the main autoantigen-immunogen in systemic lupus erythematosus (SLE), and these antinucleosome antibodies are an important marker of the disease activity. Antinucleosome (antichromatin) antibodies play a key role in the pathogenesis of SLE. Nearly all patients with SLE have antinucleosome antibodies. Anti-NCS is one of the many antinuclear antibodies (see p. 88) that indicate autoimmune diseases. Anti-NCS has a sensitivity of 100% and specificity of 97% for SLE diagnosis. Anti-NCS antibodies show the highest correlation with disease activity. Anti-NCS antibodies also show strong association with renal damage (glomerulonephritis and proteinuria) associated with SLE. Anti-NCS autoantibodies are more prevalent than anti-DNA in patients with SLE.

Histone antibodies are present in 20% to 55% of idiopathic SLE cases and 80% to 95% of drug-induced lupus erythematosus cases. They occur in less than 20% of other types of connective tissue diseases. This antibody is particularly helpful in identifying patients with drug-induced lupus erythematosus caused by drugs such as procainamide, quinidine, penicillamine, hydralazine, methyldopa, isoniazid, and acebutolol. There are several subtypes of AHA. In drug-induced lupus erythematosus, a specific AHA (anti-[(H2A-H2B)-DNA] IgG) is produced. In most of the other associated diseases (rheumatoid arthritis, juvenile rheumatoid arthritis, primary biliary cirrhosis, autoimmune hepatitis, and dermatomyositis/polymyositis), the AHAs are of other varying specificities. A variety of immune testing methods are used to identify these antinuclear antibodies including ELISA and indirect immunofluorescence methods.

PROCEDURE AND PATIENT CARE

Before
- Explain the procedure to the patient.
- Tell the patient that no fasting is required.

During
- Collect one red-top or gold-top tube of venous blood.

After
- Apply pressure to the venipuncture site.
- Assess the site for bleeding.

TEST RESULTS AND CLINICAL SIGNIFICANCE

▲ Increased Levels

Systemic lupus erythematosus: *This disease is most commonly associated with anti-NCS antibodies.*

Drug-induced lupus erythematosus: *This disease is most commonly associated with anti-HST antibodies.*
Other autoimmune diseases: *Diseases such as lupus hepatitis are occasionally associated with anti-NCS antibodies.*

RELATED TESTS

Antinuclear Antibody (ANA) (p. **88**). This is a type of antibody commonly associated with autoimmune diseases such as SLE.
Anti-DNA Antibody (p. **78**). This is useful in the diagnosis and follow-up of SLE.

Anticyclic-Citrullinated Peptide Antibody (Cyclic Citrullinated Peptide Antibody, CCP IgG, Anti-CCP)

NORMAL FINDINGS

<20 units/mL

INDICATIONS

Anti-CCP is useful in the diagnosis of patients with unexplained joint inflammation, especially when the traditional blood test, rheumatoid factor (RF) (see p. 454), is negative or below 50 units/mL.

TEST EXPLANATION

Anti-CCP is known more formally as *anticyclic-citrullinated peptide antibody* and is formed by the intermediary conversion of the amino acid ornithine to arginine. Anti-CCP appears early in the course of rheumatoid arthritis (RA) and is present in the blood of most patients with the disease. When the citrulline antibody is detected in a patient's blood, there is a high likelihood that the patient has RA. Among patients with early RA, 30% to 40% may not have elevation of RF, making the diagnosis difficult in the initial stage. If the anti-CCP is elevated, the diagnosis of RA can be made even if RF is negative. This is particularly important because aggressive treatment in the early stages of RA prevents progression of joint damage. Anti-CCP may rise years before any clinical onset of arthritis or significant elevation of RF. At a cutoff of 5 units/mL, the sensitivity and specificity of anti-CCP for RA are 67.5% and 99.3%, respectively. RF has a sensitivity of 66.3% and a lower specificity (82.1%) than anti-CCP. When the two antibodies are used together, the specificity for diagnosing RA is 99.1%. Other autoimmune inflammatory diseases are rarely associated with elevated anti-CCP levels. It may also be useful in differentiating other entities that can resemble RA, and at times, cause RF positive test results (i.e., Polymyalgia Rheumatica and Parvoviral Arthropathy).

Anti-CCP is thought to be directly involved in the pathogenesis of RA. Citrullinated proteins are found in inflamed synovial tissue of patients with RA and may elicit a humoral mechanism for the joint inflammation that highlights RA. The presence of anti-CCP in RA indicates a more aggressive and destructive form of the disease. I–t is also a marker for disease progression. Some feel that anti–CCP-positive RA and anti–CCP-negative RA are clinically different disease entities—with the former having a far worse outcome. Anti–CCP-positive RA patients have more swollen joints and show more radiologic destruction than anti–CCP-negative patients with RA.

Anti-CCP ELISA testing is well correlated among the various commercially available assays with the same antigen specificity, but the numerical normal values for each assay differ widely. These methods include semi-quantitative enzyme-linked immunosorbent assay.

PROCEDURE AND PATIENT CARE

Before

 Explain the procedure to the patient.

Tell the patient that no fasting or preparation is required.

During

- Collect a venous blood sample in a red-top tube.

After

- Apply pressure to the venipuncture site.
- Assess the site for bleeding.

TEST RESULTS AND CLINICAL SIGNIFICANCE

▲ Increased Levels

Rheumatoid arthritis: *RF and anti-CCP are part of a rheumatoid panel often performed to diagnose and monitor RA.*

RELATED TESTS

Rheumatoid Factor (RF) (p. 454). This is the most widely used test to assist in diagnosis and determining prognosis of RA.

Erythrocyte Sedimentation Rate (ESR) (p. 221). This test is used to assess RA disease activity.

C-Reactive Protein (CRP) (p. 184). This test is used to identify and assess treatment for most inflammatory diseases.

Antidiuretic Hormone (ADH, Vasopressin, Arginine Vasopressin [AVP])

NORMAL FINDINGS

1-5 pg/mL or 1-5 ng/L (SI units)

INDICATIONS

ADH levels are tested in patients suspected of having diabetes insipidus or the syndrome of inappropriate ADH (SIADH). This test is often performed in patients who complain of polyuria or polydipsia and are found to have marked variations in blood and urine osmolarity or sodium levels.

TEST EXPLANATION

ADH, also known as vasopressin, is formed by the hypothalamus and stored in the posterior pituitary gland. It controls the amount of water reabsorbed by the kidney. ADH release is stimulated by an increase in serum osmolality or a decrease in intravascular blood volume. Physical stress, surgery, and even high levels of anxiety may also stimulate ADH release. On release of ADH more water is reabsorbed from the glomerular filtrate at the level of the distal convoluted renal tubule and collecting ducts. This increases the amount of free water within the bloodstream and causes highly concentrated urine.

With low ADH levels, water is excreted, thereby producing hemoconcentration and a more dilute urine. Diabetes insipidus (DI) occurs when ADH secretion is inadequate or when the kidney is unresponsive to ADH stimulation. Inadequate ADH secretion is usually associated with central neurologic abnormalities (neurogenic DI), such as trauma, tumor, or inflammation of the brain (hypothalamus). Surgical ablation of the pituitary gland will also result in the neurogenic form of DI; such patients excrete large volumes of free water in the dilute urine. Their blood is hemoconcentrated, producing a strong thirst.

Primary renal diseases may make the renal collecting system less sensitive to ADH stimulation (nephrogenic DI). Again, in this instance, dilute urine may be produced by excretion of high volumes of free water. To differentiate ADH deficiency (neurogenic DI) from renal resistance to ADH (nephrogenic DI), a water deprivation (ADH stimulation p. 979) test is performed. Water intake is restricted during this test. Urine osmolality is measured. Vasopressin is administered. In neurogenic DI, there is no rise in urine osmolality after water restriction, but there is a rise after vasopressin is given. In nephrogenic DI, there is no rise in urine osmolality after water deprivation or vasopressin administration. The diagnosis indicated by this test can be corroborated by a serum ADH level. ADH levels are low in neurogenic DI. ADH levels are high in nephrogenic DI.

High serum ADH levels are also associated with SIADH. In response to this inappropriately high level of ADH secretion, water is reabsorbed by the kidneys greatly in excess of normal amounts. Thus the patient's blood becomes very diluted and the urine is concentrated. Blood levels of important serum ions diminish, causing severe neurologic, cardiac, and metabolic alterations. SIADH can be associated with pulmonary diseases (e.g., tuberculosis, bacterial pneumonia), severe stress (e.g., surgery, trauma), CNS tumor, infection, or trauma. Ectopic secretion of ADH from neoplasm (paraneoplastic syndrome) can cause SIADH. The most common tumors associated with SIADH include carcinomas of the lung and thymus; lymphoma; leukemia; and carcinomas of the pancreas, urologic tract, and intestine. Patients with myxedema or Addison disease also can experience SIADH. Some drugs are know to cause SIADH (see Interfering Factors).

INTERFERING FACTORS

- Patients with dehydration, hypovolemia, or stress may have increased ADH levels.
- Patients with overhydration, decreased serum osmolality, and hypervolemia may have decreased ADH levels.
- Use of a glass syringe or collection tube causes degradation of ADH.
- Drugs that *increase* ADH levels include acetaminophen, barbiturates, cholinergic agents, cyclophosphamide, diuretics (e.g., thiazides), estrogen, narcotics, nicotine, oral hypoglycemic agents (particularly sulfonylureas), and tricyclic or selective serotonin reuptake inhibitor (SSRI) antidepressants.
- Drugs that *decrease* ADH levels include alcohol, beta-adrenergic agents, morphine antagonists, and phenytoin.

PROCEDURE AND PATIENT CARE

Before

- Explain the procedure to the patient.
- Ensure that the patient is adequately hydrated. Tell the patient to fast for 12 hours.
- Evaluate the patient for high levels of physical or emotional stress.

During

- Collect a venous blood sample in a prechilled plastic anticoagulant tube while the patient is in the sitting or recumbent position.

After

- Apply pressure or a pressure dressing to the venipuncture site.
- Assess the venipuncture site for bleeding.
- The specimen is centrifuged at low temperatures in the laboratory. The serum may be frozen and sent to a reference laboratory on dry ice for testing.

TEST RESULTS AND CLINICAL SIGNIFICANCE

▲ Increased Levels

SIADH,

Central nervous system (CNS) tumors or infection,

Pneumonia or pulmonary tuberculosis,

Ectopic ADH secretion (usually from lung cancer),

Endocrinopathies, such as myxedema or Addison disease:

> *The above-noted diseases have been implicated to be associated with inappropriate high levels of ADH. Patients experience dilutional hyponatremia, hypoosmolality, and concentrated urine.*

Nephrogenic DI caused by primary renal diseases: *Because of primary renal disease, the kidneys cannot respond to ADH. The patient becomes hemoconcentrated and hyperosmolar. As a result, ADH is maximally stimulated, yet the kidneys cannot respond.*

Postoperative days 1 to 3,

Severe physical stress (e.g., trauma, pain, prolonged mechanical ventilation):

> *Stress is a potent stimulator (through the autonomic nervous system) of ADH.*

Hypovolemia,

Dehydration:

> *Decreased blood volume is a potent direct stimulator of ADH.*

Acute porphyria

▼ Decreased Levels

Neurogenic (or central) DI caused by CNS trauma, tumor, or infection,

Surgical ablation of pituitary gland:

> *The hypothalamus or pituitary ADH-secreting cells are destroyed by the above-noted disease processes.*

Hypervolemia: *Increased blood volume is an inhibitor of ADH secretion.*

Decreased serum osmolality caused by overhydration, nephrotic syndrome, psychogenic polydipsia, IV overinfusion of non–salt-containing fluid: *Decreased serum osmolality is an inhibitor of ADH secretion.*

RELATED TESTS

Water Deprivation (p. 979). This test is helpful in differentiation of the causes of polyuria (neurogenic DI, nephrogenic DI, psychogenic polydipsia).

Osmolality, Blood (p. 378). This test is a measurement of solute load in the serum.

Osmolality, Urine (p. 938). This test is a measurement of solute load in the urine.

Sodium, Blood (p. 466). This is a direct measurement of sodium level in the blood.

Sodium, Urine (p. 946). This is a direct measurement of sodium level in the urine.

Antidiuretic Hormone Suppression (see following test). This test is used to differentiate SIADH from other causes of hyponatremia or edematous states.

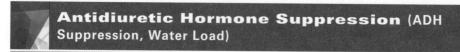

Antidiuretic Hormone Suppression (ADH Suppression, Water Load)

NORMAL FINDINGS

65% of water load excreted in 4 hours
80% of water load excreted in 5 hours
Urine osmolality (in second hour): ≤100 mmol/kg
Urine to serum (U/S) osmolality ratio: >100
Urine specific gravity: <1.003

INDICATIONS

This test is used to differentiate the syndrome of inappropriate ADH (SIADH) from other causes of hyponatremia or edematous states listed in Box 2-3.

TEST EXPLANATION

This test is used to evaluate the possibility of SIADH in patients with electrolyte abnormalities (such as hyponatremia) or edematous states. Usually this test is performed concomitantly with measurements of urine and serum osmolality. Patients with SIADH will excrete none or very little of the water load. Furthermore, their urine osmolality will never be less than 100, and the U/S ratio is greater than 100. Patients with hyponatremia, other edematous states, or chronic renal diseases will excrete up to 80% of the water load and will develop midrange osmolality results.

CONTRAINDICATIONS

- Patients with severe pain, nausea, stress, hypovolemia, or hypotension, because ADH is already near maximally stimulated.

BOX 2-3	Causes of Hyponatremia or Edema

Hyponatremia
- SIADH
- Primary (or psychogenic) polydipsia
- Adrenal insufficiency
- Excessive sodium loss (vomiting, diarrhea, diuretics, excessive sweating)
- Pseudohyponatremia associated with excessive nonionic solute load (e.g., hyperglycemia, hyperlipidemia, hyperproteinemia)
- Sick cell syndrome associated with chronic debilitating diseases

Edematous States
- Congestive heart failure
- Cirrhosis
- Nephrosis
- Myxedema

POTENTIAL COMPLICATIONS

- Water intoxication in patients with SIADH, because they are not able to excrete the water load. Symptoms would include anorexia, nausea, vomiting, abdominal cramps, confusion, irritability, convulsions, and coma.

INTERFERING FACTORS

- Patients with dehydration, hypovolemia, hypotension, or stress may have increased ADH levels.
- Drugs that *increase* ADH levels include acetaminophen, barbiturates, cholinergic agents, cyclophosphamide, estrogen, narcotics, nicotine, oral hypoglycemic agents, some diuretics (e.g., thiazides), and tricyclic antidepressants.

PROCEDURE AND PATIENT CARE

Before

- Explain the procedure to the patient.
- Instruct the patient to fast after midnight before the test.
- The test is begun early in the morning.
- Inform the patient of the early signs of water intoxication and instruct the patient to notify you if any occur.
- Place the patient in the recumbent position. The response to water loading in the upright position is reduced because this position is associated with increased ADH.
- One hour before the test administer 300 mL of water to replace fluids lost overnight. This is not part of the water load.
- Obtain a baseline serum sodium or a serum sodium level 24 hours before the test. If the sodium concentration is above a safe level (125 mmol/L), the test can proceed. If not, the test should be canceled until the sodium is brought to a safe level by water restriction or saline infusion. This precaution will minimize the risk of water intoxication.

During

- Administer water (approximately 20 mL/kg body weight up to 1500 mL) in 10 to 20 minutes.
- Collect urine every hour for 6 hours and send it for specific gravity and osmolality measurements. (Discard the first morning specimen.)
- Obtain blood for osmolality hourly or at specified times in serum (red-top) or heparinized (green-top) tube.

After

- Observe for signs of water intoxication.
- If water load clearance does not occur, be sure to instruct the patient to restrict water ingestion. Some patients must be admitted for observation.

TEST RESULTS AND CLINICAL SIGNIFICANCE

SIADH

Water excretion: none or very little of the water load
Urine osmolality: >100
Urine specific gravity: >1.020
U/S ratio: >90

Other Hyponatremic or Edematous States (see Box 2-3)

Water excretion: up to 80% of water load
Urine osmolality: <300
Urine specific gravity: >1.020
U/S ratio: <90

RELATED TESTS

Antidiuretic Hormone (p. 73). This is a serum assay for direct measurement of ADH. This test is used in the differential diagnosis of neurogenic diabetes insipidus, nephrogenic diabetes insipidus, or psychogenic polydipsia.
Osmolality, Blood (p. 378). This test is a measurement of solute load in the serum.
Osmolality, Urine (p. 938). This test is a measurement of solute load in the urine.
Sodium, Blood (p. 466). This is a direct measurement of sodium level in the blood.
Sodium, Urine (p. 946). This is a direct measurement of sodium level in the urine.
Water Deprivation (p. 979). This is a test to assist in the differential diagnosis of diabetes insipidus.

Anti-DNA Antibody (Antideoxyribonucleic Acid Antibodies, Antibody to Double-Stranded DNA, Anti–Double-Stranded DNA [Anti–ds-DNA], DNA Antibody, Native Double-Stranded DNA)

NORMAL FINDINGS

Negative: <5 international units/mL
Intermediate: 5-9 international units/mL
Positive: ≥10 international units/mL

INDICATIONS

The anti-DNA antibody test is useful for the diagnosis and follow-up of systemic lupus erythematosus (SLE).

TEST EXPLANATION

This antibody is found in approximately 65% to 80% of patients with active SLE and rarely in patients with other diseases. High titers are characteristic of SLE. Low to intermediate levels of this antibody may be found in patients with other rheumatic diseases and in those with chronic hepatitis, infectious mononucleosis, and biliary cirrhosis. The anti-DNA titer decreases with successful therapy and increases with exacerbation of SLE and especially with the onset of lupus glomerulonephritis. Near-negative values are seen in patients with dormant SLE. This test is semi-quantitative. Therefore small changes in antibody levels do not indicate disease activity.

The anti-DNA IgG antibody is a subtype of the *antinuclear antibodies* (ANAs) (p. 88). If the ANAs are negative, there is no reason to test for anti-DNA antibodies. There are two types of anti-DNA antibodies. The first and most commonly found is the antibody against double-stranded DNA (anti–ds-DNA). The second type is the antibody against single-stranded DNA (anti–ss-DNA). This is less sensitive and specific for SLE but is positive in other autoimmune diseases. These antibody-antigen complexes that occur with autoimmune disease are not only diagnostic but are major contributors to the disease process. These complexes induce the complement system, which then may cause local or systemic tissue injury.

There are several radioimmunoassay methods for measuring anti-DNA antibodies. The Farr method is the oldest and is more sensitive than the lupus erythematosus prep. It detects anti–ds-DNA and anti–ss-DNA antibodies. As a result, its specificity is not great.

INTERFERING FACTORS

- A radioactive scan performed within 1 week before the test may alter the test results.
- Drugs that may cause *increased* levels include hydralazine and procainamide.

PROCEDURE AND PATIENT CARE

Before

- Explain the procedure to the patient.
- Tell the patient that no fasting is required.

During

- Collect a venous blood sample in a red-top tube.

After

- Apply pressure or a pressure dressing to the venipuncture site.
- Assess the venipuncture site for bleeding.

TEST RESULTS AND CLINICAL SIGNIFICANCE

▲ Increased Levels

Collagen-vascular diseases
Other autoimmune diseases, such as rheumatic fever
Chronic hepatitis
Infectious mononucleosis
Biliary cirrhosis

RELATED TEST

Antinuclear Antibody (p. 88). This is another antibody associated with SLE.

Antiextractable Nuclear Antigen (Anti-ENA, Antibodies to Extractable Nuclear Antigens, Anti–Jo-1 [Antihistidyl Transfer Synthase], Antiribonucleoprotein [Anti-RNP], Anti-Smith [Anti-SM])

NORMAL FINDINGS

Negative

INDICATIONS

The anti-ENAs are used to assist in the diagnosis of systemic lupus erythematosus (SLE) and mixed connective tissue disease (MCTD) and to eliminate other rheumatoid diseases.

TEST EXPLANATION

Anti-ENAs are a type of antinuclear antibodies to certain nuclear antigens that consist of RNA and protein. The antigen is extracted from the thymus using phosphate-buffered saline solutions and therefore is sometimes referred to as saline-extracted antigen. The most common ENAs are Smith (SM) and ribonucleoprotein (RNP) types.

The anti-SM antibody is present in about 30% of patients with SLE and in about 8% of patients with MCTD diseases. However, it is not present in patients with most other rheumatoid-collagen diseases.

The anti-RNP antibody is reported in nearly 100% of patients with MCTD disease and in about 25% of patients with SLE, discoid lupus, and progressive systemic sclerosis (scleroderma). In high titers, anti-RNP is suggestive of MCTD.

The *anti–Jo-1 (antihistidyl transfer synthase)* antibody occurs in patients with autoimmune interstitial pulmonary fibrosis and in a minority of patients with aggressive autoimmune myositis. Two other antibodies to ENAs are anti–SS-A and anti–SS-B (see p. 98) and are used mainly in the diagnostic evaluation of Sjögren syndrome.

PROCEDURE AND PATIENT CARE

Before
- Explain the procedure to the patient.
- Tell the patient that no fasting is required.

During
- Collect a venous blood sample in a red-top tube.

After
- Apply pressure or a pressure dressing to the venipuncture site.
- Assess the venipuncture site for bleeding.
- Check the venipuncture site for infection. Patients with autoimmune disease are immunocompromised.

TEST RESULTS AND CLINICAL SIGNIFICANCE

▲ Increased Anti-SM Antibodies
SLE

▲ Increased Anti-RNP Antibodies
MCTD,
SLE,
Discoid lupus scleroderma:
> *The absence of anti-SM antibodies and the presence of anti-RNP antibodies help to delineate MCTD serologically from SLE and other autoimmune diseases.*

▲ Increased Anti-Jo Antibodies

Pulmonary fibrosis

Autoimmune myositis

RELATED TESTS

Antinuclear Antibody (p. 88). This is another antibody associated with SLE.

Anti-DNA Antibody (p. 78). This is another test used to diagnose SLE.

Antiglomerular Basement Membrane Antibody
(Anti-GBM Antibody, AGBM, Glomerular Basement Antibody, Goodpasture's Antibody)

NORMAL FINDINGS

Tissue

Negative: No immunofluorescence is noted on the renal or lung tissue basement membrane.

Blood (by Enzyme Immunoassay [EIA])

Negative: <20 units

Borderline: 20-100 units

Positive: >100 units

INDICATIONS

This test is used to detect the presence of circulating glomerular basement membrane antibodies commonly present in autoimmune-induced nephritis (Goodpasture syndrome).

TEST EXPLANATION

Goodpasture syndrome is an autoimmune disease characterized by the presence of circulating antibodies against an antigen in the renal glomerular basement membrane and the pulmonary alveolar basement membrane. These immune complexes activate the complement system and thereby cause tissue injury. Patients with this problem usually display a triad of glomerulonephritis (hematuria), pulmonary hemorrhage (hemoptysis), and antibodies to basement membrane antigens. This is a rare form of glomerular nephritis. About 60% to 75% of patients with immune-induced glomerular nephritis have pulmonary complications.

With the use of immunohistochemistry and now with radioimmunoassay, antibodies also can be demonstrated in the glomeruli, renal tubular basement membrane, and the pulmonary capillary basement membranes. Lung or renal biopsies are required to demonstrate these antibodies in tissue. Serum assays are a faster and more reliable method for diagnosing Goodpasture syndrome, especially in patients in whom renal or lung biopsy may be difficult or contraindicated. Furthermore, serum levels can be used in monitoring response to therapy (plasmapheresis or immunosuppression).

PROCEDURE AND PATIENT CARE

Before

Explain the procedure to the patient.

Tell the patient to fast for 8 hours before the test. Water is permitted.
If a lung biopsy or kidney biopsy will be used to collect the specimen, explain these procedures to the patient.

During

- Collect a venous blood sample in red-top tube.

After

- Apply pressure or a pressure dressing to the venipuncture site.
- Assess the venipuncture site for bleeding.

TEST RESULTS AND CLINICAL SIGNIFICANCE

Positive

Goodpasture syndrome
Autoimmune glomerulonephritis
Lupus nephritis

RELATED TESTS

Lung Biopsy (p. 738). This is a test in which lung tissue is obtained for microscopic evaluation.
Renal Biopsy (p. 751). This is a test in which renal tissue is obtained for microscopic evaluation.

Anti-Glycan Antibodies (Crohn Disease Prognostic Panel, Multiple Sclerosis Antibody Panel)

NORMAL FINDINGS

Negative

INDICATIONS

This test is used to differentiate multiple sclerosis from other neurologic causes of weakness. It also is used to differentiate Crohn disease from other forms of inflammatory bowel diseases.

TEST EXPLANATION

Glycans (sugars or carbohydrates) exist on the surface of cells, such as erythrocytes. Anti-glycan antibodies are immunologically directed to these sugar-containing components. Antibodies to glycans can be instigated by bacterial, fungal, and parasitic infections. The use of glycan arrays for systematic screening of patients with multiple sclerosis (MS) and inflammatory bowel disease (particularly Crohn disease) has been helpful in enabling the diagnosis and prognosis in these patients.

Utilizing enzyme linked immunosorbent assay (ELISA), these antibodies can be identified and quantified. When used with other antibodies associated with Crohn disease (such as anti-*Saccharomyces cerevisiae* antibody [ASCA], anti-*laminaribioside carbohydrate* antibody [ALCA], anti-*mannobioside carbohydrate* antibody [AMCA], and anti-*chitobiose carbohydrate* antibody [ACCA]), anti-glycan antibodies are supportive of Crohn disease over ulcerative colitis or irritable bowel disease. Furthermore, higher levels of these antibodies are associated with a more complicated course of disease.

Other anti-glycan antibodies are specific for MS patients, enabling differentiation between MS patients and patients with other neurologic diseases.

PROCEDURE AND PATIENT CARE

Before

Explain the procedure to the patient.
Tell the patient that no fasting is required.

During

- Collect one lavender-, pink-, or green-top tube of venous blood.

After

- Apply pressure to the venipuncture site.

TEST RESULTS AND CLINICAL SIGNIFICANCE

▲ Increased Levels

Crohn disease
Multiple sclerosis: *Both of these diseases are associated with elevated levels of anti-glycan antibodies.*

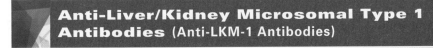

Anti-Liver/Kidney Microsomal Type 1 Antibodies (Anti-LKM-1 Antibodies)

NORMAL FINDINGS

≤20 Units (negative)
20.1-24.9 Units (equivocal)
≥25 Units (positive)

INDICATIONS

This test is used in the evaluation of patients suspected of having autoimmune hepatitis.

TEST EXPLANATION

Autoimmune liver disease (e.g., autoimmune hepatitis and primary biliary cirrhosis) is characterized by the presence of autoantibodies including smooth muscle antibodies (SMA), antimitochondrial antibodies (AMA), and anti-liver/kidney microsomal antibodies type 1 (anti-LKM-1). Subtypes of autoimmune hepatitis (AIH) are based on autoantibody reactivity patterns. For example, the presence of smooth muscle antibodies (SMA) is consistent with the diagnosis of chronic autoimmune hepatitis. The presence of anti-liver/kidney microsomal type 1 antibodies with or without SMA is consistent with autoimmune hepatitis, type 2. The presence of anti-mitochondrial antibodies is consistent with primary biliary cirrhosis.

Anti-LKM-1 antibodies serve as a serologic marker for AIH type 2 and typically occur in the absence of SMA and antinuclear antibodies. Children often have other autoantibodies (e.g., parietal cell antibodies and thyroid microsomal antibodies). These antibodies react with a short linear sequence of the recombinant antigen cytochrome monooxygenase P450 2D6. Patients with AIH type 2 more often tend to be young, female, and have severe disease that responds well to immunosuppressive therapy.

Patients with chronic hepatitis resulting from hepatitis C can also have elevated anti-LKM-1 antibodies. The diagnosis of autoimmune liver disease cannot be made on antibody testing alone. In many instances, autoimmune liver disease panel testing, including the antibodies discussed in the preceding paragraph, is performed. Testing is performed by semi-quantitative enzyme-linked immunosorbent assay/semi-quantitative indirect fluorescent antibody.

PROCEDURE AND PATIENT CARE

Before
☒ Explain the procedure to the patient.
☒ Explain the importance of performing the test in the morning.

During
• Collect a venous blood sample in a serum separator vacuum tube.

After
• Blood may be sent to a reference laboratory. Results are available in about 1 week.

TEST RESULTS AND CLINICAL SIGNIFICANCE
▲ Increased Levels

Autoimmune hepatitis: *Anti-LKM-1 antibodies react with a short linear sequence of the recombinant antigen cytochrome monooxygenase P450 2D6 within the hepatocyte.*

RELATED TESTS

Aspartate Aminotransferase (p. 119). These hepatocellular enzymes are elevated in all forms of hepatitis.
Alanine Aminotransferase (p. 39). These hepatocellular enzymes are elevated in all forms of hepatitis.
Antinuclear Antibody (p. 88). These antibodies are associated with autoimmune liver disease.
Anti–Smooth Muscle Antibody (p. 95). These antibodies are associated with autoimmune liver disease.
Antimitochondrial Antibody (p. 84). These antibodies are associated with autoimmune liver disease.

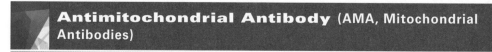

Antimitochondrial Antibody (AMA, Mitochondrial Antibodies)

NORMAL FINDINGS

No AMAs at titers >1:5 or <0.1 units

INDICATIONS

The AMA test is used primarily to aid in the diagnosis of primary biliary cirrhosis.

TEST EXPLANATION

AMA is an anticytoplasmic antibody directed against a lipoprotein in the mitochondrial membrane. Normally the serum does not contain AMA at a titer greater than 1:5. AMAs are found in 94% of patients with primary biliary cirrhosis or other autoimmune liver disease. This disease may be an autoimmune disease that occurs predominantly in young or middle-aged women. It has a slow progressive course marked by elevated liver enzymes, especially alkaline phosphatase and gamma-glutamyl transpeptidase, and a positive AMA test. Liver biopsy (see p. 734) is usually required to confirm the diagnosis because the AMA test can be positive in patients with chronic active hepatitis, drug-induced cholestasis, autoimmune hepatitis (e.g., scleroderma, systemic lupus erythematosus), extrahepatic obstruction, or acute infectious hepatitis. There are subgroups of AMA. The M-2 subgroup is highly specific for primary biliary cirrhosis. It is not useful in monitoring the course of the disease, however. For the AMA test, immunofluorescent assay (IFA) or enzyme-linked immunosorbent assay (ELISA) techniques can be used.

PROCEDURE AND PATIENT CARE

Before

✗ Explain the procedure to the patient.
✗ Tell the patient that no fasting or special preparation is required.

During

• Collect a venous blood sample in a red-top tube.

After

• Apply pressure or a pressure dressing to the venipuncture site.
• Check the venipuncture site for bleeding. Patients with jaundice often have bleeding disorders associated with vitamin K deficiency.

TEST RESULTS AND CLINICAL SIGNIFICANCE

▲ Increased Levels

Primary biliary cirrhosis: *AMA test is positive in 90% to 100% of patients.*
Chronic active hepatitis: *AMA test is positive in 30% of patients.*
Systemic lupus erythematosus,
Syphilis,
Drug-induced cholestasis,
Autoimmune hepatitis (e.g., scleroderma, systemic lupus erythematosus [SLE]),
Extrahepatic obstruction,
Acute infectious hepatitis:
    AMA test is positive in 2% to 5% of patients.

RELATED TESTS

Anti–Smooth Muscle Antibody (p. 95). This is another anticytoplasmic antibody that usually is present in patients with chronic active hepatitis and in 30% of patients with primary biliary cirrhosis.
Alkaline Phosphatase (p. 47). Although alkaline phosphatase (ALP) is found in many tissues, the highest concentrations are found in the liver, biliary tract epithelium, and bone.
Gamma-Glutamyl Transpeptidase (p. 246). This enzyme is found in the liver and is used to detect liver cell dysfunction and cholestasis.

Antimyocardial Antibody (AMA)

NORMAL FINDINGS

Negative (If positive, serum will be titrated.)

INDICATIONS

This test is used to detect an autoimmune source of myocardial injury and disease. AMAs may be detected in rheumatic heart disease, cardiomyopathy, postthoracotomy syndrome, and after myocardial infarction (MI). This test is not only used in the detection of an autoimmune cause for these conditions but also for monitoring response to treatment.

TEST EXPLANATION

A positive AMA test is associated with several forms of heart disease. AMAs may be detected before the development of clinical symptoms of heart disease. An immunologic basis has been suspected in rheumatic heart disease for a long time. Research has now documented the presence of serum antibodies against myocardial components and deposition of immunoglobulin and complement in lesional areas. Antibodies against heart muscle are also found in 20% to 40% of patients after cardiac surgery and in a smaller number of patients after MI. These antibodies are usually associated with pericarditis that follows the myocardial injury associated with cardiac surgery or MI (Dressler syndrome). AMAs have also been detected in patients with cardiomyopathy. Their role in this latter disease is unknown.

This test may be performed by indirect immunofluorescent technique. The patient's serum is added to a rat heart muscle extract. Antigen-antibody immune complexes are identified by immunofluorescent antihuman antibodies. Positive results (increased immunofluorescence) are reported in titers.

PROCEDURE AND PATIENT CARE

Before

- Explain the procedure to the patient.
- Tell the patient that no fasting or special preparation is necessary.

During

- Collect a venous blood sample in a red-top tube.

After

- Apply pressure or a pressure dressing to the venipuncture site.
- Check the venipuncture site for bleeding.

TEST RESULTS AND CLINICAL SIGNIFICANCE

▲ Increased Levels

Rheumatic heart disease,
Streptococcal infection:
> *The myocardial antigen may be associated with streptococcus because the antibody may occur in patients with other streptococcal diseases.*

Postthoracotomy (cardiac surgery) syndrome,

After MI (Dressler syndrome):

Myocardial injury occurs and the antibody develops. The antibody-antigen complex may incite the pericarditis that follows the myocardial injury.

Cardiomyopathy: *The association of cardiomyopathy and AMA is unknown. Whether the antibodies cause or contribute to the development of cardiomyopathy is being studied.*

Antineutrophil Cytoplasmic Antibody (ANCA)

NORMAL FINDINGS

Components	Reference Interval
Anti-Neutrophil Cytoplasmic Antibody, IgG	<1:20: Not significant
Myeloperoxidase Antibody	Negative: ≤19 AU/mL
	Equivocal: 20-25 AU/mL
	Positive: ≥26 AU/mL
Serine Protease 3 Antibody	Negative: ≤19 AU/mL
	Equivocal: 20-25 AU/mL
	Positive: ≥26 AU/mL

INDICATIONS

This blood test is used to assist in the diagnosis of Wegener granulomatosis (WG). It also is used to follow the course of the disease, monitor the response to therapy, and provide early detection of relapse.

TEST EXPLANATION

WG is a regional systemic vasculitis in which the small arteries of the kidneys, lungs, and upper respiratory tract (nasopharynx) are damaged by a granulomatous inflammation. Diagnosis can be made by biopsy of clinically affected tissue. Serologic testing plays a key role in the diagnosis of WG and other systemic vasculitis syndromes. Most patients with WG have circulating autoantibodies against neutrophil cytoplasm, which are useful in the diagnosis.

ANCAs are antibodies directed against cytoplasmic components of neutrophils. When ANCAs are detected with indirect immunofluorescence microscopy, two major patterns of staining are present: cytoplasmic ANCA (c-ANCA) and perinuclear ANCA (p-ANCA). Specific immunochemical assays demonstrate that c-ANCA consists mainly of antibodies to proteinase 3 (PR3) and p-ANCA consists of antibodies to myeloperoxidase (MPO). Using Semi-Quantitative Indirect Fluorescent Antibody/Semi-Quantitative Multi-Analyte Fluorescent Detection to characterize ANCA (rather than the pattern of immunofluorescence microscopy) is more specific and more clinically relevant; therefore, the terms proteinase 3-ANCA (PR3-ANCA) and myeloperoxidase-ANCA (MPO-ANCA) are used.

The PR3 autoantigen is highly specific (95% to 99%) for WG. When the disease is limited to the respiratory tract, the PR3 is positive in about 65% of patients. Nearly all patients with WG limited to the kidney do not have positive PR3. When WG is inactive, the percentage of positive drops to about 30%.

The MPO autoantigen is found in 50% of patients with WG centered in the kidney. It also occurs in patients with non-WG glomerulonephritis, such as microscopic polyangiitis (MPA).

P-ANCA antibodies can also differentiate various forms of inflammatory bowel disease. See also Anti-Glycan Antibodies (p. 82). P-ANCA are found in 50% to 70% of ulcerative colitis (UC) patients, but in only 20% of Crohn disease (CD) patients.

PROCEDURE AND PATIENT CARE

Before

 Explain the procedure to the patient.
Tell the patient that no fasting is required.

During

- Collect a venous blood sample in the tube specified by the laboratory performing the test.

After

- Apply pressure or a pressure dressing to the venipuncture site.
- Observe the venipuncture site for bleeding.

TEST RESULTS AND CLINICAL SIGNIFICANCE

▲ Increased Levels

Wegener granulomatosis,
Microscopic polyarteritis,
Idiopathic crescentic glomerulonephritis,
Ulcerative colitis,
Primary sclerosing cholangitis,
Autoimmune hepatitis,
Churg-Strauss vasculitis,
Active viral hepatitis,
Crohn disease:
  The mechanism by which these antibodies are associated with these diseases is unknown.

Antinuclear Antibody (ANA)

NORMAL FINDINGS

Negative at 1:40 dilution

INDICATIONS

ANAs are used to diagnose systemic lupus erythematosus (SLE) and other autoimmune diseases. These antibodies are primarily used to screen for SLE. Because almost all patients with SLE develop autoantibodies, a negative ANA test excludes the diagnosis. If the ANA test is positive, other antibody studies must be done to corroborate the diagnosis.

TEST EXPLANATION

Autoantibodies are directed to nuclear material (ANAs) or to cytoplasmic material (anticytoplasmic antibodies) (Tables 2-3 and 2-4). Many abnormal antibodies are present in patients with autoimmune (also called rheumatic or connective tissue) diseases. ANA is a group of protein antibodies that react against cellular nuclear material. ANA is quite sensitive for detecting SLE. Positive results occur in approximately 95% of patients with this disease; however, many other rheumatic diseases are also associated with ANA (Table 2-5). ANA, therefore, is not a specific test for SLE (Table 2-6). ANA can be tested as a specific antibody or as a group with nonspecific antigens.

ANA tests are performed using different assays (indirect immunofluorescence microscopy or by enzyme-linked immunosorbent assay [ELISA]) and results are reported as a titer with a particular type of immunofluorescence pattern (when positive). Low-level titers are considered negative, while increased titers are positive and indicate an elevated concentration of antinuclear antibodies.

ANA shows up on indirect immunofluorescence as fluorescent patterns in cells that are fixed to a slide and are evaluated under an ultraviolet microscope. Different patterns are associated with

TABLE 2-3	Common Antinuclear Antibodies and Diseases They Cause
Common Antinuclear Antibodies	**Disease**
Anti-sNP	SLE
Anti-ENA	SLE, MCTD
Anti-Smith	SLE
Anti-RNP	MCTD, SLE, PSS
Anti–Jo-1 antihistidyl	Polymyositis, dermatomyositis
Antinucleolar	PSS, SLE
Anticentromere	CREST syndrome
Anti–ss-A (Ro) and Anti–ss-B (La)	Sjögren syndrome, SLE
Rheumatoid arthritis precipitin	RA, Sjögren syndrome
Anti–scleroderma-70	PSS

CREST, Calcinosis, Raynaud, esophageal dysfunction, sclerodactyly, telangiectasia; *MCTD,* mixed connective tissue disease; *PSS,* progressive systemic sclerosis (scleroderma); *RA,* rheumatoid arthritis; *SLE,* systemic lupus erythematosus.

TABLE 2-4	Common Anticytoplasmic Antibodies and Diseases They Cause
Common Anticytoplasmic Antibody	**Disease**
Antimitochondrial	Primary biliary cirrhosis
Antineutrophil cytoplasmic	Wegener granulomatosis
Antimicrosomal	Chronic active hepatitis
Antiribosomal	SLE
Anti-RNA	Scleroderma (systemic sclerosis)

TABLE 2-5 Autoimmune Disease and Positive Antibodies	
Autoimmune Disease	**Positive Antibodies**
SLE	ANA, SLE prep, dsDNA, ssDNA, anti-DNP, SS-A
Drug-induced SLE	ANA
Sjögren syndrome	RF, ANA, SS-A, SS-B
Scleroderma	ANA, Scl-70, RNA, dsDNA
Raynaud disease	ACA, Scl-70
Mixed connective tissue disease	ANA, RNP, RF, ssDNA
Rheumatoid arthritis	RF, ANA, RANA, RAP
Primary biliary cirrhosis	AMA
Thyroiditis	Antimicrosomal, antithyroglobulin
Chronic active hepatitis	ASMA

TABLE 2-6 Disease and Percent of Patients With ANAs	
Disease	**ANA Positive (%)**
SLE	95
Progressive systemic sclerosis (scleroderma)	70
Rheumatoid arthritis	30
Sjögren syndrome	60
Dermatomyositis	30
Polyarteritis	10

a variety of autoimmune disorders. When combined with a more specific subtype of ANA (see Table 2-3), the pattern can increase specificity of the ANA subtypes for the various autoimmune diseases (Figure 2-5). An example of a positive result might be: "Positive at 1:320 dilution with a homogenous pattern." This particular test is considered positive if ANA is found in a titer with a dilution of greater than 1:32. In general, the higher the titer of a certain ANA antibody known to be associated with a certain autoimmune disease, the more likely that disease exists and the more active the disease is. As the disease becomes less active because of therapy, the ANA titers can be expected to fall.

Often the ANA test is used to screen patients with suspected SLE. If the ANA test is negative, the patient probably does not have SLE. If positive, other corroborative serologic tests are performed (see Table 2-5). About 5% of patients with SLE have a negative ANA test. In this text, the more commonly clinically used ANA subtypes are separately discussed.

INTERFERING FACTORS

▪ Drugs that may cause a *false-positive* ANA test include acetazolamide, aminosalicylic acid, chlorothiazides, chlorprothixene, griseofulvin, hydralazine, penicillin, phenylbutazone, phenytoin, procainamide, streptomycin, sulfonamides, and tetracyclines.
▪ Drugs that may cause a *false-negative* test include steroids.

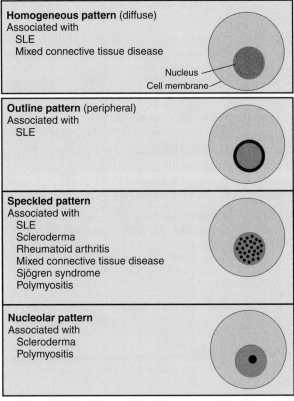

Figure 2-5 Patterns of immunofluorescent staining for antinuclear antibodies (ANAs).

PROCEDURE AND PATIENT CARE

Before

✗ Explain the procedure to the patient.
✗ Tell the patient that no fasting or preparation is required.

During

• Collect a venous blood sample in a red-top tube.

After

• Apply pressure or a pressure dressing to the venipuncture site.
• Assess the venipuncture site for bleeding.
✗ Because they are usually immunocompromised, patients with an autoimmune disease should be instructed to check for signs of infection at the venipuncture site. These patients often take steroids that further compromise their immune system.

TEST RESULTS AND CLINICAL SIGNIFICANCE

▲ Increased Levels

Systemic lupus erythematosus (SLE): *The signs and symptoms of this disease are vague and nonspecific. This disease is associated with a significant production of various autoimmune antibodies. Any organ in the patient's body can be the target of these autoantibodies. The immune complexes incite the complement system and thereby create tissue damage.*

Rheumatoid arthritis (RA): *The autoimmune response is targeted to the synovial tissues.*

Periarteritis (polyarteritis) nodosa: *The autoimmune response is targeted to the small vessels of various organs.*

Dermatomyositis,

Polymyositis:

The autoimmune response is targeted to the skeletal muscle.

Scleroderma: *The autoimmune response is targeted to the endothelium of blood vessels. Fibrosis occurs. This combined with deposit of collagen-related tissue creates the organ changes seen in the skin, gastrointestinal (GI) tract, and other internal organs.*

Sjögren syndrome: *The autoimmune response is targeted to the exocrine glands (lacrimal and salivary).*

Raynaud phenomenon: *This phenomenon is characterized by episodic digital ischemia as manifested by blanching and then cyanosis of the fingers in cold temperatures followed by rubor on rewarming. It is associated with many autoimmune diseases. The term "Raynaud disease" refers to this phenomenon without an associated autoimmune disease.*

Other immune diseases

Leukemia

Infectious mononucleosis

Myasthenia gravis

Cirrhosis

Chronic hepatitis

RELATED TESTS

Anticentromere Antibody (p. 69). This test is used to diagnose CREST syndrome.

Anti-DNA Antibody (p. 78). This test is used to diagnose SLE.

Antiextractable Nuclear Antigen (ENA) (p. 79). This test is used to diagnose SLE and mixed connective tissue disease.

Antiscleroderma Antibody (p. 93). This test is used to diagnose scleroderma.

Anti-Parietal Cell Antibody (APCA)

NORMAL FINDINGS

Negative

INDICATIONS

Anti–parietal cell antibody (APCA) testing is used to diagnose an autoimmune cause of pernicious anemia.

TEST EXPLANATION

Parietal cells exist in the proximal stomach and produce hydrochloric acid and intrinsic factor. Intrinsic factor is necessary for the absorption of vitamin B_{12} (see p. 518). Anti–parietal cell antibodies are found in nearly 90% of patients with pernicious anemia. Nearly 60% of these patients also have anti–intrinsic factor antibodies. It is thought that these antibodies contribute to the destruction of the gastric mucosa in these patients. APCA is also found in patients with atrophic gastritis, gastric ulcers, and gastric cancer.

APCA is present in other autoimmune-mediated diseases such as thyroiditis, myxedema, juvenile diabetes, Addison disease, and iron-deficiency anemia. Nearly 10% to 15% of the normal population has APCA. As one ages, the incidence of having APCA increases (especially in relatives of patients with pernicious anemia).

Laboratory testing is usually done by indirect immunofluorescence using the Fluoro-Kit. With this test system, APCA can cross-react with other antibodies, especially anticellular and antithyroid antibodies. Titer levels greater than 1:240 are considered positive.

PROCEDURE AND PATIENT CARE

Before

✗ Explain the procedure to the patient.
✗ Tell the patient that no fasting or special preparation is necessary.

During

- Collect a venous blood sample in a red-top tube.

After

- Apply pressure or a pressure dressing to the venipuncture site.
- Check the venipuncture site for bleeding.

TEST RESULTS AND CLINICAL SIGNIFICANCE

▲   Increased Levels

Pernicious anemia,
Atrophic gastritis:
   APCA and anti–intrinsic factor antibodies may destroy the parietal cell in the gastric antrum through complement fixing antibodies against the parietal cell surface.
Hashimoto thyroiditis,
Myxedema,
Insulin-dependent diabetes mellitus,
Addison disease:
   These autoimmune diseases may be interrelated in a manner that is not yet clear.

RELATED TEST

Vitamin B$_{12}$ and Methylmalonic Acid Test (p. 518). This test measures the amount of vitamin B$_{12}$ in the blood.

Antiscleroderma Antibody (Scl-70 Antibody, Scleroderma Antibody, RNA Polymerase III Antibody)

NORMAL FINDINGS

Negative

INDICATIONS

This antibody is diagnostic for scleroderma (progressive systemic sclerosis [PSS]) and is present in 45% of patients with that disease.

TEST EXPLANATION

Scl-70 antibody is an antinuclear antibody. On the fluorescent antinuclear antibody test, using the ultraviolet microscope, a specific pattern is created for the Scl-70 antibody. The pattern is a speckled group of dots throughout the nucleus (see Figure 2-5, p. 91). The test can be performed by fluorescent testing, enzyme-linked immunosorbent assay (ELISA), and enzyme immunoassay (EIA). Progressive serial dilutions are carried out.

PSS is a multisystem disorder characterized by inflammation with subsequent fibrosis of the small blood vessels in skin and visceral organs, including the heart, lungs, kidneys, and gastrointestinal (GI) tract. A collagen-like substance is also deposited into the tissue of these organs. In general, the higher the titer of Scl-70 antibody, the more likely it is that PSS exists and the more active the disease is. As the disease becomes less active because of therapy, the Scl-70 antibody titers can be expected to fall.

The absence of this antibody does not exclude the diagnosis of scleroderma. The antibody is rather specific for PSS but is occasionally seen in other autoimmune diseases, such as systemic lupus erythematosus (SLE), mixed connective tissue disease (MCTD), Sjögren syndrome, polymyositis, and rheumatoid arthritis.

RNA polymerase III antibodies are found in 11% to 23% of patients with PSS. Patients with PSS who are positive for RNA polymerase III antibodies form a distinct serologic subgroup and usually do not have any of the other antibodies typically found in PSS patients, such as anticentromere (p. 69) or anti–Scl-70. PSS patients with anti-RNA polymerase III have an increased risk of the diffuse cutaneous form of scleroderma, with a high likelihood of skin involvement and hypertensive renal disease. A positive result supports a possible diagnosis of PSS. This autoantibody is strongly associated with diffuse cutaneous scleroderma and an increased risk of acute renal crisis. A negative result indicates no detectable IgG antibodies to RNA polymerase III, but does not rule out the possibility of PSS (11% to 33% sensitivity).

INTERFERING FACTORS

- Drugs that may cause *increased* levels include aminosalicylic acid, isoniazid, methyldopa, penicillin, propylthiouracil, streptomycin, and tetracycline.

PROCEDURE AND PATIENT CARE

Before
- Explain the procedure to the patient.
- Tell the patient that no fasting is required.

During
- Collect a venous blood sample in a red-top tube.

After
- Apply pressure or a pressure dressing to the venipuncture site.
- Assess the venipuncture site for bleeding.

TEST RESULTS AND CLINICAL SIGNIFICANCE

Positive

Scleroderma (PSS),
CREST syndrome:

> *CREST is a variant of scleroderma. In both of these diseases the autoimmune response is targeted to the endothelium of blood vessels. Fibrosis occurs. This, combined with deposit of collagen-related tissue, creates the organ changes seen in the skin, GI tract, and other internal organs.*

RELATED TEST

Antinuclear Antibody (p. 88). This group of antibodies is used to diagnose systemic lupus erythematosus and other autoimmune diseases such as PSS.

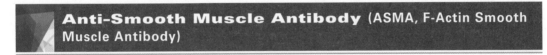

Anti–Smooth Muscle Antibody (ASMA, F-Actin Smooth Muscle Antibody)

NORMAL FINDINGS

No ASMAs at titers >1:20

INDICATIONS

The ASMA is used primarily to aid in the diagnosis of autoimmune chronic active hepatitis (CAH), which has also been referred to as "lupoid" CAH.

TEST EXPLANATION

ASMA is an anticytoplasmic antibody directed against actin, a cytoskeletal protein. Normally the serum does not contain ASMA at a titer greater than 1:20. ASMA is the most commonly recognized autoantibody in the setting of CAH. It appears in 70% to 80% of patients with CAH. Patients with some types of CAH do not test positive for ASMA antibodies. This disease may be an autoimmune disease that occurs predominantly in adult women. The clinical presentation of CAH is similar to that of viral hepatitis. That clinical picture, along with serologic and pathologic criteria, must exist for more than 6 months to be classified as CAH.

ASMA is not specific for CAH and can be positive in patients with viral infections, malignancy, multiple sclerosis, primary biliary cirrhosis, and *Mycoplasma* infections. Usually the titer of ASMA is low in these diseases. With CAH, the titer is usually higher than 1:160. The titers are not helpful in predicting prognosis, nor do they indicate response to therapy. ASMA is also used to distinguish autoimmune hepatitis from lupus erythematosus. For the ASMA test, immunofluorescent assay (IFA) or enzyme-linked immunosorbent assay (ELISA) techniques are used.

PROCEDURE AND PATIENT CARE

Before

- Explain the procedure to the patient.
- Tell the patient that no fasting or special preparation is required.

During

- Collect a venous blood sample in a red-top tube.

After

- Apply pressure or a pressure dressing to the venipuncture site.
- Check the venipuncture site for bleeding. Patients with jaundice often have bleeding disorders associated with vitamin K deficiency.

TEST RESULTS AND CLINICAL SIGNIFICANCE

▲ Increased Levels

CAH,

Mononucleosis hepatitis:

ASMA is positive in 70% to 80% of patients.

Primary biliary cirrhosis,

Viral hepatitis,

Multiple sclerosis,

Malignancy,

Intrinsic asthma:

ASMA is positive in about 30% of patients.

RELATED TESTS

Liver Enzymes, such as Alkaline Phosphatase (ALT) (p. 47) and Aspartate Aminotransferase (AST) (p. 119). These enzymes exist within the hepatocytes and are elevated in patients with hepatitis.

Antimitochrondrial Antibody (p. 84). This is an antibody that is most frequently associated with primary biliary cirrhosis. Positive titers of AMA are found in 30% of the patients with CAH.

Anti–Liver/Kidney Microsomal Type 1 Antibodies (p. 83). This antibody is helpful in the diagnosis of autoimmune hepatitis.

Antispermatozoal Antibody (Sperm Agglutination and Inhibition, Sperm Antibodies, Antisperm Antibodies, Infertility Screen)

NORMAL FINDINGS

Negative

INDICATIONS

The antispermatozoal antibody test is an infertility screening test used to detect the presence of sperm antibodies. Antibodies directed toward sperm antigens can result in diminished fertility.

TEST EXPLANATION

This test is used in the evaluation of an infertile couple usually after a postcoital test is positive. For fertilization to occur, the sperm head must first attach to the *zona pellucida* of the egg. Sperm antibodies interfere with this binding. Although there is consensus that these antibodies play a role in infertility, the percentage of sperm that must be bound by antibodies before fertility is adversely affected is less clear. The IgA antisperm antibodies to the sperm tail are associated with poor motility and poor penetration of cervical mucus. IgG antisperm antibodies are associated with blockage of sperm-ovum fusion. Semen and serum may contain sperm antibodies. Semen is the preferred specimen type for males. In cases in which semen production may present difficulties, a serum specimen can be tested instead. Serum is the preferred specimen type in females.

Positives are reported as percentage of sperm with positive bindings, the class of antibody involved (IgG, IgA, and IgM), and the site of binding (head, midpiece, tail, and/or tail tip). Greater than 50% binding is usually required to significantly lower a patient's fertility.

Not only is this test indicated for male infertility studies, but it is also used as a follow-up test when sperm agglutination is noted in the ejaculate. It is also used in men with a history of testicular trauma, biopsy, vasectomy reversal, genital tract infection, or obstructive lesions of the male ductal system. Antisperm antibodies may be found in the blood of men with blocked efferent ducts of the testes (a common cause of low sperm counts or poor sperm mobility) and in 30% to 70% of men who have had a vasectomy. Resorption of sperm from the blocked ducts results in the formation of autoantibodies to sperm as a result of sperm antigens interacting with the immune system. High titers of IgG autoantibodies are often associated with postvasectomy degeneration of the testes, which explains why 50% of men remain infertile after successful repair of a previous vasectomy.

PROCEDURE AND PATIENT CARE

Before
- Explain the procedure to the patient.

Sperm Specimen
- Inform the man that a semen specimen should be collected after avoiding ejaculation for at least 3 days.
- Give the male patient the proper container for the sperm collection.
- If the specimen is to be collected at home, be certain the patient is told that it must be taken to the laboratory for testing within 2 hours of collection.

During
- Collect a venous blood sample from both the male and the female patient in red-top tubes.

Sperm Specimen
- Collect the ejaculate in a plastic container.

Vaginal Mucus Specimen
- Collect 1 mL of cervical mucus and place it in a plastic vial.

After
- Apply pressure or a pressure dressing to the venipuncture sites.
- Check the venipuncture sites for bleeding.
- For a sperm, blood, or cervical specimen, the specimen may be placed in a plastic vial, frozen, and sent to a reference laboratory on dry ice.
- Instruct the couple when and how to obtain the test results.

TEST RESULTS AND CLINICAL SIGNIFICANCE

Infertility: *Antispermatozoal antibodies may be present in the man or the woman and may inhibit the number or motility of sperm or the ability of the sperm to penetrate the ovum.*

Blocked efferent ducts in the testes: *This is considered to be a common cause of male infertility. Reabsorption of sperm from the blocked ducts results in the formation of autoantibodies to sperm as a result of sperm antigens interacting with the immune system.*

Vasectomy: *Reabsorption of sperm from the occluded vas deferens results in the formation of autoantibodies to sperm as a result of sperm antigens interacting with the immune system.*

RELATED TESTS

Sims-Huhner Test (p. 676). This test consists of a postcoital examination of the cervical mucus to measure the ability of the sperm to penetrate the mucus and maintain motility. It is used in the diagnostic workup of infertility. This analysis is also helpful in documenting cases of suspected rape by testing the vaginal and cervical secretions for sperm.

Luteinizing Hormone and Follicle-Stimulating Hormone Assay (p. 348). These hormones are useful for determining the pituitary effect on gonadal function and spermatogenesis.

Semen Analysis (p. 671). This test is used to evaluate the quality of sperm. Semen analysis is used to evaluate an infertile couple and to document the adequacy of operative vasectomy.

Estrogen and Progesterone (pp. 226 and 416). These tests are used to indicate ovarian function and reserve.

Anti-SS-A (Ro), Anti-SS-B (La), and Anti-SS-C Antibody (Anti-Ro, Anti-La, Sjögren Antibodies)

NORMAL FINDINGS

≤29 AU/mL: Negative
30-40 AU/mL: Equivocal
≥41 AU/mL: Positive

INDICATIONS

These three antinuclear antibodies are considered antiextractable nuclear antigens (see p. 79) and are used to diagnose Sjögren syndrome.

TEST EXPLANATION

Ro, La, and SS-C antibodies are subtypes of antinuclear antibodies (ANA) (see Table 2-3, p. 89) and react to nuclear antigens extracted from human B lymphocytes. Ro and La produce a speckled immunofluorescent pattern when seen under the ultraviolet microscope. They are strongly associated with Sjögren syndrome. This disease is an immunologic abnormality characterized by progressive destruction of the lacrimal and salivary exocrine glands leading to mucosal and conjunctival dryness. This disease can occur by itself (primary) or in association with other autoimmune diseases, such as systemic lupus erythematosus (SLE), rheumatoid arthritis (RA), and scleroderma. In the latter case it is referred to as secondary Sjögren syndrome.

Anti–SS-A antibodies may be found in approximately 60% to 70% of patients with primary Sjögren syndrome. Anti–SS-B antibodies may be found in approximately 50% to 60% of patients with primary Sjögren syndrome. When anti–SS-A and SS-B antibodies are positive, Sjögren syndrome can be diagnosed accurately. These antibodies are more rarely found when secondary Sjögren syndrome is associated with RA. In fact, SS-B is only found in primary Sjögren syndrome. However, anti–SS-C is positive in about 75% of patients with RA or patients with secondary Sjögren syndrome associated with RA. Yet anti–SS-A and anti–SS-B are almost never found in patients with Sjögren syndrome associated with RA. Therefore these antibodies are also useful in differentiating primary from secondary Sjögren syndrome.

SS-A can also be found in 25% of patients with SLE. This is particularly useful in "ANA-negative" patients with SLE, because these antibodies are present in the majority of such patients. Anti–SS-B is rarely found in patients with SLE. In general, the higher the titer of anti–SS antibodies, the more likely that Sjögren syndrome exists and the more active the disease is. As Sjögren syndrome becomes less active with therapy, the anti–SS antibodies titers can be expected to fall. These antibodies can be quantified by the Semi-quantitative Multi-analyte Fluorescent Detection methodology.

PROCEDURE AND PATIENT CARE

Before

🖉 Explain the procedure to the patient.
🖉 Tell the patient that no fasting is required.

During

• Collect a venous blood sample in a red-top tube.

After

• Apply pressure or a pressure dressing to the venipuncture site.
• Assess the venipuncture site for bleeding.
• Check the venipuncture site for infection. Patients with autoimmune disease have a compromised immune system.

TEST RESULTS AND CLINICAL SIGNIFICANCE

Positive

Sjögren syndrome: *When high titers of anti–SS-A or anti–SS-B are present, Sjögren syndrome can be diagnosed with confidence.*
Rheumatoid arthritis (RA): *When high titers of anti–SS-C are present, RA with or without Sjögren syndrome can be diagnosed with confidence.*
ANA-negative SLE: *Anti–SS-A will be positive in most of these patients.*
Neonatal lupus: *Anti–SS-A will be positive in 95% of these patients.*

RELATED TESTS

Antinuclear Antibody (ANA) (p. 88). This test is used to diagnose SLE and other autoimmune diseases. The ANA ELISA screen is designed to detect antibodies against dsDNA, histone, SS-A (Ro), SS-B (La), Smith, snRNP/Sm, Scl-70, Jo-1, and centromere.
Anticentromere Antibody (p. 69). This test is used to diagnose CREST syndrome.
Anti-DNA Antibody (p. 78). This test is used to dignose SLE.

Antiextractable Nuclear Antigen (ENA) (p. 79). This test is used to diagnose SLE and mixed connective tissue disease. This is a first-line test for connective tissue disease screening.
Antiscleroderma Antibody (p. 93). This test is used to diagnose scleroderma.

Antithrombin Activity and Antigen Assay
(Antithrombin III [AT-III] Activity/Assay, Functional Antithrombin III Assay, Heparin Cofactor, Immunologic Antithrombin III, Serine Protease Inhibitor)

NORMAL FINDINGS

Antithrombin Activity

Newborn: 35%-40%
>6 months to adult: 80%-130%

Antithrombin Antigen Assay

Plasma: >50% of control value
Serum: 15%-34% lower than plasma value
Immunologic: 17-30 mg/dL
Functional: 80%-120%
Values vary according to laboratory methods.

INDICATIONS

This test is used to evaluate patients suspected of having hypercoagulable states. It is also used to help identify the cause of heparin resistance in patients receiving heparin therapy.

TEST EXPLANATION

AT-III is an alpha$_2$-globulin produced in the liver. It inhibits the serine proteases involved in coagulation (II, X, IX, XI, XII). In normal homeostasis, coagulation results from a balance between AT-III and thrombin. ATT-III is the principal plasma anticoagulant mediating inactivation of serine protease procoagulant enzymes, chiefly thrombin and coagulation factors Xa and IXa. (A deficiency of AT-III increases coagulation or the tendency toward thrombosis.) A hereditary deficiency of AT-III is characterized by a predisposition toward thrombus formation. This is passed on as an autosomal-dominant abnormality. Individuals with hereditary AT-III deficiency typically develop thromboembolic events in their early twenties. These thrombotic events are usually venous.

Acquired AT-III deficiency may be seen in patients with cirrhosis, liver failure, advanced carcinoma, nephrotic syndrome, disseminated intravascular coagulation (DIC), protein-losing enteropathies, and acute thrombosis. AT-III is also decreased as much as 30% in pregnant women and those who take estrogens. Antithrombin activity testing is ordered, along with other tests for hypercoagulable disorders (such as protein C and protein S, and lupus anticoagulant), when a patient has been experiencing recurrent venous thrombosis. Antithrombin should be measured after a blood clot has been treated and resolved because both the presence of the clot, and the therapy used to treat it, will affect antithrombin results. AT-III provides most of the anticoagulant effect of heparin. Heparin increases antithrombin activity by 1000-fold. Patients who are deficient in AT-III may be heparin resistant and require unusually high doses for an anticoagulation effect. In general, patients respond to heparin if more than 60% of normal AT-III levels exist.

There are two tests for AT-III. The first is a "functional" assay and measures AT-III activity. The second quantifies the AT-III antigen. The antithrombin activity test is performed before the antigen test, to evaluate whether the total amount of functional antithrombin activity is normal. Antithrombin activity is the primary (screening) antithrombin assay. If antithrombin activity is normal, AT III is not the cause of the hypercoagulable state. If antithrombin activity is abnormal, antithrombin antigen should be quantified.

There are two types of inherited AT-III syndromes identified by using these tests. In type 1, the antithrombin activity and quantities of antithrombin antigen are decreased. In this case, the activity is decreased because there is less antithrombin available to participate in clotting regulation. In type 2 (very rare), there is reduced antithrombin activity and normal levels of antithrombin antigen, suggesting that there is sufficient antithrombin but it is not functioning as it should.

Asymptomatic individuals with an antithrombin deficiency should receive prophylactic anticoagulation to increase their antithrombin levels before any medical/surgical interventions in which inactivity increases the risk of thrombosis. Increased levels of AT-III are not usually considered a problem and may occur in patients with acute hepatitis, obstructive jaundice, vitamin K deficiency, and kidney transplantation.

Antithrombin studies are also used as an adjunct in the diagnosis and management of carbohydrate-deficient glycoprotein syndromes (CDGS) because defective glycosylation of this AT-III in individuals with CDGS will cause hypercoagulation. Deficient AT-III may also contribute to recurrent miscarriages.

Antithrombin activity testing is also used to monitor treatment of antithrombin deficiency disorders by infusion of antithrombin concentrates. Antithrombin antigen and activity is determined using automated latex immunoassay (LIA) methodology, commonly on a Beckman Coulter ACL TOP.

INTERFERING FACTORS

- Drugs that may cause *increased* levels include anabolic steroids, androgens, oral contraceptives (containing progesterone), and sodium warfarin.
- Drugs that may cause *decreased* levels include fibrinolytics, heparin, L-asparaginase, and oral contraceptives (containing estrogen).

PROCEDURE AND PATIENT CARE

Before

- Explain the procedure to the patient.
- Tell the patient that no fasting is required.

During

- Collect a venous blood sample in a light blue- or red-top tube.

After

- Apply pressure or a pressure dressing to the venipuncture site.
- Assess the venipuncture site for bleeding. Patients receiving heparin therapy may develop a hematoma at the venipuncture site.
- Send the specimen to the laboratory immediately after collection.

TEST RESULTS AND CLINICAL SIGNIFICANCE

▲ Increased Levels

Kidney transplant,
Acute hepatitis,

Obstructive jaundice,
Vitamin K deficiency:
The exact mechanism for these levels is not known.

▼ Decreased Levels

Disseminated intravascular coagulation (DIC),
Hypercoagulation states (e.g., deep vein thrombosis),
Hepatic disorders (especially cirrhosis),
Nephrotic syndrome,
Protein-wasting diseases (malignancy),
Hereditary familial deficiency of AT-III:
These diseases are associated with specific or generalized protein/antigen deficiencies causing decreased levels of AT-III antigen/activity.

Related Tests

Coagulating Factor Concentration (p. 163). This test measures the concentration of specific coagulating factors in the blood.
Protein C, Protein S (p. 432). This is part of the evaluation of patients with coagulation disorders.
Lupus anticoagulant (p. 68 [anticardiolipin antibodies]). This test is done in many patients with thrombus.

Antithyroglobulin Antibody (Thyroid Autoantibody, Thyroid Antithyroglobulin Antibody, Thyroglobulin Antibody)

NORMAL FINDINGS

<116 IU/mL

INDICATIONS

This test is used as a marker for autoimmune thyroiditis and related diseases.

TEST EXPLANATION

Thyroglobulin autoantibodies bind thyroglobulin (Tg), a major thyroid-specific protein that plays a crucial role in thyroid hormone synthesis, storage, and release. Tg remains in the thyroid follicles until hormone production is required. Tg is not secreted into the systemic circulation under normal circumstances. However, follicular destruction through inflammation (Hashimoto's thyroiditis or chronic lymphocytic thyroiditis and autoimmune hypothyroidism), hemorrhage (nodular goiter), or rapid disordered growth of thyroid tissue (as may be observed in Graves disease or follicular cell-derived thyroid neoplasms) can result in leakage of Tg into the bloodstream. This results in the formation of autoantibodies to Tg in some individuals. Of individuals with autoimmune hypothyroidism, 30% to 50% will have detectable anti-Tg autoantibodies (Table 2-7).

The antithyroglobulin test is usually performed in conjunction with the antithyroid peroxidase antibody test (p. 104). When this is done, the specificity and sensitivity are greatly increased. Antithyroglobulin assay is a Quantitative Chemiluminescent Immunoassay. Normal results vary based on the methodology used. A small percentage of the normal population has antithyroglobulin antibodies. Normally women tend to have higher levels than men.

TABLE 2-7	Thyroid Diseases and the Incidence of Antithyroid Antibodies	
Disease	**Antithyroglobulin Antibody (%)**	**Antithyroid Peroxidase Antibody (%)**
Hashimoto thyroiditis	70	95
Graves disease	55	75
Myxedema	55	75
Nontoxic goiter	5-50	27
Thyroid cancer	20	20
Normal male	2	3
Normal female	10	15

Blood Studies

2

Tg antibodies are also used when testing Tg as a marker for follicular cell thyroid cancer. If Tg antibodies are present, Tg is then considered an inaccurate marker for recurrent/metastatic cancer.

INTERFERING FACTORS

• Normal individuals, especially elderly women, may have antithyroglobulin antibodies.

PROCEDURE AND PATIENT CARE

Before

✗ Explain the procedure to the patient.
✗ Tell the patient that no fasting is required.

During

• Collect a venous blood sample in a red-top tube.

After

• Apply pressure or a pressure dressing to the venipuncture site.
• Assess the venipuncture site for bleeding.

TEST RESULTS AND CLINICAL SIGNIFICANCE

▲ Increased Levels

Chronic thyroiditis (Hashimoto thyroiditis): *Antithyroglobulin antibodies attack the globulin in the thyroid cells. The immune complex creates an inflammatory and destructive process in the gland, which is mediated through the complement system.*

Rheumatoid arthritis (RA),

Rheumatoid-collagen disease:

   The association with other autoimmune diseases is well known; however, the mechanism of this association has not been elucidated.

Pernicious anemia: *Anti–parietal cell antibodies have been associated with the presence of antithyroglobulin antibodies.*

Thyrotoxicosis,

Hypothyroidism,

Thyroid carcinoma:

> *Thyroglobulin, which leaks out of the thyroid as a result of these destructive diseases, stimulates the immune system to produce antithyroglobulin antibodies.*

Myxedema: *The antithyroid microsomal antibodies destroy the thyroid cell, resulting in hypofunction of the gland.*

RELATED TESTS

Antithyroid Peroxidase Antibody (p. 104). This test is primarily used in the differential diagnosis of thyroid diseases, such as Hashimoto thyroiditis and chronic lymphocytic thyroiditis (in children).

Thyroid-Stimulating Immunoglobulins (p. 491). These thyroid-stimulating immunoglobulins are used to support the diagnosis of Graves disease, especially when the diagnosis is complex.

Thyroid-Stimulating Hormone (p. 486). This test is used to diagnose primary hypothyroidism and to differentiate it from secondary (pituitary) and tertiary (hypothalamus) hypothyroidism.

Thyroxine, Total (p. 497). This is one of the first tests done to assess thyroid function. It is used to diagnose thyroid function and to monitor replacement and suppressive therapy.

Triiodothyronine (p. 506). A T3 test is used to evaluate thyroid function, primarily to diagnose hyperthyroidism. It is also used to monitor thyroid replacement and suppressive medical therapy.

Antithyroid Peroxidase Antibody (Anti-TPO, TPO-Ab, Antithyroid Microsomal Antibody, Thyroid Autoantibody, Thyroid Microsomal Antibody)

NORMAL FINDINGS

Titer <9 IU/mL

INDICATIONS

This test is primarily used in the differential diagnosis of thyroid diseases, such as Hashimoto thyroiditis and chronic lymphocytic thyroiditis (in children).

TEST EXPLANATION

Thyroid microsomal antibodies are commonly found in patients with various thyroid diseases. They are present in 70% to 90% of patients with Hashimoto thyroiditis. Microsomal antibodies are produced in response to microsomes escaping from the thyroid epithelial cells surrounding the thyroid follicle. These escaped microsomes then act as antigens and stimulate the production of antibodies. These immune complexes initiate inflammatory and cytotoxic effects on the thyroid follicle. This test is often performed in conjunction with the antithyroglobulin antibody test, which greatly increases the specificity and sensitivity.

Although many different thyroid diseases are associated with elevated antimicrosomal antibody levels, the most frequent is chronic thyroiditis (Hashimoto thyroiditis in the adult and lymphocytic thyroiditis in children and young adults) (Table 2-7, p. 103). Both of these chronic inflammatory diseases have been associated with other autoimmune (collagen-vascular) diseases. Twelve percent of normal females and 1% of normal males have positive antimicrosomal antibodies.

The most sensitive assay for antimicrosomal antibodies is for the antithyroid peroxidase (anti-TPO) antibody. This assay uses enzyme immunoassays. Anti-TPO is often performed in conjunction with the antithyroglobulin antibody test (see p. 102). When this is done, the specificity and sensitivity are greatly increased.

Anti-TPO is present in almost all patients with Hashimoto thyroiditis, in more than 70% of those with Graves disease, and, to a variable degree, in patients with nonthyroid autoimmune disease. Anti-TPO correlates with the degree of lymphocytic infiltrations (inflammation) in the thyroid. Among healthy people, 5% to 10% have elevated anti-TPO levels.

PROCEDURE AND PATIENT CARE

Before
✗ Explain the procedure to the patient.
✗ Tell the patient that no fasting is required.

During
- Collect a venous blood sample in a red-top tube.

After
- Apply pressure or a pressure dressing to the venipuncture site.
- Assess the venipuncture site for bleeding.

TEST RESULTS AND CLINICAL SIGNIFICANCE

▲ Increased Levels

Chronic thyroiditis (Hashimoto thyroiditis): *Antimicrosomal antibodies attack the microsome in the thyroid cells. The immune complex creates an inflammatory and destructive process in the gland, which is mediated through the complement system.*

Rheumatoid arthritis (RA),
Rheumatoid-collagen disease:
  The association with other autoimmune diseases is well known. The mechanism of this association, however, is not well known.

Pernicious anemia: *Anti–parietal cell antibodies have been associated with the presence of antimicrosomal antibodies.*

Thyrotoxicosis,
Hypothyroidism,
Thyroid carcinoma:
  Microsomes that leak out of the thyroid as a result of the presence of these destructive diseases stimulate the immune system to produce antimicrosomal antibodies.

Myxedema: *Antithyroid microsomal antibodies destroy the thyroid cell, resulting in hypofunction of the gland.*

RELATED TEST

Antithyroglobulin Antibody (p. 102). This test is primarily used in the differential diagnosis of thyroid diseases such as Hashimoto thyroiditis.

Blood Studies

2

Apolipoproteins (Apolipoprotein A-I [Apo A-I], Apolipoprotein B [Apo B], Lipoprotein [a] [Lp(a)], Apolipoprotein E [Apo E])

NORMAL FINDINGS

Apo A-I
Adult/older adult
   Male: 75-160 mg/dL
   Female: 80-175 mg/dL
Child/adolescent
   6 months to 4 years
      Male: 67-167 mg/dL
      Female: 60-148 mg/dL
   5 to 17 years: 83-151 mg/dL
Newborn
   Male: 41-93 mg/dL
   Female: 38-106 mg/dL

Apo B
Adult/older adult
   Male: 50-125 mg/dL
   Female: 45-120 mg/dL
Child/adolescent
   Newborn: 11-31 mg/dL
   6 months to 3 years: 23-75 mg/dL
   5-17 years
      Male: 47-139 mg/dL
      Female: 41-132 mg/dL

Apo A-I/Apo B Ratio
Male: 0.85-2.24
Female: 0.76-3.23

Lipoprotein (a)
Caucasian (5th to 95th percentile)
   Male: 2.2-49.4 mg/dL
   Female: 2.1-57.3 mg/dL
African-American (5th to 95th percentile)
   Male: 4.6-71.8 mg/dL
   Female: 4.4-75 mg/dL

INDICATIONS

This test is used to evaluate the risk of atherogenic heart and peripheral vascular diseases. These levels may be better indicators of atherogenic risks than high-density lipoprotein (HDL), low-density lipoprotein (LDL), and very-low-density lipoprotein (VLDL).

TEST EXPLANATION

Apolipoproteins are the protein part of lipoproteins (e.g., HDL, LDL). In general, apolipoproteins play an important role in lipid transport in the lymphatic and the circulatory system. They also act as enzyme cofactors in lipoprotein synthesis. Apolipoproteins also act as receptor ligands to improve transport of fat particles in the cell. Apolipoprotein synthesis in the liver is controlled by a host of factors, including dietary composition, hormones (insulin, glucagon, thyroxin, estrogens, androgens), alcohol intake, and various drugs (statins, niacin, and fibric acids).

There are several types of apolipoproteins, including apo A-I, apo B, and apo E (Table 2-8). *Apolipoprotein A (apo A)* is the major polypeptide component of HDL. Low levels of apo A are associated with increased risk of coronary or peripheral artery disease (CPAD). Elevated levels may protect against CPAD.

Apo B is the major polypeptide component of LDL and chylomicrons. Apo B makes cholesterol soluble for deposition in the arterial wall. Forty percent of the protein portion of VLDL is composed of apo B. Familial hypercholesterolemia type B is caused by mutations in the Apo B gene.

Lp(a) (referred to as *Lipoprotein little a*) is a heterogenous group of lipoproteins consisting of an Apo A molecule attached to an Apo B molecule. An increased level of Lp(a) may be an independent risk factor for atherosclerosis and is particularly harmful to the endothelium. Serum concentrations of Lp(a) appear to be largely related to genetic factors; diet and lipid-lowering pharmaceuticals do not have a major impact on Lp(a) levels. Nevertheless, measurement of serum Lp(a) may contribute to a more comprehensive risk assessment in high-risk patients.

Apolipoprotein E (apo E) is involved in cholesterol transport. Through genotyping, three alleles for apo E have been identified: E2, E3, and E4. Each person gets an allele from each parent. E3/3 is the normal. E2/2 is found rarely and is associated with type III hyperlipidemia. E4/4 or E4/3 is associated with high LDL levels. The apo E4 gene has been proposed as a risk factor for Alzheimer disease. Apo E2 and E4 are associated with increased triglycerides.

Lp-PLA2 is a lipase enzyme located on the surface of circulating LDL. This protein is atherogenic. Testing is performed by immunoturbidimetric assay or nephelometry.

INTERFERING FACTORS

Apo A-I

- Physical exercise may increase apo A-I levels.
- Smoking may decrease levels.

TABLE 2-8	Summary of Apolipoproteins		
Lipoprotein	**Subcomponents**	**Lipoprotein Component**	**Associated Diseases**
Apo A	Apo A-I, Apo A-II	HDL	Low levels are a risk factor for atherogenic vascular disease.
Apo B	Apo B-100 and Apo B-48	LDL, VLDL	High levels are a risk factor for atherogenic vascular disease.
Lp(a)	Apo(a)	LDL-like proteins	High levels are a risk factor for atherogenic vascular disease.
Apo E	E2, E3, E4		Hyperlipidemia, Alzheimer disease

- Diets high in carbohydrates or polyunsaturated fats may decrease apo A-I levels.
- Drugs that may *increase* apo A-I levels include carbamazepine, estrogens, ethanol, lovastatin, niacin, oral contraceptives, phenobarbital, pravastatin, and simvastatin.
- Drugs that may *decrease* apo A-I levels include androgens, beta blockers, diuretics, and progestins.

Apo B

- Diets high in saturated fats and cholesterol may increase apo B levels.
- Drugs that may *increase* apo B levels include androgens, beta blockers, diuretics, ethanol, and progestins.
- Drugs that may *decrease* apo B levels include cholestyramine, estrogen (postmenopausal women), lovastatin, neomycin, niacin, simvastatin, and thyroxine.

Lipoprotein (a)

- Drugs that may *decrease* Lp(a) include estrogens, neomycin, niacin, and stanozolol.

Clinical Priorities

- Apolipoproteins may be better indicators of atherogenic risks than HDL, LDL, and VLDL.
- Decreased levels of apo A-I and increased levels of apo B are associated with an increased risk of CAD.
- Research has suggested that increased levels of Lp(a) are associated with a high risk of CAD.
- Test preparation requires a 12- to 14-hour fast before testing. Only water is permitted.

PROCEDURE AND PATIENT CARE

Before
- Explain the procedure to the patient.
- Instruct the patient to fast for 12 to 14 hours before testing. Only water is permitted.
- Inform the patient that smoking is prohibited.

During
- Collect a venous blood sample in a red-top tube.

After
- Apply pressure or a pressure dressing to the venipuncture site.
- Observe the venipuncture site for bleeding.

TEST RESULTS AND CLINICAL SIGNIFICANCE*

▲ Increased Apo A-I
Familial hyperalphalipoproteinemia
Pregnancy
Weight reduction

▼ Decreased Apo A-I
Coronary artery disease (CAD)
Ischemic coronary disease
Myocardial infarction (MI)

---

*The pathophysiology of these observations has not been well defined.

▲ **Increased Apo A-I—cont'd**

▼ **Decreased Apo A-I—cont'd**
Familial hypoalphalipoproteinemia
Fish eye disease
Uncontrolled diabetes mellitus
Tangier disease
Nephrotic syndrome
Chronic renal failure
Cholestasis
Hemodialysis

▲ **Increased Apo B**
Hyperlipoproteinemia (types IIa, IIb, IV, V)
Nephrotic syndrome
Pregnancy
Hemodialysis
Biliary obstruction
Coronary artery disease (CAD)
Diabetes
Hypothyroidism
Anorexia nervosa
Renal failure

▼ **Decreased Apo B**
Tangier disease
Hyperthyroidism
Inflammatory joint disease
Malnutrition
Chronic pulmonary disease
Weight reduction
Chronic anemia
Reye syndrome

▲ **Increased Lp(a)**
Premature coronary artery disease (CAD)
Stenosis of cerebral arteries
Uncontrolled diabetes mellitus
Severe hypothyroidism
Familial hypercholesterolemis
Chronic renal failure
Estrogen depletion

▼ **Decreased Lp(a)**
Alcoholism
Malnutrition
Chronic hepatocellular disease

Apo E-4 Gene
Alzheimer disease

RELATED TEST

Lipoprotein (p. 342). This is a test also used to assess the risk of atherogenic vascular disease.

Arterial Blood Gases (Blood Gases, ABG)

NORMAL FINDINGS

pH
Adult/child: 7.35-7.45
Newborn: 7.32-7.49
2 months to 2 years: 7.34-7.46
pH (venous): 7.31-7.41

Pco_2
Adult/child: 35-45 mm Hg
Child <2 years: 26-41 mm Hg
Pco_2 (venous): 40-50 mm Hg

HCO_3^-
Adult/child: 21-28 mEq/L
Newborn/infant: 16-24 mEq/L

Po_2
Adult/child: 80-100 mm Hg
Newborn: 60-70 mm Hg
Po_2 (venous): 40-50 mm Hg

O_2 Saturation
Adult/child: 95% to 100%
Elderly: 95%
Newborn: 40% to 90%

O_2 Content
Arterial: 15-22 vol %
Venous: 11-16 vol %

Base Excess
0 ± 2 mEq/L

Alveolar to Arterial O_2 Difference
<10 mm Hg

 Critical Values

pH: <7.25, >7.6
Pco_2: <20, >60
HCO_3^-: <10, >40
Po_2 (arterial): <40
O_2 saturation: 75% or lower
Base/Excess: ± 3 mEq/L

INDICATIONS

Measurement of arterial blood gasses (ABGs) provides valuable information in assessing and managing a patient's respiratory (ventilation) and metabolic (renal) acid-base and electrolyte homeostasis. It is also used to assess the adequacy of oxygenation.

TEST EXPLANATION

ABGs are used to monitor patients on ventilators, monitor critically ill nonventilator patients, establish preoperative baseline parameters, and regulate electrolyte therapy. Although O_2 saturation monitors can accurately indicate O_2, ABGs are still used to monitor O_2 flow rates in the hospital and at home. ABG measurement is often performed in conjunction with pulmonary function studies.

pH

The pH is the negative logarithm of the hydrogen ion concentration in the blood. It is inversely proportional to the actual hydrogen ion concentration. Therefore, as the hydrogen ion concentration decreases, the pH increases, and vice versa. The acids normally found in the blood include carbonic acid (H_2CO_3), dietary acids, lactic acid, and ketoacids. The pH is a measure of alkalinity (pH >7.4) and acidity pH <7.35). In respiratory or metabolic alkalosis the pH is elevated; in respiratory or metabolic acidosis the pH is decreased. The pH is usually calculated by a machine that directly measures pH.

Pco_2

The Pco_2 is a measure of the partial pressure of CO_2 in the blood. CO_2 is carried in the blood as follows: 10% in the plasma and 90% in the red blood cells (RBCs). Pco_2 is a measurement of ventilation. The faster and more deeply the patient breathes, the more CO_2 is blown off, and Pco_2 levels drop. Pco_2 is therefore referred to as the respiratory component in acid-base determination, because this value is primarily controlled by the lungs. As the CO_2 level increases, the pH decreases. The CO_2 level and the pH are inversely proportional. The Pco_2 in the blood and the cerebrospinal fluid is a major stimulant to the breathing center in the brain. As Pco_2 levels rise, breathing is stimulated. If Pco_2 levels rise too high, breathing cannot keep up with the demand to blow off or ventilate. As Pco_2 levels rise further, the brain is depressed and ventilation decreases further, causing coma.

The Pco_2 level is elevated in primary respiratory acidosis and decreased in primary respiratory alkalosis (Table 2-9). Because the lungs compensate for primary metabolic acid-base derangements, Pco_2 levels are affected by metabolic disturbances as well. In metabolic acidosis the lungs attempt to

TABLE 2-9	Normal Values for ABGs and Abnormal Values in Uncompensated Acid-Base Disturbances			
Acid-Base Disturbance	**pH**	**Pco_2 (mm Hg)**	**HCO_3^- (mEq/L)**	**Common Cause**
None (normal values)	7.35-7.45	35-45	22-26	
Respiratory acidosis	↓	↑	Normal	Respiratory depression (drugs, central nervous system trauma) Pulmonary disease (pneumonia, chronic obstructive pulmonary disease, respiratory underventilation)
Respiratory alkalosis	↑	↓	Normal	Hyperventilation (emotions, pain, respiratory overventilation)
Metabolic acidosis	↓	Normal	↓	Diabetes, shock, renal failure, intestinal fistula
Metabolic alkalosis	↑	Normal	↑	Sodium bicarbonate overdose, prolonged vomiting, nasogastric drainage

TABLE 2-10	Acid-Base Disturbances and Compensatory Mechanisms
Acid-Base Disturbance	**Mode of Compensation**
Respiratory acidosis	Kidneys will retain increased amounts of HCO_3^- to increase pH
Respiratory alkalosis	Kidneys will excrete increased amounts of HCO_3^- to lower pH
Metabolic acidosis	Lungs "blow off" CO_2 to raise pH
Metabolic alkalosis	Lungs retain CO_2 to lower pH

compensate by blowing off CO_2 to raise pH. In metabolic alkalosis the lungs attempt to compensate by retaining CO_2 to lower pH (Table 2-10).

HCO_3^- or CO_2 Content

Most of the CO_2 content in the blood is HCO_3^-. The bicarbonate ion (HCO_3^-) is a measure of the metabolic (renal) component of the acid-base equilibrium. It is regulated by the kidney. This ion can be measured directly by the bicarbonate value or indirectly by the CO_2 content (see p. 141). It is important not to confuse CO_2 content with Pco_2. CO_2 content is an indirect measurement of HCO_3^-. Pco_2 is a direct measurement of the tension of CO_2 in the blood and is regulated by the lungs.

As the HCO_3^- level increases, the pH also increases; therefore the relationship of bicarbonate to pH is directly proportional. HCO_3^- is elevated in metabolic alkalosis and decreased in metabolic acidosis (see Table 2-9). The kidneys also are used to compensate for primary respiratory acid-base derangements. For example, in respiratory acidosis the kidneys attempt to compensate by reabsorbing increased amounts of HCO_3^-. In respiratory alkalosis the kidneys excrete HCO_3^- in increased amounts in an attempt to lower pH through compensation (see Table 2-10).

Po_2

This is an indirect measure of the O_2 content of the arterial blood. Po_2 is a measure of the tension (pressure) of O_2 dissolved in the plasma. This pressure determines the force of O_2 to diffuse across the pulmonary alveoli membrane. The Po_2 level is decreased in:

1. Patients who are unable to oxygenate the arterial blood because of O_2 diffusion difficulties (e.g., pneumonia, shock lung, congestive failure)
2. Patients in whom venous blood mixes prematurely with arterial blood (e.g., congenital heart disease)
3. Patients who have underventilated and overperfused pulmonary alveoli (pickwickian syndrome; i.e., obese patients who cannot breathe properly when in the supine position or in patients with significant atelectasis)

Po_2 is one of the measures used to determine the effectiveness of O_2 therapy.

O_2 Saturation

O_2 saturation is an indication of the percentage of hemoglobin saturated with O_2. When 92% to 100% of the hemoglobin carries O_2, the tissues are adequately provided with O_2, assuming normal O_2 dissociation. As the Po_2 level decreases, the percentage of hemoglobin saturation also decreases. This decrease (see an oxyhemoglobin-dissociation curve) is linear to a certain value. However, when the Po_2 level drops below 60 mm Hg, small decreases in the Po_2 level will cause large decreases in the percentage of hemoglobin saturated with O_2. At O_2 saturation levels of 70% or lower the tissues are unable to extract enough O_2 to carry out their vital functions.

O_2 saturation is calculated by the blood gas machine using the following formula:

$$\text{Percentage of } O_2 \text{ saturation} = \frac{\text{Volume of } O_2 \text{ content Hgb}}{\text{Volume of } O_2 \text{ Hgb capacity}}$$

Pulse oximetry (see p. 1114) is a noninvasive method of determining O_2 saturation. This can be done easily and continuously. This machine measures O_2 saturation. It actually measures all forms of O_2-saturated hemoglobin, including carboxyhemoglobin (which rises during smoke inhalation or after using some inhalants). Therefore, in cases of carbon monoxide poisoning when carboxyhemoglobin is high, oximetry will indicate an inaccurately high O_2 saturation. During oximetry monitoring a small clip-like sensor is applied to the tip of the finger or earlobe. The oximeter transmits light from one side and records the amount of light on the other side, thus determining O_2 saturation.

O_2 Content

This is a calculated number that represents the amount of O_2 in the blood. The formula for calculation is

$$O_2 \text{ content} = O_2 \text{ saturation} \times \text{Hgb} \times 1.34 + Po_2 \times 0.003$$

Nearly all O_2 in the blood is bound to hemoglobin. O_2 content decreases with the same diseases that diminish Po_2.

Base Excess/Deficit

This number is calculated by the blood gas machine using the pH, Pco_2, and the hematocrit. It represents the amount of buffering anions in the blood. HCO_3^- is the largest of these. Others include hemoglobin, proteins, phosphates, and so on. Base excess is a way to take all of these anions into account when determining acid/base treatment based on the metabolic component. A negative-base excess (deficit) indicates metabolic acidosis (e.g., lactic acidosis). A positive-base excess indicates metabolic alkalosis or compensation to prolonged respiratory acidosis.

Alveolar (A) to Arterial (a) O_2 Difference (A-a Gradient)

This is a calculated number that indicates the difference between alveolar O_2 and arterial O_2. The normal value is less than 10 mm Hg (torr). If the A-a gradient is abnormally high, there is either a problem in diffusing O_2 across the alveolar membrane (thickened edematous alveoli) or unoxygenated blood is mixing with the oxygenated blood. Thickened alveolar membranes can occur in patients with pulmonary edema, pulmonary fibrosis, and acute respiratory distress syndrome (ARDS). Mixing of unoxygenated blood occurs in patients with congenital cardiac septal defects, arteriovenous (AV) shunts, or underventilated alveoli that are still being perfused (atelectasis, mucus plug, etc.).

Interpretation of ABG levels can seem difficult but is really quite easy when one follows a system of evaluation (see Table 2-9). One such system is as follows:

1. Evaluate the pH.

   If the pH is less than 7.4, acidosis is present.

   If the pH is greater than 7.4, alkalosis is present.

2. Next look at the Pco_2.

   A. If the Pco_2 is high in a patient who has been said to have acidosis (by step 1), the patient has respiratory acidosis.

   B. If the Pco_2 is low in a patient who has been said to have acidosis (by step 1), the patient has metabolic acidosis (MA) and is compensating for that situation by blowing off CO_2.

C. If the P_{CO_2} is low in a patient who has been said to have alkalosis (by step 1), the patient has respiratory alkalosis.

D. If the P_{CO_2} is high in a patient who has been said to have alkalosis (by step 1), the patient has metabolic alkalosis and is compensating for that situation by retaining CO_2.

3. Next look at the bicarbonate ion (HCO_3^-).

In patient A, HCO_3^- can be expected to be high in an attempt to compensate for the respiratory acidosis.

In patient B, HCO_3^- can be expected to be low as a reflection of the MA.

In patient C, HCO_3^- can be expected to be low to compensate for the respiratory alkalosis.

In patient D, HCO_3^- can be expected to be high as a reflection of the metabolic alkalosis.

CONTRAINDICATIONS

Arterial access should not be performed if:
- There is no palpable pulse.
- Cellulitis or open infection is present in the area considered for access.
- The Allen test is negative, indicating that there is no ulnar artery. If the radial artery is used for access, thrombosis may occur and jeopardize the viability of the hand.
- There is an AV fistula proximal to the site of proposed access.
- The patient has a severe coagulopathy.

POTENTIAL COMPLICATIONS

- Occlusion of the artery used for access. It is preferable to avoid use of end arteries such as the brachial or femoral artery.
- Penetration of other important structures anatomically juxtaposed to the artery (e.g., nerve).

INTERFERING FACTORS

- O_2 saturation can be falsely increased by the inhalation of carbon monoxide, which increases the carboxyhemoglobin level.
- In patients with chronic obstructive pulmonary disease (COPD), the stimulus to breathe is not triggered by CO_2 levels (as normal) but by O_2 levels. If a large amount of O_2 is provided to these patients, they will no longer be driven to breathe and will hypoventilate.
- Respiration can be inhibited by the use of sedative-hypnotics or narcotics. Overdosage of these drugs can cause hypoventilation in patients with normal lungs.

✓ Clinical Priorities

- Perform the Allen test to assess collateral circulation before performing the arterial puncture on the radial artery. A positive Allen test ensures collateral circulation to the hand if thrombosis of the radial artery should follow the puncture.
- Arterial puncture should not be performed on an arm with an AV fistula or shunt.
- After the arterial blood is obtained, apply pressure to the puncture site for 3 to 5 minutes to avoid hematoma formation. If the patient has an abnormal clotting time or is taking anticoagulants, apply pressure for approximately 15 minutes.

PROCEDURE AND PATIENT CARE

Before

✍ Explain the procedure to the patient.

- Notify the laboratory before drawing ABGs so that the necessary equipment can be calibrated before the blood sample arrives.
- Perform the *Allen test* to assess collateral circulation before performing the arterial puncture on the radial artery (Figure 2-6). To perform the Allen test, make the patient's hand blanch by obliterating both the radial and the ulnar pulses and then release the pressure over the ulnar artery only. If flow through the ulnar artery is good, flushing can be seen immediately. The Allen test is then positive, and the radial artery can be used for puncture. If the Allen test is negative (no flushing), repeat it on the other arm. If both arms give a negative result, choose another artery (femoral) for puncture.
- Note that the Allen test ensures collateral circulation to the hand if thrombosis of the radial artery should follow the puncture.

During

- Note that arterial blood can be obtained from any area of the body in which strong pulses are palpable, usually from the radial, brachial, or femoral artery. The artery chosen for access should have adequate collateral vessels, be easily accessible, and be surrounded by few other vital structures.
- Cleanse the arterial site carefully with an antiseptic (e.g., alcohol or povidoneiodine).
- Use a small-guage needle to collect the arterial blood in an air-free heparinzed syringe.
- After drawing the blood, remove the needle and apply pressure to the arterial site for 3 to 5 minutes.
- Expel any air bubbles in the syringe.

After

- Place the arterial blood on ice and immediately take it to the chemistry or pulmonary laboratory for analysis.
- Hold pressure or apply pressure or a pressure dressing to the arterial puncture site for 3 to 5 minutes to avoid hematoma formation.
- Assess the puncture site for bleeding. Remember that an artery rather than a vein has been accessed.
- If the patient has an abnormal clotting time or is taking anticoagulants, apply pressure for a longer period (approximately 15 minutes).

TEST RESULTS AND CLINICAL SIGNIFICANCE (see Table 2-9)

▲ Increased pH (Alkalosis)

Metabolic Alkalosis

Hypokalemia,

Hypochloremia,

Chronic and high-volume gastric suction,

Chronic vomiting,

Aldosteronism,

Use of mercurial diuretics:

Important acid hydrogen ions are lost. HCO_3^- ions are relatively high.

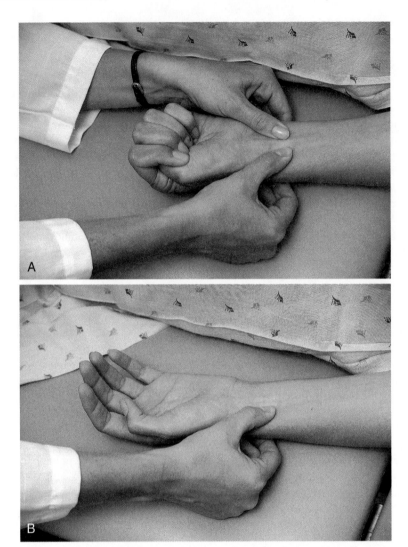

Figure 2-6 The Allen test for evaluating collateral circulation of the radial artery. **A,** Step 1, While the patient's fist is closed tightly, obliterate both the radial and ulnar arteries simultaneously. Instruct the patient to relax the hand, and watch for blanching of the palm and fingers. **B,** Step 2, Release the obstructing pressure from only the ulnar artery. Wait 15 seconds, observing the hand for flushing caused by capillary refilling. Flushing indicates a positive Allen test, verifying that the ulnar artery alone is capable of supplying the entire hand. If flushing does not occur within 15 seconds, the Allen test is negative and radial artery cannot be used.

Respiratory Alkalosis

Hypoxemic states, such as chronic heart failure (CHF), cystic fibrosis, carbon monoxide poisoning, pulmonary emboli, shock, acute severe pulmonary diseases: *With hypoxemia, breathing is accelerated. CO_2 is blown off.*

Anxiety neuroses,

Pain,

Pregnancy:

These situations are associated with hyperventilation. With hyperventilation, CO_2 is blown off.

▼ Decreased pH (Acidosis)

Metabolic Acidosis

Ketoacidosis,

Lactic acidosis:

Acid anions build up. Acidosis occurs.

Severe diarrhea,

Renal failure:

Important base ions are lost. Acid ions are relatively increased and acidosis occurs.

Respiratory Acidosis

Respiratory failure: *Pco_2 builds up, causing acidosis.*

▲ Increased Pco_2

COPD (bronchitis, emphysema),

Oversedation,

Head trauma,

Overoxygenation in a patient with COPD or pickwickian syndrome:

Reduced ventilation causes increased levels of Pco_2.

▼ Decreased Pco_2

Hypoxemia,

Pulmonary emboli:

Hypoxemia drives the respiratory center to increase ventilation. With increased ventilation, Pco_2 levels decrease.

Anxiety,

Pain,

Pregnancy:

These situations are associated with rapid ventilation. With increased ventilation, Pco_2 levels decrease.

▲ Increased HCO_3^-

Chronic vomiting or chronic high-volume gastric suction,

Aldosteronism,

Use of mercurial diuretics:

Important acid hydrogen ions are lost. HCO_3^- ions are relatively high. This causes metabolic alkalosis.

COPD: HCO_3^- ions are increased to compensate for chronic hypoventilation (high Pco_2). Compensation occurs for respiratory acidosis.

▼ Decreased HCO_3^-

Chronic and severe diarrhea,

Chronic use of loop diuretics:

Persistent loss of base ions, including HCO_3^-, occurs. Most of the CO_2 content is HCO_3^-.

Starvation,

Diabetic ketoacidosis,

Acute renal failure:

Ketoacids are built up. HCO_3^- neutralizes these acids. HCO_3^- levels therefore drop.

▲ Increased P_{O_2} and O_2 Content

Polycythemia: *The amount of hemoglobin is significantly increased. O_2 content, which saturates the hemoglobin, is also increased.*

Increased inspired O_2,

Hyperventilation:

With increased alveolar O_2 caused by breathing more rapidly or increasing the O_2 in the inspired air, the P_{O_2} and O_{22} content can be expected to increase.

▼ Decreased P_{O_2} and O_2 Content

Anemias: *The amount of hemoglobin is significantly reduced. O_2 content, which saturates the hemoglobin, is also reduced.*

Mucus plug,

Bronchospasm,

Atelectasis,

Pneumothorax,

Pulmonary edema,

ARDS,

Restrictive lung disease,

Atrial or ventricular cardiac septal defects,

Emboli:

See rationale below, under increased A-a O_2 gradient.

Inadequate O_2 in inspired air (suffocation),

Severe hypoventilation states, such as oversedation or neurologic somnolence:

Without air exchange, P_{O_2} levels fall.

▲ Increased A-a O_2 Gradient

Mucus plug,

Bronchospasm,

Atelectasis,

Pneumothorax,

Pulmonary edema,

ARDS:

Nonventilated lung tissue is still perfused. The perfused blood does not get oxygenated, however, because there is no ventilation in that area of the lung to bring O_2 to the blood. The perfused yet unoxygenated blood mixes with the oxygenated blood in the pulmonary veins. By dilution, the O_2 content of the mixed blood returning to the heart is lowered. The arterial blood is therefore lowered.

Atrial or ventricular cardiac septal defects,

Emboli:

The unoxygenated blood gains access to the oxygenated blood by direct shunting. By dilution, the O_2 content of the mixed blood returning to the heart is lowered. The arterial blood is therefore lowered.

RELATED TESTS

Pulmonary Function Tests (p. 1117). This is measurement of lung volume, which aids in the diagnosis and treatment of obstructive and restrictive lung diseases.

Fetal Scalp Blood pH (p. 239). Measurement of fetal scalp blood pH provides valuable information on fetal acid-base status. This screening test is useful clinically for diagnosing fetal distress.

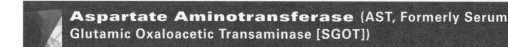

Aspartate Aminotransferase (AST, Formerly Serum Glutamic Oxaloacetic Transaminase [SGOT])

NORMAL FINDINGS

Age	Normal Value (units/L)
0-5 days	35-140
<3 yr	15-60
3-6 yr	15-50
6-12 yr	10-50
12-18 yr	10-40
Adult	0-35 units/L or 0-0.58 μkat/L (SI Units)
	(Females tend to have slightly lower levels than males)
Elderly	Slightly higher than adults

INDICATIONS

This test is used in the evaluation of patients with suspected hepatocellular diseases.

TEST EXPLANATION

This enzyme is found in very high concentrations within highly metabolic tissue, such as the heart muscle, liver cells, skeletal muscle cells, and to a lesser degree in the kidneys, pancreas, and red blood cells (RBCs). When disease or injury affects the cells of these tissues, the cells lyse. The AST is released, picked up by the blood, and the serum level rises. The amount of AST elevation is directly related to the number of cells affected by the disease or injury. Furthermore, the elevation depends on the length of time that the blood is drawn after the injury. AST is cleared from the blood in a few days. Serum AST levels become elevated 8 hours after cell injury, peak at 24 to 36 hours, and return to normal in 3 to 7 days. If the cellular injury is chronic, levels will be persistently elevated.

Because AST exists within the liver cells, diseases that affect the hepatocyte will cause elevated levels of this enzyme. In acute hepatitis, AST levels can rise 20 times the normal value. In acute extrahepatic obstruction (e.g., gallstone), AST levels quickly rise to 10 times the norm and swiftly fall. In patients with cirrhosis, the level of AST depends on the amount of active inflammation.

Serum AST levels are often compared with alanine aminotransferase (ALT) levels. The AST/ALT ratio is usually greater than 1 in patients with alcoholic cirrhosis, liver congestion, and metastatic tumor of the liver. Ratios less than 1 may be seen in patients with acute hepatitis, viral hepatitis, or infectious mononucleosis. The ratio is less accurate if AST levels exceed 10 times normal.

Patients with acute pancreatitis, acute renal diseases, musculoskeletal diseases, or trauma may have a transient rise in serum AST. Patients with RBC abnormalities such as acute hemolytic anemia and severe burns also can have elevations of this enzyme. AST levels may be decreased in patients with beriberi or diabetic ketoacidosis and in patients who are pregnant.

INTERFERING FACTORS

- Pregnancy may cause decreased AST levels.
- Exercise may cause increased levels.
- Levels are falsely decreased in patients with pyridoxine deficiency (beriberi, pregnancy), severe long-standing liver disease, uremia, or diabetic ketoacidosis.

Drugs that may cause *increased* levels include antihypertensives, cholinergic agents, coumarin-type anticoagulants, digitalis preparations, erythromycin, hepatotoxic medications, isoniazid, methyldopa, oral contraceptives, opiates, salicylates, stains, and verapamil.

PROCEDURE AND PATIENT CARE

Before

Explain the procedure to the patient.
- Avoid giving the patient any intramuscular (IM) injection.
- If possible, hold drugs that could interfere with test results for 12 hours before the test.

During

- Collect a venous sample of blood in a red-top tube. This is usually done daily for 3 days and then again in 1 week.
- Rotate the venipuncture site.
- Avoid hemolysis.
- Indicate on the laboratory slip any drugs that may cause false-positive results.
- Record the time and date of any intramuscular injection given.
- Record the exact time and date when the blood test is performed. This aids in the interpretation of the temporal pattern of enzyme elevations.

After

- Apply pressure or a pressure dressing to the venipuncture site.
- Observe the venipuncture site for bleeding.

TEST RESULTS AND CLINICAL SIGNIFICANCE

▲ Increased Levels

Liver Diseases
Hepatitis,
Hepatic cirrhosis,
Drug-induced liver injury,
Hepatic metastasis,
Hepatic necrosis (initial stages only),
Hepatic surgery,
Infectious mononucleosis with hepatitis,
Hepatic infiltrative process (e.g., tumor):
> *These diseases cause liver cell injury. The cells die and lysis of the cell occurs. The contents of the cell (including AST) are spewed out and are collected into the blood. Elevated AST levels thereby occur.*

Skeletal Muscle Diseases
Skeletal muscle trauma,
Recent noncardiac surgery,
Multiple traumas,
Severe, deep burns,
Progressive muscular dystrophy,
Recent convulsions,
Heat stroke,

Primary muscle diseases (e.g., myopathy, myositis):

> *These diseases cause muscle cell injury. The cells die and lysis of the cell occurs. The contents of the cell (including AST) are spewed out and are collected into the blood. Elevated AST levels thereby occur.*

Other Diseases

Acute hemolytic anemia,

Acute pancreatitis:

> *These diseases cause cell injury in these tissues. The cells die and lysis of the cell occurs. The contents of the cell (including AST) are spewed out and are collected into the blood. Elevated AST levels thereby occur.*

▼ Decreased Levels

Acute renal disease

Beriberi

Diabetic ketoacidosis

Pregnancy

Chronic renal dialysis

RELATED TESTS

Creatine Kinase (CK) (see p. 186). This enzyme is used similarly to AST and exists predominantly in heart and skeletal muscle.

Alanine Aminotransferase (ALT) (see p. 39). This enzyme is used similarly to AST and exists predominantly in the liver.

Lactic Dehydrogenase (LDH) (p. 329). This is an intracellular enzyme used to support the diagnosis of injury or disease involving the heart, liver, RBCs, kidneys, skeletal muscle, brain, and lungs.

Leucine Aminopeptidase (LAP) (see p. 337). This enzyme is specific to the hepatobiliary system. Diseases affecting that system will cause elevation of this enzyme.

Gamma-Glutamyl Transpeptidase (GGTP) (p. 246). This is another enzyme existing predominantly in the liver.

Alkaline Phosphatase (p. 47). This is another enzyme existing predominantly in the liver.

5'-Nucleotidase (p. 376). This is another enzyme existing predominantly in the liver.

Bilirubin

NORMAL FINDINGS

Blood

Adult/elderly/child

    Total bilirubin: 0.3-1.0 mg/dL or 5.1-17 μmol/L (SI units)

        Indirect bilirubin: 0.2-0.8 mg/dL or 3.4-12.0 μmol/L (SI units)

        Direct bilirubin: 0.1-0.3 mg/dL or 1.7-5.1 μmol/L (SI units)

Newborn total bilirubin: 1.0-12.0 mg/dL or 17.1-205 μmol/L (SI units)

Urine 0-0.02 mg/dL

 Critical Values

Adult: >12 mg/dL

Newborn: >15 mg/dL (immediate treatment required to avoid kernicterus)

INDICATIONS

This test is used to evaluate liver function. It is a part of the evaluation of adult patients with hemolytic anemias and newborns with jaundice.

TEST EXPLANATION

Bile, which is formed in the liver, has many constituents, including bile salts, phospholipids, cholesterol, bicarbonate, water, and bilirubin. Bilirubin metabolism begins with the breakdown of red blood cells (RBCs) in the reticuloendothelial system (mostly the spleen) (Figure 2-7). Hemoglobin is released from RBCs and broken down to heme and globin molecules. Heme is then catabolized to form biliverdin, which is transformed to bilirubin. This form of bilirubin is called unconjugated (indirect) bilirubin. In the liver, indirect bilirubin is conjugated with a glucuronide molecule, resulting in conjugated (direct) bilirubin. The conjugated bilirubin is then excreted from the liver cells and into the intrahepatic canaliculi, which eventually lead to the hepatic ducts, the common bile duct, and the bowel.

Jaundice is the discoloration of body tissues caused by abnormally high blood levels of bilirubin. This yellow discoloration is recognized when the total serum bilirubin exceeds 2.5 mg/dL. Jaundice results

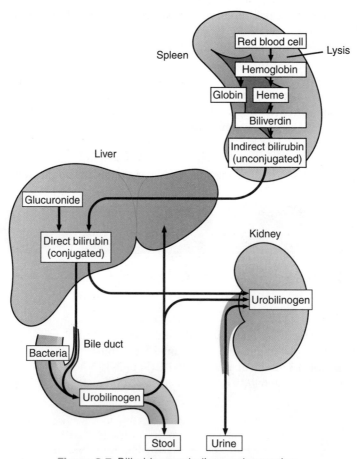

Figure 2-7 Bilirubin metabolism and excretion.

from a defect in the normal metabolism or excretion of bilirubin. This defect can occur at any stage of heme catabolism.

Physiologic jaundice of the newborn occurs if the newborn's liver is immature and does not have enough conjugating enzymes. This results in a high circulating blood level of unconjugated bilirubin, which can pass through the blood-brain barrier and deposit in the brain cells of the newborn, causing encephalopathy (kernicterus). In newborns, if bilirubin levels are greater than 15 mg/dL, immediate treatment is required to avoid mental retardation. This may include exchange transfusions. High levels of bilirubin in the newborn are often treated with light therapy.

If the defect in bilirubin metabolism occurs after addition of glucuronide, conjugated (direct) hyperbilirubinemia will result. Obstruction of the bile duct by a gallstone is the classic example of obstructed bilirubin excretion causing a direct hyperbilirubinemia.

Once the jaundice is recognized either clinically or chemically, it is important (for therapy) to differentiate whether it is predominantly caused by indirect (unconjugated) or direct (conjugated) bilirubin. This in turn will help differentiate the etiology of the defect. In general, jaundice caused by hepatocellular dysfunction (e.g., hepatitis) results in elevated levels of indirect bilirubin. This dysfunction usually cannot be repaired surgically. On the other hand, jaundice resulting from extrahepatic dysfunction (e.g., gallstones, tumor blocking the bile ducts) results in elevated levels of direct bilirubin; this type of jaundice usually can be resolved by open surgery or endoscopic surgery.

The total serum bilirubin level is the sum of the conjugated (direct) and unconjugated (indirect) bilirubin. These are separated out when "fractionation or differentiation" of the total bilirubin to its direct and indirect parts is requested from the laboratory (Figure 2-8). Normally the indirect (unconjugated) bilirubin makes up 70% to 85% of the total bilirubin. In patients with jaundice, when more than 50% of the bilirubin is direct (conjugated), it is considered a direct hyperbilirubinemia from gallstones, tumor, inflammation, scarring, or obstruction of the extrahepatic ducts. Indirect hyperbilirubinemia is diagnosed when less than 15% to 20% of the total bilirubin is direct bilirubin. Diseases that typically cause this form of jaundice include accelerated erythrocyte (RBC) hemolysis, hepatitis, or drugs.

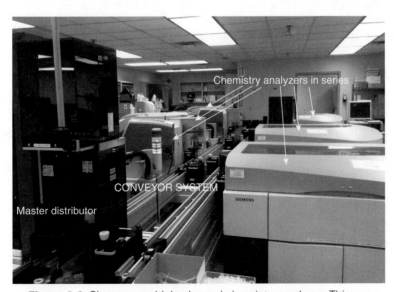

Figure 2-8 Siemens multiple channel chemistry analyzer. This is one of six chemical analyzer machines that are assembled in series and in which specimens are directed by a computerized master distributor.

Delta bilirubin is a form of bilirubin that is covalently bound to albumin. It has a longer half-life than the other bilirubins; therefore it remains elevated during the convalescent phases of hepatic disorders when the conjugated bilirubin has typically returned to normal. It can be derived by the following calculation:

$$\text{Delta bilirubin} = \text{Total bilirubin} - (\text{Direct bilirubin} + \text{Indirect bilirubin})$$

When the defect in bilirubin metabolism occurs after conjugation, elevated levels of direct (conjugated) bilirubin occur. Unlike the unconjugated form, direct bilirubin is water soluble and can be excreted into the urine. Therefore bilirubin in urine suggests disease affecting bilirubin metabolism after conjugation or defects in excretion (e.g., gallstones). There may be a small amount of bilirubin in the urine. Testing for bilirubin in the urine is a part of routine urine analysis (U/A).

INTERFERING FACTORS

- Blood hemolysis and lipemia can produce erroneous results.
- Drugs that may cause *increased* blood levels of total bilirubin include allopurinol, anabolic steroids, antibiotics, antimalarials, ascorbic acid, azathioprine, chlorpropamide (Diabinese), cholinergics, codeine, dextran, diuretics, epinephrine, meperidine, methotrexate, methyldopa, monoamine oxidase inhibitors, morphine, nicotinic acid (large doses), oral contraceptives, phenothiazines, quinidine, rifampin, salicylates, steroids, sulfonamides, theophylline, and vitamin A.
- Drugs that may cause *increased* urine bilirubin levels include allopurinol, antibiotics, barbiturates, chlorpromazine, diuretics, oral contraceptives, phenazopyridine (Pyridium), steroids, and sulfonamides.
- Drugs that may cause *decreased* blood levels of total bilirubin include barbiturates, caffeine, penicillin, and salicylates (high dose).
- Drugs that can cause *false-negative* results in urine levels include ascorbic acid (vitamin C) and indomethacin (Indocin).
- Drugs that can cause *false-positive* results in the urine level include "pyridium-like" drugs and urochromes. These drugs can color the urine yellow or orange and foil the color analysis tests. Bilirubin is not stable in urine, especially when exposed to light.

PROCEDURE AND PATIENT CARE

Before

- Explain the procedure to the patient.
- Note that fasting requirements vary among different laboratories. Some require keeping the patient on nothing by mouth (NPO) status after midnight the day of the test except for water.

During

Blood
- Collect a venous blood sample in a red-top tube.
- Use a heel puncture for blood collection in infants.
- Prevent hemolysis of blood during phlebotomy.
- Do not shake the tube, because inaccurate test results may occur.
- Protect the blood sample from bright light. Prolonged exposure (over 1 hour) to sunlight or artificial light can reduce bilirubin content.

Urine
- Note that this is a spot urine test.

- Collect at least 10 mL of urine for quick, simple testing.
- Use reagent strips (e.g., Multistix) or tablets (e.g., Icotest) for quick, simple testing.

Urine Testing With Multistix Reagent Strips
- Note that this is a firm, plastic strip with seven separate areas for testing pH, protein, glucose, ketones, bilirubin, blood, and urobilinogen.
- For testing bilirubin, obtain a fresh urine specimen and examine it as soon as possible.
- Immerse the dipstick in the well-mixed urine and then remove immediately to avoid dissolving other reagents.
- Tap the dipstick against the rim of the urine container to remove excess urine.
- Hold the strip horizontally and compare it with the color chart on the label of the bottle in the designated time period.

Urine Testing With Icotest Tablets
- Place 5 drops of urine on the special test mat.
- Add 2 drops of water. The bilirubin test is positive if the mat turns blue or purple within the designated time period.
- Note that this test is considered more sensitive than reagent strips for detecting bilirubin.

After
Blood
- Apply pressure or a pressure dressing to the venipuncture site.
- Assess the venipuncture site for bleeding. Patients with jaundice may have prolonged clotting times.

Urine
- Do not reuse reagent strips or Icotest tablets.
- Whether using strips or tablets or if sending the urine to the laboratory, note that medications may affect test results.

TEST RESULTS AND CLINICAL SIGNIFICANCE
▲ Increased Blood Levels of Conjugated (Direct) Bilirubin
Gallstones,
Extrahepatic duct obstruction (tumor, inflammation, gallstone, scarring, surgical trauma):
  These diseases cause a blockage of the bile ducts. Bile, containing bilirubin, cannot be excreted. Blood levels rise.
Extensive liver metastasis: *The intrahepatic ducts or hepatic ducts become obstructed because of tumor. Bile, containing bilirubin, cannot be excreted. Blood levels rise.*
Cholestasis from drugs: *Some drugs inhibit the excretion of bile from the hepatocyte into the bile canaliculi. Bile, containing bilirubin, cannot be excreted. Blood levels rise.*
Dubin-Johnson syndrome,
Rotor syndrome:
  Congenital defects in enzyme quantity inhibit metabolism and excretion of bilirubin. Blood levels rise.

▲ Increased Blood Levels of Unconjugated (Indirect) Bilirubin
Erythroblastosis fetalis,
Transfusion reaction,
Sickle cell anemia,

Hemolytic jaundice,

Hemolytic anemia,

Pernicious anemia,

Large-volume blood transfusion,

Resolution of large hematoma:

RBC destruction occurs. Large amounts of heme are available for catabolism into bilirubin. This quantity exceeds the liver's capability to conjugate bilirubin. Indirect (unconjugated) bilirubin levels rise.

Hepatitis,

Cirrhosis,

Sepsis,

Neonatal hyperbilirubinemia:

The diseased, injured, or immature liver cannot conjugate the bilirubin presented to it. Indirect (unconjugated) bilirubin levels rise.

Crigler-Najjar syndrome,

Gilbert syndrome:

Congenital enzyme deficiencies interrupt conjugation of bilirubin. Indirect (unconjugated) bilirubin levels rise.

▲ Increased Urine Levels of Bilirubin

Gallstones,

Extrahepatic duct obstruction (tumor, inflammation, gallstone, scarring, surgical trauma),

Extensive liver metastasis,

Cholestasis from drugs,

Dubin-Johnson syndrome,

Rotor syndrome:

Defects in bilirubin metabolism and excretion, as discussed earlier, inhibit intestinal excretion of bilirubin. The above-noted diseases are associated with direct (conjugated) hyperbilirubinemia. The conjugated bilirubin is water soluble and is excreted, in a small part, in the urine.

RELATED TESTS

Liver Enzymes such as Alkaline Phosphatase (ALP) (p. 47), Lactic Dehydrogenase (LDH) (p. 329), Aspartate Aminotransferase (AST) (p. 119), Alanine Aminotransferase (ALT) (p. 39), and 5'-Nucleotidase (p. 376). These tests are very helpful in the evaluation of the liver.

Complete Blood Cell Count (p. 174), Haptoglobin (p. 274), and other blood tests. These tests are helpful in the evaluation of hemolytic anemias.

Blood Typing (Blood Group Microarray Testing)

NORMAL FINDINGS

Compatibility

INDICATIONS

This test is used to determine the blood type of the patient before donating or receiving blood and to determine the blood type of expectant mothers to assess the risks of Rh incompatibility between mother and newborn.

TEST EXPLANATION

With blood typing, ABO and Rh antigens can be detected in the blood of prospective blood donors and potential blood recipients. This test is also used to determine the blood type of expectant mothers and newborns. A description of the ABO system, Rh factors, and blood crossmatching is reviewed here. The incidence of each blood type is noted in Table 2-11.

ABO System

Human blood is grouped according to the presence or absence of A or B antigens. The surface membranes of group A red blood cells (RBCs) contain A antigens (Figure 2-9); group B RBCs contain B antigens on their surface; group AB RBCs have both A and B antigens; and group O RBCs have neither A nor B antigens. In general, a person's serum does not contain antibodies to match the surface antigen on his or her RBCs. That is, persons with group A antigens (type A blood) will not have anti-A antibodies; however, they will have anti-B antibodies. The converse is true for persons with group B antigens. Group O blood will have both anti-A and anti-B antibodies. These antibodies against A and B blood group antigens are formed in the first 3 months of life after exposure to similar antigens on the surface of naturally occurring bacteria in the intestine.

Blood transfusions are actually transplantations of tissue (blood) from one person to another. It is important that the recipient not have antibodies to the donor's RBCs. If this were to occur, there could be a hypersensitivity reaction, which can vary from mild fever to anaphylaxis with severe intravascular hemolysis. If donor ABO antibodies are present against the recipient antigens, usually only minimal reactions occur.

Persons with group O blood are considered universal donors because they do not have antigens on their RBCs. People with group AB blood are considered universal recipients because they have no antibodies to react to the transfused blood. Group O blood is usually transfused in emergent situations in which rapid, life-threatening blood loss occurs and immediate transfusion is required. The chance of a transfusion reaction is least when type O is used. Women of childbearing potential should receive group O negative blood, and men generally receive group O positive blood when emergency transfusion prior to type-specific or crossmatched blood is required.

ABO typing is not required for autotransfusions (blood donated by a patient several weeks prior to a major operation and then transfused postoperatively). However, in most hospitals, ABO typing is performed on those patients in the event that further blood transfusion of banked blood is required.

Blood Type (ABO, Rh)	Antigens Present	Antibodies Possibly Present	Percent of General Population
O, +	Rh	A, B	35
O, −*	None	A, B, Rh	7
A, +	A, Rh	B	35
A, −	A	B, Rh	7
B, +	B, Rh	A	8
B, −	B	A, Rh	2
AB, +†	A, B, Rh	None	4
AB, −	A, B	Rh	2

TABLE 2-11 Blood Typing

*Universal donor.
†Universal recipient.

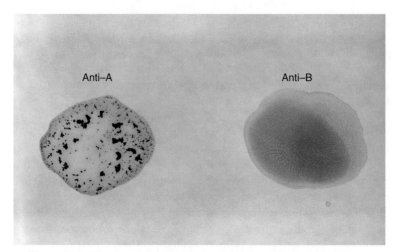

Figure 2-9 Blood typing by agglutination laboratory method. An "A" antigen that is present on the surface of the patient's red blood cell reacts with known anti-a antibody that has been added to a drop of the patient's blood. Agglutination (clumping) is visible on the left. No agglutination is noted on the right when anti-B antibody is added to a drop of the patient's blood. This patient has type A blood. In most laboratories, blood typing is automated by a machine that utilizes agglutination inhibition (see p. 2).

Rh Factors

The presence or absence of Rh antigens on the RBC's surface determines the classification of Rh positive or Rh negative. After ABO compatibility, Rh factor is the next most important antigen affecting the success of a blood transfusion. The major Rh factor is Rho(D). There are several minor Rh factors. If Rho(D) is absent, the minor Rh antigens are tested. If negative, the patient is considered Rh negative (Rh−).

Rh− persons may develop antibodies to Rh antigens if exposed to Rh positive (Rh+) blood by prior transfusions or fetal-maternal blood mixing. All women who are pregnant should have a blood typing and Rh factor determination. If the mother's blood is Rh−, the father's blood should also be typed. If his blood is Rh+, the woman's blood should be examined for the presence of Rh antibodies (by the indirect Coombs test). If the initial screening is negative (no antibodies to Rh found), the test is repeated at 28 to 30 weeks and 36 weeks of pregnancy. If these tests are also negative, the fetus is not at risk. However, if the test is positive, the fetus is at risk for hemolytic disease of the newborn (erythroblastosis fetalis). In this disease the mother is Rh− and the fetus is Rh+. Any fetal bleeding that occurs can sensitize the mother to form anti-Rh antibodies. These antibodies cross the placenta and hemolyze the fetal RBCs. Problems ranging from mild fetal anemia to in utero fetal death could occur. The severity of the hemolytic anemia can be evaluated by determining the quantity of bilirubin in the amniotic fluid (amniocentesis [p. 632]).

Hemolytic disease of the newborn can be prevented by Rh typing during pregnancy. If the mother is Rh−, she should be advised that she is a candidate for Rho-GAM (Rh immunoglobulin that "neutralizes" the Rh antigen) after the delivery. RhoGAM can reduce the chance of fetal hemolytic problems during subsequent pregnancies.

Other Blood Typing Systems

There are nine different gene codes for blood groups assayed. Most are minor and not clinically significant. However in certain clinical circumstances, these minor blood group antigens and

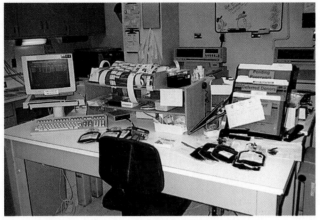

Figure 2-10 Immunohematology section of the laboratory showing the area where units of blood are processed and labeled.

BOX 2-4   Blood Tests Required on Donated Blood

- ABO typing
- Rh typing
- Rh antibody screen
- Hepatitis B surface antigen
- Hepatitis B core antigen
- Hepatitis C antibody

- Syphilis
- HIV testing antibody 1 and 2
- HIV antigen
- HTLV 1 testing
- Liver hepatocellular enzyme (ALT)

---

acquired antigens can become significant. This may occur with frequent blood transfusions or in patients with leukemia or lymphoma. Multiplex PCR microarray analysis provides identification of the many variants involving these blood group systems and is particularly helpful in the described patients.

Blood Crossmatching

Although typing for the major ABO and Rh antigens is no guarantee that a reaction will not occur, it does greatly reduce the possibility of such a reaction. Many potential minor antigens are not routinely detected during blood typing. If allowed to go unrecognized, these minor antigens also can initiate a blood transfusion reaction. Therefore blood is not only typed but also crossmatched to identify a mismatch of blood caused by minor antigens. Crossmatching consists of the mixing of the recipient's serum with the donor's RBCs in saline solution followed by the addition of Coombs serum (indirect Coombs test). Only blood products containing RBCs need to be crossmatched. Plasma products do not need to be crossmatched but should be ABO compatible because other cells (WBCs and platelets) have ABO antigens (Figure 2-10).

Homologous (donor and recipient are different people) and directed (recipient chooses the donor) blood for donation must be rigorously tested before transfusion (Box 2-4). Autologous (recipient and donor is the same person) blood for transfusions, however, is not subject to that same testing. It is important to note, however, that autologous blood transfusion is not 100% safe. As a result of the additives used for banking purposes, blood and hypersensitivity reactions can still occur.

Finally, one must be aware of graft-versus-host disease (GVHD) in which donor lymphocytes included in the blood transfusion may engraft and multiply in the recipient. These lymphocytes can react against the recipient's tissues. This is most common among immunocompromised patients. Pretransfusion radiation of the unit of blood to be transfused will avoid this problem.

INTERFERING FACTORS

- Non-ABO or non-Rh (D) minor antibodies can interfere with obtaining an adequate crossmatch.

PROCEDURE AND PATIENT CARE

Before

☒ Explain the procedure to the patient.
☒ Tell the patient that no fasting is required.

During

- Collect a venous blood sample in a red-top tube. (Tube color may vary among laboratories.)
- Avoid hemolysis.
- Label the blood tube appropriately before sending it to the laboratory.

After

- Apply pressure or a pressure dressing to the venipuncture site.
- Assess the venipuncture site for bleeding.

TEST RESULTS AND CLINICAL SIGNIFICANCE

ABO type
Rh type
Crossmatch compatibility

RELATED TESTS

Coombs Test, Indirect (p. 177). This test detects circulating antibodies against RBCs.
Amniocentesis (p. 632). This is a test of amniotic fluid, which may demonstrate some evidence of hemolytic disease of the newborn.

CA 15-3 and CA 27-29 Tumor Marker (Cancer Antigen 15-3, Cancer Antigen 27-29)

NORMAL FINDINGS

CA 15-3: <31 units/mL or <31 kunits/L (SI units)
CA 27.29: <38 units/mL or <38 kunits/L (SI units)

INDICATIONS

The CA 15-3 and CA 27-29 antigens are tumor-associated serum markers available for breast cancer monitoring.

TEST EXPLANATION

Carcinoembryonic antigen (CEA), the most widely used tumor marker, is limited by poor sensitivity and specificity for patients with breast cancer. Monoclonal antibody technology has permitted the development of CA 15-3 and CA 27-29 antigens. These antigens are not as sensitive for the diagnosis of primary breast cancer as other tumor markers are for their respective tumors. That is, CA 15-3 and CA 27-29 levels are high in only 50% of patients who have a localized breast cancer or a small tumor burden. However, 80% of patients with metastatic breast cancer do have elevated CA 15-3 levels and 65% have elevated CA 27-29 levels; therefore the usefulness of these antigen tests as a screening technique in early breast cancers (the most common cancer of women) is quite limited.

Benign breast disease and nonbreast malignancies (e.g., lung, pancreas, ovary, prostate) also can cause elevation of these antigen levels. These antigens are useful in monitoring the patient's response to therapy of metastatic breast cancer. A partial or complete response to treatment will be confirmed by declining levels. Likewise, a persistent rise in these antigen levels despite therapy strongly suggests progressive disease.

CA 15-3 and CA 27-29 have a high sensitivity but a somewhat lower specificity. Many diseases, both benign and malignant, can cause elevations in these values. Therefore they cannot be used to diagnose recurrence. However, in the patient who has symptoms, signs, or other test results that indicate recurrence, an elevation in one of these tumor markers would corroborate the diagnosis of recurrent breast cancer. These tumor markers are better suited for indicating response of metastatic disease to treatment (when already elevated). CA 15-3 was the first breast tumor marker available. It is usually performed by a reference laboratory using competitive inhibition radioimmune assay. The CA 27-29 marker is done by immunoradiometric assay.

Clinical Priorities

- CA 15-3 and 27-29 tumor markers are not used for screening of early breast cancers.
- These tumor antigens are used for monitoring the patient's response to therapy for metastatic breast cancer. Declining levels suggest a good response to therapy; rising levels suggest disease progression.

INTERFERING FACTORS

- Some of the other benign and malignant diseases associated with elevations of these antigens include cancer of the lung, ovary, pancreas, prostate, and colon; fibrocytic disease of the breast; cirrhosis; and hepatitis.

PROCEDURE AND PATIENT CARE

Before

 Explain the procedure to the patient.

Tell the patient that no fasting is required.

During

- Collect a venous blood sample in a red-top tube.
- The blood sample may be sent to a central diagnostic laboratory for determinations. The results may not be available for 7 to 10 days.

After

- Apply pressure or a pressure dressing to the venipuncture site.
- Observe the venipuncture site for bleeding.

TEST RESULTS AND CLINICAL SIGNIFICANCE

▲ Increased Levels

Metastatic breast cancer: *Breast cancer antigens on the surface of the breast cancer cell leak into the bloodstream, where they can be detected.*

RELATED TEST

Carcinoembryonic Antigen (CEA) (p. 145). This is another tumor marker used in the monitoring of breast cancer.

CA 19-9 Tumor Marker (Cancer Antigen 19-9)

NORMAL FINDINGS

< 37 units/mL or <37 kunits/L (SI units)

INDICATIONS

CA 19-9 antigen is a tumor marker used for the diagnosis of patients with pancreatic or hepatobiliary cancer, evaluation of response to treatment, and surveillance.

TEST EXPLANATION

CA 19-9 is a carbohydrate cell-surface antigen. It exists on the surface of some cancer cells. Although initially thought to be specific for colorectal cancer, it is now used primarily in the evaluation of patients with pancreatic or hepatobiliary cancers. In the diagnosis of pancreatic carcinoma, for example, the presence of a pancreatic mass or biliary obstruction and greatly elevated CA 19-9 levels would support the diagnosis of pancreatic cancer over benign pancreatitis. Hepatobiliary cancer is suspected in patients whose presenting symptoms are ascites, jaundice, and elevated CA 19-9 levels. CA 19-9 levels may not be elevated in all patients with pancreatic carcinoma. Approximately 70% of patients with pancreatic carcinoma and 65% of patients with hepatobiliary cancer have elevated levels.

CA 19-9 levels are used in the posttreatment surveillance of those who have had pancreatic or hepatobiliary cancers. In the few patients with pancreatic or biliary cancer who have a good response to surgery, chemotherapy, or radiation therapy, a decline in serum levels of CA 19-9 will confirm this response. A rapid rise in CA 19-9 levels may be associated with recurrent or progressive tumor growth. Mildly elevated levels may exist in patients with gastric cancer, colorectal cancer, hepatoma, and even in 6% to 7% of patients with non-gastrointestinal (GI) malignancies. Patients who have pancreatitis, gallstones, cirrhosis, inflammatory bowel disease (IBD), or cystic fibrosis (CF) also can have minimally elevated levels of CA 19-9.

Because of its lack of sensitivity and specificity, CA 19-9 is not effective in screening for pancreatobiliary tumors in the general population.

 Clinical Priorities

- CA 19-9 is not used as a screening test for pancreatic or hepatobiliary tumors because of its lack of sensitivity and specificity.
- CA 19-9 is used to support the diagnosis of pancreatic or hepatobiliary tumors and to monitor patients' response to treatment.

PROCEDURE AND PATIENT CARE

Before
☒ Explain the procedure to the patient.
☒ Tell the patient that no fasting is required.

During
- Collect a venous blood sample in a red-top tube.
- The blood may be sent to a central diagnostic laboratory for CA 19-9 determinations. The results may not be available for 7 to 10 days.

After
- Apply pressure or a pressure dressing to the venipuncture site.
- Observe the venipuncture site for bleeding.

TEST RESULTS AND CLINICAL SIGNIFICANCE

▲ Increased Levels
Pancreatic carcinoma,
Cholecystitis,
Colorectal cancer,
Hepatobiliary carcinoma,
Cirrhosis,
Gallstones,
Pancreatitis,
Gastric cancer,
Lung cancer,
Inflammatory bowel disease,
Rheumatoid diseases:
> *CA 19-9 antigen is released from the surface of the cancer cell and leaks into the bloodstream, where it can be detected.*

RELATED TEST

Carcinoembryonic Antigen (CEA) (p. 145). This is another tumor marker that is elevated in patients with pancreatobiliary cancer.

CA-125 Tumor Marker (Cancer Antigen-125)

NORMAL FINDINGS

0-35 units/mL or <35 kunits/L (SI units)

INDICATIONS

CA-125 is used in the detection of ovarian cancer. It is also used to determine the extent of disease and to monitor the response to treatment.

TEST EXPLANATION

This tumor marker has a high degree of sensitivity and specificity for ovarian cancer. Just as alpha-fetoprotein (AFP) and human chorionic gonadotropin (hCG) are accurate tumor markers for germ cell tumors of the ovary, CA-125 is an extremely accurate marker for nonmucinous epithelial tumors of the ovary. It is elevated in more than 80% of women with ovarian cancer.

The CA-125 marker can be used in many ways. By itself, it cannot be used to diagnose ovarian cancer, but it helps support the diagnosis of ovarian cancer. For example, a greatly elevated CA-125 level in women who have abdominal distention, ascites, and a palpable pelvic mass is strong confirmation that the underlying etiology is an epithelial ovarian malignancy.

The CA-125 serum tumor marker is also used to determine a patient's response to therapy. Comparative serial testing will show a progressive decline in CA-125 levels for patients responding to treatment. Also, CA-125 tumor markers can predict whether or not a second-look (repeat) diagnostic laparotomy will be positive. A second-look laparotomy will detect a residual tumor in 97% of patients whose CA-125 level is greater than 35 units/mL, whereas only 56% of patients with ovarian cancer whose CA-125 level is less than 35 units/mL will have a positive second-look laparotomy. A precipitous fall in CA-125 after two courses of chemotherapy is an accurate predictor of a complete response to chemotherapy and is interpreted as a good prognostic sign.

Finally, CA-125 determinations can be used in posttreatment surveillance of patients with ovarian cancer. In a patient who has had a complete response to radiation therapy, chemotherapy, or surgery, a delayed rise in the CA-125 level is an early predictor of a recurrent tumor in 93% of patients. Abnormal levels can antedate the appearance of obvious recurrent ovarian cancer by 2 to 7 months.

CA-125 is not an effective screening test for the asymptomatic general public because of its lack of specificity. It is used in "high-risk" women who have a strong family history of ovarian cancer or have a breast cancer antigen (BRCA) genetic defect (p. 1094). Elevated levels in the general population indicate that either benign or malignant disease is present in 95% of patients.

Other tumors and benign processes can cause elevated CA-125 levels as well. Diseases that affect the peritoneum, such as cirrhosis, pancreatitis, peritonitis, endometriosis, and pelvic inflammatory disease (PID), can cause elevated levels of CA-125. Other malignancies occurring in the female genital tract, pancreas, colon, lung, and breast can also be associated with elevated levels of this protein. A toftal of 1% to 2% of the normal population has CA-125 levels in excess of 3535 units/mL.

INTERFERING FACTORS

- The first trimester of pregnancy and normal menstruation may be associated with mild elevations of CA-125 levels.

- Patients with benign peritoneal diseases (e.g., cirrhosis, endometriosis) will have mildly increased levels.
- Smoking can falsely increase CA-125 levels.
- Patients who have had recent abdominal surgery may have elevated CA-125 levels for as long as 3 weeks after surgery.

 Clinical Priorities

- CA-125 is used in detecting ovarian cancer and in determining its extent and response to treatment.
- CA-125 is not an effective screening test for asymptomatic women because of its lack of specificity. It is used in "high-risk" women with a strong history of ovarian cancer.
- CA-125 levels can be used to determine the need for a second-look (repeat) diagnostic laparotomy in women being followed after ovarian cancer therapy.

PROCEDURE AND PATIENT CARE

Before
☒ Explain the procedure to the patient.
☒ Tell the patient that no fasting or sedation is required.

During
- Collect a venous of blood sample in a red-top tube.
- The blood may be sent to a central diagnostic laboratory for determination of CA-125 level.
- The results are available to the local hospital in 3 to 7 days.

After
- Apply pressure or a pressure dressing to the venipuncture site.
- Observe the venipuncture site for bleeding.
- Provide emotional support to the patient. Cancer testing is very stressful.

TEST RESULTS AND CLINICAL SIGNIFICANCE

▲ Increased Levels

Malignant Disorders
Cancer of the ovary,
Cancer of the pancreas,
Cancer of the colon,
Cancer of the lung,
Peritoneal carcinomatosis,
Cancer of the nonovarian female genital tract,
Cancer of the breast,
Lymphoma:
   The CA-125 antigen from the surface ovarian cancer cells leaks into the blood, where it can be detected.

Benign Disorders
Cirrhosis,

Peritonitis,
Pregnancy,
Endometriosis,
Pancreatitis,
Pelvic inflammatory disease (PID):
   The mechanism of elevated CA-125 in these diseases is not known.

RELATED TESTS

Carcinoembryonic Antigen (CEA) (p. 145). This tumor marker can be elevated in ovarian epithelial tumors.
Alpha-Fetoprotein (p. 54). This tumor marker is elevated in nonepithelial ovarian tumors.
Human Chorionic Gonadotropin (p. 304). This tumor marker is elevated in nonepithelial ovarian tumors.

 Calcitonin (Human Calcitonin [HCT], Thyrocalcitonin)

NORMAL FINDINGS

Basal (Plasma)

Males: ≤19 pg/mL or ≤19 ng/L (SI units)
Females: ≤14 pg/mL or ≤14 ng/L (SI units)

Calcium Infusion (2.4 mg/kg)

Males: ≤190 pg/mL or ≤190 ng/L
Females: ≤130 pg/mL or ≤130 ng/L

Pentagastrin Injection (0.5 mcg/kg)

Males: ≤110 pg/mL or ≤110 ng/L
Females: ≤30 pg/mL or ≤30 ng/L

INDICATIONS

This test is usually indicated to evaluate persons with suspected medullary carcinoma of the thyroid. Calcitonin is useful in monitoring response to therapy and predicting recurrences of medullary thyroid cancer. It is also useful as a screening test for those with a family history of medullary cancer.

TEST EXPLANATION

Calcitonin is a hormone secreted by the parafollicular or C cells of the thyroid gland. Secretion is stimulated by elevated serum calcium levels. Calcitonin contributes to calcium homeostasis. It decreases serum calcium levels by inhibiting bone resorption and increasing calcium excretion by the kidneys.

This test is usually used in the evaluation of patients who have confirmed or suspected medullary carcinoma of the thyroid. Seventy-five percent of these patients have hypersecretion of calcitonin despite normal serum calcium levels. Calcitonin is useful in monitoring response to therapy and predicting recurrences of medullary thyroid cancer. It is also useful as a screening test for those with a family history of medullary cancer and therefore at high risk (20%) for medullary cancer. This is a cancer of the thyroid with a familial tendency and if found late has a poor prognosis. This cancer is often associated with multiple endocrine neoplasia (MEN) syndromes. Routine screening for elevated calcitonin levels can detect medullary cancer early and improve chances for cure. Calcitonin can be used as a tumor marker in monitoring patients with medullary cancer of the thyroid. Increases in calcitonin levels herald progression of the cancer. Declining levels indicate tumor regression. C-cell hyperplasia, a benign calcitonin-producing disease that also has a familial tendency, is also associated with elevated calcitonin levels.

Equivocal elevations in calcitonin levels should be followed with further provocative testing using pentagastrin or calcium to stimulate calcitonin secretion. *Pentagastrin stimulation* involves an intravenous (IV) infusion with blood samples drawn before the injection and at 90 seconds, 2 minutes, and 5 minutes following the infusion. The *calcium infusion test* can be performed in a variety of ways but is most commonly administered with blood drawn to establish baseline and 5- and 10-minute postinfusion blood levels. With medullary cancer of the thyroid, the provocative tests can cause the calcitonin to rise significantly.

Elevated levels of calcitonin also may be seen in people with cancer of the lung, breast, and pancreas. This is probably a form of paraneoplastic syndrome in which there is an ectopic production of calcitonin by the nonthyroid cancer cells.

INTERFERING FACTORS

- Levels are often elevated in normal pregnant females and in newborns.
- Drugs that may cause *increased* levels include calcium, cholecystokinin, epinephrine, glucagon, pentagastrin, and oral contraceptives.

PROCEDURE AND PATIENT CARE

Before

- Explain the procedure to the patient.
- Tell the patient that an overnight fast is required. Water is permitted.

During

- Collect a venous blood sample in a heparinized green-top or a chilled red-top tube according to the laboratory's protocol.
- The specimen should be placed on ice immediately. The blood may be frozen and sent to a reference laboratory.

After

- Apply pressure or a pressure dressing to the venipuncture site.
- Assess the venipuncture site for bleeding.
- Tell the patient that results may not be available for several days if this test is sent to a reference laboratory for analysis.

TEST RESULTS AND CLINICAL SIGNIFICANCE

▲ Increased Levels

Medullary carcinoma of the thyroid,
C-cell hyperplasia:
> *Calcitonin is secreted by the thyroid in these diseases despite the calcium blood levels. These abnormalities are not responsive to the normal regulatory feedback mechanisms.*

Oat cell carcinoma of lung,
Breast carcinoma,
Pancreatic cancer:
   These cancers can act as an autonomous ectopic site of calcitonin production.
Primary hyperparathyroidism,
Secondary hyperparathyroidism as a result of chronic renal failure:
   These states are associated with high serum calcium levels. High calcitonin levels may be compensatory.
Pernicious anemia,
Zollinger-Ellison syndrome:
   Several endocrine familial and nonfamilial multiple endocrinopathies (Apudoma) may be associated with high calcitonin levels.
Alcoholic cirrhosis: *The mechanism is not well defined. Perhaps the liver cannot metabolize hormones well and high levels of calcitonin result.*
Thyroiditis

RELATED TEST

Calcium, Blood (see following test). This is a direct measurement of the serum calcium level.

 Calcium, Blood (Total/Ionized Calcium, Ca)

NORMAL FINDINGS

Age	mg/dL	mmol/L
TOTAL CALCIUM		
<10 days	7.6-10.4	1.9-2.60
Umbilical	9.0-11.5	2.25-2.88
10 days–2 years	9.0-10.6	2.3-2.65
Child	8.8-10.8	2.2-2.7
Adult*	9.0-10.5	2.25-2.62
IONIZED CALCIUM		
Newborn	4.20-5.58	1.05-1.37
2 months–18 years	4.80-5.52	1.20-1.38
Adult	4.5-5.6	1.05-1.30

 Critical Values

Total calcium: <6 or >13 mg/dL or <1.5 or >3.25 mmol/L (SI units)
Ionized calcium: <2.2 or >7 mg/dL or <0.78 or >1.58 mmol/L (SI units)

INDICATIONS

The serum calcium test is used to evaluate parathyroid function and calcium metabolism by directly measuring the total amount of calcium in the blood. Serum calcium levels are used to monitor patients

---

*Values tend to decrease in the elderly.

with renal failure, renal transplantation, hyperparathyroidism, and various malignancies. They are also used to monitor calcium levels during and after large-volume blood transfusions.

TEST EXPLANATION

Serum calcium is necessary in many metabolic enzymatic pathways. It is vital for muscle contractility, cardiac function, neural transmission, and blood clotting. The serum calcium test is used to evaluate parathyroid function and calcium metabolism by directly measuring the total amount of calcium in the blood. The bone and the teeth act as a reservoir for calcium. When blood levels decrease, parathyroid hormone (PTH) release is stimulated. This hormone acts on the reservoirs to release calcium into the blood. About one half of the total calcium exists in the blood in its free (ionized) form, and about one half exists in its protein-bound form (mostly with albumin). The serum calcium level is a measure of both. As a result, when the serum albumin level is low (as in malnourished patients), the serum calcium level will also be low, and vice versa. As a rule of thumb, the total serum calcium level decreases by approximately 0.8 mg for every 1-g decrease in the serum albumin level. Serum albumin should be measured with serum calcium.

The ionized form of calcium also can be measured by ion-selective electrode techniques or can be calculated from several available formulas. An advantage of measuring the ionized form is that it is unaffected by changes in serum albumin levels. Many laboratories do not have the equipment to perform the ionized calcium assay. Certainly, when albumin levels are variable, measurement of ionized calcium can allow more accurate calcium replacement therapy if needed. This is especially true during open heart surgery, major organ transplantation, and renal dialysis.

When the serum calcium level is elevated on at least three separate determinations, the patient is said to have hypercalcemia. Symptoms of hypercalcemia may include anorexia, nausea, vomiting, somnolence, and coma. The most common cause of hypercalcemia is hyperparathyroidism. Parathormone causes elevated calcium levels by increasing gastrointestinal (GI) absorption, decreasing urinary excretion, and increasing bone resorption. Malignancy, the second most common cause of hypercalcemia, can cause elevated calcium levels in two main ways. First, tumor metastasis (myeloma, lung, breast, renal cell) to the bone can destroy the bone, causing resorption and pushing calcium into the blood. Second, the cancer (lung, breast, renal cell) can produce a PTH-like substance that drives the serum calcium up (ectopic PTH). Excess vitamin D ingestion can increase serum calcium by increasing renal and GI absorption. Granulomatous infections such as sarcoidosis and tuberculosis are associated with hypercalcemia.

In some instances a normal serum calcium does not preclude hypercalcemia. For example, if the serum calcium is normal in a patient with reduced serum albumin (the calcium should be reduced in these patients), hypercalcemia should be suspected. A similar situation exists in patients with chronic renal failure. These patients have high phosphate levels and other anions that tend to chronically lower serum calcium. As a result, PTH is persistently stimulated to increase calcium levels. The calcium levels return to normal in time, but that "normal" level actually represents a "high" level when one considers that it should be low in these individuals. This is the classic case of secondary hyperparathyroidism.

Hypocalcemia occurs in patients with hypoalbuminemia. The most common causes of hypoalbuminemia are malnutrition (especially in alcoholics) and large-volume intravenous infusions. Because one half of the calcium is bound to albumin, when albumin is low, calcium should be expected to be low. Large blood transfusions are associated with low serum calcium levels, because the citrate additives used in banked blood for anticoagulation bind the free calcium in the recipient's bloodstream. Intestinal malabsorption, renal failure, rhabdomyolysis, alkalosis, and acute pancreatitis (because of saponification of fat) are also known to be associated with low serum calcium levels. Hypomagnesemia can be associated with refractory hypocalcemia. Symptoms of hypocalcemia include nervousness, excitability, and tetany.

INTERFERING FACTORS

- Vitamin D intoxication may cause increased calcium levels.
- Excessive ingestion of milk may cause increased levels.
- Serum pH can affect calcium values. A decrease in pH causes increased calcium levels.
- Prolonged tourniquet time will lower pH and factitiously increase calcium levels.
- There is normally a small diurnal variation in calcium, with peak levels occurring around 9 PM.
- Hypoalbuminemia is associated with decreased levels of total calcium.
- Drugs that may cause *increased* levels include alkaline antacids, androgens, calcium salts, ergocalciferol, hydralazine, lithium, PTH, thiazide diuretics, thyroid hormone, and vitamin D.
- Drugs that may cause *decreased* levels include acetazolamide, albuterol, anticonvulsants, asparaginase, aspirin, calcitonin, cisplatin, corticosteroids, estrogens, heparin, laxatives, loop diuretics, magnesium salts, oral contraceptives, and thiazide diuretic.

PROCEDURE AND PATIENT CARE

Before

- Explain the procedure to the patient.
- Tell the patient that no fasting is required; however, the serum calcium may be part of a multichemical analysis in which fasting is required for the other studies.

During

- Collect a venous blood sample in a red-top tube.
- Avoid prolonged tourniquet use.

After

- Apply pressure or a pressure dressing to the venipuncture site.
- Assess the venipuncture site for bleeding.

TEST RESULTS AND CLINICAL SIGNIFICANCE

▲ Increased Levels (Hypercalcemia)

Hyperparathyroidism,
Nonparathyroid PTH-producing tumor (e.g., lung or renal carcinoma):
   Parathormone or a similar hormone mobilizes calcium stores from the bone to the blood.
Metastatic tumor to bone,
Paget disease of bone,
Prolonged immobilization:
   Bone destruction or thinning pushes calcium from the bone and into the blood.
Milk-alkali syndrome: *With increased ingestion of milk products or antacids (which contain calcium), the serum calcium level can be elevated.*
Vitamin D intoxication: *Vitamin D works synergistically with PTH to increase serum calcium.*
Lymphoma,
Multiple myeloma,
Granulomatous infections such as sarcoidosis and tuberculosis:
   These diseases are associated with enhanced levels of vitamin D, which works synergistically with PTH to increase serum calcium.
Addison disease: *Glucocorticosteroids inhibit vitamin D activity. When steroid activity is decreased, vitamin D action is enhanced. Vitamin D works synergistically with PTH to increase serum calcium.*

Acromegaly

Hyperthyroidism

▼ Decreased Levels (Hypocalcemia)

Hypoparathyroidism: *PTH acts to increase serum calcium. If PTH levels are reduced, serum calcium declines.*

Renal failure,

Hyperphosphatemia secondary to renal failure:

Excess anions, present in patients with renal failure, bind serum calcium.

Rickets,

Vitamin D deficiency:

Vitamin D acts synergistically with PTH. PTH acts to increase serum calcium. Without that synergism, calcium levels decline.

Osteomalacia,

Hypoalbuminemia,

Malabsorption:

Less calcium is available to the blood.

Pancreatitis,

Fat embolism:

Pancreatitis is associated with saponification (binding of calcium to fats) of the peripancreatic tissue. This reduces the calcium from the blood.

Alkalosis: *High pH in the blood drives the calcium to intracellular spaces. Blood levels decline.*

RELATED TESTS

Parathyroid Hormone (p. 380). This is a measurement of PTH, which increases serum calcium levels.

Albumin (p. 424). This is a direct measurement of serum albumin. Albumin has a major effect on serum calcium metabolism.

Vitamin D (p. 520). Adequate levels of this vitamin are required for calcium absorption.

Carbon Dioxide Content (CO_2 Content, CO_2-Combining Power, Bicarbonate [HCO_3^-])

NORMAL FINDINGS

Adult/elderly: 23-30 mEq/L or 23-30 mmol/L (SI units)

Child: 20-28 mEq/L

Infant: 20-28 mEq/L

Newborn: 13-22 mEq/L

▌ Critical Values

<10 mEq/L or >40 mEq/L

INDICATIONS

The CO_2 content is a measure of CO_2 in the blood. In the peripheral venous blood this is used to assist in evaluating the pH status of the patient and to assist in evaluation of electrolytes.

TEST EXPLANATION

The serum CO_2 test is usually included with other electrolyte assessments. It is usually performed using a multiphasic testing machine that also measures sodium, potassium, chloride, blood urea nitrogen (BUN), and creatinine. *It is important not to confuse this test with Pco$_2$.* This CO_2 content measures H_2CO_3, dissolved CO_2 and the bicarbonate ion (HCO_3^-) that exists in the serum. Because the amounts of H_2CO_3 and dissolved CO_2 in the blood are so small, CO_2 content is an indirect measure of HCO_3^- anion. HCO_3^- anion is second in importance to the chloride ion in electrical neutrality (negative charge) of extracellular and intracellular fluid; it plays a major role in acid-base balance.

Levels of HCO_3^- are regulated by the kidneys. Increases occur with alkalosis, and decreases occur with acidosis. This test can be performed on arterial blood as discussed further on p. 109. When CO_2 content is measured in the laboratory with other serum electrolytes, air affects the specimen and the CO_2 partial pressure can be altered. Therefore venous blood specimens are not highly accurate for measuring true CO_2 content or HCO_3^-. It is primarily used as a rough guide for acid-base balance.

INTERFERING FACTORS

- Underfilling the tube with blood allows CO_2 to escape from the serum specimen and may significantly reduce HCO_3^- values.
- Drugs that may cause *increased* serum CO_2 and HCO_3^- levels include aldosterone, barbiturates, bicarbonates, ethacrynic acid, hydrocortisone, loop diuretics, mercurial diuretics, and steroids.
- Drugs that may cause *decreased* levels include methicillin, nitrofurantoin (Furadantin), paraldehyde, phenformin, tetracycline, thiazide diuretics, and triamterene.

PROCEDURE AND PATIENT CARE

Before

- Explain the procedure to the patient.
- Tell the patient that no fasting is required.

During

- Collect a venous blood sample in a red-top or green-top tube.

After

- Apply pressure or a pressure dressing to the venipuncture site.
- Assess the venipuncture site for bleeding.

TEST RESULTS AND CLINICAL SIGNIFICANCE

▲ Increased Levels

Severe vomiting,
High-volume gastric suction,
Aldosteronism,
Use of mercurial diuretics:
  Important acid hydrogen ions are lost. HCO_3^- ions are relatively high.
Chronic obstructive pulmonary disease (COPD): *HCO_3^- ions are increased to compensate for chronic hypoventilation (high Pco$_2$). This is compensation for respiratory acidosis.*
Metabolic alkalosis: *Metabolic alkalosis is defined by an increased amount of HCO_3^- anions in the blood.*

▼ Decreased Levels

Chronic diarrhea,
Chronic use of loop diuretics:
   Persistent loss of base ions, including HCO_3^-. Most of the CO_2 content is HCO_3^-.
Renal failure,
Diabetic ketoacidosis,
Starvation:
   Ketoacids and other anions are built up. HCO_3^- neutralizes these acids. HCO_3^- levels therefore drop.
Metabolic acidosis: *Metabolic acidosis is defined by a decreased amount of HCO_3^- anions in the blood.*
Shock: *Lactic acid builds up and is buffered by the HCO_3^-, therefore HCO_3^- levels diminish.*

RELATED TEST

Arterial Blood Gases (ABGs) (p. 109). This is a battery of arterial blood tests that are used to evaluate acid-base status. CO_2 content and HCO_3^- are components of that test.

 Carboxyhemoglobin (COHb, Carbon Monoxide [CO])

NORMAL FINDINGS

Nonsmoker: <3% saturation of total hemoglobin
Light smoker: 2%-5%
Heavy smoker: 5%-10%
Newborn: ≥12%

 Critical Values

>20%

INDICATIONS

This test is used to detect CO poisoning.

TEST EXPLANATION

This test measures the amount of serum COHb, which is formed by the combination of CO and hemoglobin (Hgb). CO combines with Hgb 200 times more readily than O_2 can combine with Hgb (oxyhemoglobin). This results in fewer Hgb bonds available to combine with O_2. Furthermore, when CO occupies the O_2-binding sites, the hemoglobin molecule is changed so as to bind the remaining O_2 more tightly. This greater affinity of CO for Hgb and change in O_2-binding strength does not allow the O_2 to readily pass from the red blood cells (RBCs) to the tissue. Less O_2 is therefore available for tissue cell respiration. This results in hypoxemia. CO poisoning is documented by Hgb analysis for COHb. A specimen should be drawn as soon as possible after exposure, because CO is rapidly cleared from the Hgb by breathing normal air. O_2 saturation studies and oximetry are inaccurate in CO-exposed patients, because they measure all forms of O_2-saturated hemoglobin, including COHb. In these circumstances the results will be normal, even though the patient is hypoxemic.

TABLE 2-12 Symptoms of CO Poisoning by Level of Hgb Saturation	
CO-Saturated Hgb (%)	**Symptoms**
10	Slight dyspnea
20	Headache
30	Irritability, disturbed judgment, memory loss
40	Confusion, weakness, dimness of vision
50	Fainting, ataxia, collapse
60	Coma
>60	Death

This test can also be used to evaluate patients with complaints of headache, irritability, nausea, vomiting, and vertigo, who may have been unknowingly exposed to CO. Its greatest use, however, is in patients exposed to smoke inhalation, exhaust fumes, and fires. Other sources of CO include tobacco smoke, petroleum and natural gas fuel fumes, automobile exhaust, unvented natural-gas heaters, and defective gas stoves. Symptoms of CO poisoning correlated with blood levels are shown in Table 2-12. CO toxicity is treated by administering high concentrations of O_2 to displace the COHb.

✓ Clinical Priorities

- CO combines with Hgb 200 times more readily than O_2 can combine with Hgb. This results in hypoxemia.
- CO poisoning is documented by the COHb test. Specimens should be drawn as soon as possible after exposure, because CO is rapidly cleared from the Hgb by breathing normal air.
- CO toxicity is treated by administration of high concentrations of O_2 to displace the COHb.
- Severe CO toxicity may be treated with hyperbaric oxygen.

PROCEDURE AND PATIENT CARE

Before

 Explain the procedure to the patient or the family.
- Obtain the patient history for possible source of CO inhalation.
- Assess the patient for signs and symptoms of mild CO toxicity (e.g., headache, weakness, dizziness, malaise, dyspnea) and moderate to severe CO toxicity (e.g., severe headache, bright-red mucous membranes, cherry-red blood). Maintain patient safety precautions if confusion is present.

During

- Collect a venous blood sample in a lavender-top or green-top tube.

After

- Apply pressure or a pressure dressing to the venipuncture site.
- Assess the venipuncture site for bleeding.

- Treat the patient as indicated by the physician. Usually the patient receives high concentrations of O_2. Severe CO toxicity may be treated with hyperbaric oxygen.
- Encourage respirations to allow the patient to clear CO from the Hgb.

TEST RESULTS AND CLINICAL SIGNIFICANCE

▲ Increased Levels

CO poisoning

RELATED TESTS

Oximetry (p. 1114). This test is used to easily and continuously monitor O_2 saturation of Hgb.
Oxygen Saturation (p. 112). This test measures the amount of Hgb saturated by O_2.

Carcinoembryonic Antigen (CEA)

NORMAL FINDINGS

<5 ng/mL or 5 mcg/L (SI units)

INDICATIONS

This tumor marker is used for determining the extent of disease and prognosis in patients with cancer (especially gastrointestinal [GI] or breast). It is also used in monitoring the disease and its treatment.

TEST EXPLANATION

CEA is a protein that normally occurs in fetal gut tissue. By birth, detectable serum levels disappear. In the early 1960s, CEA was found to exist in the bloodstream of adults who had colorectal tumors. It was originally thought to be a specific indicator of the presence of colorectal cancer. Subsequently, however, this tumor marker has been found in patients who have a variety of carcinomas (e.g., breast, pancreatic, gastric, hepatobiliary), sarcomas, and even many benign diseases (e.g., ulcerative colitis, diverticulitis, cirrhosis). Chronic smokers also have elevated CEA levels.

Because the CEA level can be elevated in both benign and malignant diseases, it is not a specific test for colorectal cancer. Furthermore, not all colorectal cancers produce CEA. Therefore CEA is not a reliable screening test for the detection of colorectal cancer in the general population. Its use is limited to determining the prognosis and monitoring the response of tumor to antineoplastic therapy in a patient with cancer. This is especially helpful in patients with breast and GI cancers. The initial pretreatment CEA level is an indicator of tumor burden and therefore prognosis. Patients with smaller and early stage tumors are likely to have low, if not normal, CEA levels. Patients with more advanced or metastatic tumors are likely to have high CEA levels. A drastic reduction of the preoperative CEA to normal levels indicates complete eradication of the tumor. Therefore this test is used to determine the efficacy of treatment.

This test also is used in the surveillance of patients with cancer. A steadily rising CEA level is occasionally the first sign of tumor recurrence. This makes CEA testing very valuable in the follow-up of patients who have already had potentially curative therapy. It is important to reiterate that many (about 20%) patients with advanced breast or GI tumors may not have elevated CEA levels.

CEA can also be detected in body fluids other than blood. Its presence in those body fluids indicates metastasis. This test is commonly performed on peritoneal fluid or chest effusions. Elevated CEA levels in these fluids indicate metastasis to the peritoneum or pleura, respectively. Likewise, elevated CEA levels in the cerebrospinal fluid (CSF) indicate central nervous system (CNS) metastasis.

INTERFERING FACTORS

- Smokers tend to have higher CEA levels than nonsmokers.
- Benign diseases (e.g., cholecystitis, colitis, diverticulitis) and especially liver diseases (e.g., hepatitis, cirrhosis) are also associated with elevated CEA levels.
- Results may vary considerably depending on the method used for quantification. Because of this, results from different laboratories cannot be compared or interchangeably interpreted.

PROCEDURE AND PATIENT CARE

Before
✗ Explain the procedure to the patient.
✗ Tell the patient that no fasting is required.

During
- Collect a peripheral blood specimen. The collecting tube varies according to the commercial laboratory. Diagnostic kits are now available so that CEA can be tested at most local hospitals.
- Indicate on the laboratory slip if the patient smokes or has diseases that can affect test results.

After
- Apply pressure or a pressure dressing to the venipuncture site.
- Observe the venipuncture site for bleeding.

TEST RESULTS AND CLINICAL SIGNIFICANCE

▲ Increased Levels

Cancer (GI, breast, lung, pancreatic, hepatobiliary): *The cancer cells produce CEA on their cell surface. By a yet unrecognized mechanism, the CEA leaks into the bloodstream. Elevated levels result.*
Inflammation (colitis, cholecystitis, pancreatitis, diverticulitis),
Cirrhosis,
Crohn disease,
Peptic ulcer:
  The mechanism by which benign diseases produce CEA is unknown.

RELATED TESTS

CA 15-3 and CA 27-29 Tumor markers (p. 130). These antigens are tumor-associated serum markers for staging breast cancer and monitoring disease treatment.
CA 19-9 Tumor Marker (p. 132). This tumor marker is elevated in pancreatobiliary tumors and colorectal tumors.

Cell Surface Immunophenotyping (Flow Cytometry Cell Surface Immunophenotyping, Lymphocyte Immunophenotyping, AIDS T-Lymphocyte Cell Markers, CD4 Marker, CD4/CD8 Ratio, CD4 Percentage)

NORMAL FINDINGS

Cells	Percent	Number of Cells/μL
T cells	60-95	800-2500
T-helper (CD4) cells	60-75	600-1500
T-suppressor (CD8) cells	25-30	300-1000
B cells	4-25	100-450
Natural killer cells	4-30	75-500

CD4/CD8 ratio: >1

INDICATIONS

This test is used to detect the progressive depletion of CD4 T lymphocytes, which is associated with an increased likelihood of clinical complications from acquired immunodeficiency syndrome (AIDS). Test results can indicate if a patient with AIDS is at risk for developing opportunistic infections. It is also used to confirm the diagnosis of acute myelocytic leukemia (AML) and to differentiate AML from acute lymphocytic leukemia (ALL).

TEST EXPLANATION

All lymphocytes originate from reticulum cells in the bone marrow. Normal hematopoietic cells undergo changes in expression of cell surface markers as they mature from stem cells into cells of a committed lineage. Monoclonal antibodies have been developed that react with lymphoid and myeloid glycoprotein antigens on the cell surface of peripheral blood cells. One kind of lymphocyte that matures in the bone marrow is called a B lymphocyte. B lymphocytes provide humoral immunity (produce antibodies). A second type of lymphocyte matures in the thymus and is called a T lymphocyte. T lymphocytes are responsible for cellular immunity. Finally, there is a group of lymphocytes that has neither T nor B markers. These are called "natural killer cells" and will chemically attack foreign or cancer cells without prior sensitization. Monoclonal antibodies against cell-surface markers are used to identify the various forms of lymphocytes. The absolute numbers and percentages are then counted using flow cytometry. This can be performed on blood or on cell suspensions of tissue.

CD4 helper cells and CD8 cells are examples of T-lymphocytes. T-lymphocytes, and especially CD4 counts, when combined with HIV RNA viral load testing (p. 294), are used to determine the time to initiate antiviral therapy. They also can be used to monitor antiviral therapy. Successful antiviral therapy is associated with an increase in CD4 counts. Worsening of disease or unsuccessful therapy is associated with decreasing T-lymphocyte counts.

There are three related measurements of CD4 T lymphocytes. The first measurement is the total *CD4-cell count.* This is measured in whole blood and is the product of the WBC count, the lymphocyte differential count, and the percentage of lymphocytes that are CD4 T cells. The second measurement, the *CD4 percentage,* is a more accurate prognostic marker. It measures the percentage of CD4 lymphocytes in the whole blood sample by combining immunophenotyping with flow cytometry. This procedure relies on detecting specific antigenic determinants on the surface of the CD4 lymphocyte by antigen-specific monoclonal antibodies labeled with a fluorescent dye. The third prognostic marker, which is also more reliable than the total CD4 count, is the *ratio of CD4 (T-helper) cells to CD8 (T-suppressor) cells.*

Of the three T-cell measurements, the total CD4 count is the most variable. There is substantial diurnal variation in this count. Because it is a calculated measurement, the combination of possible laboratory error and personal fluctuation can result in wide variations in test results. With the CD4 percentage and CD4/CD8 ratios, very little diurnal variation and laboratory error exist. The Multicenter AIDS Cohort Study suggests that the latter two measurements are more accurate than the total CD4 count. However, because the total CD4-cell count was originally thought to be the best marker, this test was used in many of the studies that now form the basis for practice recommendations. It will take time before the more accurate measurements find clinical pertinence in practice recommendations.

The pathogenesis of AIDS is largely attributed to a decrease in the T lymphocyte that bears the CD4 receptor. Progressive depletion of CD4 T lymphocytes is associated with an increased likelihood of clinical complications from AIDS. Therefore CD4 measurement is a prognostic marker that can indicate whether a patient infected with human immunodeficiency virus (HIV) is at risk for developing opportunistic infections. The measurement of CD4-cell levels is used to decide whether to initiate *Pneumocystis jiroveci* pneumonia prophylaxis and antiviral therapy and for determining the prognosis of patients with HIV infection.

Both immunodeficiency and the dosage of immunosuppressive medications used after organ transplant are also monitored with the use of this cell surface immunophenotyping. Lymphomas and other lymphoproliferative diseases are now classified and treated according to the predominant lymphocyte type identified. In some instances, the prognosis of these diseases depends on this lymphocyte phenotyping.

The U.S. Public Health Service has recommended that CD4 prognostic markers be monitored every 3 to 6 months in all persons infected with HIV. Because the CD4 counts gradually fall in virtually all such patients, periodic review of the count can be emotionally stressful for both the patient and physician. The patient confronts his or her mortality as the health care provider confronts his or her ultimate powerlessness against the relentlessly advancing infections.

As the CD4-cell measurements decrease, the probability of developing AIDS increases. Forty-eight percent of patients can be expected to develop AIDS within 6 months when their CD4 count is less than 100 cells/mm³. It is recommended that antiviral therapy be started in patients whose CD4 count is less than 500 to 600 cells/mm³. *P. jiroveci* pneumonia prophylaxis should be started when the CD4 count is less than 200 to 300 cells/mm³.

CD4 prognostic markers also can be useful in guiding the approach to the patient's symptoms. Complaints such as cough and headache are common in most people; however, in patients infected with HIV, these symptoms often raise concerns about opportunistic infections. If the CD4 cell count exceeded 500 cells/mm³ in the past 6 months, there is a very low probability that these symptoms result from opportunistic infections. Knowing this, the patient and physician can feel comfortable with routine care.

Flow cytometry is able to analyze thousands of cells in less than a minute. The flow cytometer has three components in testing: an optical, a fluid, and an electronic system. The *optical* system consists of an argon laser that emits a single wavelength of light at 488 nm (blue region). Cells are labeled with one of several fluorochromes, including fluorescein (FITC), phycoerythrin (PE), and peridinin-chlorophyll protein (PCP), as a result of monoclonal antibody–fluorochrome conjugate binding to a specific blood cell. The fluorochromes are excited by the laser and emit *green* (FITC), *orange* (PE), and *red* (PCP) light that is measured through optical filters designed to capture their specific wavelength. The *fluid* system introduces the fluorochrome-bound cells in suspension into a pressurized sheath of fluid that travels through a clear cuvette. The laser light intersects a stream of cells that pass single file through the cuvette. The *electronic* system measures electronic signals from the detectors that provide measures of the magnitude of fluorescence intensity and the extent of light scatter associated with each cell as it passes through the laser. Most clinical flow cytometers measure five parameters on each cell: two nonfluorescence measures (magnitude of forward and side scatter) and three fluorescence measures (green, orange, and red light intensity). Multiple markers can be used simultaneously to identify different cell populations.

By using a combination of monoclonal antibodies recognizing B-cell, T-cell, and myeloid antigens, it is possible to confirm the diagnosis of acute myelocytic leukemia (AML) and to differentiate AML from acute lymphocytic leukemia (ALL) if morphology and traditional immunohistochemistry are inconclusive (<15% of cases). It is also helpful in identifying mixed patterns of leukemia that may affect prognosis and treatment. Furthermore, flow cytometric cell surface immunophenotyping is extremely helpful in differentiating various forms of immunodeficiency diseases.

CONTRAINDICATIONS

- Patients who are not emotionally prepared for the prognosis that the results may indicate.

INTERFERING FACTORS

- Although diurnal variation is usually of no significance, it may have some impact when counts are low. Higher counts can be expected in the late morning hours.
- A recent viral illness can decrease total T-lymphocyte counts.
- Nicotine and very strenuous exercise have been shown to decrease lymphocyte counts. However, such data are now being questioned.
- Steroids can *increase* lymphocyte counts.
- Immunosuppressive drugs will *decrease* lymphocyte counts.

✓ Clinical Priorities

- Progressive depletion of CD4 T lymphocytes is associated with increased complications from AIDS. Examples include severe immunosuppression, life-threatening opportunistic infections, malignancies, wasting syndrome, and HIV-related encephalopathy.
- The CD4 percentage and CD4/CD8 ratio provide more accurate measurements of CD4 T lymphocytes than the total CD4 count.
- The U.S. Public Health Service recommends monitoring CD4 counts every 3 to 6 months for all persons infected with HIV.

PROCEDURE AND PATIENT CARE

Before

- Explain the procedure to the patient.
- Tell the patient that no fasting or preparation is required.
- Maintain a nonjudgmental attitude toward the patient's sexual practices.
- Allow the patient ample opportunity to express his or her concerns regarding the results.

During

- Record the time of day when the blood specimen is obtained.
- Observe universal body and blood precautions. Wear gloves when handling blood products from all patients.
- Never recap needles. Dispose of needles and syringes in a puncture-proof container.
- Collect a venous blood sample in a large green-top tube (containing sodium heparin).
- Collect a venous blood sample in a small lavender-top tube (containing ethylene diamine tetraacetic acid).

After

- Keep the specimen at room temperature. Do not refrigerate.
- The specimen must be evaluated within 24 hours.
- Often specimens are sent to a central laboratory.
- Apply pressure or a pressure dressing to the venipuncture site.
- Assess the puncture site for bleeding.
- Instruct the patient to observe the venipuncture site for infection. Patients with AIDS or organ recipients are immunocompromised and susceptible to infection.
- Encourage the patient to discuss his or her concerns regarding the prognostic information that may be provided by these results.

TEST RESULTS AND CLINICAL SIGNIFICANCE

▲ Increased Levels

Chronic lymphocytic leukemia,
B-cell lymphoma:
  These patients can be expected to have increased B-lymphocyte counts in their tumor tissue or in their peripheral blood.
T-cell lymphoma: *These patients can be expected to have increased T-lymphocyte counts in their tumor tissue or in their peripheral blood (if their bone marrow is heavily involved with tumor).*

▼ Decreased Levels

Organ transplant patients: *A decreased lymphocyte count is expected and desirable for immunosuppression of organ rejection.*
HIV-positive patients: *When CD4 counts are below 200/mm^3, the patient is at increased risk for clinical symptoms from AIDS and the opportunistic infections that accompany this disease.*
Congenital immunodeficiency: *Children with DiGeorge syndrome and thymic hypoplasia will have decreased or no B lymphocytes.*

RELATED TESTS

HIV Serology (p. 297). This test is used to detect HIV antibody or antigen in high-risk persons.
HIV Viral Load (p. 297). This test is used to determine the amount of HIV viral load in the blood of an infected patient and is an accurate marker for prognosis and disease progression.

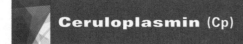

Ceruloplasmin (Cp)

NORMAL FINDINGS

Adults: 23-50 mg/dL or 230-500 mg/L (SI units)
Neonates: 2-13 mg/dL or 20-130 mg/L (SI units)

INDICATIONS

This test is an acute-phase reactant protein and can indicate an acute illness. However, its primary use is in the diagnosis of preclinical states of Wilson disease.

TEST EXPLANATION

Cp is an alpha$_2$-globulin that binds copper for transport within the bloodstream after it is absorbed from the gastrointestinal (GI) tract. Levels are decreased in most instances of Wilson disease, which is an inherited disorder. Patients who are homozygous for this disease make very little Cp. High unbound copper blood levels result and are toxic to tissues. The copper is deposited in the eye, brain, liver, and kidney. Wilson disease is fatal unless early treatment is instituted. If this disease is identified before significant copper deposits affect major organs, the ravages of the disease can be avoided. Cp levels are obtained in children at high risk for the disease. Teenagers and young adults with hepatitis, cirrhosis, or recurrent neuromuscular incoordination (signs compatible with Wilson disease) should also have this test. Early detection is important, because therapy is effective in most cases.

Cp is also an acute-phase reactant protein that becomes elevated during stress, infection, and pregnancy. However, it rises more slowly than other acute-phase reactants, such as C-reactive protein and erythrocyte sedimentation rate.

INTERFERING FACTORS

- Values are increased during pregnancy.
- Drugs that may cause *increased* levels include birth control pills, estrogen, methadone, phenytoin, and tamoxifen.

PROCEDURE AND PATIENT CARE

Before

- Explain the procedure to the patient.
- Tell the patient that no fasting is required.

During

- Collect a venous blood sample in a red-top tube.
- Keep the specimen on ice.

After

- Apply pressure or a pressure dressing to the venipuncture site.
- Assess the venipuncture site for bleeding.
- Medical follow-up and genetic counseling are indicated when Wilson disease is confirmed.

TEST RESULTS AND CLINICAL SIGNIFICANCE

▲ Increased Levels

Pregnancy,
Thyrotoxicosis,
Cancer,
Acute inflammatory reaction (e.g., infection, rheumatoid arthritis [RA]),
Biliary cirrhosis:
   These diseases induce the synthesis of Cp as an acute-phase reactant.
Copper intoxication: *Copper elevation will stimulate Cp in unaffected individuals.*

▼ Decreased Levels

Wilson disease: *Patients with this disease have homozygous or heterozygous genes and are unable to make Cp. Homozygous patients have lower Cp levels than heterozygous patients.*

Normal infants (6 months): *Young infants normally are unable to make adequate amounts of acute-phase reactant proteins (alpha$_2$-globulins) until they are 6 months of age.*

Nephrotic syndrome,

Sprue:

   These are protein-losing diseases. Cp is a protein that is lost in these diseases and therefore blood levels fall.

Kwashiorkor,

Starvation:

   Nutritional deficiencies are associated with low serum proteins, including Cp.

Menkes (kinky-hair) syndrome: *This is an inherited disorder associated with defects in the production of alpha$_2$-globulins such as Cp.*

RELATED TESTS

C-Reactive Protein (p. 184). This is a test for an acute-phase reactant protein.

Erythrocyte Sedimentation Rate (p. 221). This test provides the same information as an acute-phase reactant protein.

 Chloride, Blood (Cl)

NORMAL FINDINGS

Adult/elderly: 98-106 mEq/L or 98-106 mmol/L (SI units)
Child: 90-110 mEq/L
Newborn: 96-106 mEq/L
Premature infant: 95-110 mEq/L

 Critical Values

<80 or >115 mEq/L

INDICATIONS

This test is performed as a part of multiphasic testing for what is usually called "electrolytes." By itself, this test does not provide much information. However, with interpretation of the other electrolytes, chloride can give an indication of acid-base balance and hydration status.

TEST EXPLANATION

Chloride is the major extracellular anion. Its primary purpose is to maintain electrical neutrality, mostly as a salt with sodium. It follows sodium (cation) losses and accompanies sodium excesses in an attempt to maintain electrical neutrality. For example, when aldosterone encourages sodium reabsorption, chloride follows to maintain electrical neutrality. Because water moves with sodium and chloride, chloride also affects water balance. Finally, chloride also serves as a buffer to assist in acid-base balance. As carbon dioxide (and H cations) increases, bicarbonate must move from the intracellular space to the extracellular space. To maintain electrical neutrality, chloride will shift back into the cell.

Hypochloremia and hyperchloremia rarely occur alone and usually are part of parallel shifts in sodium or bicarbonate levels. Signs and symptoms of hypochloremia include hyperexcitability of the nervous system and muscles, shallow breathing, hypotension, and tetany. Signs and symptoms of hyperchloremia include lethargy, weakness, and deep breathing.

INTERFERING FACTORS

- Excessive infusions of saline solution can result in increased chloride levels.
- Drugs that may cause *increased* serum chloride levels include acetazolamide, ammonium chloride, androgens, chlorothiazide, cortisone preparations, estrogens, guanethidine, hydrochlorothiazide, methyldopa, and nonsteroidal antiinflammatory drugs.
- Drugs that may cause *decreased* levels include aldosterone, bicarbonates, corticosteroids, cortisone, hydrocortisone, loop diuretics, thiazide diuretics, and triamterene.

PROCEDURE AND PATIENT CARE

Before

- Explain the procedure to the patient.
- Tell the patient that no fasting is required.

During

- Collect a venous blood sample in a red-top or green-top tube.

After

- Apply pressure or a pressure dressing to the venipuncture site.
- Assess the venipuncture site for bleeding.

TEST RESULTS AND CLINICAL SIGNIFICANCE

▲   Increased Levels (Hyperchloremia)

Dehydration: *Chloride ions are more concentrated in the blood.*
Excessive infusion of normal saline solution: *Intake of chloride exceeds output, and blood levels rise.*
Metabolic acidosis,
Renal tubular acidosis,
Cushing syndrome,
Kidney dysfunction,
Hyperparathyroidism,
Eclampsia:
    Chloride urinary excretion is decreased.
Respiratory alkalosis: *Chloride is driven out of the cell in place of HCO_3^-.*

▼   Decreased Levels (Hypochloremia)

Overhydration,
Syndrome of inappropriate secretion of antidiuretic hormone (SIADH):
    Chloride is diluted.

Congestive heart failure: *Chloride is retained with sodium retention but is diluted by excess total body water.*

Vomiting or prolonged gastric suction,

Chronic diarrhea or high-output gastrointestinal (GI) fistula:

Chloride cation is high in the stomach and GI tract because of HCl acid produced in the stomach.

Chronic respiratory acidosis,

Metabolic alkalosis:

Chloride is driven into the cell to compensate for the HCO_3^- that leaves the cell to maintain pH neutrality.

Salt-losing nephritis,

Addison disease,

Diuretic therapy,

Hypokalemia,

Aldosteronism:

Chloride excretion is increased.

Burns: *Sodium and chloride losses from the massive burn can be great.*

RELATED TESTS

Sodium, Potassium, Bicarbonate (pp. 466, 409, and 141, respectively). These are other electrolytes commonly measured with chloride.

Chloride, Urine (p. 919). This is a measurement of chloride in the urine.

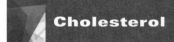

Cholesterol

NORMAL FINDINGS

Adult/elderly: <200 mg/dL or <5.20 mmol/L (SI units)

Child: 120-200 mg/dL

Infant: 70-175 mg/dL

Newborn: 53-135 mg/dL

INDICATIONS

Cholesterol testing is used to determine the risk for coronary heart disease (CHD). It is also used for evaluation of hyperlipidemias.

TEST EXPLANATION

Cholesterol is the main lipid associated with arteriosclerotic vascular disease. Cholesterol, however, is required for the production of steroids, sex hormones, bile acids, and cellular membranes. Most of the cholesterol we eat comes from foods of animal origin. The liver metabolizes the cholesterol to its free form, and cholesterol is transported in the bloodstream by lipoproteins (see p. 342). Nearly 75% of the cholesterol is bound to low-density lipoproteins (LDL), and 25% is bound to high-density lipoproteins (HDLs). Cholesterol is the main component of LDL and only a minimal component of HDL and very-low-density lipoprotein (VLDL). It is the LDL that is most directly associated with increased risk for CHD.

The purpose of cholesterol testing is to identify patients at risk for arteriosclerotic heart disease. Cholesterol testing is usually done as a part of a lipid profile, which evaluates lipoproteins and triglycerides (see pp. 342 and 504), because, by itself, cholesterol is not a totally accurate predictor of heart disease. There is considerable overlap in what are considered "normal" and "high-risk" levels. "Normal" levels have been derived from a group of patients who have no obvious evidence of CHD. However, this may not be accurate because these patients may have preclinical CHD and may not truly reflect a "no-risk" population.

There is considerable variation in cholesterol levels. Day-to-day cholesterol values in the same individual can vary by 15%. An 8% difference can even be identified within the same day. Positional changes can affect these levels. Levels can decrease by as much as 15% in the recumbent position. As a result, hospitalized patients can be expected to have lower levels than outpatients. Because of these significant variabilities, elevated results should be corroborated by repeating the study. The two results should be averaged to obtain an accurate cholesterol level for risk assessment.

Because the liver is required to metabolize ingested cholesterol products, subnormal cholesterol levels are indicative of severe liver diseases. Furthermore, because our main source of cholesterol is our diet, malnutrition is also associated with low cholesterol levels. Certain illnesses can affect cholesterol levels. For example, patients with an acute myocardial infarction (AMI) may have as much as a 50% reduction in cholesterol level for as long as 6 to 8 weeks.

Total cholesterol is used most accurately as a predictor of the risk for CHD when studied as part of the updated *Framingham Coronary Prediction* algorithm. This prediction model is used to determine a person's risk for developing an ischemic event (angina, myocardial infarction, or myocardial death) over the course of the following decade. Besides cholesterol, other factors used to estimate risk for CHD include age, lipoproteins, blood pressure, cigarette smoking history, diabetes mellitus, and gender.

This risk model uses a system whereby points are given for each factor in the model (Boxes 2-5 and 2-6). The total number of points is used to provide the patient's CHD risk. By dividing the CHD risk by age-related data (comparative risk), a risk relative to peers can be calculated. The CHD risk can be used to determine whether or not medicinal cholesterol lowering intervention is indicated.

Familial hyperlipidemias and hyperlipoproteinemias are often associated with high cholesterol.

INTERFERING FACTORS

- Pregnancy is usually associated with elevated cholesterol levels.
- Oophorectomy and postmenopausal status are associated with increased levels.
- Recumbent position is associated with decreased levels.
- Drugs that may cause *increased* levels include adrenocorticotropic hormone, anabolic steroids, beta-adrenergic blocking agents, corticosteroids, cyclosporine, epinephrine, oral contraceptives, phenytoin (Dilantin), sulfonamides, thiazide diuretics, and vitamin D.
- Drugs that may cause *decreased* levels include allopurinol, androgens, bile salt-binding agents, captopril, chlorpropamide, clofibrate, colchicine, colestipol, erythromycin, isoniazid, liothyronine (Cytomel), monoamine oxidase inhibitors, niacin, nitrates, and statins.

✓ Clinical Priorities

- Cholesterol testing is usually done as part of lipid profile testing, which also evaluates lipoproteins and triglycerides.
- Because of considerable variations in cholesterol values, elevated results should be verified by repeating the test.
- Test preparation usually requires a 12- to 14-hour fast after eating a low-fat meal. Only water is permitted.

BOX 2-5 — Coronary Disease Risk Prediction Score Sheet for Women Based on Total Cholesterol Level

Step 1:

Age	
Years	Points
30-34	−9
35-39	−4
40-44	0
45-49	3
50-54	6
55-59	7
60-64	8
65-69	8
70-74	8

Step 2:

Total Cholesterol		
(mg/dL)	(mmol/L)	Points
<160	≤4.14	−2
160-199	4.15-5.17	0
200-239	5.18-6.21	1
240-279	6.22-7.24	1
≥280	≥7.25	3

KEY:	
Color	Risk
Green	Very low
White	Low
Yellow	Moderate
Rose	High
Red	Very High

Step 3:

HDL Cholesterol		
(mg/dL)	(mmol/L)	Points
<35	≤0.90	5
35-44	0.91-1.16	2
45-49	1.17-1.29	1
50-59	1.30-1.55	0
≥60	≥1.56	−3

HDL, High-density lipoprotein.

Step 4:

Blood Pressure					
Systolic (mm Hg)	Diastolic (mm Hg)				
	<80	80-84	85-89	90-99	≥100
<120	−3 Points				
120-129		0 Points			
130-139			0 Points		
140-159				2 Points	
≥160					3 Points

NOTE: When systolic and diastolic pressures provide different estimates for point scores, use the higher number.

Step 5:

Diabetes	
	Points
No	0
Yes	4

Step 6:

Smoker	
	Points
No	0
Yes	2

Risk estimates were derived from the experience of the National Heart, Lung, and Blood Institute's Framingham Heart Study, a predominantly Caucasian population in Massachusetts, USA.

Step 7: (sum from steps 1-6)

Adding up the Points	
Age	____
Total cholesterol	____
HDL cholesterol	____
Blood pressure	____
Diabetes	____
Smoker	____
Point Total	____

HDL, High-density lipoprotein.

Step 8: (determine CHD risk from point total)

CHD Risk	
Point Total	10-Year CHD Risk (%)
≤−2	1
−1	2
0	2
1	2
2	3
3	3
4	4
5	4
6	5
7	6
8	7
9	8
10	10
11	11
12	13
13	15
14	18
15	20
16	24
≥17	≥37

CHD, Coronary heart disease.

STEP 9: (compare to women of the same age)

Comparative Risk		
Age (years)	Average 10-Year CHD Risk (%)	Low* 10-Year CHD Risk (%)
30-34	<1	<1
35-39	1	<1
40-44	2	2
45-49	5	3
50-54	8	5
55-59	12	7
60-64	12	8
65-69	13	8
70-74	14	8

CHD, Coronary heart disease.

*Low risk was calculated for a woman the same age, normal blood pressure, total cholesterol 160-199 mg/dL, HDL cholesterol 55 mg/dL, nonsmoker, no diabetes.

BOX 2-6 Coronary Disease Risk Prediction Score Sheet for Men Based on Total Cholesterol Level

Step 1:

Age	
Years	Points
30-34	−1
35-39	0
40-44	1
45-49	2
50-54	3
55-59	4
60-64	5
65-69	6
70-74	7

Step 2:

Total Cholesterol		
(mg/dL)	(mmol/L)	Points
<160	≤4.14	−3
160-199	4.15-5.17	0
200-239	5.18-6.21	1
240-279	6.22-7.24	2
≥280	≥7.25	3

KEY:	
Color	Risk
Green	Very low
White	Low
Yellow	Moderate
Rose	High
Red	Very High

Step 3:

HDL Cholesterol		
(mg/dL)	(mmol/L)	Points
<35	≤0.90	2
35-44	0.91-1.16	1
45-49	1.17-1.29	0
50-59	1.30-1.55	0
≥60	≥1.56	−2

HDL, High-density lipoprotein.

Step 4:

Blood Pressure					
Systolic (mm Hg)	Diastolic (mm Hg)				
	<80	80-84	85-89	90-99	≥100
<120	0 Points				
120-129		0 Points			
130-139			1 Point		
140-159				2 Points	
≥160					3 Points

NOTE: When systolic and diastolic pressures provide different estimates for point scores, use the higher number.

Step 5:

Diabetes	
	Points
No	0
Yes	2

Step 6:

Smoker	
	Points
No	0
Yes	2

Risk estimates were derived from the experience of the National Heart, Lung, and Blood Institute's Framingham Heart Study, a predominantly Caucasian population in Massachusetts, USA.

Step 7: (sum from steps 1-6)

Adding up the Points	
Age	_____
Total cholesterol	_____
HDL cholesterol	_____
Blood pressure	_____
Diabetes	_____
Smoker	_____
Point Total	_____

HDL, High-density lipoprotein.

Step 8: (determine CHD risk from point total)

CHD Risk	
Point Total	10-Year CHD Risk (%)
≤−1	2
0	3
1	3
2	4
3	5
4	7
5	8
6	10
7	13
8	16
9	20
10	25
11	31
12	37
13	45
≥14	≥53

CHD, Coronary heart disease.

STEP 9: (compare to men of the same age)

Comparative Risk		
Age (years)	Average 10 Year CHD Risk (%)	Low* 10 Year CHD Risk (%)
30-34	3	2
35-39	5	3
40-44	7	4
45-49	11	4
50-54	14	6
55-59	16	7
60-64	21	9
65-69	25	11
70 74	40	14

CHD, Coronary heart disease.

*Low risk was calculated for a man the same age, normal blood pressure, total cholesterol 160-199 mg/dL, HDL cholesterol 45 mg/dL, nonsmoker, no diabetes.

PROCEDURE AND PATIENT CARE

Before

✗ Instruct the patient to fast 12 to 14 hours after eating a low-fat meal before testing. Only water is permitted. Actually, cholesterol levels increase only minimally after a meal. However, early-morning fasting cholesterol levels are more easily compared when performed serially. Furthermore, lipoproteins, which are often ordered simultaneously, are affected by a previous meal. Therefore fasting is usually requested.

✗ Indicate to the patient that dietary intake for 2 weeks before testing will affect results. It is suggested that the patient eat a normal diet for at least 1 week before testing.

✗ Tell the patient that no alcohol should be consumed within 24 hours before the test.

During

- Collect a venous blood sample in a red-top tube.
- The fingerstick method is also often used for mass screening. There is less than a 5% difference in cholesterol measurements with these two methods.

After

- Apply pressure or a pressure dressing to the venipuncture site.
- Assess the venipuncture site for bleeding.
- Instruct patients with high levels regarding the following:
  - Low-cholesterol diet
    - Avoid animal fats.
    - Replace saturated fats with polyunsaturated fats.
    - Increase ingestion of fruits and vegetables.
  - Exercise
  - Appropriate body weight

TEST RESULTS AND CLINICAL SIGNIFICANCE

▲ Increased Levels

Familial hypercholesterolemia,
Familial hyperlipidemia:
   Enzymatic deficiencies in lipid metabolism are associated with elevated cholesterol.
Increased cholesterol levels are associated with hypothyroidism, uncontrolled diabetes mellitus, nephrotic syndrome, pregnancy, high-cholesterol diet, xanthomatosis, hypertension, myocardial infarction (MI), atherosclerosis, biliary cirrhosis, and extrahepatic biliary occlusion, stress, and nephrotic syndrome: *The pathophysiology of the association of cholesterol with these diseases is not well known. The association has been made by observation.*

▼ Decreased Levels

Malabsorption,
Malnutrition,
Advanced cancer:
   Most of the cholesterol is synthesized from fat eaten in the diet. When dietary intake is decreased, fat levels and subsequently cholesterol levels fall.
Decreased levels of cholesterol are also associated with hyperthyroidism, cholesterol-lowering medication, pernicious anemia, hemolytic anemia, sepsis/stress, liver disease, and acute MI (AMI): *The*

pathophysiology of the association of cholesterol with these diseases is not well known. The association has been made by observation.

RELATED TESTS

Apolipoproteins (p. 106). These polypeptides are associated with lipoproteins and have been used as accurate indicators of risk for CHD.

Lipoprotein (p. 342). HDL and LDL play an important role in the transport of lipids in the bloodstream. They, too, have been used in the assessment of risk for CHD.

Triglycerides (p. 504). This test is a measure of total triglycerides in the blood. It is a part of the lipid profile.

Cholinesterase (CHS, Pseudocholinesterase [PChE], Cholinesterase RBC, Red Blood Cell Cholinesterase, Acetylcholinesterase)

NORMAL FINDINGS

Serum cholinesterase: 8-18 units/mL or 8-18 units/L (SI units)
RBC cholinesterase: 5-10 units/mL or 5-10 units/L (SI units)
Dibucaine inhibition: 79% to 84%
(Values vary with laboratory test methods.)

INDICATIONS

This test is done to identify patients with PChE deficiency before anesthesia or to identify those who may have been exposed to phosphate poisoning.

TEST EXPLANATION

Cholinesterases hydrolyze acetylcholine and other choline esters and thereby regulate nerve impulse transmission at the nerve synapse and neuromuscular junction. There are two types of cholinesterases: *acetylcholinesterase*, also known as *true cholinesterase*, and PChE. True cholinesterase exists primarily in the red blood cells and nerve tissue. It is not in the serum. *PChE*, on the other hand, exists in the serum. Deficiencies in either of these enzymes can be acquired or congenital.

Because succinylcholine (the most commonly used muscle relaxant during anesthesia induction) is inactivated by PChE, people with an inherited PChE enzyme deficiency exhibit increased and/or prolonged effects of succinylcholine. Patients with a genetic variant of PChE may have a nonfunctioning form of PChE and will also experience prolonged effects of succinylcholine administration. Prolonged muscle paralysis and apnea will occur after anesthesia in these patients. This situation can be avoided by measuring serum cholinesterase (PChE) in all patients with a family history of prolonged apnea after surgery.

Because patients with a nonfunctioning variant of PChE will have normal total quantitative PChE levels yet still have prolonged paralytic effects of succinylcholine, a second test (dibucaine inhibition) usually is also performed. Dibucaine is a known local anesthetic that inhibits the function of normal PChE. The *dibucaine inhibition number* (DN) is the percent of PChE activity that is inhibited when dibucaine is added to the patient's serum sample. If total PChE is normal and DNs are low, the presence of a nonfunctioning PChE variant is suspected and the patient will be at risk for succinylcholine-induced prolonged paralysis. Decreased PChE enzyme activity in conjunction with a DN less than 30 suggests high risk for prolonged paralysis. Normal to decreased PChE enzyme activity in conjunction with a DN 30-79 suggests variable risk. Phenotype interpretation (homozygote or various types of heterozygosity) is based on the total PChE activity and the percent of inhibition caused by dibucaine.

A common form of acquired cholinesterase deficiency, either true or PChE, is caused by overexposure to pesticides, organophosphates, or nerve gas. The half-life of the pseudoenzyme in serum is about 8 days, and the "true" cholinesterase (AChE) of red cells is more than 3 months (determined by erythropoietic activity). Recent exposure (up to several weeks) is determined by assay of the pseudoenzyme and months after exposure by measurement of the red cell enzyme. Persons with jobs associated with chronic exposure to these chemicals are often monitored by the frequent testing of RBC cholinesterase activity. Other potential causes of reduced cholinesterase activity include chronic liver diseases, malnutrition, and hypoalbuminemia.

Increased cholinesterase activity, when found in the amniotic fluid, represents strong evidence for a *neural tube defect* (NTD). When an NTD is suspected based upon maternal serum alpha-fetoprotein (AFP) screening results or diagnosed via ultrasound, analysis of AFP and acetylcholinesterase (AChE) in amniotic fluid are useful diagnostic tools.

INTERFERING FACTORS

- Pregnancy decreases test values.
- It is important to recognize that pseudocholinesterase levels cannot be measured in postoperative patients in the recovery room if the patient is not regaining muscular function, because often one or more of the above drugs may be given during the surgery and could invalidate the results.
- Drugs that may cause *decreased* values include atropine, caffeine, codeine, estrogens, morphine sulfate, neostigmine, oral contraceptives, phenothiazines, quinidine, theophylline, steroids, and vitamin K.

PROCEDURE AND PATIENT CARE

Before
- Explain the procedure to the patient.
- Tell the patient that no fasting is required.
- If the test is done to identify the presurgical patient who may be at risk for cholinesterase deficiency, be sure the test is done several days before the planned surgery.
- It may be recommended to withhold medications that could alter test results for 12 to 24 hours before the test.

During
- Collect a venous blood sample in a red-top tube.

After
- Apply pressure or a pressure dressing to the venipuncture site.
- Assess the venipuncture site for bleeding.

TEST RESULTS AND CLINICAL SIGNIFICANCE

▲ Increased Serum Levels
Hyperlipidemia,

Nephrosis,
Diabetes:
  Increased levels are observed without any known pathophysiology.

▼ Decreased Serum Levels

Poisoning from organic phosphate insecticides: *These chemicals inhibit the activity of cholinesterases.*
Hepatocellular disease,
Malnutrition and other forms of hypoalbuminemia:
  Albumin is important in the transport and function of cholinesterases.

▲ Increased RBC Levels

Reticulocytosis
Sickle cell anemia:
  Increased RBC precursors are associated with higher levels of true cholinesterase.

▼ Decreased RBC Levels

Persons with congenital enzyme deficiency: *Cholinesterases are not synthesized.*
Poisoning from organic phosphate insecticides: *See Serum Levels.*

Chromosome Karyotype (Blood Chromosome Analysis, Chromosome Studies, Cytogenetics, Karyotype)

NORMAL FINDINGS

Female: 44 autosomes, 2 X chromosomes; karyotype: 46,XX
Male: 44 autosomes, 1 X, 1 Y chromosome; karyotype: 46,XY

INDICATIONS

This test is used to study an individual's chromosome makeup to determine chromosomal defects associated with disease or the risk for developing disease.

TEST EXPLANATION

The term "karyotyping" refers to the arrangement of cell chromosomes from the largest to the smallest to analyze their number and structure. Variations in either can produce numerous developmental abnormalities and diseases. A normal karyotype of chromosomes consists of a pattern of 22 pairs of autosomal chromosomes and a pair of sex chromosomes: XY for the male and XX for the female. Chromosomal karyotype abnormalities can be congenital or acquired. These karyotype abnormalities can occur because of duplication, deletion, translocation, reciprocation, or genetic rearrangement.

Chromosome karyotyping is useful in evaluating congenital anomalies, mental retardation, growth retardation, delayed puberty, infertility, hypogonadism, primary amenorrhea, ambiguous genitalia, chronic myelogenous leukemia, neoplasm, recurrent miscarriage, prenatal diagnosis of serious congenital diseases (especially when advanced maternal age is a factor), Turner syndrome, Klinefelter syndrome, Down syndrome, and other suspected genetic disorders. The products of conception also can be studied to determine the cause of stillbirth or miscarriage.

The most common form of karyotyping is performed by banding techniques. This technique provides a method of pairing similar chromosomes based on their size, location of the centromere (constriction that divides the chromosome into long and short arms), and other constrictions, ratio of long to short arms, satellite deoxyribonucleic acid (DNA), and banding patterns. With this method, a characteristic karyotype is determined. An extensive nomenclature system for the types has been developed.

Special chromosome studies can be performed on cells grown in special medium to identify certain chromosome abnormalities. DNA testing is now possible through the use of DNA probes and DNA linkage studies.

PROCEDURE AND PATIENT CARE

Before

- Explain the procedure to the patient.
- Determine how the specimen will be collected.
- Obtain preparation guidelines from the laboratory if indicated.
- Many patients are fearful of the test results and require considerable emotional support.
- In some states, informed consent is required.

During

- Specimens for chromosome analysis can be obtained from numerous sources. Leukocytes from a peripheral venipuncture site are the most easily obtained and most often used for this study.
- Bone marrow biopsies and surgical specimens also can sometimes be used as sources for analysis.
- During pregnancy, specimens can be collected by amniocentesis (see p. 632) and chorionic villus sampling (see p. 1088).
- Fetal tissue or products of conception can be studied as well to determine the reason for the loss of the fetus.
- Buccal mucosal cell specimens are less costly but not as accurate as other tissue for karyotyping.

After

- Aftercare depends on how the specimen was collected.
- Inform the patient that test results are generally not available for weeks to several months.
- If an abnormality is identified, the entire family line may be tested. This can be exhaustive and expensive.
- If the test results show an abnormality, encourage the patient to verbalize his or her feelings. Provide emotional support.

TEST RESULTS AND CLINICAL SIGNIFICANCE

Abnormal Findings

Chromosome abnormalities can be a cause of congenital anomalies, mental retardation, growth retardation, delayed puberty, infertility, hypogonadism, primary amenorrhea, ambiguous genitalia, chronic myelogenous leukemia, neoplasm, recurrent miscarriage, Tay-Sachs disease, sickle cell anemia, Turner syndrome, Klinefelter syndrome, and Down syndrome. See Table 2-13 for some of the commonly known abnormalities.

RELATED TESTS

Barr Body Analysis. This is an inexpensive test for detecting chromatin material (X chromatin).
Genetic Testing (p. 1093). This is another method of DNA testing.

TABLE 2-13 Common Chromosome Abnormalities	
Chromosome Abnormality	**Clinical Manifestation or Syndrome**
Trisomy 21	Down
Single X	Turner
Extra X in male (XXY)	Klinefelter
5 p deletion	Cat-cry
15 q deletion	Prader-Willi
3 q trisomy	Cornelia de Lange
Fragile X	Mental retardation
X centromere dislocation	Roberts
Philadelphia	Chronic myelogenous leukemia, acute myelogenous leukemia

Coagulating Factor Concentration (Factor Assay, Coagulating Factors, Blood-Clotting Factors)

NORMAL FINDINGS

Factor	Normal Value (% of "Normal")
II	80-120
V	50-150
VII	65-140
VIII	55-145
IX	60-140
X	45-155
XI	65-135
XII	50-150

INDICATIONS

The coagulating factor concentration test measures the concentration of specific coagulating factors in the blood.

TEST EXPLANATION

These tests measure the quantity of each specific factor suspected to be responsible for suspected defects in hemostasis. Testing is available to measure the quantity of the factors listed in Table 2-14. When these factors exist in concentrations below their "minimal hemostatic level," clotting will be impaired. These minimal hemostatic levels vary according to the factor involved.

 Deficiencies of these factors may be a result of inherited genetic defects, acquired diseases, or drug therapy. Common medical conditions associated with abnormal factor concentrations are

TABLE 2-14	Coagulation Factors			
Factor	Name	Quantitation of Minimum Hemostatic Level (mg/dL)	Abnormal Coagulation Tests Associated With Deficiency	Blood Components to Provide Specific Factor
I	Fibrinogen	60-100	PT, aPTT	C, FFP, FWB
II	Prothrombin	10-15	PT	P, WB, FFP, FWB
III	Tissue factor or thromboplastin	QNA	PT	
IV	Calcium	See calcium, p. 138		
V	Proaccelerin (labile)	5-10	PT, aPTT	FFP, FWB
VII	Stable factor	5-20	PT	P, WB, FFP, FWB
VIII	Antihemophilic factor	30	aPTT	C, FFP, VIII conc
IX	Christmas factor	30	aPTT	FFP, FWB
X	Stuart factor	8-10	PT, aPTT	P, WB, FFP, FWB
XI	Plasma thromboplastin antecedent	25	aPTT	P, WB, FFP, FWB
XII	Hageman factor	Yes	aPTT	
XIII	Fibrin stabilizing factor	No		P, C, XIII conc

aPTT, Activated partial thromboplastin time; *PT,* prothrombin time; *C,* cryoprecipitate; *FFP,* fresh frozen plasma; *FWB,* fresh whole blood (less than 24 hours old); *P,* unfrozen banked plasma; *WB,* banked whole blood; *VIII conc,* factor VIII concentrate; *XIII conc,* factor XIII concentrate.
NOTE: Recombinant factors are now available for factor VII, VIII, IX, and XIII. Concentrates are also now available for II, VII, VIII, IX, and XIII.

listed in Table 2-15). It is important to identify the exact factor or factors involved in the coagulating defect so that the appropriate blood component replacement can be administered (Table 2-14 and Figure 2-11).

The hemostasis and coagulation system is a homeostatic balance between factors encouraging clotting and factors encouraging clot dissolution. The first reaction of the body to active bleeding is blood vessel constriction. In small-vessel injury this may be enough to stop bleeding. In large-vessel injury, hemostasis is required to form a clot that will durably plug the hole until healing can occur. The primary phase of the hemostatic mechanism involves platelet aggregation to the blood vessel (Figure 2-12). Secondary hemostasis then occurs. Secondary hemostasis can be broken down into a series of four reactions that culminate in the production of thrombin and fibrin. These act to create a blood clot at the site of vascular injury. In reaction one, sometimes called the intrinsic phase of coagulation, factor XII and other proteins form a complex on the subendothelial collagen in the injured blood vessel. Through a series of reactions, activated factor XI (XIa) is formed and activates factor IX (IXa). In a complex formed by factors VIII, IX, and X, activated X (Xa) is formed.

At the same time, reaction two, the extrinsic pathway, is activated and a complex is formed between tissue factor and factor VII. Activated factor VII (VIIa) results. Factor VIIa can directly activate factor

TABLE 2-15	Conditions Associated With Abnormal Factor Concentrations	
Factor	**Increased (excess)**	**Decreased (deficiency)**
I (Fibrinogen)	Acute inflammatory reactions Trauma Coronary heart disease Cigarette smoking	Liver disease (hepatitis or cirrhosis) DIC Congenital deficiency
II (Prothrombin)	ND	Vitamin K deficiency Liver disease Congenital deficiency Warfarin ingestion
V (Proaccelerin)	ND	Liver disease DIC Fibrinolysis
VII (Proconvertin [stable factor])	ND	Congenital deficiency Vitamin K deficiency Liver disease Warfarin ingestion
VIII (Antihemophilic factor)	Acute inflammatory reactions Trauma/stress Pregnancy Birth control pills	Congenital deficiency (e.g., Hemophilia A) DIC
von Willebrand factor	ND	Congenital deficiency (e.g., von Willebrand disease) Some myeloproliferative disorders
IX (Christmas factor)	ND	Congenital deficiency (e.g., Hemophilia B) Liver disease Nephrotic syndrome Warfarin ingestion DIC Vitamin K deficiency
X (Stuart factor)	ND	Congenital deficiency Liver disease Warfarin ingestion Vitamin K deficiency
XII (Hageman factor)	ND	Congenital deficiency Liver disease DIC

DIC, Disseminated intravascular coagulation; *ND,* no common diseases states associated with excess of this factor.

X. Alternatively, VIIa can activate factors IX and X together. In reaction three, factor X is activated by the proteases generated in the two previous reactions (VIIa and IXa in concert with VIII). As an alternative, VIIa can activate factors IX and X directly. In reaction four, sometimes referred to as the common pathway, Xa converts prothrombin in the presence of factor V, calcium, and phospholipid on the platelet surface. Thrombin, in turn, converts fibrinogen to fibrin, which is polymerized into a stable clot. Thrombin also activates factor VIII to stimulate further platelet aggregation and fibrin polymerization.

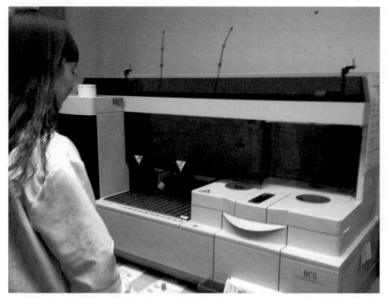

Figure 2-11 Siemens automated hemostasis analyzer. This system can analyze multiple factors involved in hemostasis.

Almost immediately, three major activators of the fibrinolytic system act on plasminogen, which had previously been absorbed into the clot, to form plasmin. Plasmin degenerates the fibrin polymer into fragments, which are cleared by macrophages.

Roman numerals have been assigned by the order in which the factor had been identified, not by their order in the above-noted hemostatic mechanism. (See Table 2-14 for a list of factor names and for routine coagulation test abnormalities associated with factor deficiency.)

Fibrinogen, like many other of the coagulation proteins, is considered an acute-phase reactant protein and is elevated in many severe illnesses. It is also considered a risk factor for coronary heart disease (CHD) and stroke. Prothrombin is a vitamin K–dependent clotting factor. Its production in the liver requires vitamin K. This vitamin is fat soluble and is dependent on bile for absorption. Bile duct obstruction or malabsorption will cause a vitamin K deficiency and result in a reduced quantity of prothrombin and other vitamin K–dependent factors (VII, IX, X). It usually takes about 3 weeks before body stores of vitamin K are exhausted.

Factor VIII is actually a complex molecule with two components. The first component is related to hemophilia A and is involved in the hemostatic mechanism as described above. The second component is the von Willebrand factor and is related to von Willebrand disease. This second component is involved in platelet adhesion and aggregation. Factor XII deficiency is a common cause of prolonged activated partial thromboplastin time (aPPT) a nonbleeding patient. Patients with factor XII deficiency have been observed to have an increased risk for myocardial infarction (MI) and venous thrombosis.

Measurement of coagulation factors in relationship to other key coagulating proteins may be helpful in determining risks of hypercoagulation. A measure of the ratio of von Willebrand factor to ADAMTS13 (a factor-cleaving protease) is an accurate predictor of thromboembolic complication after liver surgery.

Hemostasis and Fibrinolysis

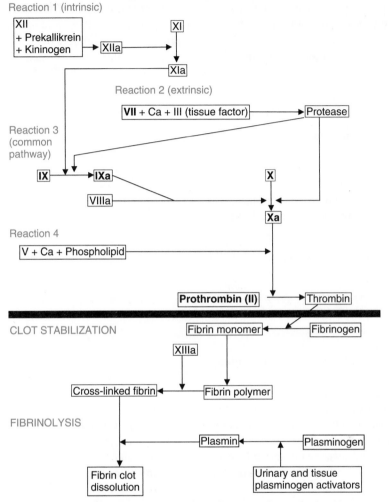

Figure 2-12 Secondary hemostasis (fibrin clot formation) and fibrinolysis (fibrin clot dissolution). Primary hemostasis involves platelet plugging of the injured blood vessel. Secondary hemostasis, as simply described here, takes place most rapidly on the platelet surface after attachment to the fractured endothelium. Four different reactions result in the formation of fibrin. As seen beneath the dark line in the figure, the fibrin clot supports the platelet clump so that the clot does not get swept away by the tremendous "shear forces" of the fast moving blood cells. Fibrinolysis follows formation of the fibrin clot in order to prevent complete occlusion of the injured blood vessel. **Bold** = Vitamin K–dependent coagulating factors.

Coagulation factor inhibitors arise in patients who are congenitally deficient in a specific factor in response to factor replacement therapy. They can also occur spontaneously without known cause or in response to a variety of medical conditions, including the postpartum state, immunologic disorders, certain antibiotic therapies, some malignancies, and old age. Inhibitors of factor VIII coagulant activity are the most commonly occurring of the specific factor inhibitors. These can be identified and quantified.

INTERFERING FACTORS

- Many of these proteins are heat sensitive, and levels will be decreased if the specimen is kept at room temperature.
- Pregnancy or the use of contraceptive medication can increase levels of several of these factors, especially VIII and IX. A mild deficiency could be masked.
- Many of these protein coagulation factors are acute-phase reactant proteins. Acute illness, stress, exercise, or inflammation could raise levels.

PROCEDURE AND PATIENT CARE

Before
🗙 Explain the procedure to the patient.
🗙 Tell the patient that no fasting is required.

During
- Collect a venous blood sample in a blue-top tube.

After
- Apply pressure or a pressure dressing to the venipuncture site.
- Assess the venipuncture site for bleeding, especially if the patient has had other episodes of clotting deficiency.
- Deliver the blood specimen to the laboratory as soon as possible.
- Freeze the specimen if testing is not going to be done immediately because these proteins are very labile.

TEST RESULTS AND CLINICAL SIGNIFICANCE

FIBRINOGEN

▲ Increased Levels
Acute inflammatory reactions,
Trauma:
    Fibrinogen is an acute-phase reactant protein.
Coronary heart disease (CHD),
Cigarette smoking:
    Elevated fibrinogen levels are merely an observation with no known pathophysiology.

▼ Decreased Levels
Liver disease (hepatitis or cirrhosis). *Fibrinogen is not made in adequate volume.*
Consumptive coagulopathy (disseminated intravascular coagulation),

Action of fibrinolysins:
Fibrinolysins act to destroy fibrinogen in the serum.

PROTHROMBIN
▼ Decreased Levels
Vitamin K deficiency,
Liver disease:
Synthesis is diminished.

PROACCELERIN
▼ Decreased Levels
Liver disease: *Synthesis is diminished.*

PROCONVERTIN STABLE FACTOR
▼ Decreased Levels
Inherited deficiency,
Vitamin K deficiency,
Liver disease,
Coumadin therapy:
Synthesis is diminished.

ANTIHEMOPHILIC FACTOR
▲ Increased Levels
Acute inflammatory reactions,
Trauma/stress,
Pregnancy:
Factor VIII is an acute-phase reactant protein.

▼ Decreased Levels
Inherited deficiency (hemophilia A): *Hemophilia A is controlled by a sex-linked gene on the X chromosome. Females are rarely affected, because the other X chromosome has a normal gene.*
Consumptive coagulation: *This factor is used up and synthesis cannot match the demand.*

VON WILLEBRAND FACTOR
▼ Decreased Levels (von Willebrand Disease)
Inherited deficiency,
Autoimmune disease:
Von Willebrand factor is reduced in quantity.

CHRISTMAS FACTOR
▼ Decreased Levels
Inherited deficiency (hemophilia B),

Liver disease,
Nephrotic syndrome,
Coumadin therapy:
  Synthesis is diminished.
Consumptive coagulation: *This factor is used up and synthesis cannot match the demand.*

STUART FACTOR
▼ Decreased Levels
This is an inherited deficiency.

HAGEMAN FACTOR
▼ Decreased Levels
Inherited deficiency,
Vitamin K deficiency,
Liver disease,
Coumadin therapy:
  Synthesis is diminished.
Consumptive coagulation: *This factor is used up and synthesis cannot match the demand.*

RELATED TESTS

Partial Thromboplastin Time, Activated (aPTT) (p. 383). This test is used to evaluate the intrinsic system and the common pathway of clot formation.
Prothrombin Time (p. 434). This test is used to evaluate the adequacy of the extrinsic system and common pathway in the clotting mechanism.
Fibrinogen (p. 241). This is a separate discussion on this coagulating factor.

Cold Agglutinins

NORMAL FINDINGS

Screen: negative
Titer: no agglutination ≤1:64

INDICATION

Cold agglutinins are used to identify and investigate cold agglutinin syndrome and unusual infections, such as *Mycoplasma pneumoniae.*

TEST EXPLANATION

Cold agglutinins are antibodies (usually IgM) to erythrocytes. All individuals have circulating antibodies directed against red blood cells, but their concentrations are often too low to trigger disease or symptoms (titers <1:64). In individuals with *cold agglutinin syndrome*, these antibodies are much higher (>1:512). At body temperatures of 28-31° C, such as those encountered during winter months, these antibodies can cause a variety of symptoms (from chronic anemia caused by intravascular hemolysis or extravascular sequestration of affected RBCs leading to acrocyanosis of the ears, fingers, or toes because of local blood stasis in the skin capillaries).

There are two forms of cold agglutinin disease, primary and secondary. The primary form has no precipitating cause. Secondary cold agglutinin disease is a result of an underlying condition, notably *Mycoplasma pneumoniae*. The Cold agglutinins test is not specific for *Mycoplasma pneumoniae* and is not recommended to diagnose the disease. It does provide supportive information, however. *Mycoplasma pneumoniae* serum antibodies (IgG and IgM) (p. 364) are also supportive of *Mycoplasma* infection.

Other possible conditions associated with cold agglutinins include influenza, mononucleosis, rheumatoid arthritis, lymphomas, HIV, Epstein-Barr virus, and cytomegalovirus. Temperature regulation is important for the performance of this test. Under no circumstances should the cold agglutinin specimen be refrigerated.

The cold agglutinin screen is performed on all specimens first to identify most of those with titer values in the normal range. If the screen is negative, no titration is required. If the screen is positive, a titer with serial saline dilutions is performed.

INTERFERING FACTORS

Some antibiotics (penicillin and cephalosporins) can interfere with the development of cold agglutinins.

PROCEDURE AND PATIENT CARE

Before

Explain the procedure to the patient.

Tell the patient that no fasting is required.

During

- Collect venous blood in a red-top tube.

After

- Apply pressure to the venipuncture site.
- Transport the specimen immediately to the laboratory.

TEST RESULTS AND CLINICAL SIGNIFICANCE

▲ Increased Levels

Mycoplasma pneumoniae infection,
Viral illness,
Infectious mononucleosis,
Multiple myeloma,
Scleroderma,
Cirrhosis,
Staphylococcemia,
Thymic tumor,
Influenza,
Rheumatoid arthritis,

Lymphoma,
Systemic lupus erythematosus,
Primary cold agglutinin disease:
  These diseases are associated with high titers of cold agglutinins of varying concentrations.

RELATED TESTS

Mycoplasma pneumonia Antibodies (p. 364). The serologic identification of IgG and IgM antibodies to *Mycoplasma* are used to support the clinical diagnosis of the infection.

 Complement Assay (C2, C3, and C4 Complement)

NORMAL FINDINGS

Total complement: 30-75 units/mL
C2: 1-4 mg/dL
C3: 75-175 mg/dL
C4: 22-45 units/mL

INDICATIONS

Measurements of complement are used primarily to diagnose hereditary deficiencies of complement peptides and monitor the activity of infectious or autoimmune diseases (systemic lupus erythematosus nephritis, membranoproliferative nephritis, or poststreptococcal nephritis).

TEST EXPLANATION

Serum complement is a group of proteins that act as enzymes to instigate a cascade-like series of reactions that lead to the synthesis of a group of proteins that facilitate the immunologic and inflammatory responses. The total complement, sometimes labeled CH50, is made by the series of reactions involving proteins C1 through C9 (classic cascade reactions). Once activated, total complement (and some precursor proteins) acts to increase vascular permeability, allowing antibodies and white blood cells (WBCs) to be delivered to the area of the immune/antigen complex. Complement also acts to increase chemotaxis (attracting WBCs to the area), phagocytosis, and immune adherence of the antibody to antigen. The end result of the complement activation cascade is the formation of the lytic membrane attack complex (MAC).

These processes are vitally important in the normal inflammatory or immunologic response. The absence of early components (C1-C4) of the complement cascade results in the inability of immune complexes to activate the cascade. Patients with deficiencies of the early complement proteins are unable to clear immune complexes. Patients with deficiencies of the late complement proteins (C5, C6, C7, C8, and C9) are unable to form the MAC. Patients with deficient complement factors have increased susceptibility to infections with encapsulated microorganisms. They may also have symptoms that suggest autoimmune disease and complement deficiency may be an etiologic factor in the development of autoimmune disease. Besides the major complement components, there are some subcomponents and "inhibitor" components involved in the system that can affect complement function.

Reduced complement levels can be congenital or acquired. Although rare, C2 deficiency is the most common inherited complement deficiency. Acquired complement deficiencies are usually instigated by ongoing inflammatory/infectious diseases. As the complement system is activated, the complement components are "consumed" or used up. If the system is persistently or overly activated, serum levels decrease. The complement system is instigated by the presence of antibody/antigen complexes. As in hereditary angioedema, complement components are used up and serum levels fall. Diseases associated with these immune complexes include serum sickness, lupus erythematosus, infectious endocarditis, renal transplant rejection, vasculitis, some forms of glomerulonephritis, and infections. As these diseases are successfully treated, complement levels can be expected to return to normal. Complement components can be increased after the onset of various acute inflammatory diseases or acute tissue damage. This is very similar to an "acute reaction" protein.

The total complement assay should be used as a screen for suspected complement deficiencies before ordering individual complement component assays. Testing is usually automated using labeled liposomes. A deficiency of an individual component of the complement cascade may result in a reduced total complement level. Specific complement factor assay can be performed by radial immunodiffusion. Complement levels can be measured in body fluids, most commonly joint fluid. Low synovial fluid complement levels are characteristic of effusions from patients with rheumatoid arthritis, systemic lupus erythematosus, and bacterial infections.

INTERFERING FACTORS

- C3 is very unstable at room temperature. If the specimen is left standing for more than 1 hour, complement levels could be falsely low. The serum should be separated out and frozen immediately when the specimen is received.

PROCEDURE AND PATIENT CARE

Before

✗ Explain the procedure to the patient.
✗ Tell the patient that no fasting or special preparation is required.

During

- Collect a venous blood sample in a red-top tube.

After

- Apply pressure or a pressure dressing to the venipuncture site.
- Observe the venipuncture site for bleeding.

TEST RESULTS AND CLINICAL SIGNIFICANCE

▲ Increased Levels

Rheumatic fever (acute),
Myocardial infarction (acute) (AMI),
Ulcerative colitis,
Inflammatory illnesses, stress, and trauma:
  Complement can develop very similarly to an acute-phase reactant protein. With these illnesses, complement is increased.
Cancer: *The pathophysiology of this observation is unknown.*

▼ Decreased Levels

Hereditary angioedema: *Hereditary angioedema is a congenital lack of a C1 "inhibitor" (often called C1 esterase). The complement system is overly activated and the complement components are consumed or used up. Serum levels fall.*

Severe liver diseases such as hepatitis or cirrhosis: *The liver is the site of synthesis of many of the complement components. Synthesis is decreased in the presence of liver disease. Serum levels fall.*

Autoimmune disease (SLE, glomerulonephritis, lupus nephritis, rheumatoid arthritis [severe and active], Sjögren syndrome),

Serum sickness (immune complex disease),

Renal transplant rejection (acute):

These diseases are associated with the increased presence of antibody/antigen complexes, which serve to act as complement activators. The complement system is overly activated and complement components are consumed. Serum levels fall.

Protein malnutrition,

Hemolytic anemia,

Malnutrition:

These diseases are associated with protein depletion. Complement is a protein and its synthesis can be expected to be reduced in these illnesses.

Infection such as gram-negative sepsis or bacterial endocarditis,

Glomerulonephritis (specifically poststreptococcal and membranoproliferative):

Alternate pathways of complement activation occur. The complement system is overly activated and complement components are consumed. Serum levels fall.

Complete Blood Cell Count and Differential Count (CBC and Diff)

The CBC and differential count (diff) are a series of tests of the peripheral blood that provide a tremendous amount of information about the hematologic system and many other organ systems. They are inexpensively, easily, and rapidly performed as a screening test. The CBC and diff include automated multimeasurement of the following studies (Figure 2-13), which are discussed separately:

Red blood cell count (see p. 439)
Hemoglobin (see p. 281)
Hematocrit (see p. 277)
Red blood cell indices (see p. 442)
    Mean corpuscular volume (MCV)
    Mean corpuscular hemoglobin (MCH)
    Mean corpuscular hemoglobin concentration (MCHC)
    Red blood cell distribution width (RDW)
White blood cell count and differential count (see p. 526)
    Neutrophils (polynucleated cells or "polys," segmented cells or "segs," band cells, stab cells)
    Lymphocytes
    Monocytes
    Eosinophils
    Basophils
Blood smear (see p. 710)

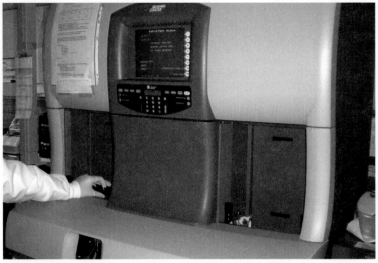

Figure 2-13 The Beckman Coulter automated CBC analyzer can perform many CBC tests in a few minutes. The automated system will notify the technologist if any significant abnormality is noted. Those findings will be corroborated by individual testing.

Platelet count (see p. 401)
Mean platelet volume (MPV) (see p. 407)

Coombs Test, Direct (Direct Antiglobulin Test [DAT])

NORMAL FINDINGS

Negative; no agglutination

INDICATIONS

This test is performed to identify immune hemolysis (lysis of red blood cells [RBCs]) or to investigate hemolytic transfusion reactions (Box 2-7).

TEST EXPLANATION

Most of the antibodies to RBCs are directed against the ABO/Rh blood grouping antigens, such as those that occur in hemolytic anemia of the newborn or blood transfusion of incompatible blood. When a transfusion reaction occurs (Box 2-8), the Coombs test can detect the patient's antibodies or complement components coating the transfused RBCs. The Coombs test is therefore useful in evaluating suspected transfusion reactions.

Non–blood-grouping antigens can develop on the RBC membrane and stimulate the formation of antibodies. Drugs such as levodopa or penicillin can do this. Also, in some autoimmune diseases, antibodies not originally directed against the patient's RBCs can attach to the RBCs and cause hemolysis, which can be detected by the direct Coombs test. Examples of the latter would include:

BOX 2-7	Symptoms of Transfusion Reaction

- Fever
- Chills
- Rash
- Flank/back pain
- Bloody urine
- Fainting or dizziness

BOX 2-8	Diagnostic Testing for Suspected Hemolytic Blood Transfusions

- Complete blood cell count (CBC)
- Electrolytes
- Blood urea nitrogen (BUN), creatinine
- Direct Coombs test (pretransfusion and posttransfusion recipient blood)
- ABO blood typing on donor and recipient blood
- RH typing on donor and recipient blood
- Blood crossmatch
- Protime
- Partial thromboplastin time (PTT)
- Fibrin split products
- Haptoglobin
- Bilirubin
- Blood cultures on donor and recipient blood
- Urine for free hemoglobin–dipstick

- Antibodies developed in reaction to drugs such as penicillin
- Autoantibodies formed in various autoimmune diseases
- Antibodies developed in some patients with advanced cancer (e.g., lymphoma)

Frequently the production of these autoantibodies against RBCs is not associated with any identifiable disease, and the resulting hemolytic anemia is therefore called idiopathic.

The direct Coombs test demonstrates that RBCs have been attacked by antibodies in the patient's bloodstream. The RBCs of patients suspected of having antibodies against RBCs are washed to eliminate any excess free gamma globulins. Coombs serum is added to the RBCs. If the RBCs have antibodies on them, Coombs serum will cause agglutination. The greater the quantity of antibodies against RBCs, the more clumping occurs. This test is read as *positive* with clumping on a scale of micro-positive to 4+. If the RBCs are not coated with autoantibodies against RBCs (immunoglobulins), agglutination will not occur; this is a *negative* test.

INTERFERING FACTORS

- Antiphospholipid antibodies (see p. 68, Anticardiolipin Antibodies) can cause a false-positive DAT.
- Drugs that may cause *false-positive* results include ampicillin, captopril, cephalosporins, chlorpromazine (Thorazine), chlorpropamide, hydralazine, indomethacin (Indocin), insulin, isoniazid (INH), levodopa, methyldopa (Aldomet), penicillin, phenytoin (Dilantin), procainamide, quinidine, quinine, rifampin, streptomycin, sulfonamides, and tetracyclines.

PROCEDURE AND PATIENT CARE

Before

🖎 Explain the procedure to the patient.
🖎 Tell the patient that no fasting is required.

During

• Collect a venous blood sample in a red-top or lavender-top tube.
• Use venous blood from the umbilical cord to detect the presence of antibodies in the newborn.

After

• Apply pressure or a pressure dressing to the venipuncture site.
• Assess the venipuncture site for bleeding.

TEST RESULTS AND CLINICAL SIGNIFICANCE

Hemolytic disease of the newborn,
Incompatible blood transfusion reaction:
   Antibodies to the patient's RBCs have been created by mixing of incompatible blood grouping antigens.
Lymphoma,
Autoimmune hemolytic anemia (rheumatoid/collagen diseases, e.g., systemic lupus erythematosus [SLE], rheumatoid arthritis [RA]):
   Autoantibodies formed in these illnesses attach to RBCs.
Mycoplasmal infection,
Infectious mononucleosis:
   In these illnesses, antibodies develop and for unknown reasons attach to the RBCs.
Hemolytic anemia after heart bypass: *Autoantibodies formed during the use of the heart/lung bypass machine attach to RBCs.*
Adult hemolytic anemia (idiopathic): *Autoantibodies not otherwise associated with any other disease attach to RBCs.*

RELATED TEST

Coombs Test, Indirect (see following test). This test is used to detect antibodies against RBCs in the serum. It is most commonly used for screening potential blood recipients.

Coombs Test, Indirect (Blood Antibody Screening, Indirect Antiglobulin Test [IAT])

NORMAL FINDINGS

Negative; no agglutination

INDICATIONS

This test is used to detect antibodies against red blood cells (RBCs) in the serum. This laboratory method is used most commonly for screening potential blood recipients.

TEST EXPLANATION

The indirect Coombs test detects circulating antibodies against RBCs. The major purpose of this test is to determine if the patient has minor serum antibodies (other than the major ABO/Rh system) to RBCs before receiving a blood transfusion. Therefore this test is the "screening" portion of the "type and screen" routinely performed for blood compatibility testing (crossmatching in the blood bank). This test is also used to detect other agglutinins, such as cold agglutinins that are associated with mycoplasmal infections.

In this test a small amount of the recipient's serum is added to donor RBCs containing known antigens on their surfaces. This is the first stage. In the second stage of the test, Coombs serum is added after the test RBCs have been washed of any free globulins. If antibodies exist in the patient's serum, agglutination occurs. In blood transfusion screening, visible agglutination indicates that the recipient has antibodies to the donor's RBCs. If the recipient has no antibodies against the donor's RBCs, agglutination will not occur; transfusion should then proceed safely without any transfusion reaction. Circulating antibodies against RBCs also may occur in an Rh-negative pregnant woman who is carrying an Rh-positive fetus.

INTERFERING FACTORS

Drugs that may cause *false-positive* results include antiarrhythmics, antituberculins, cephalosporins, chlorpromazine (Thorazine), insulin, levodopa, methyldopa (Aldomet), penicillins, phenytoin (Dilantin), quinidine, sulfonamides, and tetracyclines.

Clinical Priorities

- This test is the "screening" portion of the "type and screen" routinely performed for blood compatibility testing.
- If the recipient of the blood transfusion has antibodies to the donor's RBCs, agglutination occurs. The blood cannot be used for that recipient.
- If the recipient has no antibodies to the donor's RBCs, agglutination will not occur. Transfusion should then proceed safely without any transfusion reaction.

PROCEDURE AND PATIENT CARE

Before

- Explain the procedure to the patient.
- Tell the patient that no fasting is required.

During

- Collect a venous blood sample in a red-top tube.

After

- Apply pressure or a pressure dressing to the venipuncture site.
- Assess the venipuncture site for bleeding.
- Remember that if this antibody screening test is positive, antibody identification is then done.

TEST RESULTS AND CLINICAL SIGNIFICANCE

Incompatible crossmatched blood: *ABO/Rh antigens in the donor blood cross-react with the patient's serum.* Maternal anti-Rh antibodies,

Hemolytic disease of the newborn:

Antibodies result from previous exposure to fetal Rh+ RBCs.

Acquired immune hemolytic anemia,

Presence of specific cold agglutinin antibody: *Drugs and other illnesses are associated with the development of antibodies detected in the patient's serum.*

RELATED TEST

Coombs Test, Direct (p. 175). This test is performed to identify hemolysis or to investigate hemolytic transfusion reactions.

Cortisol, Blood (Hydrocortisone, Serum Cortisol, Salivary Cortisol)

NORMAL FINDINGS

Serum

Adult/elderly

    8 AM: 5-23 mcg/dL or 138-635 nmol/L (SI units)

    4 PM: 3-13 mcg/dL or 83-359 nmol/L (SI units)

Child 1-16 years

    8 AM: 3-21 mcg/dL

    4 PM: 3-10 mcg/dL

Newborn: 1-24 mcg/dL

Saliva

    7 AM-9 AM: 100-750 ng/dL

    3 pm-5 pm: <401 ng/dL

    11 pm-midnight: <100 ng/dL

INDICATIONS

This test is a measure of serum cortisol. It is performed on patients who are suspected to have hyperfunctioning or hypofunctioning adrenal glands.

TEST EXPLANATION

An elaborate feedback mechanism for cortisol coordinates the function of the hypothalamus, pituitary gland, and adrenal glands. Corticotropin-releasing hormone (CRH) is made in the hypothalamus. This stimulates adrenocorticotropic hormone (ACTH) production in the anterior pituitary gland. ACTH stimulates the adrenal cortex to produce cortisol. The rising levels of cortisol act as a negative feedback to curtail further production of CRH and ACTH. Cortisol is a potent glucocorticoid released from the adrenal cortex. This hormone affects the metabolism of carbohydrates, proteins, and fats. It has a profound effect on glucose serum levels. Cortisol tends to increase glucose by stimulating gluconeogenesis from glucose stores. It also inhibits the effect of insulin and thereby inhibits glucose transport into the cells.

    The best method of evaluating adrenal activity is by directly measuring plasma cortisol levels. Normally cortisol levels rise and fall during the day; this is called the diurnal variation. Cortisol levels are highest around 6 AM to 8 AM and gradually fall during the day, reaching their lowest point around midnight.

Sometimes the earliest sign of adrenal hyperfunction is only the loss of this diurnal variation, even though the cortisol levels are not yet elevated. For example, individuals with Cushing syndrome often have upper normal plasma cortisol levels in the morning and do not exhibit a decline as the day proceeds. High levels of cortisol indicate Cushing syndrome, and low levels of plasma cortisol are suggestive of Addison disease.

For this test, blood is usually collected at 8 AM and again at around 4 PM. The 4 PM value is anticipated to be one third to two thirds of the 8 AM value. Normal values may be transposed in individuals who have worked during the night and slept during the day for long periods of time.

Serum cortisol assay is measured by an automated competitive binding immunoenzymatic assay. Cortisol can be measured in the urine (p. 920). The measurement of late-night *salivary cortisol* is another effective test for Cushing syndrome. It seems to be more convenient and superior to plasma and urine for detecting cortisol in patients with mild Cushing syndrome. Salivary cortisol assay cannot be used to diagnose hypocortisolism or Addison disease because liquid chromatography-tandem mass spectrometry laboratory methods are not sensitive enough at low levels. If late-night salivary cortisol levels are elevated, the results should be confirmed with a repeat salivary cortisol measurement, a midnight blood sampling for cortisol, or a 24-hour urinary collection of free cortisol. A dexamethasone suppression test (p. 204) is another confirmation test that can be used.

INTERFERING FACTORS

- Pregnancy is associated with increased levels.
- Physical and emotional stress can elevate cortisol levels. Stress stimulates the pituitary-cortical mechanism and thereby stimulates cortisol production.
- Drugs that may cause *increased* levels include amphetamines, cortisone, estrogen, oral contraceptives, and spironolactone (Aldactone).
- Drugs that may cause *decreased* levels include androgens, aminoglutethimide, betamethasone and other exogenous steroid medications, danazol, lithium, levodopa, metyrapone, and phenytoin (Dilantin).

Clinical Priorities

- Cortisol levels are affected by a diurnal variation, with peak levels occurring around 6 AM to 8 AM and the lowest levels around midnight.
- Blood levels are usually drawn at 8 AM and again around 4 PM. The 4-PM level is usually one third to two thirds of the morning level.
- Physical and emotional stress can elevate cortisol levels.

PROCEDURE AND PATIENT CARE

Before

✒ Explain the procedure to the patient to minimize anxiety.
- Assess the patient for signs of physical stress (e.g., infection, acute illness) or emotional stress and report these to the physician.

During

Blood
- Collect a venous blood sample in a red-top or green-top tube in the morning after the patient has had a good night's sleep.
- Collect another blood sample at about 4 PM.
- Indicate the time of the venipuncture on the laboratory slip.

Saliva

1. Do not brush teeth before collecting specimen.
2. Do not eat or drink for 15 minutes before specimen collection.
3. Collect specimen between 11 PM and midnight, and record collection time.
4. Collect at least 1.5 mL of saliva in a Salivette as follows:
   a. Place swab directly into mouth by tipping container so swab falls into mouth. Do not touch swab with fingers.
   b. Keep swab in mouth for approximately 2 minutes. Roll swab in mouth, do not chew swab.
   c. Place swab back into its container without touching, and replace the cap.

After

- Apply pressure or a pressure dressing to the venipuncture site.
- Observe the venipuncture site for bleeding.

TEST RESULTS AND CLINICAL SIGNIFICANCE

▲   Increased Levels

Cushing disease,

Ectopic ACTH-producing tumors,

Stress:
> *ACTH is overproduced as a result of neoplastic overproduction of ACTH in the pituitary or elsewhere in the body by an ACTH-producing cancer. Stress is a potent stimulus to ACTH production. Cortisol rises as a result.*

Cushing syndrome (adrenal adenoma or carcinoma): *The neoplasm produces cortisol without regard to the normal feedback mechanism.*

Hyperthyroidism: *The metabolic rate is increased and cortisol levels rise accordingly to maintain the elevated glucose needs.*

Obesity: *All sterols are increased in the obese, perhaps because fatty tissue may act as a depository or site of synthesis.*

▼   Decreased Levels

Adrenal hyperplasia: *The congenital absence of important enzymes in the synthesis of cortisol prevents adequate serum levels.*

Addison disease: *As a result of hypofunctioning of the adrenal gland, cortisol levels drop.*

Hypopituitarism: *ACTH is not produced by the pituitary gland, which is destroyed by disease, neoplasm, or ischemia. The adrenal gland is not stimulated to produce cortisol.*

Hypothyroidism: *Normal cortisol levels are not required to maintain the reduced metabolic rate of hypothyroid patients.*

RELATED TESTS

Adrenocorticotropic Hormone (ACTH) Stimulation (p. 34). This test is used for the differential diagnosis of Cushing syndrome or Addison disease.

Adrenocorticotropic (ACTH) Hormone (p. 31). The serum ACTH study is a test of anterior pituitary gland function that affords the greatest insight into the causes of either Cushing syndrome (overproduction of cortisol) or Addison disease (underproduction of cortisol).

Dexamethasone Suppression (p. 204). This test is important for diagnosing Cushing syndrome and distinguishing its cause.

Cortisol, Urine (p. 920). This test is a measure of urinary cortisol. It is performed on patients who are suspected to have hyperfunctioning or hypofunctioning adrenal glands.

 C-Peptide (Connecting Peptide Insulin, Insulin C-Peptide, Proinsulin C-Peptide)

NORMAL FINDINGS

Fasting: 0.78-1.89 ng/mL or 0.26-0.62 nmol/L (SI units)
1 hour after glucose load: 5-12 ng/mL

INDICATIONS

This test is used to evaluate diabetic patients and to identify patients who secretly self-administer insulin. C-peptide is also helpful in monitoring patients with insulinomas (tumors of the insulin-secreting cells of the islets of Langerhans).

TEST EXPLANATION

C-peptide (connecting peptide) is a protein that connects the beta and alpha chains of proinsulin. In the beta cells of the islet of Langerhans of the pancreas, the chains of proinsulin are separated during the conversion of proinsulin to insulin and C-peptide. C-peptide is released into the portal vein in nearly equal amounts. Because it has a longer half-life than insulin, more C-peptide exists in the peripheral circulation. In general, C-peptide levels correlate with insulin levels in the blood, except possibly in islet cell tumors and in obese patients. The capacity of the pancreatic beta cells to secrete insulin can be evaluated by directly measuring either insulin or C-peptide. In most cases, direct measurement of insulin is more accurate. However, in some instances, direct measurement of insulin does not accurately assess the patient's insulin-generating capability. C-peptide levels more accurately reflect islet cell function in the following situations:

1. Patients with diabetes who are treated with insulin and who have antiinsulin antibodies. This most often occurs in patients treated with old bovine or pork insulin. These antibodies falsely increase insulin levels.
2. Patients who secretly administer insulin to themselves (factitious hypoglycemia). Insulin levels will be elevated. Direct insulin measurement in these patients tends to be high, because the insulin measured is self-administered exogenous insulin. But C-peptide levels in that same specimen will be low, because exogenously administered insulin suppresses endogenous insulin (and C-peptide) production.
3. Diabetic patients who are taking insulin. The exogenously administered insulin suppresses endogenous insulin production. Insulin levels only measure the exogenously administered insulin and do not accurately reflect true islet cell function. C-peptide would be a more accurate test of islet cell function. This is performed to see if the diabetes is in remission and the patient may not need exogenous insulin.
4. Distinguishing type 1 from type 2 diabetes. This is particularly helpful in newly diagnosed diabetics. A person whose pancreas does not make any insulin (type 1 diabetes) has a low level of insulin and C-peptide. A person with type 2 diabetes has a normal or high level of C-peptide.

The C-peptide test is indicated for the clinical situations described above. Further, C-peptide is used in evaluating patients who are suspected to have an insulinoma. It can differentiate patients with insulinoma from patients with factitious hypoglycemia. In the latter patients, C-peptide levels are suppressed by exogenous insulin challenge. In patients with an autonomous secreting insulinoma, C-peptide levels are not suppressed. Furthermore, C-peptide can be used to monitor treated patients with insulinoma. A rise in C-peptide levels indicates a recurrence or progression of the insulinoma. Likewise, some clinicians use C-peptide testing as an indicator of the adequacy of therapeutic surgical pancreatectomy in patients with pancreatic tumors. C-peptide can also be used to diagnose "insulin resistance" syndrome.

INTERFERING FACTORS

- Because the majority of C-peptide is degraded in the kidney, renal failure can cause increased levels of C-peptide.
- Drugs that may cause *increased* levels of C-peptide include oral hypoglycemic agents (e.g., sulfonylureas).

PROCEDURE AND PATIENT CARE

Before
Explain the procedure to the patient.
Instruct the patient to fast for 8 to 10 hours before the test. Only water is permitted.

During
- Collect a venous blood sample in a red-top tube.

After
- Apply pressure or a pressure dressing to the venipuncture site.
- Assess the venipuncture site for bleeding.

TEST RESULTS AND CLINICAL SIGNIFICANCE

▲ Increased Levels
Insulinoma: *Insulin and C-peptide are made concomitantly by the neoplastic cells.*
Pancreas transplant: *Excess C-peptide is produced by the transplanted islet cells.*
Renal failure: *C-peptide is removed from the blood by the kidneys. Diminished kidney function will lead to elevated levels.*
Administration of oral hypoglycemic agents: *Oral hypoglycemic agents stimulate insulin and C-peptide synthesis.*

▼ Decreased Levels
Factitious hypoglycemia,
Diabetes mellitus:
   The self-administered insulin suppresses endogenous insulin and C-peptide production.
Total pancreatectomy: *All islet cells have been surgically removed. C-peptide production ceases.*

RELATED TESTS

Glucose, Blood (p. 253). This is a measurement of serum glucose.
Glucagon (p. 251). This is a direct measurement of glucagon, an islet cell hormone that acts to increase serum glucose levels.

Glycosylated Hemoglobin (p. 266). This is a test to measure the amount of glycosylated hemoglobin, which is an indirect measure of the chronic state of glucose levels.

Insulin Assay (p. 315). This is a direct measurement of insulin, an islet cell hormone that acts to decrease serum glucose levels.

 C-Reactive Protein (CRP, High-Sensitivity C-Reactive Protein [hs-CRP])

NORMAL FINDINGS

<1.0 mg/dL or <10.0 mg/L (SI units)

Cardiac risk

    Low: <1.0 mg/L

    Average: 1.0 to 3.0 mg/L

    High: >3.0 mg/L

INDICATIONS

C-reactive protein (CRP) is an acute-phase reactant protein used to indicate an inflammatory illness. It is believed to be of value in predicting coronary events.

TEST EXPLANATION

CRP is a nonspecific, acute-phase reactant protein used to diagnose bacterial infectious disease and inflammatory disorders, such as acute rheumatic fever and rheumatoid arthritis. It is also elevated when there is tissue necrosis. CRP levels do not consistently rise with viral infections. CRP is a protein produced primarily by the liver during an acute inflammatory process and other diseases. A positive test result indicates the presence, but not the cause, of the disease. The synthesis of CRP is initiated by antigen-immune complexes, bacteria, fungi, and trauma. CRP is functionally analogous to immunoglobulin G, except that it is not antigen specific. CRP interacts with the complement system.

The CRP test is a more sensitive and rapidly responding indicator than the erythrocyte sedimentation rate (ESR). In an acute inflammatory change, CRP shows an earlier and more intense increase than ESR; with recovery, the disappearance of CRP precedes the return of ESR to normal. The CRP also disappears when the inflammatory process is suppressed by antiinflammatory agents, salicylates, or steroids.

This test is also useful in evaluating patients with an acute myocardial infarction (AMI). The level of CRP correlates with peak levels of the MB isoenzyme of creatine kinase (see p. 186), but CRP peaks occur 18 to 72 hours later. Failure of CRP to normalize may indicate ongoing damage to the heart tissue. Levels are not elevated in patients with angina.

Atheromatous plaques in diseased arteries typically contain inflammatory cells. Multiple prospective studies have also demonstrated that baseline CRP is a good marker of future cardiovascular events. The CRP level may be a stronger predictor of cardiovascular events than the low-density lipoprotein (LDL) cholesterol level. When used together with the lipid profile (see Lipid Panel, Appendix C), it adds prognostic information to that conveyed by the Framingham risk score.

Recent development of a *high sensitivity assay for CRP* (hs-CRP) has enabled accurate assays at even low levels. Atheromatous plaques in diseased arteries typically contain inflammatory cells. Multiple prospective studies have also demonstrated that baseline CRP is a good marker of future cardiovascular events. The CRP level may be a stronger predictor of cardiovascular events than the low-density lipoprotein (LDL) cholesterol level. When used together with the lipid profile (see Lipid Profile, Appendix C), it adds prognostic information to that conveyed by the Framingham risk score. Because of the individual variability in hs-CRP, two separate measurements are required to classify a person's risk level. In patients with stable coronary disease or acute coronary syndromes, hs-CRP measurement may be useful as an independent marker for assessing likelihood of recurrent events, including death, myocardial infarction (MI), or restenosis after percutaneous coronary intervention (PCI). hs-CRP is most commonly used when other causes of systemic inflammation have been eliminated.

Another indicator of inflammation besides CRP that is instigating considerable attention as a cardiac risk factor is *lipoprotein-associated phospholipase A$_2$* (Lp-PLA$_2$). Lp-PLA$_2$ promotes vascular inflammation through the hydrolysis of oxidized LDL within the intima, contributing directly to the atherogenic process. When combined with CRP, testing for Lp-PLA$_2$ markedly increases the predictive value in determining risk for a cardiac event, especially in patients whose cholesterol (see p. 154) is normal. The *PLAC test* is an enzyme-linked immunosorbent assay (ELISA) using two highly specific monoclonal antibodies to measure the level of Lp-PLA$_2$ in the blood.

The CRP test also may be used postoperatively to detect wound infections. CRP levels increase within 4 to 6 hours after surgery and generally begin to decrease after the third postoperative day. Failure of the levels to fall is an indicator of complications, such as infection or pulmonary infarction.

INTERFERING FACTORS

- Elevated test results can occur in patients with hypertension, elevated body mass index, metabolic syndrome/diabetes mellitus, chronic infection (gingivitis, bronchitis), chronic inflammation (rheumatoid arthritis), and low high-density lipoprotein (HDL)/high triglycerides.
- Cigarette smoking can cause increased levels.
- Decreased test levels can result from moderate alcohol consumption, weight loss, and increased activity or endurance exercise.
- Medications that may *increase* test results include estrogens and progesterones.
- Medications that may *decrease* test results include fibrates, niacin, and statins.

PROCEDURE AND PATIENT CARE

Before
- Explain the procedure to the patient.
- Tell the patient that fasting usually is not required; however, some laboratories require a 4- to 12-hour fast. Water is permitted.

During
- Collect one red-top tube of venous blood.

After
- Apply pressure or a pressure dressing to the venipuncture site.
- Assess the venipuncture site for bleeding.

TEST RESULTS AND CLINICAL SIGNIFICANCE

▲ Increased Levels

Acute, noninfectious inflammatory reaction (e.g., arthritis, acute rheumatic fever, Reiter syndrome, Crohn disease),

Collagen-vascular diseases (e.g., vasculitis syndrome, lupus erythematosus),

Tissue infarction or damage (e.g., acute myocardial infarction [AMI], pulmonary infarction, kidney or bone marrow transplant rejection, soft-tissue trauma),

Bacterial infections such as postoperative wound infection, urinary tract infection, or tuberculosis,

Malignant disease,

Bacterial infection (e.g., tuberculosis, meningitis):

> *These diseases are all associated with an inflammatory reaction that instigates the synthesis of CRP.*

Increased risk for cardiovascular ischemic events: *Inflammation of the intimal lining of a blood vessel, and particularly the coronary vessels, is associated with an increased risk for intimal injury thereby leading to distal vessel plaque occlusions.*

RELATED TESTS

Erythrocyte Sedimentation Rate (p. 221). This is also an acute-phase reactant protein. It is a nonspecific test used to detect inflammatory, infectious, and necrotic processes.

Complement Assay (p. 172). Not only are some of the complement components acute-phase reactant proteins, but CRP also interacts with this complex immune system.

Fibrinogen (p. 241). This is an important part of the hemostatic mechanism. It is also an acute-phase reactant protein.

Lipoproteins (p. 342). This is an important risk factor for heart disease.

Homocysteine (p. 301). This is an important risk factor for heart disease.

Creatine Kinase (CK, Creatine Phosphokinase [CPK])

NORMAL FINDINGS

Total CK

Adult/elderly (Values are higher after exercise.)
    Male: 55-170 units/L or 55-170 units/L (SI units)
    Female: 30-135 units/L or 30-135 units/L (SI units)
Newborn: 68-580 units/L (SI units)

Isoenzymes

CK-MM: 100%
CK-MB: 0%
CK-BB: 0%

INDICATIONS

This test is used to support the diagnosis of myocardial muscle injury (infarction). It can also indicate neurologic or skeletal muscle diseases.

TEST EXPLANATION

CK is found predominantly in the heart muscle, skeletal muscle, and brain. Serum CK levels are elevated when these muscle or nerve cells are injured. CK levels can rise within 6 hours after damage. If damage is not persistent, the levels peak at 18 hours after injury and return to normal in 2 to 3 days (Figure 2-14).

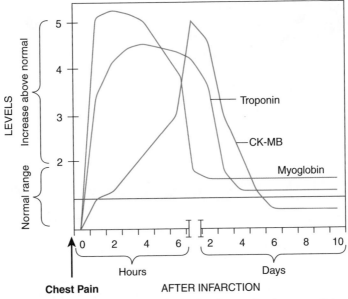

Figure 2-14 Blood studies useful in the diagnosis of myocardial infarction.

To test specifically for myocardial muscle injury, electrophoresis is performed to detect the three CK isoenzymes: CK-BB (CK1), CK-MB (CK2), and CK-MM (CK3). The CK-MB isoenzyme portion appears to be specific for myocardial cells. CK-MB levels rise 3 to 6 hours after infarction occurs. If there is no further myocardial damage, the level peaks at 12 to 24 hours and returns to normal 12 to 48 hours after infarction. CK-MB levels do not usually rise with transient chest pain caused by angina, pulmonary embolism, or congestive heart failure. One can expect to see a rise in CK-MB in patients with shock, malignant hyperthermia, myopathies, or myocarditis. Mild elevation of CK-MB (below the threshold of positive) can occur in patients with unstable angina and will signify an increased risk for an occlusive event. Very small amounts of CK-MB also exist in skeletal muscle. Severe injury to, or diseases of the skeletal muscle can also raise the CK-MB isoenzyme above normal.

The CK-MB isoenzyme level is helpful in both quantifying the degree of myocardial infarction (MI) and timing the onset of infarction. The CK-MB isoenzyme is often used to determine appropriateness of thrombolytic therapy, which is used for MI. High CK-MB levels would suggest that significant infarction has already occurred, thereby precluding the benefit of thrombolytic therapy.

Because the CK-BB isoenzyme is found predominantly in the brain and lung, injury to either of these organs (e.g., cerebrovascular accident, pulmonary infarction) will be associated with elevated levels of this isoenzyme.

The CK-MM isoenzyme normally makes up almost all of the circulatory total CK enzymes in healthy people. When the total CK level is elevated as a result of increases in CK-MM, injury to or disease of the skeletal muscle is present. Examples of this include myopathies, vigorous exercise, multiple intramuscular (IM) injections, electroconvulsive therapy, cardioversion, chronic alcoholism, or surgery. Because CK is made only in the skeletal muscle, the normal value of total CK (and therefore CK-MM) varies according to a person's muscle mass. Large muscular people may normally have a CK level in the high range of normal. Likewise, people of small stature or those with low muscle mass will be expected to have low CK levels. This is important because high normal CK levels in these patients can mask an MI.

TABLE 2-16   Timing of Appearance and Disappearance of Commonly Used Cardiac Enzymes

Enzyme	HOURS		DAYS
	Starts to Rise	Peaks	Returns to Normal
CK-MB	4	18	2
Troponin T	4-6	10-24	10
Troponin I	4-6	10-24	4

Clinical Priorities

- Avoid IM injections in patients with cardiac disease. IM injections can cause elevated CK levels.
- The CK-MB isoenzyme is helpful in both quantifying the degree of MI and timing the onset of the infarction.
- The CK-MB isoenzyme is often used to determine the appropriateness of thrombolytic therapy. High levels may indicate that significant infarction has already occurred, thus precluding a benefit from thrombolytic therapy.

Each isoenzyme has been found to have isoforms. The CK-MM isoforms MM1 and MM3 are most useful for cardiac disease. An MM3/MM1 ratio of greater than 1 suggests acute myocardial injury. A CK-MB ratio of MB2/MB1 greater than 1 also indicates acute myocardial injury.

CK is the main cardiac enzyme studied in patients with heart disease. Because its blood clearance and metabolism are well known, its frequent determination (on admission and at 12 hours and 24 hours) can accurately reflect timing, quantity, and resolution of an MI (see Figure 2-14). The clearance characteristics of commonly used cardiac enzymes are noted in Table 2-16.

New blood assays for cardiac markers have promised to rapidly and accurately detect acute MI (AMI) in the emergency room. One of these assays is troponin (see p. 508). A new assay is ischemia-modified albumin (see p. 326).

INTERFERING FACTORS

- Intramuscular (IM) injections can cause elevated CK levels.
- Strenuous exercise and recent surgery may cause increased levels.
- Early pregnancy may produce decreased levels.
- Muscle mass is directly related to a patient's normal CK level.
- Drugs that may cause *increased* levels include alcohol, amphotericin B, ampicillin, some anesthetics, anticoagulants, aspirin, captopril, clofibrate, colchicine, dexamethasone (Decadron), furosemide (Lasix), lithium, lidocaine, morphine, propranolol, statins, and succinylcholine.

PROCEDURE AND PATIENT CARE

Before

- Explain the procedure to the patient.
- Discuss with the patient the need and reason for frequent venipuncture in diagnosing MI.

- Avoid IM injections in patients with cardiac disease. These injections may falsely elevate the total CK level.
- Tell the patient that no food or fluid restrictions are necessary.

During

- Collect a venous blood sample in a red-top tube. This is usually done initially and 12 hours later, followed by daily testing for 3 days and then at 1 week.
- Rotate the venipuncture sites.
- Avoid hemolysis.
- Record the time and date of any IM injection.
- Record the exact time and date of venipuncture on each laboratory slip. This aids in the interpretation of the temporal pattern of enzyme elevations.

After

- Apply pressure or a pressure dressing to the venipuncture site.
- Observe the venipuncture site for bleeding.

TEST RESULTS AND CLINICAL SIGNIFICANCE

▲ Increased Levels of Total CK

Diseases or injury affecting the heart muscle, skeletal muscle, and brain.

▲ Increased Levels of CK-BB Isoenzyme

Diseases that affect the central nervous system (CNS) (e.g., brain injury, brain cancer, cerebrovascular accident [stroke], subarachnoid hemorrhage, seizures, shock, Reye syndrome)
Electroconvulsive therapy
Adenocarcinoma (especially breast and lung): *The pathophysiology of this observation is not known.*
Pulmonary infarction: *The lung tissue has small amounts of CK-BB. With cellular injury of this organ, the contents of the cell, including CK, spill out into the bloodstream, causing elevated CK-BB isoenzyme levels.*

▲ Increased Levels of CK-MB Isoenzyme

AMI,
Cardiac aneurysm surgery,
Cardiac defibrillation,
Myocarditis,
Ventricular arrhythmias,
Cardiac ischemia:
  Any disease or injury to the myocardium causes CK-MB to spill out of the damaged cells and into the bloodstream, producing elevated CK-MB isoenzyme levels.

▲ Increased Levels of CK-MM Isoenzyme

Rhabdomyolysis,
Muscular dystrophy,
Myositis:
  Diseases affecting skeletal muscle cause CK-MM to spill out of the damaged cells and into the bloodstream, producing elevated CK-MM isoenzyme levels.
Recent surgery,
Electromyography,

IM injections,

Trauma,

Crush injuries:

> *Injury affecting skeletal muscle causes CK-MM to spill out of the damaged cells and into the bloodstream, producing elevated CK-MM isoenzyme levels.*

Delirium tremens,

Malignant hyperthermia,

Recent convulsions,

Electroconvulsive therapy,

Shock:

> *Anoxic injury from lack of blood supply or repetitive muscular motion can cause injury to skeletal muscle. This causes CK-MM to spill out of the damaged cells and into the bloodstream, producing elevated CK-MM isoenzyme levels.*

Hypokalemia,

Hypothyroidism:

> *These diseases have a metabolic effect on skeletal muscle. Muscle injury results. This causes CK-MM to spill out of the damaged cells and into the bloodstream, producing elevated CK-MM isoenzyme levels.*

RELATED TESTS

Aspartate Aminotransferase (AST) (p. 119). Elevated levels of this enzyme may indicate cardiac injury. It is not specific to the heart, however.

Lactic Dehydrogenase (LDH) (p. 329). This intracellular enzyme is used to support the diagnosis of injury or disease involving the heart, liver, red blood cells, kidneys, skeletal muscle, brain, and lungs.

Alanine Aminotransferase (ALT) (see p. 39). This enzyme is used similarly to AST and exists predominantly in the liver.

Leucine Aminopeptidase (LAP) (see p. 337). This enzyme is specific to the hepatobiliary system. Diseases affecting that system will cause elevation of this enzyme.

Gamma-Glutamyl Transpeptidase (GGTP) (p. 246). This is another enzyme existing predominantly in the liver.

Alkaline Phosphatase (p. 47). This is another enzyme existing predominantly in the liver.

5'-Nucleotidase (p. 376). This is another enzyme existing predominantly in the liver.

Troponins (p. 508). This is a biochemical marker used to assist in the evaluation of patients with chest pain.

 Creatinine, Blood (Serum Creatinine)

NORMAL FINDINGS

Less than 2 years: 0.1-0.4 mg/dL

2 years to <6 years: 0.2-0.5 mg/dL

6 years to <10 years: 0.3-0.6 mg/dL

10 years to <18 years: 0.4-1.0 mg/dL

18 years to <41 years: Female: 0.5-1.0 mg/dL

18 years to <41 years: Male: 0.6-1.2 mg/dL

41 years to <61 years: Female: 0.5-1.1 mg/dL
41 years to <61 years: Male: 0.6-1.3 mg/dL
61 years and above: Female: 0.5-1.2 mg/dL
61 years and above: Male: 0.7-1.3 mg/dL

 Critical Values

>4 mg/dL (indicates serious impairment in renal function)

INDICATIONS

Creatinine is used to diagnose impaired renal function.

TEST EXPLANATION

This test measures the amount of creatinine in the blood. Creatinine is a catabolic product of creatine phosphate, which is used in skeletal muscle contraction. The daily production of creatine, and subsequently creatinine, depends on muscle mass, which fluctuates very little. Creatinine, as blood urea nitrogen (BUN), is excreted entirely by the kidneys and therefore is directly proportional to renal excretory function. Thus, with normal renal excretory function, the serum creatinine level should remain constant and normal. Besides dehydration, only renal disorders, such as glomerulonephritis, pyelonephritis, acute tubular necrosis, and urinary obstruction, will cause an abnormal elevation in creatinine. There are slight increases in creatinine levels after meals, especially after ingestion of large quantities of meat. Furthermore, there may be some diurnal variation in creatinine (nadir at 7 AM and peak at 7 PM).

The serum creatinine test, as with the BUN, is used to diagnose impaired renal function. Unlike the BUN, however, the creatinine level is affected minimally by hepatic function. The creatinine is used as an approximation of the glomerular filtration rate (GFR). The serum creatinine level has much the same significance as the BUN level but tends to rise later. Therefore elevations in creatinine suggest chronicity of the disease process. In general, a doubling of creatinine suggests a 50% reduction in the glomerular filtration rate. The creatinine level is interpreted in conjunction with the BUN. These tests are referred to as *renal function studies:* The BUN/creatinine ratio is a good measurement of kidney and liver function. The normal range is 6 to 25, with 15.5 being the optimal adult value for this ratio.

While serum creatinine is the most commonly used biochemical parameter to estimate GFR in routine practice, there are some shortcomings to the use of this parameter. Factors such as muscle mass and protein intake can influence serum creatinine, leading to an inaccurate estimation of GFR. Moreover, in unstable, critically ill patients, acute changes in renal function can make real-time evaluation of GFR using serum creatinine difficult. On the other hand, *cystatin C,* a protein that is produced at a constant rate by all nucleated cells, is probably a better indicator of GFR. Because of its constant rate of production, its serum concentration is determined only by glomerular filtration. Its level is not influenced by those factors that affect creatinine and BUN.

Cystatin C might predict the risk for developing *chronic kidney disease,* thereby signaling a state of "preclinical" kidney dysfunction. Several studies have found that increased levels of cystatin C are associated with the risk for death, several types of cardiovascular disease (including myocardial infarction, stroke, heart failure, peripheral arterial disease, and metabolic syndrome). For women, the average reference interval is 0.52 to 0.90 mg/L with a mean of 0.71 mg/L. For men, the average reference interval is 0.56 to 0.98 mg/L with a mean of 0.77 mg/L.

Age-Related Concerns

- The elderly and young children normally have lower creatinine levels as a result of reduced muscle mass. This may potentially mask renal disease in patients of these age groups.

INTERFERING FACTORS

- A diet high in meat content can cause transient elevations of serum creatinine.
- Drugs that may *increase* creatinine values include ACE inhibitors, aminoglycosides (e.g., gentamicin), cimetidine, heavy-metal chemotherapeutic agents (e.g., cisplatin), and other nephrotoxic drugs such as cephalosporins (e.g., cefoxitin).

PROCEDURE AND PATIENT CARE

Before
- Explain the procedure to the patient.
- Tell the patient that no fasting is required.

During
- Collect a venous blood sample in a red-top tube.
- For pediatric patients, blood is usually drawn from a heel stick.

After
- Apply pressure or a pressure dressing to the venipuncture site.
- Observe the venipuncture site for bleeding.

TEST RESULTS AND CLINICAL SIGNIFICANCE

▲ Increased Levels

Diseases affecting renal function, such as glomerulonephritis, pyelonephritis, acute tubular necrosis, urinary tract obstruction, reduced renal blood flow (e.g., shock, dehydration, congestive heart failure [CHF], atherosclerosis), diabetic nephropathy, nephritis: *With these illnesses, renal function is impaired and creatinine levels rise.*

Rhabdomyolysis: *Injury of the skeletal muscle causes myoglobin to be released in the bloodstream. Large amounts are nephrotoxic. Creatinine levels rise.*

Acromegaly,
Gigantism:
   These diseases are associated with increased muscle mass, which causes the "normal" creatinine level to be high.

▼ Decreased Levels

Debilitation,
Decreased muscle mass (e.g., muscular dystrophy, myasthenia gravis [MG]):
   These diseases are associated with decreased muscle mass, which causes the "normal" creatinine level to be low.

RELATED TESTS

Blood Urea Nitrogen (BUN) (p. 511). This is a test of renal function. Unlike creatinine, there are many nonrenal factors that can alter this test result.

Creatinine Clearance (see following test). This is a more accurate measurement of renal function. It is a direct measurement of glomerular filtration rate.

Creatinine Clearance (CrCl)

NORMAL FINDINGS

Adult (<40 years)
    Male: 107-139 mL/min or 1.78-2.32 mL/sec (SI units)
    Female: 87-107 mL/min or 1.45-1.78 mL/sec (SI units)
Values decrease 6.5 mL/min/decade of life after age 20 years with decline in glomerular filtration rate (GFR).
Newborn: 40-65 mL/min
eGFR: >60 mL/min/1.73 m^2

INDICATIONS

The creatinine clearance is used to measure the GFR of the kidney.

TEST EXPLANATION

Creatinine is a catabolic product of creatine phosphate, which is used in skeletal muscle contraction. The daily production of creatine, and subsequently creatinine, depends on muscle mass, which fluctuates very little. Creatinine is excreted entirely by the kidneys and therefore is directly proportional to the GFR (i.e., the number of milliliters of filtrate made by the kidneys per minute). CrCl is a measure of the GFR. Urine and serum creatinine levels are assessed and the clearance rate is calculated.

The amount of filtrate made in the kidney depends on the amount of blood to be filtered and on the ability of the nephron to act as a filter. The amount of blood present for filtration is decreased in renal artery atherosclerosis, dehydration, and shock. The ability of the nephron to act as a filter is decreased by diseases such as glomerulonephritis, acute tubular necrosis, and most other primary renal diseases. Significant bilateral obstruction to urinary outflow affects glomerular filtration (CrCl) only after it is long-standing.

When one kidney alone becomes diseased, the opposite kidney, if normal, has the ability to compensate by increasing its filtration rate. Therefore, with unilateral kidney disease or nephrectomy, a decrease in CrCl is not expected if the other kidney is normal.

Several nonrenal factors may influence CrCl. With each decade of age, the CrCl decreases 6.5 mL/min because of a decrease in the GFR. Because urine collections are timed, incomplete collections will falsely decrease CrCl. Muscle mass varies among people. Decreased muscle mass will give lower CrCl values. Likewise, ingestion of large amounts of meat will temporarily increase CrCl.

 Age-Related Concerns

- Adult values decrease 6.5 mL/min with each decade of life after age 20 years because of a decrease in GFR.

The CrCl test requires a 24-hour urine collection and a serum creatinine level. CrCl is then computed using the following formula:

$$\text{Creatinine clearance} = UV/P$$

where

U = number of milligrams per deciliter of creatinine excreted in the urine over 24 hours
V = volume of urine in milliliters per minute
P = serum creatinine in milligrams per deciliter

Creatinine values are often used to assess the completeness of a 24-hour urine collection. In patients with normal creatinine, the CrCl should indicate whether all the urine has been collected for the full 24 hours.

The 24-hour urine collections used to measure CC are too time consuming and expensive for routine clinical use. The GFR can be estimated (*estimated GFR [eGFR]*) using the Modification of Diet in Renal Disease (MDRD) Study equation. This is an equation that uses the serum creatinine, age, and numbers that vary depending upon sex and ethnicity to calculate the GFR with very good accuracy. The prediction equation for GFR is as follows, with Pcr being serum or plasma creatinine in mg/dL:

$$GFR \left(mL/min/1.73m^2\right) = 1.86 \times (Pcr)^{-1.154} \times (age)^{-0.203}$$
$$\times (0.742 \text{ if female}) \times (1.210 \text{ if African American})$$

The GFR is expressed in mL/min/1.73 m²

An increasing number of institutions across the country are beginning to report an eGFR on patients who are 18 years and older with every serum creatinine ordered. The eGFR calculation can be programmed into most laboratory information systems. As a result, chronic renal disease is being recognized more frequently in its early stages. Chronic kidney disease can be treated and progression to renal failure slowed or prevented. For example, if a patient with diabetes is found to have a reduced GFR of 49 at an annual examination, that patient's primary care physician can and should take steps to treat the early chronic kidney disease. This may include the use of ACE inhibitors, more aggressive treatment of high blood pressure, glycemic dietary control, and treatment of high cardiac risk factors. The eGFR can be used to calculate medication dosage in patients with decreased renal function.

Table 2-17 shows population estimates for mean (average) estimated glomerular filtration rate (eGFR) by age. There is no difference between races or sexes when eGFRs are expressed per square meter of body surface area. For diagnostic purposes, most laboratories report eGFR values above 60 as ">60 mL/min/1.73 m²," not as an exact number.

TABLE 2-17   Mean Estimated GFR (eGFR)

Age (Years)	Mean eGFR
20-29	116 mL/min/1.73 m²
30-39	107 mL/min/1.73 m²
40-49	99 mL/min/1.73 m²
50-59	93 mL/min/1.73 m²
60-69	85 mL/min/1.73 m²
70+	75 mL/min/1.73 m²

Cystatin C is a cysteine proteinase inhibitor that is produced by all nucleated cells and found in serum. Since it is formed at a constant rate and freely filtered by the kidneys, its serum concentration (like creatinine) is another accurate test that can estimate GFR.

INTERFERING FACTORS

- Exercise may cause increased creatinine values.
- Incomplete urine collection may give a falsely lowered value.
- Pregnancy increases CrCl. This is due in part to the increased load placed on the kidneys by the growing fetus.
- A diet high in meat can cause transient elevation of the serum creatinine and CrCl. When the creatinine is high, its clearance is increased. Therefore the CrCl overestimates the GFR.
- The eGFR may be inaccurate in extremes of age and in patients with severe malnutrition or obesity, paraplegia or quadriplegia, and in pregnant women.
- Drugs that may cause *increased* levels include aminoglycosides (e.g., gentamicin), cimetidine, heavy-metal chemotherapeutic agents (e.g., cisplatin), and nephrotoxic drugs such as cephalosporins (e.g., cefoxitin).
- Drugs that may cause a *decrease* in eGFR interfere with creatinine secretion (e.g., cimetidine or trimethoprim) or creatinine assay (cephalosporins). In these cases, a 24-hour creatinine clearance may be necessary to accurately estimate kidney function.

PROCEDURE AND PATIENT CARE

Before

- Explain the procedure to the patient.
- Tell the patient that no special diet is usually required.
- Note that some laboratories instruct the patient to avoid cooked meat, tea, coffee, or drugs on the day of the test. Check with the laboratory.

During

- See Box 11-2, Guidelines for 24-Hour Urine Collection, p. 907.
- Encourage the patient to drink fluids during the 24-hour collection unless this is contraindicated for medical purposes.
- Instruct the patient to avoid vigorous exercise during the 24 hours, because exercise may cause an increased CrCl.
- Make sure a venous blood sample is drawn in a red-top tube during the 24-hour collection.
- Mark the patient's age, weight, and height on the requisition sheet.

After

- Transport the urine specimen promptly to the laboratory.
- Apply pressure or a pressure dressing to the venipuncture site.

TEST RESULTS AND CLINICAL SIGNIFICANCE

▲ Increased Levels

Exercise,
Pregnancy,
High cardiac output syndromes:
   As blood flow increases to the kidney, GFR and CrCl increase.

▼ Decreased Levels

Impaired kidney function (e.g., renal artery atherosclerosis, glomerulonephritis, acute tubular necrosis),

Conditions causing decreased GFR (e.g., congestive heart failure [CHF], cirrhosis with ascites, shock, dehydration):
Conditions that are associated with decreased blood flow to the kidney will decrease GFR.

RELATED TESTS

Blood Urea Nitrogen (BUN) (p. 511). This is a test of renal function. Unlike creatinine, there are many nonrenal factors that can alter this test result.

Creatinine, Blood (p. 190). The creatinine is used to diagnose impaired renal function.

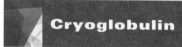

NORMAL FINDINGS

No cryoglobulins detected

INDICATIONS

This test is performed to identify cryoglobulins in patients with symptoms of purpura, arthralgia, or Raynaud phenomenon. Cryoglobulin testing is used to support the diagnosis of the diseases that are known to be associated with cryoglobulins.

TEST EXPLANATION

Cryoglobulins are abnormal immunoglobulin protein complexes that exist within the blood of patients with various diseases. These proteins will precipitate reversibly at low temperatures and will redissolve with rewarming. These cryoglobulins can precipitate within the blood vessels of the fingers when exposed to cold temperatures. This precipitation causes slugging of the blood within those blood vessels. These patients may have symptoms of purpura, arthralgia, or Raynaud phenomenon (pain, cyanosis, coldness of the fingers).

These proteins exist in varying quantities, depending on the disease entity with which they are associated. The cryoglobulins can be classified, which helps determine the underlying disease state. Type I (monoclonal) cryoglobulinemia is associated with monoclonal gammopathy of undetermined significance, macroglobulinemia, or multiple myeloma. Type II (mixed, two or more immunoglobulins of which one is monoclonal) cryoglobulinemia is associated with autoimmune disorders, such as vasculitis, glomerulonephritis, systemic lupus erythematosus, rheumatoid arthritis, and Sjögren syndrome. It may also be seen in such infections as hepatitis, infectious mononucleosis, cytomegalovirus, and toxoplasmosis. Type II cryoglobulinemia may also be essential (i.e., occurring in the absence of underlying disease). Type III (polyclonal) cryoglobulinemia is associated with the same disease spectrum as Type II cryoglobulinemia.

For this test, the blood sample is taken to the chemistry laboratory, where it is refrigerated for 72 hours. After that time the specimen is evaluated for precipitation. If precipitation is identified, it is measured and recorded. The tube is then rewarmed, and the specimen is reexamined for dissolution of that precipitation. If precipitation of the refrigerated specimen is identified and dissolved on re-warming, cryoglobulins are present. If cryoglobulin qualitative is positive, then immunofixation elec-trophoresis typing and quantitative IgA, IgG, and IgM is performed to classify the type of cryoglobu-lin that exists.

PROCEDURE AND PATIENT CARE

Before

✗ Explain the procedure to the patient.

✗ Inform the patient that an 8-hour fast may be required. This will minimize turbidity of the serum caused by ingestion of a recent (especially fatty) meal. Turbidity may make the detection of precipita-tion rather difficult.

During

• Collect a venous blood sample in a red-top tube that has been prewarmed to body temperature.

After

• Apply pressure or a pressure dressing to the venipuncture site.
• Observe the venipuncture site for bleeding.

✗ If cryoglobulins are present, warn the patient to avoid cold temperatures and contact with cold ob-jects to minimize Raynaud symptoms. Tell the patient to wear gloves in cold weather.

TEST RESULTS AND CLINICAL SIGNIFICANCE

The following is a list of diseases associated with the presence of cryoglobulins:

Connective tissue disease (e.g., lupus erythematosus, Sjögren syndrome, RA)

Lymphoid malignancies (e.g., multiple myeloma, leukemia, Waldenström macroglobulinemia, lym-phoma)

Acute and chronic infections (e.g., infectious mononucleosis, endocarditis, poststreptoccocal glomeru-lonephritis)

Liver disease (e.g., hepatitis, cirrhosis)

RELATED TESTS

Agglutinin, Febrile/Cold (pp. 233 and 170). These agglutinins are antibodies that cause red blood cells to aggregate at high or low temperatures, respectively.

Rheumatoid Factor (p. 454). This test is useful in the diagnosis of RA. Other diseases, such as SLE, may cause a positive result.

Cutaneous Immunofluorescence Antibodies
(Indirect IFA Antibodies, Anti–Basement Zone Antibodies, Anti–Cell Surface Antibodies)

NORMAL FINDINGS

No evidence of antibodies

INDICATIONS

This test is used to diagnose and monitor autoimmune-mediated dermatitis and paraneoplastic dermatitis.

TEST EXPLANATION

Autoimmune-mediated skin lesions are often associated with the presence of elevated levels of antibodies in the serum (see Antiscleroderma Antibody, p. 93) and in the skin (see Skin Biopsy, p. 760). IgG anti-basement zone (BMZ) antibodies are produced by patients with pemphigoid, epidermolysis bullosa acquisita (EBA), and bullous eruption of lupus erythematosus (LE). The titer of anti-CS antibodies generally correlates with disease activity of pemphigus. This test is useful for confirming a diagnosis of these diseases and monitoring therapeutic response. Indirect immunofluorescence (IF) testing may be diagnostic when histologic or direct IF studies are only suggestive, nonspecific, or negative.

Anti–cell surface (CS) antibodies correlate with a diagnosis of pemphigus.

Anti–basement zone (BMZ) antibodies correlate with a diagnosis of bullous pemphigoid, cicatricial pemphigoid, epidermolysis bullosa acquisita (EBA), or bullous eruption of lupus erythematosus (LE).

Results should be interpreted in conjunction with clinical information, histologic pattern, and results of direct immunofluorescence (IF) study.

PROCEDURE AND PATIENT CARE

Before

☒ Explain the procedure to the patient.
☒ Tell the patient that no fasting is required.

During

- Collect a venous blood sample in a red-top tube.

After

- Apply pressure or a pressure dressing to the venipuncture site.
- Assess the venipuncture site for bleeding.

TEST RESULTS AND CLINICAL SIGNIFICANCE

Positive

Pemphigoid
Pemphigus
Bullosa acquisita
Bullous lupus erythematosus
Paraneoplastic dermatitis:

> *In these diseases an autoimmune reaction is instigated and directed to the skin and other organs. As a result, IgG, IgA, and IgM antibody levels will increase.*

RELATED TEST

Skin Biopsy (p. 760). Cutaneous immunofluorescence antibodies can also be detected directly on skin biopsy. This test is confirmatory for autoimmune dermatitis.

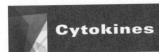

NORMAL FINDINGS

Varies by laboratory and technique

INDICATIONS

Cytokine assays are predominantly used for clinical research. Clinically, they may predominantly have the following uses:

- Measurement of acquired immunodeficiency syndrome (AIDS) progression
- Measurement of progression of inflammatory diseases, such as rheumatoid arthritis (RA) and other autoimmune diseases
- Tumor markers (e.g., breast cancer, lymphoma, and leukemia)
- Determination of risk for disease (e.g., risk for developing Kaposi sarcoma in AIDS patients)
- Determination of treatment of disease (e.g., which patients with RA may benefit from cytokine therapy)
- Determination of immune function and response
- Monitoring of patients receiving cytokine therapy or anticytokine therapy

TEST EXPLANATION

Cytokines are a group of proteins that have multiple functions but, in general, are produced by immune cells to communicate and orchestrate the immune response. The immune system has many different cells that must act together to effectively protect the body from infection, inflammation, or tumor. The cykotines are made by many different types of cells, including lymphocytes (T cells, B cells), monocytes, and eosinophils. Some cytokines stimulate each other, and some inhibit other cytokines to maintain balance. Originally, cytokines were named by their function (T cell growth factor, colony stimulating factor, etc.). As more was learned about this complex group of proteins, it became apparent that a single cytokine might act differently on different cells. Therefore naming the cytokine by function was confusing and misleading. As more cytokines have been identified, they were named *interleukins* and numbered by the sequence of discovery. Interleukins, in general, are made by leukocytes. Lymphokines and monokines are made by lymphocytes and monocytes, respectively. Other cytokines include *interferon* and *growth factors*.

Cytokines have receptors in other cells to which they attach and instigate a series of intracellular activity that may be associated with secretion, motion, or cell division. Cytokines are used therapeutically in stimulating bone marrow production of blood cells in patients with suppression (by chemotherapy) or disease of the bone marrow. They are used as potent antiinflammatory or antineoplastic agents. Some cytokines are produced at increased levels in particular disease states and are, thereby, markers for disease extent, progression, and response to therapy. For cancers that are associated with elevated cytokines, they act as "tumor markers." *Human Interferon Inducible protein 10* is a small cytokine belonging to the chemokine family that affects cellular chemotaxis, immune response, and bone marrow inhibition. This protein, when present in high quantities in an acutely ill patient, is an accurate predictor of multiple organ failure.

Any table designed to list all of the cytokines and their function quickly becomes inaccurate and imperfect. The discovery of new cytokines and new functions changes so frequently that any table is outdated in the delay to publication. Likewise, any listing of normal values will be just as quickly antiquated as methods of testing changes so frequently. It is suggested that reference to "normal values" be directed to the laboratory performing the assay.

Usually, cytokine testing is performed on serum. However, joint fluid is often tested in the evaluation of the patient with arthritis. Likewise, if inflammatory encephalitis or meningitis is considered, cerebrospinal fluid may be the specimen.

INTERFERING FACTORS

- Cells can still produce cytokines after specimen collection. It is best to freeze the specimen.
- Cytokines can degrade in the specimen container.
- Cytokines can stimulate or inhibit other cytokines while in the specimen container.

PROCEDURE AND PATIENT CARE

Before

☒ Explain the procedure to the patient.
☒ Tell the patient that no fasting or preparation is required.

During

- Collect a venous blood sample in a red-top tube.
- Usually this specimen is sent to a reference laboratory.

After

- Apply pressure to the venipuncture site.

TEST RESULTS AND CLINICAL SIGNIFICANCE

Abnormal Findings

AIDS: *The cytokine profile associated with the developing stages of AIDS or the susceptibility to AIDS related tumors has yet to be determined.*

Various malignancies (breast cancer, lymphoma, and leukemia): *Progression of these tumors may be the result or the instigator of elevated cytokines.*

Impaired immune function: *Cytokines are integral in the function of both cellular and humoral immune response. The exact cytokine profile for immune dysfunction has yet to be determined.*

Rheumatoid arthritis: *RA and other autoimmune diseases may be associated with increased cytokine levels compatible with a strong immune reaction. Measurement of certain cytokines may be important in monitoring more advanced anticytokine treatments for autoimmune diseases.*

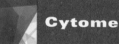

Cytomegalovirus (CMV)

NORMAL FINDINGS

No virus isolated

INDICATIONS

This test is used to identify cytomegalovirus (CMV) in suspected patients.

TEST EXPLANATION

CMV belongs to the viral family that includes herpes simplex, Epstein-Barr, and varicella-zoster viruses. CMV infection is widespread. Infections usually occur in the fetus, during early childhood, and in the young adult. Certain populations are at increased risk. Male homosexuals, transplant patients, and acquired immunodeficiency syndrome (AIDS) patients are particularly susceptible. Infections are acquired by contact with body secretions or urine. Blood transfusions are commonly implicated in the spread of CMV. As many as 35% of patients receiving multiple transfusions become infected with CMV. Most patients with acute disease have no or very few (mononucleosis-like) symptoms. Others may have mononucleosis-like symptoms of fever, lethargy, and anorexia. After infection there is an asymptomatic incubation period of about 60 days. Acute symptoms then develop. This is followed by a latent phase. Reactivation can occur at any time.

CMV is the most common congenital infection. Pregnant mothers can get the disease during their pregnancy, or a previous CMV infection can become reactivated. Approximately 10% of infected newborns exhibit permanent damage, usually mental retardation and auditory damage. Fetal infection can cause microcephaly, hydrocephaly, cerebral palsy, mental retardation, or death.

The term *TORCH* (toxoplasmosis, other, rubella, CMV, herpes) has been applied to infections with recognized detrimental effects on the fetus. The effects on the fetus may be direct or indirect (e.g., precipitating abortion or premature labor). Included in the category of "other" are infections (e.g., syphilis). All of these tests are discussed separately.

Virus culture is the most definitive method of diagnosis. However, a culture cannot differentiate an acute infection from a chronic, inactive infection. Immunofluorescence, enzyme-linked immunosorbent assay (ELISA), and latex agglutination methods of identifying anti-CMV antibodies reveal much more information about the activity of the infection. CMV immunoglobulin (Ig) G antibody levels persist for years after infection. Identification of IgM antibodies, however, indicates a relatively recent infection. Three different CMV antigens can be detected immunologically. They are called early, intermediate-early, and late antigens and indicate onset of infection. CMV inclusion bodies can be identified in the renal cells sloughed into the urine and are seen during a routine urinalysis. PCR assays demonstrate sensitive and specific detection of CMV nucleic acid.

No specific therapy is known for this infection. If the diagnosis is established early by viral culture or serology, abortion may be an option. A fourfold increase in CMV titer in paired sera drawn 10 to 14 days apart is usually indicative of an acute infection.

PROCEDURE AND PATIENT CARE

Before

✗ Explain the procedure to the patient.

During

- For culture specimens, a urine, sputum, or mouth swab is the specimen of choice. Fresh specimens are essential.
- The specimens are cultured in a virus laboratory, which takes about 3 to 7 days.
- For an antibody or antigen titer, collect blood in a gold-top or red-top tube.
- Collect a specimen from the mother with suspected acute infection as early as possible.
- Collect the convalescent specimen 2 to 4 weeks later.

After

- Apply pressure or a pressure dressing to the venipuncture site.
- Assess the venipuncture site for bleeding.

TEST RESULTS AND CLINICAL SIGNIFICANCE

CMV infection

 D-Dimer (Fragment D-Dimer, Fibrin Degradation Product [FDP], Fibrin Split Products)

NORMAL FINDINGS

<0.4 mcg/mL

INDICATIONS

The D-dimer test is used to identify intravascular clotting.

TEST EXPLANATION

The fragment D-dimer test assesses both thrombin and plasmin activity. D-dimer is a fibrin degradation fragment that is made through lysis of cross-linked (D-dimerized) fibrin. As plasmin acts on the fibrin polymer clot, fibrin degradation products and D-dimer are produced. The D-dimer assay provides a highly specific measurement of the amount of fibrin degradation that occurs. Normal plasma does not have detectable amounts of fragment D-dimer. For a discussion of other fibrin degradation products, see Thrombosis Indicators (p. 482).

This test provides a simple and confirmatory test for disseminated intravascular coagulation (DIC). Positive results of the D-dimer assay correlate with positive results of other thrombosis indicators. The D-dimer assay may be more specific than the FDP assay, but it is less sensitive. Therefore combining the FDP and the D-dimer provides a highly sensitive and specific test for recognizing DIC.

Levels of D-dimer can also increase when a fibrin clot is lysed by thrombolytic therapy. Thrombotic problems such as deep vein thrombosis (DVT), pulmonary embolism, sickle cell anemia, and thrombosis of malignancy are also associated with high D-dimer levels. D-Dimer is used as an effective screening test for DVT. It is able to accurately identify patients with DVT who are then sent for venous duplex scanning (p. 900). The d-dimer test, however, is often positive in patients who are already hospitalized. If the D-dimer test is negative, its high predictability indicates that the patient does not have PE/DVT, and further testing may not be necessary.

Finally, the D-dimer test can be used to determine the duration of anticoagulation therapy in patients with DVT. Patients with an abnormal D-dimer level 1 month after the discontinuation of anticoagulant therapy have a significant incidence of recurrent DVT. This incidence can be reduced by restarting anticoagulation therapy.

The D-dimer can be tested by immunoturbidimetric methods or latex quantitative/qualitative assay.

INTERFERING FACTORS

- The D-dimer level may be decreased in lipemic patients.
- The presence of rheumatoid factor at a level >50 IU/mL may lead to increased levels of D-dimer.

PROCEDURE AND PATIENT CARE

Before

✗ Explain the procedure to the patient.
✗ Tell the patient that no fasting is required.

During

- Collect a venous blood sample in a blue-top tube.

After

- Apply pressure or a pressure dressing to the venipuncture site.
- Assess the venipuncture site for bleeding. If the patient is receiving anticoagulants or has coagulopathies, remember that the bleeding time will be increased.

TEST RESULTS AND CLINICAL SIGNIFICANCE

▲ Increased Levels

DIC: *This is a phenomenon of rapid intramicrovascular coagulation and synchronous fibrinolysis. D-dimer is produced by the action of plasmin on the fibrin polymer clot.*

Primary fibrinolysis,

During thrombolytic or defibrination therapy:
D-dimer is produced by the action of plasmin on the fibrin polymer clot.

Deep vein thrombosis,

Pulmonary embolism,

Arterial thromboembolism,

Sickle cell anemia with or without vasoocclusive crisis:
The body's natural reaction to clot development is fibrinolysis. D-dimer is produced by the action of plasmin on the fibrin polymer clot.

Pregnancy,

Malignancy,

Surgery:
These clinical situations are associated with varying degrees of clotting and fibrinolysis. D-dimer is produced by the action of plasmin on the fibrin polymer clot.

RELATED TESTS

The following are tests used to assist in the diagnosis of DIC:

Prothrombin Time (PT) (p. 434). The PT is used to evaluate the adequacy of the extrinsic system and common pathway in the clotting mechanism.

Coagulating Factor Concentration (p. 163). This is a quantitative measurement of specific coagulation factors.

Partial Thromboplastin Time, Activated (aPTT) (p. 383). This test is used to evaluate the intrinsic system and the common pathway of clot formation. It is most commonly used to monitor heparin therapy.

Dexamethasone Suppression (DS, Prolonged/Rapid DS, Cortisol Suppression, Adrenocorticotropic Hormone [ACTH] Suppression)

NORMAL FINDINGS

Prolonged Method

Expected values (normal)

Low dose: >50% reduction of plasma cortisol and 17-hydroxycorticosteroid (17-OCHS) levels
High dose: >50% reduction of plasma cortisol and 17-OCHS levels

Rapid Method

Normal: nearly zero cortisol levels

INDICATIONS

The DS test is important for diagnosing adrenal hyperfunction (Cushing syndrome) and distinguishing its cause.

TEST EXPLANATION

An elaborate feedback mechanism for cortisol exists to coordinate the function of the hypothalamus, pituitary gland, and the adrenal glands. Corticotropin-releasing hormone (CRH) is made in the hypothalamus. This stimulates ACTH production in the anterior pituitary gland. ACTH stimulates the adrenal cortex to produce cortisol. The rising levels of cortisol act as a negative feedback and curtail further production of CRH and ACTH. Cortisol is a potent glucocorticoid released from the adrenal cortex. This hormone affects the metabolism of carbohydrates, proteins, and fats. It especially has a profound effect on glucose serum levels.

The DS test is based on pituitary ACTH secretion being dependent on the plasma cortisol feedback mechanism. As plasma cortisol levels increase, ACTH secretion is suppressed; as cortisol levels decrease, ACTH secretion is stimulated. Dexamethasone is a synthetic steroid (similar to cortisol) that will suppress ACTH secretion. Under normal circumstances this results in reduced stimulation to the adrenal glands and ultimately a drop of 50% or more in plasma cortisol and 17-OCHS levels. This important feedback system does not function properly in patients with Cushing syndrome.

In Cushing syndrome caused by bilateral adrenal hyperplasia (Cushing disease), the pituitary gland is reset upward and responds only to high plasma levels of cortisone and steroids. In Cushing syndrome caused by adrenal adenoma or cancer (which acts autonomously), cortisol secretion will continue despite a decrease in ACTH. When Cushing syndrome is caused by an ectopic ACTH-producing tumor (as in lung cancer), that tumor is also considered autonomous and will continue to secrete ACTH despite high cortisol levels. Again, no decrease occurs in plasma cortisol. Knowledge of the following defects in the normal cortisol-ACTH feedback system is the basis for understanding the DST.

Cushing Syndrome Caused by Bilateral Adrenal Hyperplasia

Low dose: no change
High dose: >50% reduction of plasma cortisol and 17-OCHS levels

Cushing Syndrome Caused by Adrenal Adenoma or Carcinoma

Low dose: no change
High dose: no change

Cushing Syndrome Caused by Ectopic ACTH-Producing Tumor

Low dose: no change
High dose: no change

The DS test also may identify depressed persons likely to respond to electroconvulsive therapy or antidepressants rather than to psychologic or social interventions. ACTH production will not be suppressed after administration of low-dose DS in these patients.

The *prolonged* DS test can be performed over a 6-day period on an outpatient basis. The rapid DS test is easily and quickly performed and is used primarily as a screening test to diagnose Cushing syndrome. It is less accurate and less informative than the prolonged DS test, but when its results are normal, the diagnosis of Cushing syndrome can safely be excluded.

INTERFERING FACTORS

- Physical and emotional stress can elevate ACTH release and obscure interpretation of test results. Stress is stimulatory to the pituitary, which thereby secretes ACTH.
- Drugs that can affect test results include barbiturates, estrogens, oral contraceptives, phenytoin (Dilantin), spironolactone (Aldactone), steroids, and tetracyclines.

PROCEDURE AND PATIENT CARE

Before

- Explain the procedure (prolonged or rapid test) to the patient.
- Obtain the patient's weight as a baseline for evaluating side effects of steroids.

During

- There are several documented methods of performing this test by varying the dose and duration of testing.

Prolonged Test

- Obtain a baseline 24-hour urine collection for corticosteroids (urine 17-OCHS [see p. 926] or urinary cortisol).
- Collect blood for determination of baseline plasma cortisol levels if indicated. Collect 24-hour urine specimens daily over a 6-day period. Because 6 continuous days of urine collections are needed, no urine specimens are discarded except for the first voided specimen on day 1, after which the collection begins.
- On day 3 administer a low dose of DS by mouth.
- On day 5 administer a high of DS by mouth.
- Administer the DS with milk or an antacid to prevent gastric irritation.
- The urine samples for cortisol and 17-OCHS do not need a preservative.
- Note that the creatinine content is measured in all the 24-hour urine collections to demonstrate their accuracy and adequacy.
- Keep the urine specimens refrigerated or on ice during the collection period.

Rapid Test

- Give the patient a dose of dexamethasone by mouth at 11 PM.
- Administer the DS with milk or an antacid to prevent gastric irritation.
- Attempt to ensure a good night's sleep. Sedative/hypnotics are used only if absolutely necessary.

- At 8 AM the next morning, draw blood for determination of the plasma cortisol level before the patient arises.
- If no cortisol suppression occurs after administration of the dose of dexamethasone, administer a higher dose to suppress ACTH production. This is referred to as the *overnight 8-mg DS suppression test.* Patients with adrenal hyperplasia will suppress. Patients with adrenal or ectopic tumors will not suppress.

After

- Evaluate the patient for evidence of gastric irritation.
- Assess the patient for steroid-induced side effects by monitoring weight, glucose levels, and potassium levels.
- Send specimens to the laboratory promptly.

TEST RESULTS AND CLINICAL SIGNIFICANCE

Adrenal Hyperfunction (Cushing Syndrome)

Cushing disease,

Ectopic ACTH-producing tumors:

> *In these illnesses, ACTH is produced without regard to the inhibitory feedback mechanism that normally exists. This is a result of neoplastic overproduction of ACTH in the pituitary or elsewhere in the body by an ACTH-producing cancer. ACTH is not suppressed. As a result, cortisol is not suppressed.*

Adrenal adenoma or carcinoma: *Neoplasms of the adrenal glands are not sensitive to the inhibitory feedback mechanism that normally exists. Therefore ACTH will be suppressed by the DS, but cortisol production (the end point of the test) is not.*

Bilateral adrenal hyperplasia: *The inhibitory feedback mechanism that normally exists in the pituitary-adrenal system is blunted. Therefore at low dexamethasone doses no change in cortisol production is seen. At high dexamethasone doses, however, the ACTH and subsequently cortisol are suppressed.*

Mental depression: *ACTH is not suppressed in individuals likely to require electroconvulsive or medicinal therapy for their depression.*

RELATED TESTS

Adrenocorticotropic Hormone (ACTH) Stimulation With Cosyntropin (p. 34). This test is used to evaluate the differential diagnosis of Cushing syndrome or Addison disease.

Adrenocorticotropic Hormone (ACTH) (p. 31). The serum ACTH study is a test of anterior pituitary gland function that affords the greatest insight into the causes of either Cushing syndrome (overproduction of cortisol) or Addison disease (underproduction of cortisol).

Cortisol, Blood (p. 179). This is a direct measurement of the cortisol blood level.

Cortisol, Urine (p. 920). This test is a measure of urinary cortisol. It is performed on patients who are suspected to have hyperfunctioning or hypofunctioning of the adrenal gland.

Diabetes Mellitus Autoantibody Panel (Insulin Autoantibody [IAA], Islet Cell Antibody [ICA], Glutamic Acid Decarboxylase Antibody [GAD Ab])

NORMAL FINDINGS

<1:4 titer; no antibody detected

INDICATIONS

This test is used in the evaluation of insulin resistance. It is also used to identify type 1 diabetes and in patients with a suspected allergy to insulin. This antibody panel is also used in surveillance of patients who have received pancreatic islet cell transplantation.

TEST EXPLANATION

Type 1 diabetes mellitus (DM) is insulin-dependent diabetes (IDDM). It is becoming increasingly recognized that this disease is an "organ specific" form of autoimmune disease that results in destruction of the pancreatic islet cells and their products. These antibodies are used to differentiate type 1 DM from type 2 non-insulin-dependent DM. Nearly 90% of patients with type 1 diabetes have one or more of these autoantibodies at the time of their diagnosis. Patients with type 2 diabetes have low or negative titers.

These antibodies often appear years before the onset of symptoms. The panel is useful to screen relatives of IDDM patients who are at risk for developing the disease. Sixty percent to 80% of first-degree relatives with both ICA and IAA will develop IDDM within 10 years. GAD Ab provides confirmatory evidence. The presence of these antibodies identifies which gestational diabetic will eventually require insulin permanently. Once recognized, preventive diabetic treatment is instituted. This may include counseling plus antibody and glucose monitoring.

The most common type of anti-insulin antibody is immunoglobulin (Ig) G, but IgA, IgM, IgD, and IgE also have been reported. Most of these insulin antibodies do not cause clinical problems, but they may complicate most insulin assays. Anti-insulin antibodies act as insulin-transporting proteins and bind the free insulin. This can reduce the amount of insulin available for glucose metabolism. They may also contribute to insulin resistance (daily insulin requirements exceeding 200 units/day for 2 days). IgM, especially, may cause insulin resistance. Insulin allergy (most common with animal insulin) may result from IgE antibodies to insulin.

Although it was common in the past for diabetic patients to develop anti-insulin antibodies after prolonged treatment with exogenous insulin, the development and therapeutic use of recombinant DNA insulin has virtually eliminated that problem. Nevertheless the presence of insulin antibodies is diagnostic of factitious hypoglycemia from surreptitious administration of insulin. This antibody panel is also used in surveillance of patients who have received pancreatic islet cell transplantation. Finally these antibodies can be used to identify late onset type 1 diabetes in those patients previously thought to have type 2 diabetes.

INTERFERING FACTORS

- When anti-insulin antibodies are measured by radiobinding assay, radioactive scans within 7 days before the test may interfere with the test result.

PROCEDURE AND PATIENT CARE

Before

- Explain the procedure to the patient.
- Tell the patient that no fasting is required.

During

- Collect a venous blood sample in a plain red-top or a blood/serum separator tube.

After

- Apply pressure to the venipuncture site.

TEST RESULTS AND CLINICAL SIGNIFICANCE

▲ Increased Levels

Insulin resistance: *The anti-insulin antibodies bind insulin and thereby diminish the amount of free insulin available for glucose metabolism.*

Allergies to insulin: *Although allergies occur most frequently with the use of animal-generated insulin, they can still occur with human insulin. A rash or lymphadenopathy may be the result of such an allergy.*

Factitious hypoglycemia: *Because most patients develop anti-insulin antibodies to exogenous insulin, the identification of these antibodies supports the secretive self-administration of insulin in a patient who denies the use of insulin.*

RELATED TESTS

C-Peptide (p. 182). This test is used to evaluate diabetic patients. It is also used to identify patients who secretly self-administer insulin.

Insulin Assay (p. 315). This test is used to diagnose insulinoma (tumor of the islets of Langerhans) and to evaluate abnormal lipid and carbohydrate metabolism. It is used in the evaluation of patients with fasting hypoglycemia.

2,3-Diphosphoglycerate (2,3-DPG in Erythrocytes)

NORMAL FINDINGS

12.3 ± 1.87 μmol/g of hemoglobin or 0.79 ± 0.12 mol/mol hemoglobin (SI units)
4.2 ± 0.64 μmol/mL of erythrocytes or 4.2 ± 0.64 mmol/L erythrocytes (SI units)
Levels are lower in newborns and even lower in premature infants.

INDICATIONS

This test is used in the evaluation of nonspherocytic hemolytic anemia.

TEST EXPLANATION

2,3-DPG is a by-product of the glycolytic respiratory pathway of the red blood cell (RBC). A congenital enzyme deficiency in this vital pathway alters the RBC shape and survival significantly. Nonspherocytic anemia is the result. Another result of the enzyme deficiency is reduced synthesis of 2,3-DPG. 2,3-DPG controls O_2 transport from the RBCs to the tissues. Deficiencies of this enzyme result in alterations of the RBC O_2 dissociation curve that controls release of O_2 to the tissues. Many anemias not a result of 2,3-DPG deficiency are associated with increased levels of 2,3-DPG as a compensatory mechanism.

Usually, 2,3-DPG levels increase in response to anemia or hypoxic conditions (e.g., obstructive lung disease, congenital cyanotic heart disease, after vigorous exercise). Increases in 2,3-DPG decrease the O_2 binding to hemoglobin so that O_2 is more easily released to the tissues when needed (lower arterial Po_2). Levels of 2,3-DPG are decreased as a result of inherited genetic defects. This genetic defect parallels sickle cell anemia and hemoglobin C diseases.

INTERFERING FACTORS

- Levels may be increased after vigorous exercise.
- High altitudes may increase 2,3-DPG levels.
- Banked blood has decreased amounts of 2,3-DPG.
- Acidosis decreases 2,3-DPG levels.

PROCEDURE AND PATIENT CARE

Before

📛 Explain the procedure to the patient.
📛 Tell the patient that no fasting is required.

During

- Collect a venous blood sample in a red-top tube.

After

- Apply pressure or a pressure dressing to the venipuncture site.
- Assess the venipuncture site for bleeding.

TEST RESULTS AND CLINICAL SIGNIFICANCE

▲ Increased Levels

Anemia: *Increased 2,3-DPG levels are compensatory to provide adequate O_2 to the tissues.*

Hypoxic heart and lung diseases (e.g., obstructive lung disease, cystic fibrosis, congenital cyanotic heart disease): *Hypoxemia stimulates the production of 2,3-DPG.*

Hyperthyroidism: *Increased metabolic processes increase O_2 requirements. This need is met by increased 2,3-DPG.*

Chronic renal failure: *Erythropoietin deficiency as a result of chronic renal failure causes anemia. Increased 2,3-DPG levels are compensatory to provide adequate O_2 to the tissues.*

Pyruvate kinase deficiency: *This enzyme is important in the glycolytic respiratory pathway of the RBC. Its function is to metabolize 2,3-DPG by-products. In the absence of this enzyme, 2,3-DPG is not metabolized and increased levels result.*

Compensation for higher altitudes: *In compensation for the reduced oxygen availability, 2,3-DPG is increased in order to shift the oxygen dissemination curve to the right, making more oxygen available to the tissues.*

▼ Decreased Levels

Polycythemia: *2,3-DPG is made in the RBC as a result of its glycolytic respiratory process. Increased numbers of RBCs will cause compensatory decreased 2,3-DPG.*

Acidosis: *Decreased 2,3-DPG is associated with metabolic or respiratory acidosis.*

After massive blood transfusion: *Banked RBCs lose their 2,3-DPG during storage.*

2,3-DPG disease: *The enzymes required for synthesis of 2,3-DPG are reduced. As a result, 2,3-DPG is reduced.*

Respiratory distress syndrome: *The pathophysiology of this observation is unknown.*

2,3-DPG mutase deficiency: *This enzyme is critical in the synthesis of 2,3-DPG. Reduced levels of this enzyme cause reduced 2,3-DPG.*

RELATED TEST

Complete Blood Cell Count (p. 174). This is a series of tests that provide information about the hematologic system and many other organ systems.

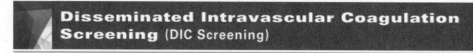

Disseminated Intravascular Coagulation Screening (DIC Screening)

NORMAL FINDINGS

No evidence of DIC

INDICATIONS

This group of tests is indicated for patients who are suspected of having acute DIC (demonstrate a coagulopathy), for patients who have chronic DIC (chronic microembolic processes), and for patients who are at great risk for DIC (patients with sepsis or advanced cancer).

TEST EXPLANATION

This is a group of tests used to detect DIC. Many pathologic conditions can instigate or are associated with DIC. The more common ones include bacterial septicemia, amniotic fluid embolism, retention of a dead fetus, malignant neoplasia, liver cirrhosis, extensive surgery (especially on the prostate or liver), extracorporeal heart bypass, extensive trauma, severe burns, and transfusion reactions.

In DIC the entire clotting mechanism is triggered inappropriately. This results in significant systemic or localized intravascular formation of fibrin clots. Consequences of this futile clotting are small blood vessel occlusion and excessive bleeding caused by consumption of the platelets and clotting factors that have been used in intravascular clotting. The fibrinolytic system is also activated to break down the clot formation and the fibrin involved in the intravascular coagulation. This fibrinolysis results in the formation of fibrin degradation products (FDPs) (see Thrombosis Indicators [p. 482]) which, by themselves, act as anticoagulants; these FDPs only serve to enhance the bleeding tendency.

Organ injury can occur as a result of intravascular clots, which cause microvascular occlusion in various organs. This may cause serious anoxic injury in affected organs. Also, RBCs passing through partly plugged vessels are injured and subsequently hemolyzed. The result may be ongoing hemolytic anemia. Figure 2-15 summarizes DIC pathophysiology and effects. Heparin is sometimes used to treat DIC because it inhibits the ongoing futile thrombin formation. This decreases the use of clotting factors and platelets, and bleeding ceases.

When a patient with a bleeding tendency is suspected of having DIC, a series of routinely performed laboratory tests are done (prothrombin time [PT], partial thromboplastin time [PTT], bleeding time, and platelet count). If results are abnormal, further testing should be performed (Table 2-18). With these tests, the hematologist can make the appropriate diagnosis confidently. All of these tests are discussed separately.

RELATED TEST

Protein C, Protein S (p. 432). This test identifies patients who are deficient in protein C and/or S. This is part of an evaluation of hypercoagulation.

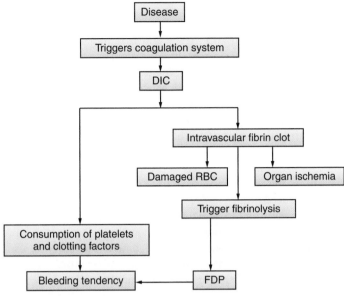

Figure 2-15 Pathophysiology of DIC, which may result in bleeding tendency, organ ischemia, and hemolytic anemia. (FDP, Fibrin degradation products; RBCs, red blood cells.)

TABLE 2-18	Disseminated Intravascular Coagulation Screening Tests
Test	**Result**
Platelet count (p. 401)	Decreased
Prothrombin time (p. 434)	Prolonged
Partial thromboplastin time (p. 383)	Prolonged
Coagulating factors (p. 163)	Decreased factors I, II, V, VIII, X, and XIII—more commonly used for diagnosis than screening
Fibrin degradation products (p. 202)	Increased
Fibrinogen (p. 241)	Decreased
D-Dimer (p. 202)	Increased
Fibrinopeptide A (p. 482)	Increased
Prothrombin fragment (p. 482)	Increased

Drug Monitoring (Therapeutic Drug Monitoring [TDM])

NORMAL FINDINGS

See Table 2-19.

INDICATIONS

TDM entails measuring blood drug levels to determine effective drug dosages and prevent toxicity. TDM is used to adjust the dosage of medications so as to maximize efficacy and minimize side effects.

TEST EXPLANATION

There are several factors that affect both efficacy and toxicity. They include patient compliance (TDM can be used to determine patient compliance), patient age and size, access to adequate care, optimal dosing, and drug pharmacology issues, including absorption, elimination, and drug interactions. Drug monitoring is helpful in patients who take other medicines that may affect drug levels or act in a synergistic or antagonistic manner with the drug to be tested. There are some medicines (e.g., antiarrhythmics, bronchodilators, antibiotics, anticonvulsants, cardiotonics) that have a very narrow therapeutic margin (i.e., the difference between therapeutic and toxic drug levels is small).

TDM is helpful if the desired therapeutic effect of the drug is not observed as expected. Dosages beyond normal may have to be prescribed. Likewise if toxic symptoms appear with standard doses, TDM can be used to determine reduced dosing.

Table 2-19 lists the therapeutic and toxic ranges for the average patient for commonly tested drug levels. This list is far from complete. These ranges may not apply to all patients because clinical response is influenced by many factors (Box 2-9). Also note that different laboratories use different units for reporting test results and normal ranges. It is important that sufficient time pass between the administration of the medication and the collection of the blood sample to allow for adequate absorption and therapeutic levels to occur.

Blood is routinely used for TDM because results indicate what is presently going on with the drug at any one particular time. Urine drug levels reflect the presence of the drug over the last several days. Therefore if data concerning drug levels at a particular time are necessary, blood testing is required.

Blood samples can be taken at the drug's *peak* level (highest concentration) or the *trough* level (lowest concentration). Peak levels are useful when testing for toxicity, and trough levels are useful for demonstrating a satisfactory therapeutic level. Trough levels are often referred to as *residual* levels. The time when the sample should be drawn after the last dose of the medication varies according to whether a peak or trough level is requested as well as the half-life (the time required for the body to decrease the drug blood level by 50%) of the drug. Table 2-20 lists the peak concentration times for some common drugs. If peak levels are higher than the therapeutic range, toxicity may be experienced. If trough levels are below the therapeutic range, drug therapy may not be successful.

PHARMACOGENETICS (GENETIC TESTING FOR DRUG MONITORING)

All drugs undergo metabolism by enzymes systems to activate a bound (proactive) drug and/or to deactivate an active drug. The effectiveness of these enzymes' systems of metabolism are determined by the genetic makeup of the patient. With pharmacogenetics, four categories of drug metabolizers can be identified:
- Poor metabolizers (PMs)
- Intermediate metabolizers (IMs)
- Extensive metabolizers (EMs)
- Ultrametabolizers (UMs)

In general, PMs and, to a lesser extent, IMs are prone to exaggerated side effects from active drugs, whereas normal doses of the same drugs tend to be ineffectual for UMs. If a proactive drug is administered and must be hydrolyzed to its active form, PMs will not benefit from normal doses, whereas UMs will experience drug benefit from even small doses.

TABLE 2-19   Drug Monitoring Data

Drug	Use	Therapeutic Level*	Toxic Level*
Acetaminophen	Analgesic, antipyretic	Depends on use	>25 mcg/mL
Amikacin	Antibiotic	15-25 mcg/mL	>250 mcg/mL
Aminophylline	Bronchodilator	10-20 mcg/mL	>20 mcg/mL
Amitriptyline	Antidepressant	120-150 ng/mL	>500 ng/mL
Carbamazepine	Anticonvulsant	5-12 mcg/mL	>12 mcg/mL
Cyclosporine	Immunosuppressant	100-400 ng/mL	>400 ng/mL
Chloramphenicol	Antiinfective	10-20 mcg/mL	>25 mcg/mL
Desipramine	Antidepressant	150-300 ng/mL	>500 ng/mL
Digitoxin	Cardiac glycoside	15-25 ng/mL	>25 ng/mL
Digoxin	Cardiac glycoside	0.8-2 ng/mL	>2.4 ng/mL
Disopyramide	Antiarrhythmic	2-5 mcg/mL	>5 mcg/mL
Ethosuximide	Anticonvulsant	40-100 mcg/mL	>100 mcg/mL
Gentamicin	Antibiotic	5-10 mcg/mL	>12 mcg/mL
Imipramine	Antidepressant	150-300 ng/mL	>500 ng/mL
Kanamycin	Antibiotic	20-25 mcg/mL	>35 mcg/mL
Lidocaine	Antiarrhythmic	1.5-5 mcg/mL	>5 mcg/mL
Lithium	Manic episodes of manic depression psychosis	0.8-1.2 mEq/L	>2 mEq/L
Methotrexate	Antitumor agent	>0.01 μmol	>10 μmol/24 hr
Nortriptyline	Antidepressant	50-150 ng/mL	>500 ng/mL
Phenobarbital	Anticonvulsant	10-30 mcg/mL	>40 mcg/mL
Phenytoin	Anticonvulsant	10-20 mcg/mL	>30 mcg/mL
Primidone	Anticonvulsant	5-12 mcg/mL	>15 mcg/mL
Procainamide	Antiarrhythmic	4-10 mcg/mL	>16 mcg/mL
Propranolol	Antiarrhythmic	50-100 ng/mL	>150 ng/mL
Quinidine	Antiarrhythmic	2-5 mcg/mL	>10 mcg/mL
Salicylate	Antipyretic, antiinflammatory, analgesic	100-250 mcg/mL	>300 mcg/mL
Sirolimus	Immunosuppressant	3-20 ng/mL	>20 ng/mL
Tacrolimus	Immunosuppressant	5-15 ng/mL	>20 ng/mL
Theophylline	Bronchodilator	10-20 mcg/mL	>20 mcg/mL
Tobramycin	Antibiotic	5-10 mcg/mL	>12 mcg/mL
Valproic acid	Anticonvulsant	50-100 mcg/mL	>100 mcg/mL

*Levels vary according to the laboratory performing the test.

BOX 2-9   Factors Influencing Blood Drug Levels

- Route of administration
- Drug metabolism
- Age
- Other disease
- Drug absorption
- Drug excretion
- Weight
- Laboratory methods
- Drug delivery (cardiovascular function)
- Dosage
- Other medications
- Patient compliance

TABLE 2-20	Peak Concentration Times for Some Common Drugs
Drug (Given by Routine Route)	**Peak (hr)**
Phenytoin	4-8
Phenobarbital	12
Lithium	1-3
Tricyclic antidepressants	2-6
Procainamide	1-2
Procainamide SR	4
Lidocaine	2
Quinidine	2
Digoxin	½-1½
Theophylline	2-3
Gentamicin	½
Vancomycin	¼-2

TABLE 2-21	Enzymes Involved in Drug Metabolism
Enzyme	**Drugs**
CYP2C9	Warfarin, phenytoin, nonsteroidal anti-inflammatory drugs
CYP2C19	Omeprazole, proguanil, amitriptyline, diazepam, propranolol
CYP2D6	Codeine, antidepressants, haloperidol, amiodarone, tamoxifen, diltiazem, amphetamine, dextromethorphan, anticonvulsants, flecainide, disopyramide
Atypical pseudocholinesterase	Succinylcholine
NAT2 (slow acetylator)	Isoniazid , hydralazine
UGT1A1	Irinotecan
GST	D-Penicillamine
TPMT	Azathioprine, mercaptopurine
CYP1A1	Polycyclic aromatic hydrocarbons
CYP1A2	Caffeine, theophylline, imipramine
CYP2 CYP2A6	Nicotine
CYP2E1	Ethanol
CYP3 CYP3A4	Amitriptyline, clarithromycin, cyclosporine, erythromycin, tacrolimus, lidocaine, nifedipine, tamoxifen

The cytochrome P (CYP) 450 system is a major family of drug-metabolizing enzymes. Several CYP450 enzymes are involved in the metabolism of a significant proportion of drugs (Table 2-21). *Cytochrome P450 genotype testing using PCR amplification* is a pharmacogenetic method of evaluating the metabolic effectiveness of the CYP450 system and provides data to categorize the patient's metabolizing ability as described in the preceding. This testing is performed on a buccal swab specimen.

Thiopurine methyltransferase (TPMT) is another metabolic enzyme system used in the metabolism of thiopurine drugs (e.g., azathioprine, 6-mercaptopurine [6MP], and 6-thoguanine). Defects in the TPMT noted on *TPMT gene mutation testing* leads to decreased methylation and decreased inactivation of 6MP. This can lead to enhanced bone marrow toxicity, which may cause myelosuppression, anemia, bleeding tendency, leukopenia, and infection.

Pharmacogenetics allows physicians to consider genetic information from patients in selecting medications and dosages of medications for a wide variety of common conditions, such as cardiac disease, psychiatric disease, and cancer.

Gas chromatography and liquid chromatography are commonly used in TDM. Mass spectrometry can be combined with other methods to improve sensitivity of TDM. Enzyme-multiplied immunoassay technique offers an alternative to the traditional spectroscopic and chromatographic method for measuring blood concentrations of drugs.

PROCEDURE AND PATIENT CARE

Before

- Explain the procedure to the patient.
- Tell the patient that no food or fluid restrictions are needed.
- For patients suspected of having symptoms of drug toxicity, the best time to draw the blood specimen is when the symptoms are occurring.
- If there is a concern regarding whether an adequate dose of the drug is achieved, it is best to obtain trough levels.

During

- Collect a venous blood sample in a tube designated by the laboratory. *Peak* levels are usually obtained 1 to 2 hours after oral intake, approximately 1 hour after intramuscular (IM) administration, and approximately 30 minutes after intravenous (IV) administration. *Residual (trough)* levels are usually obtained shortly before (0 to 15 minutes) the next scheduled dose. Consult with the pharmacy for specific times.

After

- Apply pressure or a pressure dressing to the venipuncture site.
- Assess the venipuncture site for bleeding.
- Clearly mark all blood samples with the following information: patient's name, diagnosis, name of drug, time of last drug ingestion, time of sample, and any other medications the patient is currently taking.
- Promptly send the specimen to the laboratory.

TEST RESULTS AND CLINICAL SIGNIFICANCE

Nontherapeutic levels of drugs,
Toxic levels of drugs:

> One must always be aware that TDM is only a guide to treatment. Therapy may be successful at drug levels below the therapeutic range. Levels above the therapeutic range may be necessary in some patients to obtain adequate therapy.

RELATED TEST

Toxicology Testing (p. 951). This is generally a urine test to determine the toxic effect of prescribed and nonprescribed drugs that are often used and abused in criminal behavior.

Drug Sensitivity Genotype Testing (AccuType)

NORMAL FINDINGS

No abnormal genetic abnormalities.

INDICATIONS

This test is indicated if a patient is taking a medication with no therapeutic effect or is experiencing signs of toxicity at normal therapeutic doses.

TEST EXPLANATION

The efficacy of therapeutic drugs can vary considerably among different patients. Factors that influence these variations include genetic aberrations, patient age, race, body weight or surface area, sex, tobacco use, concomitant medications, and comorbid medical conditions. It is extremely important to identify differences in drug metabolism so as to preclude the possibility of overdosing or underdosing.

Drug sensitivity genotype testing identifies genetic aberrations that encode various proteins required for drug metabolism. If the gene is abnormal, the protein may be deficient in quantity or character to properly metabolize the medication given to the patient. Various laboratories have "trade marked" their testing methods. A common test is called *AccuType Testing*.

Drug sensitivity genotype testing is available for predicting a patient's response to warfarin, clopidogrel, interferon-ribavirin (and other retroviral medications), metformin, and anti-TB drugs (rifampin/isoniazid).

PROCEDURE AND PATIENT CARE

Before

☒ Explain the procedure to the patient.
☒ Tell the patient that no food or fluid restrictions are needed.

During

- Collect a venous blood sample in a whole blood (EDTA, lavender-top tube) or a collection tube designated by the laboratory.
- Alternatively, 1 mL of saliva in an Oragene DNA self-collection kit can be submitted. The specimen should be maintained at room temperature.

After

- Apply pressure or a pressure dressing to the venipuncture site.
- Promptly send the specimen to the laboratory.

TEST RESULTS AND CLINICAL SIGNIFICANCE

Genetic aberrations that may alter drug metabolism: *As a result of knowing genetic aberrations in drug metabolism, drug dosages can be modified to provide the therapeutic dose without risks of toxicity.*

RELATED TEST

Drug Monitoring (p. 211). This test includes a more general discussion of pharmacogenetics.

Epstein-Barr Virus Testing (EBV Antibody Titer)

NORMAL FINDINGS

Titers ≤1:10 are nondiagnostic.
Titers of 1:10 to 1:60 indicate infection at some undetermined time.
Titers of ≥1:320 suggest active infection.
Fourfold increase in titer in paired sera drawn 10 to 14 days apart is usually indicative of an acute infection.

INDICATIONS

This test is used to diagnose a suspected EBV infection (infectious mononucleosis).

TEST EXPLANATION

EBV infects 80% of the U.S. population. Once infection occurs, the virus becomes dormant but can be reactivated later. EBV infection can produce infectious mononucleosis. Mononucleosis is seen most often in children, adolescents, and young adults. Clinical features include acute fatigue, fever, sore throat, lymphadenopathy, and splenomegaly. Laboratory findings of lymphocytosis, atypical lymphocytes, and transient serum heterophil antibodies are seen in patients with acute EBV infection. Most patients with infectious mononucleosis recover uneventfully and return to normal activity within 4 to 6 weeks. In Africa, EBV has been associated with Burkitt lymphoma. In China, EBV infection has been associated with nasopharyngeal carcinoma.

After recovery from primary EBV infection, patients are life-long, latent EBV carriers. Specific immunologic tests to identify EBV activity indicate that latent EBV can reactivate and become associated with a constellation of chronic signs and symptoms resembling infectious mononucleosis. Clinical manifestations of chronic EBV are variable and include nonspecific symptoms, such as profound fatigue (chronic fatigue syndrome), pharyngitis, myalgia, arthralgia, low-grade fever, headache, paresthesia, and loss of abstract thinking.

The majority of EBV infections can be recognized, however, by testing the patient's serum for heterophile antibodies (rapid latex slide agglutination test; mononucleosis [mono] rapid test, see p. 363). Other more specific immunologic tests are recommended only when a mononucleosis screening procedure is negative and infectious mononucleosis or a complication of Epstein-Barr virus infection is suspected. Also they more precisely define the acuity of the infection (Table 2-22). In cases in which EBV is suspected but the heterophile antibody is not detected, an evaluation of the EBV-specific

TABLE 2-22   Serologic Studies and the Timing of Infections

Serologic Study	Appears/Disappears	Clinical Significance
Mono spot heterophil	5 days/2 wk	Acute or convalescent infection
VCA-IgM	7 days/3 mo	Acute or convalescent infection
VCA-IgG	7 days/exists for life	Acute, convalescent, or old infection
EBNA-IgG	3 wk/exists for life	Old infection
EA-D	7 days/2 wk	Acute or convalescent infection

TABLE 2-23   EBV Antibodies and the Timing of Infections

	POSSIBLE RESULTS			
VCA IgG	VCA IgM	EBNA IgG	EA	Interpretation
−	−	−	−	No previous exposure
+	+	−	±	Acute infection
+	−	+	−	Past infection
+	±	±	±	Recent infection
+	±	+	+	Reactivation

antibody profile (e.g., EBV viral capsid antigen [VCA] IgM, EBV VCA IgG, and EBV nuclear antigen [EBNA]) may be useful (Table 2-23). The viral capsid antigen-antibodies (VCAs) can be immunoglobulin (Ig) G or IgM. The EBV nuclear antigen (EBNA) is located in the nuclei of the infected lymphocyte. Another EBV antigen is called the early antigen (EA). There are two EA antigens. One is EA-D and is commonly associated with nasopharyngeal cancer. EA-R is commonly associated with Burkitt lymphoma.

The interpretation of EBV antibody tests is based on the following assumptions:
1. Once the person becomes infected with EBV, the anti-VCA antibodies appear first.
2. Anti-EA (EA-D or EA-R) antibodies appear next or are present with anti-VCA antibodies early in the course of illness. An anti-EA antibody titer greater than 80 in a patient 2 years after acute infectious mononucleosis indicates chronic EBV syndrome.
3. As the patient recovers, anti-VCA and anti-EA antibodies decrease and anti-EBNA antibodies appear. Anti-EBNA antibody persists for life and reflects a past infection.
4. After the patient is well, anti-VCA and anti-EBNA antibodies are always present but at lower ranges. Occasionally anti-EA antibody also may be present after the patient recovers.

In an acute infection, heterophile antibodies usually appear on the mono spot within the first 3 weeks of illness, but then decline rapidly within a few weeks. The heterophile antibody, however, fails to develop in about 10% of adults, more frequently in children, and almost uniformly in infants with primary EBV infections. If EBV infection is suspected to have occurred more than a few weeks before testing, the mono spot test may be negative. Detecting anti-VCA IgG or EBNA will not be helpful because they indicate that an EBV infection has occurred sometime in the patient's life but not necessarily recently. But detecting anti-VCA IgM would indicate that the syndrome of complaints the patient experienced a few weeks prior was because of EBV.

In immunosuppressed patients (i.e., those with AIDS, transplantation, or long-term chemotherapy), EBV infection can be much more serious, instigating extranodal lymphoma and posttransplant lymphoproliferative disorders. These patients may have serologic negative tests because of their immunosuppression.

EBV specific antibodies are most frequently detected by using enzyme immunoassay or qualitative enzyme immunoassay. With qualitative/quantitative polymerase chain reaction laboratory methods, EBV viral nuclear particles can be identified and measured. This technique provides a much more direct indication of EBV infection.

PROCEDURE AND PATIENT CARE

Before

☒ Explain the procedure to the patient.
☒ Tell the patient that no fasting or special preparation is required.

During

- Collect a venous blood sample in a lavender-top or pink tube.
- Record the date of onset of illness on the laboratory slip.
- Obtain serum samples as soon as possible after the onset of illness.
- Obtain a second blood specimen 14 to 21 days later.

After

- Apply pressure or a pressure dressing to the venipuncture site.
- Observe the venipuncture site for bleeding.

TEST RESULTS AND CLINICAL SIGNIFICANCE

▲   Increased Levels

Infectious mononucleosis,
Chronic EBV carrier state:
   To make this diagnosis, one of the antibodies should be found in abnormal titers.
Chronic fatigue syndrome: *These EBV antibodies are not found in all cases.*
Burkitt lymphoma,
Nasopharyngeal cancer (only occasionally in the United States):
   These cancers are frequently associated with EBV carrier states. However, a cause-and-effect relationship has not been determined.

RELATED TEST

Mononucleosis Rapid Test (p. 363). This test is used to detect heterophil antibodies that can support the diagnosis of EBV infection (infectious mononucleosis).

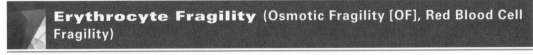

Erythrocyte Fragility (Osmotic Fragility [OF], Red Blood Cell Fragility)

NORMAL FINDINGS

Hemolysis begins at 0.5% NaCl
Hemolysis complete at 0.3% NaCl

INDICATIONS

This test is performed to detect hereditary spherocytosis and thalassemia when intravascular hemolysis is identified.

TEST EXPLANATION

Red blood cells (RBCs) are bound by a membrane that allows water to pass through while generally restricting the solutes. This process, called osmosis, causes RBCs to absorb water when in a hypotonic medium. This results in swelling and, ultimately, hemolysis as the cell bursts. The osmotic fragility test uses this fact to determine the concentration of solute inside the cell by subjecting it to salt solutions of different concentrations. The ability of the normal RBC to withstand hypotonicity results from its biconcave shape, which allows the cell to increase its volume by 70% before the surface membrane is stretched. Once this limit is reached, lysis occurs. When intravascular hemolysis is identified, OF is used to determine if the RBCs have increased fragility (tend to burst open when exposed to a higher-concentrated NaCl solution) or decreased fragility (tend to burst open in lower-concentrated, and thus more hypotonic, NaCl solution).

An osmotic fragility test primarily indicates the surface area–to–volume ratio (SAVR) of RBCs. The lower the ratio, the more fragile the RBC. OF of RBCs is defined as the ease with which the cells burst in hypotonic solutions. This is expressed in terms of the concentration of the saline solution in which the cells are hemolyzed. The numbers of cells that burst in varying concentrations of NaCl are plotted on a curve. That curve is compared to a normal curve. If the curve is shaped or shifted to the right, OF is abnormally increased (i.e., more cells lyse at higher concentrations NaCl). If the curve is abnormally shaped or shifted to the left, OF is decreased (i.e., fewer cells lyse at comparable NaCl concentrations). It is useful to record the concentration of sodium chloride solution causing 50% lysis (i.e., the median corpuscular fragility [MCF]). This value is normally 0.4% to 0.45% of NaCl. Other useful values include the concentration at which lysis begins (minimum resistance) and that at which lysis appears to be complete (maximum resistance). This test is performed by automated spectrophotometry.

Round cells (spherocytes) have increased OF compared to normal indented RBCs. In hereditary spherocytosis, there is abnormal morphology due to a lack of spectrin, a key RBC cytoskeletal membrane protein. This produces membrane instability, which forces the cell to the smallest volume—that of a sphere. This common disorder is associated with intravascular hemolysis. This is shown by increased osmotic fragility, which causes the entire curve to "shift to the right" or causes most of it to be within the normal range with a "tail" of fragile cells.

Thalassemia, on the other hand, is associated with thinner leptocytes whose OF is decreased. A single-tube osmotic fragility test has been proposed for thalassemia screening with a range of different saline concentrations. The sensitivity and specificity of a 0.36% buffered saline will provide a positive or equivocal result in nearly all patients with a thalassemia trait.

INTERFERING FACTORS

- Acute hemolysis because the osmotically labile cells are already hemolyzed and, therefore, not found in the blood specimen. Testing is recommended during a state of prolonged homeostasis with stable hematocrit.
- Dapsone can increase OF.

PROCEDURE AND PATIENT CARE

Before

Explain the procedure to the patient or child's parents.
Tell the patient that no fasting is required.

During

- Collect a venous blood sample in a green-top (sodium or lithium heparin) tube.
- Avoid hemolysis.

After

- Apply pressure or pressure dressing to the venipuncture site.
- Assess the venipuncture site for bleeding.

TEST RESULTS AND CLINICAL SIGNIFICANCE

▲ Increased Erythrocyte Fragility

Acquired hemolytic anemia,
Hereditary spherocytosis,
Hemolytic disease of the newborn,
Pyruvate kinase deficiency:
   These diseases are associated with the presence of abnormal spherocytic RBCs.
Malaria: *The plasmodium causes intravascular hemolysis and creation of rounded RBCs.*

▼ Decreased Erythrocyte Fragility

Thalassemia,
Hemoglobinopathies (C and S disease):
   This may in part be due to changes in membrane porosity or strength.
Iron deficiency anemia,
Reticulocytosis:
   The shape and relative volume of the cell area impacts OF.

RELATED TESTS

Haptoglobin (p. 274). This is an accurate marker of intravascular hemolysis.
Red Blood Cell Smear (p. 710). RBC shape is identified and quantified.

Erythrocyte Sedimentation Rate (ESR, Sed Rate Test)

NORMAL FINDINGS

Westergren Method

Male: up to 15 mm/hr
Female: up to 20 mm/hr
Child: up to 10 mm/hr
Newborn: 0-2 mm/hr

INDICATIONS

The ESR is a nonspecific test used to detect illnesses associated with acute and chronic infection, inflammation (collagen-vascular diseases), advanced neoplasm, and tissue necrosis or infarction.

TEST EXPLANATION

ESR is a measurement of the rate at which the red blood cells (RBCs) settle in saline solution or plasma over a specified time period. It is nonspecific and therefore not diagnostic for any particular organ disease or injury. Because inflammatory, neoplastic, infectious, and necrotic diseases increase the protein (mainly fibrinogen) content of plasma, RBCs have a tendency to stack up on one another, increasing their weight and causing them to descend faster. Therefore in these diseases the ESR will be increased. ESR provides the same information as an acute-phase reactant protein. That is to say that it occurs as a reaction to acute illnesses as described above.

The test can be used to detect occult disease. Many physicians use the ESR test in this way for routine patient evaluation for vague symptoms. Other physicians regard this test as so nonspecific that it is useless as a routine study. The ESR test occasionally can be helpful in differentiating disease entities or complaints. For example, in a patient with chest pain the ESR will be increased with myocardial infarction (MI) but will be normal in a patient with musculoskeletal chest pain.

The ESR is a fairly reliable indicator of the course of disease and therefore can be used to monitor disease therapy, especially for inflammatory autoimmune diseases (e.g., temporal arteritis, polymyalgia rheumatica). In general, as the disease worsens, the ESR increases; as the disease improves, the ESR decreases. If the results of the ESR are equivocal or inconsistent with clinical impressions, the C-reactive protein test is often performed.

ESR has several limitations:

1. As mentioned above, it is nonspecific.
2. It is sometimes not elevated in the face of active disease.
3. Many other factors may influence the results (see following section).

ESR elevation may lag behind other indicators early in an infection. Likewise, in the convalescent stage of a disease or infection, the ESR may remain elevated longer than other disease indicators. ESR cannot be used as an indicator of tumor burden when it is associated with neoplastic diseases, such as myeloma or breast cancer.

INTERFERING FACTORS

- Artificially low results can occur when the collected specimen is allowed to stand longer than 3 hours before the test.
- Pregnancy (second and third trimester) can cause elevated levels.
- Menstruation can cause elevated levels.
- The sedimentation tube must be perfectly vertical. Any tilt can distort results.
- Some anemias can falsely increase the ESR. There are correction nomograms available for variations in RBC count.
- Polycythemia is associated with decreased ESR.
- Diseases associated with increased proteins (e.g., macroglobulinemia) can falsely increase the ESR.
- Drugs that may cause *increased* ESR levels include dextran, methyldopa (Aldomet), oral contraceptives, penicillamine, procainamide, theophylline, and vitamin A.
- Drugs that may cause *decreased* levels include aspirin, cortisone, and quinine.

PROCEDURE AND PATIENT CARE

Before

✗ Explain the procedure to the patient.
- Hold medications that may affect test results, if indicated.

During

- Collect a venous blood sample in a yellow-top tube.
- In the laboratory, the blood is aspirated into a calibrated sedimentation tube and allowed to settle, usually for 60 minutes. The remaining clear area (plasma) is measured as the sedimentation rate.
- An alternate method is performed by measuring the distance (in millimeters) that RBCs descend (or settle) in normal saline solution in 1 hour. These processes are now automated (Figure 2-16).

After

- Transport the specimen immediately to the laboratory.
- Apply pressure or a pressure dressing to the venipuncture site.
- Assess the venipuncture site for bleeding.

TEST RESULTS AND CLINICAL SIGNIFICANCE

▲ Increased Levels

Chronic renal failure (e.g., nephritis, nephrosis): *The pathophysiology of this observation is not well defined.*

Malignant diseases (e.g., multiple myeloma, Hodgkin disease, advanced carcinomas): *Malignant diseases are often associated with increased abnormal serum proteins. Diseases associated with increased serum proteins are associated with increased ESR.*

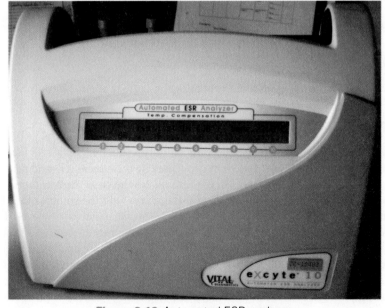

Figure 2-16 Automated ESR analyzer.

Bacterial infection (e.g., abdominal infections, acute pelvic inflammatory disease, syphilis, pneumonia),

Inflammatory diseases (e.g., temporal arteritis, polymyalgia rheumatica, rheumatoid arthritis, rheumatic fever, systemic lupus erythematosus [SLE]),

Necrotic diseases (e.g., acute myocardial infarction, necrotic tumor, gangrene of an extremity): *ESR is an acute-phase reactant protein and is elevated in the above-mentioned acute illnesses.*

Diseases associated with increased proteins (e.g., hyperfibrinogenemia, macroglobulinemia): *Diseases associated with increased serum proteins are associated with increased ESR.*

Severe anemias (e.g., iron deficiency or B_{12} deficiency): *With lower RBC volumes, the RBCs settle faster than in blood containing normal RBC volume.*

▼ Falsely Decreased Levels

Sickle cell anemia,

Spherocytosis: *Diseases that distort the RBC are associated with decreased ESR.*

Hypofibrinogenemia: *Diseases associated with decreased proteins inhibit the sedimentation of RBCs.*

Polycythemia vera: *Increased cells in the blood will inhibit the sedimentation of RBCs.*

RELATED TESTS

Complement Assay (p. 172). Some of the complement components are also acute-phase reactant proteins.

Fibrinogen (p. 241). This is an important protein involved in the hemostatic mechanism. It is also an acute-phase reactant protein.

C-Reactive Protein (p. 184). This is also an acute-phase reactant protein.

Erythropoietin (EPO)

NORMAL FINDINGS

5-35 international units/L

INDICATIONS

Erythropoietin (EPO) is used to assist in differentiating the cause of anemia or polycythemia.

TEST EXPLANATION

Erythropoietin is a glycoprotein hormone produced in the peritubular interstitial cells located in the inner cortex of the kidney. In response to decreased oxygen sensed by these renal cells and perhaps the carotid body cells, the production of EPO is increased. EPO stimulates the bone marrow to increase red blood cell (RBC) production. This improves oxygenation in the kidney, and the stimulus for EPO is reduced. This feedback mechanism is very sensitive to minimal persistent changes in oxygen levels. In patients with normal renal function, EPO levels are inversely proportional to the hemoglobin concentration.

As a hormone, EPO is often administered to patients who experience anemia as a result of chemotherapy. Occasionally, athletes abuse this hormone to improve oxygen carrying capacity and thereby improve performance.

EPO testing is performed to assist in the differential diagnosis of patients with anemia and polycythemia. EPO is elevated in patients who have a low hemoglobin because of failure of marrow production or RBC destruction (iron-deficiency or hemolytic anemia, respectively). The anemia results in reduced oxygen in the kidneys and EPO production is stimulated. However, although patients with renal diseases (or bilateral nephrectomy) are anemic, they do not have elevated EPO levels. The peritubular renal cells are damaged by renal disease. EPO levels fall and these patients experience anemia.

Patients who have polycythemia as an appropriate response to hypoxemia have elevated EPO levels. Yet patients who have malignant polycythemia vera may have reduced EPO levels. Some renal cell or adrenal carcinomas can produce elevated EPO levels that are unresponsive to the normal feedback inhibitory mechanisms.

INTERFERING FACTORS

- Pregnancy is associated with elevated EPO levels.
- The use of transfused blood decreases EPO levels.
- Drugs that *increase* EPO levels include ACTH, birth control pills, and steroids.

PROCEDURE AND PATIENT CARE

Before
Explain the procedure to the patient.

During
- Collect a venous blood sample in a red-top or gel separator tube.

After
- Apply pressure or a pressure dressing to the venipuncture site.
- Observe the venipuncture site for bleeding.

TEST RESULTS AND CLINICAL SIGNIFICANCE

▲   Increased Levels
Iron-deficiency anemia,
Megaloblastic anemia,
Hemolytic anemia,
Myelodysplasia,
Chemotherapy,
Acquired immunodeficiency syndrome (AIDS):
> *Decreased RBC production is associated with reduced oxygen carrying capacity. The specialized renal cells stimulate EPO production as a result.*

Pheochromocytoma,
Renal cell carcinoma,
Adrenal carcinoma:
> *These and other tumors can be associated with an ectopic site of EPO production.*

▼   Decreased Levels
Polycythemia vera: *Marrow erythroid production is maximal. Oxygen carrying capacity is maximized. The specialized renal cells reduce EPO production.*
Renal diseases and renal failure: *When the peritubular cells in the kidney are damaged, they cannot produce EPO. Blood levels drop.*

RELATED TESTS

Hemoglobin (p. 281). EPO is inversely proportional to hemoglobin levels.

Reticulocyte Count (p. 452). This is an important blood test that also is used in differentiating the causes of anemia and polycythemia.

Estrogen Fraction (Estriol Excretion, Estradiol, Estrone)

NORMAL FINDINGS

	Serum	Urine mcg/24 hr
Estradiol		
Child <10 years	<15 pg/mL	0-6
Adult male	10-50 pg/mL	0-6
Adult female		
Follicular phase	20-350 pg/mL	0-13
Midcycle peak	150-750 pg/mL	4-14
Luteal phase	30-450 pg/mL	4-10
Postmenopausal	≤20 pg/mL	0-4
Estriol		
Male or child <10 years	N/A	1-11
Adult female		
Follicular phase	N/A	0-14
Ovulatory phase	N/A	13-54
Luteal phase	N/A	8-60
Postmenopausal	N/A	0-11
Pregnant		
1st trimester	<38 ng/mL	0-800
2nd trimester	38-140 ng/mL	800-12,000
3rd trimester	31-460 ng/mL	5000-12,000
Total Estrogen		
Male or child <10 years	N/A	4-25
Female not pregnant	N/A	4-60
Female pregnant		
1st trimester	N/A	0-800
2nd trimester	N/A	800-5000
3rd trimester	N/A	5000-50,000

Rising estriol levels indicate normal fetal growth.

 Critical Values

Estriol levels 40% below average of two previous values demand immediate evaluation of fetal well-being during pregnancy.

INDICATIONS

Estrogen measurements are used to evaluate sexual maturity, menstrual problems, and fertility problems in females. This test is also used in the evaluation of males with gynecomastia or feminization syndromes. In pregnant women it is used to indicate fetal-placental health. In patients with estrogen-producing tumors it can be used as a tumor marker.

TEST EXPLANATION

There are three major estrogens. E_2 (estradiol) is predominantly produced in the ovary. In females there is a feedback mechanism for the secretion of E_2. Low levels of E_2 stimulate the hypothalamus to produce gonadotropin-releasing factors. These hormone factors stimulate the pituitary to produce follicle-stimulating hormone (FSH) and luteinizing hormone (LH). These two hormones stimulate the ovary to produce E_2, which peaks during the ovulatory phase of the menstrual cycle. This hormone is measured most often to evaluate menstrual and fertility problems, menopausal status, sexual maturity, gynecomastia, and feminization syndromes or as a tumor marker for patients with certain ovarian tumors.

E_1 (estrone) is also secreted by the ovary, but most is converted from androstenedione in peripheral tissues. Estrone is a more potent estrogen than estriol but is less potent than estradiol. Estrone is the major circulating estrogen after menopause.

E_3 (estriol) is the major estrogen in the pregnant female. Serial urine and blood studies of estriol excretion provide an objective assessment of placental function and fetal normality in high-risk pregnancies. Excretion of estriol increases around the eighth week of gestation and continues to rise until shortly before delivery. Estriol is produced in the placenta from estrogen precursors, which are made by the fetal adrenal gland and liver. The measurement of excreted estriol is an important index of fetal well-being. Rising values indicate an adequately functioning fetoplacental unit. Decreasing values suggest fetoplacental deterioration (failing pregnancy, dysmaturity, preeclampsia/eclampsia, complicated diabetes mellitus, anencephaly, fetal death) and require prompt reassessment of the pregnancy. If the estriol levels fall, early delivery of the fetus may be indicated.

Serial studies usually begin at approximately 28 to 30 weeks of gestation and are then repeated weekly. The frequency of these estriol determinations can be increased as needed to evaluate a high-risk pregnancy. Collection may be done daily. Although the first collection is the baseline value, all collection results are compared with previous ones, because decreasing values suggest fetal deterioration. Some physicians use an average of three previous values as a control value.

Estriol excretion studies can be done using 24-hour urine tests or blood studies. Because urinary creatinine excretion is relatively constant, creatinine clearance is often simultaneously tested to assess the adequacy of the 24-hour urine collection for estriol. A serially increasing estriol/creatinine ratio is a favorable sign in pregnancy. Plasma estriol determinations also can be used to evaluate the fetoplacental unit. These studies can conveniently and rapidly assess the quantity of free estriol in the plasma by radioimmunoassay (RIA). The plasma collected by venipuncture is an accurate reflection of the current status of the placenta and fetus. The advantage of the plasma estriol determination is that it is more easily obtained than a 24-hour urine specimen and is less affected by medications. All the estrogens can be measured by gas chromatography, but immunoassay techniques are more accurate and less affected by drugs or birth control pills.

Unfortunately only severe placental distress will decrease urinary estriol sufficiently to reliably predict fetoplacental stress. Furthermore, plasma and urinary estriol levels are normally associated with a significant daily variation, which may confuse serial results. Maternal illnesses, such as hypertension, preeclampsia, anemia, and impaired renal function, can also factitiously decrease urinary estriol levels.

Because these problems create a high number of false-positive and false-negative findings, most clinicians now use nonstress fetal monitoring (p. 569) to indicate fetal-placental health.

INTERFERING FACTORS

- Recent administration of radioisotopes may alter test results if RIA methods are used.
- Glycosuria and urinary tract infections (UTIs) can increase urine estriol levels.
- Drugs that may *increase* levels include adrenocorticosteroids, ampicillin, estrogen-containing drugs, phenothiazines, and tetracyclines.
- Drugs that may *decrease* levels include clomiphene.

PROCEDURE AND PATIENT CARE

Before

- Explain the procedure to the patient.
- If the patient is going to collect the 24-hour urine specimen at home, give her the collection bottle (with a preservative, usually boric acid) and instruct her to keep the urine refrigerated.
- Tell the patient that no food or fluid restrictions are needed.

During

Blood

- Collect a venous blood sample in a red-top tube.

24-Hour Urine

- Instruct the patient to begin the 24-hour urine collection after voiding. Discard the initial specimen and start the 24-hour collection at that point.
- Collect all urine passed during the next 24 hours. Make sure the patient knows where to store the urine container.
- Keep the specimen on ice or refrigerated during the 24-hour collection period.
- Indicate the starting time on the urine container and laboratory slip.
- Post the hours for the urine collection in a prominent place to prevent accidentally discarding the specimen.
- Instruct the patient to void before defecating so that the urine is not contaminated by feces.
- Remind the patient not to put toilet paper in the collection container.
- Encourage the patient to drink fluids during the 24 hours.
- Collect the last specimen as close as possible to the end of the 24-hour period. Add this urine to the collection.

After

- Apply pressure or a pressure dressing to the venipuncture site.
- Observe the venipuncture site for bleeding.
- Transport the 24-hour urine specimen promptly to the laboratory.
- Inform the patient how and when to obtain the results of this study.

TEST RESULTS AND CLINICAL SIGNIFICANCE

▲ Increased Levels

Feminization syndromes: *Estrogens are increased in these syndromes for a variety of reasons. The male begins to develop female secondary sex characteristics.*

Precocious puberty: *Children who develop secondary sexual characteristics at an abnormally early age often have a genetic defect in adrenal cortisol metabolism. As a result, large amounts of sex steroid precursors accumulate and are converted to estrogens by the ovary. This causes precocious secondary sexual changes.*

Ovarian tumor,

Testicular tumor,

Adrenal tumor:

Gonadal tumors (e.g., granulosa thecal cell tumors) secrete estrogens. The higher the levels, the greater the tumor burden. In these instances estrogen can act as a tumor marker that can be used to monitor the disease.

Normal pregnancy: E_3 *is the main estrogen elevated during pregnancy, although E_1 and E_2 are also elevated. Multiple pregnancies are associated with particularly high levels of E_3.*

Hepatic cirrhosis,

Liver necrosis:

Estrogens are catabolized, in part, by the liver. If liver function is deficient, estrogens and their precursors accumulate. Adult feminization can result.

Hyperthyroidism: *An estrogen-related increase in the production of thyroid-binding globulin produces an elevation of serum total T_4.*

▼ Decreased Levels

A failing pregnancy is associated with reduced placental production of E_3: *Any disease that causes fetal distress, dysmaturity, Rh isoimmunization, preeclampsia/eclampsia, anencephaly, or fetal death will be associated with reduced E_3 levels.*

Turner syndrome: *This syndrome is seen in females who are missing one X chromosome. They have gonadal dysgenesis to varying degrees.*

Hypopituitarism,

Primary and secondary hypogonadism,

Stein-Leventhal syndrome:

Diseases affecting the organs involved in the synthesis of sex hormones anywhere in the hypothalamus/pituitary/gonadal axis will be associated with reduced estrogen levels.

Menopause: *With normal age-related ovarian failure, estrogen (especially E_1) levels decline.*

Anorexia nervosa: *Reduction in fat intake reduces sterol precursors available for estrogen synthesis.*

RELATED TESTS

Luteinizing Hormone (LH) and Follicle-Stimulating Hormone (FSH) Assay (p. 348). These are measurements of gonadal stimulatory hormones.

Fetal Nonstress Test (p. 569). This is a more accurate test of placental/fetal viability.

 Ethanol (Ethyl Alcohol, Blood Alcohol, Blood EtOH)

NORMAL FINDINGS

0-50 mg/dL or 0%-0.05%

 Critical Values

>300 mg/dL or >65 mmol/L (SI units)

INDICATIONS

This test is usually performed to evaluate alcohol-impaired driving or overdose.

TEST EXPLANATION

Ethanol depresses the central nervous system and may cause reduced alertness, coma, and death. Proper collection, handling, and storage of blood alcohol are important for medicolegal cases involving sobriety testing. Legal testing must be done by specially trained people and must have a strict chain-of-custody (a paper trail that records sample movement and handling).

Samples tested for legal purposes may include blood, breath, urine, and/or saliva. The blood test is the specimen of choice. Blood is taken from a peripheral vein in living patients and from the aorta in cadavers. Results are given as mg/dL, g/100 mL or as a percentage. Each represents the same amount of alcohol. Blood alcohol concentrations (BACs) >80 mg/dL (0.08%) may cause flushing, slowing of reflexes, and impaired visual activity. Depression of the CNS occurs with BACs >0.1%, and fatalities are reported with levels >0.4%. BACs >0.1% can cause hypotension, although this is rare. This is especially important to recognize in the trauma patient in shock. Persons with BACs <0.05% are not considered under the influence of alcohol. Levels >0.05% to 0.10% are considered to be illegal and definite evidence of intoxication in most states. The American Medical Association says that a person can become impaired when the blood alcohol level hits 0.05%.

For legal purposes, when outside of a laboratory or hospital, taking a blood sample for later analysis in the laboratory is not practical or efficient. Breath testing is the most common test performed on automobile drivers. It uses the tail end sample of breath from deep in the lungs and uses a conversion factor to estimate the amount of alcohol in the blood. Blood alcohol testing may be ordered to confirm or refute findings, and/or ordered as an alternative to breath testing. Alcohol that a person drinks shows up in the breath because it gets absorbed from the intestinal tract and into the bloodstream. The alcohol is not metabolized on first pass through the liver. As the blood goes through the lungs, some of the volatile alcohol moves across the alveolar membranes and is exhaled. Conversion tables are available to calculate blood levels based on alcohol levels identified in the various nonblood specimens.

Urine testing may also be performed as an alternative to blood. Usually a patient collects and discards a urine sample and then collects a second sample 20 to 30 minutes later. Saliva alcohol testing is not as widely used, but may be used as an alternate screening test. Alcohol stays in the saliva for 6 to 12 hours. Finally hair testing is used but represents a more chronic use of alcohol.

INTERFERING FACTORS

- Elevated blood ketones (as with diabetic ketoacidosis) can cause false elevation of blood and breath test results.
- Bacteria in the urine of diabetic patients with glucosuria can metabolize the glucose to alcohol.
- Alcohols other than ethanol (e.g., isopropyl [rubbing alcohol] or methanol [grain alcohol]) will also cause testing to be positive.
- The use of alcohol-based mouthwash or cough syrup may cause false-positives on a breath test.

✓ Clinical Priorities

- This test is used to diagnose alcohol intoxication and overdose.
- Use povidone-iodine or peroxide to cleanse the venipuncture site instead of an alcohol wipe.
- Proper collection, handling, and storage of the blood sample are important for medical/legal cases involving sobriety.
- Patients should be advised of their legal rights.

PROCEDURE AND PATIENT CARE

Before

- Explain the procedure to the patient.
- Follow the institution's protocol if the specimen will be used for legal purposes.
- Patients should be advised of their legal rights. Sometimes this is best done by a law enforcement officer. The alcohol level may be used as evidence for later court proceedings.

During

- Use a povidone-iodine wipe or peroxide instead of an alcohol wipe for cleansing the venipuncture site.
- Collect a venous blood sample in a gray-top or red-top tube according to the agency's protocol.
- If a gastric or urine specimen is indicated, approximately 20 to 50 mL of fluid is necessary.
- Breath samples for analysis are taken at the end of expiration after a deep inspiration.

After

- Apply pressure or a pressure dressing to the venipuncture site.
- Assess the venipuncture site for bleeding.
- Follow the agency's protocol regarding specimen collection.
- The exact time of specimen collection should be indicated. Also, signatures of the collector and a witness may be needed in some instances for legal evidence.

TEST RESULTS AND CLINICAL SIGNIFICANCE

▲ **Increased Levels**

Alcohol intoxication or overdose: *Alcohol is rapidly absorbed from the stomach in about 1 hour. If the stomach is empty, absorption is faster. Alcohol is metabolized in the liver. A 70-kg person with normal liver function can metabolize about 15 mg of alcohol per hour.*

Factor V-Leiden (FVL, Mutation Analysis)

NORMAL FINDINGS

Negative

INDICATIONS

This test is used to diagnose factor V-Leiden thrombophilia.

TEST EXPLANATION

Factor V is an important factor in reaction 4 (common pathway) of normal hemostasis (see p. 163). The term *factor V-Leiden* refers to an inherited abnormal form of factor V in which there is a specific glutamine-to-arginine substitution at nucleotide 1691 in the gene for factor V. That genetic mutation causes a single amino acid replacement (Arg506 Gln) at one of three cleavage sites in the factor V molecule. The endogenous anticoagulant, protein C (see p. 432) normally is able to break down factor V at one of these cleavage sites. However, protein C cannot inactivate this same cleavage site on factor V-Leiden. FVL is therefore inactivated at a rate approximately ten times slower than normal factor V and persists longer in the circulation. This results in increased thrombin generation and a mild hypercoagulable state reflected by elevated levels of prothrombin fragment F1+2 and other activated coagulation markers.

Individuals heterozygous for the factor V-Leiden mutation have a slightly increased risk for venous thrombosis. Homozygous individuals have a much greater thrombotic risk (e.g., deep vein thrombosis [DVT], arterial thrombosis, or pulmonary embolism).

Individuals who are candidates for FVL testing include patients who have:

- Experienced a thrombotic event without any predisposing factors
- A strong family history of thrombotic events
- Experienced a thrombotic event before 30 years of age
- Experienced DVT during pregnancy or while taking birth control pills
- Had venous thrombosis at unusual sites (e.g., cerebral, mesenteric, portal, or hepatic veins)
- Experienced an arterial clot

Factor V-Leiden is the most common hereditary blood coagulation disorder in the United States. It is present in 5% of the Caucasian population and 1.2% of the African-American population. Only about 10% of patients who have FVL will experience a thrombotic event.

Testing for FVL is sometimes preceded by a screening coagulation test called the *activated protein C (APC) resistance test*. This is a test to identify resistance of factor V to activated protein C (APC). Protein C (see p. 432), in the presence of its cofactors thrombomodulin and thrombin, is enzymatically cleaved to its active form, activated protein C. APC is an important natural anticoagulant (to balance coagulation) that functions by inactivating the critical coagulation factors fVa and fVIIIa. In thrombotic patients (many of whom have FVL), those factors will be resistant to deactivation when exposed to APC. Pregnancy and reactive causes of increased factor VIII can also be associated with APC resistance.

APC resistance testing is performed on citrated plasma (blue tops) from thrombotic patients with a normal activated partial thromboplastin time (aPTT) before anticoagulant therapy. Briefly, a standard aPTT test (see p. 383) is performed in the absence and then in the presence of commercially available activated protein C. In the normal response, the aPTT is prolonged in the presence of APC due to the anticoagulant action of this protein. An abnormality is detected by failure to prolong the aPTT caused by "resistance to APC." The results are reported as a ratio of the APC-aPTT/aPTT with a normal result greater than 2.0. Patients with the lowest APC ratios appear to be homozygous for the abnormal factor V molecule while heterozygotes appear to have ratios intermediate between the normal range and homozygote levels.

If APC resistance is identified, the patient then may choose to undergo mutation testing by DNA analysis of the F5 gene, which encodes the factor V protein. Polymerase chain reaction/restriction enzyme digestion/gel electrophoresis or fluorescent direct mutation testing methods are commonly used. This testing should be accompanied by professional genetic counseling for the patient and family members.

PROCEDURE AND PATIENT CARE

Before

✍ Explain the procedure to the patient.

- If the patient is receiving heparin by intermittent injection, plan to draw the blood specimen for the aPTT 30 minutes to 1 hour before the next dose of heparin.
- If the patient is having FVL mutational analysis, anticoagulants will not interfere with testing.

During

- Collect a venous blood sample in one or two blue-top tubes.
- Venous blood is collected in a purple (EDTA) tube for FVL mutational analysis.
- As an alternative, genetic testing can be done on the patient's cells obtained by a smear of the oral surface of the cheek.

After

- Apply pressure or a pressure dressing to the venipuncture site.
- Assess the venipuncture site for bleeding. Remember, if the patient is receiving anticoagulants, the bleeding time will be increased.
- Results are provided to the patient by a physician and a genetic counselor.

TEST RESULTS AND CLINICAL SIGNIFICANCE

APC resistance: *These patients most probably have FVL, but other forms of thrombophilia (predisposition to thrombotic events) can cause APC resistance.*

FVL genetic mutation

Homozygous: *These patients have received a FVL gene from each parent and have a thrombotic risk that exceeds 80 times that of the normal population.*

Heterozygous: *These patients have received a FVL gene from one parent and normal factor V from the other. These individuals have a thrombotic risk for about 10 times that of the normal population.*

RELATED TESTS

Protein C, Protein S (p. 432). This test identifies patients who are deficient in either protein C and/or protein S.

Partial Thromboplastin Time, Activated (p. 383). The aPTT test is used to identify APC resistance and is a preliminary test to identify individuals with FVL.

Febrile Antibodies (Febrile Agglutinins)

NORMAL FINDINGS

Titers ≤1:80

INDICATIONS

These antibodies are used to diagnose rickettsial, Salmonella, or Brucella infections.

TEST EXPLANATION

Febrile antibodies are used to support the diagnosis and monitoring of infectious diseases such as salmonellosis, rickettsial diseases, brucellosis, and tularemia. Neoplastic diseases, such as leukemias and lymphomas, are also associated with febrile agglutinins. Appropriate antibiotic treatment of the infectious agent is associated with a drop in the titer/activity of febrile antibodies. Screening testing (EIA) is first performed and reported in dilution. If positive (>1:80), disease-specific antibodies are then quantified by immunofluorescence assay. This test is nonspecific and insensitive. More specific testing for these infective agents provides more sensitive and specific laboratory testing.

Salmonella and acute brucellosis along with the spotted group of rickettsial agents (*R. rickettsii* causing Rocky Mountain spotted fever; *R. akari* causing Rickettsialpox; and *R. conorii* causing Boutonneuse fever) can be identified. The typhus fever group of rickettsial agents (*R. typhi* causing endemic or murine typhus; *R. prowazekii* causing epidemic typhus; and Brill-Zinsser disease caused by reactivation of latent *R. prowazekii*) can also be quantified.

IgM reactivity usually indicates an acute infection. However, IgM reactivity, in the absence of IgG reactivity, may represent a false-positive reaction. Recent infection should be confirmed by demonstrating either IgG seroconversion or a fourfold or greater increase in IgG titer when acute and convalescent sera are tested in parallel.

Temperature regulation is important for the performance of these tests. Under no circumstances should the febrile agglutinin be heated before delivery to the laboratory.

PROCEDURE AND PATIENT CARE

Before

✗ Explain the procedure to the patient.
✗ Tell the patient that no fasting is required.

During

• Collect venous blood in a red-top tube.

After

• Apply pressure to the venipuncture site.
• Transport the specimen immediately to the laboratory.

ABNORMAL FINDINGS

▲ Increased levels

Salmonellosis infection,
Rickettsial disease,
Brucellosis,
Tularemia,
Leukemia,
Lymphoma,
Systemic lupus erythematosus:
> *These unusual infections and other diseases can be associated with febrile agglutination of RBCs. The specific immunoglobulin can be identified and associated with the clinical presentation to assist in the diagnosis of the infective agent.*

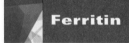

Ferritin

NORMAL FINDINGS

Male: 12-300 ng/mL or 12-300 mcg/L (SI units)
Female: 10-150 ng/mL or 10-150 mcg/L (SI units)
Child/adolescent
    Newborn: 25-200 ng/mL
    ≤1 month: 200-600 ng/mL
    2-5 months: 50-200 ng/mL
    6 months-15 years: 7-142 ng/mL

INDICATIONS

This is the most sensitive test to determine iron-deficiency anemia.

TEST EXPLANATION

The serum ferritin study is a good indicator of available iron stores in the body. Ferritin, the major iron-storage protein, is normally present in the serum in concentrations directly related to iron storage. In normal patients, 1 ng/mL of serum ferritin corresponds to approximately 8 mg of stored iron. Ferritin levels rise persistently in males and postmenopausal females. In premenopausal females, levels stay about the same. Decreases in ferritin levels indicate a decrease in iron storage associated with iron-deficiency anemia. A ferritin level of below 10 mg/100 mL is diagnostic of iron-deficiency anemia. A decrease in serum ferritin level often precedes other signs of iron deficiency, such as decreased iron levels or changes in red blood cell (RBC) size, color, and number. Only when protein depletion is severe can ferritin be decreased by malnutrition. Increased levels are a sign of iron excess, as seen in hemochromatosis, hemosiderosis, iron poisoning, or recent blood transfusions. Increases in ferritin are also noted in patients with megaloblastic anemia, hemolytic anemia, and chronic hepatitis. Furthermore, ferritin is factitiously elevated in patients with chronic disease states such as neoplasm, alcoholism, uremia, collagen diseases, or chronic liver diseases. The ferritin test is also used in patients with chronic renal failure to monitor iron stores.

A limitation of this study is that ferritin also can act as an acute-phase reactant protein and may be elevated in conditions not reflecting iron stores (e.g., acute inflammatory diseases, infections, metastatic cancer, lymphomas). Elevations in ferritin occur 1 to 2 days after onset of the acute illness and the level peaks at 3 to 5 days. If iron deficiency coexists in patients with these diseases, it may not be recognized because the levels of ferritin would be factitiously elevated by the concurrent disease.

When combined with the serum iron level and total iron-binding capacity (TIBC), this test is useful in differentiating and classifying anemias. For example, in patients with iron deficiency anemia the ferritin, iron, and transferrin saturation levels are low, whereas the TIBC and transferrin levels are high (Table 2-24). Ferritin is measured by either radioimmunoassay or enzyme immunoassay.

INTERFERING FACTORS

- Recent transfusions or recent ingestion of a meal containing a high iron content (red meats) may cause elevated ferritin levels. The iron that is ingested stimulates ferritin production to store the increased serum iron.
- Recent administration of a radionuclide can cause abnormal levels if testing is performed by radioimmunoassay.
- Hemolytic diseases may be associated with an artificially high iron content. Iron is freed from the hemoglobin that is released from the hemolyzed RBCs. Ferritin synthesis is increased to store the increased serum iron.
- Acute and chronic inflammatory conditions and Gaucher disease can falsely increase ferritin levels.
- Disorders of excessive iron storage (e.g., hemochromatosis, hemosiderosis) are associated with high ferritin levels. Ferritin synthesis is increased to store the increased serum iron.
- Iron-deficient menstruating women may have decreased ferritin levels, because their iron stores are generally low as a result of monthly menses.
- Iron preparations may *increase* ferritin levels. Ferritin synthesis is increased to store the increased serum iron.

TABLE 2-24	Iron Studies in Various Clinical States			
	Ferritin	Iron	Total Iron Binding Capacity	Transferrin Saturation
Chronic blood loss	L	L	E	L
Acute blood loss	N	L	N	L
Iron deficiency	L	L	E	L
Hemolytic anemia	E	E	L	E
Chronic disease	E	L	L	L
Hemochromatosis	E	E	L	E
Pregnancy	L	L	E	L
Estrogen therapy	N	E	E	L
Acute inflammation	E	N	L	E

E, Elevated; *L*, low; *N*, normal.

PROCEDURE AND PATIENT CARE

Before
✗ Explain the procedure to the patient.
✗ Tell the patient that no fasting is required.

During
• Collect a venous blood sample in a red-top tube.

After
• Apply pressure or a pressure dressing to the venipuncture site.
• Assess the venipuncture site for bleeding.

TEST RESULTS AND CLINICAL SIGNIFICANCE

▲ Increased Levels

Hemochromatosis,
Hemosiderosis:
   Increased iron stores in the tissues stimulate ferritin production for storage.
Megaloblastic anemia,
Hemolytic anemia:
   RBCs in anemias lyse and release iron into the bloodstream. Ferritin production is stimulated to store the excess free iron.
Alcoholic/inflammatory hepatocellular disease,
Inflammatory disease,
Advanced cancers:
   Because ferritin is an acute-phase reactant protein, its production is increased with acute diseases.
Chronic illnesses such as leukemias, cirrhosis, chronic hepatitis, or collagen-vascular diseases: *The pathophysiology of this observation is not known.*

▼ **Decreased Levels**

Iron-deficiency anemia: *When iron stores are decreased, less ferritin is required. Levels diminish.*
Severe protein deficiency: *Ferritin is a protein. In severely depleted persons, ferritin synthesis is reduced.*
Hemodialysis: *Iron stores can be reduced by dialysis. Decreased iron stores require less ferritin. Levels diminish.*

RELATED TESTS

Iron Level (p. 322). This is a direct measurement of bound iron in the blood.
Total Iron-Binding Capacity (p. 322). TIBC is a measurement of all proteins available for binding mobile iron. Transferrin represents the largest quantity of iron-binding proteins.
Transferrin (p. 322). Transferrin represents the largest quantity of iron-binding proteins.
Transferrin Receptor Assay (p. 502). This is used to differentiate iron deficiency from other anemias.

Fetal Hemoglobin Testing (Kleihauer-Betke Test)

NORMAL FINDINGS

<1% of red blood cells (RBCs)

INDICATIONS

This test is performed on pregnant women to determine the presence of and quantify the amount of fetal-maternal hemorrhage.

TEST EXPLANATION

Fetal hemoglobin may be present in the mother's blood because of fetal-maternal hemorrhage (FMH), which causes leakage of fetal cells into the maternal circulation. When large volumes of fetal blood are lost in this way, serious and potentially fatal neonatal outcomes can result. Massive FMH may be the cause of around 1 in every 50 stillbirths. No historical or clinical features allow antecedent identification of those in whom FMH may be the cause of an intrauterine death. Therefore a large proportion of patients with FMH will continue to remain undetected.

Leakage of fetal RBCs can begin anytime after the mid-first trimester. It presumably results from a breach in the integrity of the placental circulation. As pregnancy continues, more and more women will show evidence of fetal RBCs in their circulation so that by term about 50% will have detectable fetal cells. Most of these, however, are the result of very small leaks. The total fetal blood volume lost in this way is 2 mL or less in 96% to 98% of pregnancies. Small leaks are not implicated in intrauterine death.

Risk factors correlated with the increasing risk for massive FMH include maternal trauma, placental abruption, placental tumors, third trimester amniocentesis, fetal hydrops, pale fetal organs, antecedent sinusoidal fetal heart tracing, and twinning. Having one or more of these features should be an indication for fetal hemoglobin testing.

The standard method of detecting FMH is the *Kleihauer-Betke test*. This takes advantage of the differential resistance of fetal hemoglobin to acid. A standard blood smear is prepared from mother's blood. An acid bath is then used that removes all adult hemoglobin but does not remove fetal hemoglobin. Subsequent staining makes fetal cells (containing fetal hemoglobin) rose pink, although the mother's cells are only seen as "ghosts." A large number of cells (e.g., 5000) are counted under the microscope and the ratio of fetal to maternal cells is generated.

The flow cytometric method for HbF determination offers several advantages over the traditional Kleihauer-Betke method. This more objective method has been shown to improve sensitivity, precision, and linearity over traditional methods.

FMH becomes of even greater significance when the mother is Rh negative as this is the mechanism through which Rh sensitization could develop if the fetus has paternal Rh-positive blood cells. If this is known to exist, RhoGAM (RhIG, Rh immunoglobulin) antibodies directed to Rh-positive fetal cells are given to the pregnant mother (at about 28 weeks of pregnancy, and within 72 hours after a birth, miscarriage, abortion, or amniocentesis). RhoGAM is often administered if any invasive procedure is performed on the Rh-negative mother where she may be exposed to the Rh-positive fetal blood. The RhoGAM antibodies kill the fetal RBCs in the maternal bloodstream before the mother has an opportunity to develop any antibodies to fetal Rh-positive RBCs. This precludes more aggressive anti-fetal RBC occurrences in the near or remote future. By determination of the amount and volume of fetal blood loss, a dose of Rhogam can be calculated using the following formula:

$$\text{Vials of RhIG} = \frac{\text{Milliliters of fetal blood}}{30}$$

This test is often performed on women who have delivered a stillborn baby to see if FMH was a potential cause of fetal death.

INTERFERING FACTORS

- Any maternal condition (such as sickle cell disease) that involves persistence of fetal hemoglobin in the mother will cause a false positive.
- If the blood is drawn after cesarean section, a false positive could be recorded. Vaginal delivery does result in higher frequency of detection of FMH.

PROCEDURE AND PATIENT CARE

Before

🖎 Explain the procedure to the patient.

During

- Collect a venous blood sample in a red-top tube for serum testing.
- Avoid hemolysis.

After

- Apply pressure to the venipuncture site.
- Emphasize to the patient the importance of antepartal health care.
- Provide emotional support in the event this test is performed after a stillborn delivery.

TEST EXPLANATION AND CLINICAL SIGNIFICANCE

▲ Increased Levels

Feto-maternal hemorrhage (FMH): *Fetal, placental, or maternal pathology can result in leakage of fetal cells into the maternal bloodstream.*

Hereditary persistence of fetal hemoglobin: *With any hemoglobinopathy, fetal hemoglobin is often continually made in RBCs as a compensatory mechanism to insure good tissue oxygenation. This will be identified through this test and may give the false sense of FMH.*

Intrachorionic thrombi: *Placental thrombosis causes a breakdown in maternal/fetal membrane barrier. Fetal cells can cross over into the maternal circulation.*

 Fetal Scalp Blood pH

NORMAL FINDINGS

pH: 7.25-7.35
O_2 saturation: 30%-50%
Po_2: 18-22 mm Hg
Pco_2: 40-50 mm Hg
Base excess: 0 to –10 mEq/L

INDICATIONS

This test indicates fetal well-being or fetal distress.

TEST EXPLANATION

Measurement of fetal scalp blood pH provides valuable information on fetal acid-base status. This test is useful for diagnosing fetal distress.

Although the oxygen partial pressure (Po_2), carbon dioxide partial pressure (Pco_2), and bicarbonate ion (HCO_3^-) concentration can be measured with the fetal scalp blood sample, the pH is the most useful clinically. The pH normally ranges from 7.25 to 7.35 during labor; a mild decline within the normal range is noted with contractions and as labor progresses.

Fetal hypoxia causes anaerobic glycolysis, resulting in excess production of lactic acid. This causes an increase in hydrogen ion concentration (acidosis) and a decrease in pH. Acidosis reflects the effect of hypoxia on cellular metabolism. A high correlation exists between low pH levels and low Apgar scores.

Fetal oxygen saturation can be measured by oximetry, see p. 1114.

CONTRAINDICATIONS

- Patients with premature membrane rupture, because infection can be instilled into the uterus
- Patients with active cervical infection (e.g., gonorrhea, herpes, human immunodeficiency virus [HIV]), because the active infection can be spread to the fetus

POTENTIAL COMPLICATIONS

- Continued bleeding from the puncture site
- Hematoma
- Ecchymosis
- Infection

Clinical Priorities

- The fetal scalp pH indicates fetal well-being or fetal distress.
- Fetal hypoxia causes anaerobic glycolysis, resulting in excess production of lactic acid. This causes a decrease in pH.
- A high correlation exists between a low pH and low Apgar scores.

PROCEDURE AND PATIENT CARE

Before

📋 Explain the procedure to the patient.
- Obtain an informed consent for this procedure.
📋 Tell the patient that no fasting or sedation is required.

During

- Note the following procedural steps:
  1. Amnioscopy is performed with the mother in the lithotomy position.
  2. The cervix is dilated, and the endoscope (amnioscope) is introduced into the cervical canal.
  3. The fetal scalp is cleansed with an antiseptic and dried with a sterile cotton ball.
  4. A small amount of petroleum jelly is applied to the fetal scalp to cause droplets of fetal blood to bead.
  5. After the skin on the scalp is pierced with a small metal blade, beaded droplets of blood are collected in long, heparinized capillary tubes.
  6. The tube is sealed with wax and placed on ice to retard cellular respiration, which can alter the pH.
  7. The physician performing the procedure applies firm pressure to the puncture site to retard bleeding.
  8. Scalp blood sampling can be repeated as necessary.
- Note that this study is performed by a physician in approximately 10 to 15 minutes.
📋 Tell the patient that she may be uncomfortable during the cervical dilation.

After

📋 Inform the patient that she may have vaginal discomfort and menstrual-type cramping.
- After delivery assess the newborn and identify and document the puncture site(s).
- Cleanse the fetal scalp puncture site with an antiseptic solution and apply an antibiotic ointment.

TEST RESULTS AND CLINICAL SIGNIFICANCE

▲   Increased Levels

Fetal distress: *Fetal hypoxia causes anaerobic glycolysis, resulting in excess production of lactic acid. This causes an increase in hydrogen ion concentration (acidosis) and a decrease in pH.*

RELATED TEST

Arterial Blood Gases (p. 109). This test provides valuable information in assessing and managing a patient's respiratory (ventilation) and metabolic (renal) acid-base and electrolyte homeostasis. It is also used to assess adequacy of oxygenation.

Fetal Oxygen Saturation (p. 1114). This is useful in monitoring fetal well-being during labor and delivery.

Fibrinogen (Factor I, Quantitative Fibrinogen)

NORMAL FINDINGS

Adult: 200-400 mg/dL or 2-4 g/L (SI units)
Newborn: 125-300 mg/dL

Critical Values

Values of <100 mg/dL can be associated with spontaneous bleeding.

INDICATIONS

Fibrinogen is used primarily to aid in the diagnosis of suspected bleeding disorders. This testing is used to detect increased or decreased fibrinogen (factor I) concentration of acquired or congenital origin. It is also used for monitoring severity and treatment of disseminated intravascular coagulation and fibrinolysis.

TEST EXPLANATION

Fibrinogen is essential to the blood-clotting mechanism. It is part of the "common pathway" (fourth reaction) in the coagulation system. Fibrinogen is converted to fibrin by the action of thrombin during the coagulation process. Fibrinogen, which is produced by the liver, is also an acute-phase reactant protein. It rises sharply during tissue inflammation or tissue necrosis.

High levels of fibrinogen have been associated with an increased risk for coronary heart disease (CHD), stroke, myocardial infarction (MI), and peripheral arterial disease. Reduced levels can be seen in patients with liver disease, malnourished states, and consumptive coagulopathies (e.g., disseminated intravascular coagulation [DIC]). Large-volume blood transfusions are also associated with low levels, because banked blood does not contain fibrinogen. Reduced levels of fibrinogen will cause prolonged prothrombin (PT) and partial thromboplastin (PTT) times. Electromagnetic mechanical clot or viscosity detection is the most commonly performed laboratory method used in quantification.

INTERFERING FACTORS

- Blood transfusions within the past month may affect test results.
- Diets rich in omega-3 and omega-6 fatty acids reduce fibrinogen levels.
- Drugs that may cause *increased* levels include estrogens and oral contraceptives.
- Drugs that may cause *decreased* levels include anabolic steroids, androgens, asparaginase, phenobarbital, streptokinase, urokinase, and valproic acid.

PROCEDURE AND PATIENT CARE

Before

 Explain the procedure to the patient.
 Tell the patient that no fasting is required.

During

- Collect one tube of venous blood in a blue-top tube.

After

- Apply pressure or a pressure dressing to the venipuncture site.
- Assess the venipuncture site for bleeding.

TEST RESULTS AND CLINICAL SIGNIFICANCE

▲ Increased Levels

Acute inflammatory reactions (e.g., rheumatoid arthritis [RA], glomerulonephritis),
Trauma,
Acute infection such as pneumonia:
  Fibrinogen is an acute-phase reactant protein.
Coronary heart disease (CHD),
Stroke,
Peripheral vascular disease,
Cigarette smoking:
  Elevated fibrinogen levels are merely an observation with no known pathophysiology.
Pregnancy: *Pregnancy is associated with increased serum proteins (including fibrinogen).*

▼ Decreased Levels

Liver disease (hepatitis, cirrhosis): *Fibrinogen is not made in adequate volume.*
Consumptive coagulopathy (DIC),
Fibrinolysins:
  Primary and secondary fibrinolysins act to destroy fibrinogen within the serum.
Congenital afibrinogenemia: *A genetic defect precludes the synthesis of fibrinogen.*
Advanced carcinoma,
Malnutrition:
  Severe protein depletion is associated with reduced levels of fibrinogen (a protein).
Large-volume blood transfusion: *Fibrinogen does not exist in normal levels in banked blood. The more that is transfused, the more the native fibrinogen is diluted.*

RELATED TESTS

Prothrombin Time (PT) (p. 434). The PT is used to evaluate the adequacy of the extrinsic system and common pathway in the clotting mechanism.

Partial Thromboplastin Time (PTT) (p. 383). This test is used to evaluate the intrinsic system and the common pathway of clot formation. It is most commonly used to monitor heparin therapy.

Coagulating Factor Concentration (p. 163). This is a quantitative measurement of specific coagulation factors.

Thrombosis Indicators (p. 482). These tests are most commonly used to support the diagnosis of DIC.

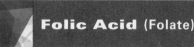

Folic Acid (Folate)

NORMAL FINDINGS

5-25 ng/mL or 11-57 mmol/L (SI units)

INDICATIONS

This test quantifies the folate level in the blood. It is used in patients who have megaloblastic anemia. It is also used to assess nutritional status, especially in alcoholics.

TEST EXPLANATION

Folic acid, one of the B vitamins, is necessary for normal function of red blood cells (RBCs) and white blood cells (WBCs). It is needed for the adequate synthesis of certain purines and pyrimidines, which are precursors of deoxyribonucleic acid (DNA). It is also used in the synthesis of several amino acids. Vitamin B_{12} is necessary for conversion of inactive 5-methyltetrahydrofolate to the active tetrahydrofolate, the active form of folate. As with vitamin B_{12}, the folate level depends on adequate dietary ingestion and normal intestinal absorption of this vitamin.

The finding of a low serum folate means that the patient's recent diet has been subnormal in folate content and/or that recent absorption of folate has been subnormal. In time, folate levels will also drop in the tissues. Tissue folate is best tested by determining the content of folate in RBCs. A low RBC folate can mean either that there is tissue folate depletion due to folate deficiency requiring folate therapy, or alternatively, that the patient has primary vitamin B_{12} (see p. 518) deficiency blocking the ability of cells to take up folate. In the latter case, the proper therapy would be with vitamin B_{12} rather than with folic acid. For these reasons it is advisable to determine RBC folate in addition to serum folate.

Folic acid blood levels are performed to assess folate availability in pregnancy, to evaluate hemolytic disorders, and to detect anemia caused by folic acid deficiency (in which the RBCs are abnormally large, causing a megaloblastic anemia). These RBCs have a shortened life span and impaired oxygen-carrying capacity. If low, RBC folate is measured.

The main causes of folic acid deficiency include dietary deficiency (usually in the alcoholic patient), malabsorption syndrome, pregnancy, and certain anticonvulsant drugs. Decreased folic acid levels are seen in patients with folic acid deficiency anemia (megaloblastic anemia), hemolytic anemia, malnutrition, malabsorption syndrome, malignancy, liver disease, sprue, and celiac disease. Some drugs (e.g., anticonvulsants, antimalarials, alcohol, aminopterin, methotrexate) are folic acid antagonists and interfere with nucleic acid synthesis.

Elevated levels of folic acid may be seen in patients with pernicious anemia. Because there is not an adequate amount of vitamin B_{12} in these patients to metabolize folic acid, levels of folate rise in pernicious anemia. The folic acid test should be done in conjunction with tests for vitamin B_{12} levels.

The folate test is often part of the workup in alcoholic patients to assess nutritional status. Folate must be depleted for at least 5 months before megaloblastic anemia occurs.

Radioimmunoassay (RIA), enzyme immunoassay (EIA), quantitative chemiluminescent immunoassay, or automated competitive-binding receptor assay techniques are commonly used methods of folic acid measurement.

INTERFERING FACTORS

- A folate-deficient patient who has received a blood transfusion may have a falsely normal result.
- Because RIA is the method of choice for folic acid determination, radionuclide administration should be avoided for at least 24 hours.
- *Drugs that may cause *decreased* folic acid levels include* alcohol, aminopterin, aminosalicylic acid, ampicillin, antimalarials, chloramphenicol, erythromycin, estrogens, methotrexate, oral contraceptives, penicillin derivatives, phenobarbital, phenytoin, and tetracyclines.

PROCEDURE AND PATIENT CARE

Before

☒ Explain the procedure to the patient.
☒ Tell the patient that no fasting is usually required. (However, some laboratories prefer an 8-hour fast.)
☒ Instruct the patient not to consume alcoholic beverages before the test.
- Draw the specimen before starting folate therapy.

During

- Collect a venous blood sample in a red-top tube.
- Avoid hemolysis. Folate in the RBCs can falsely raise serum folate levels when hemolysis of the RBC occurs.
- Indicate on the laboratory slip any medications that may affect test results.

After

- Apply pressure or a pressure dressing to the venipuncture site.
- Assess the venipuncture site for bleeding.
- Transport the blood to the laboratory immediately after collection.

TEST RESULTS AND CLINICAL SIGNIFICANCE

▲   Increased Levels

Pernicious anemia: *When there is an inadequate amount of vitamin B_{12} to metabolize folic acid, levels of folate rise.*
Vegetarianism: *Increased ingestion of folate-containing vegetables can lead to increased levels of folic acid.*
Recent massive blood transfusion: *Folate in the hemolyzed RBCs of banked blood can falsely raise serum folate levels.*

▼   Decreased Levels

Malnutrition: *Inadequate intake of folic acid is the most common cause of folate deficiency. This is most common in alcoholics. Alcohol also reduces folic acid absorption.*
Malabsorption syndrome (e.g., sprue, celiac disease): *Folic acid, like vitamin B_{12}, is absorbed in the small intestine. In malabsorption, folic acid is not absorbed. Serum and tissue levels decline.*
Pregnancy: *Folic acid deficiency in pregnancy probably results from a combination of inadequate intake and increased demand placed by the fetus on the maternal source of folic acid.*
Folic acid deficiency (megaloblastic) anemia,
Hemolytic anemia:
   These anemias are the result of folic acid deficiency. The large megaloblastic RBCs cannot conform to small capillaries. Instead, they fracture and hemolyze. The shortened life span ultimately leads to anemia.
Malignancy,
Liver disease,
Chronic renal disease:
   The pathophysiology for these observations is not known.

RELATED TESTS

Vitamin B_{12} (p. 518). This is a measurement of the level of vitamin B_{12} in the serum. This test should be performed with a folic acid test.

Complete Blood Cell Count (CBC) (p. 174). This is performed routinely and can identify megaloblastic anemia.

 Galectin-3 (GAL-3)

NORMAL FINDINGS

≤22.1 ng/mL

INDICATIONS

This test is helpful in determining the prognosis of congestive heart failure.

TEST EXPLANATION

Heart failure progresses primarily by dilatation of the ventricular cardiac chamber through remodeling in fibrosis as a response to cardiac injury and/or overload. Galectin-3 (GAL-3) is a biomarker that appears to be actively involved in both the inflammatory and fibrotic pathways involved in remodeling. GAL-3 is a carbohydrate-binding lectin whose expression is associated with inflammatory cells, including macrophages, neutrophils, and mast cells. GAL-3 has been linked to cardiovascular physiologic processes, including myofibroblast proliferation, tissue repair, and cardiac remodeling in the setting of heart failure. Concentrations of GAL-3 have been used to predict adverse remodeling after a variety of cardiac insults.

Elevated GAL-3 results indicate an increased risk for adverse outcomes. Elevated levels are associated with increased risk of mortality and prolongation of the symptoms associated with congestive heart failure. Unlike natriuretic peptides, such as beta natriuretic peptides (BNP) (p. 367), GAL-3 is not useful in the diagnosis of heart failure. Testing was performed by quantitative 2-site manual enzyme-linked immunosorbent assay (ELISA).

INTERFERING FACTORS

- Hemolysis increases GAL-3 levels.
- Heterophil antibodies (p. 363) increase GAL-3 levels.

PROCEDURE AND PATIENT CARE

Before

🖉 Explain the procedure to the patient.
🖉 Tell the patient that no fasting is required.

During

- Collect a venous blood sample in an EDTA (usually lavender) containing tube.

After

- Apply pressure to the venipuncture site.
- Assess the venipuncture site for bleeding.
- Continue with aggressive medical care for suspected CHF.

TEST RESULTS AND CLINICAL SIGNIFICANCE

▲ Increased Levels

Congestive heart failure: *Congestive heart failure is associated with cardiac remodeling. As a result, GAL-3 is secreted into the bloodstream.*

RELATED TESTS

Chest X-Ray (p. 1014). This test may demonstrate an enlarged heart, commonly associated with congestive heart failure. Pulmonary edema can also be noted.

Echocardiography (p. 877). This test is accurate in determining cardiac remodeling and enlarged cardiac ventricles.

Beta Natriuretic Peptides (p. 367). Natriuretic peptides are used to identify and stratify patients with congestive heart failure (CHF).

Gamma-Glutamyl Transpeptidase (GGTP, g-GTP, Gamma-Glutamyl Transferase [GGT])

NORMAL FINDINGS

Male and female >45 years: 8-38 units/L or 8-38 international units/L (SI units)
Female <45 years: 5-27 units/L or 5-27 international units/L (SI units)
Elderly: slightly higher than adult
Child: similar to adult
Newborn: 5 times higher than adult

INDICATIONS

This is a sensitive indicator of hepatobiliary disease. It is also used as an indicator of heavy and chronic alcohol use.

TEST EXPLANATION

The enzyme GGTP participates in the transfer of amino acids and peptides across the cellular membrane and possibly participates in glutathione metabolism. The highest concentrations of this enzyme are found in the liver and biliary tract. Lesser concentrations are found in the kidney, spleen, heart, intestine, brain, and prostate gland. Men may have higher GGTP levels than women because of the additional levels in the prostate. Very small amounts have been detected in endothelial cells of capillaries. This test is used to detect liver cell dysfunction, and it is highly accurate in indicating even the slightest degree of cholestasis. This is the most sensitive liver enzyme for detecting biliary obstruction, cholangitis, or cholecystitis. As with leucine aminopeptidase and 5'-nucleotidase, the elevation of GGTP generally parallels that of alkaline phosphatase; however, GGTP is more sensitive. Also, as with 5'-nucleotidase and leucine aminopeptidase, GGTP is not increased in bone diseases as is alkaline phosphatase. A normal GGTP level with an elevated alkaline phosphatase level would imply skeletal disease. An elevated GGTP and elevated alkaline phosphatase level would imply hepatobiliary disease. GGTP is also not elevated in childhood or pregnancy as alkaline phosphatase (ALP) usually is.

Another important clinical value of GGTP is that it can detect chronic alcohol ingestion. It is, therefore, very useful in the screening and evaluation of alcoholic patients. GGTP is elevated in approximately 75% of patients who chronically drink alcohol.

Why this enzyme is elevated after an acute myocardial infarction (AMI) is not clear. It may represent the associated hepatic insult (if elevation occurs in the first 7 days) or the proliferation of capillary endothelial cells in the granulation tissue that replaces the infarcted myocardium. The elevation usually occurs 1 to 2 weeks after infarction.

INTERFERING FACTORS

- Values may be decreased in late pregnancy.
- Drugs that may cause *increased* levels include alcohol, phenobarbital, and phenytoin (Dilantin).
- Drugs that may cause *decreased* levels include clofibrate and oral contraceptives.

PROCEDURE AND PATIENT CARE

Before

- Explain the procedure to the patient.
- Tell the patient that an 8-hour fast is recommended. Only water is permitted.

During

- Collect a venous blood sample in a red-top tube.

After

- Apply pressure or a pressure dressing to the venipuncture site.
- Assess the venipuncture site for bleeding. Patients with liver dysfunction often have prolonged clotting times.

TEST RESULTS AND CLINICAL SIGNIFICANCE

▲   Increased Levels

Liver diseases (e.g., hepatitis, cirrhosis, hepatic necrosis, hepatic tumor or metastasis, hepatotoxic drugs, cholestasis, jaundice): *Liver and biliary cells contain GGTP. When injured or diseased, these cells lyse and the GGTP leaks into the bloodstream.*

Myocardial infarction (MI): *The pathophysiology is not clear. It may be associated with hepatic insult or the proliferation of capillary endothelial cells in the granulation tissue that replaces the infarcted myocardium.*

Alcohol ingestion: *The pathophysiology is not clear. It may be associated with hepatic insult.*

Pancreatic diseases (e.g., pancreatitis, cancer of the pancreas): *Pancreatic cells contain GGTP. When injured or diseased, these cells lyse and the GGTP leaks into the bloodstream.*

Epstein-Barr virus (EBV) (infectious mononucleosis), cytomegalovirus infections, and Reye syndrome: *The pathophysiology is not clear. It may be associated with subclinical hepatitis that can occur with these infections.*

RELATED TESTS

Alanine Aminotransferase (ALT) (p. 39). This liver enzyme is elevated in hepatocellular disease.

Alkaline Phosphatase (ALP) (p. 47). This test is used to detect and monitor diseases of the liver or bone.

Aspartate Aminotransferase (AST) (p. 119). This liver enzyme is elevated in hepatocellular disease.

5'-Nucleotidase (p. 376). This liver enzyme is elevated in diseases affecting the biliary tree.

Creatine Phosphokinase (CPK) (p. 186). This enzyme is similar to AST and exists predominantly in the heart and the skeletal muscle.

Lactic Dehydrogenase (LDH) (p. 329). This intracellular enzyme is used to support the diagnosis of injury or disease involving the heart, liver, red blood cells, kidneys, skeletal muscle, brain, and lungs.

Leucine Aminopeptidase (LAP) (p. 337). This enzyme is specific to the hepatobiliary system. Diseases affecting that system will cause elevation of this enzyme.

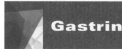

Gastrin

NORMAL FINDINGS

Adult: 0-180 pg/mL or 0-180 ng/L (SI units)
Child: 0-125 pg/mL
Levels are higher in elderly patients.

INDICATIONS

This test is used in the evaluation of patients with peptic ulcers to diagnose Zollinger-Ellison (ZE) syndrome or G-cell hyperplasia.

TEST EXPLANATION

Gastrin is a hormone produced by the G cells located in the distal part of the stomach (antrum). Gastrin is a potent stimulator of gastric acid. In normal gastric physiology an alkaline environment (created by food or antacids) stimulates the release of gastrin. Gastrin then stimulates the parietal cells of the stomach to secrete gastric acid. The pH environment in the stomach is thereby reduced. By negative feedback, this low-pH environment suppresses further gastrin secretion.

ZE syndrome (gastrin-producing pancreatic tumor) and G-cell hyperplasia (overfunctioning of G cells in the distal stomach) are associated with high serum gastrin levels. Patients with these tumors have aggressive peptic ulcer disease. Unlike the patient with routine peptic ulcers, the patient with ZE syndrome or G-cell hyperplasia has a high incidence of complicated and recurrent peptic ulcers. It is important to identify this latter group of patients to institute more appropriate, aggressive medical and surgical therapy. The serum gastrin level will be normal in patients with routine peptic ulcers and greatly elevated in patients with ZE syndrome or G-cell hyperplasia.

It is important to note, however, that patients who are taking antacid peptic ulcer medicines, have had peptic ulcer surgery, or have atrophic gastritis will have a high serum gastrin level (in response to alkalinity in the stomach). However, levels usually are not as high as in patients with ZE syndrome or G-cell hyperplasia.

Not all patients with ZE syndrome exhibit increased levels of serum gastrin. Some may have "top" normal gastrin levels, which makes these patients difficult to differentiate from patients with routine peptic ulcer disease. ZE syndrome or G-cell hyperplasia can be diagnosed in these "top" normal patients by gastrin stimulation tests using calcium or secretin. Patients with these diseases will have greatly increased serum gastrin levels associated with the infusion of these drugs.

INTERFERING FACTORS

- Peptic ulcer surgery creates a persistent alkaline environment, which is the strongest stimulant to gastrin.
- Ingestion of high-protein food can result in an increase in serum gastrin two to five times the normal level.
- Diabetic patients taking insulin may have falsely *elevated* levels in response to hypoglycemia.
- Drugs that may *increase* serum gastrin include antacids and H_2-blocking agents (e.g., esomeprazole, lansoprazole, omeprazole, pantoprazole, rabeprazole). These medications create an alkaline environment, which is the strongest stimulant to gastrin.
- Calcium or insulin can *increase* gastrin levels by acting as a gastrin stimulant.
- Other drugs that may *increase* gastrin levels include catecholamines and caffeine.
- Drugs that may *decrease* levels include anticholinergics and tricyclic antidepressants.

PROCEDURE AND PATIENT CARE

Before

- Explain the procedure to the patient.
- Instruct the patient to fast for 12 hours before the test. Water is permitted.
- Tell the patient to avoid alcohol for at least 24 hours before the test.

During

- Collect a venous blood sample in a red-top tube.
- For the *calcium infusion test*, administer calcium gluconate intravenously. A preinfusion serum gastrin level is then compared with specimens taken every 30 minutes for 4 hours.
- For the *secretin test*, administer secretin intravenously. Preinjection and postinjection serum gastrin levels are taken at 15-minute intervals for 1 hour after injection.
- Indicate on the laboratory slip any drugs that may affect test results.

After

- Apply pressure or a pressure dressing to the venipuncture site.
- Observe the venipuncture site for bleeding.

TEST RESULTS AND CLINICAL SIGNIFICANCE

▲ Increased Levels

ZE syndrome: *This syndrome is associated with a pancreatic islet cell gastrin-producing tumor.*

G-cell hyperplasia: *The G cells in the antrum of the stomach are hyperplastic and produce increased amounts of gastrin.*

Pernicious anemia,

Atrophic gastritis:

   An achlorhydric alkaline environment exists in these illnesses. This is a strong stimulant to gastrin secretion.

Gastric carcinoma: *Cancer of the stomach usually exists in an achlorhydric alkaline environment. This is a strong stimulant to gastrin secretion.*

Chronic renal failure: *Gastrin is metabolized by the kidney. Without adequate kidney function, gastrin levels increase.*

Pyloric obstruction or gastric outlet obstruction: *The stomach becomes distended. Gastric distention is a potent stimulant to gastrin production.*

Retained antrum after gastric surgery: *Antral tissue mistakenly left on the duodenal stump after gastric resection is constantly bathed in duodenal alkaline juices. This is a strong stimulant to gastrin secretion.*

RELATED TEST

Gastric Analysis. This is an older test of gastric juices that is used to diagnose ZE syndrome and to determine the adequacy of antipeptic medical and surgical therapy.

Gliadin Antibodies (Endomysial Antibodies, Tissue Transglutaminase Antibodies)

NORMAL FINDINGS

	Age	Normal
Gliadin IgA/IgG	0-2 years	<20 EU
	3 years and older	<25 EU
Endomysial IgA	All ages	Negative
Tissue transglutaminase IgA	All ages	<20 EU

INDICATIONS

This test is used to diagnose celiac disease and sprue by identifying antibodies to gliadin and gluten in affected patients.

TEST EXPLANATION

Gliadin and gluten are proteins found in wheat and wheat products. Patients with celiac disease cannot tolerate ingestion of these proteins or any products containing wheat. These proteins are toxic to the mucosa of the small intestine and cause characteristic pathologic lesions. These patients experience severe intestinal malabsorption symptoms. The only treatment is for the patient to abstain from wheat and wheat-containing products.

When an affected patient ingests wheat-containing foods, gluten and gliadin build up in the intestinal mucosa. These gliadin and gluten proteins (and their metabolites) cause direct mucosal damage. Furthermore, IgA immunoglobulins (antigliadin, antiendomysial, and antitissue transglutaminase [tTG-ab]) are made, appearing in the gut mucosa and in the serum of severely affected patients. The identification of these antibodies in the blood of patients with malabsorption is helpful in supporting the diagnosis of celiac sprue or dermatitis herpetiformis. However, a definitive diagnosis of celiac disease can be made only when a patient with malabsorption is found to have the pathologic intestinal lesions characteristic of celiac disease. Also, the patient's symptoms must be improved with a gluten-free diet. Both are needed for the diagnosis. Because of the high specificity of endomyosial antibodies (EMA) for celiac disease, the test may obviate the need for multiple small bowel biopsies to verify the diagnosis. This may be particularly advantageous in the pediatric population, including the evaluation of children with failure to thrive.

In patients with known celiac disease, these antibodies can be used to monitor disease status and dietary compliance. Furthermore, these antibodies identify successful treatment, as they will become negative in patients on a gluten-free diet.

INTERFERING FACTORS

- Other gastrointestinal (GI) diseases such as Crohn disease, colitis, and severe lactose intolerance can be associated with *elevated* gliadin antibodies.

PROCEDURE AND PATIENT CARE

Before

☒ Explain the procedure to the patient.
☒ Tell the patient that no fasting is required.
- Obtain a list of foods that have been ingested in the last 48 hours.
- Assess how much malabsorption symptoms the patient has been experiencing in the last few weeks.

During

- Collect a venous blood sample in a red-top tube.

After

- Apply pressure to the venipuncture site.
- Assess the venipuncture site for bleeding.

TEST RESULTS AND CLINICAL SIGNIFICANCE

Celiac disease,
Celiac sprue,
Nontropical sprue:
    Antibodies to gluten and gliadin are formed in affected and are present in the blood.
Dermatitis herpetiformis: *This is a chronic, extremely itchy rash consisting of papules and vesicles. It is associated with sensitivity of the intestine to gluten in the diet (celiac sprue).*

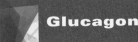

Glucagon

NORMAL FINDINGS

50-100 pg/mL or 50-100 ng/L (SI units)

INDICATIONS

This is a direct measurement of glucagon in the blood. It is used to diagnose a glucagonoma. It is also useful in the evaluation of some diabetic patients. Finally, pancreatic function can be investigated with the use of this test.

TEST EXPLANATION

Glucagon is a hormone secreted by the alpha cells of the pancreatic islets of Langerhans. Glucagon is secreted in response to hypoglycemia and increases the blood glucose by breaking down glycogen to glucose in the liver. It also increases glucose in other tissues by inhibiting passage of glucose into cells and by encouraging efflux of glucose from the cell. Glucagon oxidizes triglycerides to fatty acids and glycerol that forms glucose. As serum glucose levels rise in the blood, glucagon is inhibited by a negative feedback mechanism.

Elevated glucagon levels may indicate the diagnosis of a glucagonoma (i.e., an alpha islet cell neoplasm). Glucagon deficiency occurs with extensive pancreatic resection or with burned-out pancreatitis. Arginine is a potent stimulator of glucagon. If the glucagon levels fail to rise even with arginine infusion, the diagnosis of glucagon deficiency as a result of pancreatic insufficiency is confirmed.

Normally glucagon decreases after ingestion of a carbohydrate-loaded meal through an elaborate negative feedback mechanism. This does not occur in patients with diabetes. Furthermore, in the insulin-dependent diabetic, glucagon stimulation caused by hypoglycemia does not occur. Arginine stimulation is performed to differentiate pancreatic insufficiency and diabetes. The diabetic will have an exaggerated elevation of glucagon with arginine administration. In pancreatic insufficiency, glucagon is not stimulated with arginine. In diabetic patients, hypoglycemia fails to stimulate glucagon release, as occurs in a nondiabetic person.

Because glucagon is thought to be metabolized by the kidneys, renal failure is associated with high glucagon levels and, as a result, high glucose levels. When rejection of a transplanted kidney occurs, one of the first signs of rejection may be increased serum glucose levels. Quantitative radioimmunoassay is commonly used for quantification of glucagon levels.

INTERFERING FACTORS

- Test results may be invalidated if a patient has undergone a radioactive scan within the previous 48 hours and glucagon is measured by radioimmunoassay (RIA). Administration of radionuclides can affect results.
- Levels may be elevated after prolonged fasting, stress, or moderate to intense exercise.
- Drugs that may cause *increased* levels include some amino acids (e.g., arginine), cholecystokinin, danazol, gastrin, glucocorticoids, insulin, nifedipine, and sympathomimetic amines.
- Drugs that may cause *decreased* levels include atenolol, propranolol, and secretin.

PROCEDURE AND PATIENT CARE

Before
- Explain the procedure to the patient.
- Tell the patient that fasting is necessary for 10 to 12 hours before the test. Only water is permitted.

During
- Collect a venous blood sample in a lavender-top tube.

After
- Apply pressure or a pressure dressing to the venipuncture site.
- Assess the venipuncture site for bleeding.
- Place the specimen on ice and send it to the laboratory immediately.

TEST RESULTS AND CLINICAL SIGNIFICANCE

▲ Increased Levels

Familial hyperglucagonemia: *There is a genetic defect that causes a predominance of a glucagon precursor.*

Glucagonoma: *There are several syndromes, including the more common multiple endocrine neoplasia, that are associated with glucagonomas.*

Diabetes mellitus (DM): *Inappropriate elevations in glucagon levels in hyperglycemic type I diabetic patients indicate that paradoxical glucagon release may contribute to disease severity.*

Chronic renal failure: *Glucagon is metabolized by the kidney. With loss of that function, glucagon and glucose levels rise.*

Severe stress, including infection, burns, surgery, and acute hypoglycemia: *Stress stimulates catecholamine release. This in turn stimulates glucagon secretion.*

Acromegaly: *Growth hormone is a stimulator of glucagon.*

Hyperlipidemia: *The pathophysiology of this observation is not well established.*

Acute pancreatitis: *The contents of the pancreatic cells (including glucagon) are spilled into the bloodstream as they are injured during the inflammation.*

Pheochromocytoma: *Catecholamines are potent stimulators to glucagon secretion.*

▼ Decreased Levels

Idiopathic glucagon deficiency: *The pathophysiology of this process is not well understood. An autoantibody process may be the cause.*

Diabetes mellitus (DM): *In diabetic patients, low glucagon levels (undetectable or in the lower quartile of the normal range) in the presence of hypoglycemia indicate impairment of hypoglycemic counterregulation. These patients may be particularly prone to recurrent hypoglycemia.*

Cystic fibrosis,

Chronic pancreatitis:
The chronically diseased pancreas cannot produce glucagon.

Postpancreatectomy: *In the absence of pancreatic tissue, glucagon secretion will not occur.*

Cancer of pancreas: *Pancreatic tissue destroyed by tumor will not secrete glucagon.*

RELATED TEST

Glucose, Blood (see following test). This test is commonly used to diagnose diabetes. Glucagon levels are inversely related to blood glucose levels.

Glucose, Blood (Blood Sugar, Fasting Blood Sugar [FBS])

NORMAL FINDINGS

Cord: 45-96 mg/dL or 2.5-5.3 mmol/L (SI units)

Premature infant: 20-60 mg/dL or 1.1-3.3 mmol/L

Neonate: 30-60 mg/dL or 1.7-3.3 mmol/L

Infant: 40-90 mg/dL or 2.2-5.0 mmol/L

Child <2 years: 60-100 mg/dL or 3.3-5.5 mmol/L

Child >2 years to adult:

Fasting: 70-110 mg/dL or <6.1 mmol/L (Fasting is defined as no caloric intake for at least 8 hours.)

Casual: ≤200 mg/dL or <11.1 mmol/L (Casual is defined as any time of day.)

Elderly: increase in normal range after age 50 years

Critical Values

Adult male: <50 and >450 mg/dL
Adult female: <40 and >450 mg/dL
Infant: <40 mg/dL
Newborn: <30 and >300 mg/dL

INDICATIONS

This test is a direct measurement of the blood glucose level. It is most commonly used in the evaluation of diabetic patients.

TEST EXPLANATION

Through an elaborate feedback mechanism, glucose levels are controlled by insulin and glucagon. Glucose levels are low in the fasting state. In response, glucagon, which is made in the alpha cells of the pancreatic islets of Langerhans, is secreted. Glucagon breaks glycogen down to glucose in the liver and glucose levels rise. If the fasting persists, protein and fatty acids are broken down under glucagon stimulation. Glucose levels continue to rise.

Glucose levels are elevated after eating. Insulin, which is made in the beta cells of the pancreatic islets of Langerhans, is secreted. Insulin attaches to insulin receptors in muscle, liver, and fatty cells, in which it drives glucose into these target cells to be metabolized to glycogen, amino acids, and fatty acids. Blood glucose levels diminish. Many other hormones (e.g., adrenocorticosteroids, adrenocorticotropic hormone [ACTH], epinephrine, growth, thyroxine) can also affect glucose metabolism.

The serum glucose test is helpful in diagnosing many metabolic diseases. Serum glucose levels must be evaluated according to the time of day they are performed. For example, a glucose level of 135 mg/dL may be abnormal if the patient is in the fasting state, but this level would be within normal limits if the patient had eaten a meal within the last hour. Glycosylated hemoglobin (p. 266) is now being performed more frequently to identify diabetes because this blood test represents blood sugar levels over the last 120 days. That being said, the diagnosis of diabetes should be confirmed with a repeat of the same tests initially performed but on a different day to guard against laboratory error.

In general, true glucose elevations indicate diabetes mellitus (DM), however, there are many other possible causes of hyperglycemia. Similarly, hypoglycemia has many causes. The most common cause is inadvertent insulin overdose in patients with brittle diabetes. If diabetes is suspected based on elevated fasting blood levels, a glycosylated hemoglobin or glucose tolerance test can be performed.

Glucose determinations must be performed frequently in new diabetic patients to monitor closely the insulin dosage to be administered. Finger stick blood glucose determinations are usually performed before meals and at bedtime. Results are compared with a sliding-scale insulin chart ordered by the physician to provide coverage with subcutaneous regular insulin.

For diabetic patients who experience recurrent episodes of severe hypoglycemia or who require more than three doses of insulin per day, minimally invasive glucose monitoring is available. A small, sterile, disposable glucose-sensing device is inserted into the subcutaneous tissue (usually the arm). This sensor measures the change in glucose in the interstitial fluid. This information is recorded in a small beeper-sized monitor for 3 to 4 days. The monitor is taken to the doctor's office, where it is connected to a standard personal computer. Specialized software then downloads the stored information and a more effective insulin regimen can be developed.

INTERFERING FACTORS

- Many forms of stress (e.g., trauma, general anesthesia, infection, burns, myocardial infarction [MI]) can cause increased serum glucose levels.
- Caffeine may cause increased levels.
- Many pregnant women experience some degree of glucose intolerance. If significant, it is called gestational diabetes.
- Most intravenous (IV) fluids contain dextrose, which is quickly converted to glucose. Most patients receiving IV fluids will have increased glucose levels.
- Drugs that may cause *increased* levels include antidepressants (tricyclics), antipsychotics, beta-adrenergic blocking agents, corticosteroids, cyclosporins, IV dextrose infusion, dextrothyroxine, diazoxide, diuretics, epinephrine, estrogens, glucagon, isoniazid, lithium, niacin, phenothiazines, phenytoin, salicylates (acute toxicity), and triamterene.
- Drugs that may cause *decreased* levels include acetaminophen, alcohol, alpha-glucosidase inhibitors, anabolic steroids, biguanides, clofibrate, disopyramide, gemfibrozil, incretin mimetics, insulin, monoamine oxidase inhibitors, meglitinides, pentamidine, propranolol, sulfonylureas, and thiazolidinediones.

✓ Clinical Priorities

- Serum glucose levels must be evaluated according to the time of day they are obtained. Increased levels follow a recent meal.
- Glucose determinations must be performed frequently in new diabetic patients to determine appropriate insulin therapy. Finger stick blood glucose determinations are usually performed before meals and at bedtime.
- Many forms of stress can cause increased serum glucose levels.
- Many drugs affect glucose levels.

PROCEDURE AND PATIENT CARE

Before

Explain the procedure to the patient.
For fasting blood sugar determination, the patient must fast for 8 hours. Water is permitted.
To prevent starvation, which may artificially raise the glucose levels, the patient should not fast longer than 8 hours.
- Withhold insulin or oral hypoglycemics until after blood is obtained.

During

- Collect a venous blood sample in a red-top or gray-top tube.
- Glucose levels can also be evaluated by a finger stick blood test using either a visually read test or a reflectance meter. The advantage of the visually read test is that it does not require an expensive machine. However, the patient must be able to visually interpret the color of the reagent strip. Using reflectance meters (e.g., Glucometer, Accu Check bG, Stat Tek) improves the accuracy of the blood glucose determination.

After

- Apply pressure or a pressure dressing to the venipuncture site.

- Observe the venipuncture site for bleeding.
- Be certain that the patient receives a meal after fasting blood work.

TEST RESULTS AND CLINICAL SIGNIFICANCE

▲ Increased Levels (Hyperglycemia)

Diabetes mellitus (DM): *This disease is defined by glucose intolerance and hyperglycemia. A discussion of the many possible etiologies is beyond the scope of this manual.*

Acute stress response: *Severe stress, including infection, burns, and surgery, stimulates catecholamine release. This in turn stimulates glucagon secretion, which causes hyperglycemia.*

Cushing syndrome: *Blood cortisol levels are high. This in turn causes hyperglycemia.*

Pheochromocytoma: *Catecholamine stimulates glucagon secretion, which causes hyperglycemia.*

Chronic renal failure: *Glucagon is metabolized by the kidney. With loss of that function, glucagon and glucose levels rise.*

Glucagonoma: *Glucagon is autonomously secreted, causing hyperglycemia.*

Acute pancreatitis: *The contents of the pancreatic cells (including glucagon) are spilled into the bloodstream as the cells are injured during the inflammation. The glucagon causes hyperglycemia.*

Diuretic therapy: *Certain diuretics cause hyperglycemia.*

Corticosteroid therapy: *Cortisol causes hyperglycemia.*

Acromegaly: *Growth hormone stimulates glucagon, which causes hyperglycemia.*

▼ Decreased Levels (Hypoglycemia)

Insulinoma: *Insulin is autonomously produced without regard to biofeedback mechanisms.*

Hypothyroidism: *Thyroid hormones affect glucose metabolism. With diminished levels of this hormone, glucose levels fall.*

Hypopituitarism: *Many pituitary hormones (adrenocorticotropic hormone [ACTH], growth hormone) affect glucose metabolism. With diminished levels of these hormones, glucose levels fall.*

Addison disease: *Cortisol affects glucose metabolism. With diminished levels of this hormone, glucose levels fall.*

Extensive liver disease: *Most glucose metabolism occurs in the liver. With decreased liver function, glucose levels decrease.*

Insulin overdose: *This is the most common cause of hypoglycemia. Insulin is administered at too high of a dose (especially in brittle diabetes) and glucose levels fall.*

Starvation: *With decreased carbohydrate ingestion, glucose levels diminish.*

RELATED TESTS

Diabetes Mellitus (DM) Autoantibody Panel (p. 206). This test is used in the evaluation of insulin resistance. It is also used to identify type I diabetes and patients with a suspected allergy to insulin. This antibody panel is also used in surveillance of patients who have received pancreatic islet cell transplants.

Glucose, Urine (p. 924). Testing for glucose in the urine is a part of routine urinalysis. If present, glucose in the urine reflects the degree of glucose elevation in the blood. Urine glucose tests are also used to monitor the effectiveness of therapy for DM.

Glycosylated Hemoglobin (p. 266). This is an accurate method of indicating average glucose levels over the past 100 to 120 days before the test.

Glucose Tolerance (p. 261). This is a test of a patient's capability to handle a glucose load.

Glucose, Postprandial (p. 257). This is a timed glucose measurement after a carbohydrate meal.

Glucagon (p. 251). This is a direct measurement of glucagon, which acts to increase glucose in the blood.
Insulin Assay (p. 315). This is a direct measurement of insulin, which acts to decrease glucose in the
  blood.

Glucose, Postprandial (2-Hour Postprandial Glucose
[2-Hour PPG], 2-Hour Postprandial Blood Sugar, 1-Hour Glucose
Screen for Gestational Diabetes Mellitus, O'Sullivan Test)

NORMAL FINDINGS
2-Hour PPG
0-50 years: <140 mg/dL or <7.8 mmol/L (SI units)
50-60 years: <150 mg/dL
60 years and older: <160 mg/dL

1-Hour Glucose Screen for Gestational Diabetes
<140 mg/dL

INDICATIONS
The 2-hour PPG test is a measurement of the amount of glucose in the patient's blood 2 hours after a
meal is ingested (postprandial). It is used to diagnose diabetes mellitus (DM).

TEST EXPLANATION
For this study, a meal acts as a glucose challenge to the body's metabolism. Insulin is normally secreted
immediately after a meal in response to the elevated blood glucose level, causing the level to return to
the premeal range within 2 hours. In patients with diabetes the glucose level usually is still elevated 2
hours after the meal. The PPG is an easily performed screening test for DM. If the results are greater
than 140 and less than 200 mg/dL, a glucose tolerance test may be performed to confirm the diagnosis.
If the 2-hour PPG is greater than 200 mg/dL, the diagnosis of DM is confirmed. Also, a glucose tolerance or glycosylated hemoglobin test can be performed to corroborate and better evaluate the disease.

  The 1-hour glucose screen is used to detect gestational DM, which is the most common medical
complication of pregnancy. Gestational diabetes is a carbohydrate intolerance first recognized during pregnancy and affects 3% to 8% of pregnant women, with up to half of these women developing
overt diabetes later in life. The detection and treatment of gestational diabetes may reduce the risk
for several adverse perinatal outcomes (e.g., excessive fetal growth and birth trauma, fetal death,
neonatal morbidity).

  Screening for gestational diabetes is performed with a 50-100 g oral glucose load followed by a glucose level determination 1 hour later. This is called the *O'Sullivan test.* Screening is done between 24
and 28 weeks of gestation. However, patients with risk factors such as a previous history of gestational
diabetes may benefit from earlier screening. Patients whose serum glucose level equals or exceeds 140
mg/dL may be evaluated by a 3-hour glucose tolerance test.

INTERFERING FACTORS
• Stress can increase glucose levels through the catecholamine effect of increasing serum glucose.

- If the patient eats a small snack or eats candy during the 2-hour interval, glucose levels will be falsely elevated.
- If the patient is not able to eat the entire test meal or vomits some or all of the meal, levels will be falsely decreased.

PROCEDURE AND PATIENT CARE

Before

🖉 Explain the procedure to the patient.
- Usually a fasting blood glucose is done before the meal is given. This acts as a baseline glucose level (see p. 253).
🖉 For the 2-hour PPG, instruct the patient to fast for 12 hours before testing. Instruct the patient to eat the entire meal (with at least 75 g of carbohydrates) and then not to eat anything else until the blood is drawn 2 hours later.
- For the 1-hour glucose screen for gestational diabetes, give the fasting or nonfasting patient a 50-g oral glucose load.
🖉 Instruct the patient not to smoke during the test.
🖉 Inform the patient that he or she should rest during the 1- or 2-hour interval, because exercise can increase glucose levels.

During

- Collect a venous blood sample in a red-top or gray-top tube 1 or 2 hours after the patient has eaten the test meal.

After

- Apply pressure or a pressure dressing to the venipuncture site.
- Observe the venipuncture site for bleeding.

TEST RESULTS AND CLINICAL SIGNIFICANCE

▲ Increased Levels

Diabetes mellitus (DM): *This disease is defined by glucose intolerance and hyperglycemia. A discussion of the many possible etiologies is beyond the scope of this manual.*

Gestational diabetes mellitus (DM): *This disease is defined by glucose intolerance and hyperglycemia during pregnancy.*

Malnutrition: *Malnourished patients have very poor glucose tolerance when they start to eat. The pathophysiology and theories of this observation are not well defined and are multiple.*

Hyperthyroidism: *Thyroid hormone is an ancillary hormone that affects glucose metabolism and acts to increase glucose levels.*

Acute stress response: *Severe stress, including infection, burns, and surgery, stimulates catecholamine release. This in turn stimulates glucagon secretion, which causes hyperglycemia.*

Cushing syndrome: *Blood cortisol levels are high. This in turn causes hyperglycemia.*

Pheochromocytoma: *Catecholamine stimulates glucagon secretion, which causes hyperglycemia.*

Chronic renal failure: *Glucagon is metabolized by the kidney. With loss of kidney function, glucagon and glucose levels rise.*

Glucagonoma: *Glucagon is autonomously secreted, causing hyperglycemia.*

Diuretic therapy: *Certain diuretics cause hyperglycemia.*

Corticosteroid therapy: *Cortisol causes hyperglycemia.*

Acromegaly: *Growth hormone stimulates glucagon, which causes hyperglycemia.*

Extensive liver disease: *Most glucose metabolism occurs in the liver. With decreased function of the liver, glucose levels decrease.*

▼ Decreased Levels

Insulinoma: *Insulin is autonomously produced without regard to biofeedback mechanisms.*

Hypothyroidism: *Thyroid hormone affects glucose metabolism. With diminished levels of this hormone, glucose levels fall.*

Hypopituitarism: *Many pituitary hormones (adrenocorticotropic hormone [ACTH], growth hormone) affect glucose metabolism. With diminished levels of these hormones, glucose levels fall.*

Addison disease: *Cortisol affects glucose metabolism. With diminished levels of this hormone, glucose levels fall.*

Insulin overdose: *This is the most common cause of hypoglycemia. Insulin is administered at too high of a dose (especially in brittle diabetes), and glucose levels fall.*

Malabsorption or maldigestion: *The test meal is not absorbed and glucose levels do not increase.*

RELATED TESTS

Glucose, Blood (p. 253). This test is a direct measurement of the blood glucose level. It is most commonly the initial test in the evaluation of diabetic patients.

Glycosylated Hemoglobin (p. 266). This is an accurate method of indicating glucose tolerance in the recent past.

Glucose Tolerance (p. 261). This is a test of a patient's capability to handle a glucose load.

Glucose-6-Phosphate Dehydrogenase (*G6PD Screen, G6PD Quantification, Glucose-6-Phosphate Dehydrogenase Deficiency [G-6-PD] DNA Sequencing*)

NORMAL FINDINGS

Negative (quantification)

12.1 ± 2 IU/g of hemoglobin

146-376 units/trillion RBC

G6PD sequencing: no mutation noted

INDICATIONS

This test is used to identify G-6-PD deficiency in patients who have developed hemolysis after taking certain oxidizing drugs. It is especially useful in males of certain ethnic populations who are susceptible to this genetic defect.

TEST EXPLANATION

G-6-PD is an enzyme used in glucose metabolism. G-6-PD deficiency causes precipitation of oxidized (forms Heinz bodies) hemoglobin. This may result in hemolysis of variable severity. This disease is a sex-linked, recessive trait carried on the X chromosome. The full effect of this genetic defect is not seen if the normal gene is present on a second X chromosome to oppose the genetic defect.

In males there is no second X gene and the genetic defect is unopposed. Affected males inherit this abnormal gene from their mothers, who are usually asymptomatic. In these males the disease is most severe.

In rare cases when females have the defective gene on both X chromosomes, the disease is equally severe. Most commonly, however, women act as a "carrier" of the gene in that they have the defective gene on one X chromosome and have a normal gene for G-6-PD on the other X chromosome. These women have variable expressions of the disease from no symptoms to moderate symptoms if under a significant degree of stimulation. Most mutations identified are classified according to the following scheme: Class I—severe enzyme deficiency with chronic non-spherocytic hemolytic anemia; Class II—severe enzyme deficiency with <10% normal activity; Class III—mild to moderate enzyme deficiency (10%-60% normal activity); and Class IV—very mild to almost normal enzyme activity (>60% normal activity with no clinical consequences).

In the United States, G-6-PD is found mainly in African Americans. About 10% to 15% of that population is affected by the disease. Also, those of Mediterranean descent (Italians, Greeks, Sephardic Jews) are at risk for the genetic defect.

G-6-PD is an important enzyme involved in the pentose pathway of glucose metabolism that produces NADPH in the RBC. Most of the glucose in a young RBC is metabolized to produce NADH by the Embden-Meyerhof pathway. As the RBC ages, the pentose pathway becomes the dominant pathway of glucose metabolism. The NADPH in turn maintains the supply of reduced glutathione, which is used to neutralize free oxidative radicals that damage the RBC. Glutathione protects the RBC against potentially destructive oxidizing states such as infection, pharmacologic agents, or certain foods (e.g., fava beans). If NADPH is present through the action of G-6-PD, the RBC is not susceptible to oxidizing agents. When the reductive effects of glutathione are deficient, as in patients with G-6-PD deficiency, proteins precipitate on the RBC membrane, leading to RBC destruction and hemolysis. Patients with severe G-6-PD deficiency can have chronic or intermittent hemolysis. Persons with mild deficiency do not have hemolysis without exposure to the oxidizing drugs or oxidizing events. With the administration of an oxidizing drug, hemolysis can start as early as the first day and usually by the fourth day. The most common oxidizing drugs known to precipitate hemolysis and anemia in G-6-PD deficiency are antimalarials, sulfa drugs, nitrofurantoin, aspirin, and phenacetin (Box 2-10). Acute bacterial or viral or acidosis can also precipitate a hemolytic process in these patients.

This test is used to diagnose G-6-PD deficiency in suspected individuals. The quantification is used as a screening test. There are several different testing methods available for G-6-PD screening and testing. G-6-PD enzyme assay direct quantitation is most definitive.

Glucose-6-phosphate dehydrogenase deficiency (G6PD) *DNA sequencing* by polymerase chain reaction/sequencing can most accurately make the diagnosis of this disease. Combined with quantification, the

BOX 2-10	Drugs That Precipitate Hemolysis in G-6-PD–Deficient Patients	
• Acetanilid	• Methylene blue	• Quinidine
• Antimalarials	• Nalidixic acid	• Sulfa
• Antipyretics	• Nitrofurantoin	• Sulfonamides
• Ascorbic acid	• Phenacetin	• Thiazide diuretics
• Aspirin	• Phenazopyridine	• Tolbutamide
• Dapsone	• Primaquine	• Vitamin K (water soluble)

disease course can be accurately determined. As in all genetic diseases, pretesting counseling and informed consent are recommended.

INTERFERING FACTORS

- With the dye reduction and glutathione screening testing, reticulocytosis associated with a hemolytic episode may be associated with falsely high levels of G-6-PD.

PROCEDURE AND PATIENT CARE

Before

Explain the procedure to the patient.
Tell the patient that no fasting is required.

During

- Collect a venous blood sample in a lavender-top or green-top tube.
- Avoid hemolysis.

After

- Apply pressure or a pressure dressing to the venipuncture site.
- Assess the venipuncture site for bleeding.
- If the test indicates a G-6-PD deficiency, give the patient a list of drugs that may precipitate hemolysis. Instruct patients with the Mediterranean type of this disease not to eat fava beans. Teach patients to read labels on any over-the-counter (OTC) drugs for the presence of agents (e.g., aspirin, phenacetin) that may cause hemolytic anemia.

TEST RESULTS AND CLINICAL SIGNIFICANCE

▲ Increased Levels

Reticulocytosis (e.g., pernicious anemia or chronic blood loss): *With the dye reduction and glutathione screening testing, reticulocytosis associated with a hemolytic episode may be associated with falsely high levels of G-6-PD.*

▼ Decreased Levels

G-6-PD deficiency

Glucose Tolerance (GT, Oral Glucose Tolerance [OGT])

NORMAL FINDINGS

Serum

Fasting: <110 mg/dL or <6.1 mmol/L (SI units)
30 minutes: <200 mg/dL or <11.1 mmol/L
1 hour: <200 mg/dL or <11.1 mmol/L
2 hours: <140 mg/dL or <7.8 mmol/L
3 hours: 70-115 mg/dL or <6.4 mmol/L
4 hours: 70-115 mg/dL or <6.4 mmol/L

Urine

Negative

INDICATIONS

This test is used to assist in the diagnosis of diabetes mellitus (DM). It is also used in the evaluation of patients with hypoglycemia.

TEST EXPLANATION

In the past, The National Diabetes Data Group (NDDG) has defined criteria sufficient for the diagnosis of diabetes mellitus (Table 2-25). These include any one the following:

1. Sufficient clinical symptoms (polydipsia, polyuria, ketonuria, weight loss) plus random blood glucose >200 mg/dL.
2. Elevated FBG >126 mg/dL on more than one occasion.
3. A 2-hour blood glucose >200 mg/dL during oral GT testing.

These criteria should be reconfirmed by repeat testing on a different day in the absence of unequivocal hyperglycemia and metabolic decompensation. A diagnosis of diabetes mellitus could be made on the basis of the results from two tests—fasting blood glucose (p. 253) and GTT—performed on separate days that are close in time. The American Diabetes Association (ADA), the International Diabetes Federation, and the European Association for the Study of Diabetes all indicate that two abnormal glycosylated hemoglobin assays (p. 266) should be used whenever possible instead of the fasting glucose and GTT.

The GT test, then, is used when diabetes is suspected (retinopathy, neuropathy, diabetic-type renal diseases), but the criteria for the diagnosis cannot be met without the data obtained by the GT test. This test is not part of routine screening for diabetes. The GT test may be used for the following:

- Patients with a family history of diabetes
- Patients who are massively obese
- Patients with a history of recurrent infections

TABLE 2-25	National Diabetes Data Group's Reclassification of Diabetic Patients	
NDDG Classification	**Diagnosis***	**Old Classification**
Diabetes mellitus (insulin and noninsulin dependent)	Unequivocal signs/symptoms FBC >126 more than once; GT at 2 hours >200 more than once	Overt diabetes
Impaired GT	Blood glucose between 140 and 200 mg/dL 2 hours after oral glucose load	Latent (chemical) diabetes
Previous abnormality of glucose tolerance	Normal GT test but previous abnormal GT test	Subclinical diabetes
Potential abnormality of GT	Genetic predisposition to diabetes (family history)	Prediabetes
Gestational diabetes mellitus	Onset of unequivocal diabetes or GT test results exceeding pregnancy criteria†	Diabetes of pregnancy

GT, Glucose tolerance; *FBG*, fasting blood glucose.
*Glucose levels are recorded in mg/100 mL.
†Onset or recognition of criteria during pregnancy but not before.

- Patients with delayed healing of wounds (especially on the lower legs or feet)
- Women who have a history of stillbirths, premature births, or large babies
- Patients who have transient glycosuria or hyperglycemia during pregnancy or following myocardial infarction (MI), surgery, or stress

In the GT test, the patient's ability to tolerate a standard oral glucose load (75 g) is evaluated by obtaining serum and urine specimens for glucose level determinations before glucose administration and then at 30 minutes, 1 hour, 2 hours, 3 hours, and sometimes 4 hours after the administration. Normally there is a rapid insulin response to the ingestion of a large oral glucose load. This response peaks in 30 to 60 minutes and returns to normal in about 3 hours. Patients with an appropriate insulin response are able to tolerate the dose quite easily, with only a minimal and transient rise in serum glucose levels within 1 to 2 hours after ingestion. Glucose will not spill over into the urine in normal patients.

Patients with diabetes will not be able to tolerate this load. As a result, their serum glucose levels will be greatly elevated from 1 to 5 hours (Figure 2-17). Also, glucose can be detected in their urine.

Gestational diabetes also can be diagnosed by the GT test. Generally the diagnosis of diabetes can be made if two or more of the results exceed the following:

- Fasting: 105 mg/dL
- 1 hour: 190 mg/dL
- 2 hours: 165 mg/dL
- 3 hours: 145 mg/dL

The American Diabetes Association recommends that pregnant women who have not previously had an abnormal GT result should be screened between 24 and 28 weeks of gestation with a 50-g dose of glucose. This is called the *O'Sullivan test*. A glucose level of 130-140 mg/100 mL one hour later should be followed by a 3-hour GTT.

GI absorption can vary among individuals. For that reason, some centers prefer to administer an intravenous (IV) glucose load rather than depend on gastrointestinal (GI) absorption. Also, occasionally a patient is unable to tolerate the oral glucose load (e.g., patients with prior gastrectomy, short-bowel syndrome, malabsorption). In these instances an intravenous glucose tolerance (IV GT) test can be performed by administering the glucose load intravenously. The values for the IV GT test differ slightly from those of the oral GT test because IV glucose is absorbed faster.

Glucose intolerance also may exist in patients with oversecretion of hormones that have an ancillary affect on glucose, such as patients with Cushing syndrome, pheochromocytoma, acromegaly, aldosteronism, or hyperthyroidism. Patients with chronic renal failure, acute pancreatitis, myxedema, type IV

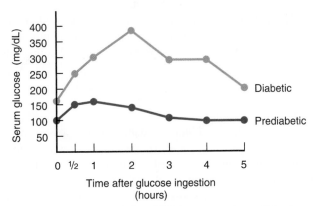

Figure 2-17 Glucose tolerance (GT) test curve for a diabetic and a prediabetic patient.

lipoproteinemia, infection, or cirrhosis can also have an abnormal GT test. Certain drugs, as mentioned below, can cause abnormal GT results.

The GT test is also used to evaluate patients with hypoglycemia. This hypoglycemia may occur as late as 5 hours after the initial glucose load.

CONTRAINDICATIONS

- Patients with serious concurrent infections or endocrine disorders, because glucose intolerance will be observed even though these patients may not be diabetic.
- Patients who vomit part or all of the glucose meal, which invalidates the test.

POTENTIAL COMPLICATIONS

- Dizziness, tremors, anxiety, sweating, euphoria, or fainting may occur during testing. If these symptoms occur, a blood specimen is obtained. If the glucose level is too high, the test may need to be stopped and insulin administered.

INTERFERING FACTORS

- Smoking during the testing period stimulates glucose production because of the nicotine.
- Stress (e.g., from surgery, infection) can increase glucose levels.
- Exercise during the test can affect glucose levels.
- Fasting or reduced caloric intake before the GT test can cause glucose intolerance.
- Drugs that may cause glucose intolerance include antihypertensives, antiinflammatory drugs, aspirin, beta blockers, furosemide, nicotine, oral contraceptives, phenothiazines, psychiatric drugs, steroids, and thiazide diuretics.

PROCEDURE AND PATIENT CARE

Before

- Explain the procedure to the patient.
- Educate the patient about the importance of having adequate food intake with adequate carbohydrates (150 g) for at least 3 days before the test.
- Instruct the patient to fast for 12 hours before the test.
- Instruct the patient to discontinue drugs (including tobacco) that could interfere with test results.
- Give the patient written instructions explaining the pretest dietary requirements.
- Obtain the patient's weight to determine the appropriate glucose loading dose (especially in children).

During

- Obtain fasting blood and urine specimens.
- Administer the prescribed oral glucose solution, usually 75 g of glucose or dextrose for nonpregnant patients or 100 g for pregnant patients. There are several commercial preparations available. The glucose load may be diluted in as much as 300 mL of lemon juice/water mixture.
- Give pediatric patients a carbohydrate load based on their body weight.
- Instruct the patient to ingest the entire glucose load.
- Tell the patient that he or she cannot eat anything until the test is completed. However, encourage the patient to drink water. No other liquids should be taken during the testing period.

✐ Inform the patient that tobacco, coffee, and tea are not allowed, because they cause physiologic stimulation.
- Collect a venous blood sample in a gray-top tube at 30 and 60 minutes and at hourly periods.
- Collect urine specimens at hourly periods.
- During the testing period, assess the patient for reactions such as dizziness, sweating, weakness, and giddiness. (These are usually transient.) If the symptoms are persistent, obtain a serum glucose level.
- For the IV GT test, administer the glucose load intravenously over 3 to 4 minutes.

After
- Apply pressure or a pressure dressing to the venipuncture sites.
- Mark on the tubes the time that the specimens are collected.
- Send all specimens promptly to the laboratory.
- Allow the patient to eat and drink normally.
- Administer insulin or oral hypoglycemics if ordered.
- Assess the venipuncture sites for bleeding.

TEST RESULTS AND CLINICAL SIGNIFICANCE

▲ Increased Levels

Diabetes mellitus (DM): *This disease is defined by glucose intolerance and hyperglycemia. A discussion of the many possible etiologies is beyond the scope of this manual.*

Acute stress response: *Severe stress, including infection, burns, and surgery, stimulates catecholamine release. This in turn stimulates glucagon secretion, which causes hyperglycemia and glucose intolerance.*

Cushing syndrome: *Blood cortisol levels are high. This causes hyperglycemia and glucose intolerance.*

Pheochromocytoma: *Catecholamines stimulate glucagon secretion, which causes hyperglycemia and glucose intolerance.*

Chronic renal failure: *Glucagon is metabolized by the kidney. With loss of that function, glucagon and glucose levels rise.*

Glucagonoma: *Glucagon is autonomously secreted, causing hyperglycemia.*

Acute pancreatitis: *The contents of the pancreatic cells (including glucagon) are spilled into the bloodstream as the cells are injured during the inflammation. The glucagon causes hyperglycemia.*

Diuretic therapy: *Certain diuretics cause hyperglycemia.*

Corticosteroid therapy: *Cortisol causes hyperglycemia and glucose intolerance.*

Acromegaly: *Growth hormone stimulates glucagon, which causes hyperglycemia and glucose intolerance.*

Myxedema: *Usually these patients have a flat GT curve, but they may have a "diabetic curve."*

Somogyi response to hypoglycemia: *This is a reactive hyperglycemia following hypoglycemia that may occur from an exaggerated insulin response to the glucose load.*

After gastrectomy: *These patients can dump most of the glucose load into the small intestines in just minutes because the normal pylorus is absent. This can cause rapid absorption of glucose into the bloodstream and cause a false elevation in glucose level during the early part of the test.*

RELATED TESTS

Diabetes Mellitus (DM) Autoantibody Panel (p. 206). This test is used in the evaluation of insulin resistance. It is also used to identify type 1 diabetes and patients with a suspected allergy to insulin. This antibody panel is also used in surveillance of patients who have received pancreatic islet cell transplants.

Glucose, Blood (p. 253). This is the primary screening test to diagnose diabetes.

Glucose, Urine (p. 924). Testing for glucose in the urine is a part of routine urinalysis. If present, it reflects the degree of glucose elevation in the blood. Urine glucose tests are also used to monitor the effectiveness of therapy for diabetes mellitus.

Glycosylated Hemoglobin (p. 266). This is an accurate method of indicating glucose tolerance in the recent past.

Glucagon (p. 251). This is a direct measurement of glucagon, which acts to increase glucose in the blood.

Insulin Assay (p. 315). This is a direct measurement of insulin, which acts to decrease glucose in the blood.

Glycosylated Hemoglobin (GHb, GHB, Glycohemoglobin, Hemoglobin A_{1c} [HbA_{1c}], Diabetic Control Index, Glycated Protein)

NORMAL FINDINGS

Nondiabetic adult/child: 4%-5.9%
Good diabetic control: <7%
Fair diabetic control: 8%-9%
Poor diabetic control: >9%
Values vary according to laboratory methods.

INDICATIONS

This test is used to diagnose and monitor diabetes treatment. It measures the amount of HbA_{1c} in the blood and provides an accurate long-term index of the patient's average blood glucose level.

TEST EXPLANATION

In adults about 98% of the hemoglobin in the red blood cell (RBC) is hemoglobin A. About 7% of hemoglobin A consists of a type of hemoglobin (HbA_1) that can combine strongly with glucose in a process called glycosylation. When glycosylation occurs, it is not easily reversible.

HbA_1 is actually made up of three components: A_{1a}, A_{1b}, and A_{1C}. HbA_{1c} is the component that combines most strongly with glucose. Therefore, HgA_{1c} is the most accurate measurement because it contains the majority of glycosylated hemoglobin. If the total HbA_1 is measured, its value is 2% to 4% higher than the HbA_{1c} component.

As the RBC circulates, it combines its HbA_1 with some of the glucose in the bloodstream to form glycohemoglobin (GHb). The amount of GHb depends on the amount of glucose available in the bloodstream over the RBC's 120-day life span. Therefore determination of the GHb value reflects the average blood sugar level for the 100- to 120-day period before the test. The more glucose the RBC is exposed to, the greater the GHb percentage. One important advantage of this test is that the sample can be drawn at any time, because it is not affected by short-term variations (e.g., food intake, exercise, stress, hypoglycemic agents, patient cooperation). It is also possible for very high short-term blood glucose levels to cause an elevation of GHb. Usually, however, the degree of glucose elevation results not from a transient high level but from a persistent, moderate elevation over the entire life of the RBC.

Like GHb, the glucose can nonenzymatically bind to proteins in proportion to the mean blood glucose level. The *glycated protein* is stable until the degradation of the protein. Recall that the average life span of an RBC (and the GHb within) is 120 days. The GHb, therefore, may not reflect more recent changes in glucose levels. Because the turnover rate of proteins is much faster than that of hemoglobin, the measurement of serum *glycated proteins* (such as *glycated albumin*) or *fructosamine* provides more recent information about glucose levels. Glycated proteins reflect an average blood glucose level of the past 15 to 20 days. Although an initial single glycated protein result may not separate good glucose control from poor control, serial testing provides a much better indication of glucose control.

The GHb or glycated proteins tests are particularly beneficial for the following:

1. Evaluating the success of diabetic treatment and patient compliance.
2. Comparing and contrasting the success of past and new forms of diabetic therapy.
3. Determining the duration of hyperglycemia in patients with newly diagnosed diabetes.
4. Providing a sensitive estimate of glucose imbalance in patients with mild diabetes.
5. Individualizing diabetic control regimens.
6. Providing a sense of reward for many patients when the test shows achievement of good diabetic control.
7. Evaluating the diabetic patient whose glucose levels change significantly from day to day (brittle diabetes).
8. Differentiating short-term hyperglycemia in nondiabetics (e.g., recent stress or myocardial infarction [MI]) and diabetics (in whom the glucose has been persistently elevated).
9. Differentiating short-term hyperglycemia in nondiabetics (e.g., recent stress or myocardial infarction [MI]) and diabetics (in whom the glucose has been persistently elevated).

A diagnosis of diabetes mellitus can be made on the basis of the results from two tests—fasting blood glucose (p. 253) and GTT—performed on separate days that are close in time. The American Diabetes Association (ADA), the International Diabetes Federation, and the European Association for the Study of Diabetes all indicate that two abnormal GHb assays should be used whenever possible instead of the fasting glucose and GTT.

By a relatively simple calculation, GHb can be correlated accurately with the daily *mean plasma glucose (MPG)* level, the average glucose level throughout the day. This has been very helpful for diabetics and their health care professionals in determining and evaluating daily glucose goals. There is a linear relationship between A_{1c} (GHb) and PG:

$$MPG = (35.6 \times GHb) - 77.3$$

with a Pearson correlation coefficient (r) of 0.82. Each 1% change in GHb represents a change of approximately 35 mg/dL MPG or 2 mmol/L (Table 2-26). At present there are several ongoing studies designed to identify and document the accuracy of simple mathematical equations design to easily convert GHb to MPG.

The results of the glycosylated hemoglobin assay will be inaccurate in patients with conditions that involve high red blood cell turnover (e.g., hemolytic anemia) or who have had recent blood transfusions.

TABLE 2-26   Correlation Between GHb and MPG

A_{1c} (%)	Approximate Mean Plasma Glucose (mg/dL)	Interpretation
4	65	Nondiabetic range
5	100	Nondiabetic range
6	135	Nondiabetic range
7	170	ADA target
8	205	Action suggested

INTERFERING FACTORS

- Hemoglobinopathies can affect results, because the quantity of hemoglobin A (and, as a result, HbA_1) varies considerably in these diseases.
- Falsely elevated values occur when the RBC life span is lengthened because the HbA_1 has a longer period available for glycosylation.
- Abnormally low levels of proteins may falsely indicate normal glycated fructosamine levels despite the reality of high glucose levels.
- Ascorbic acid may cause *falsely low* levels of glycated fructosamine.

PROCEDURE AND PATIENT CARE

Before
- Explain the procedure to the patient.
- Tell the patient that fasting is not indicated.

During
- Collect a venous blood sample in a gray-top or lavender-top tube.

After
- Apply pressure or a pressure dressing to the venipuncture site.
- Assess the venipuncture site for bleeding.

TEST RESULTS AND CLINICAL SIGNIFICANCE

▲ Increased Levels

Newly diagnosed diabetic patient: *This test is not used to diagnose new diabetics because the range of "normal" is so broad; it is best used to assess glycemic control during treatment.*

Poorly controlled diabetic patient,

Nondiabetic hyperglycemia (e.g., acute stress response, Cushing syndrome, pheochromocytoma, glucagonoma, corticosteroid therapy, acromegaly):
Patients with these illnesses tend to have persistently elevated glucose levels that cause an elevated GHb and glycated proteins.

Patients with splenectomy: *In these patients RBC survival is prolonged. More time for hemoglobin glycosylation is available. GHb and glycated proteins levels increase.*

Pregnancy: *In some women with gestational diabetes or prediabetes, persistently high levels of glucose occur that cause elevated GHb and glycated proteins levels.*

▼ Decreased Levels

Hemolytic anemia,

Chronic blood loss:
RBC survival is shortened. Therefore there is less time for glycosylation, and GHb and glycated proteins levels decrease.

Chronic renal failure: *These patients have reduced hemoglobin levels as a result of lack of erythropoietin, which is produced in the kidney. HbA_1 is also decreased.*

RELATED TESTS

Glucose, Blood (p. 253). This is the primary screening test for diabetes.

Glucose, Urine (p. 924). Testing for glucose in the urine is a part of routine urinalysis. If glucose is present in the urine, it reflects the degree of glucose elevation in the blood. Urine glucose tests are also used to monitor the effectiveness of therapy for diabetes mellitus (DM).

Glucose Tolerance (p. 261). This is a test of a patient's capability to handle a glucose load.

Glucose, Postprandial (p. 257). This is a timed glucose measurement after a carbohydrate meal.

Glucagon (p. 251). This is a direct measurement of glucagon, which acts to increase glucose in the blood.

Insulin Assay (p. 315). This is a direct measurement of insulin, which acts to decrease glucose in the blood.

Growth Hormone (GH, Human Growth Hormone [HGH], Somatotropin Hormone [SH])

NORMAL FINDINGS

Men: <5 ng/mL or <5 mcg/L (SI units)
Women: <10 ng/mL or <10 mcg/L
Children:
    Newborn: 5-23 ng/mL (mcg/L [SI units])
    1 week: 2-27 ng/mL (mcg/L [SI units])
    1-12 mos: 2-10 ng/mL (mcg/L [SI units])
    >1 year female: 0-10 ng/mL (mcg/L [SI units])
    >1 year male: 0-6 ng/mL (mcg/L [SI units])

INDICATIONS

This test is used to identify GH deficiency in adolescents with short stature, delayed sexual maturity, or other growth deficiencies. It is also used to document the diagnosis of GH excess in patients with gigantism or acromegaly. GH is used to identify and follow patients with ectopic growth hormone produced by neoplasms. Finally, it is often used as a screening test for pituitary hypofunction.

TEST EXPLANATION

GH, or somatotropin, is secreted by the acidophil cells in the anterior pituitary gland and plays a central role in modulating growth from birth until the end of puberty. There is an elaborate feedback mechanism associated with the secretion of GH. The hypothalamus secretes growth hormone–releasing hormone, which stimulates GH release from the pituitary. GH exerts its effects on many tissues through a group of peptides called somatomedins. The most commonly tested somatomedin is *somatomedin C* (p. 317), which is produced by the liver and has a major effect on cartilage. High levels of somatomedins stimulate the production of somatostatin from the hypothalamus. Somatostatin inhibits further secretion of GH from the pituitary. GH is secreted during sleep, exercise, and ingestion of protein and in response to hypoglycemia.

In the total absence of GH, linear growth occurs at one half to one third of the normal rate. GH also plays a role in the control of body anabolism throughout life by increasing protein synthesis, increasing the breakdown of fatty acids in adipose tissue, and increasing the blood glucose level.

If GH secretion is insufficient during childhood, limited growth and dwarfism may result. Also, a delay in sexual maturity may occur in adolescents with reduced GH levels. Conversely, overproduction of GH during childhood results in gigantism, with the person reaching nearly 7 to 8 feet in height. An excess of GH during childhood (after closure of long bone end plates) results in acromegaly, which is characterized by an increase in bone thickness and width but no increase in height.

GH tests are also used to confirm hypopituitarism or hyperpituitarism. GH assay is the most widely used test for GH deficiency or excess. Because GH secretion is episodic, random assays for GH are not adequate determinants of GH deficiency. Normal GH levels overlap significantly with deficient levels. Low GH levels may indicate deficiency or may be normal for certain individuals at certain times of the day. To negate time variables in GH testing, GH should be drawn 60 to 90 minutes after deep sleep. Levels increase during sleep. Also, strenuous exercise can be performed for 30 minutes in an effort to stimulate GH production. GH levels drawn at the end of the exercise period are expected to be maximal. These two methods are helpful in evaluating GH deficiency.

To negate the common variations in GH secretion, screening for *insulin-like growth factor (IGF-1) or somatomedin C* provides a more accurate reflection of the mean plasma concentration of GH. If the IGF-1 is normal, the patient virtually never has acromegaly. IGF-1 is not helpful in evaluating patients with GH deficiency because levels are affected by nutritional status, liver and thyroid function, and age. These proteins are not affected by the time of day or food intake as is GH, because they circulate bound to proteins that are durable and long lasting.

A *GH stimulation test* (p. 272) can be performed to evaluate the body's ability to produce GH in cases of suspected GH deficiency. The *growth hormone suppression test* is used to identify gigantism in children or acromegaly in the adult. If GH can be suppressed to less than 2 ng/mL, neither of these conditions exists. The most commonly used suppression test is the oral glucose tolerance test (p. 261). Through a rise in glucose, GH normally is suppressed. In acromegalic patients, only a slight or no decrease in GH occurs.

INTERFERING FACTORS

- Random measurements of GH are not adequate determinants of GH deficiency, because hormone secretion is episodic.
- A radioactive scan performed within the week before the test may affect test results if levels are determined by radioimmunoassay (RIA).
- GH secretion is increased by stress, exercise, diet, and low blood glucose levels.
- ✗ Drugs that may cause *increased* levels include amphetamines, arginine, dopamine, estrogens, glucagon, histamine, insulin, levodopa, methyldopa, and nicotinic acid.
- ✗ Drugs that may cause *decreased* levels include corticosteroids and phenothiazines.

PROCEDURE AND PATIENT CARE

Before
- ✗ Explain the procedure to the patient.
- The patient should not be emotionally or physically stressed, because this can increase GH levels.
- It is preferred that patients be well rested and are kept on nothing by mouth (NPO) status after midnight the morning of the test. Water is permitted.

During
Growth Hormone
- Collect a venous blood sample red-top tube.
- Because approximately two thirds of the total production of GH occurs during sleep, its secretion also can be measured during hospitalization by obtaining blood samples while the patient is sleeping.

Growth Hormone Suppression Test
- Obtain peripheral venous access with normal saline solution (NSS).
- Obtain baseline GH and glucose levels as described above.
- Administer the prescribed glucose dose.
- Obtain GH and glucose levels at 10, 60, and 120 minutes after glucose ingestion.

After

- Apply pressure or a pressure dressing to the venipuncture site.
- Assess the venipuncture site for bleeding.
- Indicate the patient's fasting status and the time the blood is collected on the laboratory slip. Include the patient's recent activity (e.g., sleeping, walking, eating).
- Because the half-life of GH is only 20 to 25 minutes, send the blood to the laboratory immediately after collection.

TEST RESULTS AND CLINICAL SIGNIFICANCE

▲ Increased Levels

Gigantism,
Acromegaly:
   These two syndromes are caused by excess GH.
Anorexia nervosa: *Starvation stimulates GH secretion.*
Stress,
Major surgery,
Hypoglycemia,
Starvation,
Deep-sleep state,
Exercise:
   These situations stimulate GH secretion.
Hypoglycemia: *Hypoglycemia stimulates GH secretion.*

▼ Decreased Levels

GH deficiency,
Pituitary insufficiency:
   GH is produced in the pituitary. Diseases, tumors, ischemia, or trauma to the pituitary or hypothalamus causes GH deficiency.
Dwarfism: *This is a result of GH deficiency in children.*
Hyperglycemia: *Elevated glucose levels inhibit GH secretion.*
Failure to thrive: *This is a result of GH deficiency in infants.*
Delayed sexual maturity: *This is a result of GH deficiency in adolescents.*

RELATED TESTS

Growth Hormone (GH) Stimulation (p. 272). This is a test designed to stimulate the secretion of GH. It is required to accurately diagnose GH deficiency.
Somatomedin C (p. 317). Somatomedin C levels parallel GH levels. However, they are not affected by the many factors that cause significant variations in GH results.

Growth Hormone Stimulation (GH Provocation, Insulin Tolerance [IT], Arginine)

NORMAL FINDINGS

GH levels >10 ng/mL or >10 mcg/L (SI units)

INDICATIONS

The GH stimulation test is used to identify patients who are suspected of having GH deficiency. A normal patient can have low GH levels, but if GH is still low after GH stimulation, the diagnosis can be more accurately made.

TEST EXPLANATION

Because GH secretion is episodic, random measurement of plasma GH is not adequate to make the diagnosis of GH deficiency. To diagnose GH deficiency, GH stimulation tests are indicated. One of the most reliable GH stimulators is insulin-induced hypoglycemia, in which the blood glucose declines to less than 40 mg/dL. Other GH stimulants include vigorous exercise and drugs (e.g., arginine, glucagon, levodopa, clonidine). Glucagon is more widely used for GH stimulation because of safety concerns with insulin-induced hypoglycemia.

Pituitary GH deficiency cannot be diagnosed by identifying a deficiency of GH to just one stimulant, because as many as 20% of normal patients will fail to respond to the stimulant. Therefore a double-stimulated test is usually performed: arginine infusion is followed by insulin-induced hypoglycemia. Arginine is an amino acid that stimulates GH secretion; hypoglycemia also stimulates GH secretion. A GH concentration over 10 mg/L after stimulation effectively excludes GH deficiencies. Hypothyroidism should be excluded before GH stimulation testing.

GH also can be stimulated by vigorous exercise. This may entail running or stair-climbing for 20 minutes. Blood samples of GH are obtained at 0, 20, and 40 minutes. GH-releasing factor can also be used to stimulate GH. At present the best method of identifying patients deficient in GH is a positive stimulation test followed by a positive response to a therapeutic GH trial. GH deficiency is also suspected when bone age, as determined by x-ray films of the long bones (see p. 1006), indicates delayed growth according to chronologic age.

Only minor discomfort is associated with this test and results from the insertion of the intravenous (IV) line and the hypoglycemic response induced by the insulin injection. This may include postural hypotension, somnolence, diaphoresis, and nervousness. This procedure is usually performed by a nurse under physician supervision. This test takes approximately 2 hours to perform.

CONTRAINDICATIONS

- Patients with epilepsy, because seizures can be induced by the hypoglycemia
- Patients with cerebrovascular disease, because hypoglycemia may induce stroke
- Patients with myocardial infarction (MI), because the stress associated with the hypoglycemia may cause angina or an MI
- Patients with low basal plasma cortisol levels, because they cannot respond to or compensate for the hypoglycemia

POTENTIAL COMPLICATIONS

- Hypoglycemia may be so significant and severe as to cause ketosis, acidosis, and shock. With close observation, this is unlikely.

PROCEDURE AND PATIENT CARE

Before

✍ Explain the procedure very carefully to the patient and, if appropriate, to the parents.

✍ Instruct the patient to remain on nothing by mouth (NPO) status after midnight on the morning of the test. Water is permitted.

During

- Note the following procedural steps:
  1. A saline lock IV line is inserted for the administration of medications and the withdrawal of frequent blood samples.
  2. Baseline blood levels are obtained for GH, glucose, and cortisol.
  3. Venous samples for GH are obtained 0, 60, and 90 minutes after injection of arginine and/or insulin or glucagon.
  4. Blood glucose levels are monitored at 15- to 30-minute intervals with the glucometer. The blood sugar should drop to less than 40 mg/dL for effective measurement of GH reserve.
- Monitor the patient for signs of hypoglycemia, postural hypotension, somnolence, diaphoresis, and nervousness.
- Ice chips are often given during the test for patient comfort.

After

- Observe the venipuncture site for bleeding.
- ✍ Inform the patient and family that results may not be available for approximately 7 days. Some laboratories run GH tests only once a week.
- After the test, give the patient cookies and punch or an IV glucose infusion.
- Send the blood to the laboratory immediately after collection, because the half-life of growth hormone is only 20 to 25 minutes.

TEST RESULTS AND CLINICAL SIGNIFICANCE

▼ Decreased Levels

Pituitary deficiency,
GH deficiency:

> *Diseases (e.g., tumor, infarction, trauma) of the pituitary can result in failure of the pituitary to secrete either GH or all the pituitary hormones. GH stimulation tests will fail to stimulate GH secretion.*

RELATED TESTS

Somatomedin C (p. 317). Somatomedin C levels parallel GH levels. However, they are not affected by the many factors that cause significant variations in GH results.

Growth Hormone (p. 269). This test is a direct quantitative assay for GH.

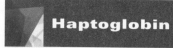
Haptoglobin

NORMAL FINDINGS
Adult: 50-220 mg/dL or 0.5-2.2 g/L (SI units)
Newborn: 0-10 mg/dL or 0-0.1 g/L (SI units)

 Critical Values

<40 mg/dL

INDICATIONS
This test is used to identify the presence of intravascular hemolysis. This protein is decreased when significant hemolysis occurs. It is nonspecific for indicating the type of hemolytic anemia.

TEST EXPLANATION
The serum haptoglobin test is used to detect intravascular destruction (lysis) of red blood cells (RBCs). This is called hemolysis. Haptoglobins are glycoproteins produced by the liver. These haptoglobins are powerful, free hemoglobin–binding proteins. In hemolytic anemias associated with the hemolysis of RBCs, the released hemoglobin is quickly bound to haptoglobin and the new complex is rapidly catabolized. This results in a diminished amount of free haptoglobin in the serum; this decrease cannot be readily compensated for by normal liver production. As a result, the patient demonstrates a transient reduced level of haptoglobin in the serum. Megaloblastic anemias can reduce the haptoglobin level because of the increased destruction of megaloblastic RBC precursors in the bone marrow.

Haptoglobins are also decreased in patients with primary liver disease not associated with hemolytic anemias. This occurs because the diseased liver is unable to produce these glycoproteins. Hematoma can reduce haptoglobin levels by the absorption of hemoglobin into the blood and by binding hemoglobin with haptoglobin.

Elevated haptoglobin concentrations are found in many inflammatory diseases, and therefore haptoglobin can be used as a nonspecific acute-phase reactant protein in much the same way as the erythrocyte sedimentation rate (see p. 221). That is, levels of haptoglobin increase with severe infection, inflammation, tissue destruction, acute myocardial infarction (AMI), burns, and some cancers.

INTERFERING FACTORS
- A slight decrease in haptoglobin levels is noted in normal pregnancy.
- Ongoing infection can cause falsely elevated test results.
- Drugs that may cause *increased* haptoglobin levels include androgens and steroids.
- Drugs that may cause *decreased* levels include chlorpromazine, diphenhydramine, indomethacin, isoniazid, nitrofurantoin, oral contraceptives, quinidine, and streptomycin.

PROCEDURE AND PATIENT CARE
Before
- Explain the procedure to the patient.
- Tell the patient that no fasting is required.

During

- Collect a venous blood sample in a red-top tube.
- Avoid hemolysis, which may alter test results.

After

- Apply pressure or a pressure dressing to the venipuncture site.
- Assess the venipuncture site for bleeding.

TEST RESULTS AND CLINICAL SIGNIFICANCE

▲ Increased Levels

Collagen-rheumatic diseases,

Infection (e.g., pyelonephritis, urinary tract infection [UTI], pneumonia),

Tissue destruction (e.g., myocardial infarction [MI]),

Nephritis,

Ulcerative colitis,

Neoplasia:

The above and many other diseases can cause an elevation of haptoglobin, an acute-phase reactant protein.

Biliary obstruction: *Haptoglobin, after attaching to hemoglobin, is excreted by the liver in the bile. Obstruction will diminish that excretion.*

▼ Decreased Levels

Hemolytic anemia (e.g., erythroblastosis fetalis, autoimmune hemolytic anemias, hemoglobinopathies [sickle cell], paroxysmal nocturnal hemoglobinuria, drug-induced hemolytic anemia, or uremia): *Hemolysis occurs, freeing hemoglobin in the plasma. The free hemoglobin is tightly bound to haptoglobin. The complex is catabolized and excreted. Haptoglobin cannot be replaced fast enough and levels in the blood fall.*

Transfusion reactions: *ABO antibodies bind to ABO antigens on the RBC membrane and cause hemolysis. Hemoglobin is liberated from the RBC. The free hemoglobin is tightly bound to haptoglobin. The complex is catabolized and excreted. Haptoglobin cannot be replaced fast enough and levels in the blood fall.*

Prosthetic heart valves: *The mechanical trauma of the valve on the RBC causes hemolysis, and hemoglobin is liberated from the RBC. The free hemoglobin is tightly bound to haptoglobin. The complex is catabolized and excreted. Haptoglobin cannot be replaced fast enough and levels in the blood fall.*

Primary liver disease: *The diseased liver cannot make adequate amounts of haptoglobin. The liver is the sole source of haptoglobin.*

Hematoma,

Tissue hemorrhage:

The free hemoglobin in the hematoma binds the haptoglobin. The complex is catabolized and excreted. Haptoglobin cannot be replaced fast enough and levels in the blood fall.

 Heinz Body Preparation

NORMAL FINDINGS

No Heinz bodies detected

INDICATIONS

This test is used to detect Heinz bodies that occur as a result of oxidative denaturation of the hemoglobin molecule.

TEST EXPLANATION

Heinz bodies are water-insoluble precipitates of oxidated-denatured proteins or hemoglobin that form within red blood cells. They occur as a result of exposure to oxidative chemicals and drugs. Mutations of hemoglobin (particularly Hb Koln), thalassemias, and defects in the hemoglobin-reductive defense system against oxidation (G6PD deficiency or pyruvate kinase deficiency) lead to an enhanced tendency toward oxidative hemolysis. The diagnosis of these problems can be established by the detection of Heinz bodies in red blood cells (RBCs) by obtaining a Heinz body preparation.

Heinz bodies are often associated with hemolytic anemias and the presence of spherocytosis. The pathophysiology of these anemias starts with oxidative injury to hemoglobin. As a result, red cell inclusions (Heinz bodies) of variable size and usually eccentric location adhere to the red cell membrane. Smooth movement of the membrane over the cytosol is reduced. These RBCs are selectively blocked from leaving the splenic cords and entering the sinuses. Splenic macrophages attack these RBCs and cause hemolysis. This process can be severe enough to cause intravascular destruction as well, producing hemoglobinemia and hemoglobinuria. Most often the clinical picture includes a normocytic anemia associated with splenomegaly.

Agents that commonly induce oxidation of hemoglobin include: nitrofurantoin, sulfasalazine, *p*-aminosalicylic acid, acetaminophen, phenazopyridine, phenacetin, dapsone, and other sulfones. Diets high in pickled or smoked foods, nitrates, recreational drugs, mothballs, and industrial chemicals can also oxidize hemoglobin.

For Heinz body detection, fresh blood is incubated with a supravital stain (such as methyl violet or Nile blue) and examined by microscopy for presence of stained inclusions close to the red cell membrane (Heinz bodies). These RBC granules can be quantified by several different methods, but are most commonly counted microscopically. It is important not to confuse Heinz bodies with other RBC granules, such as Howell Jolly bodies.

PROCEDURE AND PATIENT CARE

Before

☒ Explain the procedure to the patient.
☒ Tell the patient that no fasting is required.

During

- Collect a venous blood sample in a lavender-top (EDTA), pink-top (K$_2$EDTA), or green-top tube (sodium or lithium heparin).

After

- Apply pressure or a pressure dressing to the venipuncture site.
- Assess the venipuncture site for bleeding.

TEST RESULTS AND CLINICAL SIGNIFICANCE

▲ Increased Levels

Unstable hemoglobinopathies (e.g., Hb Gun Hill),

Red cell enzymopathies (e.g., G6PD),
Thalassemia,
Heinz body hemolytic anemia:
   These hemolytic anemias are highlighted by the presence of Heinz bodies in RBCs.

RELATED TESTS

Red Blood Cell Count (p. 439). RBC count is used to identify hemolytic anemia that may be highlighted
   by Heinz bodies.
Haptoglobin (p. 274). The serum haptoglobin test is used to detect intravascular hemolysis of RBCs.

Hematocrit (Hct, Packed Red Blood Cell Volume, Packed Cell Volume [PCV])

NORMAL FINDINGS

Male: 42%-52% or 0.42-0.52 volume fraction (SI units)
Female: 37%-47% or 0.37-0.47 volume fraction (SI units)
Pregnant female: >33%
Elderly: values may be slightly decreased.
Child/adolescent
   Newborn: 44%-64%
   2-8 weeks: 39%-59%
   2-6 months: 35%-50%
   6 months-1 year: 29%-43%
   1-6 years: 30%-40%
   6-18 years: 32%-44%

 Critical Values

<21% or >65%

 Age-Related Concerns

- Values in children are age specific, with normal values varying throughout the first 18 years.
- Values are slightly decreased in the elderly.

INDICATIONS

The Hct is an indirect measurement of red blood cell (RBC) number and volume. It is used as a rapid
measurement of RBC count. It is repeated serially in patients with ongoing bleeding or as a routine part
of the complete blood cell count. It is an integral part of the evaluation of anemic patients.

TEST EXPLANATION

The Hct is a measure of the percentage of the total blood volume that is made up by the RBCs. The
height of the RBC column is measured after centrifugation. It is compared to the height of the column of

the total whole blood. The ratio of the height of the RBC column compared with the original total blood column is multiplied by 100%. This is the Hct value. It is routinely performed as part of a complete blood cell count. The Hct closely reflects the hemoglobin (Hgb) and RBC values. The Hct in percentage points usually is approximately three times the Hgb concentration in grams per deciliter when RBCs are of normal size and contain normal amounts of Hgb.

Normal values vary according to gender and age. Women tend to have lower values than men, and Hct values tend to decrease with age. Abnormal values indicate the same pathologic states as abnormal RBC counts and Hgb concentrations. Decreased levels indicate anemia (reduced number of RBCs). Increased levels can indicate erythrocytosis (Figure 2-18).

Like other RBC values, the Hct can be altered by many factors other than RBC production. For instance, in dehydrated patients the total blood volume is contracted. The RBCs make up a greater proportion of the total blood volume, and the Hct measurement is therefore falsely high. Likewise, if the RBC is morphologically increased in size, the RBCs will make up a greater proportion of the total blood volume, and Hct will again be falsely high.

The Hct can be measured in a capillary tube (by skin puncture) by placing the blood in the tube, which is then spun in a microcentrifuge. The percentage of the RBC portion of the column to the whole column is the Hct. This value is most often calculated by automated cell counting machines.

Decisions concerning the need for blood transfusion are usually based on the Hgb or the Hct. In an otherwise healthy person, transfusion is not considered as long as the Hgb is above 8 g/dL or the Hct is above 24%. In younger people who can safely and significantly increase their cardiac output, a Hct of 18% may be acceptable. In an older individual with an already compromised oxygen-carrying capacity (caused by cardiopulmonary diseases), transfusion may be recommended when the Hct level is below 30%.

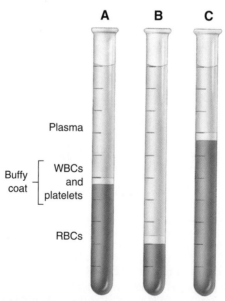

Figure 2-18 Tubes showing hematocrit levels of normal blood, blood with evidence of anemia, and blood with evidence of polycythemia. Note the buffy coat located between the packed red blood cells (RBCs) and the plasma. **A,** A normal percentage of RBCs. **B,** Anemia (low percentage of RBCs). **C,** Polycythemia (high percentage of RBCs).

INTERFERING FACTORS

- Abnormalities in RBC size may alter Hct values. Larger RBCs are associated with higher Hct levels, because the larger RBCs take up a greater percentage of the total blood volume.
- Extremely elevated white blood cell (WBC) counts decrease Hct, which would falsely indicate anemia.
- Hemodilution and dehydration may affect the Hct level (see previous discussion).
- Pregnancy usually causes slightly decreased values because of chronic hemodilution.
- Living at high altitudes causes increased Hct values as a result of a physiologic response to the decreased oxygen available.
- Values may not be reliable immediately after hemorrhage because the percentage of total blood volume taken up by the RBC has not changed. Not until the total blood volume is replaced with fluids will the Hct decrease.

 Drugs that may cause *decreased* levels include chloramphenicol and penicillin.

✔ Clinical Priorities

- Normal values vary according to gender and age.
- Pregnancy usually causes slightly decreased values because of chronic hemodilution.
- The Hct (in percentage points) is usually three times the Hgb concentration (in grams per deciliter) when RBCs are of normal size and contain normal amounts of Hgb.
- In dehydration the Hct is falsely elevated. In overhydration the value is decreased.

PROCEDURE AND PATIENT CARE

Before

Explain the procedure to the patient.
Tell the patient that no fasting is required.

During

- Collect a venous blood sample in a lavender-top tube; only 0.5 mL is required when using capillary tubes.
- Avoid hemolysis.

After

- Apply pressure or a pressure dressing to the venipuncture site.
- Assess the venipuncture site for bleeding.

TEST RESULTS AND CLINICAL SIGNIFICANCE

▲ Increased Levels

Erythrocytosis: *The number of RBCs is increased. This can result from illnesses or as a physiologic response to external situations.*

Congenital heart disease: *Cyanotic heart diseases cause chronically low Po$_2$ levels. In response, the RBCs increase in number. Therefore the Hct increases.*

Polycythemia vera: *This is a result of the bone marrow inappropriately producing great numbers of RBCs, causing the Hct to increase.*

Severe dehydration (e.g., severe diarrhea, burns): *With depletion of extracellular fluid, the total blood volume decreases, but the number of RBCs stays the same. Therefore the percentage of total blood volume that is taken up by the RBCs increases and the Hct increases.*

Severe chronic obstructive pulmonary disease (COPD): *Chronic states of hypoxia cause stimulation of RBC production as a physiologic response to increased oxygen-carrying capacity. Therefore the Hct increases.*

▼ Decreased Levels

Anemia: *This is a term given to the state associated with reduced RBC numbers. Because the Hct is an indirect reflection of RBC numbers, the Hct will also be reduced. Many different types of diseases are associated with anemia.*

Hemoglobinopathy: *Patients with Hgb disorders or other blood dyscrasias have a reduced number and survival of RBCs. Therefore the Hct is decreased.*

Cirrhosis: *This is a chronic state of fluid overload. The RBCs are diluted and make up a smaller percentage of the total blood volume. Therefore the Hct decreases.*

Hemolytic anemia (e.g., erythroblastosis fetalis, hemoglobinopathies, drug-induced hemolytic anemias, paroxysmal nocturnal hemoglobinuria): *The RBC survival is diminished in hemolytic anemia. The number of RBCs decreases and therefore the Hct is decreased.*

Hemorrhage: *With active bleeding, the number of RBCs decreases and therefore the Hct is decreased. It takes time (several hours), however, for the Hct to fall. Only when the blood volume is replenished with fluid does the Hct diminish.*

Dietary deficiency: *With certain vitamin or mineral deficiencies (e.g., iron), the RBC number or size is decreased. Therefore the Hct is decreased.*

Bone marrow failure: *With reduced synthesis of the RBCs, the Hct will decrease.*

Prosthetic valves: *The prosthetic valve causes mechanical trauma to the RBCs. RBC survival is diminished, so RBC numbers diminish and Hct decreases.*

Renal disease: *Erythropoietin is made in the kidney and is a strong stimulant to RBC production. With a reduced level of erythropoietin, the RBC numbers diminish and the Hct is decreased.*

Normal pregnancy: *In pregnancy, normally there is increased blood volume because of a chronic state of overhydration. Combined with a relative "malnourished" state, the Hct is diminished by a decrease in the number of RBCs and the percentage of total blood volume they make up.*

Rheumatoid/collagen-vascular diseases (e.g., rheumatoid arthritis, lupus): *Chronic illnesses are associated with a reduced production of RBCs. Therefore the Hct is decreased.*

Lymphoma,

Multiple myeloma,

Leukemia,

Hodgkin disease:
  Hematologic cancers are often associated with bone marrow failure of RBC production. The number of RBCs diminishes and the Hct decreases.

RELATED TESTS

Hemoglobin (p. 281). This is a measurement of the concentration of Hgb in the blood. It is closely associated with the RBC count and Hct value.

Red Blood Cell Count (p. 439). This is a measurement of the number of RBCs per cubic millimeter of blood. It is closely associated with the Hgb and Hct values.

Red Blood Cell Indices (p. 442). These provide data about the size and Hgb content of the RBC.

Hemoglobin (Hgb, Hb)

NORMAL FINDINGS

Male: 14-18 g/dL or 8.7-11.2 mmol/L (SI units)
Female: 12-16 g/dL or 7.4-9.9 mmol/L
    Pregnant female: >11 g/dL
Elderly: Values are slightly decreased.
Child/adolescent
    Newborn: 14-24 g/dL
    0-2 weeks: 12-20 g/dL
    2-6 months: 10-17 g/dL
    6 months-1 year: 9.5-14 g/dL
    1-6 years: 9.5-14 g/dL
    6-18 years: 10-15.5 g/dL

 Critical Values

<7 g/dL or >21 g/dL

 Age-Related Concerns

- Values in children are age specific, with normal values varying throughout the first 18 years.
- Values are slightly decreased in the elderly.

INDICATIONS

This test is a measure of the total amount of Hgb in the blood. It is used as a rapid indirect measurement of the red blood cell (RBC) count. It is repeated serially in patients with ongoing bleeding or as a routine part of the complete blood cell count (CBC). It is an integral part of the evaluation of anemic patients.

TEST EXPLANATION

The Hgb concentration is a measure of the total amount of Hgb in the peripheral blood. The test is normally performed as part of a CBC. Hgb serves as a vehicle for oxygen and carbon dioxide transport. The oxygen-carrying capacity of the blood is determined by the Hgb concentration. Hgb also acts as an important acid-base buffer system.

    As with the RBC count, normal values vary according to gender and age. Women tend to have lower values than men and Hgb values tend to decrease with age. The Hgb closely reflects the hematocrit (Hct) and RBC values. The Hct in percentage points usually is approximately three times the Hgb concentration in grams per deciliter when RBCs are of normal size and contain normal amounts of Hgb.

Abnormal values indicate the same pathologic states as abnormal RBC counts and Hct concentrations. Decreased levels indicate anemia (reduced number of RBCs). Increased levels can indicate erythrocytosis. In addition, however, changes in plasma volume are more accurately reflected by the Hgb concentration. Dilutional overhydration decreases the concentration, whereas dehydration tends to cause an artificially high value. Slight decreases in the values of Hgb and Hct during pregnancy reflect the expanded blood volume because of a chronic state of overhydration; the number of cells is actually increased during pregnancy. Hgb is usually measured by an automated cell counter. There is very little variability (2% to 3%) with most well-kept machines.

Hgb is made up of heme (iron surrounded by protoporphyrin) and globin consisting of an alpha- and a beta-polypeptide chain. Abnormalities in the globin structure are called hemoglobinopathies (e.g., sickle cell disease, hemoglobin C disease). Some diseases are caused by abnormalities in globin chain synthesis (such as thalassemia). In these diseases the RBC counts can be low, the RBC survival can be diminished, and the RBC-carrying capacity can be reduced.

Too little Hgb puts a strain on the cardiopulmonary system to maintain good oxygen-carrying capacity. With critically low hemoglobin levels, patients are at great risk for angina, heart attack, congestive heart failure, and stroke. When Hgb levels are too high because of increased numbers of RBCs, intravascular sludging occurs, leading to stroke and other organ infarction. Decisions concerning the need for blood transfusion are usually based on the Hgb or the Hct. In an otherwise healthy person, transfusion is not considered as long as the Hgb is above 8 g/dL or the Hct is above 24%. In younger people who can safely and significantly increase their cardiac output, an Hgb level of 6 g/dL may be acceptable. In an older individual with an already compromised oxygen-carrying capacity (cardiopulmonary diseases), transfusion may be recommended when the Hgb level is below 10.

INTERFERING FACTORS

- Slight Hgb decreases normally occur during pregnancy because of the dilution effect of the expanded blood volume.
- There is a slight diurnal variation in Hgb levels.
- Hgb levels are highest around 8 AM and are lowest around 8 PM. This may vary as much as 1 g/dL.
- Heavy smokers have higher Hgb levels than nonsmokers.
- Living in high altitudes causes increased Hgb values as a result of a physiologic response to the decreased oxygen available at these high altitudes.
- Drugs that may cause *increased* levels include gentamicin and methyldopa (Aldomet).
- Drugs that may cause *decreased* levels include antibiotics, antineoplastic drugs, aspirin, indomethacin (Indocin), rifampin, and sulfonamides.

Clinical Priorities

- Dilutional overhydration decreases the Hgb concentration. Dehydration tends to cause an artificially high value.
- The Hct (in percentage points) is usually three times the Hgb concentration (in grams per deciliter) when RBCs are of normal size and contain a normal amount of Hgb.
- Living at high altitudes causes increased Hgb values as a result of a physiologic response to decreased oxygen levels.

PROCEDURE AND PATIENT CARE

Before

☒ Explain the procedure to the patient.
☒ Tell the patient that no fasting is required.

During

- Collect a venous blood sample in a lavender-top tube.
- Avoid hemolysis.
- List on the laboratory slip any drugs that may affect test results.

After

- Apply pressure or a pressure dressing to the venipuncture site.
- Observe the venipuncture site for bleeding.

TEST RESULTS AND CLINICAL SIGNIFICANCE

▲ Increased Levels

Erythrocytosis: *The number of RBCs is increased as a result of illnesses or as a physiologic response to external situations (e.g., high altitude).*

Congenital heart disease: *Cyanotic heart diseases cause chronically low Po₂ levels. In response, the RBCs increase in number. Therefore the Hgb increases.*

Severe chronic obstructive pulmonary disease: *Chronic states of hypoxia cause stimulation of RBC production as a physiologic response to increased oxygen-carrying capacity. Therefore the Hgb increases.*

Polycythemia vera: *This is a result of the bone marrow inappropriately producing great numbers of RBCs. Therefore the Hgb increases.*

Severe dehydration (e.g., severe diarrhea, burns): *With depletion of extracellular fluid, the total blood volume decreases, but the number of RBCs stays the same. Therefore the percentage of total blood volume that is taken up by the RBCs increases and Hgb increases.*

▼ Decreased Levels

Anemia: *This is a term given to the state associated with reduced RBC numbers. Because the Hgb is an indirect reflection of RBC numbers, the Hgb will also be reduced. Many different types of diseases are associated with anemia.*

Hemoglobinopathy: *Patients with Hgb disorders or other blood dyscrasias have reduced RBC number and RBC survival. Therefore the Hgb is decreased.*

Cirrhosis: *This is a chronic state of fluid overload. The RBCs are diluted and make up a smaller percentage of the total blood volume. Therefore the Hgb decreases.*

Hemolytic anemia (e.g., erythroblastosis fetalis, hemoglobinopathies, drug-induced hemolytic anemias, transfusion reactions, or paroxysmal nocturnal hemoglobinuria): *The RBC survival is diminished in hemolytic anemia. The number of RBCs decreases and the Hgb decreases.*

Hemorrhage: *With active bleeding, the number of RBCs decreases and the Hgb decreases. It takes time (several hours), however, for the Hgb to fall. Only if the blood volume is replenished with fluid does the Hgb diminish.*

Dietary deficiency: *With certain vitamin or mineral deficiencies (e.g., iron), the RBC number or size is decreased. Therefore the Hgb is decreased.*

Bone marrow failure: *With reduced synthesis of the RBCs, the Hgb will decrease.*

Prosthetic valves: *The prosthetic valve causes mechanical trauma to the RBCs. RBC survival is diminished. RBC numbers diminish and Hgb decreases.*

Renal disease: *Erythropoietin is made in the kidney and is a strong stimulant to RBC production. With a reduced level of erythropoietin, the RBC numbers diminish and the Hgb is decreased.*

Normal pregnancy: *In pregnancy, normally there is increased blood volume because of a chronic state of overhydration. Combined with a relative "malnourished" state, the Hgb is diminished by a decrease in the number of RBCs and the percentage of total blood volume they make up.*

Rheumatoid/collagen-vascular diseases (e.g., rheumatoid arthritis [RA], lupus, sarcoidosis): *Chronic illnesses are associated with a reduced production of RBCs. Therefore the Hgb is decreased.*

Lymphoma,

Multiple myeloma,

Neoplasia,

Leukemia,

Hodgkin disease:
   Hematologic cancers are often associated with bone marrow failure of RBC production. The number of RBCs diminishes and the Hgb decreases.

Splenomegaly: *With an enlarged functioning spleen, RBCs are sequestered and eliminated from the functioning vascular system.*

RELATED TESTS

Hematocrit (p. 277). This is a measurement of the percentage of the total blood volume taken up by the RBCs. It is closely associated with Hgb values and RBC count.

Red Blood Cell Count (p. 439). This is a measurement of the number of RBCs per cubic millimeter of blood. It is closely associated with Hgb and Hct values

Red Blood Cell Indices (p. 442). These provide data about the size and Hgb content of the RBC.

Hemoglobin Electrophoresis (Hgb Electrophoresis)

NORMAL FINDINGS

Adult/elderly: percentage of total hemoglobin
   Hgb A_1: 95%-98%
   Hgb A_2: 2%-3%
   Hgb F: 0.8%-2%
   Hgb S: 0%
   Hgb C: 0%
   Hgb E: 0%
Children (Hgb F)
   Newborn (Hgb F): 50%-80%
   <6 months: <8%
   >6 months: 1%-2%

INDICATIONS

Hgb electrophoresis is a test that enables abnormal forms of Hgb (hemoglobinopathies) to be detected and quantified. This test is used to diagnose sickle cell anemia, thalassemia, and other hemoglobinopathies.

TEST EXPLANATION

Although many different Hgb variations have been described, the more common types are A_1, A_2, F, S, E, and C. Each major Hgb type is electrically charged to varying degrees. When the Hgb from lysed red blood cells (RBCs) is placed on electrophoresis paper in an electromagnetic field, the Hgb variants migrate at different rates and therefore spread apart from each other. The migration of the various forms of Hgb makes up a series of bands on the paper. The bands therefore correspond to the various forms of Hgb present. The pattern of bands is compared to normal and to well-known abnormal patterns. A diagnosis can then be made. Each band can be quantitated as a percentage of the total Hgb, indicating the severity of any recognized abnormality.

The form *Hgb A_1* constitutes the major component of Hgb in the normal RBC. *Hgb A_2* is only a minor component (2% to 3%) of the normal Hgb total. *Hgb F* is the major Hgb component in the fetus but usually exists in only minimal quantities in the normal adult. Levels of Hgb F greater than 2% in patients over 3 years of age are considered abnormal. Hgb F is able to transport oxygen when only small amounts of oxygen are available (as in fetal life). In patients requiring compensation for prolonged chronic hypoxia (as in congenital cardiac abnormalities), Hgb F may be found in increased levels to assist in the transport of the available oxygen.

Hgb S and *Hgb C* are abnormal forms of Hgb that occur predominantly in American blacks. Hemoglobin E occurs predominantly in Southeast Asians. Hgb S is associated with sickle cell anemia. Hgb S is a relatively insoluble variant. When little oxygen is available, it assumes a crescent (sickle) shape that greatly distorts the RBC morphology. Vascular sludging is a consequence of the localized sickling and may lead to organ infarction. The duration of survival of the sickled RBC is diminished, and these patients also have anemia. RBCs containing Hgb C have a decreased life span and are more readily lysed than normal RBCs. Mild to severe hemolytic anemia may result. The Hgb contents of some common disorders affecting hemoglobin, as determined by electrophoresis, are indicated in Table 2-27.

Hgb E is produced less efficiently by RBC precursors; if there is an increased Hgb E content in the RBCs, those cells will have a low mean corpuscular volume (MCV, p. 442).

Quantifying abnormal hemoglobins is helpful in determining the zygosity of a familial hemoglobinopathy. Furthermore quantification of abnormal hemoglobin proteins provides a method of monitoring treatments designed to increase more effective hemoglobin variants and decrease abnormal variants. Hemoglobin quantification can be performed by high-performance liquid chromatography (HPLC) and polymerase chain reaction (PCR) analysis.

TABLE 2-27	Hemoglobin Content of Some Common Hemoglobinopathies						
	PERCENTAGE RANGE						
	Hgb A	Hgb A_2	Hgb F	Hgb S	Hgb H	Hgb C	Hgb E
Sickle cell disease	0	2-3	2	95-98	0	0	0
Sickle cell trait	50-65	2-3	2	35-45	0	0	0
Hemoglobin C disease	0	2-3	2	0	0	90-100	0
Three gene deletion alpha-thalassemia (Hgb H disease)	65-90	0.3-1.5	0.4-4.5	0	0-30	0	0
Beta-thalassemia major	0	0-15	85-100	0	0	0	0
Beta-thalassemia trait	50-85	4-8	1-5	0	0	0	0
Hgb E disease	0	0	0	0	0	0	100

INTERFERING FACTORS

- Blood transfusions within the previous 12 weeks may alter test results.
- Glycosylated Hgb can blur the peak of Hgb F and cause falsely low levels of Hgb F.

PROCEDURE AND PATIENT CARE

Before

Explain the procedure to the patient.
Tell the patient that no fasting is required.

During

- Collect a venous blood sample in a lavender-top tube.

After

- Apply pressure or a pressure dressing to the venipuncture site.
- Assess the venipuncture site for bleeding.

TEST RESULTS AND CLINICAL SIGNIFICANCE

▲ Increased Levels

Sickle cell disease,
Hemoglobin H disease,
Thalassemia major,
Sickle cell trait,
Thalassemia minor,
Hemoglobin C trait or disease,
Hemoglobin E trait or disease:
  These hemoglobinopathies have a "classic" Hgb electrophoresis pattern that is diagnostic for the respective disease.

RELATED TEST

Hemoglobin (p. 281). This is a direct measurement of the Hgb that exists in the "average" RBC.

Hepatitis Virus Studies (Hepatitis-Associated Antigen [HAA], Australian Antigen)

NORMAL FINDINGS

Negative

INDICATIONS

This group of tests is used to diagnose and to identify the serologic type and current status of hepatitis. It is important to diagnose and identify the type of hepatitis as soon as possible so that the patient can be immediately treated and appropriately isolated.

TEST EXPLANATION

Hepatitis is an inflammation of the liver caused by viruses, alcohol ingestion, drugs, toxins, or overwhelming bacterial sepsis. The three common viruses now recognized to cause disease are hepatitis A, hepatitis B, and hepatitis C (also called non-A/non-B) viruses. Hepatitis D and E viruses are much less common in the United States. Hepatitis D can infect the liver only by entering into a hepatitis B virus, which it uses as a carrying vehicle. Therefore hepatitis D cannot cause disease unless patients have hepatitis B virus in their bloodstream in the active, chronic, or carrier forms. The various types of hepatitis cannot be differentiated on the basis of their clinical presentation. The clinical presentations are similar in that they all include low-grade fever, malaise, anorexia, and fatigue. Most often they are all associated with elevations of hepatocellular enzymes such as aspartate aminotransferase (AST), alanine aminotransferase (ALT), and lactic dehydrogenase (LDH).

Hepatitis A virus (HAV) was originally called *infectious hepatitis.* It has a short incubation period of 2 to 6 weeks and is highly contagious. During active infection, HAV is excreted in the stool and transmitted via oral-fecal contamination of food and drink. Most infections are not associated with symptoms severe enough to warrant medical evaluation. Immune globulin (IgG) and IgM antibodies to HAV are routinely used when HAV infection is suspected.

The first HAV antibody to appear is the IgM antibody *(HAV-Ab/IgM)* in approximately 3 to 4 weeks after exposure or just before hepatocellular enzyme elevations occur. These IgM levels usually return to normal in approximately 8 weeks. The next antibody to HAV to rise is IgG *(HAV-Ab/IgG),* which appears approximately 2 weeks after the IgM begins to increase and slowly returns to normal levels. The IgG antibody can remain detectable for more than 10 years after the infection. If the IgM antibody is elevated in the absence of the IgG antibody, acute hepatitis is suspected. If however IgG is elevated in the absence of IgM elevation, a convalescent or chronic stage of HAV viral infection is indicated.

These antibodies may not be positive soon after infection occurs, which can delay the investigation of the infectious outbreaks. The HAV virus can be detected directly by measuring *HAV RNA* in the sera of patients suspected of acute infection.

Hepatitis B virus (HBV) is commonly known as *serum hepatitis.* It has a long incubation period of 5 weeks to 6 months. HBV is most frequently transmitted by blood transfusion; however, it also can be contracted via exposure to other body fluids. HBV may cause a severe and unrelenting form of hepatitis culminating in liver failure and death. The incidence is increased among blood transfusion recipients, male homosexuals, dialysis patients, transplant patients, intravenous drug abusers, and patients with leukemia or lymphoma. Hospital personnel are also at increased risk for infection, mostly as a result of needle stick contamination.

HBV, also called the Dane particle, is made up of an inner core surrounded by an outer capsule. The outer capsule contains the *hepatitis B surface antigen (HBsAg),* formerly called Australian antigen. The inner core contains *HBV core antigen (HBcAg).* The *hepatitis B e-antigen (HBeAg)* is also found within the core. Antibodies to these antigens are called HBsAb, HBcAb, and HBeAb. The tests used to detect these antigens and antibodies include (Table 2-28):

1. *Hepatitis B surface antigen (HBsAg).* This is the most frequently and easily performed test for hepatitis B, and it is the first test to become abnormal. HBsAg rises before the onset of clinical symptoms, peaks during the first week of symptoms, and returns to normal by the time jaundice subsides. HBsAg generally indicates active infection by HBV. If the level of this antigen persists in the blood, the patient is considered to be a carrier.

2. *Hepatitis B surface antibody (HBsAb).* This antibody appears approximately 4 weeks after the disappearance of the surface antigen and signifies the end of the acute infection phase. HBsAb

TABLE 2-28	Hepatitis Testing	
Serologic Findings	**Appearance/Disappearance**	**Application**
HAV-Ab/IgM	4-6 wk/3-4 mo	Acute HAV infection
HAV-Ab/IgG	8-12 wk/10 yr	Previous HAV exposure/immunity
HBeAg	1-3 wk/6-8 wk	Acute HBV infection
HBeAb	4-6 wk/4-6 yr	Acute HBV infection ended
HBsAg	4-12 wk/1-3 mo	Acute HBV infection
HBsAb total	3-10 mo/6-10 yr	Previous HBV infection/immunity indicated
HBVc-Ab/IgM	2-12 wk/3-6 mo	Acute HBV infection
HBVc-Ab total	3-12 wk/life	Previous HBV infection/convalescent stage
HCV-Ab/IgG	3-4 mo/2 yr	Previous HCV infection
HDV Ag	1-3 days/3-5 days	Acute HDV infection
HDV-Ab/IgM	10 days/1-3 mo	Acute HDV infection
HDV-Ab total	2-3 mo/7-14 mo	Chronic HDV infection

also signifies immunity to subsequent infection. Concentrated forms of this agent constitute the hyperimmunoglobulin given to patients who have come in contact with HBV-infected patients (e.g., contact by an inadvertent needle prick from a needle previously used on a patient with HBV infection). HBsAb is the antibody that denotes immunity after administration of hepatitis B vaccine.

3. *Hepatitis B core antigen (HBcAg).* No tests are currently available to detect this antigen.
4. *Hepatitis B core antibody (HBcAb).* This antibody appears approximately 1 month after infection with HBsAg and declines (although it remains elevated) over several years. HBcAb is also present in patients with chronic hepatitis. The HBcAb level is elevated during the time lag between the disappearance of HBsAg and the appearance of HBsAb. This interval is called the "core window." During the core window, HBcAb is the only detectable marker of a recent hepatitis infection.
5. *Hepatitis B e-antigen (HBeAg).* This antigen generally is not used for diagnostic purposes but rather as an index of infectivity. The presence of HBeAg correlates with early and active disease, as well as with high infectivity in acute HBV infection. The persistent presence of HBeAg in the blood predicts the development of chronic HBV infection.
6. *Hepatitis B e-antibody (HBeAb).* This antibody indicates that an acute phase of HBV infection is over, or almost over, and that the chance of infectivity is greatly reduced.

Hepatitis B DNA can be quantified and is a direct measurement of the HBV viral load. A one- or two-log decrease in viral load in a hepatitis B–infected patient means antiviral therapy is working. A one- or two-log increase in a similar patient means an antiviral has stopped working and that viral resistance may have developed. High levels of HBV-DNA, ranging from 100,000 to more than 1 billion viral copies per milliliter, indicate a high rate of HBV replication. Low or undetectable levels, about 300 copies per milliliter or less, indicate an "inactive" infection. The World Health Organization established the international unit or copies per milliliter (mL), written as international units/mL or copies/mL, to measure HBV DNA. Detection of HBV DNA serves as an important supplementary test to serology in a number of clinical settings. It is helpful in the early detection of HBV infection, monitoring of disease, and determining low levels of viremia in patients with nonreplicative HBV disease and chronic hepatitis. Because the intent of treatment is to eliminate HBV, accurate measurement of low viral load is very important.

Hepatitis C virus (HCV) (non-A/non-B [NANB] hepatitis) is transmitted in a manner similar to HBV. Most cases of hepatitis are caused by blood transfusion. HCV is found in as many as 8% of blood donors worldwide. The incubation period is 2 to 12 weeks after exposure. The clinical manifestations of the illness parallel those of HBV. However, unlike with HBV, HCV infection is chronic in more than 60% of infected persons. Although the disease course is variable, it is slowly progressive. Twenty percent of HCV patients develop cirrhosis and hepatocellular cancers associated with this chronic infection.

The screening test for detecting HCV infection is the detection of *anti-HCV antibodies* to HCV recombinant core antigen, *NS3* gene, NS4 antigen, and NS5 antigen. The antibodies can be detected within 4 weeks of infection. With *HCV-RNA testing*, the HCV virion can be directly detected and quantified (viral load). Real-time PCR is used for HBV DNA testing. HCV RNA viral load is quantitated by using RT-PCR methods and is usually expressed as units per milliliter or copies per milliliter. Although a higher viral load may not necessarily be a sign of more severe or more advanced disease, it does correlate with likelihood to respond to treatment. HCV RNA tests can also be used to monitor response to hepatitis C treatment.

Hepatitis D virus (HDV) is known to cause *delta hepatitis.* As stated earlier, the HDV must enter the HBV to gain access to the liver and be infective. The patient must have HBV in the blood from a past or synchronously occurring infection. In the United States this is most commonly transmitted through tainted blood. The *HDV antigen* can be detected by immunoassay within a few days after infection. The IgM and total antibodies to HDV are also detected early in the disease. A persistent elevation of these antibodies indicates a chronic or carrier state.

Hepatitis E virus (HEV) was initially included in the non-A/non-B virus group but was isolated several years ago as an etiologic virus of short incubation. No antigen or antibody tests are currently widely available and accurate for the serologic identification of this infecting agent.

PROCEDURE AND PATIENT CARE

Before
☒ Explain the procedure to the patient.
☒ Tell the patient that no fasting is required.

During
- Collect a venous blood sample in a red-top tube.
- Usually a hepatitis profile that includes several HBV antigens and antibodies is performed.

After
- Apply pressure or a pressure dressing to the venipuncture site.
- Assess the venipuncture site for bleeding.
- Handle the specimen as if it were capable of transmitting hepatitis.
- Immediately discard the needle in the appropriate receptacle.
- Send the specimen to the laboratory promptly.
☒ Advise patients with suspected hepatitis that they should refrain from intimate contact with another person. Until the serology indicates otherwise, the person should be considered infective.

TEST RESULTS AND CLINICAL SIGNIFICANCE

▲ Increased Levels

Hepatitis A,
Hepatitis B,
Hepatitis C (non-A, non-B hepatitis),
Hepatitis D,
Hepatitis E:
   These viral forms of hepatitis can exist in an acute, chronic, carrier, or chronic active phase.

RELATED TESTS

Aspartate Aminotransferase (AST) (p. 119), Alanine Aminotransferase (ALT) (p. 39), Lactic Dehydrogenase (LDH) (p. 329). These hepatocellular enzymes are elevated during the acute phase and
chronic active phase of hepatitis.

Hexosaminidase (Hexosaminidase A, Hex A, Total Hexosaminidase, Hexosaminidase A and B)

NORMAL FINDINGS

Hexosaminidase A: 7.5-9.8 units/L (SI units)
Total hexosaminidase: 9.9-15.9 units/L (SI units)
(Check with the laboratory because of wide variety of testing methods.)

INDICATIONS

Hex A is used to identify patients affected by Tay-Sachs disease and unaffected persons who may be
carriers of this deadly genetic defect.

TEST EXPLANATION

Tay-Sachs disease (TSD) is a lysosomal storage disease (GM2 gangliosidoses) first characterized by
loss of motor skills in infancy and early childhood. Death usually occurs by age 4 to 8 years. TSD is
a result of a mutation in an autosomal recessive gene carried on chromosome 15. An affected person
must inherit a defective gene from each parent to have TSD. One out of 25 Ashkenazi (Eastern European) Jews is a carrier for this genetic mutation. There are 80 different genetic mutations that inhibit
the function of this important gene (p. 1097). This gene encodes the synthesis of an enzyme called
hexosaminidase. Without this enzyme, lysosomes of GM2 accumulate, particularly in the central
nervous system.

   Two clinically important isoenzymes of hexosaminidase have been detected in the serum: hexosaminidase A (made up of one alpha subunit and one beta subunit) and hexosaminidase B (made up of two
beta subunits). Any genetic mutation that affects the alpha unit will cause a deficiency of hexosaminidase A, resulting in TSD. A mutation that affects the beta unit will cause a deficiency in hexosaminidase
A and B. Sandhoff disease, an uncommon variant of Tay-Sachs, occurs with deficiency of both of these
enzymes. Other genetic mutations of this same gene can cause chronic GM2-gangliosidosis, a disease
similar to TSD that becomes apparent later in life (adolescence).

Because TSD is uniformly untreatable and fatal, a significant effort has gone into the development of biochemical testing to identify carriers of the genetic mutation (persons who carry one of the recessive genetic defective genes). Hex A has been found to be abnormally low in carriers, whereas hex B is high. Therefore testing for total hexosaminidase is not useful. A carrier has a 25% chance of having a child with TSD if the other biologic parent is also a carrier. Pregnancy should occur only with thorough genetic counseling. In communities in which the Ashkenazi Jewish population is high, hex A screening has been very effective for identifying carriers. Further, hex A is used to diagnose TSD in infants, young children, and adults. Genetic testing (p. 1093) is useful to corroborate the identification of an affected person or a carrier.

If a couple at risk for producing offspring with TSD chooses to proceed with pregnancy, amniocentesis (p. 632) can be performed. The amniotic fluid and or cells obtained by chorionic villus sampling can be tested for hex A. Cells obtained during amniocentesis can also be tested for the precise genetic mutation.

INTERFERING FACTORS

- Hemolysis of the blood sample can cause inaccurate test results.
- Pregnancy can cause markedly increased values. For this reason, blood tests are not done during pregnancy.
- Oral contraceptives can *falsely increase* levels.

PROCEDURE AND PATIENT CARE

Before

- Explain the procedure to the patient. Emphasize the importance of this test to Jewish couples of Eastern European ancestry who plan to have children. Explain that both must carry the defective gene to transmit TSD to their offspring.
- Professional genetic counseling should be provided to every person considering undergoing this test.
- Patients should be made aware of the possible effects on their lives if hex A levels are found to be reduced.
- Check with the laboratory regarding withholding contraceptives.

During

- Collect a venous blood sample in a red-top tube. Avoid hemolysis.
- Note that pregnant women can be evaluated by amniocentesis (p. 632) or chorionic villus biopsy (p. 1088).
- Note that infants may have blood obtained by heelstick. Neonates often have blood drawn through the umbilical cord.

After

- If only one partner is a carrier, reassure the couple that their offspring cannot inherit TSD.
- Arrange genetic counseling if both partners are carriers of TSD and pregnancy is desired.

TEST RESULTS AND CLINICAL SIGNIFICANCE

▼ Decreased Hexosaminidase

Tay-Sachs disease: *The synthesis of hex A is prevented by a genetic mutation in the gene encoded for production of the alpha unit of that enzyme. GM2 gangliosides accumulate in neural tissue, causing neurologic and mental deterioration.*

▼ Decreased Hexosaminidase A and B

Sandhoff disease: *The synthesis of hex A and B is prevented by a genetic mutation in the gene encoded for production of the beta unit of those enzymes. GM2 gangliosides accumulate in neural tissue, causing neurologic and mental deterioration.*

RELATED TESTS

Genetic Testing (p. 1093). By testing for a mutation at the site of the gene known to be involved in TSD, more definitive corroborative evidence of disease state and carrier status can be obtained.

Amniocentesis (p. 632). Through this technique, fetal cells and fluid can be obtained and tested for hex A.

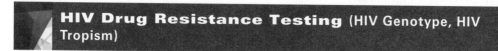

HIV Drug Resistance Testing (HIV Genotype, HIV Tropism)

NORMAL FINDINGS

No detectable HIV-1 genotypic mutations conferring resistance to an antiviral drug

INDICATIONS

This test is used for the identification of key HIV genotypic mutations that are associated with resistance to highly active antiretroviral therapy (HAART).

TEST EXPLANATION

There are several factors that affect the success of HIV antiviral medications. These include patient compliance, access to adequate care, optimal dosing, and drug pharmacology issues, including absorption, elimination, and drug interactions. Another significant factor that determines a patient's response to anti-viral HIV drugs is the percentage of a HIV viral population that is resistant to the nucleotide reverse-transcriptase inhibitors, non-nucleotide reverse-transcriptase inhibitors, and protease inhibitors that may be administered to destroy the HIV virus. HIV resistance to therapy develops in 78% of patients. In these patients, genotypic mutations arising in the drug-targeted HIV viral gene loci occur because of evolutionary pressure from antiviral therapy and results in antiviral resistance that may compromise HAART in HIV-infected patients receiving HAART. This information can be identified based on HIV genotyping or the identification of HIV tropism. When combination therapy fails, detection and analysis of HIV genotypic mutations or tropism can guide necessary changes to antiretroviral therapy and decrease HIV viral load, thereby improving patient outcome.

HIV tropism is laboratory methodology that sets up a vector construct that when the patient's nucleic acid is inserted, the ability of the HIV virus to infect the cell is determined. This is a phenotype assay that is biologically driven. This assay is sensitive and correlates well to clinical outcomes. Unfortunately, this testing is expensive and labor intensive. HIV genotyping is an alternative to HIV tropism.

HIV genotyping is able to detect changes in the viral genome that are associated with drug resistance. By amplification and analysis of drug-targeted HIV gene sequence, identification of changes in nucleotide bases and associated amino acid codons that may cause antiviral drug resistance can be identified. Such genotypic changes are deemed as mutations by comparing the sequence data of the patient's HIV strain to those of a "wild-type" HIV strain. The significance of these genotypic mutations in relation to antiviral resistance is then determined by a set of interpretive rules.

Results of any genotypic mutation found would include:

- "Susceptible" result indicates no reduced susceptibility.
- "Possible resistance" result indicates that the mutation(s) detected has or have been associated with diminished virologic response in some but not all patients.
- "Resistant" result indicates that the mutation(s) detected has or have been associated with a maximum reduction in susceptibility of the virus.
- "Insufficient evidence" result indicates that current scientific data are insufficient to determine if the mutation(s) detected is or are associated with decreased susceptibility of the virus to the specific antiviral drug.
- "Unable to genotype" result indicates that the sequence data obtained are of poor quality to determine the presence or absence of genotypic resistant mutations in the patient's HIV strain. One possible cause of such poor sequence data is low HIV viral load (i.e., <1000 copies/mL).

HIV genotyping is particularly useful when failure to the most active antiviral therapy is suspected by decreasing CD4 counts (p. 147). HIV genotyping can also be performed in conjunction with *HIV drug sensitivity testing*. HIV sensitivity testing estimates the ability of a cloned copy of the patient's virus to replicate in a cell culture in the presence of a particular antiviral drug. This same testing can help determine the amount of drug needed to inhibit viral replication. It is generally reported as the concentration of drug required to inhibit (inhibiting concentration, IC) viral replication by 50%, or the IC_{50}. This is particularly helpful when considering the use of expensive drugs or when frequent hypersensitivity to a particular drug is possible.

INTERFERING FACTORS

- If the plasma HIV-1 RNA viral load is less than 1000 HIV-1 RNA copies per mL of plasma, genotyping may be inaccurate.
- Minor HIV-1 populations that are less than approximately 20% of the total population may not be identified by this test.

PROCEDURE AND PATIENT CARE

Before

☒ Explain the procedure to the patient.

☒ Tell the patient that no fasting or preparation is required.

- Maintain a nonjudgmental attitude toward the patient's sexual practices. Allow the patient ample time to express his or her concerns regarding the results.

During

- Observe universal body and blood precautions. Wear gloves when handling blood products from all patients.
- Obtain venous blood in lavender (EDTA) or pink (K_2EDTA) tube.
- Never recap needles. Dispose of needles and syringes required for obtaining the blood specimen in a puncture-proof container designed for this purpose.

After

- Immediately transport the specimen to the laboratory.
- Specimens are sent to a central laboratory.
- Apply pressure to the venipuncture site.
- Instruct the patient to observe the venipuncture site for infection. Patients with AIDS are immunocompromised and susceptible to infection.

TEST RESULTS AND CLINICAL SIGNIFICANCE

Drug Resistance

This assay has been optimized for genotypic analysis for drug resistance of HAART of HIV-1 subtype B (the majority of HIV-1 isolates reported in the United States and Europe).

RELATED TESTS

HIV Serologic and Virologic Testing (p. 297). These tests are used to detect HIV infection.

HIV RNA Quantification (see following test). This is a measure of the HIV viral load in an HIV-infected patient.

HIV RNA Quantification (HIV Viral Load)

NORMAL FINDINGS

Undetected

INDICATIONS

This test is used to determine the amount of human immunodeficiency virus (HIV) viral load in the blood of an infected patient. This test is an accurate marker for prognosis, disease progression, response to antiviral treatment, and indication for antiretroviral prophylactic treatment.

TEST EXPLANATION

Quantitation of HIV RNA in the blood of patients infected with HIV can be used as a confirmatory or supplementary test after serologic tests (p. 297) are positive. Quantification is also helpful when confirmatory tests are indeterminate or cannot be accurately interpreted. Virologic testing is helpful in differentiating newborn HIV infection from passive transmission of HIV antibodies from a HIV infective mother. Finally HIV RNA quantification testing determines HIV "viral load." Determining viral load is used:

- To determine a baseline viral level before initiating anti–HIV-1 drug therapy
- To identify HIV-1 drug resistance while on anti-HIV therapy
- To identify noncompliance with anti–HIV-1 drug therapy
- To monitor HIV-1 disease progression while on or off anti–HIV-1 drug therapy
- To recommend the initiation of antiretroviral treatment (Table 2-29). To determine the course of the disease because it is more accurate than any other test, including CD4 T-cell counts (p. 147).
- To determine patient survival (Table 2-30).

HIV viral load is determined by quantifying the amount of genetic material of the virus in the blood. There are several different laboratory methods of measuring HIV viral load. It is important that the

TABLE 2-29	Recommendations for Antiretroviral Therapy Based on Viral Load and CD4 Count		
	HIV RNA VIRAL LOAD (COPIES/mL)		
CD4 Count (×10⁵/L)	**<5000**	**5000-30,000**	**>30,000**
<350	Recommend therapy	Recommend therapy	Recommend therapy
351-500	Consider therapy	Recommend therapy	Recommend therapy
>500	Defer therapy	Consider therapy	Recommend therapy
Symptomatic		Recommend therapy	

(Note: CD4 Count is expressed as $\times 10^5/L$)

TABLE 2-30	Utilizing the Viral Load to Predict Disease Course				
	HIV RNA VIRAL LOAD (COPIES/mL)				
	<500	**501-3000**	**3001-10,000**	**10,001-30,000**	**>30,000**
Percent developing AIDS	5.4	16.6	31.7	55.2	80
Percent dying from AIDS	0.9	6.3	18.1	34.9	69.5

same method be used in monitoring the course of the disease. Because results vary according to the testing methods, it is important to know which method is used when considering whether to initiate treatment. A common method uses a reverse-transcriptase polymerase chain reaction (RT-PCR) using gene amplification. This method can quantify HIV-1 or -2 RNA to ranges of less than 50 copies/mL.

In general, it is recommended to determine the baseline viral load by obtaining two measurements 2 to 4 weeks apart after HIV infection. Monitoring may continue with testing every 3 to 4 months in conjunction with CD4 counts. Both tests provide data used to determine when to start antiviral treatment. The viral load test can be repeated every 4 to 6 weeks after starting or changing antiviral therapy. Usually antiviral treatment is continued until the HIV viral load is less than 500 copies/mL. It is important to recognize that a *nondetectable* result does not mean no virus is left in the blood after treatment; it means that the viral load has fallen below the limit of detection by the test. However the clinical implications of a viral load below 50 copies/mL remain unclear. Possible causes of such a result include very low plasma HIV-1 viral load present (e.g., in the range of 1 to 19 copies/mL), very early HIV-1 infection (i.e., less than 3 weeks from time of infection), or absence of HIV-1 infection (i.e., false-positive). A significant (greater than threefold) rise of viral load should warrant consideration of alteration of therapy.

In general, this test is not recommended as a screening/confirmatory test for suspected HIV infection. However, clinicians may recommend the quantification of viral load (DNA or RNA) for screening of infants born to HIV-infected mothers.

INTERFERING FACTORS

- Incorrect handling and processing of the specimen can cause inconsistent results.
- Recent flu shots may temporarily *increase* viral levels.
- Concurrent infections can cause inconsistent results.
- Variable compliance to therapy may alter test results.

Clinical Priorities

- Do not give test results over the phone. Increasing viral load results can have devastating consequences.
- Because test results vary according to the laboratory test method, it is important to use the same laboratory method for monitoring the course of the disease.
- Viral loads are usually repeated after starting or changing antiviral therapy. A significant rise in viral load should warrant immediate reevaluation of therapy.

PROCEDURE AND PATIENT CARE

Before

✗ Explain the procedure to the patient.
✗ Tell the patient that no fasting or preparation is required.
- Maintain a nonjudgmental attitude toward the patient's sexual practices. Allow the patient ample time to express his or her concerns regarding the results.

During

- Observe universal body and blood precautions. Wear gloves when handling blood products from all patients.
- Collect a blood sample in a lavender-top (EDTA) tube. If the test is sent out, the plasma is separated out and at least 2.5 mL is frozen and sent.
- Never recap needles. Dispose of needles and syringes required for obtaining the blood specimen in a puncture-proof container designed for this purpose.

After

- Immediately transport the specimen to the laboratory.
- Specimens are often sent to a central laboratory.
- Apply pressure to the venipuncture site.
✗ Instruct the patient to observe the venipuncture site for infection. Patients with AIDS are immunocompromised and susceptible to infection.
✗ Do not give results over the telephone. Increasing viral load may have devastating consequences.
✗ Encourage the patient to discuss his or her concerns regarding the prognostic information that may be obtained by these results.

TEST RESULTS AND CLINICAL SIGNIFICANCE

▲ Increased Levels

HIV infection: *Generally, the level of HIV viral load parallels the course of HIV disease. Reduction in viral loads can be expected with successful therapy.*

RELATED TESTS

HIV Serology (p. 297). This test is used to diagnose HIV infection.

Lymphocyte Immunophenotyping (p. 147). This test is used to measure CD4 lymphocyte counts. This is another marker for disease prognosis, response to treatment, and also an indicator for starting prophylactic antiretroviral treatment.

HIV Drug Resistance Testing (p. 292). HIV drug sensitivity testing estimates the ability of a cloned copy of the patient's virus to replicate in a cell culture in the presence of a particular antiviral drug. It can help determine the amount of drug needed to inhibit viral replication.

HIV Serologic and Virologic Testing (AIDS Serology, Acquired Immunodeficiency Serology, AIDS Screen, Human Immunodeficiency Virus [HIV] Antibody Test, Western Blot Test, p24 Direct Antigen, HIV-RNA Viral Test)

NORMAL FINDINGS

No evidence of HIV antigen or antibodies

INDICATIONS

These tests are used to detect HIV infection.

TEST EXPLANATION

There are two active types of human immunodeficiency viruses, types 1 and 2. HIV 1 is most prevalent type within the United States and Western Europe, whereas HIV 2 is mostly limited to Western African nations. Serologic testing identifies antibodies developed as a result of HIV 1 or 2 infections. Virologic tests identify RNA (or DNA) specific to HIV. Virologic tests can identify HIV infection in the first 11 days after infection. Serologic tests can identify HIV infection only after about 3 weeks. This 3-week time period is called the "seroconversion window." Serologic testing for HIV is divided into "screening tests" and "confirmatory" tests (Box 2-11).

In the past serologic screening of patients suspected of having HIV-1 or -2 infection usually began with a HIV antibody "screening test" using a qualitative chemiluminescent immunoassay. If positive, a confirmatory test was required to make the diagnosis of HIV infection. HIV serologic qualitative screening tests (for HIV-1 and -2) were used to screen high- and low-risk individuals or for donor blood products (Table 2-31 and Box 2-12). Because these rapid screening qualitative antibody immunoassays do not detect viral antigens, they could not detect infection in its earliest stage (before antibodies are

BOX 2-11	Serologic Testing for HIV

Screening Tests	Confirmatory/Discriminatory Tests
HIV-1 p24 antigen	WB HIV-1 antibody
HIV-1 antibody	WB HIV-2 antibody
HIV-2 antibody	Immunoblot–HIV-2 antibody
HIV-1/HIV-2 antibody	Immunofluorescence HIV-1 antibody (IFA)
Combined HIV-1/HIV-2 + HIV-1 p 24 antigen	HIV RNA NAAT qualitative testing
Rapid HIV-1 antibody	
Rapid HIV-2 antibody	
Rapid HIV-1/HIV-2 antibody	

WB, Western blot.

formed). Because some persons who undergo HIV testing do not return to learn their test results, there has been a strong push toward the "point of service" rapid HIV antibody serologic screening testing in which results can be available in less than 1 hour. This is particularly helpful in urgent or emergent care points of service in which HIV transmission could occur from blood or body fluid contamination. Furthermore, rapid antibody testing is helpful during labor in women whose HIV status is unknown.

Point-of-care home kits are available that provide anonymous registration and pretest counseling via a toll-free call. Sample collection in the privacy of one's home, laboratory processing, and post-test counseling are components of this home-testing process. The procedure involves pricking a finger with a special device, placing drops of blood on a specially treated card, and then mailing the card to a licensed laboratory to be tested. Test results are available to the client within 3 business days for the Express Kit and 7 days for the Standard Kit after shipment of the sample to the laboratory.

Confirmatory tests for HIV-1 and -2 antibodies include the Western blot assay and the indirect immunofluorescence assay (IFA). The Western blot assay can recognize either HIV-1 or -2 antibodies. The Western blot is associated with lower sensitivity during the time of seroconversion. However, when positive, the Western blot is very accurate. IFA assay can also discriminate between HIV-1 and -2 antibodies. It is more sensitive than the Western blot assay. These are often done as multi-spot or immunoblot testing.

The *p24 direct serologic antigen assay* detects the viral protein p24 in the peripheral blood of HIV-infected individuals, in which it exists either as a free (core) antigen or complexed to anti-p24 antibodies. The p24 antigen may be detectable as early as 16 days after infection. The p24 antigen test can be used to assess the antiviral activity of anti-HIV therapies. The p24 antigen test can also be used to differentiate active neonatal HIV infection from passive HIV antibody present from the mother's blood. It is also used to detect HIV infection before antibody seroconversion, detect HIV in donor blood, and monitor therapy.

The use of oral fluids for serologic HIV testing is as an alternative to serum testing. These new HIV-1 antibody tests use *oral mucosal transudate* (OMT), a serum-derived fluid that enters saliva from the gingival crevice and across oral mucosal surfaces. Another noninvasive alternative to blood testing is *urine testing for HIV*. Only a spot urine collection is required. Testing urine for HIV antibodies is

TABLE 2-31	Centers for Disease Control HIV Screening Recommendations
Who	**How Often**
All adults ages 18-64	Once in a lifetime
All adults with known risk factors	Yearly
All pregnant women	Once
Pregnant women at risk for HIV	Second test in third trimester
Newborns if mother is HIV+ or HIV status is unknown	Frequent repeated testing through first 6 months of life

BOX 2-12   Risk Factors for HIV Infection

- Sexually active male homosexuals
- Bisexual males
- Women with at-risk male partner
- Women with multiple male partners
- IV drug abusers
- Persons receiving blood products containing HIV
- Infants of HIV+ mothers or mothers of unknown HIV status

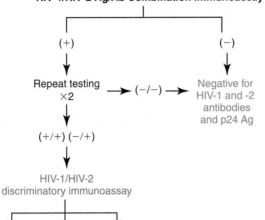

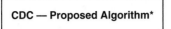

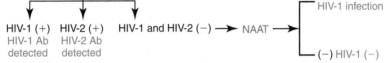

CDC — Proposed Algorithm*

HIV-1/HIV-2 Ag/Ab Combination Immunoassay

(+)

(−)

Repeat testing
×2 → (−/−) → Negative for
HIV-1 and -2
antibodies
and p24 Ag

(+/+) (−/+)

HIV-1/HIV-2
discriminatory immunoassay

HIV-1 (+)   HIV-2 (+)   HIV-1 and HIV-2 (−) → NAAT →
HIV-1 Ab   HIV-2 Ab
detected   detected

(+) Acute
HIV-1 infection

(−) HIV-1 (−)

*An IgM-sensitive Ab immunoassay if the Ag/Ab combination assay is not available.

Figure 2-19 CDC proposed HIV testing algorithm. (Reprinted with permission from the Association of Public Health Laboratories [APHL] 2011.)

valuable, especially when venipuncture is inconvenient, difficult, or unacceptable. Insurance companies also commonly use it. It is important to note that all urine HIV tests are detecting antibodies and not the HIV particles. Urine does not contain the virus and is not a body fluid capable of infecting others.

HIV antigen/antibody (Ag/Ab) combination assays are now available that can detect HIV infection on average 5 to 7 days earlier than assays that only detect antibodies. Reducing the seroconversion window has always been an important goal in HIV diagnostics because individuals with acute HIV infection have high viral loads and are highly infectious. As discussed, in the past, the two-step immunoassay (IA)/rapid test screen followed by the Western blot confirmation approach had been the gold standard for HIV diagnosis. With the development of the newer Ag/Ab combination test, the CDC has proposed another algorithm for HIV testing (Figure 2-19).

The serologic tests described in the preceding detect HIV infection based on demonstration of antibodies to HIV or to HIV viral antigen protein (p. 297). HIV viral RNA particles can be detected (by qualitative testing for HIV RNA) and quantified (by HIV RNA quantification-viral load, see p. 294) using *Nucleic Acid Amplification Tests (NAATs)* methods. Although too expensive to use as screening tests, NAAT testing can identify HIV 11 days after infection. HIV-RNA tests can be used as confirmatory or discriminatory tests, especially when other confirmatory tests are indeterminate or cannot be accurately interpreted. NAAT testing is helpful in differentiating newborn HIV infection from passive transmission of HIV antibodies from an HIV-infective mother.

A person with positive HIV test results does not have AIDS until he or she develops the clinical features of diminished immune ability. Positive confirmatory HIV antibody test results are required under laws in many states to be reported to the departments of health of the respective states in which the patients reside.

INTERFERING FACTORS

- False-positive results can occur in patients who have autoimmune disease, lymphoproliferative disease, leukemia, lymphoma, syphilis, or alcoholism.
- False-positives can occur in noninfected pregnant women.
- HIV-2 infection can cause a positive HIV-1 and -2 screening antibody test and an indeterminate WB HIV-1 confirmatory test.
- False-negative results can occur in the early incubation stage or end stage of AIDS.

Clinical Priorities

- Do not relay the test results over the telephone. Positive results may have devastating consequences, including loss of job, insurance, relationships, and housing.
- Encourage patients with positive test results to inform their sexual partners so they can be tested.
- Inform patients with positive test results that subsequent sexual contact will put partners at high risk for contracting AIDS.

PROCEDURE AND PATIENT CARE

Before

- Explain the procedure to the patient.
- Obtain an informed consent as required by law.
- Tell the patient that no fasting or preparation is required.
- Maintain a nonjudgmental attitude toward the patient's sexual practices and allow the patient ample time to express his or her concerns regarding the results.

During

- Observe universal blood and body precautions. Wear gloves when handling blood products from all patients.
- For routine HIV testing, collect a venous blood sample in a red-top tube. The blood is often sent to an outside laboratory for testing, although testing kits are becoming increasingly available in hospital laboratories and even in homes.
- If the patient wishes to remain anonymous, use a number with the patient's name; be sure to record it accurately.
- Note that if the serologic test is reactive (i.e., test is positive twice consecutively), the Western blot test is performed on the same blood sample.

After

- Apply pressure or a pressure dressing to the venipuncture site.
- Assess the site for bleeding.
- Instruct the patient to observe the venipuncture site for infection. Patients with AIDS are immunocompromised and susceptible to infection.
- Follow the institution's policy regarding test result reporting.
- Do not give results over the telephone. Remember that positive results may have devastating consequences.

Explain to the patient that a positive Western blot test merely implies exposure to and presence of the AIDS virus within the body. It does not mean that the patient has clinical AIDS. Not all patients with positive results on an antibody test will acquire the disease.

Encourage patients testing positive to identify their sexual contacts so that they can be informed and tested.

Inform the patient that subsequent sexual contact will put new partners at high risk for contracting AIDS.

Provide patient education regarding safe sexual practices.

TEST RESULTS AND CLINICAL SIGNIFICANCE

▲ Increased Levels

AIDS,

AIDS-related complex:

It is important to be aware that HIV infection occurs several years before development of AIDS. There is some evidence that the disease can be prevented with aggressive early treatment of HIV infection.

RELATED TESTS

Cell Surface Immunophenotyping (p. 147). This test quantifies the number of CD4 and CD8 lymphocytes in an HIV-positive patient. These tests are predictive of the disease course and prognosis.

HIV Viral Load (p. 294). This test is used to determine the amount of HIV viral load in the blood of an infected patient and is an accurate marker for prognosis and disease progression.

Homocysteine (HCY)

NORMAL FINDINGS

4-14 μmol/L

INDICATIONS

Homocysteine is an important predictor of coronary, cerebral, and peripheral vascular disease. When a strong familial predisposition or early-onset vascular disease is noted, homocysteine testing should be performed to determine if genetic or acquired homocysteine excess exists. Because elevated homocysteine levels are associated with vitamin B_{12} or folate deficiency, this is a reasonable test to use for the detection and surveillance of malnutrition.

TEST EXPLANATION

Homocysteine is an intermediate amino acid formed during the metabolism of methionine. Increasing evidence suggests that elevated blood levels of homocysteine may act as an independent risk factor for ischemic heart disease, cerebrovascular disease, and peripheral arterial disease. Homocysteine appears to promote the progression of atherosclerosis by causing endothelial damage, promoting low-density lipoprotein (LDL) deposition, and promoting vascular smooth muscle growth. Screening for

Blood Studies

2

hyperhomocysteinemia (levels >15 μmol/L) should be considered in individuals with progressive and unexplained atherosclerosis despite normal lipoproteins and in the absence of other risk factors. It is also recommended in patients with an unusual family history of atherosclerosis, especially at a young age. A person with an elevated homocysteine level is also at a five-times increased risk for stroke, dementia, and Alzheimer disease. Elevated levels also appear to be a risk factor for osteoporotic fractures in older men and women.

Dietary deficiency of vitamins B_6, B_{12}, or folate is the most common nongenetic cause of elevated homocysteine. These vitamins are essential cofactors involved in the metabolism of homocysteine to methionine. Because of the relationship of homocysteine to these vitamins, homocysteine blood levels are helpful in the diagnosis of deficiency syndromes associated with these vitamins. In patients with megaloblastic anemia, homocysteine levels may be elevated before results of the more traditional tests become abnormal. Therefore using homocysteine as an indicator may result in earlier treatment and thus improvement of symptoms in patients with these vitamin deficiencies. Some practitioners recommend homocysteine testing in patients with known poor nutritional status (alcoholics, drug abusers) and the elderly. Homocysteine is elevated in children with inborn errors of methionine metabolism.

Some researchers believe that elevated levels of homocysteine can be treated by administration of vitamins B_6 and B_{12}, and folate. Several research reports recommend this vitamin therapy for homocysteine levels greater than 14 μmol/L.

Genetic defects encoding the synthesis of the enzymes responsible for the metabolism of homocysteine to cysteine or the remethylation of homocysteine to methionine are the most common familial cause of hyperhomocysteinemia. Afflicted children suffer from homocystinuria and experience very premature and accelerated atherosclerosis during childhood.

Both fasting and post–methionine loading levels of homocysteine can be measured. In most laboratories, total homocysteine concentrations are measured. A major disadvantage in homocysteine testing is that methods are not standardized. With the more recent development of *enzyme immunoassay (EIA)*, results will be more standardized. However, newer testing kits simplifying high-performance liquid chromatography with fluorescence detection are simple and accurate. In general, homocysteine levels lower than 12 are considered optimal, levels from 12 to 15 are borderline, and levels greater than 15 are associated with high risk for vascular disease. When blood levels are elevated, urine levels of homocysteine are also increased.

CONTRAINDICATIONS

- Patients whose creatinine levels exceed 1.5 mg/dL: Elevated creatinine levels indicate malfunctioning kidneys that cannot effectively filter methionine (a protein).

INTERFERING FACTORS

- Levels may increase with age.
- Patients with renal impairment have elevated levels of homocysteine because of poor excretion of the protein.
- Men usually have higher levels of homocysteine than women do. This is most likely because of higher creatinine values and greater muscle mass.
- Patients with a low intake of B vitamins have higher levels of homocysteine. The B vitamins help to break down and recycle homocysteine.
- Smoking is associated with increased homocysteine levels.

⌶ Drugs that may cause *increased* levels include azaribine, carbamazepine, methotrexate, nitrous oxide, theophylline, and phenytoin.

⌶ Drugs that are associated with *decreased* levels include folic acid, oral contraceptives, and tamoxifen.

PROCEDURE AND PATIENT CARE

Before

☒ Explain the procedure to the patient.

☒ Instruct the patient to fast for 10 to 12 hours before the test. Meats contain elevated levels of homocysteine.

During

- Obtain the fasting blood sample in a collection tube that contains EDTA, heparin, or sodium citrate (blue-top or lavender-top tube).
- For *methionine loading,* the patient ingests approximately 100 mg/kg of methionine after fasting for 10 to 12 hours. A blood sample is obtained. Repeat blood samples are collected at 2, 4, 8, 12, and 24 hours to compare levels of B vitamins and amino acids in the plasma.

After

- In the laboratory, the blood should be spun down within 30 minutes to avoid false elevation caused by release of homocysteine from red blood cells (RBCs).
- Apply pressure or a pressure dressing to the venipuncture site.
- Assess the venipuncture site for bleeding.

TEST RESULTS AND CLINICAL SIGNIFICANCE

▲ Increased Levels

Cardiovascular disease,

Cerebrovascular disease,

Peripheral vascular disease:

> As a direct effect of homocysteine on the vascular wall, intimal injury and plaque formation occurs. Accentuated smooth muscle vascular constriction serves to further diminish the vessel lumen, thereby compounding the vascular occlusive results. Ischemic events in the cerebral, coronary, and peripheral tissues occur earlier, more severely, and more frequently.

Cystinuria,

Vitamin B_6 or B_{12} deficiency,

Folate deficiency:

> Deficient quantity of metabolic enzymes or metabolic cofactors (vitamin B_{12} or folate) diminishes metabolism of homocysteine. Blood levels and subsequently urine levels increase.

Malnutrition: *Malnourished patients have low vitamin B_{12} and folate intake. Because these vitamins are essential to the metabolism of homocysteine, blood levels increase.*

RELATED TESTS

Vitamin B_{12} (p. 518) and Folate (p. 242). Blood levels of these substances are easily determined. The results have an impact on levels of homocysteine.

Lipoproteins (p. 342). Lipoproteins are also important predictors of cardiac atherosclerotic risks.

Cholesterol (p. 154) and Triglycerides (p. 504). These, too, are important predictors of cardiac atherosclerotic risks.

Apolipoproteins (p. 106). This test is used to measure apolipoprotein levels. This may be a better indicator of atherogenic risks than total high-density lipoprotein (HDL) or total LDL.

Human Chorionic Gonadotropin (hCG, Pregnancy Tests, hCG Beta Subunit)

NORMAL FINDINGS

Negative: <5 IU/L
Indeterminate: 5-25 IU/L
Positive: >25 IU/L

INDICATIONS

That test is used to diagnose pregnancy. It is also helpful in monitoring high-risk pregnancies. It can be used as a tumor marker for hCG-producing cancers.

TEST EXPLANATION

All pregnancy tests are based on the detection of human chorionic gonadotropin (hCG), which is secreted by the placental trophoblast after the ovum is fertilized. hCG appears in the blood and urine of pregnant women as early as 10 days after conception. In the first few weeks of pregnancy, hCG rises markedly, and serum levels are higher than urine levels. After about 1 month, hCG is about the same in either specimen.

hCG is made up of alpha and beta subunits. The alpha subunit is the same for many other glycoprotein hormones, including TSH, FSH, and LH. The beta subunit is specific for hCG. Immunologic tests are performed by using commercially prepared antibodies against the hCG and its subunits (particularly the beta subunit). Most of these laboratory methods use sandwich type immunoassay. In this technique, a monoclonal antibody directed to the alpha and beta subunit of hCG is applied to a bound solid phase substrate. The specimen (urine or serum) is applied to the bound solid phase substrate. Simultaneously or sequentially, a labeled monoclonal antibody directed to the beta subunit is bound to that same surface. The free antibody is washed away and the residual bound beta subunit identified by its particular label represents the quantity of the beta subunit of hCG that exists within the patient's specimen.

With the development of hCG sandwich-type immunoassay, very small levels of hCG can be detected, and pregnancy can be determined 3 to 7 days after conception. Furthermore, this method of EIA eliminates any crossover reactivity with other non-hCG glycoprotein hormones and thereby increases accuracy and specificity. The diagnostic cutoff for pregnancy is >25 IU/L. Values between 5 and 25 IU/L are indeterminate for pregnancy. Results can be confirmed with a repeat test in 72 hours. Values in pregnancy should double every 3 days for the first 6 weeks. When an embryo is first large enough to be visible on transvaginal ultrasound (p. 887), the patient generally will have hCG concentrations between 1000 and 2000 IU/L. If the hCG value is high and gestational contents are not visible in the uterus, ectopic pregnancy is suggested.

There are qualitative serum and urine hCG assays and quantitative serum hCG assays (Table 2-32). All assays use the same sandwich immunoassays. There are different point-of-care testing devices for hospital/laboratory use and for use by the general public. In the tests for the public, the patient's urine is tested. The urine is applied to a testing apparatus and the color change is compared to a standard. If the color matches that standard, pregnancy is present. Other tests kits use the development of a line or plus symbol that may appear indicating pregnancy. These tests take only a few minutes to perform and

TABLE 2-32   Recommended Uses for hCG Testing

Test Name	Recommended Use
Qualitative beta hCG	Rapid pregnancy test
Quantitative hCG	More accurate pregnancy test
	Used to monitor high-risk pregnancy
Quantitative hCG (tumor marker)	Monitor patients with hCG secreting tumors

obtain results. They are best if performed a few days after all missed menses. However, they can be positive on the day of an expected menses.

hCG is synthesized in the placenta and maintains the corpus luteum, and, hence, progesterone production, during the first trimester. Thereafter the placenta produces steroid hormones, diminishing the role of hCG. Concentrations of hCG fall, leveling off around week 20, significantly above prepregnancy levels. After delivery, miscarriage, or pregnancy termination, hCG falls until prepregnancy levels are reached. Increased total hCG levels in the first and second trimester are associated with Down syndrome, whereas decreased levels may occur in trisomy 18.

Normally hCG is not present in nonpregnant women. In a very small number of women (less than 5%), hCG exists in minute levels. The presence of hCG does not necessarily indicate a normal pregnancy. Ectopic pregnancy, hydatidiform mole of the uterus, recent abortion, and choriocarcinoma of the uterus can all produce hCG. However, hCG levels in ectopic pregnancy fail to double appropriately, and decreased levels eventually result relative to the values expected in normal pregnancies of similar gestational age.

Outside of pregnancy, hCG may be secreted by seminomatous and non-seminomatous testicular tumors, ovarian germ cell tumors, gestational trophoblastic disease (e.g., hydatidiform mole), and benign or malignant nontesticular teratomas. Rarely other tumors including hepatic, neuroendocrine, breast, ovarian, pancreatic, cervical, and gastric cancers may secrete hCG. In tumors, hCG is a valuable marker that can be used to identify and monitor tumor activity. Serial measurement of hCG following treatment is used to monitor therapeutic response in these tumors and will detect persistent or recurrent neoplastic disease.

INTERFERING FACTORS

- Tests performed too early in the pregnancy, before there is a significant hCG level, may give false-negative results.
- Hematuria and proteinuria in the urine may cause false-positive results.
- Hemolysis of blood may interfere with test results.
- Urine pregnancy tests can vary according to the dilution of the urine. hCG levels may be undetectable in a dilute urine specimen but may be detectable in a concentrated urine specimen.
- Drugs that may cause *false-negative* urine results include diuretics (by causing dilute urine) and promethazine.
- Drugs that may cause *false-positive* results include anticonvulsants, antiparkinsonian drugs, hypnotics, and tranquilizers (especially promazine and its derivatives).

PROCEDURE AND PATIENT CARE

Before

- Explain the procedure to the patient.
- If a urine specimen will be collected, give the patient a urine container the evening before so that she can provide a first-voided (most concentrated) morning specimen. This specimen generally contains the greatest concentration of hCG.

During

- Collect the first-voided urine specimen for urine testing.
- Collect a venous blood sample in a red-top tube for serum testing.
- Avoid hemolysis.

After

- Apply pressure or a pressure dressing to the venipuncture site.
- Assess the venipuncture site for bleeding.
- Emphasize to the patient the importance of antepartal health care.

TEST RESULTS AND CLINICAL SIGNIFICANCE

▲ Increased Levels

Pregnancy,
Ectopic pregnancy:

> *Highest beta hCG levels (>30,000 milli-international units/mL) are recorded in pregnancy. Lowest amounts are generally seen in ectopic pregnancy.*

Hydatidiform mole of uterus,
Choriocarcinoma of uterus,
Germ cell (choriocarcinoma, teratomas, embryonal cell) tumors of testes or ovaries,
Other tumors (poorly differentiated tumors, such as hepatoma and lymphoma):

> *hCG is produced in these patients in variable amounts. The extent of tumor burden and ability to secrete hCG affect hCG levels. The serial monitoring of hCG in these tumors is probably more important than the initial test result.*

▼ Decreased Levels

Threatened abortion,
Incomplete abortion,
Dead fetus:

> *These conditions are all associated with diminished viability of the placenta, which produces the hCG associated with pregnancy.*

Human Lymphocyte Antigen (HLA Antigen, HLA-B27 Antigen, Human Leukocyte A Antigen, White Blood Cell Antigens, Histocompatibility Leukocyte A Antigen)

NORMAL FINDINGS

Negative

INDICATIONS

HLA testing is used in histocompatibility testing for organ or other tissue transplantation. These antigens are present with certain diseases, so the test is used to support their diagnosis. These antigens can identify patients who are allergic to certain medications. Finally HLA testing is used in paternity investigations.

TEST EXPLANATION

The HLA antigens exist on the surface of white blood cells (WBCs) and on the surface of all nucleated cells in other tissues. These antigens can be detected most easily on the cell surface of lymphocytes. The presence or absence of these antigens is determined by the genes on chromosome 6. There are four genes at this locus. Each gene controls the presence or absence of HLA A, B, C, and D. There is probably a fifth genetic locus that is closely related to D and is called DR.

The HLA system of antigens (particularly D) has been used to indicate tissue compatibility with tissue transplantation. If the HLA antigens of the donor are not compatible with the recipient, the recipient will make antibodies to those antigens, accelerating rejection. Survival of the transplanted tissue is increased if HLA matching is good. Prior HLA sensitization causes antibodies to form in the blood of a transplant recipient and shortens the survival of red blood cells (RBCs) or platelets when transfused.

The HLA system has also been used to assist in the diagnosis of certain other diseases. For example, HLA B27 is present in 80% of patients with Reiter syndrome. When a patient presents with recurrent and multiple arthritic complaints, the presence of HLA-B27 supports the diagnosis of Reiter syndrome. HLA-B27 is found in 5% to 7% of normal patients. Other HLA-disease associations are listed in Table 2-33.

The HLA-B 1502 allele is associated with hypersensitivity to carbamazepine, phenytoin, and fosphenytoin used to treat epilepsy, manic/bipolar disorders, and neuropathic pain. Hypersensitivity to carbamazepine is a leading cause of Stevens-Johnson syndrome and toxic epidermal necrolysis (SJS/TEN).

Because HLA antigens are genetically determined, they are useful in *paternity investigations*. This is particularly helpful if the reputed father or child has an unusual HLA genotype. A common HLA genotype in either the father or child increases the likelihood that there are many potential fathers of that child.

Although this test has been performed using serologic methods, PCR using other laboratory methods such as Luminexx technology are primarily utilized. It is important when requesting HLA testing, that the order indicates the specific HLA antigen test to be performed.

TABLE 2-33   HLV and Diseases

HLA Antigen	Disease
B27	Reiter syndrome
	Ankylosing spondylitis
	Yersinia enterocolitica arthritis
	Anterior uveitis
	Graves disease
B8	Celiac disease
	Chronic active hepatitis
	Multiple sclerosis
	Myasthenia gravis
	Dermatitis herpetiformis
B17	Psoriasis
Bw15 + B8	Juvenile diabetes
DR3 or DR4	Diabetes associated with beta cell autoantibodies
A3	Hemochromatosis
DR4	Rheumatoid arthritis
DR7, DRw3, B8	Gluten enteropathy

PROCEDURE AND PATIENT CARE

Before

Explain the procedure to the patient.

Tell the patient that no fasting or special preparation is required.

During

- Collect a venous blood sample in a green-top tube.

After

- Apply pressure or a pressure dressing to the venipuncture site.
- Assess the venipuncture site for bleeding.

TEST RESULTS AND CLINICAL SIGNIFICANCE

Positive for HLA Antigens

Ankylosing spondylitis,
Reiter syndrome,
Yersinia enterocolitica arthritis,
Anterior uveitis,
Graves disease,
Celiac disease/gluten enteropathy,
Chronic active hepatitis,
Multiple sclerosis,
Myasthenia gravis,
Dermatitis herpetiformis,
Psoriasis,
Juvenile diabetes/diabetes associated with beta cell autoantibodies,
Hemochromatosis,
Rheumatoid arthritis (RA):

> *Specific HLA antigens are present in these diseases in varying frequencies. The association of these HLA antigens with the pathophysiology of these diseases is not known.*

Human Placental Lactogen ([hPL], Human Chorionic Somatomammotropin [HCS])

NORMAL FINDINGS

Weeks of Pregnancy	hPL Concentration (mg/L = mcg/mL)
Up to 20	0.05-1
Up to 22	1.5-3
Up to 26	2.5-5
Up to 30	4-6.5
Up to 34	5-8
Up to 38	5.5-9.5
Up to 42	5-7

INDICATIONS

This test is used to evaluate the adequacy of the placenta in high-risk pregnancies.

TEST EXPLANATION

The human placenta produces several hormones that are homologous to hormones of the anterior pituitary. Human placental lactogen (hPL), whose task is to maintain the pregnancy, is structurally similar to both human prolactin and growth hormone. Not surprisingly, hPL demonstrates both lactogenic and growth-stimulating activity.

Serum levels of hPL rise very early in normal pregnancy and continue to increase until a plateau is reached at approximately the 35th week postconception. As such, assays for maternal serum levels of hPL are useful in monitoring placental function. Measurements of hPL are also used in pregnancies complicated by hypertension, proteinuria, edema, postmaturity, placental insufficiency, or possible miscarriage.

A decreasing serum concentration of hPL is pathognomonic for a malfunction of the placenta that may cause intrauterine growth restriction, an intrauterine death of the fetus, or an imminent miscarriage. Pregnant women experiencing hypertonia also show low serum concentrations of hPL. Because of the short biologic half-life of hPL in serum, the determination of hPL always gives a very accurate picture of the present situation.

Increased serum concentrations of hPL are found in women suffering from diabetes mellitus (DM) and, because of the higher placental mass, in multiple pregnancies. In contrast to estriol, the hPL concentration only depends on the placental mass and not on the fetal function. The simultaneous determination of hPL and estriol can be helpful in the differential evaluation of the placental function.

No single endocrine test has proved to be effective in all cases. Of the current endocrine factors, serum unconjugated estriol (p. 226) would appear to be the best predictor of fetal distress or well-being. However, estriol interpretation is limited because values experience short-term and daily fluctuations. When following high-risk pregnancies, the delivery decision should not be based on a single factor. Rather, the decision to deliver should be based on the estriol values, hPL, and monitoring of the fetal heart rate in response to contractions or stress (p. 566).

Quantitative (and qualitative) analysis is performed by radial immunodiffusion (RID). ELISA test kits are available and are accurate.

INTERFERING FACTORS

- Prior nuclear medicine scans because a radioimmunoassay may be used for the determination of hPL.

PROCEDURE AND PATIENT CARE

Before

- Explain the procedure to the patient.
- Tell the patient that no fasting is required.

During

- Collect a venous blood sample in a red-top tube.
- Indicate the date of the last menstrual period on the laboratory slip.

After

- Apply pressure to the venipuncture site.
- Explain the possibility that serial testing is often required.

TEST RESULTS AND CLINICAL SIGNIFICANCE

▲   Increased Levels

Multiple pregnancies,
Placental site trophoblastic tumor,
Intact molar pregnancy,
Diabetes:
   These diseases are commonly associated with increased placental mass and hPL as a result.
Rh incompatibility

▼   Decreased Levels

Placental insufficiency,
Toxemia,
Preeclampsia,
Hydatidiform mole,
Choriocarcinoma:
   All of the above noted diseases are associated with a reduced function of the placenta. As a result hPL is reduced. Pathophysiology of this finding is not clear.

RELATED TESTS

Estrogen Fractions (p. 226). Estrogen fractions are an accurate predictor of the status of the placenta and fetus.
Fetal Contraction Stress Test (p. 566) and Fetal Nonstress Test (p. 569). These are tests of the adequacy of the fetal-placental unit.
Progesterone (p. 416). Progesterone can be used to monitor the status of the placenta.

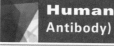

Human T-Cell Lymphotrophic Virus ([HTLV] I/II Antibody)

NORMAL FINDINGS

Negative

INDICATIONS

Testing for this virus is helpful in the diagnosis of certain types of leukemias.

TEST EXPLANATION

Several forms of HTLV, a human retrovirus, affect humans. HTLV-I is associated with adult T-cell leukemia/lymphoma. HTLV-II is associated with adult hairy-cell leukemia and neurologic disorders such as tropical spastic paraparesis. Humans can be infected with these viruses, however, and not develop any malignancy or diseases.

The human immunodeficiency viruses (HIVs), which are known to be the cause of acquired immunodeficiency syndrome (AIDS), are also retroviruses; however, HTLV infection is not associated with AIDS. HTLV transmission is similar, though, to HIV transmission (e.g., body fluid contamination, intravenous drug use, sexual contact, breastfeeding).

Infection by these viruses results in the appearance of specific antibodies against the viruses that can be detected by serologic tests. Blood and organ donors are routinely tested for the presence of anti-HTLV-I/II antibodies by enzyme immunoassays (EIA), which are highly sensitive but lack specificity. For accurate diagnosis of HTLV-I/II infection, all initially EIA-positive results should be verified by a confirmatory test, such as Western blot or line immunoassay. HTLV-I and -II can also be directly detected by real-time amplification of the specific HTLV genomic DNA sequences from the blood of infected patients.

PROCEDURE AND PATIENT CARE

Before

- Explain the procedure to the patient.
- Tell the patient that no fasting is required.

During

- Collect a venous blood sample in a red-top tube.

After

- Apply pressure or a pressure dressing to the venipuncture site.
- Assess the venipuncture site for bleeding.

TEST RESULTS AND CLINICAL SIGNIFICANCE

▲ Increased Levels

Acute HTLV infection,
Adult T-cell leukemia,
Hairy cell leukemia,
Tropical spastic paraparesis:
 The pathophysiology of the association of these illnesses with HTLV infection is not known.

21-Hydroxylase Antibodies

NORMAL FINDINGS

<1 U/mL

INDICATION

This study is used to determine an autoimmune cause of Addison's disease.

TEST EXPLANATION

Chronic primary adrenal insufficiency (Addison's disease) is most commonly caused by the insidious autoimmune destruction of the adrenal cortex and is characterized by the presence of adrenal cortex autoantibodies in the serum. It can occur sporadically or in combination with other autoimmune endocrine diseases. This antibody may precipitate this disease. Measurement of this antibody is used in the investigation of causes of adrenal insufficiency.

PROCEDURE AND PATIENT CARE

Before

Explain the procedure to the patient.
Tell the patient that no fasting is required.

During

- Collect a venous blood sample in a red-top tube.

After

- Apply pressure or a pressure dressing to the venipuncture site.

TEST RESULTS AND CLINICAL SIGNIFICANCE

Autoimmune adrenal insufficiency,
Autoimmune polyglandular syndrome:
  These diseases are commonly associated with autoimmune-instigated antibodies.

RELATED TESTS

Cortisol (p. 179). This blood test indicates the function of the adrenal gland. In Addison disease this will be diminished.
Adrenocorticotropic Hormone (ACTH) (p. 31). This blood test helps in the diagnosis of Addison disease and Cushing syndrome.

Immunoglobulin Quantification

NORMAL FINDINGS

Results vary by age and methods.
IgG (mg/dL)
  Adults: 565-1765
  Children: 250-1600
IgA (mg/dL)
  Adults: 85-385
  Children: 1-350
IgM (mg/dL)
  Adult: 55-375
  Children: 20-200
IgD and IgE: minimal

INDICATIONS

Serum protein quantification is used to detect and monitor the course of hypersensitivity diseases, immune deficiencies, autoimmune diseases, chronic infections, malignancies, and intrauterine fetal infections.

TEST EXPLANATION

Proteins within the blood are made up of albumin and globulin. Several types of globulin exist, one of which is gamma globulin. Antibodies are made up of gamma globulin protein and are called *immuno-globulins*. There are many classes of immunoglobulins (antibodies). *Immunoglobulin G (IgG)* constitutes approximately 75% of the serum immunoglobulins; therefore it constitutes the majority of circulating blood antibodies. *IgA* constitutes approximately 15% of the immunoglobulins within the body and is present primarily in secretions of the respiratory and gastrointestinal tracts, saliva, colostrum, and tears. IgA is also present to a smaller degree in the blood. *IgM* is an immunoglobulin primarily responsible for ABO blood grouping and rheumatoid factor; it is also involved in the immunologic reaction to many infections. IgM does not cross the placenta, therefore an elevation of IgM in a newborn indicates in utero infection such as rubella, cytomegalovirus (CMV), or sexually transmitted disease (STD). *IgE* often mediates an allergic response and is measured to detect allergic diseases. *IgD*, which constitutes the smallest part of the immunoglobulins, is rarely evaluated or detected.

Laboratory methods to identify specific light chain monoclonal proteins associated with specific neoplastic and non-neoplastic diseases are increasingly becoming available. Although *electrophoresis* is usually required to interpret an elevated immunoglobulin class as polyclonal versus monoclonal, *immunofixation* is usually required to characterize a monoclonal protein. If there is a discrete M-peak, the monoclonal protein can be monitored with quantitative immunoglobulins (in the blood or urine with immunonephelometry).

Increased serum immunoglobulin concentrations occur because of polyclonal or oligoclonal immunoglobulin proliferation in hepatic disease (hepatitis, liver cirrhosis), connective tissue diseases, and both acute and chronic infections. Elevation of immunoglobulins may occur in monoclonal gammopathies such as multiple myeloma, primary systemic amyloidosis, monoclonal gammopathies of undetermined significance, and related disorders. Decreased immunoglobulin levels are found in patients with acquired or congenital immune deficiencies. Specific immunologic testing can indicate the etiologic agents of infection or allergy. It can be used to monitor therapy and recurrence. Testing can determine the type of connective tissue disease, its severity, clinical course, and response to therapy.

INTERFERING FACTORS

- Drugs that may cause *increased* immunoglobulin levels are many. A few of the commonly used ones include therapeutic gamma globulin, hydralazine, isoniazid (INH), phenytoin (Dilantin), procainamide, and tetanus toxoid and antitoxin.

PROCEDURE AND PATIENT CARE

Before

- Explain the procedure to the patient.
- Tell the patient that no fasting or special preparation is required.

During

- Collect a venous blood sample in a red-top tube.
- Indicate on the laboratory slip if the patient has received any vaccinations or immunizations within the past 6 months.

After

- Apply pressure or a pressure dressing to the venipuncture site.
- Observe the venipuncture site for bleeding.

TEST RESULTS AND CLINICAL SIGNIFICANCE

▲ Increased IgA Levels

Chronic liver diseases (e.g., primary biliary cirrhosis),
Chronic infections,
Inflammatory bowel disease:
> *The pathophysiology of these observations is not well known.*

▼ Decreased IgA Levels

Ataxia,
Telangiectasia,
Congenital isolated deficiency:
> *These illnesses are caused by isolated IgA or combined immunoglobulin deficiencies.*

Hypoproteinemia (e.g., nephrotic syndrome, protein-losing enteropathies): *The hypoproteinemia that results from these diseases causes the IgA deficiency.*
Drug immunosuppression (steroids, dextran): *The production of IgA is diminished.*

▲ Increased IgG Levels

Chronic granulomatous infections (e.g., tuberculosis, Wegener granulomatosis, sarcoidosis),
Hyperimmunization reactions,
Chronic liver disease,
Multiple myeloma (monoclonal IgG type),
Autoimmune diseases (e.g., rheumatoid arthritis, Sjögren disease, systemic lupus erythematosus [SLE]):
> *All the above conditions stimulate IgG synthesis. The pathophysiology of this observation is not known.*

Intrauterine devices: *These devices work by creating a subclinical localized inflammatory reaction that is harmful to the sperm. Part of that reaction is the synthesis of IgG.*

▼ Decreased IgG Levels

Wiskott-Aldrich syndrome,
Agammaglobulinemia:
> *These diseases are a result of a genetic deficiency that results in inadequate synthesis of IgG and other immunoglobulins.*

Acquired immunodeficiency syndrome (AIDS): *This creates a deficiency throughout the entire immune system. IgG and other immunoglobulins are diminished.*
Hypoproteinemia (e.g., nephrotic syndrome, protein-losing enteropathies): *The hypoproteinemia that results from these diseases causes the IgG deficiency.*
Drug immunosuppression (steroids, dextran): *The production of IgG is diminished.*
Non-IgG multiple myeloma,
Leukemia:
> *IgG production is diminished because the marrow is taken over by tumor cells.*

▲ Increased IgM Levels

Waldenström macroglobulinemia: *This is a malignancy similar to myeloma in which IgM is secreted at high levels by the malignant lymphoplasma cells. It is very similar diagnostically to IgM myeloma.*
Chronic infections (e.g., hepatitis, mononucleosis, sarcoidosis): *These infections stimulate the humoral response and many of the immunoglobulins, including IgM.*

Blood Studies

2

Autoimmune diseases (e.g., SLE, rheumatoid arthritis): *The pathophysiology is not well known. It is assumed that these antibodies somehow contribute to the disease process.*

Acute infections: *IgM is the first immunoglobulin to respond to an infectious agent (viral, bacterial, parasitic).*

Chronic liver disorders (e.g., biliary cirrhosis): *The pathophysiology is not well defined.*

▼ Decreased IgM Levels

Agammaglobulinemia: *This disease is a result of a genetic deficiency in which the synthesis of IgM and other immunoglobulins is inadequate.*

AIDS: *This creates a deficiency throughout the entire immune system. IgM and other immunoglobulins are diminished.*

Hypoproteinemia (e.g., nephrotic syndrome, protein-losing enteropathies): *The hypoproteinemia that results from these diseases causes the IgM deficiency.*

Drug immunosuppression (steroids, dextran): *The production of IgM is diminished.*

IgG or IgA multiple myeloma,

Leukemia:
IgM production is diminished because the marrow is taken over by tumor cells.

▲ Increased IgE Levels

Allergy reactions (e.g., hayfever, asthma, eczema, anaphylaxis): *Allergic reactions stimulate the production of IgE antibodies.*

Allergic infections (e.g., aspergillosis, parasites)

▼ Decreased IgE Levels

Agammaglobulinemia: *This can be specific for IgE or may include the deficient production of all the immunoglobulins.*

RELATED TESTS

Protein (p. 424). This is a quantification of all the components that make up the serum proteins, including albumin, alpha 1 and 2, beta 1 and 2, and gamma globulins. This test can also detect abnormal proteins created by neoplasms and infections.

Prealbumin (p. 412). This is a quantification of prealbumin, which is a component of proteins. This test is used to assess a person's nutritional status. It is also used to indicate the status of liver function.

Insulin Assay

NORMAL FINDINGS

Adult: 6-26 µU/mL or 43-186 pmol/L (SI units)
Newborn: 3-20 µU/mL

 Critical Values

>30 µU/mL

INDICATIONS

This test is used to diagnose insulinoma (tumor of the islets of Langerhans) and to evaluate abnormal lipid and carbohydrate metabolism. It is used in the evaluation of patients with fasting hypoglycemia.

TEST EXPLANATION

Insulin regulates blood glucose levels by facilitating the movement of glucose out of the bloodstream and into the cells. Insulin secretion is primarily reactive to the blood glucose level. Normally, as the blood glucose level increases, the insulin level also increases; as the glucose level decreases, insulin release stops.

Some investigators believe that measuring the ratio of the blood sugar and insulin on the same specimen obtained during the oral glucose tolerance (GT) test is more reliable than measuring insulin levels alone. Combined with the oral GT test, the insulin assay can show characteristic curves. For example, patients with juvenile diabetes have low fasting insulin levels and display flat GT insulin curves, because there is little or no increase in insulin levels. Patients who are mildly diabetic have normal fasting insulin levels and display GT curves with a delayed rise.

Type 2 diabetes (adult onset) is characterized by an excess of insulin production in response to GT testing. This hyperresponse of insulin may precede hyperglycemia by many years, allowing the patient time and opportunity to take action to reduce the incidence of outright diabetes through diet management and lifestyle changes.

When combined with a fasting blood sugar, insulin assay is very accurate in detecting insulinoma. After the patient fasts for 12 to 14 hours, the insulin/glucose ratio should be less than 0.3. Patients with insulinoma have ratios greater than this. To increase the sensitivity and specificity of these combined tests for insulinoma, Turner and others have proposed the "amended" insulin/glucose ratios using variable mathematic "fudge" factors:

$$\frac{\text{Serum insulin level} \times 100}{\text{Serum glucose} - 30 \text{ mg}/100 \text{ mL}}$$

A Turner amended ratio greater than 50 suggests insulinoma.

Insulin is quantified utilizing immunoassay laboratory methodology such as quantitative electrochemiluminescent immunoassay. Results will vary considerably according to the technique used.

INTERFERING FACTORS

- Most patients treated with insulin for diabetes develop insulin antibodies within a few months. These antibodies can interfere with insulin radioimmune assay (RIA) results by competing with the insulin antibodies used in the insulin assay.
- Food intake and obesity may cause increased insulin levels.
- Recent administration of radioisotopes may affect test results by interfering with the RIA method to detect insulin.
- Drugs that may cause *increased* insulin levels include corticosteroids, levodopa, and oral contraceptives.

PROCEDURE AND PATIENT CARE

Before

- Explain the procedure to the patient.
- Keep the patient on nothing by mouth (NPO) status for 8 hours.

During

- Collect a venous blood sample in a red-top tube and pack it in ice.
- Avoid hemolysis.
- If the serum insulin level will be measured during the GT test, collect the blood sample before oral ingestion of the glucose load and at designated intervals after glucose ingestion (based on the laboratory's protocol).

After

- Apply pressure or a pressure dressing to the venipuncture site.
- Observe the venipuncture site for bleeding.
- Transport the specimen immediately to the laboratory.

TEST RESULTS AND CLINICAL SIGNIFICANCE

▲ Increased Levels

Insulinoma: *This is a tumor of the beta cells in the islets of Langerhans of the pancreas. This is diagnosed in patients who have hyperinsulinemia despite hypoglycemia. These patients have persistently high C-peptide levels despite glucose levels of below 30 mg/dL. The amended Turner insulin/glucose ratio exceeds 50.*

Cushing syndrome: *The elevated glucose caused by the cortisol overproduction in patients with this syndrome acts as a constant stimulant to insulin.*

Acromegaly: *The elevated glucose level caused by growth hormone overproduction in the patient with acromegaly acts as a constant stimulant to insulin.*

Obesity: *These patients have a persistently high insulin level.*

Fructose or galactose intolerance: *These complex sugars cannot be metabolized normally and, like glucose, stimulate insulin production.*

▼ Decreased Levels

Diabetes: *Insulin-dependent diabetes is, in part, caused by lack of endogenous insulin.*

Hypopituitarism: *This disease is associated with reduced thyroid and adrenal function along with reduced growth hormone levels. This leads to reduced glucose levels. Insulin production is diminished.*

RELATED TESTS

Glucose Tolerance (p. 261). This is a test of a patient's capability to handle a glucose load.

Glucose, Postprandial (p. 257). This is a timed glucose measurement after a carbohydrate meal.

C-Peptide (p. 182). This test is used to evaluate diabetic patients. It is also used to identify patients who secretly self-administer insulin.

Insulin Antibody (p. 206). This test is used in the evaluation of insulin resistance. It is also used to identify type 1 diabetes. It is used when allergy to insulin is suspected.

Insulin-like Growth Factor (IGF-1, Somatomedin C, Insulin-like Growth Factor Binding Proteins [IGF BP])

NORMAL FINDINGS

Adult: 42-110 ng/mL

Child

Age (yr)	Girls (ng/mL)	Boys (ng/mL)
0-8	5-128	2-118
9-10	24-158	15-148
11-13	65-226	55-216
14-15	124-242	114-232
16-17	94-231	84-211
18-19	66-186	56-177

INDICATIONS

This is a screening test to identify patients with growth hormone (GH) deficiency, pituitary insufficiency, and acromegaly. These levels depend on the levels of GH.

TEST EXPLANATION

Growth hormone (GH) exerts its effects on many tissues through a group of peptides called *somatomedins*. The most commonly tested somatomedin is insulin-like growth factor (IGF-1).

Great variation in GH secretion occurs during the day. A random GH assay result may significantly overlap between normal and abnormal values. To diminish the common variations in GH secretion, screening for IFG-1 provides a more accurate reflection of the mean plasma concentration of GH. Somatomedins are not affected (as GH is) by the time of day, food intake, or exercise because they circulate bound to proteins that are durable or long-lasting. As a result there is no overlap of results of IGF-1 between normal and abnormal values. Normally there is a large increase during the pubertal growth spurt.

Levels of IGF-1 depend on levels of GH. As a result, IGF-1 levels are low when GH levels are deficient. (See GH [p. 269] for a discussion of causes of and diseases associated with GH deficiency.) Nonpituitary causes of reduced IGF-1 levels include malnutrition, severe chronic illnesses, severe liver disease, hypothyroidism, renal failure, inflammatory bowel disease, and Laron dwarfism. Abnormally low test results require an abnormally reduced or absent GH during a GH-stimulation test (p. 272) to make the diagnosis of GH deficiency.

Pediatricians commonly use *insulin-like growth factor binding proteins* (IGF BPs) to even further diminish the impact of the variables affecting GH and somatomedin levels. Specifically IGF BP 2 and IGF BP 3 are the most commonly measured. However, if GH deficiency is strongly suspected yet documentation using GH or somatomedins is questionable, IGF BP determinations are helpful. IGF BP 3 is less age dependent and is the most accurate (97% sensitivity and specificity). These proteins help to evaluate GH deficiencies and GH-resistant syndromes (e.g., Laron dwarfism). Finally these binding proteins are very useful in predicting responses to therapeutic exogenous GH administration.

The causes of short stature and the initial tests for patients with short stature are listed in Box 2-13 and Table 2-34, respectively.

INTERFERING FACTORS

- A radioactive scan performed a week before the test may affect test results, because somatomedin C is often measured by radioimmunoassay (RIA). Results may be confounded by the prior administration of radioisotopes.
- Estrogens may cause *decreased* levels.

BOX 2-13	Causes of Short Stature

- GH deficiency
- Gonadal dysgenesis
- Russell-Silver dwarfism
- Hypothyroidism
- Pseudohypoparathyroidism
- Laron-type dwarfism
- Cushing syndrome
- Bone/cartilage dysplasia
- Idiopathic

TABLE 2-34	Initial Tests for Patients With Short Stature

Test	Reason for Test
Thyroxine	Rule out hypothyroidism
Somatomedin C	Rule out GH deficiency
GH	Rule out GH deficiency
GH stimulation	Rule out GH deficiency
X-ray films of wrists	Document growth retardation
Calcium (serum levels)	Rule out pseudohypoparathyroidism
Phosphate (serum levels)	Rule out rickets
Bicarbonate (serum levels)	Rule out renal tubular acidosis
Blood urea nitrogen (BUN)	Rule out renal failure
Complete blood cell count	Rule out anemia or nutritional or chronic disorders
Sedimentation rate	Rule out inflammatory bowel diseases
Chromosomal karyotype	Rule out chromosomal abnormalities (gonadal dysgenesis)

PROCEDURE AND PATIENT CARE

Before

- Explain the procedure to the patient.
- Tell the patient that an overnight fast before the test is preferred.

During

- Collect a venous blood sample red-top tube.

After

- Apply pressure or a pressure dressing to the venipuncture site.
- Assess the venipuncture site for bleeding.

TEST RESULTS AND CLINICAL SIGNIFICANCE

▲ Increased Levels

Gigantism,

Acromegaly:
These two syndromes are caused by excess GH levels, which increase somatomedin C.
Stress,
Major surgery,
Hypoglycemia,
Starvation,
Deep-sleep state,
Exercise:
The above conditions stimulate GH secretion, which increases somatomedin C.
Hypoglycemia: *Hypoglycemia stimulates GH, which stimulates somatomedin C.*

▼ Decreased Levels

GH deficiency: *Somatomedin C is dependent on GH levels.*
Pituitary insufficiency: *GH is produced in the pituitary. Diseases, tumors, ischemia, or trauma to the pituitary or hypothalamus causes GH deficiency. Somatomedin C is dependent on GH levels.*
Dwarfism: *This is a result of GH and somatomedin C deficiency in children.*
Laron type dwarfism: *This syndrome is associated with GH receptor resistance. Somatomedin C secretion does not occur.*
Hyperglycemia: *Elevated glucose levels inhibit GH and somatomedin C secretion.*
Failure to thrive: *This is a result of GH and somatomedin C deficiency in infants.*
Delayed sexual maturity: *This is a result of GH and somatomedin C deficiency in adolescents.*
Malnutrition,
Malabsorption,
Anorexia nervosa:
These diseases lead to hypoproteinemia. Because somatomedin C is a protein, levels will be reduced with hypoproteinemia.
Severe liver disease: *Somatomedin C is made in the liver. With severe liver disease, somatomedin levels fall.*
Hypothyroidism: *Somatomedin C levels fall in hypothyroid patients.*

RELATED TESTS

Growth Hormone Stimulation (p. 272). This is a test designed to stimulate the secretion of GH. It is required to accurately make the diagnosis of GH deficiency.
Growth Hormone (p. 269). This is a direct quantitative assay for GH.

Intrinsic Factor Antibody (IF ab)

NORMAL FINDINGS

Negative

INDICATIONS

The intrinsic factor antibody is used to diagnose pernicious anemia (PA). It is particularly helpful when the hematologic picture is not fully developed.

TEST EXPLANATION

Pernicious anemia is one of the major causes of vitamin B_{12} deficiency and megaloblastic anemia. It is a disease of the stomach in which secretion of intrinsic factor is severely reduced or absent, resulting in malabsorption of B_{12}. In view of its association with a variety of antibodies, including parietal cell antibody (see p. 92) and at least two types of anti–intrinsic factor antibody, pernicious anemia appears to be an autoimmune process. Antibodies to intrinsic factor are found in very high percentage of children with juvenile pernicious anemia (PA).

Approximately 50% to 75% of adult patients have intrinsic factor antibodies. There are two types of this antibody. Type I, blocking antibody, the more common, prevents the binding of vitamin B_{12} and intrinsic factor. Type II antibody, binding antibody, is less specific for PA and affects the binding of intrinsic factor in the ileum. The blocking antibody is extremely specific for PA and is more sensitive than binding antibody. In the context of a low or borderline B_{12} result, where other clinical and hematologic findings are compatible with a diagnosis of B_{12} deficiency, the presence of intrinsic factor blocking antibody can be taken as confirmation of this diagnosis and, at the same time, as an indication of its cause. A negative result, on the other hand, cannot rule out the possibility of pernicious anemia because blocking antibody is not demonstrable in nearly 50% of all patients with this disorder.

The diagnosis of PA rarely requires vitamin B_{12} absorption testing (Schilling Test). Testing for antiparietal cell antibodies and intrinsic factor antibodies is easier, quicker, and in most cases more accurate. Rapid testing can be performed easily with radioimmunoassay methods.

INTERFERING FACTORS

- IF antibody levels are decreased if an injection of vitamin B_{12} is administered within 48 hours of testing. This is because the administration of vitamin B_{12} is also associated with other binding sites in addition to IF, thus binding IF ab and lowering levels.

PROCEDURE AND PATIENT CARE

Before

- Explain the procedure to the patient.
- Tell the patient that no fasting or special preparation is necessary.
- Ensure that no parenteral B_{12} has been administered in the last 48 hours.

During

- Collect a venous blood sample in a red-top tube.

After

- Apply pressure or a pressure dressing to the venipuncture site.
- Check the venipuncture site for bleeding.

TEST RESULTS AND CLINICAL SIGNIFICANCE

▲ Increased Levels

Pernicious anemia: *Anti–intrinsic factor antibodies may destroy the parietal cell in the gastric antrum through complement fixing antibodies against the parietal cell surface.*

RELATED TESTS

Schilling Test. With the use of this test, the ability to absorb vitamin B_{12} is evaluated. This test is also used in the evaluation of patients with pernicious anemia. This test is no longer a major part of the diagnosis of PA.

Anti–Parietal Cell Antibody (p. 92). This test is used to diagnose PA serologically.

Vitamin B_{12} (p. 518). This test is a direct measurement of B_{12} serum levels, known to be reduced in PA.

Iron Level (Fe), Total Iron-Binding Capacity (TIBC), Transferrin, Transferrin Saturation

NORMAL FINDINGS

Iron

Male: 80-180 mcg/dL or 14-32 µmol/L (SI units)
Female: 60-160 mcg/dL or 11-29 µmol/L (SI units)
Newborn: 100-250 mcg/dL
Child: 50-120 mcg/dL

TIBC

250-460 mcg/dL or 45-82 µmol/L (SI units)

Transferrin

Adult male: 215-365 mg/dL or 2.15-3.65 g/L (SI units)
Adult female: 250-380 mg/dL or 2.50-3.80 g/L (SI units)
Newborn: 130-275 mg/dL
Child: 203-360 mg/dL

Transferrin Saturation

Males: 20% to 50%
Females: 15% to 50%

INDICATIONS

These tests are used to evaluate iron metabolism in patients when iron deficiency, overload, or poisoning is suspected.

TEST EXPLANATION

Serum Iron

Abnormal levels of iron are characteristic of many diseases, including iron-deficiency anemia and hemochromatosis. As much as 70% of the iron in the body is found in the hemoglobin of the red blood cells (RBCs). The other 30% is stored in the form of ferritin (see p. 234) and hemosiderin. Iron is supplied by the diet. About 10% of the ingested iron is absorbed in the small intestine and transported to the plasma. There the iron is bound to a globulin protein called *transferrin* and carried to the bone marrow for incorporation into hemoglobin. Transferrin exists in relationship to the need for iron. When iron stores are low, transferrin levels increase, whereas transferrin is low when there is too much iron.

Usually about one third of the transferrin is being used to transport iron. Because of this, the blood serum has considerable extra iron-binding capacity, which is the *Unsaturated Iron Binding Capacity (UIBC)*. The TIBC equals UIBC plus the serum iron measurement. Some laboratories measure UIBC, some measure TIBC, and some measure transferrin. The serum iron determination is a measurement of the quantity of iron bound to transferrin.

Iron-deficiency anemia is a result of reduced stored iron. It has many causes, including (1) insufficient iron intake, (2) inadequate gut absorption, (3) increased requirements (as in growing children and late pregnancy), and (4) loss of blood (as in menstruation, bleeding peptic ulcer, colon neoplasm). Iron deficiency results in a decreased production of hemoglobin, which in turn results in a small, pale (microcytic, hypochromic) RBC. A decrease in the mean corpuscular volume and mean corpuscular hemoglobin concentration (see p. 442) is also seen. A decreased serum iron level, elevated total iron-binding capacity (TIBC), and low transferrin saturation value are characteristic of iron-deficiency anemia.

Acute iron poisoning due to accidental or intentional overdose is characterized by a serum iron level that exceeds the total iron binding capacity (TIBC). Chronic iron overload or poisoning is called hemochromatosis or hemosiderosis. Excess iron is usually deposited in the brain, liver, and heart and causes severe dysfunction of these organs. Massive blood transfusions also may cause elevated serum iron levels, although only transiently. Transfusions should be avoided before serum iron level determinations.

Because serum iron levels may vary significantly during the day, the blood specimen should be drawn in the morning, especially when the results are used to monitor iron replacement therapy. The patient should refrain from eating for approximately 12 hours to avoid artificially high iron measurements caused by eating food with a high iron content.

TIBC and Transferrin

TIBC is a measurement of all proteins available for binding mobile iron. Transferrin represents the largest quantity of iron-binding proteins. Therefore TIBC is an indirect yet accurate measurement of transferrin. Ferritin is not included in TIBC, because it binds only stored iron. During iron overload, transferrin levels stay about the same or decrease, whereas the other less common iron-carrying proteins increase in number. In this situation, TIBC is less reflective of true transferrin levels. TIBC is increased in 70% of patients with iron deficiency.

Transferrin is a negative acute-phase reactant protein. That is, in various acute inflammatory reactions, transferrin levels diminish. Transferrin also is diminished in patients with chronic illnesses such as malignancy, collagen-vascular diseases, or liver diseases. Hypoproteinemia is also associated with reduced transferrin levels. Pregnancy and estrogen therapy are associated with increased transferrin levels.

TIBC is usually measured by adding excess iron to the patient's serum. This saturates all the transferrin. Excess iron is removed. The iron that is left is a direct measurement of TIBC and an indirect measurement of transferrin. Many laboratories do not perform TIBC measurements; in this case, transferrin is measured directly.

TIBC varies minimally with iron intake. TIBC is more a reflection of liver function (transferrin is produced by the liver) and nutrition than of iron metabolism. TIBC values often are used to monitor the course of patients receiving hyperalimentation.

TIBC and Transferrin Saturation

The percentage of transferrin and other mobile iron-binding proteins saturated with iron is calculated by dividing the serum iron level by the TIBC.

$$\text{Transferrin saturation (\%)} = \frac{\text{Serum iron level} \times 100\%}{\text{TIBC}}$$

The normal value for transferrin saturation is 20% to 50%. Calculation of transferrin saturation is helpful in determining the cause of abnormal iron and TIBC levels. Transferrin saturation is decreased to below 15% in patients with iron deficiency anemia. It is increased in patients with hemolytic, sideroblastic, or megaloblastic anemias and also in patients with iron overload or iron poisoning. Increased intake or absorption of iron (as in hemochromatosis) leads to elevated iron levels. In such cases the TIBC is unchanged; as a result, the percentage of transferrin saturation is very high. Unsaturated iron binding capacity (UIBC) has been proposed as an inexpensive alternative to transferrin saturation.

Chronic illness (e.g., infections, neoplasia, cirrhosis) is characterized by a low serum iron level, decreased TIBC, and normal transferrin saturation. Pregnancy is marked by high levels of protein, including transferrin. Because iron requirements are high, it is not unusual to find low serum iron levels, high TIBC, and a low percentage of transferrin saturation in late pregnancy.

CONTRAINDICATIONS

- Patients with hemolytic diseases, because they may have an artificially high iron content. The iron in the hemolyzed RBCs leaks out into the bloodstream.

INTERFERING FACTORS

- Recent blood transfusions may increase serum iron.
- Recent ingestion of a meal containing high iron content may increase serum iron.
- Hemolytic diseases may be associated with an artificially high iron content.
- Drugs that may cause *increased* iron levels include chloramphenicol, dextran, estrogens, ethanol, iron preparations, methyldopa, and oral contraceptives.
- Drugs that may cause *decreased* iron levels include adrenocorticotropic hormone (ACTH), cholestyramine, chloramphenicol, colchicine, deferoxamine, methicillin, and testosterone.
- Drugs that may cause *increased* TIBC levels include fluorides and oral contraceptives.
- Drugs that may cause *decreased* TIBC levels include ACTH and chloramphenicol.

PROCEDURE AND PATIENT CARE

Before
- Explain the procedure to the patient.
- Keep the patient fasting for 12 hours before the blood test. Water is permitted.
- Assess the patient for a history of recent blood transfusion and recent meals high in iron content. Both may affect test results.

During
- Collect a venous blood sample in a red-top tube. The specimen should always be obtained using a 20-gauge or larger needle.
- Avoid hemolysis, because the iron contained in the RBC will pour out into the serum and cause artificially high iron levels.

After
- Apply pressure or a pressure dressing to the venipuncture site.
- Assess the venipuncture site for bleeding.

TEST RESULTS AND CLINICAL SIGNIFICANCE

▲ Increased Serum Iron Levels

Hemosiderosis or hemochromatosis: *These two forms of iron deposits are created by serum iron excesses. They can be acquired or result from a genetic defect in iron metabolism.*

Iron poisoning: *Increased iron intake increases serum iron levels.*

Hemolytic anemia: *The iron in the hemoglobin of the hemolyzed RBCs leaks out into the bloodstream.*

Massive blood transfusions: *There is about 1 mg of iron in each milliliter of packed RBCs.*

Hepatitis or hepatic necrosis: *The pathophysiology of this observation is not well established.*

Lead toxicity: *The lead overload may displace the iron stores.*

▼ Decreased Serum Iron Levels

Insufficient dietary iron: *Because all body iron is from dietary intake, a persistently reduced intake will lead to reduced serum levels.*

Chronic blood loss (irregular menses, uterine cancer, GI cancer, inflammatory bowel disease, diverticulosis, urologic tract [hematuria] cancer, hemangioma, arteriovenous malformation): *Chronic blood loss depletes the iron because most of the iron in the body exists in the hemoglobin of the RBCs.*

Inadequate intestinal absorption of iron (e.g., malabsorption, short-bowel syndrome): *Because all body iron is from dietary intake, a persistently reduced intake will lead to reduced serum levels.*

Pregnancy (late): *Fetal requirements deplete the mother's body store of iron.*

Iron-deficiency anemia: *This anemia results when iron and iron stores become depleted.*

Neoplasia: *Iron levels are depleted in these patients for several reasons.*

▲ Increased TIBC or Transferrin Levels

Estrogen therapy,
Pregnancy (late),
Polycythemia vera,
Iron-deficiency anemia:
  The pathophysiology of the observation in the above-listed diseases is not clear.

▼ Decreased TIBC or Transferrin Levels

Malnutrition,
Hypoproteinemia:
  Transferrin is a protein. Its levels can be expected to decrease as protein is depleted from the body.
Inflammatory diseases,
Cirrhosis:
  Transferrin is a negative acute-phase reactant protein. That is, in various acute inflammatory reactions, transferrin levels diminish.
Hemolytic anemia,
Pernicious anemia,
Sickle cell anemia:
  These anemias are associated with elevated iron levels and decreased TIBC. The pathophysiology of the latter is not clear.

▲ Increased Transferrin Saturation or TIBC Saturation

Hemochromatosis or hemosiderosis,
Increased iron intake (oral or parenteral):
  Increased iron levels saturate the transferrin.

Hemolytic anemias: *The iron is increased (see previous discussion). Increased iron levels saturate the transferrin.*

▼ Decreased Transferrin Saturation or TIBC Saturation

Iron-deficiency anemia,

Chronic illnesses (e.g., malignancy, other chronic illnesses): *Iron levels are low, and transferrin levels are increased.*

RELATED TEST

Ferritin (p. 234). This is a measure of iron stores and is the most accurate indicator of iron deficiency.

Ischemia-Modified Albumin (IMA)

NORMAL FINDINGS

<85 international units/mL

INDICATIONS

This test is performed on patients with chest pain to determine if the pain is caused by cardiac ischemia.

TEST EXPLANATION

When albumin is exposed to an ischemic environment its N terminal is altered causing an alteration of the albumin called ischemia-modified albumin (IMA). This has become particularly helpful in identifying cardiac ischemia. When combined with troponins (p. 508), myoglobin (p. 365), and ECG, the diagnosis of an ischemic cardiac event can be corroborated or ruled out. IMA is produced continually during the period of ischemia. Blood levels will rise within 10 minutes of the initiation of the ischemic event and stay elevated for 6 hours after ischemia has resolved.

Normally, the N terminal of albumin can easily bind heavy metals, such as cobalt. In contrast, IMA cannot bind cobalt. This reality forms the basis for IMA testing. In the Cobalt Binding Test, cobalt is added to the patient's serum. Unbound cobalt levels are measured. Higher levels of unbound cobalt indicate greater concentrations of IMA, which in turn indicates cardiac ischemia.

IMA may also be elevated in patients with pulmonary embolus or acute stroke. False positives can occur in other clinical circumstances such as advance cancers, acute infections, and endstage renal or liver disease.

PROCEDURE AND PATIENT CARE

Before

 Explain the procedure to the patient.

Tell the patient that no food or fluid restrictions are necessary.

During

- Collect a venous blood sample in a yellow-top (serum separator) tube. This is usually done after the initial onset of chest pain, then 12 hours later, and then daily testing for 3 to 5 days.
- Rotate the venipuncture sites.

- Record the exact time and date of venipuncture on each laboratory slip. This aids in the interpretation of the temporal pattern of blood level elevations.

After
- Apply pressure or a pressure dressing to the venipuncture site.
- Observe the venipuncture site for bleeding.

TEST RESULTS AND CLINICAL SIGNIFICANCE
▲ Increased Levels
Myocardial ischemia,
Brain ischemia,
Pulmonary ischemia:
  Myocardial ischemia produces free radicals that alter normal albumin to become IMA.

RELATED TESTS
Creatine Phosphokinase MB (p. 186). Elevation of CPK-MB on this blood test is closely linked to myocardial muscle. It is elevated early in myocardial injury. Its usefulness is limited in patients who have had chest pain for more than 24 hours.

Myoglobin (p. 365). This protein is a nonspecific indicator of cardiac disease. However, it is also elevated with skeletal muscle disease or trauma.

Electrocardiogram (ECG) (p. 544). This is the electrodiagnostic test most commonly used to detect myocardial injury and infarction.

Troponins (p. 508). This test is a specific indicator of cardiac muscle injury. It is also helpful in predicting the possibility of future cardiac events.

 Lactic Acid (Lactate)

NORMAL FINDINGS
Venous blood: 5-20 mg/dL or 0.6-2.2 mmol/L (SI units)
Arterial blood: 3-7 mg/dL or 0.3-0.8 mmol/L (SI units)

 Critical Values

>4 mmol/L (SI units)

INDICATIONS
Measurement of lactic acid is helpful to document and quantify the degree of tissue hypoxemia associated with shock or localized vascular occlusion. It is also a measurement of the degree of success associated with treatment of those conditions.

TEST EXPLANATION
Under conditions of normal oxygen availability to tissues, glucose is metabolized to CO_2 and H_2O for energy. When oxygen to the tissues is diminished, anaerobic metabolism of glucose occurs, and lactate

(lactic acid) is formed instead of CO_2 and H_2O. To compound the problem of lactic acid buildup, when the liver is hypoxic, it fails to clear the lactic acid. Lactic acid accumulates, causing lactic acidosis (LA). Therefore blood lactate is a fairly sensitive and reliable indicator of tissue hypoxia. The hypoxia may be caused by local tissue hypoxia (e.g., mesenteric ischemia, extremity ischemia) or generalized tissue hypoxia such as exists in shock. Lactic acid blood levels are used to document the presence of tissue hypoxia, determine the degree of hypoxia, and monitor the effect of therapy. Type I LA is caused by diseases that increase lactate but are not hypoxia related, such as glycogen storage diseases or liver diseases, or by drugs. LA caused by hypoxia is classified as type II. Shock, convulsions, and extremity ischemia are the most common causes of type II LA. Type III LA is idiopathic and is most commonly seen in nonketotic patients with diabetes. The pathophysiology of lactic acid accumulation in type III LA is not known.

INTERFERING FACTORS

- The prolonged use of a tourniquet or clenching of hands increases lactate levels.
- Vigorous exercise can *increase* levels.
- Drugs that *increase* lactic acid levels include aspirin, cyanide, ethanol, nalidixic acid, and phenformin.

PROCEDURE AND PATIENT CARE

Before
- Explain the procedure to the patient.
- Tell the patient that no fasting is required.

During
- Instruct the patient to avoid making a fist before and while blood is being withdrawn.
- Avoid the use of a tourniquet if possible.
- Collect a venous blood or arterial blood sample in a red-top tube.

After
- Apply pressure or a pressure dressing to the venipuncture site.
- Observe the venipuncture site for bleeding.

TEST RESULTS AND CLINICAL SIGNIFICANCE

▲ Increased Levels

Shock,

Tissue ischemia:
Anaerobic metabolism occurs in hypoxemic organs and tissues. As a result, lactic acid is formed, causing increased blood levels.

Carbon monoxide poisoning: *Carbon monoxide binds hemoglobin more tightly than oxygen. Therefore no oxygen is available to the tissues for normal aerobic metabolism. Anaerobic metabolism occurs and lactic acid is formed, resulting in increased blood levels.*

Severe liver disease,

Genetic errors of metabolism:
Acquired and genetic diseases associated with inefficient aerobic glucose metabolism causes increased amounts of lactic acid to be synthesized. Therefore blood levels rise.

Diabetes mellitus (nonketotic): *Lactic acid levels rise in patients with poorly controlled diabetes most likely because of inefficient aerobic glucose metabolism, causing increased production of this product.*

RELATED TEST

Arterial Blood Gases (p. 109). This is a measure of acid-base balance of the blood. An increased level of lactic acid is associated with metabolic acidosis.

Lactic Dehydrogenase (LDH, Lactate Dehydrogenase)

NORMAL FINDINGS

Total LDH

Newborn: 160-450 units/L
Infant: 100-250 units/L
Child: 60-170 units/L at 30° C
Adult/elderly: 100-190 units/L at 37° C (lactate → pyruvate) or 100-190 units/L (SI units)

Isoenzymes

Adult/elderly:
  LDH-1: 17% to 27%
  LDH-2: 27% to 37%
  LDH-3: 18% to 25%
  LDH-4: 3% to 8%
  LDH-5: 0% to 5%

INDICATIONS

This is an intracellular enzyme used to support the diagnosis of injury or disease involving the heart, liver, red blood cells (RBCs), kidneys, skeletal muscle, brain, and lungs.

TEST EXPLANATION

The enzyme LDH is found in the cells of many body tissues, especially the heart, liver, RBCs, kidneys, skeletal muscle, brain, and lungs. Because LDH is widely distributed through the body, the total LDH level is not a specific indicator of any one disease or indicative of injury to any one organ. When disease or injury affects the cells containing LDH, the cells lyse and LDH is spilled into the bloodstream where it is identified in higher than normal levels. The LDH is a measure of total LDH. Actually five separate fractions (isoenzymes) make up the total LDH. Each tissue contains a predominance of one or more LDH enzymes (Table 2-35).

In general, isoenzyme LDH-1 comes mainly from the heart; LDH-2 comes primarily from the reticuloendothelial system; LDH-3 comes from the lungs and other tissues; LDH-4 comes from the kidney, placenta, and pancreas; and LDH-5 comes mainly from the liver and striated muscle. In normal persons, LDH-2 makes up the greatest percentage of total LDH.

Specific patterns of LDH isoenzymes are considered classic for certain diseases. For example:
- *Isolated elevation of LDH-1* (above LDH-2) indicates myocardial injury.
- *Isolated elevation of LDH-5* indicates hepatocellular injury or disease.
- *Elevation of LDH-2 and LDH-3* indicates pulmonary injury or disease.

TABLE 2-35	Lactic Dehydrogenase Isoenzymes in Tissue of Origin
Tissue	**Lactic Dehydrogenase Isoenzyme**
Heart	1, 2
Red blood cell	1
Skeletal muscle	5
Lung	3, 2
Reticuloendothelial system	2
Kidney	4
Liver	5
Pancreas, placenta	4

- *Elevation of all LDH isoenzymes* indicates multiorgan injury (e.g., myocardial infarction [MI] with congestive heart failure [CHF] causing pulmonary and hepatic congestion along with decreased renal perfusion). Advanced malignancy and diffuse autoimmune inflammatory diseases such as lupus can also cause this pattern.

With myocardial injury, the serum LDH level rises within 24 to 48 hours after an MI, peaks in 2 to 3 days, and returns to normal in approximately 5 to 10 days. This makes the serum LDH level especially useful for a delayed diagnosis of MI (e.g., when the patient reports having had severe chest pain 4 days earlier). The LDH-1 is generally not as useful as troponin (p. 508) or creatine kinase-MB (p. 186) for the detection of MI, unless the MI occurred 24 hours or more prior to the assay.

It is important to note that two diseases causing elevated LDH may coexist and that one may obscure the other. For example, a patient who has one disease (e.g., pulmonary infarction or congestive heart failure) may also be having an acute MI. The elevation in LDH-1 may be obscured by the elevation of LDH-2 or LDH-3.

LDH is also measured in other body fluids. Elevated urine levels of total LDH indicate neoplasm or injury to the urologic system. When the LDH in an effusion (pleural, cardiac, peritoneal) is greater than 60% of the serum total LDH (i.e., effusion LDH/serum LDH ratio >0.6), the effusion is said to be an *exudate* and not a transudate.

INTERFERING FACTORS

- Hemolysis of blood will cause false-positive LDH levels because LDH exists in the RBCs. Lysis of these cells causes the LDH to pour out into the specimen blood and falsely elevate the LDH level.
- Strenuous exercise may cause elevation of total LDH and specifically LDH-1, LDH-2, and LDH-5.
- Drugs that may cause *increased* LDH levels include alcohol, anesthetics, aspirin, clofibrate, fluorides, mithramycin, narcotics, and procainamide.
- Drugs that may cause *decreased* levels include ascorbic acid.

Clinical Priorities

- Because LDH is widely distributed throughout the body, the total LDH level is not a specific indicator of any disease or organ injury. Isoenzymes are more specific and helpful diagnostically.
- When LDH-1 is greater than LDH-2, myocardial injury is strongly suspected. This may be referred to as a "flipped LDH."
- Isolated elevations of LDH-5 usually indicate hepatocellular injury or disease.
- Values vary markedly across the life span.

PROCEDURE AND PATIENT CARE

Before

☒ Explain the procedure to the patient.
☒ Tell the patient that no fasting is required.
☒ Inform the patient if he or she will be receiving frequent venipuncture for the evaluation of a myocardial infarction.

During

- Collect a venous blood sample in a red-top tube.
- Record the date and time when blood was drawn on the laboratory slip for an accurate evaluation of the temporal pattern of enzyme elevations.

After

- Apply pressure or a pressure dressing to the venipuncture site.
- Assess the venipuncture site for bleeding.

TEST RESULTS AND CLINICAL SIGNIFICANCE

▲ Increased Levels

MI: *These patients classically have significant elevations in LDH-1 and, to a lesser degree, LDH-2.*

Pulmonary disease (e.g., embolism, infarction, pneumonia, CHF): *These patients classically have significant elevations in LDH-2 and LDH-3.*

Hepatic disease (e.g., hepatitis, active cirrhosis, neoplasm): *These patients classically have significant elevations in LDH-5.*

RBC disease (e.g., hemolytic or megaloblastic anemia, RBC destruction from prosthetic heart valves): *These patients classically have significant elevations in LDH-1.*

Skeletal muscle disease and injury (e.g., muscular dystrophy, recent strenuous exercises, muscular trauma): *These patients classically have significant elevations in LDH-5.*

Renal parenchymal disease (e.g., infarction, glomerulonephritis, acute tubular necrosis, kidney transplantation rejection): *These patients classically have significant elevations in LDH-1.*

Intestinal ischemia and infarction: *These patients classically have significant elevations in LDH-5.*

Neoplastic states,

Testicular tumors (seminoma, dysgerminomas): *These patients classically have significant elevations in LDH-1.*

Lymphoma and other reticuloendothelial system (RES) tumors: *These patients classically have significant elevations in LDH-3 and LDH-2.*

Advanced solid tumor malignancies: *These patients classically have significant elevations in all LDH isoenzymes.*

Pancreatitis: *These patients classically have significant elevations in LDH-4.*

Diffuse disease or injury (e.g., heat stroke, collagen disease, shock, hypotension): *These patients classically have significant elevations in all LDH isoenzymes.*

RELATED TESTS

Aspartate Aminotransferase (AST) (p. 119). This is another enzyme existing predominantly in the liver.

Gamma-Glutamyl Transpeptidase (GGTP) (p. 246). This is another enzyme existing predominantly in the liver.

Alkaline Phosphatase (p. 47). This is another enzyme existing predominantly in the liver.

5'-Nucleotidase (p. 376). This is another enzyme existing predominantly in the liver.

Creatine Phosphokinase (CPK) (p. 186). This enzyme is used predominantly to evaluate heart and skeletal muscle.

Alanine Aminotransferase (ALT) (p. 39). This enzyme is used similarly to aspartate aminotransferase and exists predominantly in the liver.

Leucine Aminopeptidase (LAP) (p. 337). This enzyme is specific to the hepatobiliary system. Diseases affecting that system will cause elevation of this enzyme.

 Lactose Tolerance

NORMAL FINDINGS

Blood
Adult/elderly: rise in plasma glucose levels greater than 20 mg/dL; no abdominal cramps or diarrhea

Breath
Greater than 50 ppm hydrogen increase over baseline

INDICATIONS

This test is used to identify patients who have lactose intolerance caused by lactase insufficiency, intestinal malabsorption, maldigestion, or bacterial overgrowth in the small intestine. This test is performed on adults who complain of diarrhea and in infants who have failure to thrive, persistent diarrhea, or vomiting.

TEST EXPLANATION

This test is performed to detect lactose intolerance. Lactose is a disaccharide typically found in dairy products; during digestion, lactose is broken down into glucose and galactose by the intestinal enzyme lactase. Because lactose-intolerant patients have an absence of lactase, lactose digestion will not occur. Likewise, patients with other causes of malabsorption or maldigestion also will not absorb lactose. Glucose plasma will not rise after the ingestion and the small bowel is flooded with a high lactose load. Bacterial catabolism of the lactose occurs within the intestine. This creates excess hydrogen ions and methane (flatus). It also has a strong cathartic effect. Symptoms of lactose intolerance include flatulence, abdominal cramping, abdominal bloating, diarrhea, and failure to thrive in infants. Although all adults have some degree of lactase reduction, severe lactose intolerance can occur in patients with inflammatory bowel disease, short-gut syndrome, and other malabsorption syndromes. Lactase deficiency can be congenital and become apparent in the newborn.

The incidence of primary lactose deficiency is greater than 50% in several ethnic groups, such as Mediterranean, black African, and Asian. Northern European and North American Caucasians are the only population groups able to maintain small-intestinal lactase activity throughout life.

In this test a lactose load is given. If lactase is not present in sufficient quantities, lactose is not metabolized to glucose and galactose. Plasma levels of glucose do not rise as expected. Therefore lower-than-expected serum glucose levels suggest no absorption. Patients who have malabsorption without lactase deficiency will also fail to elevate the blood glucose levels, not because the lactose was not broken down but because the glucose could not be absorbed. These patients can be evaluated by following the lactose tolerance test with a glucose tolerance test. That is, after a positive lactose tolerance test, the patient returns and is given 25 g of a glucose/galactose preparation. A normal increase in glucose indicates that the patient can absorb glucose and that the problem is, indeed, lactase insufficiency.

There is also a breath test portion to this test in which the exhaled air is analyzed for hydrogen content. This is called the *lactose breath test* (or *hydrogen breath test*). The bacteria in the colon produce hydrogen when exposed to unabsorbed food, particularly the lactose load that was not absorbed in the small intestine. Large amounts of hydrogen may also be produced when the colonic bacteria move back into the small intestine, a condition called bacterial overgrowth of the small bowel. In this instance, the bacteria are exposed to the lactose load, which has not had a chance to completely traverse the small intestine to be fully digested and absorbed. Large amounts of the hydrogen produced by the bacteria are absorbed into the blood flowing through the wall of the small intestine and colon. This hydrogen-containing blood travels to the lungs, where the hydrogen is released and exhaled in the breath in measurable quantities.

Prior to lactose hydrogen breath testing, individuals must fast for at least 12 hours. At the start of the test, the individual blows into a hydrogen analyzer. The individual then ingests a small amount of the test sugar (lactose, sucrose, sorbitol, fructose, lactulose, etc., depending on the purpose of the test). Additional samples of breath are collected and analyzed for hydrogen every 15 minutes for 1 to 5 hours. When rapid intestinal transit is present, the test dose of nondigestible lactulose reaches the colon more quickly than normal, and therefore hydrogen is produced by the colonic bacteria soon after the sugar is ingested. When bacterial overgrowth of the small bowel is present, ingestion of lactulose results in two separate periods during the test in which hydrogen is produced, an earlier period caused by the bacteria in the small intestine and a later one caused by the bacteria in the colon.

INTERFERING FACTORS

- Enterogenous steatorrhea (i.e., malabsorption) will diminish absorption of glucose from the gut even if the lactose is broken down by normal levels of lactase.
- Strenuous exercise will reduce the glucose levels and possibly give a false-positive result.
- Diabetics may have a rise in glucose levels that exceed 20 mg/dL despite lactase insufficiency.
- Smoking may increase blood glucose levels and cause false-positive results.
- Ethnicity has a major impact on primary lactose deficiency.
- Antibiotics can decrease the bacteria in the intestine and may cause false-negative breath tests. They should not be taken for 1 month before testing.

Clinical Priorities

- This test can identify patients with lactose intolerance caused by lactase deficiency.
- Lactase deficiency may be the cause of vomiting, diarrhea, malabsorption, and failure to thrive in *infants.*
- Although most *adults* have some degree of lactase reduction, severe lactose intolerance can occur in patients with inflammatory bowel diseases, short-gut syndrome, and other malabsorption syndromes.
- Smoking may increase blood glucose levels and cause false-positive results.
- Ethnicity has a major impact on primary lactose deficiency.

PROCEDURE AND PATIENT CARE

Before

☒ Explain the procedure to the patient. Inform the patient that four blood samples will be needed.
☒ Instruct the patient to fast for 8 hours before testing.
☒ Instruct the patient to avoid strenuous exercise for 8 hours before testing because it may factitiously affect the blood glucose level.
☒ Inform the patient that smoking is prohibited before testing. This may falsely increase the blood glucose level.

During

- Obtain a venous blood sample in a gray-top tube from the fasting patient.
- Provide a specified dose of lactose for the patient. Usually 100 g of lactose is diluted with 200 mL of water for ingestion in adults.
- Note that pediatric doses of lactose are based on weight.
- Collect three more blood samples at 30, 60, and 120 minutes after the ingestion of lactose.
☒ Tell the patient that the only discomfort is the venipuncture; however, patients with lactase deficiency may have symptoms such as cramps and diarrhea.
- If the breath test is being done, the exhaled air is evaluated for hydrogen content before ingestion of lactose and every 15 minutes thereafter. Hydrogen levels are recorded for 2 hours.

After

- Apply pressure or a pressure dressing to the venipuncture site.
- Observe the venipuncture site for bleeding.
- Note that patients with abnormal test results may require a monosaccharide tolerance test (e.g., glucose or galactose tolerance test).

TEST RESULTS AND CLINICAL SIGNIFICANCE

▼ Decreased Levels

Lactase insufficiency: *Lactase quantities are insufficient to break down the lactose load. Glucose is not absorbed, and serum glucose levels do not rise.*
Enterogenous diarrhea: *Despite normal breakdown of lactose, the glucose is not absorbed because of malabsorption disease of the gut. Serum glucose levels do not rise.*

RELATED TEST

Glucose Tolerance (p. 261). This test is used to assist in the diagnosis of diabetes mellitus (DM). It is also used in the evaluation of patients with hypoglycemia. Because it differentiates the lactase-deficient patient from the patient with enterogenous malabsorption diarrhea, this test is helpful in the evaluation of patients suspected of having lactose intolerance.

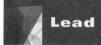

Lead

NORMAL FINDINGS

<10 mcg/dL

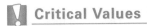 **Critical Values**

Pediatrics (≤15 years): ≥20 mcg/dL
Adults (≥16 years): ≥70 mcg/dL

INDICATIONS

This test is used to identify and monitor lead poisoning.

TEST EXPLANATION

Lead is a heavy metal found in the environment that is a heavy metal toxin. Although lead is now banned from household paints, it is still found in paint used before 1980. Lead is found in dirt from areas adjacent to homes painted with lead-based paints. Water transported through lead or lead-soldered pipe will contain some lead with higher concentrations found in water that is weakly acidic.

Lead inhibits aminolevulinic acid dehydratase and ferrochelatase, both of which catalyze synthesis of heme. The end result is decreased hemoglobin synthesis and anemia. Lead also is an electrophile that avidly forms covalent bonds with the sulfhydryl group of cysteine in proteins. Thus proteins in all tissues exposed to lead will have lead bound to them. The most common sites affected are epithelial cells of the gastrointestinal tract and epithelial cells of the proximal tubule of the kidney. The brain is also a common depository for excess lead.

Signs and symptoms in adults may include a decline in mental status, muscle weakness, headaches, memory loss, mood disorders, and miscarriage or premature birth in pregnant women. Children may demonstrate irritability, anorexia, weight loss, and learning difficulties.

Lead poisoning is a preventable condition that results from environmental exposure to lead. This exposure, indicated by elevated blood lead levels, can result in permanent damage of almost all parts of the body. However, its effects are most pronounced on the central nervous system and kidneys causing symptoms ranging from mild learning disabilities and behavioral problems to encephalopathy. Children less than 6 years of age are the most likely to be exposed and affected by lead. Blood lead levels are the best test for detecting and evaluating recent acute and chronic exposure. Blood lead samples are used to screen for exposure and to monitor the effectiveness of treatment. Lead in the human body can also be measured in blood, urine, bones, teeth, or hair. Blood tests are usually performed. Lead assay is performed on a quantitative inductively coupled plasma-mass spectrometer (hematofluorometry). If one test is elevated, it should be repeated.

At critically high levels, immediate medical evaluation is recommended and chelation therapy is considered when symptoms of lead toxicity are present. Although blood lead has the highest correlation with lead poisoning, lead can be detected in the urine, nails, and hair. These other specimens are used to corroborate blood analysis or document past lead exposure. If the hair is collected and segmented in a time sequence (based on length from root), the approximate time of exposure can be assessed.

PROCEDURE AND PATIENT CARE

Before
✍ Explain the procedure to the patient.
✍ Tell the patient that no fasting is required.

During

- Collect a venous blood in a royal blue-top tube. A tan-top (lead only) Becton-Dickinson tube can be used.
- A fingerstick can be performed to obtain nearly 1 mL of blood.
- In addition to the venous blood sample or the fingerstick, a few mL of EDTA whole blood can be collected.
- Usually the blood sample is sent to a central diagnostic laboratory. The results are available to the local hospital in 7 to 10 days.

After

- Apply pressure to the venipuncture site.

TEST RESULTS AND CLINICAL SIGNIFICANCE

Lead exposure: *This heavy metal still presents a risk of poisoning to intercity children living around aging interior paint and lead water pipes.*

RELATED TESTS

Zinc Protoporphyrin (p. 534). This test is used to screen for lead poisoning.

Legionnaires Disease Antibody

NORMAL FINDINGS

No *Legionella* antibody titer

INDICATIONS

This test is indicated in patients suspected to have Legionnaires disease and who have negative cultures and smears identifying *Legionella*.

TEST EXPLANATION

Legionnaires disease was originally described as a fulminating pneumonia caused by *Legionella pneumophila,* a tiny, gram-negative, rod-shaped bacterium. Nearly half of the clinical cases have been caused by serogroup type 1. This organism can also cause an influenza type of illness called "Pontiac fever."

The diagnosis of Legionnaires disease can be made by culturing this organism from suspected infected fluid, such as blood, sputum, or pleural fluid, or from lung tissue. Sputum for this test is best obtained by transtracheal aspiration or from bronchial washings. However, growing this organism in culture is difficult. A negative culture does not mean that the patient does not have Legionnaires disease. Another method of diagnosis is by directly identifying the organism in a microscopic smear of infected fluid with the use of direct fluorescent antibody methods. If positive, this allows for rapid identification of *Legionella.* However, this is difficult also because the concentration may not be high enough to see the bacterium in the specimen.

The most common and easiest method for diagnosis is detection of the antibody directed against the Legionnaires bacterium in the patient's blood. This is done if the culture or direct fluorescent tests are negative. The indirect fluorescent antibody assay or enzyme-linked immunosorbent assay (ELISA) methods are commonly used. A presumptive diagnosis of Legionnaires disease can be made in a symptomatic person when a single antibody titer is 1:256 or greater. Another way to make the diagnosis is to perform the antibody test 1 and 3 weeks after the onset of symptoms. A fourfold rise in titer to at least 1:128 between the acute (1-week) and the convalescent (3-week) phases is diagnostic. Unfortunately it may take 4 to 6 weeks for serologic tests to be positive. The patient would be seriously ill by then. *Legionella* antigens in the urine may be identified a few days after the onset of the clinical symptoms, but the sensitivity is very low (about 30%).

PROCEDURE AND PATIENT CARE

Before
☒ Explain the procedure to the patient.
☒ Tell the patient that no fasting is required.

During
• Collect a venous blood sample in a red-top tube.

After
• Apply pressure or a pressure dressing to the venipuncture site.
• Observe the venipuncture site for bleeding.

TEST RESULTS AND CLINICAL SIGNIFICANCE

▲ **Increased Levels**

Legionnaires disease

Leucine Aminopeptidase (LAP, Aminopeptidase Cytosol)

NORMAL FINDINGS

Blood
Male: 80-200 units/mL or 19.2-48.0 units/L (SI units)
Female: 75-185 units/mL or 18.0-44.4 units/L (SI units)

Urine
2-18 units/24 hr

INDICATIONS

This test is used for diagnosing liver disorders. It aids in the differential diagnosis of patients with high levels of alkaline phosphatase.

TEST EXPLANATION

LAP is an intracellular enzyme that exists in the hepatobiliary system and, to a much smaller degree, in the pancreas and the small intestine. When disease or injury affects those organs, the cells lyse and LAP is spilled out into the bloodstream. Produced almost exclusively by the liver, LAP is used in diagnosing liver disorders and in the differential diagnosis of increased levels of alkaline phosphatase (ALP). LAP levels tend to parallel ALP levels in hepatic disease. LAP is a sensitive indicator of cholestasis; however, unlike ALP, LAP remains normal in bone disease. LAP can be detected in both the blood and the urine. Patients with elevated serum LAP levels will show elevations in urine levels. When the urine LAP level is elevated, however, the blood level may have already returned to normal.

INTERFERING FACTORS

- Pregnancy may cause increased values if tested by the enzyme method. Although there is not a quantitative increase in this "LAP-like" enzyme, its activity is increased. This causes a false increase in the LAP if tested by the enzyme method.
- Drugs that may cause *increased* LAP levels include estrogens and progesterones.

PROCEDURE AND PATIENT CARE

Before

- Explain the procedure to the patient.
- Tell the patient that no fasting is required.

During

- Collect venous blood in a red-top tube.
- If a urine sample is needed, follow the procedure for a 24-hour urine collection (see Box 11-2, p. 907).

After

- Apply pressure or a pressure dressing to the venipuncture site.
- Assess the venipuncture site for bleeding. Patients with liver dysfunction often have prolonged clotting times.

TEST RESULTS AND CLINICAL SIGNIFICANCE

▲ Increased Levels

Hepatobiliary disease (e.g., hepatitis, cirrhosis, hepatic necrosis, hepatic ischemia, hepatic tumor, hepatotoxic drugs, cholestasis, gallstones): *LAP is an enzyme that exists in the liver and biliary cells. Disease or injury of these tissues will cause the cells to lyse. LAP will spill out into the bloodstream, and levels will rise.*

RELATED TESTS

Creatine Phosphokinase (CPK) (p. 186). This enzyme is used similarly to aspartate aminotransferase (AST) and exists predominantly in heart and skeletal muscle.

Alanine Aminotransferase (ALT) (p. 39). This enzyme is used similarly to AST and exists predominantly in the liver.

Lactic Dehydrogenase (LDH) (p. 329). This is an intracellular enzyme used to support the diagnosis of injury or disease involving the heart, liver, red blood cells (RBCs), kidneys, skeletal muscle, brain, and lungs.

Aspartate Aminotransferase (AST) (p. 119). This is another enzyme existing predominantly in the liver.

Gamma-Glutamyl Transpeptidase (GGTP) (p. 246). This is another enzyme that exists predominantly in the liver.

Alkaline Phosphatase (p. 47). This is another enzyme existing predominantly in the liver.

5'-Nucleotidase (p. 376). This is another enzyme existing predominantly in the liver.

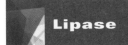

NORMAL FINDINGS

0-160 units/L or 0-160 units/L (SI units) (values are method dependent)

Indications

This test is used in the evaluation of pancreatic disease.

TEST EXPLANATION

The most common cause of an elevated serum lipase level is acute pancreatitis. Lipase is an enzyme secreted by the pancreas into the duodenum to break down triglycerides into fatty acids. As with amylase, lipase appears in the bloodstream following damage to or disease affecting the pancreatic acinar cells.

Because lipase was thought to be produced only in the pancreas, elevated serum levels were considered to be specific to pathologic pancreatic conditions. It is now apparent that other conditions can be associated with elevated lipase levels. Lipase is excreted through the kidneys. Therefore elevated lipase levels are often found in patients with renal failure. Intestinal infarction or obstruction also can be associated with lipase elevation. However, the lipase elevations in nonpancreatic diseases are less than three times the upper limit of normal as compared with pancreatitis, in which they are often 5 to 10 times normal values. Other conditions such as cholangitis, mumps, cholecystitis, or peptic ulcer are more rarely associated with elevated lipase levels.

In acute pancreatitis, elevated lipase levels usually parallel serum amylase levels. The lipase levels usually rise a little later than amylase levels (24 to 48 hours after the onset of pancreatitis) and remain elevated for 5 to 7 days. Because they peak later and remain elevated longer than the serum amylase levels, serum lipase levels are more useful in the late diagnosis of acute pancreatitis. Lipase levels are less useful in more chronic pancreatic diseases (e.g., chronic pancreatitis, pancreatic carcinoma).

INTERFERING FACTORS

- Drugs that may cause *increased* lipase levels include bethanechol, cholinergics, codeine, indomethacin, meperidine, methacholine, and morphine.
- Drugs that may cause *decreased* levels include calcium ions.

Clinical Priorities

- This test is useful in evaluating pancreatitis. Lipase elevations are often 5 to 10 times normal values in pancreatitis.
- In acute pancreatitis, elevated lipase levels usually parallel serum amylase levels. Because lipase levels peak later and remain elevated longer than amylase levels, they are more useful in the late diagnosis of acute pancreatitis.

PROCEDURE AND PATIENT CARE

Before

- Explain the procedure to the patient.
- Instruct the patient to remain on nothing by mouth (NPO) status, except for water, for 8 to 12 hours before the test.

During

- Collect a venous blood sample in a red-top tube.

After

- Apply pressure or a pressure dressing to the venipuncture site.
- Observe the venipuncture site for bleeding.

TEST RESULTS AND CLINICAL SIGNIFICANCE

▲ Increased Levels

Pancreatic diseases (e.g., acute pancreatitis, chronic relapsing pancreatitis, pancreatic cancer, pancreatic pseudocyst): *Lipase exists in the pancreatic cell and is released into the bloodstream when disease or injury affects the pancreas.*

Biliary diseases (e.g., acute cholecystitis, cholangitis, extrahepatic duct obstruction): *Although the pathophysiology of these observations is not well understood, it is suspected that lipase exists inside the cells of the hepatobiliary system. Disease or injury of these tissues would cause the lipase to leak into the bloodstream and cause levels to be elevated.*

Renal failure: *Lipase is excreted by the kidney. If excretion is poor, as in renal failure, lipase levels will rise.*

Intestinal diseases (e.g., bowel obstruction, infarction): *Lipase exists in the mucosal cells lining the bowel (mostly in the duodenum). Injury through obstruction or ischemia will cause the cells to lyse. Lipase will leak into the bloodstream and cause levels to be elevated.*

Salivary gland inflammation or tumor: *Like amylase, salivary glands contain lipase, although to a much lesser degree. Tumors, inflammation, or obstruction of salivary ducts will cause the cells to lyse. Lipase will leak into the bloodstream and cause levels to be elevated.*

Peptic ulcer disease: *The pathophysiology of this observation is not well understood. Certainly, in perforated peptic disease the lipase in the gastrointestinal (GI) contents leaks out into the peritoneum, where it is picked up by the bloodstream. Lipase levels rise.*

RELATED TEST

Amylase (p. 61). Disease affecting the pancreas also will cause elevations of this enzyme.

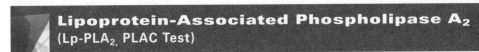

Lipoprotein-Associated Phospholipase A$_2$
(Lp-PLA$_2$, PLAC Test)

NORMAL FINDINGS

Average value for females: 174 ng/mL (range: 120-342)
Average value for males: 251 ng/mL (range: 131-376)

INDICATIONS

This test helps predict the risk of cardiovascular disease.

TEST EXPLANATION

Lipoprotein-associated phospholipase A$_2$ (Lp-PLA$_2$) promotes vascular inflammation through the hydrolysis of oxidized LDL within the intima, contributing directly to the atherogenic process. Lp-PLA$_2$ is an independent predictor of cardiovascular disease. When combined with CRP (p. 184), testing for Lp-PLA$_2$ markedly increases the predictive value in determining risk for a cardiac event, especially in patients whose Adult Treatment Panel III (ATP III) cardiac risks are moderate. Lp-PLA$_2$ levels >200 ng/mL would warrant reclassifying the patient to the next highest ATP risk category, which would require more aggressive use of cholesterol-lowering agents. Lp-PLA$_2$ may play an important role in the progression of atherosclerosis and overall plaque stability. Lp-PLA$_2$ may be an effective target for anti-atheromatous therapies in the future.

Lp-PLA$_2$ is also an accurate aid in assessing the risk for ischemic stroke associated with atherosclerosis at all levels of blood pressure. The PLAC test is an enzyme-linked immunosorbent assay (ELISA) using two highly specific monoclonal antibodies to measure the level of Lp-PLA$_2$ in the blood.

PROCEDURE AND PATIENT CARE

Before
☒ Explain the procedure to the patient.
☒ Tell the patient that fasting usually is not required

During
• Collect one red-top tube of venous blood.

After
• Apply pressure or a pressure dressing to the venipuncture site.

TEST RESULTS AND CLINICAL SIGNIFICANCE

Atherosclerosis: *Not recommended for cardiovascular disease risk assessment in asymptomatic adults. May aid in CVD risk stratification in specific populations.*

RELATED TESTS

C-Reactive Protein (p. 184). This protein also indicates an inflammatory component to vascular disease, thereby increasing the risk of an ischemic event.
Lipoproteins (p. 342). This test is considered to be another predictor of heart/vascular disease.

Lipoproteins (High-Density Lipoproteins [HDL, HDL-C] Low-Density Lipoproteins [LDL, LDL-C], Very Low–Density Lipoproteins [VLDL], Lipoprotein Electrophoresis, Lipoprotein Phenotyping, Lipid Fractionation, Non-HDL Cholesterol, Lipid Profile)

NORMAL FINDINGS

HDL

Male: >45 mg/dL or >0.75 mmol/L (SI units)
Female: >55 mg/dL or >0.91 mmol/L (SI units)

Risk for Heart Disease	HDL mg/dL (SI Units)	
	Male	Female
Low	60 (1.55)	70 (1.81)
Moderate	45 (1.17)	55 (1.42)
High	25 (0.65)	35 (0.90)

LDL

Adult: <130 mg/dL
Children: <110 mg/dL

VLDL

7-32 mg/dL

INDICATIONS

Lipoproteins are considered to be an accurate predictor of heart disease. As part of the lipid profile, these tests are performed to identify persons at risk for developing heart disease and to monitor therapy if abnormalities are found (Box 2-14).

TEST EXPLANATION

Lipoproteins are proteins in the blood whose main purpose is to transport cholesterol, triglycerides, and other insoluble fats. They are used as markers indicating the levels of lipids within the bloodstream. Lipoproteins can be classified by their measured density.

BOX 2-14	Blood Tests Used to Assess Risk for Coronary Vascular Disease

- Total Cholesterol
- High-Density Cholesterol
- Low-Density Cholesterol
- Triglycerides
- Apolipoprotein B
- Lipoprotein (a)

- Apolipoprotein E Genotyping
- Fibrinogen
- C Reactive Protein
- Homocysteine
- Insulin, Fasting

General categories of lipoproteins, listed in order from larger and less dense (more fat than protein) to smaller and denser (more protein, less fat) are as follows:

- Chylomicrons—carry triacylglycerol (fat) from the intestines to the liver, skeletal muscle, and to adipose tissue.
- Very low–density lipoproteins (VLDL)—carry (newly synthesized) triacylglycerol from the liver to adipose tissue.
- Intermediate-density lipoproteins (IDL)—are intermediate between VLDL and LDL. They are not usually detectable in the blood.
- Low-density lipoproteins (LDL)—carry cholesterol from the liver to cells of the body. Sometimes referred to as the "bad cholesterol" lipoprotein.
- High density lipoproteins (HDL)—collects cholesterol from the body's tissues (and vascular endothelium) and brings it back to the liver. Removing lipids from the endothelium (reverse cholesterol transport) provides a protective effect against heart disease. Therefore HDL is referred to as the "good cholesterol" lipoprotein.

The "lipid profile" usually measures total cholesterol (discussed separately on p. 154), triglycerides, HDL, LDL, and VLDL. Through the use of *segmented gradient gel electrophoresis (SGGE)*, lipoproteins could be subclassified to more accurately indicate cardiovascular risks and familial risks of heart disease. Levels of lipoproteins are genetically influenced; however, these levels can be altered by diet, lifestyle, and medications.

Clinical and epidemiologic studies have shown that total HDL cholesterol is an independent, inverse risk factor for coronary artery disease (CAD). Low levels (<35 mg/dL) are believed to increase a person's risk for CAD, while high levels (>60 mg/dL) are considered protective. When HDL and total cholesterol measurements are combined in a ratio fashion (Table 2-36), the accuracy of predicting CAD is increased. The total cholesterol/HDL ratio should be at least 5:1, with 3:1 being ideal.

SGGE identified five subclasses of HDL (2a, 2b, 3a, 3b, and 3c), but only 2b is cardioprotective. HDL 2b is the most efficient form of HDL in reverse cholesterol transport. Patients with low total HDL levels often have low levels of HDL 2b. When levels of total HDL are between 40 and 60, cardioprotective levels of HDL 2b are minimal. However, when levels of total HDL are greater than 60, levels of HDL 2b predominate, and efficient reverse cholesterol transport takes place. This protects the coronary arteries from disease. The other subclasses of HDL are not capable of reverse cholesterol transport and therefore are not cardioprotective. Levels of HDL 2b can be increased by niacin supplements but not by statins (i.e., HMG-CoA reductase inhibitors [simvastatin, lovastatin]).

LDLs ("bad" cholesterol) are also cholesterol rich. However, most cholesterol carried by LDLs can be deposited into the lining of the blood vessels and is associated with an increased risk for arteriosclerotic

TABLE 2-36	**Risk for Coronary Heart Disease Based on Ratio of Cholesterol to High-Density Lipoproteins**	
	TOTAL CHOLESTEROL/ HIGH-DENSITY LIPOPROTEINS	
Risk for Coronary Heart Disease	**Male**	**Female**
One half average	3.4	3.3
Average	5.0	4.4
Two times average (moderate)	10.0	7.0
Three times average (high)	24.0	11.0

heart and peripheral vascular disease. Therefore high levels of LDLs are atherogenic. Target LDL levels vary according to the risk profile of the patient (Table 2-37). For example, the optimal LDL level should be less than 70 mg/dL in patients at high risk for heart disease. The LDL level can be calculated using a modified Friedwald formula:

$$LDL = \text{Total cholesterol} - (HDL + [\text{Triglycerides} \div 5])$$

There are other formulas for deriving LDL, which may account for different sets of normal values. The formula is inaccurate if the triglycerides exceed 400 mg/dL. More recently, laboratory chromogenic methods in which various detergents are used to separate out LDL allow for a more accurate measurement of LDL. This method uses a unique detergent to solubilize only the non-LDL lipoprotein particles and a second detergent solubilizes the remaining LDL particles, which are then measured by a chromogenic coupler that provides color formation.

With the use of SGGE, LDL has been divided into seven classes based on particle size. These subclasses include (from largest to smallest) LDL I, LDL IIa, LDL IIb, LDL IIIa, LDL IIIb, LDL IVa, and LDL IVb. The most commonly elevated forms of LDL (IIIa and IIIb) are small enough to get between the endothelial cells and cause atheromatous disease. The larger LDL particles (LDL I, LDL IIa, and LDL IIb) cannot get into the endothelial layer and therefore are not associated with increased risk for disease. LDL IVa and IVb, however, are very small and are associated with aggressive arterial plaques that are particularly vulnerable to ulceration and vascular occlusion. Nearly all patients with levels of LDL IVa and IVb greater than 10% of total LDL have vascular events within months.

LDL patterns can be identified, and they are associated with variable risks of coronary artery disease (CAD). LDL pattern A is seen in patients with mostly large LDL particles and does not carry increased risks for CAD. LDL pattern B is seen in patients with mostly small LDL particles and is associated with

TABLE 2-37   National Cholesterol Education Program Therapy 2004 Guidelines for Low-Density Lipoproteins

Risk Category	LDL-C Goal	Initiate TLC	Consider Drug Therapy
High risk: CHD (10-year risk: >20%)	<100 mg/dL (Optional: <70 mg/dL)	≥100 mg/dL	≥100 mg/dL (Optional: <100 mg/dL)
Moderately high risk: 2+ risk factors (10-year risk: 10%-20%)	<130 mg/dL	≥130 mg/dL	≥130 mg/dL (Optional: 100-129 mg/dL)
Moderate risk: 2+ risk factors (10-year risk: <10%)	<130 mg/dL	≥130 mg/dL	≥160 mg/dL
Lower risk: 0-1 risk factor	<160 mg/dL	≥160 mg/dL	≥190 mg/dL (Optional: 160-189 mg/dL)

CHD, Coronary heart disease; *LDL-C,* low density lipoprotein cholesterol; *TLC,* therapeutic lifestyle changes (reduced intake of saturated fats and cholesterol, drug therapy, increased fiber, weight reduction, and increased physical activity).
Risk factors: cigarette smoking, hypertension, low HDL cholesterol, family history, and age.
10-year risk: Data from the Framingham Heart Study used to estimate risk of CHD (age, gender, HDL cholesterol, total cholesterol, systolic B/P, use of B/P medications).

an increased risk for CAD. An intermediate pattern is noted in a large number of patients; they have small and large LDL particles and experience an intermediate risk for CAD. LDL levels can be lowered with diet, exercise, and statins.

Because LDL particles vary in size and composition, the amount of cholesterol they carry (LDL-C) is not a reliable measure of the number of LDL particles (LDL-P) and a patient's risk for CHD. Direct measurement of the number of LDL particles (i.e., LDL-P) by Nuclear Magnetic Resonance (NMR) Spectroscopy provides prognostic information that is independent of LDL-C. Direct measurement by LDL-P has proved to be a better predictor of CHD events than LDL-C.

VLDLs, though carrying a small amount of cholesterol, are the predominant carriers of blood triglycerides. To a lesser degree, VLDLs are also associated with an increased risk for CAD because they can be converted to LDL by lipoprotein lipase in skeletal muscle. The VLDL value is sometimes expressed as a percentage of total cholesterol. Levels in excess of 25% to 50% are associated with increased risk for coronary disease.

The Adult Treatment Panel III (ATP III) of the National Cholesterol Education Program issued an evidence-based set of guidelines on cholesterol management. The goal for high-risk patients (those with known coronary artery disease or > 2 risk factors) is an LDL lower than 70 mg/dL. All ATP reports have identified low-density lipoprotein cholesterol (LDL-C) as the primary target of cholesterol lowering therapy. Many prospective studies have shown that high serum concentrations of LDL-C are a major risk factor for coronary heart disease (CHD). Moreover, lowering LDL-C levels will reduce the risk for major coronary events.

The World Health Organization adopted the Fredrickson classification of lipid disorders to identify particular lipoprotein patterns (phenotypes) that are associated with certain inherited or acquired diseases or syndromes. Fredrickson's classification (Table 2-38), through the use of electrophoresis, simply identifies which lipoproteins are raised.

There are a variety of methods used to measure the lipoprotein classes. All require serum separation, usually by ultracentrifugation. In the past, lipoproteins were measured through the use of electrophoresis. Immunologic, catalase reagent, and chemical kits are now available for accurately quantifying lipoproteins.

TABLE 2-38   Primary Hyperlipidemias (WHO/Fredrickson Classification)

Fredrickson Classification	Elevated Lipoprotein	Associated Clinical Disorders
I	Chylomicrons	Lipoprotein lipase deficiency, apolipoprotein CII deficiency, uncontrolled diabetes mellitus (DM)
IIa	LDL	Familial hypercholesterolemia, nephrosis, hypothyroidism, familial combined hyperlipidemia
IIb	LDL, VLDL	Familial combined hyperlipidemia
III	Intermediate-density lipoproteins	Dysbetalipoproteinemia, DM, alcoholism
IV	VLDL	Familial hypertriglyceridemia, familial combined hyperlipidemia, diabetes mellitus
V	Chylomicrons, VLDL	Diabetes, nephrosis, malnutrition

INTERFERING FACTORS

- Smoking and alcohol ingestion decrease HDL levels.
- Binge eating can alter lipoprotein values.
- HDL values are age- and sex-dependent.
- HDL values, like cholesterol, tend to decrease significantly for as long as 3 months following myocardial infarction (MI).
- HDL is elevated in patients with hypothyroid and diminished in those with hyperthyroid.
- High triglyceride levels can make LDL calculations inaccurate.
- Drugs that may cause altered lipoprotein levels include:
  - Beta blockers: increase triglycerides, decrease HDL-C, decrease LDL size, decrease HDL 2b
  - Alpha-blockers: decrease triglycerides, increase HDL-C, increase LDL size, increase HDL 2b
  - Dilantin: increases HDL-C
  - Steroids: in general, increase triglycerides
  - Estrogens: increase triglycerides

✓ Clinical Priorities

- Lipoproteins are considered to be predictors of heart disease. Blood levels should be collected after a 12- to 14-hour fast.
- HDL is often called good cholesterol, because it removes cholesterol from the tissues and transports it to the liver for excretion. High levels are associated with a decreased risk for coronary heart disease.
- LDL is often called bad cholesterol, because it carries cholesterol and deposits it into the peripheral tissues. High levels are associated with an increased risk for CHD.

PROCEDURE AND PATIENT CARE

Before

Instruct the patient to fast for 12 to 14 hours before testing. Only water is permitted.
Inform the patient that dietary indiscretion within the previous few weeks may influence lipoprotein levels.

During

- Collect a venous blood sample in a red-top tube.

After

- Apply pressure or a pressure dressing to the venipuncture site.
- Observe the venipuncture site for bleeding.
Instruct patients with high lipoprotein levels regarding diet, exercise, and appropriate body weight.

TEST RESULTS AND CLINICAL SIGNIFICANCE

▲ Increased HDL

Familial HDL lipoproteinemia: *Genetically, the patient is predetermined to have high HDL levels.*
Excessive exercise: *HDL can rise with chronic exercise for 30 minutes three times a week. When the exercise greatly exceeds that minimum, HDL can become significantly elevated.*

▼ **Decreased HDL**

Metabolic syndrome: *This syndrome is associated with an atherogenic lipid profile (ALP) that includes decreased HDL, increased triglycerides, elevated fasting glucose, high blood pressure, and abdominal obesity measured by waist circumference.*

Familial low HDL: *Genetically, the patient is predetermined to have low HDL levels. As a result, these patients are at high risk for CHD.*

Hepatocellular disease (e.g., hepatitis, cirrhosis): *HDL is made in the liver. Without liver function, HDL is not made and levels fall.*

Hypoproteinemia (e.g., nephrotic syndrome, malnutrition): *With loss of proteins, HDL is not made and levels fall. When the hypoproteinemia is severe, however, and oncotic pressures fall, the production of lipoproteins could be stimulated and actually rise. Elevation of HDL occurs only late in the disease.*

▲ **Increased LDL and VLDL**

Familial LDL lipoproteinemia: *Genetically, the patient is predetermined to have high LDL levels.*

Nephrotic syndrome: *The loss of proteins diminishes the plasma oncotic pressures. This appears to stimulate hepatic lipoprotein synthesis of LDL and possibly to diminish lipoprotein disposal of the same.*

Glycogen storage diseases (e.g., von Gierke disease): *VLDL synthesis is increased and excretion is diminished. VLDL and LDL levels rise.*

Hypothyroidism: *VLDL and LDL catabolism is diminished. VLDL and LDL levels rise. This is a common cause of lipid abnormalities, especially among women.*

Alcohol consumption: *Hyperlipidemias are known to occur in persons who drink excessive quantities of alcohol. However, there also may be a genetic factor associated with this observation.*

Chronic liver disease (e.g., hepatitis, cirrhosis): *The liver catabolizes LDL. Without that catabolism, blood levels increase.*

Hepatoma: *The normal inhibition of LDL synthesis by eating dietary fats does not occur. LDL synthesis continues unabated. LDL levels rise.*

Gammopathies (e.g., multiple myeloma): *High levels of gamma globulins (IgG and IgM) attach to the VLDL and LDL molecule and thereby decrease their catabolism.*

Familial hypercholesterolemia type IIa: *LDL receptors are altered, and LDL is produced at increased rates.*

Cushing syndrome: *VLDL synthesis is increased. VLDL is converted to LDL.*

Apoprotein CII deficiency: *This genetic defect is associated with a deficiency of lipoprotein lipase. As a result, VLDL and other lipoproteins (chylomicrons) accumulate.*

▼ **Decreased LDL and VLDL**

Familial hypolipoproteinemia: *Genetically, the patient is predetermined to have low VLDL or LDL levels.*

Hypoproteinemia (e.g., malabsorption, severe burns, malnutrition): *Early in the course of this process, LDLs are low. However, later the LDL and VLDL levels can actually rise.*

Hyperthyroidism: *Catabolism of LDL and VLDL is increased and levels fall.*

RELATED TESTS

Cholesterol (p. 154). This is a measure of total cholesterol in the blood. It is a part of the lipid profile.

Triglycerides (p. 504). This is a measure of total triglyceride in the blood. It is a part of the lipid profile.

Apolipoproteins (p. 106). This test is used to measure apolipoprotein levels. This may be a better indicator of atherogenic risks than total HDL or total LDL.

Luteinizing Hormone (LH, Lutropin) and Follicle-Stimulating Hormone (FSH) Assay

NORMAL FINDINGS

Values may vary depending on assay method.

	Luteinizing Hormone (international units/L)	Follicle-Stimulating Hormone (international units/L)
ADULT		
Male	1.24-7.8	1.42-15.4
Female		
Follicular phase	1.68-15	1.37-9.9
Ovulatory peak	21.9-56.6	6.17-17.2
Luteal phase	0.61-16.3	1.09-9.2
Postmenopause	14.2-52.3	19.3-100.6
CHILD (AGE 1-10 YEARS)		
Male	0.04-3.6	0.3-4.6
Female	0.03-3.9	0.68-6.7

INDICATIONS

LH/FSH levels are helpful in the determination of menopause. Furthermore, they are integral in the evaluation of suspected gonadal failure. Infertility evaluations also include these tests.

TEST EXPLANATION

LH and FSH are glycoproteins produced in the anterior pituitary gland in response to stimulation by gonadotropin-releasing hormone (GNRH), previously called luteinizing-releasing hormone. GNRH is stimulated when circulating levels of estrogen (in females) or testosterone (in males) are low. Through a feedback mechanism, GNRH is stimulated by the hypothalamus, which in turn stimulates the production and release of LH and FSH. These two hormones then act on the ovary or testes. In the female, FSH stimulates the development of follicles in the ovary. In the male, FSH stimulates Sertoli cell development. In the female, LH stimulates follicular production of estrogen, ovulation, and formation of a corpus luteum. In the male, LH stimulates testosterone production from the Leydig cells. In the end, estrogen or testosterone is produced, which in turn inhibits FSH and LH. FSH is necessary for maturation of the ovaries and testes. FSH and LH are necessary for sperm production. In the female these hormones are secreted differently at different times in the menstrual cycle. The midcycle peak of FSH is necessary for follicle/ovum formation. LH also must peak about that same time to stimulate ovulation or corpus luteal formation that could potentially support an embryo if fertilization were to occur.

Earlier bioassays could not distinguish FSH from LH. Therefore they were often measured together. For that matter, early bioassays often included thyroid-stimulating hormone and human chorionic gonadotropin. Now with the use of better methodology such as quantitative electrochemiluminescent or liquid chromatography–tandem mass spectrometry, these hormones can each be measured separately and accurately.

LH is secreted in a pulsatile manner. One specimen may not accurately indicate total body levels of this hormone. Often several specimens of blood are obtained 20 to 30 minutes apart, and the blood is pooled or results of each are averaged. The variable nature of LH can be diminished by measuring LH in a 24-hour urine sample. The disadvantage is that LH values can be falsely low because of dilution with large urine volumes. Spot urine tests have become very useful in the evaluation and treatment of infertility. Because LH is rapidly excreted into the urine, the plasma LH surge that precedes ovulation by 24 hours can be recognized quickly and easily. This is used to indicate the period when the woman is most fertile. The best time to obtain a urine specimen is between 11 AM and 3 PM. Usually the woman begins to test her urine on the 10th day following the onset of her menses and continues to do so daily. Home kits using a color change as an end point are now marketed to make this process even more convenient.

These hormones are used in the evaluation of infertility. Performing an LH assay is an easy way to determine if ovulation has occurred. An LH surge in blood levels indicates that ovulation has taken place. Under the influence of LH, the corpus luteum develops from the ruptured Graafian follicle. Daily samples of serum LH around the middle of the woman's cycle can detect the LH surge, which is thought to occur on the day of maximal fertility.

These assays (particularly FSH) also determine whether a gonadal insufficiency is primary (problem with the ovary/testicle) or secondary (caused by pituitary insufficiency resulting in reduced levels of FSH and LH). Elevated levels of FSH and LH in patients with gonadal insufficiency indicate primary gonadal failure, as may be seen in women with polycystic ovaries or during menopause. In secondary gonadal failure, LH and FSH levels are low as a result of pituitary failure or some other pituitary-hypothalamic impairment, stress, malnutrition, or physiologic delay in growth and sexual development.

FSH and LH assays are often done to diagnose menopause. LH hormones are also used to study testicular dysfunction in men and to evaluate endocrine problems related to precocious puberty in children. The use of these hormone assays can also help in the evaluation of disorders of sexual differentiation, such as Klinefelter syndrome.

INTERFERING FACTORS

- Recent use of radioisotopes may affect test results if the testing method is performed by radioimmunoassay. The previously administered radioisotope may interfere with the results.
- Human chorionic gonadotropin (hCG) and thyroid-stimulating hormone (TSH) may interfere with some immunoassay methods because of the similarities of part of the hormone molecule. Therefore patients with hCG-producing tumors and those with hypothyroid should be expected to have falsely high LH levels.
- Drugs that may *increase* LH or FSH levels include anticonvulsants, cimetidine, clomiphene, digitalis, levodopa, naloxone, and spironolactone.
- Drugs that may *decrease* LH levels include digoxin, estrogens, oral contraceptives, progesterones, steroids, testosterone, and phenothiazines.

✔ Clinical Priorities

- Levels of FSH and LH vary in the female patient according to phases in the menstrual cycle.
- These hormones are valuable in the evaluation of infertility. Daily samples of LH around a woman's midcycle can detect the LH surge, which is thought to occur on the day of maximum fertility.
- Spot urine tests have become useful in evaluating and treating infertility. Home test kits are now available for detecting LH in the urine.
- FSH and LH assays are often performed to diagnose menopause so hormone replacement can be started.

PROCEDURE AND PATIENT CARE

Before
☒ Explain the procedure to the patient.
☒ Tell the patient that no food or fluid restrictions are needed.

During
Blood
- Collect a venous blood sample in a red-top tube.
- Indicate the date of the last menstrual period on the laboratory slip. Note if the woman is postmenopausal.

Urine
- Collect a 24-hour specimen; a preservative may be used.
- Keep the specimen refrigerated during the collection period.
- Note that the patient may also perform LH assays at home using a home urine test or a 24-hour urine test.
- If a spot urine test is performed, follow the directions accompanying the kit.

After
- Apply pressure or a pressure dressing to the venipuncture site.
- Assess the venipuncture site for bleeding.

TEST RESULTS AND CLINICAL SIGNIFICANCE

▲ Increased Levels

Gonadal failure (e.g., physiologic menopause, ovarian dysgenesis [Turner syndrome], testicular dysgenesis [Klinefelter syndrome], castration, anorchia, hypogonadism, polycystic ovaries, complete testicular feminization syndrome): *Decreased levels of estrogen or testosterone occur with gonadal failure. Through a feedback mechanism, FSH and LH secretion is stimulated maximally.*

Precocious puberty: *One cause of precocious puberty is oversecretion of FSH and LH.*

Pituitary adenoma: *Some pituitary adenomas secrete FSH or LH without regard to any feedback mechanism.*

▼ Decreased Levels

Pituitary failure: *FSH and LH are produced in the anterior pituitary. The first indication of pituitary failure is reduction of FSH/LH and the resulting gonadal failure.*

Hypothalamic failure: *GNRH is produced in the hypothalamus and stimulates FSH/LH production. Failure of that portion of the brain to produce GNRH will cause reduced FSH/LH levels.*

Stress,

Anorexia nervosa,

Malnutrition:
   The pathophysiology of these observations is not clear.

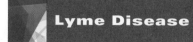

Lyme Disease

NORMAL FINDINGS

Lyme antibody EIA (Lyme Index Value [LIV])
   <0.90 = negative

0.91-1.09 = equivocal

>1.10 = positive

Western Blot

>5 different IgG antibodies reactive = positive

>2 different IgM antibodies reactive = positive

PCR

Negative

INDICATIONS

This test is used to diagnose Lyme disease.

TEST EXPLANATION

Lyme disease was first recognized in Lyme, Connecticut in 1975. It is caused by a spirochete called *Borrelia burgdorferi*. This is the most common tick-borne disease. The spirochete is spread by a bite from a black-legged tick (*Ixodes pacificus*) or deer tick (*Ixodes scapularis*).

Clinical presentation of Lyme disease can either be localized or disseminated. Characteristic of early localized disease is the presence of erythema migrans, a round or oval erythematous skin lesion with a bull's-eye pattern that develops at the site of the tick bite; it is usually present 7 to 14 days after the tick bite and should be ≥5 cm in largest diameter for a firm Lyme disease diagnosis. Disseminated disease that may affect the musculoskeletal, cardiac, or nervous system can follow erythema chronicum migrans (ECM) within days or weeks and is considered early-stage disseminated disease. Meningoencephalitis, cranial or peripheral neuropathies, myocarditis, atrioventricular nodal block, or arthritis are some of the inflammatory changes that may occur. Lyme carditis may overlap temporally with neurologic Lyme disease (late-stage disseminated disease).

Cultures of the ECM can isolate the spirochete in half of the cases. However, it is difficult to culture and takes a long time to grow. Cultures of the blood or CSF are even less helpful. Currently screening serologic studies are performed for the detection of Lyme disease. Enzyme-linked immunosorbent assay (EIA) is the best diagnostic test for Lyme disease. This test determines titers of specific IgM and specific IgG antibodies to the *B. burgdorferi* spirochete. Levels of specific IgM antibody peak during the third to sixth week after disease onset and then gradually decline. Titers of specific IgG antibodies are generally low during the first several weeks of illness, reach maximal levels in 4 to 6 months, and often remain elevated for years.

Lyme disease can be confused with various viral infections. In these patients a single titer of specific IgM antibody may suggest the correct diagnosis. Acute and convalescent sera can be tested to verify the diagnosis. The Food and Drug Administration (FDA) recommends that all samples with positive or equivocal results in the *Borrelia burgdorferi* antibody EIA (screening) should be tested by Western blot. Positive or equivocal EIA screening test results should not be interpreted as truly positive until verified with a confirmatory Western blot assay. The Western blot antibody assay can identify specifically the IgG or the IgM antibody. The Western blot assay is considered positive for IgG if five or more of the 10 significant electrophoretic bands are considered positive for *Borrelia burgdorferi* specific IgG antibody. The Western blot IgM antibody assay is considered positive if two or more out of three significant electrophoretic bands are considered positive for *Borrelia burgdorferi* IgM antibody. However, the screening test and/or Western blot for *B. burgdorferi* antibodies may be falsely negative in early stages of Lyme disease, including the period when erythema migrans is apparent.

It is important to note that the diagnosis of Lyme disease can be made with certainty only when the clinical picture of the acute disease and the serologic results both support the diagnosis. Without the clinical picture, serologic tests are often falsely positive and the diagnosis is incorrectly made. The Centers for Disease Control and Prevention (CDC) requires the following for the diagnosis to be made with certainty:

- Isolation of *B. burgdorferi* from an infected tissue or specimen

- Identification of IgM and IgG antibodies to *B. burgdorferi* in the blood or CSF
- Acute and convalescent blood samples with significant positive antibody titers

Patients with suspected Lyme disease should have the serologic test repeated if the initial test is negative. Amplification of *Borrelia* genomic DNA by real-time PCR testing can be performed on cerebrospinal fluid or urine to support the diagnosis. Ticks, after about 36 hours of attachment, may be tested by molecular methods to identify *B. burgdorferi*.

INTERFERING FACTORS

- Previous infection with *B. burgdorferi* can cause positive serologic results. These patients no longer have Lyme disease.
- Other spirochete diseases (syphilis, leptospirosis) can cause false-positive results.

PROCEDURE AND PATIENT CARE

Before

Explain the procedure to the patient.
Tell the patient that no fasting or special preparation is required.

During

- Collect a venous blood sample in a red-top tube.

After

- Apply pressure or a pressure dressing to the venipuncture site.
- Assess the venipuncture site for bleeding.

TEST RESULTS AND CLINICAL SIGNIFICANCE

Lyme disease. *At present there is significant controversy whether positive serologic testing with vague symptoms is associated with a chronic form of Lyme disease. At present the clinical manifestations of the acute disease and the serologic tests are required for the diagnosis.*

Magnesium (Mg)

NORMAL FINDINGS

Adult: 1.3-2.1 mEq/L or 0.65-1.05 mmol/L (SI units)
Child: 1.4-1.7 mEq/L
Newborn: 1.4-2 mEq/L

 Critical Values

<1 or >9 mEq/L

INDICATIONS

This test is used to identify magnesium deficiency or overload.

TEST EXPLANATION

Most of the magnesium is found in the body intracellularly. About half is in the bone. Most of the magnesium is bound to an adenosine triphosphatase (ATP) molecule and is important in phosphorylation of ATP (main source of energy for the body). Therefore this electrolyte is critical in nearly all metabolic processes. Furthermore, magnesium acts as a cofactor that modifies the activity of many enzymes. Carbohydrate, protein, and nucleic acid synthesis and metabolism depend on magnesium.

Most organ functions, including neuromuscular tissue, also depend on magnesium. It is important to monitor magnesium levels in cardiac patients. Low magnesium levels may increase cardiac irritability and aggravate cardiac arrhythmias. Hypermagnesemia retards neuromuscular conduction and is demonstrated as cardiac conduction slowing (widened PR and Q-T intervals with wide QRS), diminished deep-tendon reflexes, and respiratory depression.

As intracellular elements, body levels of potassium, magnesium, and calcium (in order of quantity) are closely linked. The intracellular electrical charge must be maintained. When the level of one of these positive electrically charged elements is low, another positively charged element is driven into the intracellular space to maintain electrical neutrality. Extracellular and blood levels therefore decrease. A total body reduction in one of those elements creates a comparable blood reduction in the others. Magnesium is closely related to calcium in that it increases the intestinal absorption of calcium. Magnesium is also important in calcium metabolism. Often hypocalcemia will respond to magnesium replacement.

Magnesium deficiency occurs in patients who are malnourished because of malabsorption or maldigestion or lack of food intake. This becomes especially significant in postoperative patients, who may not eat for 5 to 7 days and whose metabolism (and therefore the need for magnesium) is accelerated. Alcohol abuse increases magnesium loss in the urine. Moderate hypomagnesemia occurs with diabetes, hypoparathyroidism, hyperthyroidism, and hyperaldosteronism. Toxemia of pregnancy is also believed to be associated with reduced magnesium levels. Symptoms of magnesium depletion are mostly neuromuscular (i.e., weakness, irritability, tetany, EKG changes, delirium, and convulsions).

Increased magnesium levels most commonly are associated with ingestion of magnesium-containing antacids. Most of the serum magnesium is excreted by the kidney; therefore chronic renal diseases also cause elevated magnesium levels. Several drug interactions also can result in decreased or increased magnesium levels. Because magnesium is an intracellular cation, hemolysis of the collected blood sample should be avoided. Hemolysis will create falsely elevated levels of magnesium. Symptoms of increased magnesium levels include lethargy, nausea and vomiting, and slurred speech.

INTERFERING FACTORS

- Hemolysis should be avoided when collecting this specimen. Magnesium is an intracellular ion, and lysis of red blood cells (RBCs) will release great quantities of magnesium into the blood and cause falsely high results.
- Drugs that *increase* magnesium levels include antacids, aminoglycoside antibiotics, calcium-containing medication, laxatives, lithium, loop diuretics, and thyroid medication.
- Drugs that *decrease* magnesium levels include some antibiotics, diuretics, and insulin.

PROCEDURE AND PATIENT CARE

Before

- Explain the procedure to the patient.
- Tell the patient that no special diet or fasting is required.

During

- Collect a venous blood sample in a red-top or green-top tube.
- Avoid hemolysis.

After

- Apply pressure or a pressure dressing to the venipuncture site.
- Assess the venipuncture site for bleeding.

TEST RESULTS AND CLINICAL SIGNIFICANCE

▲ Increased Levels

Renal insufficiency: *Magnesium is excreted by the kidneys. With end-stage renal failure, excretion is reduced and magnesium accumulates in the blood. See discussion below regarding decreased magnesium levels in tubular diseases of the kidney.*

Addison disease: *Aldosterone enhances magnesium excretion. With reduced aldosterone, magnesium excretion is diminished.*

Ingestion of magnesium-containing antacids or salts: *Magnesium is absorbed from the intestines. Blood levels rise.*

Hypothyroidism: *The pathophysiology of this observation is not clear.*

▼ Decreased Levels

Malnutrition,

Malabsorption:

> *The major source of magnesium is dietary intake and absorption from the intestines. When either is inhibited, magnesium levels in the blood fall. In malabsorption, all fat-soluble vitamins are lost. Vitamin D levels diminish, and hypocalcemia follows. Magnesium levels therefore fall in light of the low calcium (see above).*

Hypoparathyroidism: *In this disease, calcium levels are reduced. Calcium enhances intestinal absorption of magnesium, and with low calcium levels, magnesium is not well absorbed, so blood levels diminish. In hyperparathyroidism, calcium levels are high and magnesium levels increase.*

Alcoholism: *Ethanol increases magnesium losses in the urine.*

Chronic renal tubular disease: *Magnesium is reabsorbed in the renal tubule. Diseases affecting this area of the kidney (e.g., tubular necrosis) or drugs that are toxic to the renal tubule (e.g., aminoglycosides) will allow increased losses of magnesium in the urine.*

Diabetic acidosis: *With treatment of this disease, magnesium levels fall. As insulin is given to these patients to drive glucose into the cells, magnesium follows and blood levels drop.*

 Maternal Screen Testing (Maternal Triple Screen, Maternal Quadruple Screen)

NORMAL FINDINGS

Low probability of fetal defects

INDICATIONS

This is a series of tests that are provided to pregnant women in early pregnancy as a screening test to identify potential birth defects or serious chromosomal/genetic abnormalities.

TEST EXPLANATION

These screening tests may indicate the potential for the presence of fetal defects (particularly trisomy 21 [Down syndrome] or trisomy 18). They may also indicate increased risk for neural tube defects (e.g., myelomeningocele, spina bifida) or abdominal wall defects (omphalocele or gastroschisis).

The incidence of these abnormalities is directly related to maternal age. In the United States maternal screening is routinely offered to all pregnant women, usually in their second trimester of pregnancy. Patients must understand that this is a screening test, not a diagnostic test. If the screening tests are positive, more accurate definitive testing, such as chorionic villus sampling (CVS) in early pregnancy or amniocentesis in mid-pregnancy, is recommended. Most pregnant women greater than 35 years of age routinely have CVS or amniocentesis without maternal screening. FISH CVS or amniotic fluid testing (see Laboratory Genetics, p. 1104) for aneuploidy provides rapid detection of chromosome abnormalities.

Several variations of this test are available:
- Double test: Measures two markers, hCG (p. 304) and alpha-fetoprotein (AFP, p. 54).
- Triple test (maternal triple screen test): Measures three markers, human chorionic gonadotropic (hCG), AFP, and estriol (p. 226) AFP is produced in the yolk sac and fetal liver. Unconjugated estriol and hCG are produced by the placenta.
- Quadruple test: Measures four markers, hCG, AFP, estriol, and inhibin A.
- Fully integrated screen test: Measures AFP, estriol, fetal nuchal translucency (p. 888), beta and total hCG, and pregnancy-associated plasma protein-A (PAPP-A, p. 414).

The maternal triple screen test offers a 50% to 80% chance of detecting pregnancies with trisomy 21 as compared with AFP alone, which has only a 30% chance of detection. The Quadruple screen is now routinely recommended and is combined with fetal nuchal translucency [FNT] (see Pelvic Ultrasonography, p. 887). These tests are most accurately performed during the second trimester of pregnancy, more specifically between the 14th and 24th weeks (ideal 16-18 weeks). The use of ultrasound to accurately indicate gestational age improves the sensitivity and specificity of maternal serum screening.

First trimester screening for genetic defects is an option for pregnant women. This testing would include FNT combined with the beta subunit of hCG (beta-hCG, p. 304), and pregnancy-associated plasma protein-A (PAPP-A, p. 414). A low level of PAPP-A may indicate an increased risk for having a stillborn baby. These tests have detection rates comparable to standard second-trimester triple screening.

First trimester (11-13 weeks) screening offers several potential advantages over second-trimester screening. When test results are negative, it may help reduce maternal anxiety earlier. If results are positive, it allows women to take advantage of first trimester prenatal diagnosis by CVS at 10 to 12 weeks or early pregnancy amniocentesis. Detecting problems earlier in the pregnancy may allow women to prepare for a child with health problems. It also affords women greater privacy and less health risk if they elect to terminate the pregnancy. In first trimester testing, open neural tube defects cannot be determined

With trisomy 21, second trimester absolute maternal serum levels of AFP and unconjugated estriol are about 25% lower than normal levels and maternal serum hCG is approximately two times higher than the normal hCG level. The results of the screening are expressed in *multiples of median (MoM)*. AFP and urinary estriol (E_3) values during pregnancies with trisomy 21 are lower than those associated with normal pregnancies, which means that values below the mean are below 1 MoM. The hCG value for trisomy 21 is greater than 1 MoM. The MoM, fetal age, and maternal weight are used to calculate the possible risk for chromosomal abnormalities (e.g., trisomy 21). All of the previously named maternal screening tests are discussed elsewhere in this book. For the sake of thoroughness, Inhibin A is discussed here.

Inhibin A is normally secreted by the granulosa cells in the ovaries and inhibits the production of follicle-stimulating hormone (FSH) by the pituitary gland. Inhibin A is a glycoprotein of placental origin in pregnancy similar to hCG. Levels in maternal serum remain relatively constant through the 15th to 18th week of pregnancy. Inhibin A is important in the control of fetal development. Maternal serum levels of inhibin A are twice as high in pregnancies affected by trisomy 21 as in unaffected pregnancies. The discovery of this fact led to the inclusion of inhibin A in the serum screening tests for trisomy 21. Inhibin A concentrations are significantly lower in women with normal pregnancies than in women with pregnancies that result in spontaneous abortions. Furthermore circulating concentrations of inhibin A appear to reflect tumor mass for certain forms of ovarian cancer. More accurate diagnostic testing is required if screening tests are abnormal.

Pregnancy-associated plasma protein-A (PAPP-A) is discussed on p. 414.

It is important to recognize that maternal screening provide only an estimation of risk and not a diagnosis. A negative result indicates that the estimated risk falls below the screen cutoff. A positive result indicates that the estimated risk exceeds the screen cutoff. Neither is a diagnosis of normal or abnormal, respectively. Maternal screen can be performed sequentially. The cutoffs of risks differ depending on the timing of testing. For example for Down syndrome, *Sequential Maternal Screening*, Part 1 (performed in the first trimester), serum results are negative when the calculated risk is less than 1/50 (2%). If Part 1 is negative, an additional specimen is submitted in the second trimester. With *Sequential Maternal Screening*, Part 2, serum results are negative when the calculated risk is less than 1/270 (0.37%). Negative results mean that the risk is less than the established cutoff; they do not guarantee the absence of Down syndrome. Results are positive when the risk is greater than the established cutoff (i.e., >1/50 in Sequential Maternal Screening, Part 1, and greater than 1/270 in Sequential Maternal Screening, Part 2). Positive results are not diagnostic. When both Sequential Maternal Screening Part 1 and Part 2 are performed with a screen cutoff of 1/270, the combination of maternal age, nuchal translucency (NT), pregnancy-associated plasma protein A (PAPP-A), alpha-fetoprotein (AFP), unconjugated estriol (uE3), human chorionic gonadotropin (hCG), and inhibin A has an overall detection rate of approximately 90% with a false-positive rate of approximately 3% to 4%. In practice, both the detection rate and false-positive rate vary with maternal age. These numbers change when looking at risk for other abnormalities, such as trisomy 18 or neural tube defects.

PROCEDURE AND PATIENT CARE

Before

- Explain the procedure to the patient.
- Allow the patient to express her concerns and fears regarding the potential for birth defects.

During

- Most of these tests can be done with a venous blood sample in a red-top tube. hCG and estriol can also be tested by collecting a urine sample.

After

- Provide the results to the patient and (other family members as per patient desires) during a personal consultation.
- Allow the patient to express her concerns if the results are positive.
- Assist the patient in scheduling and obtaining more accurate diagnostic testing if the results are positive.

TEST RESULTS AND CLINICAL SIGNIFICANCE
Positive Serum Screening Tests
Trisomy 21,
Trisomy 18,
Neural tube defects,
Abdominal wall defects:
> Increased serum markers are associated with potential for birth defects. AFP markers are decreased in trisomy chromosomal defects, however. Low levels of PAPP-A may be associated with stillbirths.

RELATED TESTS
Alpha-Fetoprotein (p. 54). This test is one of the commonly performed screening tests for possible birth defects.

Pelvic Ultrasonography (p. 887). This test includes a description of fetal nuchal translucency, an accurate screening test for chromosomal abnormalities.

Human Placental Lactogen (p. 308). This is an accurate test to indicate the presence of fetal distress, disease, or growth restriction.

Pregnancy-Associated Plasma Protein-A (p. 414). This is a maternal screening test for potential birth abnormalities.

Metanephrine, Plasma Free

NORMAL FINDINGS
Normetanephrine: 18-111 pg/mL
Metanephrine: 12-60 pg/mL
(Results will vary among laboratories.)

Indications
This test is used to identify pheochromocytoma of the adrenal or extraadrenal glands.

TEST EXPLANATION
Pheochromocytomas, although rarely a cause of hypertension, are dangerous tumors that should be investigated. These tumors produce several catecholamines that can cause episodic or persistent hypertension that is unresponsive to treatment. The current diagnosis of pheochromocytoma depends on biochemical evidence of catecholamine production by the tumor. The best test to establish the diagnosis has not been determined.

Until recently, urinary vanillylmandelic acid (VMA) and catecholamine measurements (see p. 975) were used. Urinary testing is not as sensitive as plasma testing. The low prevalence of these tumors among the tested population and the inadequate sensitivity and specificity of urinary testing made diagnosis of pheochromocytoma cumbersome and time-consuming. The development of high-performance liquid chromatography (HPLC) has allowed for more sensitivity in measuring plasma-free metanephrine levels. This is a blood test that measures the amount of metanephrine and normetanephrine, which are metabolites of epinephrine and norepinephrine, two catecholamines.

The high sensitivity of plasma-free metanephrine testing provides a high negative predictive value to the test. This means that if the concentrations of the free metanephrines in the blood are normal, it is very unlikely that a patient has a pheochromocytoma. False positives do occur, though rarely. The diagnostic superiority of plasma metanephrines over plasma or urinary catecholamines and urinary VMA is clear. In about 80% of patients with pheochromocytoma, the magnitude of increase in plasma-free metanephrines is so large that the tumor can be confirmed with close to 100% probability. Intermediate concentrations of normetanephrine and metanephrine are considered indeterminate.

Urinary testing may clarify indeterminate findings. However, comparison of plasma metanephrines and urine metanephrines requires caution because different catecholamine metabolites are measured. Testing for some urinary catecholamines may be more specific than for plasma-free metanephrines, meaning that false positives are less common with urinary testing.

When interpreting results, the following may be helpful:

- Any sample in which the concentrations of *both* normetanephrine and metanephrine are less than the upper reference range limit should be considered normal, and the presence of pheochromocytoma is highly unlikely.
- Any sample where the concentrations of *either* normetanephrine or metanephrine exceed their respective upper reference range limits should be considered elevated.
- Whenever the normetanephrine or metanephrine concentration exceeds the indeterminate range, the presence of pheochromocytoma is highly probable and should be located via imaging techniques.

INTERFERING FACTORS

- Increased levels of metanephrines may be caused by caffeine or alcohol.
- Vigorous exercise, stress, and starvation may cause increased metanephrine levels.
- Drugs that may cause *increased* metanephrine levels include epinephrine- or norepinephrine-containing drugs, levodopa, lithium, and nitroglycerin.
- Acetaminophen can interfere with HPLC testing of metanephrines and should be avoided for 48 hours before testing.

PROCEDURE AND PATIENT CARE

Before

- Explain the procedure to the patient.
- Explain the dietary and medicinal restrictions.

During

- Identify and minimize factors contributing to patient stress and anxiety. Physical exertion and emotional stress may alter metanephrine test results.
- The patients may be asked to lie down and rest quietly for 15 to 30 minutes before sample collection.
- The blood sample may be collected while supine.
- Collect a venous blood sample in a chilled lavender-top (EDTA) or pink-top (K2EDTA) tube. Invert to mix with preservatives.

After

- Apply pressure to the venipuncture site.
- Send the specimen to the laboratory as soon as the test is completed.

TEST RESULTS AND CLINICAL SIGNIFICANCE

▲ Increased Levels

Pheochromocytoma: *This is a neuroendocrine tumor of the medulla of the adrenal glands (originating in the chromaffin cells) that secretes excessive amounts of catecholamines that are subsequently metabolized to metanephrines.*

RELATED TEST

Vanillylmandelic Acid and Catecholamines (p. 975). This 24-hour urine test for VMA and catecholamines is performed primarily to diagnose hypertension secondary to pheochromocytoma, neuroblastomas, and other rare adrenal tumors.

 Methemoglobin (Hemoglobin M)

NORMAL FINDINGS

0.06-0.24 g/dL or 9.3-37.2 μmol/L (SI units)
0.4%-1.5% of total hemoglobin

 Critical Values

>40% of total hemoglobin

Indications

This test is used to identify methemoglobinemia in hypoxemic children and adults.

TEST EXPLANATION

Methemoglobin is continuously formed in the red blood cells (RBCs). During the production of normal adult deoxygenated hemoglobin, methemoglobin is reduced to normal adult deoxygenated hemoglobin by nicotinamide adenine dinucleotide dependent reductase enzyme (NADH). If oxygenation of the iron component in the protohemoglobin occurs without subsequent reduction of the heme iron back to its Fe^{+2} form as exists in normal hemoglobin, excess methemoglobin accumulates. The oxidized iron form in methemoglobin is unable to combine with oxygen to carry the oxygen to the peripheral tissues. Therefore the oxyhemoglobin dissociation curve is "shifted to the left" resulting in cyanosis and hypoxia. Elderly, pediatric, or chronically hypoxemic patients are particularly sensitive to methemoglobin production.

Methemoglobinemia can be congenital or, more commonly, is acquired. Hemoglobin M disease is a genetic defect that results in a group of abnormal hemoglobins that are methemoglobins. Another genetic mutation can cause a deficiency in NADH methemoglobin reductase enzyme that is required to deoxygenate methemoglobin to normal adult hemoglobin. These forms of methemoglobinemia occur in infants, are usually severe, are not amenable to treatment, and are often fatal.

Acquired methemoglobinemia is a result of ingestion of nitrates (e.g., from well water), or drugs such as phenacetin, sulfonamides, isoniazid, local anesthetics containing benzocaine, sulfonamide antibiotics, silver nitrate, and Pyridium. Several over-the-counter local anesthetics used for toothache or hemorrhoidal pain contain benzocaine. The acquired form of the disease commonly occurs in older individuals and results in an acute crisis that is effectively treated with ascorbic acid or methylene blue. However, methylene blue is contraindicated in G6PD deficiency.

INTERFERING FACTORS

- Tobacco use and carbon monoxide poisoning are associated with increased methemoglobin levels.
- Drugs that may cause *increased* levels include some antibiotics, isoniazid, local anesthetics, and sulfonamides.

PROCEDURE AND PATIENT CARE

Before

Explain the procedure to the patient.
Tell the patient that no fasting is required.

During

- Collect a venous blood sample in a green-top (heparin) tube.
- Methemoglobin is very unstable. Place the specimen in an ice slush immediately after collection.
- Avoid hemolysis.

After

- Apply pressure to the venipuncture site.
- Be prepared to provide oxygen support and close monitoring in the event the patient is becoming increasingly hypoxic.

TEST RESULTS AND CLINICAL SIGNIFICANCE

Hereditary methemoglobinemia: *Cyanosis will start in early infancy.*
Acquired methemoglobinemia:

Both forms are associated with hypoxemia. Both can be improved with ascorbic acid and in some cases, methylene blue.

Microglobulin (Beta-$_2$ Microglobulin [B$_2$M], Alpha 1 Microglobulin, and Retinol-Binding Protein)

NORMAL FINDINGS

Beta-$_2$ Microglobulin

Blood: 0.7-1.8 mcg/mL
Urine: ≤300 mcg/L
CSF: ≤2.4 mg/L

Alpha 1 Microglobulin

Urine:
<50 years: <13 mg/g creatinine
≥50 years: <20 mg/g creatinine

Retinol-Binding Protein (RBP)

Urine: <163 mcg/24 hours

INDICATIONS

This test is used to evaluate patients with malignancies, chronic infections, inflammatory diseases, and renal diseases.

TEST EXPLANATION

Beta-$_2$ microglobulin (B_2M) is a protein found on the surface of all cells. It is an HLA major histocompatibility antigen that exists in increased numbers on the cell surface and particularly on lymphatic cells. Production of this protein increases with cell turnover. B_2M is increased in patients with malignancies (especially B-cell lymphoma, leukemia, or multiple myeloma), chronic infections, and in patients with chronic severe inflammatory diseases. It is an accurate measurement of myeloma tumor disease activity, stage of disease, and prognosis and, as such, is an important tumor marker. This tumor marker is best determined in the blood.

B_2M, *alpha 1 microglobulin*, and *retinol-binding proteins* pass freely through glomerular membranes and are near completely reabsorbed by renal proximal tubules cells. Because of extensive tubular reabsorption, under normal conditions very little of these proteins appear in the final excreted urine. Therefore an increase in the urinary excretion of these proteins indicates proximal tubule disease or toxicity and/or impaired proximal tubular function. In patients with a urinary tract infection, these proteins indicate pyelonephritis. These proteins are helpful in differentiating glomerular from tubular renal disease. In patients with aminoglycoside toxicity, heavy metal nephrotoxicity, or tubular disease, protein urine levels are elevated. Excretion is increased 100 to 1000 times normal levels in cadmium-exposed workers. This test is used to monitor these workers. Periodic testing is performed on these patients to detect kidney disease at its earliest stage. To date there are no convincing studies to indicate that one protein has better clinical utility than the other.

B_2M is particularly helpful in the differential diagnosis of renal disease. If blood and urine levels are obtained simultaneously, one can differentiate glomerular from tubular disease. In glomerular disease, because of poor glomerular filtration, blood levels are high and urine levels are low. In tubular disease, because of poor tubular reabsorption, the blood levels are low and urine levels are high. Blood levels increase early in kidney transplant rejection.

Urinary excretion of these proteins can be determined from either a 24-hour collection or a random urine collection. The 24-hour collection is traditionally considered the gold standard. For random or spot collections, the concentration of alpha-1-microglobulin is divided by the urinary creatinine concentration. This corrected value adjusts alpha-1-microglobulin for variabilities in urine concentration.

Increased CSF levels of B_2M indicate central nervous system involvement with leukemia, lymphoma, HIV, or multiple sclerosis.

Quantitative chemiluminescent immunoassay or nephelometry methods are used to identify these proteins in the urine or serum.

INTERFERING FACTORS

- Results could be affected by recent nuclear imaging when B_2M testing is performed by radioimmunoassay.
- B_2M is unstable in acid urine.

PROCEDURE AND PATIENT CARE

Before

🖐Explain the procedure to the patient to minimize anxiety.

During

Blood

- Collect a venous blood sample in a red-top tube.

Urine

🖐See Box 11-2, Guidelines for a 24-Hour Urine Collection, p. 907.

🖐Encourage the patient to drink fluids during the 24 hours unless this is contraindicated for medical purposes.

- If a single random urine collection is requested, collect specimen for protein and creatinine testing to adjust for urine concentration.

After

- Apply pressure to the venipuncture site.
- Send the urine collection to the laboratory.

TEST RESULTS AND CLINICAL IMPLICATIONS

▲ Increased Urine Levels

Renal tubule disease,

Drug-induced renal toxicity,

Heavy metal–induced renal disease:

In primary renal tubular disease, these proteins cannot be reabsorbed by the renal tubule. They therefore are elevated in excreted urine.

Lymphomas, leukemia, myeloma:

In patients with advanced disease, glomerular filtration of these proteins exceeds the ability of renal tubules to reabsorb them. Thus they are elevated in excreted urine.

▲ Increased Serum Levels

Lymphomas, leukemia, myeloma,

Glomerular renal disease,

Renal transplant rejection:

Glomerular filtration of these proteins is diminished and serum levels rise.

Viral infections, especially HIV and cytomegalovirus,

Chronic inflammatory processes:

Inflammation is associated with increased cell turnover. Thus shedding increases levels of these proteins into the serum.

RELATED TESTS

Microalbumin (p. 931). Like the above-noted proteins, microalbumin is a marker for renal disease.

Blood Urea Nitrogen (p. 511). This is a measure of renal function.

Creatinine (p. 190). This is a measure of renal function.

Mononucleosis Rapid Test (Mononuclear Heterophil Test, Heterophil Antibody Test, Monospot Test)

NORMAL FINDINGS

Negative (<1:28 titer)

INDICATIONS

This is a rapid slide test designed to assist in the diagnosis of infectious mononucleosis.

TEST EXPLANATION

The mononucleosis rapid test is performed to make the diagnosis of infectious mononucleosis (IM), a disease caused by the Epstein-Barr virus (EBV). Usually young adults are affected by mononucleosis. The clinical presentation is fever, pharyngitis, lymphadenopathy, and splenomegaly. Detectable levels of the IM heterophile antibody can usually be expected to occur between the sixth and tenth day following the onset of symptoms. The level usually increases through the second or third week of illness and, thereafter, can be expected to persist, gradually declining over a 12-month period. The IM heterophile antibody has been associated with several diseases other than IM. These include leukemia, Burkitt lymphoma, pancreatic carcinoma, viral hepatitis, cytomegalovirus infections, and others.

Several heterophil agglutination tests are available, but the most frequently performed is the rapid slide test for infectious mononucleosis (previously called the Monospot test). In most tests, a suspension of polystyrene latex particles is coated with a highly purified antigen from bovine red cell membranes. The degree of purity of the antigen is such that it only reacts with infectious mononucleosis heterophile antibodies. If infectious mononucleosis heterophile antibodies are present in serum, the latex suspension changes its uniform appearance and a clear agglutination becomes evident, indicating an EBV virus infection. EBV immunologic quantification (p. 312) is available when IM is suspected but the Mono Spot is negative.

The diagnosis of infectious mononucleosis must include the following criteria:

- Clinical presentation compatible with infectious mononucleosis
- Hematologic presentation compatible with that of infectious mononucleosis (lymphocytosis)
- Atypical lymphocytes in significant numbers
- Positive serologic test for infectious mononucleosis

PROCEDURE AND PATIENT CARE

Before

Explain the procedure to the patient.
Tell the patient that no fasting or special preparation is required.

During

- Collect a venous blood sample in a red-top tube.

After

- Apply pressure or a pressure dressing to the venipuncture site.
- Observe the venipuncture site for bleeding.

TEST RESULTS AND CLINICAL SIGNIFICANCE

▲ Increased Levels

Infectious mononucleosis,

Chronic EBV infection,

Chronic fatigue syndrome,

Burkitt lymphoma,

Some forms of chronic hepatitis:

> *The above diseases are often associated with abnormal quantities of heterophil agglutinating antibodies similar to those formed in patients with infectious mononucleosis.*

RELATED TEST

Epstein-Barr Virus Testing (p. 217). These tests are recommended only when a mononucleosis screening procedure is negative and infectious mononucleosis or a complication of Epstein-Barr virus infection is suspected. Also they more precisely define the acuity of the infection.

Mycoplasma pneumoniae Antibodies, IgG and IgM

NORMAL FINDINGS

IgG

≤0.9 (negative)

0.91-1.09 (equivocal)

≥1.1 (positive)

IgM

≤0.9 (negative)

0.91-1.09 (equivocal)

≥1.1 (positive)

IgM by IFA

Negative (reported as positive or negative)

INDICATIONS

This test is used to support the clinical diagnosis of disease associated with *Mycoplasma pneumoniae*.

TEST EXPLANATION

Several diseases have been associated with the mycoplasmal pneumoniae infection, including pharyngitis, tracheobronchitis, pneumonia, and inflammation of the tympanic membrane. *Mycoplasma pneumoniae* accounts for approximately 20% of all cases of pneumonia. Classically it causes a disease that has been described as primary atypical pneumonia. The disease is of insidious onset with fever, headache, and malaise for 2 to 4 days before the onset of respiratory symptoms. Most patients do not require hospitalization. Symptomatic infections attributable to this organism most commonly occur in children and young adults. These infections may be associated with cold agglutinin syndrome (p. 170).

Positive IgM results are consistent with acute infection, although there may be some cross-reactivity associated with other mycoplasma infections. A single positive IgG result only indicates previous immunologic exposure. Negative results do not rule out the presence of *Mycoplasma pneumoniae–* associated disease because the specimen may have been drawn before the appearance of detectable antibodies. If a *Mycoplasma* infection is clinically suspected, a second specimen should be submitted at least 14 days later. The continued presence or absence of antibodies cannot be used to determine the success or failure of therapy.

After serologic combinations to identify IgG/IgM antibody complexes, serial dilutions are performed and the color changes are measured photometrically. The color intensity of the dilutions depends on the antibody concentration in the serum sample. The IgM complex can be identified by immunofluorescent assay (IFA).

PROCEDURE AND PATIENT CARE

Before
☒ Explain the procedure to the patient.
☒ Tell the patient that no fasting is required.

During
- Collect venous blood in a red-top tube.

After
- Apply pressure to the venipuncture site.
- Transport the specimen immediately to the laboratory. Avoid undue cooling of the specimen, which may lead to agglutination.

TEST RESULTS AND CLINICAL SIGNIFICANCE

Mycoplasma infection: *With the combination of positive antibodies and a compatible clinical picture, the diagnosis of Mycoplasma infection can be confidently made.*

RELATED TESTS

Cold Agglutinins (p. 170). This test identifies antibodies to RBCs that cause agglutination when exposed to cold temperatures. Although other diseases are also associated with the presence of these antibodies, *Mycoplasma* infections are considered predominant.

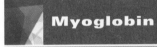
Myoglobin

NORMAL FINDINGS
<90 mcg/L or <90 mcg/L (SI units)

INDICATIONS
This test is used in the early evaluation of a patient with suspected acute myocardial infarction (MI). It is also used to assist in the diagnosis of disease or injury of skeletal muscle.

TEST EXPLANATION

Myoglobin is an oxygen-binding protein found in cardiac and skeletal muscle. Measurement of myoglobin provides an early index of damage to the myocardium, such as occurs in myocardial infarction (MI) or reinfarction. Increased levels, which indicate cardiac muscle injury or death, occur in about 3 hours. Although this test is more sensitive than creatine phosphokinase (CPK) isoenzymes, it is not as specific. Trauma, inflammation, or ischemic changes to the noncardiac skeletal muscles can also cause elevated levels of myoglobin. The benefit of myoglobin over CPK-MB (see p. 186) is that it may become elevated earlier in some patients. This may prove beneficial because thrombolytic therapy should be started within the first 6 hours after an MI.

As already indicated, disease or trauma of the skeletal muscle also causes elevations in myoglobin. With sudden and severe muscle injury, myoglobin can reach very high levels. Because myoglobin is excreted in the urine and is nephrotoxic, urine levels must be monitored in patients with high levels. To screen for myoglobin, the routine urine dipstick for hemoglobin can be used.

INTERFERING FACTORS

- Recent administration of radioactive substances may affect test results determined by radioimmunoassay (RIA) methods. The recently administered radioisotope may interfere with testing.
- Increased myoglobin levels can occur after intramuscular (IM) injections. The injection can cause localized muscle injury and instigate an inflammatory response that could elevate myoglobin levels.

PROCEDURE AND PATIENT CARE

Before
☒ Explain the procedure to the patient.
☒ Tell the patient that no fasting is required.

During
- Collect a venous blood sample in a red-top tube.

After
- Apply pressure or a pressure dressing to the venipuncture site.
- Observe the venipuncture site for bleeding.

TEST RESULTS AND CLINICAL SIGNIFICANCE

▲ Increased Levels

MI: *Injury to cardiac muscle causes the cells to lyse and expel the myoglobin into the bloodstream.*
Skeletal muscle inflammation (myositis): *Injury to skeletal muscle causes the cells to lyse and expel the myoglobin into the bloodstream.*
Malignant hyperthermia,
Muscular dystrophy,
Skeletal muscle ischemia,
Skeletal muscle trauma,
Rhabdomyolysis:

All of these diseases affect the skeletal muscles. This causes the muscle cells to lyse and expel the myoglobin into the bloodstream.

Seizures: *Persistent seizure activity injures skeletal muscle tissue. This causes the muscle cells to lyse and expel the myoglobin into the bloodstream.*

▼ **Decreased Levels**

Polymyositis: *In some cases, antimyoglobin antibodies exist and diminish myoglobin in the blood.*

RELATED TESTS

Creatine Phosphokinase (CPK) (p. 186). This test is very useful in the evaluation of MI.

Lactic Dehydrogenase (LDH) (p. 329). This enzyme is also elevated when injury to muscle tissue occurs.

Troponins (p. 508). This test is a specific indicator of cardiac muscle injury.

Natriuretic Peptides (Atrial Natriuretic Peptide [ANP], Brain Natriuretic Peptide [BNP], C-type Natriuretic Peptide [CNP], B-Type Natriuretic Peptide [BNP], Ventricular Natriuretic Peptide, CHF Peptides)

NORMAL FINDINGS

ANP 22-77 pg/mL or 22-77 ng/L (SI units)
BNP <100 pg/mL or <100 ng/L (SI units)
CNP: yet to be determined

 Critical Values

>100 pg/mL

INDICATIONS

Natriuretic peptides are used to identify and stratify patients with congestive heart failure (CHF).

TEST EXPLANATION AND RELATED PHYSIOLOGY

Natriuretic peptides (NPs) are used to identify and stratify patients with congestive heart failure (CHF). NPs are neuroendocrine peptides that oppose the activity of the renin-angiotensin system. There are three major NPs: ANP, BNP, and CNP. ANP is synthesized in the cardiac atrial muscle. The main source of BNP is the membrane granules in the cardiac ventricle, although it was initially found in porcine brain. CNP was first localized in the nervous system but later found to be produced by the endothelial cells. The cardiac peptides are continuously released by the heart muscle cells in low levels. But, the rate of release can be increased by a variety of neuroendocrine and physiologic factors, including hemodynamic load, to regulate cardiac preload and afterload. Because of these properties, BNP and ANP have been implicated in the pathophysiology of hypertension, CHF, and atherosclerosis. Both ANP and BNP are released in response to atrial and ventricular stretch, respectively, and will cause vasorelaxation, inhibition of aldosterone secretion from the adrenal gland

and renin from the kidney, thereby increasing natriuresis and reduction in blood volume. CNP has a vasorelaxation effect but does not stimulate natriuresis.

BNP, in particular, correlates well to left ventricular pressures. As a result, BNP is a good marker for CHF. BNP levels, by themselves, are more accurate than any historical or physical findings or laboratory values in identifying congestive heart failure as the cause of dyspnea. The diagnostic accuracy of BNP at a cutoff of 100 pg/mL was 83.4% in research studies.

The higher the levels of BNP are, the more severe the CHF. This test is used in urgent care settings to aid in the differential diagnosis of shortness of breath (SOB). If BNP is elevated, the SOB is because of CHF. If BNP levels are normal, the SOB is pulmonary and not cardiac. This is particularly helpful in evaluating SOB in patients with cardiac and chronic lung disease.

Furthermore, BNP is a helpful prognosticator and is used in CHF risk stratification. CHF patients whose BNP levels do not rapidly return to normal with treatment experience a significantly higher risk for mortality in the ensuing months than do those whose BNP levels rapidly normalize with treatment. In early rejection of heart transplants, BNP levels can be elevated. Measurement of plasma BNP concentration is evolving as a very efficient and cost effective mass screening technique for identifying patients with various cardiac abnormalities. This measurement is important regardless of etiology and degree of left ventricular (LV) systolic dysfunction that can potentially develop into obvious heart failure and carry a high risk for a cardiovascular event.

In some laboratories, BNP is measured as an *N-terminal fragment of pro–brain (B-type) natriuretic peptide (NT–pro-BNP)*. The clinical information provided by either the BNP or the pro-BNP is about the same and the tests are used interchangeably. In most clinical laboratories, BNP is performed by automated systems using chemiluminescence (e.g., Beckman Coulter). Screening diabetics for BNP elevation to determine the risk for cardiac diseases is used because of the low cost of performing the test as compared with an echocardiogram. BNP is also elevated in patients with prolonged systemic hypertension and those with acute myocardial infarction (MI).

INTERFERING FACTORS

- BNP levels are generally higher in healthy women than healthy men.
- BNP levels are higher in older patients.
- BNP levels are elevated in patients who have had cardiac surgery for 1 month postoperatively. This does not reflect the presence of CHF.
- There are several different methods of measuring BNP. Normal values vary whether or not the whole protein of a BNP fragment protein is measured.
- Natrecor (nesiritide), a recombinant form of the endogenous human peptide used to treat CHF, will *increase* plasma BNP levels for several days.

PROCEDURE AND PATIENT CARE

Before
- Explain the procedure to the patient.
- Tell the patient that no fasting is required.

During
- Collect a venous blood sample in an EDTA (usually lavender) containing tube.

After
- Apply pressure to the venipuncture site.

- Assess the venipuncture site for bleeding.
- Continue with aggressive medical care for suspected CHF.

TEST RESULTS AND CLINICAL SIGNIFICANCE

▲ Increased Levels

Congestive heart failure,
Myocardial infarction,
Systemic hypertension,
Heart transplant rejection,
Cor pulmonale:

> *These diseases are all associated with increased ventricular and/or atrial cardiac pressure. As a result, cardiac natriuretic peptides are secreted, causing a relaxation of blood vessels (vasodilation), an increase in the excretion of sodium (natriuresis) and fluid (diuresis), and a decrease in injurious neurohormones (endothelin, aldosterone, angiotensin II). All of these actions work in concert on the vessels, heart, and kidney to decrease the fluid load on the heart, allowing the heart to function better and improving cardiac performance.*

RELATED TEST

Chest X-Ray (p. 1014). This test provides information about the heart, lungs, bony thorax, mediastinum, and great vessels.

Neuron-Specific Enolase (NSE)

NORMAL FINDINGS

<8.6 mcg/L

INDICATIONS

This test is used as a marker in patients with neuron-specific enolase-secreting tumors (e.g., carcinoids, small cell lung carcinoma, neuroblastomas). It is also used as an auxiliary tool in the assessment of comatose patients: the higher the NSE level, the more injury to the central nervous system.

TEST EXPLANATION

NSE is a glycolytic enzyme that catalyzes the conversion of phosphoglycerate to phosphoenol pyruvate. It is present in neuronal, neuroendocrine, and amine precursor uptake decarboxylation (APUD) cells. NSE, in serum or cerebrospinal fluid (CSF), is often elevated in diseases, which result in neuronal destruction. Measurement of NSE in serum of CSF therefore can assist in the differential diagnosis of a variety of neuron-destructive and neurodegenerative disorders. NSE might also have utility as a prognostic marker in neuronal hypoxic injury.

Elevated NSE concentrations are observed in patients with neuroblastoma, pancreatic islet cell carcinoma, medullary thyroid carcinoma, pheochromocytoma, and other neural crest–derived or neuroendocrine tumors. NSE levels are frequently increased in patients with small cell lung cancer (SCLC) and infrequently in patients with non-SCLC. When increased, NSE can be used to monitor disease progression and management in SCLC. Levels of NSE occasionally can be elevated in benign disorders, such as pneumonia and benign hepatobiliary diseases.

NSE values can vary significantly among methods and assays. Serial follow-up should be performed with the same assay. If assays are changed, patients should have new baseline values. Immunometric assays are most commonly used.

INTERFERING FACTORS

- Hemolysis can lead to significant artifactual NSE elevations because erythrocytes contain NSE.

PROCEDURE AND PATIENT CARE

Before

☒ Explain the procedure to the patient.
☒ Tell the patient that no fasting is required.

During

- Collect a venous blood sample in a red-top tube.

After

- Apply pressure to the venipuncture site.

TEST RESULTS AND CLINICAL SIGNIFICANCE

▲ Increased Levels

Small cell lung cancer,
Neuroblastoma,
APUD-omas,
Creutzfeldt-Jakob disease:

> Any neuronal based tumor or neuronal injured tissue will secrete excess NSE in the blood or CSF (if the disease affects the central nervous system). In doing so, NSE is a measure of tumor burden or neuronal injury or disease.

RELATED TEST

Magnetic Resonance Imaging (p. 1106). This noninvasive diagnostic procedure provides invaluable information about the brain, central nervous system, bones, joints, breasts, and so on.

Neutrophil Antibody Screen (Granulocyte Antibodies, Polymorphonucleocyte Antibodies [PMN ab], Antigranulocyte Antibodies, Antineutrophil Antibodies, Neutrophil Antibodies)

NORMAL FINDINGS

Negative for neutrophil antibodies.

INDICATIONS

This test is performed to identify antibodies to white blood cells (WBCs) if blood transfusion is associated with an immune reaction.

TEST EXPLANATION

Neutrophil antibodies are directed toward WBCs. They develop during blood transfusions. Patients who experience a transfusion reaction despite complete compatibility testing before blood administration should have a neutrophil antibody screen to see if WBC incompatibility is the source of the reaction. This test is most commonly a part of post-transfusion antibody screening, which is a battery of testing performed if a transfusion reaction is suspected (see Boxes 2-15 and 2-16).

Most commonly, the recipient has antibodies to the donor WBCs and will experience a fever during transfusion. More severe, however, is the reaction when the donor plasma contains antibodies to the recipient's WBCs. This nonhemolytic reaction can lead to severe transfusion reactions, including acute pulmonary failure (transfusion-related acute lung injury [TRALI]) and multiorgan system failure. The majority of TRALI cases can be triggered by passive transfer of human lymphocyte antigen (HLA) or neutrophil-specific antibodies from the donor to the recipient. TRALI is the leading cause of transfusion-related mortality rates and accounts for 13% of all transfusion deaths.

INTERFERING FACTORS

- Recent administration of dextran may stimulate the induction of WBC antibodies.
- Recent administration of intravenous (IV) contrast media may stimulate the induction of WBC antibodies.
- Blood transfusion in the past 3 months can instigate WBC antibodies to donor blood.

BOX 2-15 Symptoms of a Transfusion Reaction		
• Fever	• Rash	• Bloody urine
• Chills	• Flank/back pain	• Fainting or dizziness

BOX 2-16 Adverse Transfusion Reactions	
Immune Mediated	**Non–Immune Mediated**
• Acute hemolytic reaction	• Fluid overload
• Delayed serologic reaction	• Hypothermia
• Febrile nonhemolytic reaction	• Iron and electrolyte overload
• Allergic reaction	• Coagulation and immune dilution
• Anaphylactic allergic reaction	• Infectious hepatitis
• Acute lung injury	• Human immune deficiency virus
	• Cytomegalovirus
	• Bacteria

PROCEDURE AND PATIENT CARE

Before

☒ Explain the procedure to the patient.
☒ Tell the patient that no fasting is required.

During

- Collect a venous blood sample in a red-top or lavender-top tube.
- Indicate on the request slip that the patient has had a blood transfusion reaction.

After

- Apply pressure to the venipuncture site.

TEST RESULTS AND CLINICAL SIGNIFICANCE

Blood transfusion reaction: *In recipient's or donor's blood, a positive result indicates presence of neutrophil antibodies, identifying the transfusion reaction as a result of these antibodies.*

RELATED TESTS

Coombs Test, Direct (p. 175). This test is performed to identify hemolysis (lysis of red blood cells [RBCs]) or to investigate hemolytic transfusion.

Coombs Test, Indirect (p. 177). This test is used to detect antibodies against RBCs in the serum. It is most commonly used for screening potential blood recipients.

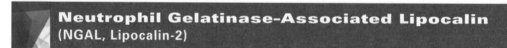

Neutrophil Gelatinase-Associated Lipocalin
(NGAL, Lipocalin-2)

NORMAL FINDING

No rise in NGAL from baseline. (Results vary according to testing methods.)

INDICATIONS

NGAL is a predictor for acute kidney injury (AKI), previously referred to as acute renal failure, and chronic kidney disease (CKD).

TEST EXPLANATION

There are no early markers for acute or chronic renal disease. Serum creatinine levels rise only after there has been significant renal impairment and injury. It is important to note that the earlier renal disease or injury is identified, the more successfully it can be treated. Early treatment also helps to lower the morbidity associated with the disease. This is particularly important in patients who have serious nonrenal disease (e.g., heart surgery, renal transplant, sepsis). In these patients, severe acute kidney injury (AKI) increases morbidity and mortality of hospitalized patients.

NGAL is a member of the lipocalin family of proteins, which bind and transport small lipophilic molecules. NGAL is generally expressed in low concentrations from the renal tubules, but it increases greatly in the presence of epithelial injury and inflammation. A marked elevation in NGAL indicates that renal injury has occurred and aggressive supportive treatment should be instituted. NGAL concentrations rise 48 hours before a rise in creatinine is noted. NGAL can be detected in both urine and blood within two hours of a renal insult.

NGAL can be measured in the urine, plasma, or serum samples with ELISA test kits. Results are available in less than 1 hour in a standard laboratory with conventional ELISA equipment. This is particularly helpful in an intensive care environment. By itself, the absolute baseline laboratory result is not as important as are the succeeding results. Normal values vary according to which laboratory method is used and the patient's baseline GFR. NGAL varies inversely with the GFR. Urine or blood samples can also be analyzed using an established and validated enzyme immunoassay (EIA).

NGAL measurements are being used increasingly in a variety of clinical situations leading to AKI (such as during cardiac surgery, kidney transplantation, contrast nephropathy, and hemolytic uremic syndrome, and in the intensive care setting). It is also useful in conditions leading to CKD (such as lupus nephritis, glomerulonephritis, obstruction, dysplasia, polycystic kidney disease, IgA nephropathy, renal dysplasia, obstructive uropathy, and glomerular and cystic diseases).

PROCEDURE AND PATIENT CARE

Before

- Explain the procedure to the patient.
- Tell the patient that no fasting is required.

During

- Collect a venous blood sample in a red-top tube.
- Collect urine specimens at the same time each day, for consecutive days.

After

- Apply pressure or a pressure dressing to the venipuncture site.
- Observe the venipuncture site for bleeding.
- Results are compared to previous day's testing.

TEST RESULTS AND CLINICAL SIGNIFICANCE

▲ Increased Levels

Primary or secondary renal disease: *Levels of NGAL increase with renal injury.*

RELATED TEST

Serum Creatinine (p. 190). This is a late marker for impaired renal function.

Newborn Metabolic Screening

NORMAL FINDINGS
Negative

 Critical Values

Positive for any one of the tests

INDICATIONS
Newborn metabolic screening is the practice of testing every newborn for certain harmful or potentially fatal disorders that are not otherwise apparent at birth.

TEST EXPLANATION
Newborn screening tests take place before the newborn leaves the hospital. Babies are tested to identify serious or life-threatening (and for the most part preventable or treatable) diseases before symptoms begin. These diseases are usually rare. However, if they are not accurately diagnosed and treated, they can cause mental retardation, severe illness, and premature death in newborns. Many of these are metabolic disorders, often called "inborn errors of metabolism." Other disorders that may be detected through screening are endocrine or hematologic. In most states, this testing is mandatory.

Within 48 hours of a child's birth, a sample of blood is obtained from a "heel stick," and the blood is analyzed. The sample, called a "blood spot," is tested at a reference laboratory. It is generally recommended that the sample be taken *after* the first 24 hours of life. Some tests, such as the one for phenylketonuria (PKU), may not be as sensitive until the newborn has ingested an ample amount of the amino acid phenylalanine, which is a constituent of both human and cow's milk, and after the postnatal thyroid surge has subsided. This is generally after about 2 days.

With the use of *Tandem mass spectrometry* (tandem MS), multiple blood tests can be performed quickly and efficiently. When directed to newborn blood screening, the use of these specialized instruments can detect abnormally elevated proteins associated with certain metabolic disorders. They are capable of screening for more than 20 inherited metabolic disorders with a single test in only a few minutes. Tandem MS is very accurate and can measure very small amounts of similar material with excellent precision. For example, PKU (see below) tandem MS has been shown to reduce the false-positive rate (false alarms) for this disorder more than tenfold compared to the best alternative method available. The disorders listed below are the ones typically included in newborn screening programs:

PKU: An inherited disease, PKU is characterized by deficiency of the enzyme phenylalanine hydroxylase, which converts phenylalanine to tyrosine. Phenylalanine is an essential amino acid necessary for growth; however, any excess must be degraded by conversion to tyrosine. An infant with PKU lacks the ability to make this necessary conversion. Thus phenylalanine accumulates in the body and spills over into the urine. If the amount of phenylalanine is not restricted in infants with PKU, progressive mental retardation results. A low-phenylalanine diet will need to be followed throughout childhood and adolescence and perhaps into adult life. (Incidence: 1 in 10,000 to 25,000.)

Congenital hypothyroidism: Affected babies without treatment experience retarded growth and brain development. If the disorder is detected early, a baby can be treated with oral doses of thyroid hormone to permit normal development. (Incidence: 1 in 4000.)

Galactosemia: Babies with galactosemia lack the enzyme that converts galactose into glucose, a sugar the body is able to use. As a result, milk and other dairy products must be eliminated from the diet. Otherwise, galactose can build up and cause blindness, severe mental retardation, growth deficiency, and even death. (Incidence: 1 in 60,000 to 80,000.) There are several less severe forms of galactosemia that may be detected by newborn screening. These may not require any intervention.

Sickle cell anemia: Sickle cell disease is an inherited blood disease in which red blood cells stretch into abnormal "sickle" shapes (see p. 464). This can cause episodes of pain, damage to vital organs (such as the lungs and kidneys), and even death. Young children with sickle cell anemia are especially prone to certain dangerous bacterial infections. The screening test can also detect other disorders affecting hemoglobin (the oxygen-carrying substance in the blood). (Incidence: about 1 in every 500 African American births and 1 in every 1000 to 1400 Hispanic American births.)

Biotinidase deficiency: Babies with this condition do not have enough biotinidase, an enzyme that recycles biotin (one of the B vitamins) in the body. This deficiency may cause seizures, poor muscle control, immune system impairment, hearing loss, mental retardation, coma, and even death. If the deficiency is detected early, however, problems can be prevented by biotin administration. (Incidence: 1 in 126,000.)

Congenital adrenal hyperplasia: This is actually a group of disorders resulting in a deficiency of adrenal hormones. It can affect the development of the genitals and may cause death. Lifelong treatment through hormone supplementation manages the condition. (Incidence: 1 in 12,000.)

Maple syrup urine disease (MSUD): Babies with MSUD are missing an enzyme needed to process the amino acids leucine, isoleucine, and valine (present in protein-rich foods such as milk, meat, and eggs) that are essential for the body's normal growth. When these are not processed properly, they can build up in the body, causing urine to smell like maple syrup or sweet, burnt sugar. These babies usually have little appetite and are extremely irritable. If not detected and treated early, MSUD can cause mental retardation, physical disability, and even death. A carefully controlled diet free of high-protein foods can prevent these outcomes. (Incidence: 1 in 250,000.)

Homocystinuria: This metabolic disorder results from a deficiency in cystathionine β-synthase, responsible for the metabolism of methionine and homocysteine. If untreated, it can lead to dislocated lenses of the eyes, mental retardation, skeletal abnormalities, and hypercoagulability. However, a special diet combined with dietary supplements may help prevent most of these problems. (Incidence: 1 in 50,000 to 150,000.)

Tyrosinemia: Babies with this disorder cannot metabolize tyrosine. If it accumulates in the body, it can cause mild retardation, language skill difficulties, liver problems, and even death from liver failure. A special diet and sometimes a liver transplant are needed to treat the condition. Early diagnosis and treatment seem to offset long-term problems. (Incidence: not yet determined.)

Cystic fibrosis: This is an inherited disorder expressed in the lung and gastrointestinal tract that causes cells to release thick mucus leading to chronic respiratory disease, problems with digestion, and poor growth. There is no known cure; treatment involves trying to prevent the serious lung infections associated with it and providing adequate nutrition. (Incidence: 1 in 2000 white babies.)

Toxoplasmosis: Toxoplasmosis is a parasitic infection that can be transmitted through the mother's placenta to an unborn child. The disease-causing organism, which is found in undercooked meat, can invade the brain, eye, and muscle, possibly resulting in blindness and mental retardation. (Incidence: 1 in 1000.)

These are not the only metabolic disorders that can be detected through newborn screening. Certain other rare disorders can also be detected and include Duchenne's muscular dystrophy, human immune deficiency virus (HIV) infection, and neuroblastoma. Hematologic disorders, such as glucose-6-phosphate dehydrogenase (G6PD) deficiency and thalassemia, can also be identified.

Most, but not all, states require newborns' hearing to be screened before they are discharged from the hospital. The hearing test involves placing a tiny earphone in the baby's ear and measuring his or her response to sound. A child develops critical speaking and language skills in the first few years of life, and if a hearing loss is discovered early, developmental effects on language skills can be avoided.

INTERFERING FACTORS

- Premature infants may have false-positive results because of delayed development of liver enzymes.
- Infants tested before 24 hours of age may have false-*negative* results.
- Feeding problems (e.g., vomiting) may cause false-*negative* results.

PROCEDURE AND PATIENT CARE

Before

🖎 Inform the parents about the purpose and method of the test.
- Assess the infant's feeding patterns before performing the test. An inadequate amount of protein ingested before performing the test can cause false-*negative* results.

During

- Place a few drops of blood from a heel stick in each circle on the filter paper.
- Indicate on the laboratory slip the infant's name, mother's name, hospital, present date and time, date and time of birth, and primary health care provider.

After

🖎 Inform the parents that if test results are positive they will be notified by their health care provider, and further testing/treatment will be recommended (depending on the particular condition).

TEST RESULTS AND CLINICAL SIGNIFICANCE

Metabolic diseases,
Endocrine diseases,
Hematologic diseases:
　The detection of these disorders before they become clinically apparent may allow opportunities for treatment before there are significant mental or physical harm to the newborn.

　5'-Nucleotidase

NORMAL FINDINGS

0.0-1.6 units at 37° C or 0.0-1.6 units at 37° C (SI units)

INDICATIONS

5'-Nucleotidase is used to support the diagnosis of hepatobiliary obstructive disease. It is especially useful in helping confirm that an elevated alkaline phosphatase (ALP) is the result of liver pathology rather than pathology of another tissue origin.

TEST EXPLANATION

5'-Nucleotidase is an enzyme specific to the liver. The 5'-nucleotidase level is elevated in patients with liver diseases, especially those associated with cholestasis. It provides information similar to ALP. However, ALP is not specific to the liver. Diseases of the bone, sepsis, pregnancy, and other disease can produce ALP elevation. When there is doubt regarding the cause of an elevated ALP, a 5'-nucleotidase test is recommended. If that enzyme is elevated along with the ALP, the pathologic source is certainly the liver. If the 5'-nucleotidase is normal in the face of an elevated ALP, the pathologic source is outside the liver (bone, kidney, spleen). Gamma-glutamyl transpeptidase (GGTP) is used similarly, as it is also specific to the liver. GGTP and ALP can also be elevated from drug-induced cholestasis; 5'-nucleotidase cannot.

INTERFERING FACTORS

Drugs that may cause *increased* 5'-nucleotidase levels include hepatotoxic agents.

PROCEDURE AND PATIENT CARE

Before

☒ Explain the procedure to the patient.
☒ Tell the patient that no fasting is required.

During

- Collect a venous blood sample in a red-top tube.

After

- Apply pressure or a pressure dressing to the venipuncture site.
- Assess the venipuncture site for bleeding. Patients with liver dysfunction often have prolonged clotting times.

TEST RESULTS AND CLINICAL SIGNIFICANCE

▲ Increased Levels

Bile duct obstruction,
Cholestasis:
> *The 5'-nucleotidase test is most specific for pathologic conditions that cause intrahepatic or extrahepatic biliary obstruction.*

Hepatitis,
Cirrhosis,
Hepatic necrosis,
Hepatic ischemia,
Hepatic tumor,
Hepatotoxic drugs:
> *To a lesser degree, hepatocellular disease is associated with elevations of this enzyme.*

RELATED TESTS

Gamma-Glutamyl Transpeptidase (GGTP) (p. 246). This is another enzyme that, when elevated, specifically points to hepatic pathology.

Alkaline Phosphatase (ALP) (p. 47). This is an enzyme that exists in the liver and other organs. It is not specific to the liver.

 Osmolality, Blood (Serum Osmolality)

NORMAL FINDINGS

Adult/elderly: 285-295 mOsm/kg H_2O or 285-295 mmol/kg (SI units)
Child: 275-290 mOsm/kg H_2O

 Critical Values

<265 mOsm/kg H_2O
>320 mOsm/kg H_2O

INDICATIONS

This test is used to gain information about fluid status and electrolyte imbalance. It is also helpful in evaluating illnesses involving antidiuretic hormone (ADH).

TEST EXPLANATION

Osmolality measures the number of dissolved particles in serum/plasma per unit volume. As the amount of free water in the blood increases or the number of particles decreases per unit volume of serum, osmolality decreases. As the amount of water in the blood decreases or the number of particles per unit volume increases, osmolality increases. Osmolality increases with dehydration and decreases with overhydration.

There is an elaborate feedback mechanism that controls osmolality. Increased osmolality will stimulate secretion of ADH. This will result in increased water reabsorption in the kidney, more concentrated urine, and less concentrated serum. A low serum osmolality will suppress the release of ADH, resulting in decreased water reabsorption and large amounts of dilute urine. The simultaneous use of urine osmolality (p. 938) helps in the interpretation and evaluation of problems involving osmolality.

The serum osmolality test is useful in evaluating fluid and electrolyte imbalance. The test is very helpful in the evaluation of seizures, ascites, hydration status, acid-base balance, suspected antidiuretic hormone (ADH) abnormalities, and suspected poisoning. Osmolality is also helpful in identifying the presence of organic acids, sugars, and ethanol.

The osmolality can be predicted based on calculations of serum sodium, glucose, and BUN—the three most important solutes in the blood.

The equation is:

$$Osmolality = 2 \times Na + \frac{Glu}{18} + \frac{BUN}{2.8}$$

The normal range of serum osmolality is 285 to 295 mOsm/L. The measured osmolality should not exceed the predicted by more than 10 mOsm/L. A difference of more than 10 mOsm/L is considered an *osmolal gap* or *delta gap*. Causes for a serum osmolal gap include mannitol, ethanol, methanol, ethylene glycol, and other toxins in very high concentration, usually small molecules. Another measure providing similar data is the ratio of serum sodium to osmolality. Normally the ratio of serum sodium, in mEq/L, to serum osmolality, in mOsm/kg, is between 0.43 and 0.5. The ratio may be distorted in drug intoxication.

Osmolality may have a role in evaluation of coma patients. Values greater than 385 mOsm/kg H_2O are associated with stupor in patients with hyperglycemia. When values of 400 to 420 are detected, grand mal seizures can occur. Values greater than 420 can be lethal. The simultaneous use of urine osmolality (p. 938) helps in the interpretation and evaluation of problems with osmolality.

Clinical Priorities

- This test provides valuable information about fluid and electrolyte balance.
- Osmolality increases with dehydration and decreases with overhydration.
- The simultaneous measurement of urine osmolality helps in interpreting and evaluating problems with fluid balance.

PROCEDURE AND PATIENT CARE

Before
 Explain the procedure to the patient.
Tell the patient that no fasting is required.

During
- Collect a venous blood sample in a red-top tube.
- For pediatric patients, draw blood from a heel stick.

After
- Apply pressure or a pressure dressing to the venipuncture site.
- Observe the venipuncture site for bleeding.

TEST RESULTS AND CLINICAL SIGNIFICANCE

▲ Increased Levels

Hypernatremia,
Hyperglycemia,
Hyperosmolar nonketotic hyperglycemia,
Ketosis,
Azotemia:
All of the above illnesses are associated with an increase in the number of particles dissolved in the blood.
Dehydration: *Decreased replacement of ongoing water losses leads to dehydration and a rise in the serum osmolality.*
Mannitol therapy,
Ingestion of ethanol, methanol, or ethylene glycol:

These drugs stimulate free water loss from the kidneys and excretion in the urine. As a result, the serum osmolality is increased. Furthermore, their by-products cause an increase in the number of solutes in the blood and thereby increase the osmolality.

Uremia,

Diabetes insipidus,

Renal tubular necrosis,

Severe pyelonephritis:

The above illnesses are associated with poor urine concentration. Free water is lost and serum osmolality increases.

▼ Decreased Levels

Overhydration: *The provision of free water above the ongoing losses creates a situation in which there is excess free water in the blood. Serum osmolality decreases.*

Syndrome of inappropriate ADH (SIADH) secretion: *Several illnesses can create this syndrome. ADH is inappropriately secreted despite factors that normally would inhibit its secretion. As a result, large quantities of water are reabsorbed by the kidney. The serum becomes dilute and osmolality decreases.*

Paraneoplastic syndromes associated with carcinoma (lung, breast, colon): *These cancers act as an autonomous ectopic source for the secretion of ADH. The pathophysiology is the same as described above for SIADH.*

RELATED TESTS

Urine Osmolality (p. 938). This is a measurement of the concentration of dissolved particles in the urine. When measured with the serum osmolality, greater insight is obtained about problems of fluid balance.

Antidiuretic Hormone (ADH) (p. 73). This is a direct measurement of ADH in the blood.

Antidiuretic Hormone (ADH) Suppression (p. 76). This test is very helpful in the evaluation of ADH abnormalities.

Parathyroid Hormone (PTH, Parathormone)

NORMAL FINDINGS

Assay	Assay Includes	Conventional Normal Values (pg/mL)	SI Units (ng/L)
PTH intact (whole)	Intact PTH	10-65	10-65
PTH N-terminal	N-terminal	8-24	8-24
	Intact PTH		
PTH C-terminal	C-terminal		
	Intact PTH	50-330	50-330
	Midmolecule		

INDICATIONS

PTH is measured to assist in the evaluation of hypercalcemia or hypocalcemia. It is routinely monitored in patients with chronic renal failure (CRF).

TEST EXPLANATION

PTH is the only hormone secreted by the parathyroid gland in response to hypocalcemia. When calcium serum levels return to normal, PTH levels diminish. PTH, therefore, is one of the major factors affecting calcium metabolism. This test is useful in establishing a diagnosis of hyperparathyroidism and distinguishing nonparathyroid from parathyroid causes of hypercalcemia. Increased PTH levels are seen in patients with hyperparathyroidism (primary, secondary, or tertiary); in patients with nonparathyroid, ectopic PTH-producing tumors (pseudohyperparathyroidism); or as a normal compensatory response to hypocalcemia in patients with malabsorption or vitamin D deficiency.

Primary hyperparathyroidism is most often caused by a parathyroid adenoma and only rarely from parathyroid cancer. These patients have high PTH and calcium levels. Secondary hyperparathyroidism is the exaggerated response of the parathyroid gland to kidney insensitivity to PTH in CRF patients. CRF patients have chronically low serum calcium levels in reaction to persistently high levels of phosphate that the kidney fails to excrete. In response to this persistently low calcium, the parathyroid is constantly stimulated to produce PTH to attempt to maintain a normal calcium level. This is called secondary hyperparathyroidism. These patients have high PTH and normal to slightly low calcium levels. Occasionally a patient with CRF overshoots the compensatory process and autonomously develops unnecessarily high PTH production that leads to hypercalcemia. This is called tertiary hyperparathyroidism. These patients have high PTH and high calcium levels.

It is important to measure serum calcium (see p. 138) simultaneously with PTH. Most laboratories have a PTH/calcium nomogram already made up indicating what PTH level is considered normal for each calcium level.

Decreased PTH levels are seen in patients with hypoparathyroidism or as a compensatory response to hypercalcemia in patients with metastatic bone tumors, sarcoidosis, vitamin D intoxication, or milk-alkali syndrome. Of course, surgical ablation of the parathyroid glands is another cause of hypoparathyroidism.

Whole (intact) PTH is metabolized to several different fragments, including an amino or N-terminal, a midregion or midmolecule, and a carboxyl or C-terminal. The intact PTH and the N-terminal are metabolically active. These can all be measured by immunoassay. The intact PTH and all fragments generally provide accurate information concerning the level of PTH in the blood. The intact PTH is probably most often tested as it is most reliable.

INTERFERING FACTORS

- Recent injection of radioisotopes may interfere with this test if radioimmunoassay (RIA) methods are used. However, RIA is not a frequently used method of measuring PTH fragments.
- Drugs that *increase* PTH include anticonvulsants, isoniazid, lithium, phosphates, rifampin, and steroids.
- Drugs that *decrease* PTH include cimetidine, pindolol, and propranolol.

✓ Clinical Priorities

- This test is routinely monitored in patients with CRF. These patients have chronically low serum calcium levels in reaction to persistently high phosphate levels that the kidney fails to excrete.
- It is important to measure serum PTH and serum calcium levels at the same time. These values are important for a differential diagnosis. Most laboratories have PTH/calcium nomograms indicating normal PTH levels for each calcium level.
- PTH levels are affected by a diurnal variation. Levels are highest around 2 AM and lowest around 2 PM. Usually an 8 AM blood specimen is drawn. If the patient works nights, the laboratory should be notified so that changes in the diurnal variation can be factored in.

PROCEDURE AND PATIENT CARE

Before

✗ Explain the procedure to the patient.

- Keep the patient on nothing by mouth (NPO) status except for water after midnight on the day of the test.

During

- Obtain an 8 AM blood specimen, because diurnal rhythm affects PTH levels. (Check with the laboratory if the patient works at night.) PTH levels are highest around 2 AM and lowest around 2 PM.
- Collect a venous blood sample in a red-top tube. Note that some laboratories require blood in an iced plastic syringe.
- Obtain a serum calcium level determination at the same time if ordered. The serum PTH and serum calcium levels are important for a differential diagnosis.

After

- Indicate on the laboratory slip the time the blood was drawn, because a diurnal rhythm affects test results.
- Apply pressure or a pressure dressing to the venipuncture site.
- Check the venipuncture site for bleeding.
- Most PTH specimens are sent to a central laboratory. The specimen should be kept cold and transported on dry ice.

TEST RESULTS AND CLINICAL SIGNIFICANCE

▲ Increased Levels

Hyperparathyroidism secondary to adenoma or carcinoma of the parathyroid gland: *PTH is autonomously produced by the parathyroid gland. PTH levels are elevated.*

Non–PTH-producing tumors (paraneoplastic syndrome) commonly noted with lung, kidney, or breast carcinoma: *These tumors produce a "PTH-related protein" that acts like PTH and increases serum calcium. Because it is structurally similar to PTH, it is measured with PTH testing and gives a falsely high PTH result.*

Congenital renal defect: *These patients have a congenital kidney nonresponsiveness to "normal" quantities of PTH. As a result, calcium decreases despite normal quantities of PTH. The parathyroid is called on to produce even greater quantities of PTH. This is also called pseudohyperparathyroidism.*

Hypocalcemia: *PTH elevation is the result of a physiologic compensation for low serum calcium.*

Chronic renal failure: *These patients cannot excrete phosphates. As a result, serum calcium levels diminish. PTH elevation is the result of a physiologic compensation for low serum calcium. This is secondary hyperparathyroidism. Occasionally a patient with CRF develops parathyroid hyperplasia that leads to PTH levels in excess of the amount required for physiologic homeostasis. This is called tertiary hyperparathyroidism.*

Malabsorption syndrome: *These patients do not absorb calcium or fat-soluble vitamins such as vitamin D. Serum calcium falls. PTH elevation is the result of a physiologic compensation for low serum calcium.*

Vitamin D deficiency and rickets: *Vitamin D is integral to the absorption of calcium from the gut. With inadequate levels, serum calcium decreases. PTH elevation is the result of a physiologic compensation for low serum calcium.*

▼ Decreased Levels

Hypoparathyroidism caused by surgical ablation or immunoablation: *PTH is not produced at levels necessary to maintain normal calcium levels.*

Hypercalcemia: *Reduced PTH is a normal physiologic response to high serum calcium.*

Metastatic bone tumor: *Tumor in the bone can mobilize large quantities of calcium. Reduced PTH is a normal physiologic response to high serum calcium.*

Hypercalcemia of malignancy (most often with lung, breast, or lymphoma cancer): *For unknown reasons, serum calcium levels become very high in these cancer patients. They do not have bone metastasis or PTH-related proteins. Reduced PTH is a normal physiologic response to high serum calcium.*

Sarcoidosis: *These patients can develop elevated serum calcium levels. Reduced PTH is a normal physiologic response to high serum calcium.*

Vitamin D intoxication: *These patients have high serum calcium levels as a result of vitamin D stimulating maximal calcium intestinal absorption. Reduced PTH is a normal physiologic response to high serum calcium.*

Milk-alkali syndrome: *These infants are given cooked whole milk that is very high in calcium. They develop high serum calcium levels. Reduced PTH is a normal physiologic response to high serum calcium.*

DiGeorge syndrome: *These immunodeficient children also have hypocalcemia that may be due to hypoparathyroidism.*

RELATED TESTS

Calcium, Blood (p. 138). This is a direct measurement of serum calcium. This test should be done simultaneously with a PTH test to improve interpretation of PTH levels.

Phosphate (p. 391). This is a direct measurement of the inorganic phosphate levels in the serum, which are affected by PTH.

Partial Thromboplastin Time, Activated (aPTT, Partial Thromboplastin Time [PTT])

NORMAL FINDINGS

aPTT: 30-40 seconds
PTT: 60-70 seconds
Patients receiving anticoagulant therapy: 1.5-2.5 times control value in seconds

 Critical Values

aPTT: >70 seconds
PTT: >100 seconds

INDICATIONS

The PTT test is used to assess the intrinsic system and the common pathway of clot formation. It is also used to monitor heparin therapy.

TEST EXPLANATION

Hemostasis and the coagulation system represent a homeostatic balance between factors encouraging clotting and factors encouraging clot dissolution. The first reaction of the body to active bleeding is blood vessel constriction. In small vessel injury this may be enough to stop bleeding. In large vessel injury, hemostasis is required to form a clot that will durably plug the hole until healing can occur. The primary phase of the hemostatic mechanism involves platelet aggregation to blood vessel (see Figure 2-12 on p. 167). Next, secondary hemostasis occurs. The first phase of reactions is called the intrinsic system. Factor XII and other proteins form a complex on the subendothelial collagen in the injured blood vessel. Through a series of reactions, activated factor XI (XIa) is formed and activates factor IX (IXa). In a complex formed by factors VIII, IX, and X, activated X (Xa) is formed.

At the same time the extrinsic system is activated and a complex is formed between tissue thromboplastin (factor III) and factor VII. Activated factor VII (VIIa) results. VIIa can directly activate factor X. Alternatively, VIIa can activate IX and X together.

The final step is a common pathway in which prothrombin is converted to thrombin on the surface of the aggregated platelets. The main purpose of thrombin is to convert fibrinogen to fibrin, which is then polymerized into a stable gel. Factor XIII crosslinks the fibrin polymers to form a stable clot.

Almost immediately three major activators of the fibrinolytic system act on plasminogen, which had previously been absorbed into the clot, to form plasmin. Plasmin degenerates the fibrin polymer into fragments that are cleared by macrophages.

The PTT evaluates factors I (fibrinogen), II (prothrombin), V, VIII, IX, X, XI, and XII. When the PTT is combined with the prothrombin time, nearly all of the hemostatic abnormalities can be recognized. When any of these factors exists in inadequate quantities, as in hemophilia A and B or consumptive coagulopathy, the PTT is prolonged. Because factors II, IX, and X are vitamin K–dependent factors, biliary obstruction, which precludes GI absorption of fat and fat-soluble vitamins (e.g., vitamin K), can reduce their concentration and thus prolong the PTT. Because coagulation factors are made in the liver, hepatocellular diseases will also prolong the PTT.

Heparin has been found to inactivate prothrombin (factor II) and to prevent the formation of thromboplastin. These actions prolong the intrinsic clotting pathway for approximately 4 to 6 hours after each dose of heparin. Therefore heparin is capable of providing therapeutic anticoagulation. The appropriate dose of heparin can be monitored by the PTT. PTT test results are given in seconds along with a control value. The control value may vary slightly from day to day because of the reagents used.

Recently activators have been added to the PTT test reagents to shorten normal clotting time and provide a narrow normal range. This shortened time is called the activated PTT. The normal aPTT is 30 to 40 seconds. Desired ranges for therapeutic anticoagulation are 1.5 to 2.5 times normal (e.g., 70 seconds). The aPTT specimen should be drawn 30 to 60 minutes before the patient's next heparin dose is given. If the aPTT is less than 50 seconds, therapeutic anticoagulation may not have been achieved and more heparin is needed. An aPTT greater than 100 seconds indicates that too much heparin is being given; the risk for serious spontaneous bleeding exists when the aPTT is this high. The effects of heparin can be reversed by the parenteral administration of 1 mg of protamine sulfate for every 100 units of the heparin dose.

Heparin's effect, unlike that of warfarin, is immediate and short lived. When a thromboembolic episode (e.g., pulmonary embolism, arterial embolism, thrombophlebitis) occurs, immediate and complete anticoagulation is most rapidly and safely achieved by heparin administration. This drug is often given during cardiac and vascular surgery to prevent intravascular clotting during clamping of the vessels. Often small doses of heparin (5000 units subcutaneously every 12 hours) are given to prevent thromboembolism in high-risk patients. This dose alters the PTT very little, and the risk for spontaneous bleeding is minimal.

INTERFERING FACTORS

- Drugs that may *prolong* PTT test values include antihistamines, ascorbic acid, chlorpromazine, heparin, and salicylates.

Clinical Priorities

- The PTT is used to monitor heparin therapy. Heparin's effect is immediate and short lived.
- If too much heparin is given, its effects can be reversed by parenteral administration of protamine sulfate.
- Patients receiving heparin need to be evaluated for bleeding tendencies. These include bruising, petechiae, low-back pain, and bleeding gums. Blood may be detected in the urine and stool.

PROCEDURE AND PATIENT CARE

Before

- Explain the procedure to the patient.
- If the patient is receiving heparin by intermittent injection, plan to draw the blood specimen for the aPTT 30 minutes to 60 minutes before the next dose of heparin.
- If the patient is receiving a continuous heparin infusion, draw the blood at any time.

During

- Collect a venous blood sample in one or two blue-top tubes.

After

- Apply pressure or a pressure dressing to the venipuncture site.
- Assess the venipuncture site for bleeding. Remember, if the patient is receiving anticoagulants or has coagulopathies, the bleeding time will be increased.
- Assess the patient to detect possible bleeding. Check for blood in the urine and all other excretions and assess the patient for bruises, petechiae, and bleeding gums.
- If severe bleeding occurs, note that the anticoagulant effect of heparin can be reversed by parenteral administration of protamine sulfate.

TEST RESULTS AND CLINICAL SIGNIFICANCE

▲ Increased Levels

Congenital clotting factor deficiencies (e.g., von Willebrand disease, hemophilia, hypofibrinogenemia): *These hereditary illnesses are associated with very little, if any, of the respective clotting factors. As a result, the PTT is prolonged.*

Cirrhosis of liver,

Vitamin K deficiency: *The liver makes most of the clotting factors. For synthesis of some of those clotting factors, vitamin K is required. In the above illnesses the clotting factors of the intrinsic system and common pathways are inadequate in quantity. As a result, the PTT is prolonged.*

Disseminated intravascular coagulation (DIC): *Key clotting factors involved in the intrinsic system are consumed.*

Heparin administration: *Heparin inhibits the intrinsic system at several points. As a result, the PTT is prolonged.*

Coumarin administration: *Although coumarin has a greater impact on the prothrombin time, it does inhibit the function of factors II, IX, and X. As a result, the PTT is prolonged.*

▼ **Decreased Levels**

Early stages of DIC: *Circulating procoagulants exist in the early stages of DIC. These act to shorten or decrease the PTT.*

Extensive cancer (e.g., ovarian, pancreatic, colon): *The pathophysiology of this association is not well known.*

RELATED TESTS

Prothrombin Time (p. 434). This test is used to evaluate the adequacy of the extrinsic system and common pathway in the clotting mechanism.

Coagulating Factor Concentration (p. 163). This is a quantitative measurement of specific coagulation factors.

Parvovirus B19 Antibody

NORMAL FINDINGS

Negative for immunoglobulin (Ig)M- and IgG-specific antibodies to parvovirus B19

INDICATIONS

This test is performed on children who have vague symptoms of fever, arthralgias, and rash suggestive of erythema infectiosum. It is also becoming a part of routine testing for proposed organ donors.

TEST EXPLANATION

The parvovirus group includes several species-specific viruses of animals. Parvovirus B19 is known to be a human pathogen. Many of the severe manifestations of B19 viremia relate to the ability of the virus to infect and lyse red blood cells (RBCs) precursors in the bone marrow. The name "B19" was derived from the code number of the human serum in which the virus was discovered.

Erythema infectiosum is the most common manifestation of B19 infection and occurs predominantly in children. This pathogen is also referred to as "fifth disease," because it was classified in the late nineteenth century as the fifth in a series of six exanthems of childhood. This infection is also sometimes referred to as "academy rash." The typical presentation is a self-limiting, mild illness with a low-grade fever, malar rash, and occasionally arthralgia. Normally the rash begins on the face and may also develop on the arms and legs. Outbreaks of erythema infectiosum appear most often during the winter and spring months.

Parvovirus B19 has also been associated with a number of other clinical problems, including:

- Flulike illness associated with joint inflammation, rash, and occasionally purpura in young adults.
- Increased risk for abortion or stillbirth caused by hydrops fetalis and fetal loss in some infected pregnant women.
- Transient aplastic crisis in patients with chronic hemolytic anemia. In immunocompromised patients (acquired immunodeficiency syndrome [AIDS] patients, organ donors), this virus can be so severe as to cause aplastic anemia and bone marrow failure. With increasing frequency, this antibody test is being used for all potential organ donors.
- Chronic severe anemia in patients with immunodeficiency related to infection with human immune deficiency virus (HIV), congenital immunodeficiency, acute lymphocytic leukemia during maintenance chemotherapy, and recipients of bone marrow transplants.

Because of the recently discovered spectrum of diseases caused by parvovirus B19, laboratory diagnosis has come into great demand. Serologic testing for parvovirus B19–specific IgM and IgG antibodies can be detected by enzyme-linked immunosorbent assay (ELISA) and indirect fluorescent antibody immunofluorescence methods. Acute infections can be determined by B19-compatible symptoms and the presence of IgM antibodies that remain detectable up to a few months. Past infection or immunity is documented by IgG antibodies that persist indefinitely with IgM antibodies. Fetal infection may be recognized by hydrops fetalis and the presence of B19 DNA in amniotic fluid or fetal blood.

PROCEDURE AND PATIENT CARE

Before
☒ Explain the procedure to the patient.
☒ Tell the patient that no fasting or special preparation is necessary.

During
• Collect a venous blood sample according to the laboratory protocol.

After
• Apply pressure or a pressure dressing to the venipuncture site.
• Assess the venipuncture site for bleeding.
☒ Inform the patient that it normally requires approximately 2 to 3 days to receive test results.

TEST RESULTS AND CLINICAL SIGNIFICANCE

▲ Increased Levels

Erythema infectiosum (fifth disease),
Joint arthralgia and arthritis:
These diseases are self-limiting and elevate antibodies through the course of viremia.
Hydrops fetalis,
Fetal loss:
These obstetric disasters could be due to maternal infection with parvovirus.
Transient aplastic anemia,
Chronic anemia,
Bone marrow failure:
These problems occur mostly in patients who are immunocompromised. In such patients the viremia is much more significant. RBC precursors are target cells for the virus.

Pepsinogen

NORMAL FINDINGS

Pepsinogen I: 28-100 ng/mL
Pepsinogen II: <22 ng/mL

INDICATIONS

This test is used to identify pernicious anemia (PA), gastric atrophy, or peptic disease. It is also used to identify precancerous changes in those at great risk for gastric carcinoma.

TEST EXPLANATION

Pepsinogens are secreted in the stomach and are made in the oxyntic gland mucosa of the proximal stomach. When exposed to gastric acid, pepsinogen is converted to pepsin, an active enzyme that is proteolytic and promotes digestion. Patients with gastric atrophy, pernicious anemia (PA), or those who have had gastrectomy have low levels of pepsinogen I. Pepsinogen I levels are slightly elevated in gastric ulcer, higher in gastroduodenal ulcer, and significantly elevated in duodenal ulcer. Patients with Zollinger-Ellison syndrome exhibit greatly elevated levels. Pepsinogen I has been used as a subclinical marker of increased risk for stomach cancer. Pepsinogen I can also be measured in the urine.

Pepsinogen II is made by oxyntic gland mucosa cells that are in the distal stomach and proximal duodenum. Because PA generally affects the proximal stomach, diminished levels of pepsinogen I with normal levels of pepsinogen II are strongly supportive of PA.

Pepsinogens are measured by immunoassay techniques in the blood and urine.

PROCEDURE AND PATIENT CARE

Before

☒ Explain the test to the patient.

☒ Instruct the patient to fast for 10 to 12 hours before collection of the specimen.

☒ Tell the patient that antacids or other medications affecting stomach acidity or gastrointestinal motility should be discontinued, if possible, for at least 48 hours before collection. Verify with the laboratory or health care provider.

During

• Collect a venous blood sample in a red-top tube.

After

• Apply pressure or a pressure dressing to the venipuncture site.
• Deliver the blood specimen to the laboratory as soon as possible.
• The specimen is usually frozen because most testing is performed in a central laboratory.

TEST RESULTS AND CLINICAL SIGNIFICANCES

▼ Decreased Values

Pernicious anemia,

Gastric atrophy,

Chronic gastritis:
   These diseases are associated with gastric mucosal atrophy. Therefore pepsinogen I synthesis will be reduced.

Peptic ulcer disease: *The exact pathophysiology of this finding is not clear. It might be related to the reactive inflammatory changes associated with active ulcer disease.*

RELATED TESTS

Intrinsic Factor Antibody (p. 320). This antibody is used to diagnosis pernicious anemia (PA).

Anti-Parietal Cell Antibody (p. 92). These antibodies are associated with PA.

Vitamin B$_{12}$ (p. 518). Deficient levels are associated with PA.

Pheochromocytoma Suppression and Provocative Testing (Clonidine suppression test [CST], Glucagon stimulation test)

NORMAL FINDINGS

Glucagon Stimulation
Norepinephrine: <3 times basal levels

Clonidine Suppression
Norepinephrine: >50% reduction in basal levels or <500 pg/mL
Epinephrine: >50% reduction in basal levels or <275 pg/mL

INDICATIONS
These tests are used to identify pheochromocytoma when catecholamine levels are not assuredly diagnostic.

TEST EXPLANATION
In patients with significantly high blood pressure that is refractory to treatment, the diagnosis of pheochromocytoma (PH) is often considered. PHs usually arise from the adrenal glands and are often difficult to detect. Pheochromocytomas release chemicals called catecholamines, causing high blood pressure that is excessive and resistant to treatment. The definitive diagnosis of pheochromocytoma rests primarily on the demonstration of excessive catecholamine production, best achieved with a resting plasma catecholamine assay. When basal catecholamine plasma levels are excessive (norepinephrine >2000 pg/mL) in nonstressed patients, the diagnosis of PH is certain. However, when basal levels are far less than 2000 pg/mL, the diagnosis of PH is far less certain. Plasma catecholamine levels are not often helpful unless the blood specimen is obtained during a hypertensive paroxysm. Urine metanephrines (p. 975) are best tested at times other than hypertensive episodes.

When the diagnosis of PH is not certain, suppression and provocative tests may be necessary. Plasma catecholamines *(epinephrine and norepinephrine)* are particularly useful during suppression or provocative tests.

Normally, glucagon (less commonly metoclopramide and naloxone) is used as a provocative agent. Glucagon stimulates the release of catecholamines. In the presence of pheochromocytoma, the agents can cause the tumor to release excessive catecholamines into the bloodstream. The glucagon stimulation test has been superseded in recent years by the clonidine suppression test because it can provoke dangerous increases in blood pressure in patients with pheochromocytomas.

Clonidine is normally a potent suppressor of catecholamine production. Yet it has little to no suppressive effect on catecholamines in patients with pheochromocytoma. Suppressive testing is much safer than provocative testing because there is no real chance of a hypertensive paroxysm. The clonidine suppression test (CST) is nearly 100% accurate.

CONTRAINDICATIONS
- Patients with hypovolemia should not have suppression testing because they could experience a precipitous drop in blood pressure.

POTENTIAL COMPLICATIONS

- Drowsiness during CST
- Hypotension during CST, especially in patients treated aggressively for hypertension
- Extremely high blood pressure during provocative testing: If a patient develops a sudden increase in blood pressure, intravenous medication may be administered in an attempt to control the blood pressure.

INTERFERING FACTORS

- False suppression with CST may occur in patients with low basal catecholamine levels.
- Drugs that may cause *false-positive* suppression tests include antidepressants and beta-blockers.

PROCEDURE AND PATIENT CARE

Before

- Explain the procedure to the patient.
- Identify and explain the medications being administered before testing.
- The patient must be reclining calmly for 30 minutes before testing.

During

- Collect a venous blood sample from an antecubital vein in a heparinized tube for determination of basal catecholamine levels (epinephrine and norepinephrine).
- Monitor vital signs closely throughout the testing period.

Glucagon provocative test

- Administer a prescribed dose of glucagon intravenously.
- Two minutes later, obtain a blood specimen as described above.
- Be prepared to treat a severe hypertensive episode.

Clonidine suppression test

- Administer a prescribed dose of clonidine orally.
- Three hours later, obtain a blood specimen as described above.

After

- Monitor vital signs for at least 1 hour after conclusion of the procedure.

TEST RESULTS AND CLINICAL SIGNIFICANCE

Pheochromocytoma: *This is a rare catecholamine-secreting tumor of the adrenal gland derived from chromaffin cells. These tumors can also arise outside the adrenal gland and are termed extraadrenal pheochromocytomas or paragangliomas. They may precipitate life-threatening hypertension or cardiac arrhythmias.*

RELATED TEST

Vanillylmandelic Acid (p. 975). This 24-hour urine test for VMA and catecholamines is performed primarily to diagnose hypertension secondary to pheochromocytoma. It is also used to detect the presence of neuroblastomas and other rare adrenal tumors.

Phosphate (PO₄), Phosphorus (P)

NORMAL FINDINGS

Adult: 3.0-4.5 mg/dL or 0.97-1.45 mmol/L (SI units)
Elderly: values slightly lower than adult
Child: 4.5-6.5 mg/dL or 1.45-2.10 mmol/L (SI units)
Newborn: 4.3-9.3 mg/dL or 1.4-3.0 mmol/L (SI units)

 Critical Values

<1 mg/dL

INDICATIONS

This test is performed to assist in the interpretation of studies investigating parathyroid and calcium abnormalities. It is usually done to measure phosphate levels and ensure that adequate blood levels exist.

TEST EXPLANATION

Phosphorus in the body is in the form of a phosphate. Phosphorus and phosphate will be used interchangeably throughout this and other discussions. Most of the phosphate in the body is a part of organic compounds. Only a small part of total body phosphate is inorganic phosphate (i.e., not part of another organic compound). It is the inorganic phosphate that is measured when a "phosphate," "phosphorus," "inorganic phosphorus," or "inorganic phosphate" is requested. Most of the body's inorganic phosphorus is intracellular and combined with calcium within the skeleton; however, approximately 15% of the phosphorus exists in the blood as a phosphate salt. The organic phosphate (not measured by this test) is used to synthesize part of the phospholipid compounds in the cell membrane, adenosine triphosphatase (ATP) for energy source in metabolism, nucleic acids, or enzymes (e.g., 2,3-diphosphoglycerate). The inorganic phosphate (measured in this test) contributes to electrical and acid-base homeostasis.

Dietary phosphorus is absorbed in the small bowel. The absorption is very efficient, and only rarely is hypophosphatemia caused by gastrointestinal (GI) malabsorption. Antacids, however, can bind phosphorus and decrease intestinal absorption. Renal excretion of phosphorus should equal dietary intake to maintain a normal serum phosphate level. Phosphate levels vary significantly during the day, with lowest values occurring around 10 AM and highest values occurring 12 hours later.

Phosphorus levels are determined by calcium metabolism, parathormone (parathyroid hormone [PTH]), renal excretion, and, to a lesser degree, intestinal absorption. Because an inverse relationship exists between calcium and phosphorus, a decrease of one mineral results in an increase in the other. Therefore, serum phosphorus levels depend on calcium metabolism and vice versa. The regulation of phosphate by PTH is such that PTH tends to decrease phosphate reabsorption in the kidney. PTH and vitamin D, however, tend to stimulate phosphate absorption weakly within the gut.

Hypophosphatemia may have four general causes: shift of phosphate from extracellular to intracellular, renal phosphate wasting, loss from the gastrointestinal tract, and loss from intracellular stores. Hyperphosphatemia is usually secondary to increased intake or an inability of the kidneys to excrete phosphate.

INTERFERING FACTORS

- Recent carbohydrate ingestion, including intravenous (IV) glucose administration, causes decreased phosphorus levels, because phosphorus enters the cell with glucose.
- Laxatives or enemas containing sodium phosphate can *increase* phosphorus levels.
- Drugs that may cause *increased* levels include methicillin, steroids, some diuretics (furosemide and thiazides), and vitamin D (excessive).
- Drugs that may cause *decreased* levels include antacids, albuterol, anesthesia agents, estrogens, insulin, oral contraceptives, and mannitol.

PROCEDURE AND PATIENT CARE

Before

- Explain the procedure to the patient.
- Keep the patient on nothing by mouth (NPO) status after midnight on the day of the test.
- If indicated, discontinue IV fluids with glucose for several hours before the test.

During

- Collect a venous blood sample in a red-top tube.
- Avoid hemolysis. Handle the tube carefully. Hemolysis can falsely elevate the phosphate level because phosphate is an intracellular ion. Cellular lysis of red blood cells (RBCs) will cause the intracellular phosphate to spill into the blood.
- Use a heel stick to draw blood from infants.

After

- Take the specimen to the laboratory immediately.
- Indicate on the laboratory slip the time the blood was obtained.
- Apply pressure or a pressure dressing to the venipuncture site.
- Check the venipuncture site for bleeding.

TEST RESULTS AND CLINICAL SIGNIFICANCE

▲ Increased Levels (Hyperphosphatemia)

Hypoparathyroidism: *Renal reabsorption is enhanced.*

Renal failure: *Renal excretion of phosphates is diminished.*

Increased dietary or IV intake of phosphorus: *The increased intake obviously leads to transiently elevated phosphate levels.*

Acromegaly: *Renal reabsorption is enhanced.*

Bone metastasis: *The phosphate stores in the bones are mobilized by the destructive bone tumors.*

Sarcoidosis: *Intestinal absorption of phosphates is increased because of the vitamin D effect produced by granulomatous infections.*

Hypocalcemia: *Calcium and phosphates exist in an inverse relationship. When one is elevated, the other is low.*

Acidosis: *When the pH is reduced, phosphates are driven out of the cell and into the bloodstream as part of a buffering system.*

Rhabdomyolysis,
Advanced lymphoma or myeloma,
Hemolytic anemia:
　　Cell lysis associated with the above diseases causes intracellular phosphate to pour out into the bloodstream. Phosphate levels rise.

▼　Decreased Levels (Hypophosphatemia)

Inadequate dietary ingestion of phosphorus: *This is very rare, because phosphate reabsorption in the intestine is so efficient.*
Chronic antacid ingestion: *Antacids bind the phosphate in the intestine and preclude absorption.*
Hyperparathyroidism: *PTH increases urinary excretion of phosphates.*
Hypercalcemia: *Calcium and phosphate levels have an inverse relationship. When one is elevated, the other is low.*
Chronic alcoholism: *The pathophysiology of this observation is probably due to multiple causes. It may be in part nutritional and in part because of magnesium deficiency.*
Vitamin D deficiency (rickets): *Renal tubules fail to reabsorb phosphates.*
Treatment of hyperglycemia,
Hyperinsulinism (childhood):
　　Insulin tends to drive phosphates into the cells.
Malnutrition: *Rarely is malnutrition a cause of phosphate deficiency, because phosphate is so efficiently absorbed through the intestine. However, when malnutrition is associated with a deficiency of fat-soluble vitamins such as vitamin D, phosphate renal reabsorption is diminished. Phosphate levels decrease.*
Alkalosis: *Phosphate acts as a buffer. When pH increases, phosphate levels in the blood diminish because of an intracellular shift.*
Gram-negative sepsis

RELATED TESTS

Parathyroid Hormone (p. 380). This is a measurement of parathyroid hormone, which raises serum phosphate and calcium levels.
Calcium, Blood (p. 138). This is a direct measurement of serum calcium. This test should be done simultaneously with phosphate measurements.

Phosphatidylinositol Antigen (PI-Linked Antigen)

NORMAL FINDINGS

RBCs
　　Type I (normal expression): 99%-100%
　　Type II (partial deficient): 0%-0.99%
　　Type III (deficient): 0%-0.01%
Granulocytes: 0%-0.01%
Monocytes: 0%-0.05%

INDICATIONS

The PI-linked antigen is useful for screening and confirming the diagnosis of paroxysmal nocturnal hemoglobinuria (PNH). It is also used to monitor the disease.

TEST EXPLANATION

Paroxysmal nocturnal hemoglobinuria (PNH) is an acquired hematologic disorder of the bone marrow stem cell that is characterized by nocturnal hemoglobinuria, chronic hemolytic anemia, thrombosis, and pancytopenia, and in some patients by acute or chronic myeloid malignancies. These patients have dark urine caused by ongoing hemolysis. PNH appears to be a hematopoietic stem cell disorder that affects erythroid, granulocytic, and megakaryocytic cell lines. The abnormal cells in PNH have been shown to lack glycosylphosphatidylinositol (GPI)-linked proteins in RBCs and WBCs. Mutations in the *phosphatidylinositol glycan A (PIGA) gene* have been identified consistently in patients with PNH, thus confirming the biologic defect in this disorder.

Flow cytometric immunophenotyping of peripheral blood (WBC and RBC) is performed to determine the presence or absence of PI-linked antigens (CD14, FLAER, and/or CD59 antigens) using monoclonal antibodies directed against them. These proteins are absent on the cells of patients with PNH. Certain GPI-anchored proteins protect red blood cells from destruction; others are involved in blood clotting, whereas others are involved in fighting infection. Therefore the majority of the disease manifestations (i.e., hemolytic anemia, thrombosis, and infection) result from a deficiency of these GPI-anchored proteins.

Individuals without PNH have normal expression of all PI-linked antigens—CD14 (monocytes), CD16 (neutrophils and NK cells), CD24 (neutrophils), and CD59 (RBCs). Other GPI-linked antigens noted to be absent in PNH include CD55, and CD59. In addition, FLAER, a fluorescently labeled inactive variant of aerolysin, binds directly to the GPI anchor and can be used to evaluate the expression of the GPI linkage.

PROCEDURE AND PATIENT CARE

Before
☒ Explain the procedure to the patient.
☒ Tell the patient that no fasting is required.

During
• Collect a venous blood sample in a yellow (ACD)-top tube.

After
• Apply pressure or a pressure dressing to the venipuncture site.

TEST RESULTS AND CLINICAL SIGNIFICANCE

▼ **Decreased Levels**

PNH: *These GPI linked antigens are reduced or absent in patients with PNH. Determining which antigen is most significantly reduced will highlight the disease manifestations.*

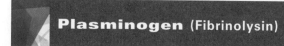

Plasminogen (Fibrinolysin)

NORMAL FINDINGS

2.4-4.4 Committee on Thrombolytic Agents (CTA) units/mL

INDICATIONS

This test is used to diagnose suspected plasminogen deficiency in patients who present with multiple thromboembolic episodes.

TEST EXPLANATION

Plasminogen is a protein involved in the fibrinolytic process of intravascular blood clot dissolution (see Figure 2-12 on p. 167). Plasminogen is converted to plasmin by proteolytic cleavage. This reaction can be catalyzed by urokinase, streptokinase, or tissue plasminogen activator (t-PA). Plasmin can destroy fibrin and dissolve clots. This fibrinolytic system helps maintain a normal homeostatic balance between coagulation and anticoagulation.

Plasminogen levels are occasionally measured during fibrinolytic therapy (for coronary and peripheral arterial occlusion) and are diminished. Decreased levels of plasminogen are also found in hyperfibrinolytic states (e.g., disseminated intravascular coagulation [DIC], primary fibrinolysis), because the plasminogen is used up. Because plasminogen is made in the liver, patients with cirrhosis or other severe liver diseases can be expected to have decreased levels. There are also rare cases of hereditary deficiencies of this protein. Decreased plasminogen levels put a patient at great risk for arterial or venous thrombosis.

Pregnancy and especially eclampsia are associated with increased levels of plasminogen. Patients with inflammatory conditions that may be associated with increased levels of C-reactive protein also may have concomitant mild elevations of plasminogens, which are acute-phase reactant proteins.

PROCEDURE AND PATIENT CARE

Before
☒ Explain the procedure to the patient.
☒ Tell the patient that no fasting is required.

During
- Collect a venous blood sample in a blue-top tube containing sodium citrate.
- Avoid excessive agitation of the blood sample.

After
- Apply pressure or a pressure dressing to the venipuncture site.
- Assess the venipuncture site for bleeding, especially if the patient is suspected of having a hyperfibrinolytic process (e.g., DIC).

TEST RESULTS AND CLINICAL SIGNIFICANCE

▲ Increased Levels

Pregnancy: *The pathophysiology of this observation is not well known. It may relate to amniotic proteins gaining access to the maternal circulation.*

▼ Decreased Levels

Hyperfibrinolytic state (e.g., DIC, fibrinolysis)
Primary liver disease: *Plasminogen is made in the liver. With severe liver disease, synthesis will not occur.*
Syndrome associated with hypercoagulation (e.g., venous and arterial clotting): *This syndrome can occur with many different types of diseases (e.g., colon cancer).*

Congenital deficiencies of plasminogen: *Although rare, such deficiencies can occur and place the patient at great risk for thromboembolic episodes.*

Malnutrition: *With severe malnutrition, protein depletion is so great that it interrupts plasminogen production.*

Plasminogen Activator Inhibitor 1 Antigen/ Activity (PAI-1)

NORMAL FINDINGS

Antigen assay: 2-46 ng/mL
Activity: <31.1 IU/mL

INDICATIONS

Plasminogen activator inhibitor 1 (PAI-1) is the principal inactivator of the fibrinolytic system. High levels are associated with a number of atherosclerotic risk factors.

TEST EXPLANATION

PAI-1 is a protein that inhibits plasminogen activators. During fibrinolysis, tissue plasminogen activator (tPA) converts plasminogen into plasmin. Plasmin plays a critical role in fibrinolysis by degrading fibrin (see Figure 2-12 on p. 167). PAI-1 is the primary inhibitor of tPA and urokinase plasminogen activator (uPA) in the blood. PAI-1 limits the production of plasmin and keeps fibrinolysis in check.

Elevated levels of PAI-1 are associated with a predisposition to thrombosis, including veno-occlusive disease after bone marrow transplantation or high-dose chemotherapy. Familial thrombosis has been associated with inherited elevation of plasma PAI-1 activity. Increased levels of PAI-1 have also been reported in a number of conditions including malignancy, liver disease, the postoperative period, septic shock, the second and third trimesters of pregnancy, obesity, coronary heart disease, and in patients with restenosis after coronary angioplasty. Increased levels may reduce the effectiveness of antithrombolytic therapy. Patients with insulin resistance syndrome and diabetes mellitus tend to have increased PAI-1 levels.

Low plasma levels of the active form of PAI-1 have been associated with abnormal clinically significant bleeding. Complete deficiency of PAI-1, either congenital or acquired, is associated with bleeding manifestations that include hemarthroses, hematomas, menorrhagia, easy bruising, and postoperative hemorrhage. Most laboratory tests are not capable of accurately quantifying low concentrations of PAI-1; therefore PAI-1 deficiency is difficult to identify.

PAI-1 is an acute phase reactant, and it will fluctuate in the face of an acute infection. Furthermore there is a top normal diurnal variation associated with PAI-1 levels. PAI-1 antigen can be measured directly by ELISA or by PCR genotyping. PAI-1 activity can be measured by bio-immunoassay. Results vary by methodology.

INTERFERING FACTORS

- Because PAI-1 is an acute-phase reactant, it can become transiently elevated by infection, inflammation, or trauma.

- Levels increase during pregnancy.
- PAI-1 has a circadian rhythm with highest concentration occurring in the morning and lowest concentrations in the afternoon and evening.

PROCEDURE AND PATIENT CARE

Before
- Explain the procedure to the patient.
- Tell the patient that no fasting is required.

During
- Collect a venous blood sample in a blue-top tube. Discard the first several milliliters of blood if PAI-1 is the only test being drawn. If multiple tests are being drawn, fill the blue-top tube after any red-top tube.
- Gently invert the blood tube several times after collection.

After
- Apply pressure or a pressure dressing to the venipuncture site.
- Assess the venipuncture site for bleeding, especially if the patient has a bleeding disorder.
- Deliver the tube immediately to the laboratory.

TEST RESULTS AND CLINICAL SIGNIFICANCE

▲ Increased Levels

Acute coronary syndrome,
Coronary artery disease,
Restenosis after coronary angioplasty:
   Inhibition of fibrinolysis increases the risk for thrombosis.
Infection,
Inflammation,
Trauma:
   PAI-1 is an acute-phase reactant and can be transiently elevated in these conditions.
Pregnancy: *Pregnancy is associated with increased proteins, including PAI-1.*
Diabetes mellitus,
Insulin resistance syndrome:
   The association of elevated PAI-1 with these diseases is observational. The pathophysiology is unknown.

▼ Decreased Levels

Bleeding disorders: *Excessive degradation of fibrin increases the risk for bleeding.*

RELATED TESTS

Plasminogen (p. 394). This test is used to diagnose suspected plasminogen deficiency in patients who present with multiple thromboembolic episodes.
Protein S/C (p. 432). This test identifies patients who are deficient in protein C and/or S. This is part of the evaluation of patients with coagulation disorders.
Factor V-Leiden (p. 231). This test is used to diagnose factor V-Leiden thrombophilia and is used in the evaluation of increased thrombosis.

Platelet Aggregation

NORMAL FINDINGS

Vary with platelet agonist used

INDICATIONS

This test is a measure of platelet function and aids in the evaluation of bleeding disorders.

TEST EXPLANATION

Platelet aggregation is important in hemostasis. A clump of platelets surrounds an area of acute blood vessel endothelial injury. Normal platelets adhere to this area of injury, and through a series of chemical reactions, they attract other platelets to the area. This is platelet aggregation, the first step in hemostasis. After this step the normal coagulation factor cascade occurs. Certain diseases that affect either platelet number or function can inhibit platelet aggregation and thereby prolong bleeding times. Congenital syndromes, uremia, myeloproliferative disorders, and drugs are associated with abnormal platelet aggregation. If blood is passed through a heart-lung or dialysis pump, platelet injury can occur and aggregation capability can be reduced.

Many agonists are used to stimulate platelet aggregation in the laboratory. Platelet aggregation is measured by determining the turbidity of platelet-rich plasma. As platelet aggregation is stimulated in vitro, turbidity decreases and light transmission through the specimen increases. This test is performed with an optical device called an aggregometer. Usually the patient's blood specimen is spun to a platelet-rich component. Next, an agonist to platelet aggregation, such as adenosine diphosphate, collagen, epinephrine, or ristocetin, is added. Turbidity is then measured within the aggregometer, and a curve indicating light transmission per unit of time is plotted. Normal curves have been identified for any one agonist that is used.

This is a very sensitive test, and it can be significantly affected by a number of variables, including:
1. Concentration of sodium citrate
2. Platelet count
3. Storage temperature
4. Concentration of the agonist addition
5. Reaction temperature
6. Degrees of lipemia, hemoglobinemia, or bilirubinemia

INTERFERING FACTORS

- Factors that may cause *increased* platelet aggregation include blood storage temperature, hyperbilirubinemia, hemoglobinemia, hyperlipidemia, and platelet count.
- Drugs that may cause *decreased* platelet aggregation include aspirin, antibiotics, nonsteroidal antiinflammatory agents, and thienopyridine antiplatelet drugs, such as ticlopidine (Ticlid) and clopidogrel (Plavix).

PROCEDURE AND PATIENT CARE

Before

- Explain the procedure to the patient.
- Tell the patient that no fasting is required.

During

- Collect a venous blood sample in a blue-top tube.
- If the patient is receiving any drugs that may interfere with platelet aggregation or has any diseases such as jaundice, hyperlipidemia, or hemolysis, this should be listed on the laboratory request slip.

After

- Apply pressure or a pressure dressing to the venipuncture site.
- Assess the venipuncture site for bleeding.
- Remember that abnormalities in platelet aggregation can prolong bleeding time, and a significant hematoma at the venipuncture site may occur.

TEST RESULTS AND CLINICAL SIGNIFICANCE

Prolonged Platelet Aggregation

Various congenital disorders (e.g., Wiskott-Aldrich syndrome, Bernard-Soulier syndrome, von Willebrand disease): *Platelet aggregation is diminished in autosomal recessive diseases.*

Connective tissue disorder (e.g., lupus erythematosus): *The pathophysiology of these observations is not understood.*

Recent cardiopulmonary or dialysis bypass: *Platelet injury develops as the platelets are passing through this machinery. The injured platelets are less likely to function normally in regard to aggregation.*

Uremia: *Not only is there a reduced platelet number in uremic patients, but a reduced aggregation capability has also been observed.*

Various myeloproliferative diseases, including leukemia, myeloma, and dysproteinemia: *The pathophysiology of these observations is not clear. It may be related to abnormal antibodies affecting the platelet membrane.*

Drugs (e.g., aspirin): *Drugs can have an immediate, and in some cases long-lasting, negative effect on platelet aggregation.*

RELATED TESTS

Platelet Count (p. 401). This is a direct measurement of platelet number.

Platelet Antibody (see following test). This test identifies antibodies directed against platelets.

Platelet Volume, Mean (p. 407). This is a measurement of the size of the platelets. It is helpful in the evaluation of thrombocytopenia.

 Platelet Antibody (Antiplatelet Antibody Detection)

NORMAL FINDINGS

No antiplatelet antibodies identified

INDICATIONS

This test is used to evaluate thrombocytopenia and exclude an immune-associated etiology.

TEST EXPLANATION

Immune-mediated destruction of platelets may be caused by either autoantibodies directed against antigens located on the same person's platelets or alloantibodies that develop after exposure to transfused platelets received from a donor. These antibodies are usually directed to an antigen on the platelet membrane, such as human leukocyte antigen (HLA) (see p. 306) or platelet-specific antigen (e.g., PLA1, PLA2). Many different laboratory techniques can be used to demonstrate the antiplatelet antibodies. These tests can directly identify the immunoglobulin with the use of radioimmunoassay (RIA) or immunofluorescence. Quantitative measurements are possible with cytofluorometry. Other tests identify complement binding on the affected platelet membrane. Most antiplatelet antibody testing is now performed using immunologic assays.

Antibodies directed to platelets will cause early destruction of the platelets and subsequent thrombocytopenia. Immunologic thrombocytopenia includes the following:

1. *Idiopathic thrombocytopenia purpura (ITP)* is a term that describes a group of disorders characterized by immune-mediated destruction of the platelets within the spleen or other reticuloendothelial organs. Platelet-associated immunoglobulin (Ig)G antibodies are detected in 90% of these patients.

2. *Posttransfusion purpura* is a rare syndrome characterized by the sudden onset of severe thrombocytopenia a few hours to a few days after transfusion of red blood cells (RBCs) or platelets. This is usually associated with an antibody to AB, B, and O (ABO), HLA, or PLA antigens on the RBC. In most situations the blood recipient has previously been sensitized to a PLA1 antigen during previous transfusions or during previous pregnancy. Once these antibodies form, they destroy the donor's PLA1-positive platelets and the recipient's PLA-negative platelets.

3. *Maternal-fetal platelet antigen incompatibility* (neonatal thrombocytopenia) occurs when the fetal platelet contains a PLA1 antigen that is absent in the mother. Just like Rh RBC incompatibility, the mother creates anti-PLA1 antibodies that cross the placenta and destroy the fetal platelets. The mother is not thrombocytopenic. Neonatal thrombocytopenia can also occur if the mother has ITP autoantibodies that are passed through the placenta and destroy the fetal platelets.

4. *Drug-induced thrombocytopenia.* While a host of drugs are known to induce autoimmune-mediated thrombocytopenia, heparin is the most common and causes heparin-induced thrombocytopenia (HIT). There are two types of HIT, type I and II, that may develop. Type I HIT is generally considered a benign condition and is not antibody mediated. In type II HIT, thrombocytopenia is usually more severe and is antibody mediated. Type II HIT is caused by an IgG antibody and usually occurs after 6 to 8 days of intravenous heparin therapy. Although platelet counts may be low, bleeding is unusual. Rather, paradoxic thromboembolism is the most worrisome complication and may be attributable to platelet activation caused by the anti–H-PF4 antibody complex instigating platelet aggregation.

   HIT occurs in about 1% to 5% of patients taking heparin for 5 to 10 days, and heparin-induced thrombosis occurs in one third to one half of these patients. Cessation of heparin is mandatory, and alternative anticoagulation is initiated. The diagnosis is suspected based on clinical symptoms, recent heparin administration, and low platelet counts. The diagnosis is confirmed by identifying *heparin-induced thrombocytopenia antibodies (HITA)*. This test uses an enzyme-linked immunosorbent assay to detect HIT-specific antibodies to heparin-PF4 complex. This assay can detect IgG, IgM, and IgA antibodies, and has a sensitivity of approximately 80% to 90%.

   Other drugs known to cause antiplatelet antibodies include cimetidine, analgesics (salicylates, acetaminophen), antibiotics (cephalosporins, penicillin derivatives, sulfonamides), quinidine-like drugs, diuretics (e.g., chlorothiazide), and others (e.g., digoxin, propylthiouracil, disulfiram [Antabuse]).

PROCEDURE AND PATIENT CARE

Before

☒ Explain the procedure to the patient.

☒ Tell the patient that no fasting is required.

During

- Collect a venous blood sample in a red-top tube. The amount of blood required depends on the initial platelet count.

After

- Apply pressure or a pressure dressing to the venipuncture site.
- Ensure adequate hemostasis in all patients with suspected thrombocytopenia.
- A platelet count is usually done 1 to 2 hours after platelet transfusion. This not only documents the posttransfusion platelet count, but it also eliminates a large proportion of posttransfusion immune thrombocytopenia reactions.

TEST RESULTS AND CLINICAL SIGNIFICANCE

▲ Increased Levels

Immune thrombocytopenia,
Idiopathic thrombocytopenia purpura,
Neonatal thrombocytopenia,
Posttransfusion purpura,
Drug-induced thrombocytopenia:

The pathophysiology of these diseases is described in the Test Explanation section.

RELATED TESTS

Platelet Count (p. 401). This is a direct measurement of platelet number.
Platelet Aggregation (p. 398). This is a test of platelet function.
Platelet Volume, Mean (p. 407). This is a measurement of the size of the platelets. It is helpful in the evaluation of thrombocytopenia.

 Platelet Count (Thrombocyte Count)

NORMAL FINDINGS

Adult/elderly: 150,000-400,000/mm^3 or 150-400 × 10^9/L (SI units)
Child: 150,000-400,000/mm^3
Infant: 200,000-475,000 mm^3
Premature infant: 100,000-300,000/mm^3
Newborn: 150,000-300,000/mm^3

 Critical Values

<20,000 or >1 million/mm^3

INDICATIONS

The platelet count is an actual count of the number of platelets (thrombocytes) per cubic milliliter of blood. It is performed on patients who develop petechiae (small hemorrhages in the skin), spontaneous bleeding, increasingly heavy menses, or thrombocytopenia. It is used to monitor the course of the disease or therapy for thrombocytopenia or bone marrow failure.

TEST EXPLANATION

Platelets are formed in the bone marrow from megakaryocytes. They are small, round, nonnucleated cells whose main role is maintenance of vascular integrity. In blood vessel injury, hemostasis is required to form a clot that will durably plug the hole until healing can occur. The primary phase of the hemostatic mechanism involves platelet aggregation. From there, the platelets help initiate the coagulation factor cascade. Most of the platelets exist in the bloodstream. A smaller percentage (25%) exists in the liver and spleen. Survival of platelets is measured in days (average of 7 to 9 days).

Platelet activity is essential to blood clotting. Counts of 150,000 to 400,000/mm³ are typically considered normal. Counts of less than 100,000/mm³ are generally considered to indicate *thrombocytopenia; thrombocytosis* (thrombocythemia) is generally said to exist when counts are greater than 400,000/mm³. Vascular thrombosis with tissue or organ infarction is the major complication of thrombocythemia. Common diseases associated with spontaneous thrombocytosis are iron deficiency anemia and malignancy (leukemia, lymphoma, solid tumors such as of the colon). Thrombocytosis may also occur with polycythemia vera, postsplenectomy syndromes, and a variety of acute/chronic infections or inflammatory processes. It should be noted that even patients with elevated platelet counts can experience a bleeding tendency because the function (platelet aggregation) of those platelets may be abnormal.

Spontaneous hemorrhage may occur with thrombocytopenia. If thrombocytopenia is severe, the platelets are often hand counted. Spontaneous bleeding is a serious danger when platelet counts fall below 20,000/mm³. Petechiae and ecchymosis will also occur at that degree of thrombocytopenia. With counts above 40,000/mm³, spontaneous bleeding rarely occurs, but prolonged bleeding from trauma or surgery may occur with counts at this level.

Causes of thrombocytopenia include:

1. Reduced production of platelets (secondary to bone marrow failure or infiltration of fibrosis, tumor, etc.)
2. Sequestration of platelets (secondary to hypersplenism)
3. Accelerated destruction of platelets (secondary to antibodies, infections, drugs, prosthetic heart valves)
4. Consumption of platelets (secondary to disseminated intravascular coagulation [DIC])
5. Platelet loss from hemorrhage
6. Dilution with large volumes of blood transfusions containing very few, if any, platelets

INTERFERING FACTORS

- Living in high altitudes may cause increased platelet levels.
- Because platelets can clump together, automated counting is subject to at least a 10% to 15% error.
- Strenuous exercise may cause increased levels.
- Decreased levels may be seen before menstruation.
- Drugs that may cause *increased* levels include estrogens and oral contraceptives.
- Drugs that may cause *decreased* levels include chemotherapeutic agents, chloramphenicol, colchicine, histamine-2–(H₂)-blocking agents (cimetidine, Zantac), hydralazine, indomethacin, isoniazid (INH), quinidine, streptomycin, sulfonamides, thiazide diuretics, and tolbutamide (Orinase).

PROCEDURE AND PATIENT CARE

Before

☒ Explain the procedure to the patient.
☒ Tell the patient that no fasting is required.

During

- Collect a peripheral venous blood sample in a lavender-top tube.

After

- Apply pressure or a pressure dressing to the venipuncture site.
- Assess the venipuncture site for bleeding.
- If the results indicate that the patient has a serious platelet deficiency:
  1. Observe the patient for signs and symptoms of bleeding.
  2. Check for blood in the urine and all excretions.
  3. Assess the patient for bruises, petechiae, bleeding from the gums, epistaxis, and low-back pain.
  4. Reassess all venipuncture sites for signs of hematoma formation.

TEST RESULTS AND CLINICAL SIGNIFICANCE

▲ Increased Levels (Thrombocytosis)

Malignant disorders (leukemia, lymphoma, solid tumors such as of the colon): *The pathophysiology of this observation is not known.*

Polycythemia vera: *This is a hyperplasia of all the marrow cell lines, including platelets.*

Postsplenectomy syndrome: *The spleen normally extracts aging platelets from the bloodstream. With surgical splenectomy, that job is less effectively done by other organs (liver, etc.). As a result, the platelet count increases.*

Rheumatoid arthritis: *The pathophysiology of this observation is not known.*

Iron-deficiency anemia or following hemorrhagic anemia: *Iron is not needed for platelet production. Anemia causes maximal stimulation of cellular production by the marrow. Red blood cells (RBCs) may not be so easily produced in light of iron deficiency. The platelet, however, can easily respond even in the presence of iron deficiency.*

▼ Decreased Levels (Thrombocytopenia)

Hypersplenism: *The spleen normally extracts aging platelets from the bloodstream. An enlarged spleen, however, extracts more platelets, both aging and new. The platelet count diminishes.*

Hemorrhage: *The platelets are lost in the bleeding process. If not replaced by transfusion of platelets, it will take some time (hours to days) for the marrow to produce an adequate number of platelets. This problem is exacerbated with treatment that replenishes blood volume and RBC count. This treatment dilutes the remaining platelets and further decreases the platelet count.*

Immune thrombocytopenia (e.g., idiopathic thrombocytopenia, neonatal, posttransfusion, or drug-induced thrombocytopenia): *Antibodies directed against antigens on the platelet cell membrane destroy the platelet and the count decreases.*

Leukemia and other myelofibrosis disorders: *The marrow is replaced by neoplastic or fibrotic tissue. Megakaryocyte function and numbers diminish. Platelets are not produced, and the count drops.*

Thrombotic thrombocytopenia: *This disease and others such as HELLP (hemolysis [H], elevated liver enzymes [EL], low platelet count [LP]) syndrome are highlighted by thrombocytopenia, hemolytic anemia, and other hematologic abnormalities.*

Graves disease: *In a small number of these patients, thrombocytopenia occurs. The pathophysiology of this observation is not known.*

Inherited disorders (e.g., Wiskott-Aldrich, Bernard-Soulier, Zieve syndromes): *The pathophysiology of this observation is not known.*

DIC: *The pathophysiology of thrombocytopenia is not clear. In part, however, it is thought that ongoing thrombosis "consumes" the platelets much like coagulating factors are "consumed." DIC usually develops concurrently with other severe disease (e.g., gram-negative sepsis) that can also produce thrombocytopenia.*

Systemic lupus erythematosus: *The pathophysiology of this observation is not known.*

Pernicious anemia: *Unlike iron, vitamin B_{12} is necessary for platelet production. A deficiency of this vitamin or folate will diminish the production of platelets.*

Some hemolytic anemias: *Often the same disease process that produces the hemolysis (e.g., hemolytic-uremic syndrome) also destroys the platelets. The platelet count falls.*

Cancer chemotherapy: *Cytotoxic drugs often affect the bone marrow. Platelets are not produced at adequate levels, and the count drops.*

Acute/chronic infections: *Bacterial, viral, and rickettsial infections can cause thrombocytopenia, especially when the patient is immunocompromised (e.g., acquired immunodeficiency syndrome [AIDS]).*

RELATED TESTS

Platelet Aggregation (p. 398). This is a test of platelet function.

Platelet Antibody (p. 399). This test identifies antibodies directed against platelets.

Platelet Function Assay (see following test). This test is used to identify platelet dysfunction in patients with normal platelet counts with prolonged bleeding.

Platelet Volume, Mean (p. 407). This is a measurement of the size of the platelets. It is helpful in the evaluation of thrombocytopenia.

Platelet Function Assay (Platelet Closure Time, PCT, Aspirin Resistance Tests)

NORMAL FINDINGS

CADP 64-120 seconds

CEPI 89-193 seconds

11-Dehydro-Thromboxane B2

   Males: 0-1089 pg/mg of creatinine

   Females: 0-1811 pg/mg of creatinine

INDICATIONS

This test is used to identify platelet dysfunction in patients who are suspected of having a bleeding abnormality. This test can identify abnormalities in the ability of platelets to aggregate or instigate the hemostatic cascade. It is used for patients with a family or personal history of acute excessive bleeding.

TEST EXPLANATION

Platelet dysfunction may be acquired, inherited, or induced by platelet-inhibiting agents. It is clinically important to assess platelet function as a potential cause of a bleeding diathesis (epistaxis, menorrhagia, postoperative bleeding, or easy bruising). The most common causes of platelet dysfunction are related to uremia, liver disease, von Willebrand disease (vWD), and exposure to such agents as acetyl salicylic acid (ASA, aspirin). The bleeding time (BT) test was a commonly performed test to evaluate platelet function. BT is labor intensive and expensive, and its accuracy is heavily dependent on operator skills. Its results cannot be reproduced and quantified. Platelet aggregation studies (p. 398) have similar accuracy problems. As a result, more clinical laboratories are using the *platelet closure time* (PCT) to more accurately quantify platelet function. Furthermore PCT can differentiate aspirin affects from other causes of platelet dysfunction (Figure 2-20).

Closure times are performed on a system in which the process of platelet adhesion and aggregation following a vascular injury is simulated in vitro. Anticoagulated whole blood is passed over membranes at a standardized flow rate, creating high shear rates that result in platelet attachment, activation, and aggregation on the membrane. A hole in the membrane is occluded when a stable platelet plug develops. The time required to obtain full occlusion of the aperture is reported as the PCT in seconds. The test is sensitive to platelet adherence and aggregation abnormalities, and allows the discrimination of aspirin-like defects and intrinsic platelet disorder. If a collagen/epinephrine (CEPI) CEPI membrane is used during testing, intrinsic platelet dysfunction can be identified. If a collagen/adenosine-5′-diphosphate (CADP) membrane is used during testing, the impact of aspirin on platelets can be determined. This test also can be used to determine resistance of aspirin's therapeutic anticoagulation effects on platelets. This is one of several *aspirin resistance tests* that are performed to determine the effectiveness of aspirin on inhibiting platelet aggregation and thereby protecting patient from vascular thromboembolic disease (Table 2-39).

Another aspirin resistance test is measurement of 11-dehydro-thromboxane B2 (11-dTXB2) in the urine. Thromboxane A2 is produced by the enzyme cyclo-oxygenase-1 (COX1) by activated platelets and still further stimulates platelet activation, platelet aggregation, and vasoconstriction.

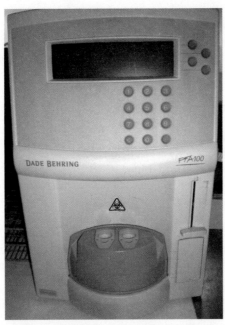

Figure 2-20 Dade Behring automated platelet function analyzer capable of determining platelet hemostatic function and the effect of medications on that function.

TABLE 2-39 Platelet Closure Time

	Normal	ASA Effect	Intrinsic Platelet Disorders
CEPI membrane	Normal	Abnormal	Abnormal
CADP membrane	Normal	Normal	Abnormal

CADP, Collagen/adenosine–5'-diphosphate; *CEPI,* collagen/epinephrine.

11-Dehydro-thromboxane B2 (11-dTXB2) is the stable, inactive metabolite of thromboxane A2. Urinary 11-dTXB2 therefore is an indication of platelet activation and aggregation. Elevated values are associated with increased risk of acute ischemic stroke and myocardial infarction. Effective aspirin therapy should reduce the level of this metabolite in the urine. If not, the patient may be aspirin resistant and may be more safely treated with an alternative therapy, including increasing the dosage of aspirin or placing the patient on another antiplatelet medication. A positive test for aspirin resistance raises the possibility that the patient may be clopidogrel (Plavix) resistant as well.

Urinary 11-dTXB2 offers an advantage over blood aspirin resistance tests because it is not subject to interference from in vitro platelet activation caused by local vein trauma or insufficient anticoagulation during blood sample collection.

INTERFERING FACTORS

- Low hematocrit or platelet count can decrease PCT.
- Aspirin and nonsteroidal antiarthritic agents (NSAIDS) can *increase* test results. These medications prevent blood from clotting by blocking the production of thromboxane A2, a chemical that platelets produce that instigates platelet aggregation. Aspirin accomplishes this by inhibiting the enzyme cyclooxygenase-1 (COX-1) that produces thromboxane A2.
- Thienopyridines can *increase* test results. When ADP attaches to ADP receptors on the surface of platelets, the platelets clump. The thienopyridines (e.g., ticlopidine [Ticlid] and clopidogrel [Plavix]) block the ADP receptor, which prevents ADP from attaching to the receptor and the platelets from clumping.

PROCEDURE AND PATIENT CARE

Before

- Explain the procedure to the patient.
- Tell the patient that no fasting is required.
- Obtain a drug history to determine whether the patient has recently had aspirin, anticoagulants, or any other medications that may affect test results.

During

- Collect a venous blood sample in a blue-top (citrate anticoagulated) tube.
- For urinary 11-dTXB2, randomly collect 10 mL urine. No preservative is necessary.

After

- Apply pressure or a pressure dressing to the puncture site.
- Assess the puncture site for bleeding.

TEST RESULTS AND CLINICAL SIGNIFICANCE

▲ Prolonged Times or Increased Values

Intrinsic Platelet Defects

Some myelodysplastic syndromes
Some myeloid leukemia
Some myeloproliferative disorders
Bernard-Soulier syndrome
Glanzmann thromboasthenia
Hermansky-Pudlak syndrome
Hereditary telangiectasia

Platelet/Blood Vessel Interaction Defects

von Willebrand disease
Collagen vascular disease
Cushing syndrome
Henoch-Schönlein syndrome
Uremia
Connective tissue disorder
Vascular disorders
> *These diseases are highlighted by a defect in the interaction of the platelet and the injured blood vessel, creating an inability of the platelets to aggregate.*

▲ Elevated B2 (11-dTXB2)

Thrombo-embolic disease: *Platelets are over activated, thereby secreting elevated B2 (11-dTXB2) levels.*

RELATED TEST

Platelet Count (p. 401). This is a quantitative measure of the number of circulating platelets. Thrombocytopenia is a common cause of excessive bleeding.

Platelet Volume, Mean (Mean Platelet Volume [MPV])

NORMAL FINDINGS

7.4-10.4 fL

INDICATIONS

This test is helpful in the evaluation of platelet disorders, especially thrombocytopenia.

TEST EXPLANATION

The MPV is a measure of the volume of a large number of platelets determined by an automated analyzer. MPV is to platelets as mean corpuscular volume (see p. 442) is to the red blood cells (RBCs).

The MPV varies with total platelet production. In cases of thrombocytopenia despite a normal reactive bone marrow (e.g., hypersplenism), the normal bone marrow releases immature platelets in an attempt to maintain a normal platelet count. These immature platelets are larger, and the MPV is increased. When bone marrow production of platelets is inadequate, the platelets that are released are small. This will be reflected as a low MPV; this makes the MPV useful in the differential diagnosis of thrombocytopenic disorders. However, because of variable results, the use of the MPV has decreased.

PROCEDURE AND PATIENT CARE

Before
☒ Explain the procedure to the patient.
☒ Tell the patient that no fasting is required.

During
• Collect a venous blood sample in a lavender-top tube.

After
• Apply pressure or a pressure dressing to the venipuncture site.
• Assess the venipuncture site for bleeding.
• If the patient is known to have a low platelet count:
    1. Observe the patient for signs and symptoms of bleeding.
    2. Check for blood in the urine and all excretions.
    3. Assess the patient for bruises, petechiae, bleeding of the gums, epistaxis, and low-back pain.

TEST RESULTS AND CLINICAL SIGNIFICANCE

▲ Increased Levels
Valvular heart disease,
Immune thrombocytopenia (e.g., idiopathic thrombocytopenia, neonatal, posttransfusion, or drug induced-thrombocytopenia),
Massive hemorrhage:
> *The above illnesses are all associated with thrombocytopenia and a normally reactive bone marrow that will produce a great number of immature platelets in an attempt to maintain a normal platelet count. These immature platelets are large and increase the MPV.*

Vitamin B_{12} or folate deficiency: *Megaloblastic changes affect the megakaryocyte just as the erythroid line is affected. The platelets that are produced are larger and may even be nucleated. The MPV is increased.*

Myelogenous leukemia: *Large, abnormal platelets are formed by neoplastic megakaryocytes if they are involved in the leukemic process. The MPV will increase.*

▼ Decreased Levels
Aplastic anemia,
Chemotherapy-induced myelosuppression:
> *When bone marrow production of platelets is inadequate, the platelets that are released are small. MPV will be reduced.*

Wiskott-Aldrich syndrome: *This syndrome is characterized by eczema, immune deficiency, thrombocytopenia, and small platelets.*

RELATED TESTS

Platelet Aggregation (p. 398). This is a test of platelet function.
Platelet Antibody (p. 399). This test identifies antibodies directed against platelets.
Platelet Count (p. 401). This is a direct measurement of the number of platelets.

Potassium, Blood (K)

NORMAL FINDINGS

Adult/elderly: 3.5-5.0 mEq/L or 3.5-5.0 mmol/L (SI units)
Child: 3.4-4.7 mEq/L
Infant: 4.1-5.3 mEq/L
Newborn: 3.9-5.9 mEq/L

 Critical Values

Adult <3 or >6.1 mEq/L
Newborn <2.5 or >8 mEq/L

INDICATIONS

This test is routinely performed in most patients evaluated for any type of serious illness. Furthermore, because this electrolyte is so important to cardiac function, it is a part of all complete routine evaluations, especially in patients who take diuretics or heart medications.

TEST EXPLANATION

Potassium is the major cation within the cell. The intracellular potassium concentration is approximately 150 mEq/L, whereas the normal serum potassium concentration is approximately 4 mEq/L. This ratio is the most important determinant in maintaining membrane electrical potential, especially in neuromuscular tissue. Because the serum concentration of potassium is so small, minor changes in concentration have significant consequences. Potassium is excreted by the kidneys. There is no reabsorption of potassium from the kidneys. Therefore, if potassium is not adequately supplied in the diet (or by intravenous [IV] administration in the patient who is unable to eat), serum potassium levels can drop rapidly.

Potassium is an important part of protein synthesis and maintenance of normal oncotic pressure and cellular electrical neutrality as indicated above. It contributes to the metabolic portion of acid-base balance in that the kidneys can shift potassium for hydrogen ions to maintain a physiologic pH.

Serum potassium concentration depends on many factors, including:

1. *Aldosterone* (and, to a lesser extent, glucocorticosteroids). This hormone tends to increase renal losses of potassium.
2. *Sodium reabsorption.* As sodium is reabsorbed, potassium is lost.
3. *Acid-base balance.* Alkalotic states tend to lower serum potassium levels by causing a shift of potassium into the cell. Acidotic states tend to raise serum potassium levels by reversing that shift.

Symptoms of *hyperkalemia* include irritability, nausea, vomiting, intestinal colic, and diarrhea. The electrocardiogram may demonstrate peaked T waves, a widened QRS complex, and a depressed ST segment.

Signs of *hypokalemia* are related to a decrease in contractility of smooth, skeletal, and cardiac muscles, which results in weakness, paralysis, hyporeflexia, ileus, increased cardiac sensitivity to digoxin, cardiac arrhythmias (dysrhythmias), flattened T waves, and prominent U waves. This electrolyte has profound effects on the heart rate and contractility. The potassium level should be carefully followed in patients with uremia, Addison disease, and vomiting and diarrhea and in patients taking steroid therapy and potassium-depleting diuretics. Potassium must be closely monitored in patients taking digitalis-like drugs, because cardiac arrhythmias may be induced by hypokalemia and digoxin.

INTERFERING FACTORS

- Opening and closing of the hand with a tourniquet in place may increase potassium levels.
- Hemolysis of blood during venipuncture or during laboratory processing causes increased levels.
- Drugs that may cause *increased* potassium levels include aminocaproic acid, antibiotics, antineoplastic drugs, captopril, epinephrine, heparin, histamine, isoniazid (INH), lithium, mannitol, potassium-sparing diuretics, potassium supplements, and succinylcholine.
- Drugs that may cause *decreased* levels include acetazolamide, aminosalicylic acid, glucose infusions, amphotericin B, carbenicillin, cisplatin, diuretics (potassium wasting), insulin, laxatives, lithium carbonate, penicillin G sodium (high doses), phenothiazines, salicylates (aspirin), and sodium polystyrene sulfonate (Kayexalate).

✔ Clinical Priorities

- This electrolyte has profound effects on the heart rate and contractility. Potassium levels must be carefully monitored in patients taking digitalis-like drugs and diuretics, because cardiac arrhythmias may be induced by hypokalemia.
- Intravenous potassium may be indicated to prevent cardiac arrhythmias for hypokalemia in the adult. Potassium is infused at a slow rate to prevent irritation to the veins.
- Serum potassium levels are affected by acid-base balance. Alkalotic states lower potassium levels and acidotic states raise levels.
- Hemolysis of blood during venipuncture or laboratory processing can cause elevations.

PROCEDURE AND PATIENT CARE

Before
- Explain the procedure to the patient.
- Tell the patient that no special diet or fasting is required.

During
- Instruct the patient to avoid opening and closing the hand after a tourniquet is applied.
- Collect a venous blood sample in a red-top or green-top tube.
- Avoid hemolysis.

After
- Apply pressure or a pressure dressing to the venipuncture site.
- Assess the venipuncture site for bleeding.
- Evaluate the patient with increased or decreased potassium levels for cardiac arrhythmias.
- Monitor patients taking digoxin and diuretics for hypokalemia.
- If indicated, administer resin exchanges (e.g., Kayexalate enema) to correct hyperkalemia.

TEST RESULTS AND CLINICAL SIGNIFICANCE

▲ Increased Levels (Hyperkalemia)

Excessive dietary intake,

Excessive IV intake:

> Because the amount of potassium in the serum is so small, minimal but significant increases in potassium intake can cause elevations in the serum level.

Acute or chronic renal failure: *This is the most common cause of hyperkalemia. Potassium excretion is diminished, and potassium levels rise.*

Addison disease,

Hypoaldosteronism,

Aldosterone-inhibiting diuretics (e.g., spironolactone, triamterene):

> Aldosterone excretion is absent. Aldosterone enhances potassium excretion. Without that effect, potassium excretion is diminished and potassium levels rise.

Crush injury to tissues,

Hemolysis,

Transfusion of hemolyzed blood,

Infection:

> Potassium exists in high levels in the cell. With cellular injury and lysis, the potassium within the cell is released into the bloodstream.

Acidosis: *To maintain physiologic pH during acidosis, hydrogen ions are driven from the blood and into the cell. To maintain electrical neutrality, potassium is expelled from the cell. Potassium levels rise.*

Dehydration: *The potassium becomes more concentrated in dehydrated patients, and serum levels appear to be elevated. When the patient is rehydrated, potassium levels may in fact be reduced.*

▼ Decreased Levels (Hypokalemia)

Deficient dietary intake,

Deficient IV intake:

> The kidneys cannot reabsorb potassium to compensate for the reduced potassium intake. Potassium levels decline.

Burns,

Gastrointestinal (GI) disorders (e.g., diarrhea, vomiting, villous adenomas):

> Excessive potassium is lost because of ongoing fluid and electrolyte losses as indicated above.

Diuretics: *These medications act to increase renal excretion of potassium. This is especially important for cardiac patients who take diuretics and digitalis preparations. Hypokalemia can exacerbate the ectopy that digoxin may instigate.*

Hyperaldosteronism: *Aldosterone enhances potassium excretion.*

Cushing syndrome: *Glucocorticosteroids have an "aldosterone-like" effect.*

Renal tubular acidosis: *Renal excretion of potassium is increased.*

Licorice ingestion: *Licorice has an "aldosterone-like" effect.*

Alkalosis: *To maintain physiologic pH during alkalosis, hydrogen ions are driven out of the cell and into the blood. To maintain electrical neutrality, potassium is driven into the cell. Potassium levels fall.*

Insulin administration: *In patients with hyperglycemia, insulin is administered. Glucose and potassium are driven into the cell. Potassium levels drop.*

Glucose administration: *In a normal person, insulin is secreted in response to glucose administration. Glucose and potassium are driven into the cell. Potassium levels drop.*

Ascites: These patients have a decreased renal blood flow from reduced intravascular volume that results from the collection of fluid. The reduced blood flow stimulates the secretion of aldosterone, which increases potassium excretion. Furthermore, these patients are often taking potassium-wasting diuretics.

Renal artery stenosis: These patients have a reduced renal blood flow. The pathophysiology is as described above.

Cystic fibrosis: These patients have increased potassium loss in secretions and sweat.

Trauma/surgery/burns: The body's response to trauma is mediated, in part, by aldosterone, which increases potassium excretion.

RELATED TESTS

Sodium, Blood (p. 466), and Chloride, Blood (p. 152). These electrolytes are often measured with potassium. Metabolically, they are all intermingled.

Potassium, Urine (p. 942). This is used to identify increased potassium excretion.

 Prealbumin (PAB, Thyroxine-Binding Prealbumin [TBPA], Thyretin, Transthyretin)

NORMAL FINDINGS

Blood

Adult/elderly: 15-36 mg/dL or 150-360 mg/L (SI units)

Child
   <5 days: 6-21 mg/dL
   1-5 years: 14-30 mg/dL
   6-9 years: 15-33 mg/dL
   10-13 years: 22-36 mg/dL
   14-19 years: 22-45 mg/dL

Urine (24-Hour)

0.017-0.047 mg/day

CSF

Approximately 2% of total cerebrospinal fluid (CSF) protein

 Critical Values

Serum prealbumin levels <10.7 mg/dL indicate severe nutritional deficiency.

INDICATIONS

This test is used to indicate a person's nutritional status. It is also used to indicate liver function status.

TEST EXPLANATION

Prealbumin is one of the major plasma proteins. Because prealbumin can bind thyroxine, it is also called thyroxine-binding prealbumin. However, prealbumin is secondary to thyroxine-binding globulin in the transportation of triiodothyronine (T_3) and thyroxine (T_4). Prealbumin also plays a role in the transport and metabolism of vitamin A. Prealbumin is measured by immunoassay.

Because prealbumin levels in serum fluctuate more rapidly in response to alterations in synthetic rate than do those of other serum proteins, clinical interest in the quantification of serum prealbumin has centered on its usefulness as a marker of nutritional status. Its half-life of 1.9 days is much less than the 21-day half-life of albumin (see p. 424). Because of prealbumin's short half-life, it is a sensitive indicator of any change affecting protein synthesis and catabolism. Therefore prealbumin is frequently ordered to monitor the effectiveness of total parenteral nutrition (TPN).

Prealbumin is significantly reduced in hepatobiliary disease because of impaired synthesis. Serum levels of prealbumin are better indicators of liver function than albumin levels. Prealbumin is also a negative acute-phase reactant protein; serum levels decrease in inflammation, malignancy, and protein-wasting diseases of the intestines or kidneys. Because zinc is required for synthesis of prealbumin, low levels occur with zinc deficiency. Increased levels of prealbumin occur in Hodgkin disease and chronic kidney disease.

Because of the low quantity of prealbumin in the serum, this protein is not often visualized on serum protein electrophoresis. However, because prealbumin crosses the blood-brain barrier, it is found in the CSF and can be seen on CSF electrophoresis (see discussion of lumbar puncture on p. 651).

INTERFERING FACTORS

- Coexistent inflammation may make test result interpretation impossible.
- Drugs that may cause *increased* levels include anabolic steroids, androgens, estrogen, and prednisolone.
- Drugs that may cause *decreased* levels include amiodarone, estrogens, and oral contraceptives.

Clinical Priorities

- Clinical interest in prealbumin has centered on its usefulness as a marker of nutritional status. Its half-life of 1.9 days is much less than the 21-day half-life of albumin.
- Prealbumin is frequently indicated to monitor the effectiveness of TPN.
- Because prealbumin is a negative acute-phase reactant protein, serum levels may decrease with inflammatory processes and may make test result interpretation impossible.

PROCEDURE AND PATIENT CARE

Before
- Explain the procedure to the patient.
- Tell the patient that no food or fluid restrictions are needed.
- If the patient is to collect a 24-hour urine specimen, provide a collection bottle.

During
- Collect a venous blood sample in a red-top tube.

After
- Apply pressure or a pressure dressing to the venipuncture site.
- Observe the venipuncture site for bleeding.
- Transport the 24-hour urine specimen to the laboratory promptly.
- Inform the patient how and when to obtain the results of this study.

TEST RESULTS AND CLINICAL SIGNIFICANCE

▲ Increased Levels

Some cases of nephrotic syndrome: *The major characteristic of the nephrotic syndrome is proteinuria that causes hypoproteinemia. Because prealbumin is so rapidly made, a disproportionate percentage of prealbumin can exist in the blood when other proteins take somewhat longer to produce.*

Hodgkin disease: *The pathophysiology of this observation is not known.*

Pregnancy: *The estrogen effect stimulates protein (prealbumin) synthesis.*

▼ Decreased Levels

Malnutrition,

Liver damage:

   The synthesis of prealbumin is diminished.

Burns: *There is acute loss of protein from the burn and chronically from the constant loss of serum through the burn.*

Inflammation: *Prealbumin is a negative acute-phase reactant protein. That is, in the presence of inflammation, prealbumin levels diminish.*

RELATED TESTS

Protein (p. 424). This is a quantification of all the components that make up the serum proteins, including albumin, alpha$_1$, alpha$_2$, beta$_1$, beta$_2$, and gamma globulins. This test can also detect abnormal proteins created by neoplasms and/or infections.

Immunoglobulin Quantification (p. 312). This is a quantification of the components that make up immunoglobulin, which is a gamma globulin.

Pregnancy-Associated Plasma Protein-A (PAPP-A)

NORMAL FINDINGS

Down syndrome

   Calculated screen risks <1:230 are reported as screen negative.

   Risks ≥1:230 are reported as screen positive.

Trisomy 18

   Calculated screen risks <1:100 are reported as screen negative.

   Risks ≥1:100 are reported as screen positive.

INDICATIONS

This test is a part of routine maternal screening for potential birth abnormalities.

TEST EXPLANATION

Pregnancy-associated plasma protein-A (PAPP-A) is made by the trophoblasts during pregnancy and released into the maternal circulation during pregnancy. Women with low blood levels of PAPP-A at 8 to 14 weeks of gestation have an increased risk of intrauterine growth restriction, trisomy 18 or 21, premature delivery, preeclampsia, and stillbirth. This protein rapidly rises in the first trimester of normal pregnancy. However, in Down-affected pregnancy, serum levels are half that of unaffected pregnancies. Furthermore, low first-trimester levels of PAPP-A in maternal serum are associated with adverse fetal outcomes, including fetal death in utero and intrauterine growth retardation.

This test is commonly used in conjunction with other pregnancy/maternal screening test (p. 354). Most first-trimester maternal screens include nuchal translucency (p. 888) measurement (a sonographic marker shown to be effective in screening fetuses for Down syndrome) and a blood draw analyte such as human chorionic gonadotropin (p. 304) or PAPP-A. A mathematical model is used to calculate a risk estimate by combining the analyte values, NT measurement, and maternal demographic information. The laboratory establishes a specific cutoff for each condition, which classifies each screen as either screen-positive or -negative.

A screen-negative result indicates that the calculated screen risk is below the established cutoff of 1:230 for Down syndrome and 1:100 for trisomy 18. A negative screen does not guarantee the absence of trisomy 18 or Down syndrome. Screen-negative results typically do not warrant further evaluation. When a Down syndrome risk cutoff of 1:230 is used for follow-up, the combination of maternal age, pregnancy-associated plasma protein A, human chorionic gonadotropin, and nuchal translucency has an overall detection rate of approximately 85% with a false-positive rate of 5% to 10%. A screen-positive result indicates that the value obtained exceeds the established cutoff. A positive screen does not provide a diagnosis, but indicates that further evaluation should be considered.

PAPP-A is present in unstable atherosclerotic plaques, and circulating levels are elevated in acute coronary syndromes, which may reflect the instability of the plaques. PAPP-A is an independent marker of unstable angina and acute myocardial infarction (heart attack). It is also a risk factor in predicting death after an acute myocardial event.

PAPP-A exists in a bound (to eosinophil major basic protein [pro-MBP]) and free form. In general, the bound form is most accurately predictive of pregnancy outcome, whereas the free form is the most accurate predictor in coronary atherosclerotic disease.

INTERFERING FACTORS

- All serum markers are adjusted for maternal weight (to account for dilution effects in heavier mothers). The estimated risk calculations and screen results are dependent on accurate information for gestation, maternal age, and weight. Inaccurate information can lead to significant alterations in the estimated risk.

PROCEDURE AND PATIENT CARE

Before

- Explain the procedure to the patient.
- Allow the patient to express her concerns and fears regarding the potential for birth defects.

During

- Most of these tests can be done with a venous blood sample in a red-top tube. hCG and estriol can also be tested by collecting a urine sample.

After

- Provide the results to the patient (and other family members if the patient desires) during a personal consultation.
- Allow the patient to express her concerns if the results are positive.
- Assist the patient in scheduling and obtaining more accurate diagnostic testing if the results are positive.

TEST RESULTS AND CLINICAL SIGNIFICANCE

Positive screening tests (trisomy 21, trisomy 18, neural tube defects, abdominal wall defects): *This is an indication of risk, not a diagnosis. This is a screening test only. Further diagnostic testing would be required if positive.*

Coronary atherosclerotic disease: *By observation, unstable coronary plaques are associated with elevated PAPP-A levels.*

RELATED TESTS

Maternal Screen Testing (p. 354).
Human Chorionic Gonadotropin (p. 304).
Pelvic Ultrasonography (p. 887). These tests are used in screening for maternal/fetal abnormalities.

 Progesterone Assay

NORMAL FINDINGS*

Progesterone Level (ng/dL[†])

Child:
    <9 years: <20
    10-15 years: <20
Adult
    Male: 10-50
    Female
      Follicular phase: <50
      Luteal phase: 300-2500
      Postmenopausal: <40
Pregnancy (trimester)
    First: 725-4400
    Second: 1950-8250
    Third: 6500-22,900

INDICATIONS

This test is used in the evaluation of women who are having difficulty becoming pregnant or maintaining a pregnancy. It is also used to monitor "high-risk" pregnancies.

TEST EXPLANATION

Progesterone acts primarily on the endometrium. It initiates the secretory phase of the endometrium in anticipation of implantation of a fertilized ovum. Normally progesterone is secreted by the ovarian corpus luteum following ovulation. In pregnancy, progesterone is produced by the corpus luteum for the first few weeks. After that the placenta begins to make progesterone. Both serum progesterone levels

---

*Considerable variation according to method used and laboratory.
[†]Extraction/radioimmunoassay.

and the urine concentration of progesterone metabolites (pregnanediol) are significantly increased during the latter half of a normal ovulatory cycle. Progesterone levels provide information about the occurrence and timing of ovulation.

Because progesterone levels rise rapidly after ovulation, this study is useful in documenting whether ovulation has occurred and, if so, its exact time. This is very useful information in women who have difficulty becoming pregnant. A series of measurements can help define the day of ovulation. Plasma progesterone levels start to rise after ovulation along with luteinizing hormone (LH), and they continue to rise for approximately 6 to 10 days. The levels then fall and menses occurs. Blood samples drawn at days 8 and 21 of the menstrual cycle normally will show a large increase in progesterone levels in the latter specimen, indicating that ovulation has occurred. Serum progesterone levels can provide comparable information and are sometimes measured in lieu of endometrial biopsy (see p. 726) to determine the phase of the menstrual cycle.

During pregnancy, progesterone levels normally rise because of the placental production of progesterone. Repeated assays can be used to monitor the status of the placenta in cases of "high-risk" pregnancy. Hormone assay for progesterone is used today to monitor progesterone supplementation in patients with an inadequate luteal phase to maintain an early pregnancy.

INTERFERING FACTORS

- Recent use of radioisotopes may affect test results if testing is done by radioimmunoassay (RIA).
- Hemolysis caused by rough handling of the sample may affect test results.
- Drugs that may interfere with test results include estrogen, clomiphene, and progesterone.

✔ Clinical Priorities

- Progesterone levels provide information about the occurrence and timing of ovulation. This is useful information in women having difficulty becoming pregnant.
- Hormone assays for progesterone are used to monitor progesterone supplementation in women with an inadequate luteal phase to maintain an early pregnancy.
- During pregnancy, progesterone levels normally rise because of placental production of progesterone. Repeated assays can be used to monitor placental states in "high-risk" pregnancies. Decreasing values are seen when placental viability is threatened.

PROCEDURE AND PATIENT CARE

Before
- Explain the procedure to the patient.
- Tell the patient that no fasting is required.

During
- Collect a venous blood sample in a red-top tube.
- Indicate the date of the last menstrual period on the laboratory slip.

After
- Apply pressure or a pressure dressing to the venipuncture site.
- Assess the venipuncture site for bleeding.

TEST RESULTS AND CLINICAL SIGNIFICANCE

▲ Increased Levels

Ovulation: *This occurs with the normal development of a corpus luteum, which makes progesterone.*

Pregnancy: *A healthy placenta produces progesterone to maintain the pregnancy.*

Luteal cysts of ovary: *The corpus luteum produces progesterone in the nonpregnant female and in the early stages of pregnancy. Cysts can also produce progesterone for prolonged periods of time.*

Hyperadrenocorticalism,

Adrenocortical hyperplasia:

> *Adrenal cortical hormones are secreted at increased rates. 17-Hydroxyprogesterone is a precursor of these cortical hormones.*

Choriocarcinoma of ovary: *This tumor produces progesterone.*

Molar pregnancy: *Hydatidiform mole can produce progesterone, although at lower levels than pregnancy.*

▼ Decreased Levels

Preeclampsia,

Toxemia of pregnancy,

Threatened abortion,

Placental failure,

Fetal death:

> *All of the above obstetric emergencies are associated with decreased placental viability. Progesterone is made by the placenta during pregnancy. Decreasing values are seen when placental viability is threatened.*

Ovarian neoplasm: *Ovarian epithelial cancers can destroy the functional ovarian tissue. Progesterone levels may decrease.*

Amenorrhea,

Ovarian hypofunction:

> *Without ovulation, a corpus luteum will not develop. Progesterone will not be secreted and progesterone and pregnanediol levels will be lower than expected.*

RELATED TEST

Pregnanediol (p. 944). Pregnanediol is a catabolic metabolite of progesterone that is excreted via the kidneys into the urine.

Prolactin Level (PRL)

NORMAL FINDINGS

Adult male: 3-13 ng/mL
Adult female: 3-27 ng/mL
Pregnant female: 20-400 ng/mL

INDICATIONS

Prolactin levels are used to diagnose and monitor prolactin-secreting pituitary adenomas.

TEST EXPLANATION

Prolactin is a hormone secreted by the anterior pituitary gland (adenohypophysis). In females, prolactin promotes lactation. Its role in males has not been demonstrated. Prolactin secretion is controlled by prolactin-inhibiting and prolactin-releasing factors secreted by the hypothalamus. Thyroid-releasing hormone (TRH) can also stimulate prolactin production. During sleep, prolactin levels increase twofold to threefold, attaining circulating levels equaling those of pregnant women. With breast stimulation, pregnancy, nursing, stress, or exercise, a surge of this hormone occurs. Prolactin is elevated in patients with prolactin-secreting pituitary acidophilic or chromophobic adenomas. To a lesser extent, moderately high prolactin levels have been observed in women with secondary amenorrhea (i.e., postpubertal), galactorrhea, primary hypothyroidism, polycystic ovary syndrome, and anorexia. Paraneoplastic tumors (e.g., lung cancer) may cause ectopic secretion of prolactin as well. In general, very high prolactin levels are more likely to be related to pituitary adenoma than to other causes.

The prolactin level is helpful for monitoring the disease activity of pituitary adenomas. Several *prolactin stimulation tests* (with TRH or chlorpromazine) and *prolactin suppression tests* (with levodopa) have been designed to help differentiate pituitary adenoma from some other causes of prolactin overproduction. Prolactin levels are used to evaluate functional and organic disease of the hypothalamus, primary hypothyroidism, section compression of the pituitary stalk, chest wall lesions, renal failure, and ectopic tumors.

Hyperprolactinemia often results in loss of libido; galactorrhea; oligomenorrhea or amenorrhea and infertility in premenopausal women; and loss of libido, impotence, infertility, and hypogonadism in men. Prolactin values that exceed the reference values may result from macroprolactin (prolactin bound to immunoglobulin). *Macroprolactin* blood levels should be evaluated if signs and symptoms of hyperprolactinemia are absent or pituitary imaging studies are not informative. Macroprolactin can be inversely computed by measuring the percent of manometric prolactin. If the percent of monomeric prolactin is less than 40% of the total, macroprolactinemia exists and the patient does not have true elevated prolactin levels.

INTERFERING FACTORS

- Stress from illness, trauma, surgery, or even the fear of a blood test can elevate prolactin levels. In patients who are fearful of venipuncture, it is best to place a saline lock and draw the blood specimen 2 hours later.
- Drugs that may cause *increased* values include antipsychotic drugs (risperidone phenothiazines), antinausea/antiemetic drugs, serotonin reuptake (antidepressants of all classes), ergot derivatives, some illegal drugs (e.g., cannabis), oral contraceptives, reserpine, opiates, histamine antagonists, monoamine oxidase inhibitors, estrogens/progesterone, several antihypertensive drugs, anticonvulsants (valproic acid), anti-tuberculous medications, and antihistamines.
- Drugs that may cause *decreased* values are clonidine, dopamine, ergot alkaloid derivatives, and levodopa.

PROCEDURE AND PATIENT CARE

Before

- Explain the procedure to the patient.
- Tell the patient no fasting or special preparation is required.
- Inform the patient that this blood sample should be drawn in the morning.
- Record the use of any medication that may affect results.

During

- Obtain a venous blood sample in a red-top tube.
- Transfer the specimen to the laboratory as soon as possible. If a delay occurs, the specimen should be placed on ice.

After

- Apply pressure or a pressure dressing to the venipuncture site.
- Assess the venipuncture site for bleeding.

TEST RESULTS AND CLINICAL SIGNIFICANCE

▲ Increased Levels

Galactorrhea: *Voluminous galactorrhea can be caused by elevated prolactin levels. A small-volume nipple discharge is quite common and not pathologic unless it is bloody.*

Amenorrhea: *Patients who have had normal menses and then stop having menses may be found to have elevated prolactin levels. Many are subsequently found to have prolactin-secreting pituitary adenomas.*

Prolactin-secreting pituitary tumor: *Most of these are benign adenomas of the acidophilic type.*

Infiltrative diseases of hypothalamus and pituitary stalk (e.g., granuloma, sarcoidosis),

Metastatic cancer of pituitary gland:

> *The pathologic destruction of the hypothalamus or pituitary can destroy the prolactin-inhibiting regulatory mechanisms.*

Hypothyroidism: *Patients with hypothyroidism because of thyroid failure have elevated TRH levels. TRH also stimulates prolactin production.*

Paraneoplastic syndrome: *These cancers are associated with ectopic production of prolactin.*

Stress (e.g., anorexia nervosa, surgery, strenuous exercise, trauma, severe illness): *The pathophysiology of these observations is not known.*

Empty sella syndrome: *These patients have a large sella turcica noted on x-ray films but do not have a pituitary adenoma, yet they often have elevated prolactin levels.*

Polycystic ovary syndrome: *The pathophysiology of this observation is not well known.*

Renal failure: *These patients probably have a reduced clearance of prolactin.*

▼ Decreased Levels

Pituitary apoplexy (Sheehan syndrome): *Women who have severe hemorrhage after obstetric delivery experience circulatory collapse. Their pituitary glands become infarcted. Prolactin levels are diminished along with other pituitary hormones.*

Pituitary destruction by tumor (craniopharyngioma): *Any disease that destroys the pituitary gland will, of course, be associated with reduced prolactin levels.*

 Prostate Specific Antigen (PSA)

NORMAL FINDINGS

0 to 2.5 ng/mL is low.
2.6 to 10 ng/mL is slightly to moderately elevated.
10 to 19.9 ng/mL is moderately elevated.
20 ng/mL or more is significantly elevated.

INDICATIONS

This test is used as a screening method for early detection of prostatic cancer. When the PSA test is combined with a rectal examination, nearly 90% of clinically significant cancers can be detected. This test is also used to monitor the disease after treatment.

TEST EXPLANATION

PSA is a glycoprotein found in high concentrations in the prostatic lumen. Significant barriers such as prostate glandular tissue and vascular structure are interposed between the prostatic lumen and the bloodstream. These protective barriers can be broached when disease such as cancer, infection, and benign hypertrophy exists. PSA can be detected in all males; however, levels are greatly increased in patients with prostatic cancer.

Elevated PSA levels are associated with prostate cancer. Levels greater than 4 ng/mL have been found in more than 80% of men with prostate cancer. The higher the levels, the greater the tumor burden. The PSA assay is also a sensitive test for monitoring response to therapy. Successful surgery, radiation, or hormone therapy is associated with a marked reduction in the PSA blood level. Significant elevation in PSA subsequently indicates the recurrence of prostatic cancer. PSA is more sensitive and specific than other prostatic tumor markers, such as prostatic acid phosphatase (PAP). Also, PSA is more accurate than PAP in monitoring response to therapy and recurrence of tumor after therapy.

There is considerable controversy regarding the use of PSA screening among asymptomatic men. The US Preventative Services Task Force (USPSTF) and other professional societies have indicated that mortality from prostate cancer is not significantly reduced by annual PSA screening. Furthermore most feel that "PSA screening identified" prostate cancer is not an aggressive cancer and is not associated with a significant increase in mortality. Approximately 80% of PSA screening testing is falsely positive. A positive screening test often triggers a biopsy and even potential life-threatening surgery with very little benefit. However, PSA screening in high-risk men such as those of African-American descent, genetic predisposition (e.g., BRCA genetic mutation), or strong family history should be offered annual PSA testing and digital rectal examinations.

It is important to be aware that some patients with early prostate cancer will not have elevated levels of PSA. It is equally important to recognize that PSA levels above 4 are not always associated with cancer. The PSA is limited by a lack of specificity within the "diagnostic gray zone" of 4 to 10 ng/mL. PSA levels also may be minimally elevated in patients with benign prostatic hypertrophy (BPH) and prostatitis. In an effort to increase the accuracy of PSA testing, other measures of PSA (Box 2-17) have been proposed.

- *PSA velocity:* PSA velocity is the change in PSA levels over time. A sharp rise in the PSA level raises the suspicion of cancer and may indicate a fast-growing cancer. Men who had a PSA velocity above 0.35 ng/mL per year had a higher relative risk for dying from prostate cancer than men who had a PSA velocity less than 0.35 ng/mL per year.

BOX 2-17   Strategies for Enhancing PSA Specificity
- Volume-adjusted PSA - PSA density - Age-specific PSA - % Free PSA

- *Age-adjusted PSA* (Table 2-40): Age is an important factor in increasing PSA levels. Men younger than age 50 should have a PSA level below 2.4 ng/mL, whereas a PSA level up to 6.5 ng/mL would be considered normal for men in their 70s.
- *PSA density:* PSA density considers the relationship of the PSA level to the size of the prostate. The use of PSA density to interpret PSA results is controversial because cancer might be overlooked in a man with an enlarged prostate. PSA density is an adjustment that divides the PSA measurement by the gland volume. Several formulas have been created to partially correct for gland volume. One such volume adjusted formula is:

$$\text{Predicated PSA} = 0.12 \times \text{Gland volume (in cubic centimeters)}$$
$$\text{as determined by ultrasound}$$

- *Free versus bound PSA:* PSA circulates in the blood in two forms: free or bound to a protein molecule. With benign prostate conditions (such as BPH), there is more free PSA, while cancer produces more of the bound form. If a man's attached PSA is high but his free PSA is not, the presence of cancer is more likely. When the %FPSA is less than 25%, there is a high likelihood of cancer (Table 2-41).
- *Alteration of PSA cutoff level:* Some researchers have suggested lowering the cutoff levels that determine if a PSA measurement is normal or elevated. For example, a number of studies have used cutoff levels of 2.5 or 3.0 ng/mL (rather than 4.0 ng/mL).
- *Prostate-specific proteins:* Patterns of prostate proteins are being studied to determine if a biopsy is necessary when a person has a slightly elevated PSA level or an abnormal DRE. *Prostatic specific membrane antigen* may, with further study, represent an excellent marker for prostate cancer. It is more frequently present than PSA in more advanced cancer. Another protein of interest is *Early Prostate Cancer Antigen (EPCA).* Unlike the PSA, this protein is not found in normal prostate cells. Instead, EPCA occurs in relatively large amounts only in prostate cancer cells. Early testing suggests that EPCA may be more accurate than PSA in identifying

TABLE 2-40   Age-Specific Reference Ranges for Serum PSA

Age Range (years)	REFERENCE RANGE (ng/mL)		
	Blacks	**Caucasians**	**Japanese**
40-49	0.0-2	0.0-2.5	0.0-2
50-59	0.0-4	0.0-3.5	0.0-3
60-69	0.0-4.5	0.0-4.5	0.0-4
70-79	0.0-5.5	0.0-6.5	0.0-5

TABLE 2-41   Probability of Cancer Based on Percent Free PSA

Percent Free PSA	Probability of Cancer (%)
0-10	56
10-15	28
15-20	20
20-25	16
>25	8

prostate cancer. Furthermore, EPCA levels are significantly higher in patients whose cancers spread outside the prostate compared with those with disease confined to the gland. EPCA-1 is a tissue-based test and EPCA-2 is a blood-based test. Patients with an EPCA-2 cutoff level of 30 ng/mL or higher are considered to be at risk for prostate cancer.

- *Prostate cancer specific biomarkers*: These biomarkers are made up of RNA that is present in prostate cancer cells at very high levels because of overexpression of particular genes. These biomarkers can be detected in the urine of patients with prostate cancer after a short period of professional prostate massage. The most commonly tested marker is the prostate cancer gene 3 (PCA3). Other genetic markers tested include GOLPH2, SPINK1, and TMPRSS2-ERG. These biomarkers are not elevated in noncancerous prostate disease. Furthermore these biomarkers are not influenced by patient age or prostate volume.

PSA is used in the staging of men with known prostate cancer. Men with PSA levels below 10 ng/mL are most likely to have localized disease and respond well to local therapy (radical prostatectomy or radiation therapy). Routine metastatic staging tests are generally not required for men with clinically localized prostate cancer when their PSA is less than 20 ng/mL.

PSA is used to follow up men after treatment for prostate cancer. Periodic PSA testing should follow any form of treatment for prostate cancer, since PSA levels can indicate need for further treatment. Following curative radical prostatectomy or radiation therapy, PSA levels should probably be 0 to 0.5 ng/mL. The pattern of PSA rise after local therapy for prostate cancer can help distinguish between local recurrence and distant spread. Patients with elevated PSA levels more than 24 months after local treatment and with a PSA doubling time after 12 months are likely to have recurrence.

PSA can be measured by electrochemiluminescent immunoassay, immunohistochemistry, or radio-immunoassay. Newer, comparably accurate, chemical tests are being used to improve the worldwide use of PSA screening testing.

INTERFERING FACTORS

- Rectal examinations are well known to falsely elevate PAP levels, and they may also minimally elevate the PSA. To avoid this problem, the PSA should be drawn before rectal examination of the prostate or several hours afterward.
- Prostatic manipulation by biopsy or transurethral resection of the prostate (TURP) will significantly elevate the PSA levels. The blood test should be done before surgery or 6 weeks after manipulation.
- Ejaculation within 24 hours of blood testing will be associated with elevated PSA levels.
- Recent urinary tract infection or prostatitis can cause elevations of PSA as much as five times baseline for as long as 6 weeks.
- Finasteride (Propecia, Proscar) and diethylstilbesterol (DES) may cause *decreased* levels of PSA.

PROCEDURE AND PATIENT CARE

Before
- Explain the procedure to the patient.
- Tell the patient that no fasting is required.

During
- Collect a venous blood sample in a red-top tube.
- The use of the %FPSA demands strict sample handling not required with the total PSA. Appropriate sample handling is necessary for accurate and consistent assay performance. Check with the laboratory for specific guidelines.

Blood Studies

2

After

- Apply pressure or a pressure dressing to the venipuncture site.
- Observe the venipuncture site for bleeding.

TEST RESULTS AND CLINICAL SIGNIFICANCE

▲ Increased Levels

Prostate cancer,
BPH,
Prostatitis:

The PSA in the cytoplasm of the diseased prostate is expelled into the bloodstream, and PSA levels are elevated.

RELATED TEST

Prostatic Acid Phosphatase (PAP) (p. 25). This is another tumor marker for prostate cancer. It is less specific and less sensitive than the PSA test, and its use is diminishing.

Protein (Protein Electrophoresis, Immunofixation Electrophoresis [IFE], Serum Protein Electrophoresis [SPEP], Albumin, Globulin, Total Protein)

NORMAL FINDINGS

Adult/elderly
 Total protein: 6.4-8.3 g/dL or 64-83 g/L (SI units)
 Albumin: 3.5-5 g/dL or 35-50 g/L (SI units)
 Globulin: 2.3-3.4 g/dL
  $Alpha_1$ globulin: 0.1-0.3 g/dL or 1-3 g/L (SI units)
  $Alpha_2$ globulin: 0.6-1 g/dL or 6-10 g/L (SI units)
  Beta globulin: 0.7-1.1 g/dL or 7-11 g/L (SI units)
Children
 Total protein
  Premature infant: 4.2-7.6 g/dL
  Newborn: 4.6-7.4 g/dL
  Infant: 6-6.7 g/dL
  Child: 6.2-8 g/dL
 Albumin
  Premature infant: 3-4.2 g/dL
  Newborn: 3.5-5.4 g/dL
  Infant: 4.4-5.4 g/dL
  Child: 4-5.9 g/dL
No protein abnormality on electrophoresis

INDICATIONS

The measurement of proteins is a part of most routine screening tests. Protein electrophoresis, however, is used to identify protein abnormalities caused by a wide spectrum of diseases, including infections, inflammation, and hematologic malignancy.

TEST EXPLANATION

Proteins are constituents of muscle, enzymes, hormones, transport vehicles, hemoglobin, and several other key functional and structural entities within the body. They are the most significant components contributing to the osmotic pressure within the vascular space. This osmotic pressure keeps fluid within the vascular space, minimizing extravasation of fluid.

Albumin and globulin constitute most of the protein within the body and are measured together as the total protein. *Albumin* is a protein that is formed within the liver. It makes up approximately 60% of the total protein. The major effect of albumin within the blood is to maintain colloidal osmotic pressure. Furthermore, albumin transports important blood constituents such as drugs, hormones, and enzymes. Albumin is synthesized within the liver and is therefore a measure of hepatic function. When disease affects the liver cell, the hepatocyte loses its ability to synthesize albumin. The serum albumin level is greatly decreased. Because the half-life of albumin is 12 to 18 days, however, severe impairment of hepatic albumin synthesis may not be recognized until after that period.

Globulins represent all non-albumin proteins. Their role in maintaining osmotic pressure is far less than that of albumin. Alpha$_1$ globulins are mostly alpha$_1$ antitrypsin. Some transporting proteins, such as thyroid and cortisol-binding globulin, also contribute to this electrophoretic zone. Alpha$_2$ globulins include serum haptoglobins (which bind hemoglobin during hemolysis), ceruloplasmin (which is a carrier for copper), prothrombin, and cholinesterase (which is an enzyme used in the catabolism of acetylcholine). Beta$_1$ globulins include lipoproteins, transferrin, plasminogen, and complement proteins; beta$_2$ globulins include fibrinogen. Gamma globulins are the immunoglobulins (antibodies) (p. 312). To a lesser degree, globulins also act as transport vehicles.

Serum albumin and some globulins are measures of nutrition. Malnourished patients, especially after surgery, have a greatly decreased level of serum proteins. Burn patients and those who have protein-losing enteropathies and uropathies, have low levels of protein despite normal synthesis. Pregnancy, especially in the third trimester, is usually associated with reduced total proteins.

In some diseases, albumin is selectively diminished, and globulins are normal or increased to maintain a normal total protein level. For example, in collagen vascular diseases (e.g., lupus erythematosus), capillary permeability is increased. Albumin, a molecule that is generally smaller than most globulins, is selectively lost into the extravascular space. Another group of diseases similarly associated with low albumin, high globulin, and normal total protein levels is chronic liver diseases. In these diseases the liver cannot produce albumin, but globulin is adequately made in the reticuloendothelial system. In both of these types of diseases the albumin level is low, but the total protein level is normal because of increased globulin levels. These changes, however, can be detected if one measures the *albumin/globulin ratio*. Normally this ratio exceeds 1.0. The diseases just described that selectively affect albumin levels are associated with lesser ratios. Increased total protein levels, particularly the globulin fraction, occur with multiple myeloma and other gammopathies. It is important to note that proteins can be factitiously elevated in dehydrated patients. This is particularly well documented by measurement of the albumin level. Albumin, globulin, and other proteins can be quantitated individually. See specific protein tests.

Serum protein electrophoresis (SPEP) can separate the various components of blood protein into bands or zones according to their electrical charge. Several well-established electrophoretic patterns have been identified and can be associated with specific diseases (Table 2-42). If a spike is detected, immunofixation techniques can be added to the electrophoretic strip. In general, polyclonal spikes are associated with infectious or inflammatory diseases in which monoclonal specific spikes are often neoplastic. Immunofixation is used to indicate deficiencies or excesses as seen with macroglobulinemia, monoclonal gammopathy of undetermined significance (MGUS), and multiple myeloma.

TABLE 2-42 Protein Electrophoresis Patterns in Specific Diseases

Pattern	Electrophoresis	Disease
Acute reaction	↓ Albumin ↑ Alpha$_2$ globulin	Acute infections, tissue necrosis, burns, surgery, stress, myocardial infarction
Chronic inflammation	sl. ↓ Albumin sl. ↑ Gamma globulin N Alpha$_2$ globulin	Chronic infection, granulomatous diseases, cirrhosis, rheumatoid-collagen diseases
Nephrotic syndrome	↓↓ Albumin ↑↑ Alpha$_2$ globulin N ↑ Beta globulin	Nephrotic syndrome
Far-advanced cirrhosis	↓ Albumin ↑ Gamma globulin Incorporation of beta and gamma peaks	Far-advanced cirrhosis
Polyclonal gamma globulin elevation	↑↑ Gamma globulin with a broad peak	Cirrhosis, chronic infection, sarcoidosis, tuberculosis, endocarditis, rheumatoid-collagen diseases
Hypogammaglobulinemia	↓ Gamma globulin with normal other globulin levels	Light-chain multiple myeloma
Monoclonal gammopathy	Thin spikes in the beta (IgA, IgM) and gamma globulins	Myeloma, Waldenström macroglobulinemia, gammopathies

↓, Decreased; ↑, increased; *sl.* ↓, slightly decreased; *sl.* ↑, slightly increased; *N*, normal; ↓↓, greatly decreased; ↑↑, greatly increased.

Immunofixation is also able to determine whether a monoclonal spike is caused by light-chain or other protein abnormalities.

With immunofixation, a monospecific antibody is placed in contact with the gel after the proteins have been separated by electrophoresis. The resulting protein-antibody complexes are subsequently specifically stained for visualization after being precipitated out. The pathologist can then identify and classify specific immunoglobulin spikes. Specific monoclonal protein studies can be performed on the urine or blood. Monoclonal immunoglobulin heavy chain (gamma, alpha, mu, delta, or epsilon) and/or light chains (kappa or lambda) can be identified. With sensitive nephelometric assay specific light chain disease can be identified (Figures 2-21 through 2-25).

This test is also used to follow the course of the disease or treatment in patients with known monoclonal immunoglobulinopathies. For example, with successful treatment for neoplastic gammopathies, IFE, upon repetition, can demonstrate reduction in the specific immunoglobulin. Finally, this test is helpful in defining more clearly the immune status of a patient whose immune status may be compromised.

Protein electrophoresis is also used to evaluate the major protein fractions found in urine. Normally only small amounts of albumins are seen. Urinary protein electrophoresis is useful in classifying the type of renal damage, if present. Immunofixation is useful in characterizing M-components observed in the protein electrophoresis and in identifying light-chain disease. These electrophoresis techniques can be provided to the CSF or any body fluid.

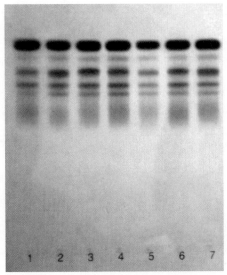

Figure 2-21 Normal automated serum protein electrophoresis for patients 1 through 7. Note dense albumin electrophoresis on top followed by globulins toward the bottom.

Serum Protein Electrophoresis

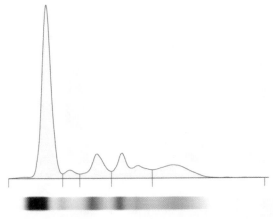

Fractions	%	Ref. %
Albumin	64.0	60.5 - 72.5
Alpha 1	2.6	1.6 - 3.4
Alpha 2	9.4	6.6 - 11.2
Beta	12.5	9.0 - 13.6
Gamma	11.5	8.5 - 13.1

Figure 2-22 Normal automated serum protein electrophoresis in graphic form for patient 1.

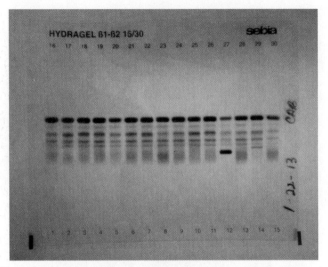

Figure 2-23 Abnormal automated serum protein electrophoresis for patients 1 through 10. Note dense migration of the paraprotein for patient 4.

Serum Protein Electrophoresis

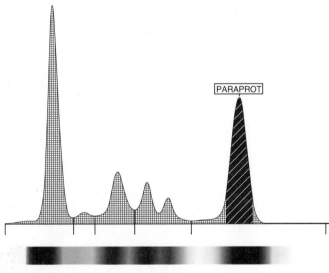

Fractions	%		Ref. %	g/dl	Ref g/dL
Albumin	41.9	<	56.2 - 69.4	3.94	3.31 - 4.94
Alpha 1	2.4		1.5 - 4.4	0.23	0.07 - 0.31
Alpha 2	12.3		7.0 - 13.6	1.16	0.58 - 0.87
Beta	11.6		8.3 - 13.7	1.09	0.62 - 1.12
Gamma	31.8	>	8.3 - 17.7	2.99	0.49 - 1.36
PARAPROT	28.4			2.67	

Figure 2-24 Normal automated serum protein electrophoresis in graphic form for patient 4. An abnormal globulin paraprotein is noted.

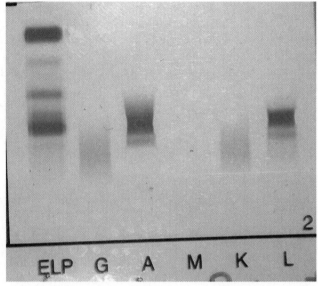

Figure 2-25 Abnormal immunofixation immunoglobulin electro-phoresis for patient 4. ELP equals protein electrophoresis pattern. Note the dense migration pattern in the lower portion of the ELP column. G equals IgG antibody; A equals IgA antibody; M equals IgM antibody; K equals kappa chains; L equals lambda chains. This patient has an IgA and lambda chain gammopathy.

INTERFERING FACTORS

- Prolonged application of tourniquet can increase both fractions of total proteins.
- Sampling of peripheral venous blood proximal to an IV administration site can result in an inaccurately low protein level. Likewise, massive IV infusion of crystalloid fluid can result in acute hypoproteinemia.
- Drugs that can cause *increased* protein levels include anabolic steroids, androgens, corticosteroids, dextran, growth hormone, insulin, phenazopyridine, and progesterone.
- Drugs that can cause *decreased* protein levels include ammonium ions, estrogens, hepatotoxic drugs, and oral contraceptives.

PROCEDURE AND PATIENT CARE

Before

- Explain the procedure to the patient.
- Tell the patient that no fasting or special preparation is required.

During

Blood

- Collect venous blood in a gold-top tube. The blood used for immunoglobulin electrophoresis can be reused.
- Indicate on the laboratory slip if the patient has received any vaccinations or immunizations within the past 6 months. Also, list any drugs that may affect test results.

Urine

☒ See Box 11-2, Guidelines for a 24-Hour Urine Collection, p. 907.

☒ Encourage the patient to drink fluids during the 24 hours unless this is contraindicated for medical purposes.

• Place the 24-hour urine collection in a plastic container and keep on ice. Use a preservative.

After

• Apply pressure to the venipuncture site.

TEST RESULTS AND CLINICAL SIGNIFICANCE

▲ Increased Albumin Levels

Dehydration: *As intravascular volume diminishes, albumin concentration measurements must increase mathematically.*

▼ Decreased Albumin Levels

Malnutrition: *Lack of amino acids available for building proteins contributes to this observation. Probably the liver dysfunction (albumin synthesis) associated with malnutrition also contributes to the low albumin levels.*

Pregnancy: *Albumin levels progressively decrease until delivery.*

Liver disease (e.g., hepatitis, extensive metastatic tumor, cirrhosis, hepatocellular necrosis): *The liver is the site of synthesis of albumin. If production of albumin is inadequate, levels can be expected to fall.*

Protein-losing enteropathies (e.g., malabsorption syndromes such as Crohn disease, sprue, Whipple disease): *Large volumes of protein are lost from the intestines because absorption is inadequate. Albumin levels will fall.*

Protein-losing nephropathies (e.g., nephrotic syndrome, nephrosis): *Large volumes of albumin can be lost through the kidneys. This loss may be selective for albumin (lipoid nephrosis) or drain out all components of proteins (glomerulonephritis).*

Third-space losses (e.g., ascites, third-degree burns): *Large amounts of albumin can be lost in the serum that weeps from chronic open burns. Albumin readily accumulates in the peritoneum of patients with ascites.*

Overhydration: *As the blood volume increases, albumin concentration measurements decrease mathematically.*

Increased capillary permeability (e.g., collagen-vascular diseases such as lupus erythematosus): *Albumin can seep out of the microvascular spaces in the tissues and cause edema or in the kidneys and cause proteinuria. The serum albumin decreases.*

Inflammatory disease: *Diseases associated with inflammation, necrosis, infarction, or burns cause an increase in acute-phase reactant proteins. These are mostly globulins. Therefore the globulin component of proteins increases and albumin decreases.*

Familial idiopathic dysproteinemia: *This is a genetic disease in which albumin is significantly reduced (and globulins are increased).*

▲ Increased Alpha₁ Globulin Levels

Inflammatory disease: *Alpha$_1$-antitrypsin is an acute-phase reactant protein that is increased with diseases associated with inflammation, necrosis, infarction, malignancy, or burns.*

▼ Decreased Alpha₁ Globulin Levels

Juvenile pulmonary emphysema: *These patients have a genetic decrease or absence of alpha$_1$ antitrypsin, which is important to normal pulmonary function.*

▲ Increased Alpha₂ Globulin Levels

Inflammatory disease: *Haptoglobin and ceruloplasmin are alpha₂ globulins. These proteins are acute-phase reactant proteins that are increased with diseases associated with inflammation, necrosis, infarction, malignancy, or burns.*

▼ Decreased Alpha₂ Globulin Levels

Hemolysis: *Haptoglobin is an alpha₂ globulin and is decreased when hemolysis occurs.*
Wilson disease: *Ceruloplasmin is an alpha₂ globulin. It is decreased in Wilson disease.*
Severe liver dysfunction: *Haptoglobulin is an alpha₂ globulin that is made in the liver. It is decreased when liver function is inadequate.*

▲ Increased Beta Globulin Levels

Hypercholesterolemia (which can occur by itself or in association with biliary cirrhosis, hypothyroidism, or nephrosis): *Beta lipoprotein is a beta globulin and is increased in hypercholesterolemia.*
Iron-deficiency anemia: *Transferrin is a beta globulin and is increased in this form of anemia.*
Estrogen therapy: *Estrogen causes increased production of these proteins.*

▼ Decreased Beta Globulin Levels

Malnutrition: *Transferrin is a beta globulin and is decreased in malnutrition.*
Consumptive coagulopathy: *Several proteins used in the coagulation process are beta globulins. They are consumed in disorders of unrestricted coagulation.*

▲ Increased Gamma Globulin Levels

Multiple myeloma,
Waldenström macroglobulinemia:
   These cancers are characterized by production of gamma globulin from neoplastic plasma cells or lymphocytes. The total gamma globulin zone may not be increased but a monoclonal spike in one portion is often seen.
Chronic inflammatory disease (e.g., rheumatoid arthritis, systemic lupus erythematosus [SLE]): *These diseases are associated with autoantibodies, and patients will have a gamma globulin spike.*
Malignancy (e.g., Hodgkin's disease, lymphoma, leukemia): *These diseases may be associated with elevated gamma globulins.*
Hyperimmunization: *A small spike can occur in the IgA portion of the gamma band.*
Cirrhosis: *Most patients have gamma and some have beta globulin spikes associated with this disease. The pathophysiology is not well known.*
Acute and chronic infection: *Infection is associated with an antibody response and therefore an increase in immunoglobulins (gamma globulins).*
Light chain disease

▼ Decreased Gamma Globulin Levels

Genetic immune disorders: *A host of immune deficiencies are associated with reduced or absent immunoglobulins.*
Secondary immune deficiency: *Several conditions (e.g., steroid use, nephrotic syndrome, severe gram-negative infection, lymphoma, leukemia) are associated with deficient levels of immunoglobulins.*

▲ Increased Blood Monoclonal Immunoglobulins

Multiple myeloma,

Waldenström's macroglobulinemia:
> *These diseases are highlighted by rapid cellular duplication of mononuclear antibody-producing cells.*

▲ Increased Blood Polyclonal Immunoglobulins

Amyloidosis,
Autoimmune diseases,
Chronic infection/inflammation,
Chronic liver disease:
> *These diseases highlighted by inflammatory reactions are associated with the development of many antibodies.*

▲ Increased Urine Monoclonal Immunoglobulins

Multiple myeloma,
Waldenström's macroglobulinemia:
> *These diseases are highlighted by rapid cellular duplication of mononuclear antibody producing cells.*

See also Table 2-42.

RELATED TESTS

Immunoglobulin Quantification (p. 312). This is a measurement of each various immunoglobulin and a determination of its clonality.

Protein C, Protein S

NORMAL FINDINGS

Protein S: 60%-130% of normal activity
Protein C: 70%-150% of normal activity
(Protein C decreases with age and in females)

Indications

This test identifies patients who are deficient in protein C and/or S. This is part of the evaluation of patients with coagulation disorders.

TEST EXPLANATION

The plasma coagulation system is tightly regulated between thrombosis and fibrinolysis. This precise regulation is important. The protein C–protein S system is an important inhibitor of coagulation. Protein C inhibits the activation of factors VIII and V (see Figure 2-12, p. 167). This inhibitory function of protein C is enhanced by protein S. Congenital deficiencies of these vitamin K–dependent proteins may cause spontaneous intravascular thrombosis. Furthermore dysfunctional forms of the proteins result in a hypercoagulable state. In addition nearly 50% of hypercoagulable states are caused by the presence of a factor V (factor V-Leiden, p. 231) that is resistant to protein C inhibition. Acquired deficiencies are less commonly symptomatic.

When protein C is tested, protein S activity also should be tested because the decreased activity of protein C may be the result of decreased protein S. When decreased protein C activity is noted, protein C resistance (the presence of factor V-Leiden) should be tested.

These proteins are vitamin K dependent and are decreased in patients who are taking Coumadin, as well as those with liver diseases or severe malnutrition. Of the total plasma protein S, approximately 60% circulates bound to C4bBP compliment protein, whereas the remaining 40% circulates as "free" protein S. Only free protein S has an anticoagulant function. Because compliment regulatory proteins are acute phase reactants, autoimmune diseases and other inflammatory diseases are associated with increased binding of protein S, causing an acquired protein S deficiency. Affected patients may experience hypercoagulable events.

Measurement of plasma free protein S antigen is performed as the initial testing for protein S deficiency. When the free protein S antigen level is below the age- and sex-adjusted normal range, quantification for total plasma protein S antigen is indicated.

INTERFERING FACTORS

- Decreased protein C may occur in the postoperative states.
- Pregnancy or the use of exogenous sex hormones is associated with decreases in proteins C and S. These low levels of protein S in pregnancy do not cause thrombosis by themselves.
- The concentration of citrate in the collection tube varies and can affect activity results.
- Active clotting states, such as DVT, can lower levels of protein S and C.
- 🍷 Drugs that can decrease levels include vitamin K inhibitors such as coumadin.

PROCEDURE AND PATIENT CARE

Before
- Explain the procedure to the patient.
- Tell the patient that fasting is not usually required.

During
- Collect a venous blood sample in a blue-top tube. If more than one blood test is to be obtained, draw the blood for proteins C or S second to avoid contamination with tissue thromboplastin that may occur in the first tube. If only blood for protein C or S is being drawn, draw a red top first (and throw it away) and then draw the blood for this study in a blue top tube (two-tube method of blood draw).
- Place the tube in an ice bath.

After
- Apply pressure to the venipuncture site.
- If the patient is found to be deficient in either protein, encourage the patient's family to be tested as they too may be similarly affected.

TEST RESULTS AND CLINICAL SIGNIFICANCE

▼ Decreased Levels

Inherited deficiency of protein C or protein S: *Protein S or C defect that may not be recognized until adulthood.*
Disseminated intravascular coagulation (DIC),
Hypercoagulable states,
Pulmonary emboli,
Arterial or venous thrombosis:
   These thrombotic diseases, when recurrent, may be the result of a protein C or S deficiency.

Vitamin K deficiency: *Protein C and S are dependent on vitamin K for their synthesis. If vitamin K is not available because of malnutrition, biliary disease, or malabsorption, these proteins will not be produced in adequate levels. Because several coagulation factors are also vitamin K-dependent, a hypercoagulable event may not occur.*

Sickle cell disease: *This condition alone does not produce a thrombophilic state.*

Autoimmune diseases,

Inflammation:

These proteins may be "used-up" in the inflammatory process.

Coumadin-induced skin necrosis: *This occurs in the feet, buttocks, thighs, breasts, upper extremities, and genitalia. The lesions usually begin as maculopapular lesions several days after initiation of warfarin and progress into bullous, hemorrhagic, necrotic lesions. Patients with protein C deficiency are at high risk for warfarin-induced skin necrosis during initiation of therapy with warfarin. Approximately one third of patients with warfarin-induced skin necrosis have protein C deficiency.*

RELATED TEST

Disseminated Intravascular Coagulation (DIC) Screening (p. 210). This group of tests is indicated for patients with coagulopathies, such as DIC.

Prothrombin Time (PT, Pro-Time, International Normalized Ratio [INR])

NORMAL FINDINGS*

11.0-12.5 seconds; 85%-100%
Full anticoagulant therapy: >1.5-2 times control value; 20%-30%
INR: 0.8-1.1

 Possible Critical Values

>20 seconds
INR: >5

INDICATIONS

The PT is used to evaluate the adequacy of the extrinsic system and common pathway in the clotting mechanism.

TEST EXPLANATION

The hemostasis and coagulation system is a homeostatic balance between factors encouraging clotting and the factors encouraging clot dissolution. The first reaction of the body to active bleeding is blood vessel constriction. In small vessel injury, this may be enough to stop bleeding. In large vessel injury, hemostasis is required to form a clot that will durably plug the hole until healing can occur. The primary phase of the hemostatic mechanism involves platelet aggregation to blood

---

* Findings depend on reagents used for PT.

vessel (see Figure 2-12 on p. 167). Next, secondary hemostasis occurs. The first phase of reactions is called the intrinsic system. Factor XII and other proteins form a complex on the subendothelial collagen in the injured blood vessel. Through a series of reactions, activated factor XI (XIa) is formed and activates factor IX (IXa). In a complex formed by factors VIII, IX, and X, activated X (Xa) is formed.

At the same time, the extrinsic system is activated and a complex is formed between tissue thromboplastin (factor III) and factor VII (which is exposed after cellular injury). Activated factor VII (VIIa) results. Factor VIIa can directly activate factor X. Alternatively, VIIa can activate IX and X together.

In the third phase, factor X is activated by the proteases formed by the two prior reactions and by activated factor IX. This reaction is a common pathway that provides the link between the intrinsic and the extrinsic systems. In the fourth and final phase, prothrombin is converted into thrombin by activated factor X in the presence of factor V, phospholipid, and calcium.

Thrombin not only converts fibrinogen to fibrin in "clot stabilization" but also stimulates platelet aggregation and activates factors V, VIII, and XIII. Once fibrin is formed, it is then polymerized into a stable gel. Factor XIII cross-links the fibrin polymers to form a stable clot.

Almost immediately three major activators of the fibrinolytic system act on plasminogen, which was previously absorbed into the clot, to form plasmin. Plasmin degenerates the fibrin polymer into fragments, which are cleared by macrophages.

The PT measures the clotting ability of factors I (fibrinogen), II (prothrombin), V, VII, and X (i.e., the extrinsic system and common pathway). When these clotting factors exist in deficient quantities, the PT is prolonged. Many diseases and drugs are associated with decreased levels of these factors. These include the following:

1. *Hepatocellular liver disease* (e.g., cirrhosis, hepatitis, and neoplastic invasive processes). Factors I, II, V, VII, IX, and X are produced in the liver. With severe hepatocellular dysfunction, synthesis of these factors will not occur, and serum concentration of these factors will be decreased.

2. *Obstructive biliary disease* (e.g., bile duct obstruction secondary to tumor or gallstones or intrahepatic cholestasis secondary to sepsis or drugs). As a result of the biliary obstruction, the bile necessary for fat absorption fails to enter the gut, and fat malabsorption results. Vitamins A, D, E, and K are fat soluble and also are not absorbed. Because the synthesis of factors II, VII, IX, and X depends on vitamin K, these factors will not be adequately produced, and serum concentrations will fall. *Hepatocellular liver disease* can be differentiated from obstructive biliary disease by determination of the patient's response to parenteral vitamin K administration. If the PT returns to normal after 1 to 3 days of vitamin K administration (10 mg intramuscularly twice a day), one can safely assume that the patient has obstructive biliary disease that is causing vitamin K malabsorption. If, on the other hand, the PT does not return to normal with the vitamin K injections, one can assume that severe hepatocellular disease exists and that the liver cells are incapable of synthesizing the clotting factors no matter how much vitamin K is available.

3. *Oral anticoagulant administration.* The coumarin derivatives dicumarol and warfarin (Coumadin, Panwarfin) are used to prevent coagulation in patients with thromboembolic disease (e.g., pulmonary embolism, thrombophlebitis, arterial embolism). These drugs interfere with the production of vitamin K–dependent clotting factors, which results in a prolongation of PT, as already described. The adequacy of coumarin therapy can be monitored by following the patient's PT. For anticoagulation, the INR typically should be between 2.0 and 3.0 for patients with atrial fibrillation, and between 3.0 and 4.0 for patients with mechanical heart valves. However, the ideal INR must be individualized for each patient (Table 2-43).

TABLE 2-43 **Preferred International Normalized Ratio (INR) According to Indication for Anticoagulation**

Indication	Preferred INR
Deep-vein thrombosis prophylaxis	1.5-2
Orthopedic surgery	2-3
Deep-vein thrombosis	2-3
Atrial fibrillation	2-3
Pulmonary embolism	2.5-3.5
Prosthetic valve prophylaxis	3-4

PT test results used to be given in seconds, along with a control value. The control value usually varied somewhat from day to day because the reagents used varied. The patient's PT value was supposed to be approximately equal to the control value. Some laboratories used to report PT values as percentages of normal activity, because the patient's results were compared with a curve representing normal clotting time. A normal PT result was 85% to 100%.

To have uniform PT results for physicians in different parts of the country and the world, the World Health Organization has recommended that PT results include the use of the *international normalized ratio (INR)* value. The reported INR results are independent of the reagents or methods used. Many hospitals are now reporting PT times in both absolute and INR numbers. Factors such as weight, body mass index, age, diet, and concurrent medications are known to affect warfarin dose requirements during anticoagulation therapy.

Warfarin interferes with the regeneration of reduced vitamin K from oxidized vitamin K in the VKOR (vitamin K oxidoreductase) complex. A recently identified gene for the major subunit of VKOR, called VKORC1, has been identified and may explain up to 44% of the variance in warfarin dose requirements. Furthermore, warfarin is metabolized in part by the cytochrome P-450 enzyme CYP2C9. The CYP2C9*2 and CYP2C9*3 genetic mutations have been shown to decrease the enzyme activity of these metabolizing enzymes, which has led to warfarin sensitivity and, in serious cases, bleeding complications. A *warfarin pharmacogenomic test panel* is available that can identify any mutations in the VKORC1-1639, CYP2C9*2, or CYP2C9*3 genes. The warfarin pharmacogenomic test can be used as part of an algorithm to determine the best initial warfarin dose and does not replace the need for routine PT testing for the calculation of the INR.

Point-of-care home testing is now available for patients who require long-term anticoagulation with warfarin. This is useful for patients with prosthetic cardiac valves, chronic atrial fibrillation, or recurrent venous thromboembolism, and is especially helpful for patients who do not live close to a testing facility. Like glucose monitoring, a finger stick is performed. A drop of blood is placed on the testing strip and inserted into the handheld testing device. The PT and INR are provided in a few minutes. The treating physician is notified by phone and any therapeutic changes can be instigated the same day.

Coumarin derivatives are slow acting, but their action may persist for 7 to 14 days after discontinuation of the drug. The action of a coumarin drug can be reversed in 12 to 24 hours by slow parenteral administration of vitamin K (phytonadione). The administration of plasma will even more rapidly reverse the coumarin effect. The action of coumarin drugs can be enhanced by drugs such as aspirin, quinidine, sulfa, and indomethacin. Barbiturates, chloral hydrate, and oral contraceptives cause increased coumarin drug binding and therefore may decrease the effects of coumarin drugs.

INTERFERING FACTORS

- Alcohol intake can prolong PT times. Alcohol diminishes liver function. Many factors are made in the liver. Lesser quantities of coagulation factors result in prolonged PT times.
- A diet high in fat or leafy vegetables may shorten PT times. Absorption of vitamin K is enhanced. Vitamin K–dependent factors are made at increased levels, thereby shortening PT times.
- Diarrhea or malabsorption syndromes can prolong PT times. Vitamin K is malabsorbed, and as a result, factors II, VII, IX, and X are not made.
- Drugs that may cause *increased* levels include allopurinol, aminosalicylic acid, barbiturates, beta-lactam antibiotics, chloral hydrate, cephalothins, cholestyramine, cimetidine, clofibrate, colestipol, ethyl alcohol, glucagon, heparin, methyldopa, neomycin, oral anticoagulants, propylthiouracil, quinidine, quinine, salicylates, and sulfonamides.
- Drugs that may cause *decreased* levels include anabolic steroids, barbiturates, chloral hydrate, digitalis, diphenhydramine, estrogens, griseofulvin, oral contraceptives, and vitamin K.

PROCEDURE AND PATIENT CARE

Before

- Explain the procedure to the patient.
- Tell the patient that no fasting is required.
- If the patient is receiving warfarin, obtain the blood specimen before the patient is given the daily dose of warfarin. The daily dose may be increased, decreased, or kept the same depending on the PT test results for that day.

During

- Collect a venous blood sample in a blue-top tube.
- List on the laboratory slip any drugs the patient is taking that may affect test results.

After

- Apply pressure or a pressure dressing to the venipuncture site.
- Assess the venipuncture site for bleeding. Remember, hemostasis will be delayed if the patient is taking warfarin or if the patient has any coagulopathies.
- If the PT is greatly prolonged, evaluate the patient for bleeding tendencies (i.e., check for blood in the urine and all excretions and assess the patient for bruises, petechiae, and low-back pain). Back pain may be a symptom of retroperitoneal bleeding.
- If severe bleeding occurs, the anticoagulant effect of warfarin can be reversed by the slow parenteral administration of vitamin K (phytonadione). If coagulation must be returned to near normal more quickly, plasma can be given.
- Because of drug interactions, instruct the patient not to take any medication unless specifically ordered by the physician.

 Home Care Responsibilities

- Coumadin levels will be regulated by PT and INR values.
- Inform patients to evaluate themselves for bleeding tendencies. Patients should assess themselves for bruises, petechiae, low-back pain, and bleeding gums. Blood may be detected in the urine and stool.
- Because of many drug interactions, instruct patients on coumadin therapy not to take any other medications unless approved by their physician.

TEST RESULTS AND CLINICAL SIGNIFICANCE

▲ Increased Levels (Prolonged PT)

Liver disease (e.g., cirrhosis, hepatitis): *Coagulation factors are made in the liver. With liver disease, synthesis is inadequate and the PT is increased.*

Hereditary factor deficiency: *A genetic defect causes a decrease in a coagulation factor. The PT is increased. Factors II, V, VII, or X could be similarly affected.*

Vitamin K deficiency: *Vitamin K–dependent factors (II, VII, IX, X) are not made. The PT is increased.*

Bile duct obstruction: *Fat-soluble vitamins, including vitamin K, are not absorbed. Vitamin K–dependent factors (II, VII, IX, X) are not made. The PT is increased.*

Coumarin ingestion: *Synthesis of the vitamin K–dependent coagulation factors is inhibited. The PT is increased.*

Disseminated intravascular coagulation (DIC): *Coagulation factors are consumed in the intravascular coagulation process. The PT is increased.*

Massive blood transfusion: *Coagulation is inhibited by the anticoagulant in the banked blood. Furthermore, with massive bleeding the factors are diluted out by the "factor-poor" banked blood.*

Salicylate intoxication

RELATED TESTS

Partial Thromboplastin Time (p. 383). This test is used to evaluate the intrinsic system and the common pathway of clot formation. It is most commonly used to monitor heparin therapy.

Coagulating Factor Concentration (p. 163). This is a quantitative measurement of specific coagulation factors.

Rabies-Neutralizing Antibody

NORMAL FINDINGS

<1:16

INDICATIONS

This test is performed after vaccination to document seroprotection in animal care workers. It is also used to determine exposure to rabies and in the diagnosis of rabies.

TEST EXPLANATION

Identification and documentation of the presence of rabies-neutralizing antibody is important for veterinary health care workers and others who are at risk or may have been exposed to the rabies virus. This test is performed on persons who are at great risk for animal bites (veterinarians and their staff, zoo workers, those who work with animals in laboratories) and on those who have received the human diploid cell rabies vaccine (HDCV). A rabies titer of greater than 1:16 is considered protective.

Rabies antibody is also used in diagnosing rabies in patients suspected of being exposed to the virus. A fourfold rise in antibody titer over several weeks in a person not previously exposed to the HDCV indicates rabies exposure. If the patient has received HDCV and has been bitten by an animal suspected of having rabies infection, a very high antibody titer may support the diagnosis. The presence of antibody in the cerebrospinal fluid (CSF) is also supportive of the diagnosis, because usually there are not antibodies in the CSF after the HDCV vaccine, but there are antibodies after a bite from a rabies-infected animal. In patients who may have been exposed to rabies, the human rabies immunoglobulin (HRIG) is given after the antibody titers have been obtained. Half of the HRIG is given into the area of the bite, and half is administered as an intramuscular (IM) injection into the gluteal region. At the same time the first of the HDCV shots are administered to begin vaccination. Four subsequent IM injections are administered over the next 28 days. One can expect to see increases in rabies antibody levels in about 10 days, but protective levels may not be present for several weeks. Postexposure protocols exist to determine the proper handling of the patient and animal, depending on the real risk for the animal's infection.

The rabies antibody is identified by the direct fluorescent antibody method. More recently immunofluorescence has been used.

PROCEDURE AND PATIENT CARE

Before
Explain the procedure to the patient.
Tell the patient that no fasting or special preparation is required.

During
- Collect a venous blood sample in a red-top tube.

After
- Apply pressure or a pressure dressing to the venipuncture site.
- Assess the venipuncture site for bleeding.

TEST RESULTS AND CLINICAL SIGNIFICANCE

Exposure to rabies vaccine: *This causes a relatively low titer of 1:16 or greater.*
Recent bite exposure to rabies virus: *This causes a progressive rise in titer to levels of 1:200 to 1:160,000.*
Active rabies in patient or animal: *Antibody titers are extremely high in patients who present with encephalitis and brain stem dysfunction. These patients rarely recover from the disease.*

Red Blood Cell Count (RBC Count, Erythrocyte Count)

NORMAL FINDINGS

($RBC \times 10^6/\mu L$ or $RBC \times 10^{12}/L$ [SI units])
Adult/elderly
    Male: 4.7-6.1
    Female: 4.2-5.4
Child
    2-8 weeks: 4.0-6.0
    2-6 months: 3.5-5.5
    6 months-1 year: 3.5-5.2
    1-6 years: 4.0-5.5
    6-18 years: 4.0-5.5
Newborn: 4.8-7.1

INDICATIONS

The RBC count is closely related to the hemoglobin (p. 281) and hematocrit (p. 277) levels and represents different ways of evaluating the number of RBCs in the peripheral blood. It is repeated serially in patients with ongoing bleeding or as a routine part of the complete blood cell count. It is an integral part of the evaluation of anemic patients.

TEST EXPLANATION

This test is a count of the number of circulating RBCs in 1 mm^3 of peripheral venous blood. The RBC count is routinely performed as part of a complete blood cell count. Within each RBC are molecules of hemoglobin that permit the transport and exchange of oxygen to the tissues and carbon dioxide from the tissues. The RBC is produced by the erythroid elements in the bone marrow. Under the stimulation of erythropoietin, RBC production is increased. Normally RBCs survive in the peripheral blood for approximately 120 days. During that time the RBC is transported through the bloodstream. In the smallest of capillaries the RBC must fold and bend to conform to the size of these tiny vessels. Toward the end of the RBC's life, the cell membrane becomes less pliable; the aged RBC is then lysed and extracted from the circulation by the spleen. Abnormal RBCs have a shorter life span and are extracted earlier. Intravascular RBC trauma, such as that caused by artificial heart valves or peripheral vascular atherosclerotic plaques, also shortens the RBC's life. An enlarged spleen, such as that caused by portal hypertension or leukemia, may inappropriately destroy and remove normal RBCs from the circulation.

Normal RBC values vary according to gender and age. Women tend to have lower values than men, and RBC counts tend to decrease with age. When the value is decreased below the range of the expected normal value, the patient is said to be anemic. Low RBC values are caused by many factors, including:

1. Hemorrhage (as in GI bleeding or trauma)
2. Hemolysis (as in glucose-6-phosphate dehydrogenase deficiency, spherocytosis, or secondary splenomegaly)
3. Dietary deficiency (as of iron or vitamin B$_{12}$)
4. Genetic aberrations (as in sickle cell anemia or thalassemia)
5. Drug ingestion (as of chloramphenicol, hydantoins, or quinidine)
6. Marrow failure (as in fibrosis, leukemia, or antineoplastic chemotherapy)
7. Chronic illness (as in tumor or sepsis)
8. Other organ failure (as in renal disease)

RBC counts greater than normal can be physiologically induced as a result of the body's requirements for greater oxygen-carrying capacity (e.g., at high altitudes). Diseases that produce chronic hypoxia (e.g., congenital heart disease) also provoke this physiologic increase in RBCs. Polycythemia vera is a neoplastic condition causing uncontrolled production of RBCs.

Like the hemoglobin and hematocrit values, the RBC count can be altered by many factors other than RBC production. For instance, in dehydrated patients the total blood volume is contracted. The RBCs will be more concentrated, and the RBC count will be falsely high. Likewise, in overhydrated patients the blood concentration is diluted and the RBC count per millimeter will be falsely low. In most hospitals and laboratories the RBC count is done by an automated counting machine with an error range of about 4% to 5%.

INTERFERING FACTORS

- Normal RBC decreases are seen during pregnancy as a result of normal body fluid increases that dilute the RBCs. Also, there is an element of nutritional deficiency that is often associated with pregnancy that may play a role in the anemia of pregnancy.

- Living in high altitudes causes increased RBC counts as a result of a physiologic response to the decreased oxygen available at these high altitudes.
- Hydration status: As stated above, dehydration factitiously increases the RBC count, and overhydration decreases the RBC count.
- Drugs that may cause *increased* RBC levels include erythropoietin and gentamicin.
- Drugs that may cause *decreased* RBC levels include those that decrease marrow production or cause hemolysis.

PROCEDURE AND PATIENT CARE

Before
- Explain the procedure to the patient.
- Tell the patient that no fasting is required.

During
- Collect a venous blood sample in a lavender-top tube.
- Thoroughly mix the blood with the anticoagulant by tilting the tube.
- Avoid hemolysis.

After
- Apply pressure or a pressure dressing to the venipuncture site.
- Observe the venipuncture site for bleeding.

TEST RESULTS AND CLINICAL SIGNIFICANCE

▲ Increased Levels

Erythrocytosis: *The number of RBCs increases as a result of illnesses or as a physiologic response to external situations (e.g., high altitude).*

Congenital heart disease: *Cyanotic heart diseases cause chronically low Po_2 levels. In response, the RBCs increase in number.*

Severe chronic obstructive pulmonary disease (COPD): *Chronic states of hypoxia cause stimulation of RBC production as a physiologic response to increase oxygen-carrying capacity.*

Polycythemia vera: *This is a result of the bone marrow inappropriately producing great numbers of RBCs.*

Severe dehydration (e.g., severe diarrhea or burns): *With depletion of extracellular fluid, the total blood volume decreases, but the number of RBCs stays the same. Because the blood is more concentrated, the number of RBCs per cubic millimeter is increased.*

Hemoglobinopathies,

Thalassemia trait:

    In response to the decreased oxygen-carrying capacity of abnormal hemoglobin, more RBCs may be produced to provide adequate oxygen-carrying capacity.

▼ Decreased Levels

Anemia: *This is a state associated with reduced RBC numbers. Many different types of diseases are associated with anemia.*

Hemoglobinopathy: *Patients with hemoglobin disorders or other blood dyscrasias may have a reduced RBC number and survival.*

Cirrhosis: *This is a chronic state of fluid overload. The RBCs are diluted, and the number of RBCs per cubic millimeter is reduced.*

Hemolytic anemia (e.g., erythroblastosis fetalis, hemoglobinopathies, drug-induced hemolytic anemias, transfusion reactions, paroxysmal nocturnal hemoglobinuria): *The RBC survival is diminished in hemolytic anemia. The number of RBCs decreases.*

Hemorrhage: *With active bleeding the number of RBCs decreases. It takes time (several hours), however, for the RBC count to fall. Only if the blood volume is replenished with fluid will the RBC count diminish.*

Dietary deficiency: *With certain vitamin or mineral deficiencies (e.g., iron, vitamin B_{12}), the RBC size or number is decreased.*

Bone marrow failure: *This results in reduced synthesis of RBC.*

Prosthetic valves: *Prosthetic valves cause mechanical trauma to the RBC. The RBC survival time is shortened and numbers diminish.*

Renal disease: *Erythropoietin is made in the kidney and is a strong stimulant to RBC production. With reduced levels of erythropoietin, the RBC numbers diminish.*

Normal pregnancy: *Normally there is increased blood volume during pregnancy because of a chronic state of overhydration. Combined with a relative "malnourished" state, the RBC count per cubic millimeter of blood is diminished.*

Rheumatoid/collagen-vascular diseases (e.g., rheumatoid arthritis, lupus, sarcoidosis): *Chronic illnesses are associated with reduced production of RBCs.*

Lymphoma,

Multiple myeloma,

Leukemia,

Hodgkin disease:
Hematologic cancers are often associated with bone marrow failure of RBC production.

RELATED TESTS

Hematocrit (p. 277). This is a measurement of the percentage of the total blood volume taken up by the RBCs. It is closely associated with the hemoglobin value and the RBC count.

Hemoglobin (p. 281). This is a measurement of the concentration of hemoglobin in the blood. It is closely associated with the RBC count and hematocrit value.

Red Blood Cell Indices (see following test). These indices provide information about the size and hemoglobin content of the RBC.

Red Blood Cell Indices (RBC Indices, Mean Corpuscular Volume [MCV], Mean Corpuscular Hemoglobin [MCH], Mean Corpuscular Hemoglobin Concentration [MCHC], Blood Indices, Erythrocyte Indices, Red Blood Cell Distribution Width [RDW])

NORMAL FINDINGS

Mean Corpuscular Volume (MCV)
Adult/elderly/child: 80-95 fL (femtoliter)
Newborn: 96-108 fL

Mean Corpuscular Hemoglobin (MCH)
Adult/elderly/child: 27-31 pg
Newborn: 32-34 pg

Mean Corpuscular Hemoglobin Concentration (MCHC)

Adult/elderly/child: 32-36 g/dL (or 32%-36%)

Newborn: 32-33 g/dL (or 32%-33%)

Red Blood Cell Distribution Width (RDW)

Adult: variation of 11%-14.5%

INDICATIONS

The RBC indices provide information about the size (MCV and RDW), hemoglobin content (MCH), and hemoglobin concentration (MCHC) of RBCs. This test is useful in classifying anemias.

TEST EXPLANATION

This test is routinely performed as part of an automated complete blood cell count. The results of the RBC, hematocrit, and hemoglobin tests (see pp. 439, 277, and 281, respectively) are necessary to calculate the RBC indices. When investigating anemia, it is helpful to categorize the anemia according to the RBC indices, as shown in Box 2-18. Cell size is indicated by the terms "normocytic," "microcytic,"

BOX 2-18	Categorization of Anemia According to Red Blood Cell Indices

Normocytic,* Normochromic† Anemia
- Iron deficiency (detected early)
- Chronic illness (e.g., sepsis, tumor)
- Acute blood loss
- Aplastic anemia (e.g., whole-body radiation)
- Acquired hemolytic anemias (e.g., from a prosthetic cardiac valve)
- Renal disease (because of the loss of erythropoietin)

Microcytic,‡ Hypochromic§ Anemia
- Iron deficiency (detected late)
- Thalassemia
- Lead poisoning

Microcytic, Normochromic Anemia
- Chronic illness

Macrocytic,¶ Normochromic Anemia
- Vitamin B_{12} or folic acid deficiency
- Phenytoin ingestion
- Chemotherapy
- Some myelodysplastic syndromes
- Myeloid leukemia
- Ethanol toxicity
- Thyroid dysfunction

*Normal RBC size.
†Normal color (normal hemoglobin content).
‡Smaller than normal RBC size.
§Less than normal color (decreased hemoglobin content).
¶Larger than normal RBC size.

and "macrocytic." Hemoglobin content is indicated by the terms "normochromic," "hypochromic," and "hyperchromic." Additional information about the RBC size, shape, color, and intracellular structure is described in the blood smear study (see p. 710).

Mean Corpuscular Volume

The MCV is a measure of the average volume, or size, of a single RBC and is therefore used in classifying anemias. MCV is derived by dividing the hematocrit by the total RBC count:

$$MCV = \frac{Hematocrit\,(\%) \times 10}{RBC\,(million/mm^3)}$$

Normal values vary according to age and gender. When the MCV value is increased, the RBC is said to be abnormally large, or *macrocytic*. This is most frequently seen in megaloblastic anemias (e.g., vitamin B_{12} or folic acid deficiency). When the MCV value is decreased, the RBC is said to be abnormally small, or *microcytic*. This is associated with iron-deficiency anemia or thalassemia. It is important to recognize that a significant number of patients with disorders associated with a variation in MCV may, in fact, not have an abnormality in MCV. For example, only 65% of patients with iron-deficiency anemia will have a reduced MCV. Furthermore, the normal values for MCV and all of the other RBC indices vary considerably. Each laboratory must develop its own normal index values.

Mean Corpuscular Hemoglobin

The MCH is a measure of the average amount of hemoglobin within an RBC. MCH is derived by dividing the total hemoglobin concentration by the number of RBCs:

$$MCH = \frac{Hemoglobin\,(g/dL) \times 10}{RBC\,(million/mm^3)}$$

Because macrocytic cells generally have more hemoglobin and microcytic cells have less hemoglobin, the causes for these values closely resemble those for the MCV value. This has been documented with the use of automated counting instruments. The MCH adds very little information to the other indices.

Mean Corpuscular Hemoglobin Concentration

The MCHC is a measure of the average concentration or percentage of hemoglobin within a single RBC. MCHC is derived by dividing the total hemoglobin concentration by the hematocrit:

$$MCHC = \frac{Hemoglobin\,(g/dL) \times 100}{Hematocrit\,(\%)}$$

When values are decreased, the cell has a deficiency of hemoglobin and is said to be *hypochromic* (frequently seen in iron-deficiency anemia and thalassemia). When values are normal, the anemia is said to be *normochromic* (e.g., hemolytic anemia). RBCs cannot be considered *hyperchromic*. Only 37 g/dL of hemoglobin can fit into the RBC. Alteration in RBC shape (spherocytosis, acute transfusion reactions, erythroblastosis fetalis) may cause automated counting machines to indicate MCHC levels above normal.

Red Blood Cell Distribution Width

The RDW is an indication of the variation in RBC size. It is calculated by a machine using the MCV and RBC values. Variations in the width of the RBCs may be helpful when classifying certain types of anemia. The RDW is essentially an indicator of the degree of *anisocytosis*, a blood condition characterized by RBCs of variable and abnormal size.

The newer electronic cell counting machines are able to sort out RBCs according to size and compare those sizes to a histogram. Normally all the RBCs are about the same size with very little variation. This creates a histogram with a single narrowed peak. Certain diseases change the size of some of the RBCs, whereas the less abnormal RBCs are less affected. For example, with folic acid deficiency or iron deficiency, the newer RBCs are more significantly affected than the older cells and therefore will be of significantly different size. This creates a histogram with multiple peaks indicating large numbers of cells at variable sizes.

INTERFERING FACTORS

- Abnormal RBC size may affect the MCH and MCHC.
- Extremely elevated WBC counts (>50,000) may increase the MCV and MCH indices when processed by automated counters.
- Large RBC precursors, for example, reticulocytes (see p. 452), cause an abnormally high MCV. This commonly occurs in response to anemias when the bone marrow is not pathologic.
- Marked elevation in lipid levels (>2000 mg/dL) causes automated cell counters to indicate high hemoglobin levels. MCV, MCHC, and MCH will be calculated falsely high.
- The presence of cold agglutinins also falsely elevates MCHC, MCH, and MCV.
- Drugs that may *increase* MCV results include azathioprine, phenytoin, and zidovudine.

PROCEDURE AND PATIENT CARE

Before
- Explain the procedure to the patient.
- Tell the patient that no fasting is required.

During
- Collect a venous blood sample in a lavender-top tube.
- Avoid hemolysis.
- Transport the specimen to the hematology laboratory, in which the blood is passed through automated machines that calculate the RBC indices.

After
- Apply pressure or a pressure dressing to the venipuncture site.
- Assess the venipuncture site for bleeding.

TEST RESULTS AND CLINICAL SIGNIFICANCE

▲ Increased MCV

Pernicious anemia (vitamin B_{12} deficiency),
Folic acid deficiency:
> *These are the most common causes of macrocytic anemia. These vitamin deficiencies may be caused by malnutrition, malabsorption, competitive parasites, or enzyme deficiencies that impair utilization of these vitamins.*

Antimetabolite therapy: *This form of chemotherapy for cancer treatment and, in lesser doses, for arthritis treatment, acts as vitamin B_{12} and folate inhibitors and can cause a macrocytic anemia.*

Alcoholism: *This is probably more related to malnutrition.*

Chronic liver disease: *The pathophysiology of this observation is multifactorial and includes poor nutrition, erythropoietin alterations, and the effects of chronic illness.*

▼ Decreased MCV

Iron-deficiency anemia,
Thalassemia,
Anemia of chronic illness:
> *These are the most common diseases associated with microcytosis.*

▲ Increased MCH

Macrocytic anemias: *The MCH is increased if the size of the RBC is large.*

▼ Decreased MCH

Microcytic anemia,
Hypochromic anemia:
> *The MCH is decreased if the size of the RBC is small or the hemoglobin is diminished.*

▲ Increased MCHC

Spherocytosis: *The automated cell counter's false perception of an elevation in the MCHC is caused by a variation in the shape of the RBC. The RBC can hold only 37 g/dL of hemoglobin. There can be no "real" hyperchromatism.*

Intravascular hemolysis: *This is caused by free hemoglobin in the blood. The automated counter sees the free hemoglobin and incorporates that into its calculations.*

Cold agglutinins: *Cold agglutinins cause the misperception of increased MCV and decreased hematocrit. The automated machine calculates a falsely high MCHC.*

▼ Decreased MCHC

Iron-deficiency anemia,
Thalassemia:
> *These are the most common causes of hypochromatism. Thalassemia minor (heterozygous) may not be clinically evident except by measurement of RBC count, MCV, and MCHC.*

▲ Increased RDW

Iron-deficiency anemia,
B_{12} vitamin or folate-deficiency anemia:
> *Increased variation in RDW is caused by a combination of factors in these diseases. RBC fragmentation alters RBC size and shape. Furthermore, new cells produced when the deficiency was greatest will be markedly different in size and shape than the older RBCs that were produced before the deficiencies were as severe.*

Hemoglobinopathies (e.g., sickle cell or C disease): *Fragmentation increases RDW variation. Furthermore, different RBCs have different amounts of pathologic hemoglobin and therefore will be affected by fragmentation to varying degrees.*

Hemolytic anemias: *Fragmentation increases RDW variation.*

Posthemorrhagic anemias: *The marrow's response to bleeding is to release premature RBCs into the bloodstream. These are larger than mature RBCs and contribute to RDW variation.*

RELATED TESTS

Hematocrit (p. 277). This is a measurement of the percentage of the total blood volume taken up by the RBCs. It is closely associated with the hemoglobin value and the RBC count.

Hemoglobin (p. 281). This is a measurement of the concentration of hemoglobin in the blood. It is closely associated with the RBC count and hematocrit value.

Red Blood Cell (RBC) Count (p. 439). This is a measurement of the number of RBCs per cubic millimeter of blood. It is closely associated with the hemoglobin and hematocrit values.

Renin Assay, Plasma (Renin Activity, Plasma Renin Activity [PRA], Plasma Renin Concentration [PRC])

NORMAL FINDINGS
Plasma Renin Assay

Adult/elderly
  Upright position, sodium depleted (sodium-restricted diet)
    Ages 20-39 years: 2.9-24 ng/mL/hr
    >40 years: 2.9-10.8 ng/mL/hr
  Upright position, sodium replaced (normal-sodium diet)
    Ages 20-39 years: 0.1-4.3 ng/mL/hr
    >40 years: 0.1-3 ng/mL/hr
Child
  0-3 years: <16.6 ng/mL/hr
  3-6 years: <6.7 ng/mL/hr
  6-9 years: <4.4 ng/mL/hr
  9-12 years: <5.9 ng/ml/hr
  12-15 years: <4.2 ng/mL/hr
  15-18 years: <4.3 ng/mL/hr

Renal Vein

Renin ratio of involved kidney to uninvolved kidney: <1.4

INDICATIONS

PRA is used to evaluate hypertension. It is helpful in the differential diagnosis of aldosteronism.

TEST EXPLANATION

Renin is an enzyme released by the juxtaglomerular apparatus of the kidney into the renal veins in response to hyperkalemia, sodium depletion, decreased renal blood perfusion, or hypovolemia. Renin activates the renin-angiotensin system, which produces angiotensins I, II, and III (p. 63), powerful vasoconstrictors that also stimulate aldosterone production from the adrenal cortex. Angiotensin and aldosterone increase the blood volume, blood pressure, and serum sodium (Figure 2-26). After release of renin from the kidney into the bloodstream, angiotensinogen, an alpha$_2$ globulin that is made in the liver, is converted into angiotensin I. This is then converted into angiotensin II in the lung.

Renin is not actually measured in this test. Plasma renin activity (PRA) measures enzyme ability to convert angiotensinogen to angiotensin I and is limited by the availability of angiotensinogen. The PRA test actually measures, by radioimmunoassay, the rate of angiotensin I generation per unit time. This is a commonly used renin assay. The specimen must be drawn under ideal circumstances, handled by

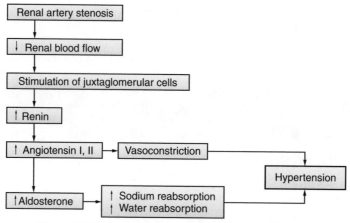

Figure 2-26 Physiology of renovascular hypertension.

TABLE 2-44	Differential Diagnosis Using Renin and Aldosterone Risk	
Disease	**Renin (PRA)**	**Aldosterone**
Conn syndrome	Low	High
Renal artery stenosis (or occlusion)	High	High
Primary renal disease	High	High
Increased salt intake	Low	Low
Salt restriction	High	High
Hypokalemia	Low	Low
Sodium-losing diuretic therapy	High	High
Addison disease	High	Low
Cushing syndrome	Low	High
Essential hypertension	Low	Normal

the local laboratory correctly, and transferred to the central laboratory in a timely manner. Even then, results may vary significantly.

The PRA is a screening procedure for the detection of essential, renal, or renovascular hypertension. The PRA may be supplemented by other tests, such as the renal vein renin assay. A determination of the PRA and a simultaneous measurement of the plasma aldosterone level are used in the differential diagnosis of primary versus secondary hyperaldosteronism (Table 2-44). Patients with primary hyperaldosteronism (adrenal adenoma overproducing aldosterone or Conn syndrome) will have increased aldosterone production associated with decreased renin activity. The aldosterone/renin ratio is ≥20.

Patients with secondary hyperaldosteronism (caused by renovascular occlusive disease or primary renal disease) will have increased levels of aldosterone and plasma renin.

Renal vein assays for renin are used to diagnose and lateralize renovascular hypertension, that is, hypertension that is related to inappropriately high renin levels from a diseased kidney or a hypoperfused kidney. The renal veins can be identified using injection of a radiopaque dye into the inferior vena cava. A catheter is placed into each renal vein, and blood is withdrawn from each vein. PRA is determined in each sample. If hypertension is caused by renal artery stenosis or renal pathology, the renal vein renin level of the affected kidney should be 1.5 or more times greater than that of the unaffected kidney or peripheral venous sample. If the levels are the same, the hypertension is not caused by a renovascular source. This is very helpful in determining whether a stenosis seen on a renal angiogram is significantly contributing to hypertension. Any stenosis identified on an arteriogram would not be considered severe enough to cause renin-related hypertension if renin levels from the renal vein were not at least 1.4 times those of the opposite kidney. Another cause for the patient's elevated blood pressure should be considered.

The *renin stimulation test* can be performed to more clearly diagnose and distinguish primary and secondary hyperaldosteronism. In this test, PRA is obtained while the patient is in the recumbent position and on a low-salt diet. The PRA is then repeated with the patient on the same diet while the patient is standing erect. In primary hyperaldosteronism the blood volume is greatly expanded. A change in position or reduced salt intake will not result in decreased renal perfusion or sodium level. Therefore renin levels do not increase. In secondary hyperaldosteronism (or normal persons with essential hypertension), the renal perfusion decreases while in the upright position and sodium levels decrease with decreased intake. Therefore renin levels increase.

The PRA is assessed as part of the *captopril test* (a screening test for renovascular hypertension). Patients with renovascular hypertension have greater falls in blood pressure and increases in PRA after administration of angiotensin-converting enzyme (ACE) inhibitors than do those with essential hypertension. For the captopril test, the patient receives an oral dose of captopril (ACE inhibitor) after a baseline PRA test, and blood pressure measurements are then taken. Subsequent blood pressure measurements and a repeat PRA test at 60 minutes are used for test interpretation. This is an excellent screening procedure to determine the need for a more invasive radiographic evaluation (such as digital subtraction renal arteriography [p. 988] or bilateral renal arteriography [p. 988]).

CONTRAINDICATIONS

- Patients who are allergic to shellfish or iodinated dye, because of potential allergic reaction to the radiopaque dye during renal vein renin assay

POTENTIAL COMPLICATIONS

- Allergic reactions to iodinated dye can occur during the renal vein renin assay. The reaction may vary from mild flushing, itching, and urticaria to severe, life-threatening anaphylaxis (evidenced by respiratory distress, drop in blood pressure, shock). In the unusual event of anaphylaxis, the patient may be treated with diphenhydramine (Benadryl), steroids, and epinephrine. Oxygen and endotracheal equipment should be on hand for immediate use.

INTERFERING FACTORS

- Renin is increased during pregnancy by virtue of increased substrate proteins concomitantly present in the serum during testing.
- Renin is increased with reduced salt intake. Reduced sodium acts as a direct stimulant to renin production.
- Renin is increased by ingestion of large amounts of licorice. Licorice has an aldosterone-like effect. This increases sodium reabsorption in the kidney and raises blood pressure, which in turn inhibits renin production.
- There is a diurnal variation in renin production. Values are higher early in the day.

- Renin levels are increased when the patient is in an upright position. Normally the upright position decreases renal perfusion because the blood pools in the veins of the lower extremities. This decreased renal perfusion is a strong stimulant to renin production. Renin levels are decreased in the recumbent position for the same reason (i.e., renal perfusion is increased in the recumbent position and renin levels diminish).
- Spironolactone interferes with renin testing and should be discontinued 4 to 6 weeks before testing.
- Drugs that *increase* levels of renin include ACE inhibitors, antihypertensives, diuretics, estrogens, oral contraceptives, and vasodilators.
- Drugs that *decrease* renin levels include beta blockers, clonidine, licorice, NSAIDs, potassium, and reserpine.

Clinical Priorities

- There is a diurnal variation in renin production. Renin levels are higher in the morning. A morning blood sample is usually drawn.
- Renin levels are affected by body position. Levels are higher in the upright position and decreased in the recumbent position.
- Renin levels are increased with reduced salt intake, because reduced sodium levels are a stimulus to renin production.

PROCEDURE AND PATIENT CARE

Before
- Explain the procedure to the patient.
- Instruct the patient to maintain a normal diet with a restricted amount of sodium (approximately 3 g/day) for 3 days before the test.
- Instruct the patient to discontinue licorice and any medications that may interrupt renin activity for 2 to 4 weeks before the test as ordered by the physician.
- Plan to draw a morning (8:00 AM to 10 AM) sample, because renin values are higher in the morning.
- For stimulation tests, instruct the patient to significantly reduce sodium intake (supplemented with potassium) for 3 days before testing.

During
- The test may be performed with the patient in an upright position.
- For the more commonly performed stimulation test, the blood is drawn in the recumbent and upright positions.
- Ensure that the patient stands or sits upright for 2 hours before the blood is drawn.
- If a recumbent sample is ordered, have the patient remain in bed in the morning until the blood sample has been obtained.
- It is best to release the tourniquet immediately before obtaining the blood specimen, because stasis can lower renin levels.
- Collect a venous blood sample and place it in a chilled lavender-top tube with ethylene diamine tetraacetic acid (EDTA) as an anticoagulant. Heparin can falsely decrease results.
- Gently invert the blood tube to allow adequate mixing of the blood sample and the anticoagulant.
- Record the patient's position, dietary status, and time of day on the laboratory slip.

- Place the tube of blood on ice, and immediately send it to the laboratory.
- In the laboratory, the blood will be centrifuged and the serum frozen.

After

- Apply pressure or a pressure dressing to the venipuncture site.
- Observe the venipuncture site for bleeding.
- Tell the patient that usually a normal diet and medications may be resumed.

TEST RESULTS AND CLINICAL SIGNIFICANCE

▲ Increased Levels

Essential hypertension: *A small percentage of these patients have renin hypertension.*

Malignant hypertension: *A large percentage of these patients with aggressive hypertensive episodes have secondary hyperaldosteronism (usually because of renal vascular occlusion or stenosis).*

Renovascular hypertension: *Renal artery stenosis or occlusion decreases the renal blood flow, which is a strong stimulant to renin production.*

Chronic renal failure: *Diseases of the kidney can stimulate the production of renin.*

Salt-losing GI disease (vomiting or diarrhea): *These patients develop hyponatremia, which is a strong stimulant to renin production.*

Addison disease: *These patients are hyponatremic, which is a strong stimulant to renin production.*

Renin-producing renal tumor: *Tumors of the juxtaglomerular apparatus are rare. They can produce renin.*

Bartter syndrome: *This syndrome is associated with potassium wasting in the kidney, high renin levels, and high aldosterone levels. This is caused by a tubular defect in sodium reabsorption.*

Cirrhosis: *These patients have increased total body water, which dilutes sodium. Sodium levels are chronically low, which is a stimulant for renin production.*

Hyperkalemia: *This is a direct stimulant for renin production.*

Hemorrhage/hypovolemia: *Any form of hypotension (including cardiogenic or septic shock) is associated with a reduction in the renal blood flow, which is a strong stimulant to renin production.*

▼ Decreased Levels

Primary hyperaldosteronism: *This is usually caused by an adrenal adenoma, and aldosterone levels are high. Aldosterone inhibits further renin production.*

Steroid therapy: *Glucocorticosteroids also have an aldosterone effect, which acts to increase serum sodium levels, decrease potassium levels, and increase blood volume. These responses all tend to diminish renin levels.*

Congenital adrenal hyperplasia: *An enzyme defect in cortisol synthesis causes an accumulation of cortisol precursors, some of which have strong aldosterone-like activity. These act to increase serum sodium levels, decrease potassium levels, and increase blood volume, all of which tend to diminish renin levels.*

Hypervolemia: *This tends to diminish renin levels.*

RELATED TEST

Aldosterone (p. 43). This is a direct measurement of aldosterone level. It is used to evaluate hypertension and aldosteronism.

Angiotensin (p. 63). This is a direct measurement of angiotensin I and II. These levels will correlate with renin levels.

Reticulocyte Count (Retic Count)

NORMAL FINDINGS

Reticulocyte Count
Adult/elderly/child: 0.5%-2% of total number of RBCs
Infant: 0.5%-3.1% of total number of RBCs
Newborn: 2.5%-6.5% of total number of RBCs

Reticulocyte Index
1.0

INDICATIONS

The reticulocyte count is an indication of the ability of the bone marrow to respond to anemia and make RBCs. It is used to classify and monitor therapy of anemias.

TEST EXPLANATION

The reticulocyte count is a test for determining bone marrow function and evaluating erythropoietic activity. This test is also useful in classifying anemias. A reticulocyte is an immature red blood cell (RBC) that can be readily identified under a microscope by staining the peripheral blood smear with Wright or Giemsa stain. It is an RBC that still has some microsomal and ribosomal material left in the cytoplasm. It sometimes takes a few days for that material to be cleared from the cell. Normally there are a small number of reticulocytes in the bloodstream.

The reticulocyte count gives an indication of RBC production by the bone marrow. Increased reticulocyte counts indicate the marrow is releasing an increased number of RBCs into the bloodstream, usually in response to anemia. A normal or low reticulocyte count in a patient with anemia indicates that the marrow response to the anemia by way of production of RBCs is inadequate and perhaps is contributing to or is the cause of the anemia (as in aplastic anemia, iron deficiency, vitamin B_{12} deficiency, depletion of iron stores). An elevated reticulocyte count found in patients with a normal hemogram indicates increased RBC production compensating for an ongoing loss of RBCs (hemolysis or hemorrhage).

Because the reticulocyte count is a percentage of the total number of RBCs, a normal to low number of reticulocytes can appear high in the anemic patient, because the total number of mature RBCs is low. To determine if a reticulocyte count indicates an appropriate erythropoietic (RBC marrow) response in patients with anemia and a decreased hematocrit, the reticulocyte index is calculated as follows:

$$\text{Reticulocyte index} = \text{Reticulocyte count (\%)} \times \frac{\text{Patient's hematocrit}}{\text{Normal hematocrit}}$$

The reticulocyte index in a patient with a good marrow response to the anemia should be 1.0. If it is below 1.0, even though the reticulocyte count is elevated, the bone marrow response is inadequate in its ability to compensate (as seen in iron deficiency, vitamin B_{12} deficiency, marrow failure). In these clinical situations, if iron or vitamin B_{12} is administered, the reticulocyte count will rise significantly to the point that the index equals or exceeds 1.0.

INTERFERING FACTORS

- Pregnancy may cause an increased reticulocyte count.
- Howell-Jolly bodies are blue stippling material in the RBC that occurs in severe anemia or hemolytic anemia. The RBCs containing these Howell-Jolly bodies look like reticulocytes and can be miscounted by some automated counter machines as reticulocytes; this gives a falsely high number of reticulocytes.

PROCEDURE AND PATIENT CARE

Before

☒ Explain the procedure to the patient.
☒ Tell the patient that no fasting is required.

During

- Collect a venous blood sample in a lavender-top tube.

After

- Apply pressure or a pressure dressing to the venipuncture site.
- Observe the venipuncture site for bleeding.

TEST RESULTS AND CLINICAL SIGNIFICANCE

▲ Increased Levels

Hemolytic anemia (e.g., immune hemolytic anemia, hemoglobinopathies, hypersplenism, trauma from a prosthetic heart valve): *The RBC survival is decreased and RBCs are destroyed at a faster rate than normal. The marrow attempts to compensate for the shortened RBC survival by producing large numbers of RBCs, some of which are immature RBCs called reticulocytes.*

Hemorrhage (3 to 4 days later): *In response to significant blood loss, the marrow attempts to compensate by producing large numbers of RBCs, some of which are immature RBCs called reticulocytes.*

Hemolytic disease of the newborn: *Immune-mediated destruction of RBCs reduces RBC survival. The marrow attempts to compensate for the shortened RBC survival by producing large numbers of RBCs, some of which are immature RBCs called reticulocytes.*

Treatment for iron, vitamin B_{12}, or folate deficiency: *After replacement treatment for anemia caused by nutritional deficiency, the marrow responds by increasing production of RBCs, some of which are immature RBCs called reticulocytes.*

▼ Decreased Levels

Pernicious anemia and folic acid deficiency,
Iron-deficiency anemia:
  These nutritional deficiencies suppress marrow production of RBCs, including reticulocytes.
Aplastic anemia,
Radiation therapy,
Malignancy,
Marrow failure,
Adrenocortical hypofunction,

Anterior pituitary hypofunction:
The marrow fails to produce RBCs and reticulocytes.
Chronic diseases: *In patients with chronic diseases, marrow production of RBCs and reticulocytes is reduced.*

RELATED TESTS

Hemoglobin (p. 281) and Hematocrit (p. 277). These are indirect measurements of the RBCs.
Red Blood Cell (RBC) Count (p. 439). This is a direct count of the total number of RBCs.

 Rheumatoid Factor (RF, Rheumatoid Arthritis [RA] Factor)

NORMAL FINDINGS

Negative (<60 units/mL by nephelometric testing)
Elderly patients may have slightly increased values.

INDICATIONS

The RF test is useful in the diagnosis of RA.

TEST EXPLANATION

RA is a chronic inflammatory disease that affects most joints, especially the metacarpal and phalangeal joints, the proximal interphalangeal joints, and the wrists; however, any synovial joint can be involved. The American College of Rheumatology has defined criteria for the diagnosis of RA. They include:

- Morning stiffness for at least 6 weeks
- Pain in at least one joint for the preceding 6 weeks
- Swelling in at least one joint for the preceding 6 weeks
- Symmetric bilateral joint swelling
- Presence of subcutaneous nodules
- Radiographic changes compatible with RA

In this disease, abnormal immunoglobulin (Ig) G antibodies produced by lymphocytes in the synovial membranes act as "antigens." Other IgG and IgM antibodies in the patient's serum react with the fc component of the abnormal synovial antigenic IgG to produce immune complexes. These immune complexes activate the complement system and other inflammatory systems to cause joint damage. The reactive IgM and sometimes IgG and IgA make up what is called the RF. IgG and IgA can also react to the synovial "IgG antigen." Tissues other than the joints, including blood vessels, lungs, nerves, and heart, may also be involved in the autoimmune inflammation.

Tests for RF are directed toward identification of the IgM antibodies. The exact role, if any, that RF plays in the pathophysiology of the disease is not well known. Approximately 80% of patients with RA have positive RF titers. To be considered positive, RF must be found in a dilution of greater than 1:80; when RF is found in titers of less than 1:80, diseases such as systemic lupus erythematosus (SLE), scleroderma, and other autoimmune conditions should be considered. Although the normal value is "no rheumatoid factor identifiable at low titers," a small number of normal patients will have RF present in a very low titer. Furthermore, a negative RF does not exclude the diagnosis of RA. When the

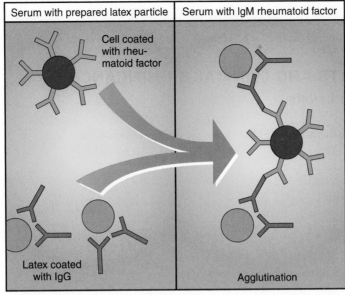

| Serum with prepared latex particle | Serum with IgM rheumatoid factor |

Cell coated with rheumatoid factor

Latex coated with IgG

Agglutination

Figure 2-27 Example of rheumatoid factor test by agglutination.

nephelometric testing procedure is used, the normal value is considered to be less than 60 units/mL. RF is not a useful disease marker, because it does not disappear in patients who are experiencing a remission of symptoms.

There are many serologic methods for detecting RF. The sheep cell agglutination test or the latex fixation test was most easily performed in the past. Better quantitation is now obtained by nephelometry. In the sheep cell agglutination test, rabbit IgG is placed on the sheep red blood cells (RBCs). When this is mixed with the patient's serum (which has been serially diluted), visual agglutination occurs if any RF is present. In the latex fixation test, human IgG is placed on a synthetic latex particle and mixed with the patient's serum. Visual agglutination is then detected if RF is present (Figure 2-27).

Other autoimmune diseases (see Table 2-5 on p. 90), such as SLE or Sjögren syndrome, also may cause a positive RF test. RF is occasionally seen in patients with tuberculosis, chronic hepatitis, infectious mononucleosis, and subacute bacterial endocarditis as well.

INTERFERING FACTORS

- Elderly patients often have false-positive results.
- Hemolysis or lipemia can be associated with false-positive results.

PROCEDURE AND PATIENT CARE

Before
☒ Explain the procedure to the patient.
☒ Tell the patient that no fasting or other preparation is required.

During
- Collect a venous blood sample in a red-top tube.

After

- Apply pressure or a pressure dressing to the venipuncture site.
- Observe the venipuncture site for bleeding.

TEST RESULTS AND CLINICAL SIGNIFICANCE

▲ Increased Levels

RA,
Other autoimmune disease (e.g., SLE, Sjögren syndrome, scleroderma),
Chronic viral infection,
Subacute bacterial endocarditis,
Tuberculosis,
Chronic active hepatitis,
Dermatomyositis,
Infectious mononucleosis,
Leukemia,
Biliary cirrhosis,
Syphilis,
Renal disease:
   The pathophysiology of these observations is not known.

RELATED TESTS

Anti-DNA Antibody (p. 78), Anti-SS Antibody (p. 98), Antiextractable Nuclear Antigen (p. 79), and Antinuclear Antibody (p. 88). These antibodies are also present in some cases of RA.

 Ribosome P Antibodies (Ribosomal P Ab, Anti-Ribosome P Antibodies)

NORMAL FINDINGS

<1 u

INDICATIONS

Ribosome P antibodies are used as an adjunct in the evaluation of patients with lupus erythematosus (LE).

TEST EXPLANATION

This antibody test should not be confused with anti-extractable nuclear antibodies (antiribonucleoprotein antibody, p. 79). Antibodies to ribosome P proteins are considered highly specific for LE, and have been reported in patients with central nervous system (CNS) involvement (i.e., lupus psychosis). This antibody is therefore an aid in the differential diagnosis of neuropsychiatric symptoms in patients with LE. Because patients with LE may manifest signs and symptoms of CNS diseases including neuropsychiatric symptoms, the presence of antibodies to ribosome P protein may be useful in the differential diagnosis of such patients. Most patients with LE do not have detectable levels of antibodies to ribosome P protein. But when they do, CNS involvement should be considered. This test is performed using immunofluorescent antibodies.

PROCEDURE AND PATIENT CARE

Before

☒Explain the procedure to the patient.
☒Tell the patient that no fasting is required.

During

- Collect a venous blood sample in a red-top tube.

After

- Apply pressure to the venipuncture site.
- Check the venipuncture site for infection. Patients with autoimmune disease have a compromised immune system.

TEST RESULTS AND CLINICAL SIGNIFICANCE

Lupus erythematosus: *Although sera from patients with lupus erythematosus (LE) can react with ribosomal protein antigens, it seems to be particularly common in patients with CNS involvement in this autoimmune disease.*

RELATED TESTS

Antichromatin Antibody (p. 70). These antibodies are present in LE.
Antiextractable Nuclear Antigen (p. 79). These antigens are used in the diagnosis of LE.
Antinuclear Antibody (p. 88). These antibodies are used in the diagnosis of LE and other autoimmune diseases.

Rubella Antibody (German Measles, Hemagglutination Inhibition [HAI])

NORMAL FINDINGS

Method	Result	Interpretation
HAI	<1:8	No immunity to rubella
HAI	>1:20	Immunity to rubella
Latex agglutination (LA)	Negative	No immunity to rubella
Enzyme-linked immunosorbent assay (ELISA) IgM	<0:9 international units/mL	No infection
ELISA IgM	>1.1 international units/mL	Active infection
ELISA IgG	<7 international units/mL	No immunity to rubella
ELISA IgG	>10 international units/mL	Immunity to rubella

 Critical Values

Evidence of susceptibility in pregnant women with recent exposure to rubella

INDICATIONS

Screening for rubella antibodies is performed to detect immunity to rubella (the causative agent for German measles). This is important for pregnant women or health care providers working with pregnant women. It is also used to diagnose rubella in newborns, children, and adults.

TEST EXPLANATION

These tests detect the presence of IgG and/or IgM antibodies to rubella. They become elevated a few days to a few weeks (depending on the method of testing) after the onset of the rash. IgM tends to disappear after about 6 weeks. IgG, however, persists at low but detectable levels for years (Table 2-45).

These antibodies become elevated in patients with active rubella infection or with past infections. In the past decade, children have been vaccinated with rubella to prevent the effects of the disease and to minimize infection. Rubella testing documents immunity to rubella. Rubella immunity testing is suggested for all health care workers. Most importantly, however, it is done to verify the presence or absence of rubella immunity in pregnant women, because congenital rubella infection in the first trimester of pregnancy is associated with congenital abnormalities (heart defects, brain damage, deafness), abortion, or stillbirth.

The term *TORCH* (*t*oxoplasmosis, *o*ther, *r*ubella, *c*ytomegalovirus, *h*erpes) has been applied to infections with recognized detrimental effects on the fetus. The effects on the fetus may be direct or indirect (e.g., precipitating abortion or premature labor). Included in the category of "other" are infections (e.g., syphilis). All of these tests are discussed separately.

If the woman's titer is greater than 1:10 to 1:20, she is not susceptible to rubella. If the woman's titer is 1:8 or less, she has little or no immunity to rubella. Pregnant women should be strongly advised to stay away from any small children, especially those with symptoms of an upper respiratory tract infection (prodromal symptoms of rubella). In addition, all health care personnel associated with maternal and child care should be screened for rubella. Immunization, if required, is not done during pregnancy but should be done before pregnancy or after delivery for nonimmune women.

A change in the HAI titer (measures IgG and IgM) from the acute to the chronic phase in a patient with a rash is the most useful method of demonstrating that the rash was related to a rubella infection. With a rubella rash, diagnosis of rubella is confirmed by obtaining an acute sample (approximately 3 days after the onset of the rash) and a convalescent sample (approximately 2 to 3 weeks later). A four-fold increase in the acute to the convalescent titer indicates that the rash was caused by an active rubella infection. Alternatively, in a pregnant woman with a rash suspected to be from rubella, an IgM antibody titer can be measured. If the titer is positive, recent infection has occurred. IgM titers appear 1 to 2 days after onset of the rash and disappear 5 to 6 weeks after infection.

Antirubella antibody testing is also used to diagnose rubella in infants (congenital rubella). Rubella is suspected in low-birth-weight (LBW) infants. Although IgG antibodies can be passed from mother to fetus, IgM antirubella antibodies cannot pass through the placenta. If an infant has IgM antibodies, acute

TABLE 2-45　Rubella Antibody Testing	
Indication	**Antibody**
Evaluate immune status	IgG
Identify active infection	IgM or IgG, acute and convalescent
Identify congenital infection	IgM

congenital or newborn rubella is suspected. Antibody testing is often used in children with congenital abnormalities that may have resulted from congenital rubella infection. This test is also recommended for anyone with a rash that may be related to rubella.

The HAI method tests for IgG and IgM. LA detects IgG only and is often used as a simple screen for immunity. Enzyme-linked immunosorbent assay (ELISA) methods for detecting IgG and IgM are now the standard for rubella testing. They provide a more accurate testing method and antibody quantities can be determined.

PROCEDURE AND PATIENT CARE

Before
Explain the purpose of the test to the patient.

During
- Collect a venous blood sample in a red-top tube.

After
- Apply pressure or a pressure dressing to the venipuncture site.
- Assess the venipuncture site for bleeding.
Inform the patient when to return for a follow-up HAI titer if indicated.

TEST RESULTS AND CLINICAL SIGNIFICANCE

Active rubella infection
Previous rubella infection leading to immunity

Rubeola Antibody

NORMAL FINDINGS

Negative

INDICATIONS

This test is used to diagnose rubeola infection (measles). It is more commonly used, today, to document immunity to infection by prior vaccination or clinical disease.

TEST EXPLANATION

Rubeola is a RNA paramyxovirus that is known to cause the measles (not German measles—see Rubella). Upper respiratory symptoms, fever, conjunctivitis, a rash, and Koplik spots on the buccal mucosa highlight the disease. Since the 1970s, children have been vaccinated to prevent this disease. Although it is usually a self-limiting disease, the virus can easily be spread (by respiratory droplets) to nonimmune pregnant women and cause preterm delivery or spontaneous abortion.

Testing for rubeola includes indirect immunofluorescence serologic identification of IgG and IgM antibodies. The first represents a previous infection. The latter indicates an acute infection. A fourfold rise in IgM indicates a current infection.

This test is used to diagnose measles in patients with a rash or viral syndrome when the diagnosis cannot be made clinically. Even more importantly, however, this test is used to establish and document immunity (active—by previous measles infection, or passive—by previous vaccination). Populations commonly tested to document immunity include college students, health care workers, and pregnant women.

PROCEDURE AND PATIENT CARE

Before

🖎 Explain the purpose of the test to the patient.

During

• Collect a venous blood sample in a red-top tube.

After

• Apply pressure to the venipuncture site.

🖎 Inform the patient when to return for a follow-up rubeola titer if indicated.

🖎 If the results are negative for immunity, recommend immunization. For women of childbearing age, vaccination should precede future pregnancy.

TEST RESULTS AND CLINICAL SIGNIFICANCE

Active rubeola infection: *These patients may not have the "classic" clinical signs of measles and diagnosis can be made with certainty through the identification of IgM antibodies in the patient's serum.*

Previous rubeola infection leading to immunity: *These patients have IgG antibodies but do not have IgM antibodies. They are protected from the disease because of previous active infection or vaccination.*

RELATED TEST

Rubella Antibody (p. 457). This test is used to diagnose German measles and to document immunity to the same.

 Septin 9 DNA Methylation Assay (Methylated Septin 9, mSEPT9, ColoVantage)

TYPE OF TEST

Blood

NORMAL FINDINGS

0.0005-50 ng DNA

INDICATIONS

This test is used to screen asymptomatic patients for colorectal cancer. Its use as a screening modality has not been established, but its main benefit may be in the early detection of colorectal cancer in patients who refuse colonoscopy or stool testing.

TEST EXPLANATION

Because of the inconvenience and discomfort associated with routine colorectal cancer screening (see colonoscopy, p. 591; stool for occult blood testing, p. 857), about half of Americans 50 to 75 years old do not follow recommended colorectal cancer (CRC) screening guidelines, leaving 40 million individuals unscreened. This precludes the opportunity for the early detection of an intestinal cancer. Recently a blood test for the detection of methylated DNA from the septin 9 (SEPT9) gene has been developed that, when positive, is very sensitive for the presence of a colorectal cancer. Using real-time methylated PCR, septin can be isolated and quantified from extracted nucleic acid in the plasma. This test has been validated in several clinical studies and shows a strong association between detection of mSEPT9 in blood plasma and the presence of colorectal cancer. Although more expensive than stool for occult blood testing, this real-time PCR laboratory blood test outperforms the stool test without the unpleasantness of a stool collection and may improve compliance for screening for colorectal cancer. Although the SEPT9 methylated DNA test may perform comparably to colonoscopy in detecting CRCs, it lacks the advantage of being potentially able to remove any precancerous polyps, thereby decreasing subsequent risks of cancer. Furthermore, Sept9 does not perform well for adenoma detection.

A positive test result means that there is an increased likelihood for the presence of a colorectal cancer or polyp. Individuals with positive test results are encouraged to undergo a diagnostic colonoscopy. Not all individuals with colorectal cancer will have a positive test result. Therefore individuals with a negative result should follow usual colorectal cancer screening guidelines.

PROCEDURE AND PATIENT CARE

Before

☒ Explain the procedure to the patient.
☒ Tell the patient that no fasting or special preparations are required.

During

• Collect a venous blood sample in a lavender (EDTA) tube.

After

• Apply pressure to the venipuncture site.

TEST RESULTS AND CLINICAL SIGNIFICANCE

▲ Increased Levels

Colorectal cancer,
Colorectal polyps:

> *Although it is clear that CRC screening reduces mortality by detecting the disease in its earliest stages when it is most effectively treated, only one half of Americans age 50 and older currently undergo any kind of screening. Reasons for not complying with colonoscopy include the time-consuming nature of the procedure and concern about invasiveness. In addition to the challenges of patient compliance with stool testing, such as the requirement for multiple samples and the handling of specimens, the performance of these tests is quite variable. Newer stool-based tests such as the immunochemical FOBT (FIT), have demonstrated sensitivity for adenoma detection.*

RELATED TESTS

Colonoscopy (p. 591). This is an endoscopic study of the entire colon and rectum that is the most effective screening study for the detection of early colorectal cancer.

Stool for Occult Blood (p. 857). Testing the stool for occult blood or DNA is an alternative accurate method of screening for early colorectal cancer.

Apt Test (p. 848). This is a method of identifying blood in newborn stool and differentiating the newborn's from the mother's blood.

 Serotonin (5-Hydroxytryptamine, 5-HT) **and Chromogranin A**

NORMAL FINDINGS

Chromogranin A: ≤225 ng/mL
Serotonin: ≤230 ng/mL

INDICATIONS

This test is used in conjunction with, or as an alternative to, 5-HIAA (p. 928) or serum chromogranin A measurements as a first-line test in the diagnosis of carcinoid syndrome or symptoms such as flushing. It is also used to monitor patients with known or treated carcinoid tumors.

TEST EXPLANATION

Serotonin is synthesized from the essential amino acid tryptophan chiefly in the gastrointestinal enterochromaffin cells (EC-cells). Many different stimuli can release serotonin from EC-cells. After it is secreted, in concert with other gut hormones, serotonin increases GI blood flow, motility, and fluid secretion. On first pass through the liver, 30% to 80% of serotonin is metabolized, predominantly to 5-hydroxyindoleacetic acid (5-HIAA), which is then excreted by the kidneys.

The main diseases that may be associated with measurable increases in serotonin are neuroectodermal tumors, in particular tumors arising from EC-cells. These tumors are collectively referred as *carcinoids*. They are subdivided into *foregut carcinoids*, arising from respiratory tract, stomach, pancreas, or duodenum (approximately 15% of cases); *midgut carcinoids*, occurring in the jejunum, ileum, or appendix (approximately 70% of cases); and *hindgut carcinoids*, which are found in the colon or rectum (approximately 15% of cases). In patients with more advanced tumors, serotonin is elevated in nearly all patients with midgut tumors, but only in approximately 50% of those with foregut carcinoids, and in no more than 20% of individuals with hindgut tumors. Foregut and hindgut tumors often have low or absent serotonin.

Carcinoids display a spectrum of aggressiveness with no clear distinguishing line between benign and malignant. The majority of carcinoid tumors do not cause significant clinical symptoms. Most symptoms are caused by elevated serotonins (carcinoid syndrome). The carcinoid syndrome consists of flushing, diarrhea, right-sided valvular heart lesions, and bronchoconstriction. The carcinoid syndrome is usually caused by midgut tumors. Because midgut tumors drain into the liver, nearly all of the serotonin is metabolized on first pass. Carcinoid symptoms, therefore, do not usually occur until liver or other distant metastases have developed that bypass the hepatic metabolism.

Diagnosis of carcinoid tumors with symptoms suggestive of carcinoid syndrome rests on measurements of serum serotonin, urinary 5-HIAA (p. 928), and serum chromogranin A (a peptide that is cosecreted alongside serotonin by the neuroectodermal cells). Metastasizing midgut carcinoid tumors usually produce blood or serum serotonin concentrations greater than 1,000 ng/mL. Only a minority of patients with carcinoid tumors will have elevated serotonin blood levels because the liver rapidly metabolizes the serotonin. It is usually impossible to diagnose small carcinoid tumors (>95% of cases) without any symptoms suggestive of carcinoid syndrome by measurement of serotonin, 5-HIAA, or chromogranin A. It is only after carcinoid tumors metastasize that serotonins become detectable because the blood that drains the metastatic carcinoid tumors carries serotonin from the metastatic tumors but does not pass through the liver for metabolism. In most cases, if a person has true carcinoid syndrome symptoms, serotonin levels are significantly elevated. If none of three analytes are elevated, carcinoids can be excluded as a cause of those symptoms.

Disease progression can be monitored in patients with serotonin-producing carcinoid tumors by measurement of serotonin or chromogranin A in the blood. However, at levels greater than approximately 5000 ng/mL, there is no longer a linear relationship between tumor burden and blood serotonin levels. Urinary 5-HIAA and serum chromogranin A continue to increase in proportion to the tumor burden.

Chromogranin A also acts as a useful diagnostic marker for other neuroendocrine neoplasms, including carcinoids, pheochromocytomas, neuroblastomas, medullary thyroid carcinomas, some pituitary tumors, functioning and nonfunctioning islet-cell tumors, and other amine precursor uptake and decarboxylation (APUD) tumors. It can also serve as a sensitive means for detecting residual or recurrent disease in treated patients. Carcinoid tumors, in particular colon and rectal carcinoids, almost always secrete chromogranin A. Other neuroendocrine tumors, such as small cell carcinoma of the lung or prostate carcinoma, may also display elevated chromogranin A levels.

After being extracted from the serum by reversed-phase solid-phase extraction, serotonin is analyzed using liquid chromatography/tandem mass spectrometry and quantified using a stable isotope-labeled internal standard. Chromogranin A is measured in a homogeneous automated immunofluorescent assay. This assay uses technology based on time-resolved amplified cryptae emission.

INTERFERING FACTORS

- Drugs that may cause *increased* serotonin levels include lithium, MAO-inhibitors, methyldopa, morphine, and reserpine.
- Drugs that may *decrease* serotonin levels include selective serotonin reuptake inhibitors (e.g., fluoxetine).
- Drugs that may cause *increased* chromogranin A levels include proton pump inhibitors (e.g., omeprazole) and should be discontinued 2 weeks before testing.

PROCEDURE AND PATIENT CARE

Before
- Explain the procedure to the patient.
- Tell the patient that no fasting or special preparations are required.

During
- Collect venous blood in a red-top tube and deliver to the laboratory as soon as possible. Because most circulating 5-HT is contained in platelets, the preferred specimens for measurement either include all or most of the platelets (i.e., whole blood and platelet-rich plasma) or consist of serum from completely clotted specimens, a process that releases nearly all 5-HT from platelets.
- Note that testing is usually performed at a reference laboratory.

After
- Apply pressure to the venipuncture site.

TEST EXPLANATION AND CLINICAL SIGNIFICANCE

▲   **Increased Levels**

Carcinoid tumors,
Neuroendocrine tumors,
Pheochromocytoma,
Small cell lung cancer:

These tumors are associated with increased replication of enterochromaffin cells, which produced these proteins that are then detected in the blood. For primary intestinal carcinoid tumors, elevated levels of these proteins may only occur with metastatic disease.

RELATED TESTS

5-Hydroxyindoleacetic Acid (p. 928). This urinary test measures the quantity of 5-hydroxyindoleacetic acid, a metabolite of serotonin that is excreted in the urine. Its use is similar to serotonin and chromogranin A.

Sickle Cell Screen (Sickledex, Hemoglobin S [Hgb S])

NORMAL FINDINGS

Negative

INDICATIONS

This test is used to screen for sickle cell disease or trait.

TEST EXPLANATION

Both sickle cell disease (homozygous for Hgb S) and sickle cell trait (heterozygous for Hgb S) can be detected by this screening study. Sickle cell anemia results from a genetic homozygous defect and is caused by the presence of Hgb S instead of Hgb A (Figure 2-28). When Hgb S becomes deoxygenated, it tends to bend in a way that causes the red blood cells (RBCs) to assume a sickle shape. These sickled RBCs cannot pass freely through the capillaries, thus they cause plugging of the microvascular tree. This may compromise the blood supply to various organs. Hgb S is found in varying quantities in 8% to 10% of the black population.

The *Sickledex test is* a blood test that is positive (turbid or cloudy test fluid) if greater than 10% of the hemoglobin is Hgb S. This is only a screening test, and its sensitivity varies according to the method used by the laboratory. Double heterozygosity for sickle trait when combined with another hemoglobinopathy (e.g., Hgb C disease) can cause a sickling disease. The definitive diagnosis of sickle cell disease or trait is made by Hgb electrophoresis (p. 284) or high-performance liquid chromatography, in which Hgb S can be identified and quantified. Immunoassay methods using monoclonal antibodies are also being used to quantify Hgb S.

Because sickle cell and Hgb C and E diseases are all associated with genetic abnormalities that affect the Beta globin gene (HBB), PCR *Beta globin gene testing* can now be performed on amniotic fluid, thereby identifying the disease in the fetal state.

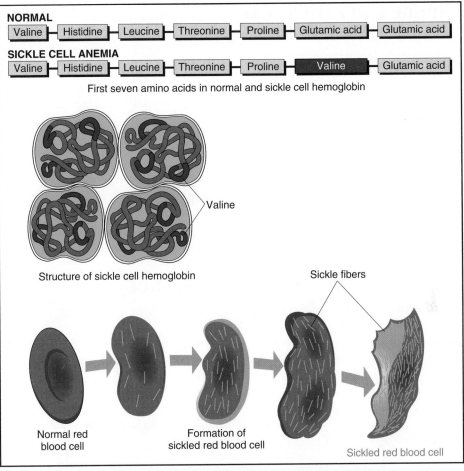

Figure 2-28 Sickle cell anemia. Sickle cell hemoglobin (Hgb) is produced by a recessive allele of the gene encoding the beta chain of Hgb. It represents a single amino acid change from a glutamic acid to valine at the sixth position in the chain. In the folded beta chain the sixth position contacts the alpha chain, and the amino acid change causes the hemoglobin to aggregate into long chains, altering the shape of the cell.

INTERFERING FACTORS

- Any blood transfusions within 3 to 4 months before the sickle cell test may cause false-negative results, because the donor's normal Hgb may dilute the recipient's abnormal Hgb S.
- Polycythemia may cause false-negative results.
- Infants less than 3 months of age may have false-negative results, because even infants with sickle cell disease have a significant amount of Hgb F in their RBCs at that age. Hgb F will not cause sickling. After 6 months of age the Hgb S variant increases in numbers in these infants. It is then that the test will be positive.
- Drugs that may cause *false-negative results* include phenothiazines.

PROCEDURE AND PATIENT CARE

Before

 Explain the procedure to the patient.

Tell the patient that no fasting is required.

During

- Collect a venous blood sample in a lavender-top tube.

After

- Apply pressure or a pressure dressing to the venipuncture site.
- Check the venipuncture site for bleeding.
- If the test is positive, Hgb electrophoresis should be performed.
- If the test is positive, genetic counseling should follow.

 Inform patients with sickle cell anemia that they should avoid situations in which hypoxia may occur (e.g., strenuous exercise, air travel in unpressurized aircraft, travel to high-altitude regions).

TEST RESULTS AND CLINICAL SIGNIFICANCE

▲ Increased Levels

Sickle cell trait,

Sickle cell anemia:

In these clinical situations more than 25% of the Hgb is of the S variation. Sickling will occur.

RELATED TEST

Hemoglobin Electrophoresis (p. 284). This test can identify and measure Hgb S. Sickle cell disease can be differentiated from the trait.

Sodium, Blood (Na)

NORMAL FINDINGS

Adult/elderly: 136-145 mEq/L or 136/145 mmol/L (SI units)
Child: 136-145 mEq/L
Infant: 134-150 mEq/L
Newborn: 134-144 mEq/L

⚠ Critical Values

<120 or >160 mEq/L

INDICATIONS

This test is a part of the routine laboratory evaluation of most patients. It is one of the tests automatically performed when "serum electrolytes" are requested. This test is used to evaluate and monitor fluid and electrolyte balance and therapy.

TEST EXPLANATION

Sodium is the major cation in the extracellular space, in which there are serum levels of approximately 140 mEq/L. The concentration of sodium intracellularly is only 5 mEq/L. Therefore sodium salts are the major determinants of extracellular osmolality. The sodium content in the blood is a result of a balance between dietary sodium intake and renal excretion. Nonrenal (e.g., sweat) sodium losses normally are minimal.

Many factors regulate sodium balance. Aldosterone causes conservation of sodium by stimulating the kidneys to reabsorb sodium and decreasing renal losses. Natriuretic hormone, or third factor, is stimulated by increased sodium levels. This hormone decreases renal absorption and increases renal losses of sodium. Antidiuretic hormone (ADH), which controls the reabsorption of water at the distal tubules of the kidney, affects sodium serum levels by dilution or concentration.

Physiologically, water and sodium are closely interrelated. As free body water is increased, serum sodium is diluted and the concentration may decrease. The kidney compensates by conserving sodium and excreting water. If free body water were to decrease, the serum sodium concentration would rise; the kidney would then respond by conserving free water. Aldosterone, ADH (vasopressin), and natriuretic factor all assist in these compensatory actions of the kidney to maintain appropriate levels of free water.

An average dietary intake of approximately 90 to 250 mEq/day is needed to maintain sodium balance in adults. Symptoms of *hyponatremia* may begin when sodium levels are below 125 mEq/L. The first symptom is weakness. When sodium levels fall below 115 mEq/L, confusion and lethargy occur and may progress to stupor and coma if levels continue to decline. Symptoms of *hypernatremia* include dry mucous membranes, thirst, agitation, restlessness, hyperreflexia, mania, and convulsions.

INTERFERING FACTORS

- Recent trauma, surgery, or shock may cause increased levels because renal blood flow is decreased. Renin and angiotensin stimulate the secretion of aldosterone, which stimulates increased renal absorption of sodium.
- Drugs that may cause *increased* levels include anabolic steroids, antibiotics, carbenicillin, clonidine, corticosteroids, cough medicines, estrogens, laxatives, methyldopa, and oral contraceptives.
- Drugs that may cause *decreased* levels include angiotensin-converting enzyme (ACE) inhibitors, captopril, carbamazepine, diuretics, haloperidol, heparin, nonsteroidal antiinflammatory drugs, sodium-free intravenous (IV) fluids, sulfonylureas, triamterene, tricyclic antidepressants, and vasopressin.

PROCEDURE AND PATIENT CARE

Before
- Explain the procedure to the patient.
- Tell the patient that food or fluid is not restricted.

During
- Collect a venous blood sample in a red-top or green-top tube.
- If the patient is receiving an IV infusion, obtain the blood from the opposite arm.

After
- Apply pressure or a pressure dressing to the venipuncture site.
- Assess the venipuncture site for bleeding.

TEST RESULTS AND CLINICAL SIGNIFICANCE

▲ Increased Levels (Hypernatremia)

Increased Sodium Intake

Increased dietary intake: *If sodium (usually in the form of salt) is ingested at high quantities without adequate free water, hypernatremia will occur.*

Excessive sodium in IV fluids: *The normal kidney can excrete about 450 to 500 mEq of sodium per day. If intake of sodium exceeds that amount in a patient without ongoing losses or a prior sodium deficit, sodium levels can be expected to rise.*

Decreased Sodium Loss

Cushing syndrome: *Corticosteroids have an "aldosterone-like" effect. See below.*

Hyperaldosteronism: *Aldosterone stimulates the kidneys to absorb sodium at the level of the renal tubule.*

Excessive Free Body Water Loss

Gastrointestinal (GI) loss (without rehydration): *If free water is lost, residual sodium becomes more concentrated.*

Excessive sweating: *Although sweat does contain some sodium, most is free water. This causes the serum sodium to become more concentrated. If the water loss is replaced without any sodium, sodium dilution and hyponatremia can occur.*

Extensive thermal burns: *If the burn is extensive, serum and a great amount of free water are lost through the open wounds. Sodium becomes more concentrated. As fluid is replaced and the body physiologically responds by stimulating ADH, sodium can be diluted and hyponatremia may occur.*

Diabetes insipidus: *The deficiency of ADH and the inability of the kidney to respond to ADH causes large free water losses. Sodium becomes concentrated.*

Osmotic diuresis: *With osmotic diuresis (excluding hyperglycemia, see below), water may be lost at a rate that exceeds sodium loss. In those situations, sodium levels increase as a result of greater concentration. If, however, free water is therapeutically provided, sodium levels may become dilute and hyponatremia may occur.*

▼ Decreased Levels (Hyponatremia)

Decreased Sodium Intake

Deficient dietary intake: *Sodium intestinal absorption is highly efficient. Salt deficiency is rare.*

Deficient sodium in IV fluids: *If IV replacement therapy provides sodium at a level less than minimal physiologic losses or less than ongoing losses, residual sodium will become diluted.*

Increased Sodium Loss

Addison disease: *Aldosterone and corticosteroid hormone levels are inadequate. Sodium is not reabsorbed by the kidneys and is lost in the urine.*

Diarrhea, vomiting, or nasogastric aspiration: *Sodium in the GI contents is lost with the fluid. Hyponatremia is magnified if IV fluid replacement does not contain adequate amounts of sodium.*

Intraluminal bowel loss (ileus, mechanical obstruction): *Great amounts of extracellular fluid are "third spaced" into the lumen of the dilated bowel. This fluid contains sodium. Hyponatremia is magnified if IV fluid replacement does not contain adequate amounts of sodium.*

Diuretic administration: *Many diuretics work by inhibiting sodium reabsorption by the kidney. Sodium levels can diminish.*

Chronic renal insufficiency: *The kidney loses its reabsorptive capabilities. Large quantities of sodium are lost in the urine.*

Large-volume aspiration of pleural or peritoneal fluid: *Sodium concentration is the same as serum in these fluids. The aspiration of these fluids is compensated by secretion of ADH, which acts to increase renal absorption of free water. Sodium becomes diluted.*

Increased Free Body Water

Excessive oral water intake: *Psychogenic polydipsia can dilute sodium.*

Hyperglycemia: *Each 60 mg/100 mL increase of glucose above normal decreases the sodium 1 mEq/L, because the osmotic effect of the glucose pulls in free water from the extracellular space and dilutes sodium. Also, sodium ketotic salts are lost in the urine. Sodium levels diminish further.*

Excessive IV water intake: *When IV therapy provides less sodium than maintenance and ongoing losses, sodium will be diluted. If sodium-free IV therapy is given to a patient who has a significant sodium deficit, sodium dilution will occur with rehydration.*

Congestive heart failure,

Peripheral edema:

These conditions are associated with increased free water retention. Sodium is diluted.

Ascites,

Peripheral edema,

Pleural effusion,

Intraluminal bowel loss (ileus or mechanical obstruction):

These conditions are associated with third-space losses of sodium.

Syndrome of inappropriate or ectopic secretion of ADH: *Oversecretion of ADH stimulates the kidney to reabsorb free water. Sodium is diluted.*

RELATED TESTS

Sodium, Urine (p. 946). This measurement of sodium in the urine is helpful in assessing sodium and water balance.

Aldosterone (p. 43). More than any other hormone, aldosterone has a significant effect on sodium blood levels.

Antidiuretic Hormone (ADH) (p. 73). By affecting free body water excretion, sodium levels become diluted or concentrated.

Squamous Cell Carcinoma Antigen (SCC Antigen)

NORMAL FINDINGS

≤2.2 ng/mL

INDICATIONS

This test is used to determine the stage and prognosis of squamous cell carcinomas. It is also used to monitor the treatment of carcinomas and a variety of nonmalignant conditions.

TEST EXPLANATION

Squamous cell carcinoma (SCC) antigen is a glycoprotein that is expressed in normal epithelium and epithelial tissues. Although the neutral forms of SCC normally remain inside the cell, acidic SCC antigen is released and often elevated in patients who have squamous cell carcinomas or other nonmalignant squamous cell lesions. It can occur in several cancers (e.g., uterine, cervical, oral cavity, esophageal, lung, anal canal, skin). SCC antigen may be involved in the malignant behavior of squamous cell cancers. Consequently, serum concentrations of SCC antigen can be used to monitor various SCCs after surgical removal. Concentrations that remain persistently elevated or begin to increase following tumor removal suggest persistent or recurrent disease. There may be an association between serum SCC antigen concentrations and tumor stage, size, and tumor aggressiveness.

A variety of nonmalignant benign diseases of the skin (e.g., eczema, erythrodermic epidermitis, pemphigus, and psoriasis), lungs (e.g., TB, adult respiratory distress syndrome, sarcoidosis, presence of pleural effusion), and other common conditions may result in increased serum concentrations of SCC antigen. Thus, SCC antigen results alone should not be interpreted as evidence of the presence or absence of malignant disease.

PROCEDURE AND PATIENT CARE

Before

- Explain the procedure to the patient.
- Tell the patient that no fasting is required.

During

- Collect a venous blood sample in a red-top tube.
- The blood sample may be sent to a central diagnostic laboratory and results may not be available for 7 to 10 days.

After

- Apply pressure or a pressure dressing to the venipuncture site.

TEST RESULTS AND CLINICAL SIGNIFICANCES

▲ Increased Values

Squamous cell carcinoma: *Cancers of the cervix, head, neck, esophagus, lung, anus, and skin are associated with increased SSC antigen.*

Dermatitis,

Pulmonary disease:

> *Benign diseases are associated with increased levels of SSC antigen, but to a lesser extent than squamous cell carcinoma.*

RELATED TEST

Carcinoembryonic Antigen (p. 145). This is a tumor marker used in evaluating several cancers.

***Streptococcus* Serologic Testing** (Antistreptolysin O Titer [ASO], Antideoxyribonuclease-B Titer, [Anti-DNase – B, ADB], *Streptococcus* Group B Antigen Detection, Streptozyme)

NORMAL FINDINGS

Antistreptolysin O Titer

Adult/elderly: ≤160 Todd units/mL

Child:
   Newborn: similar to mother's value
   6 months-2 years: ≤50 Todd units/mL
   2-4 years: ≤160 Todd units/mL
   5-12 years: 170-330 Todd units/mL

Antideoxyribonuclease-B Titer (Anti-DNase-B [ADB], ADNase-B)

Adult: ≤85 Todd units/mL or titer ≤1:85
Children:
   Preschool: ≤60 Todd units/mL or titer ≤1:60
   School age: ≤170 Todd units/mL or titer ≤1:170

Streptozyme

Titer <1:100

Streptococcus Group B Antigen

None detected.

INDICATIONS

This test is used to identify antecedent infection by group A streptococcal bacteria.

TEST EXPLANATION

Infections by group A *Streptococcus* are unique because they can be followed by a serious nonpurulent complication (such as rheumatic fever, scarlet fever, or glomerulonephritis). Serologic tests are used primarily to determine if a previous group A *Streptococcus* infection (pharyngitis, pyodermia, or pneumonia) has caused a poststreptococcal disease. These poststreptococcal diseases occur following the infection and after a period of latency during which the patient is asymptomatic. The latency period for glomerulonephritis is approximately 10 days, and for rheumatic fever is about 20 days.

These antibodies are directed against streptococcal extracellular products that are primarily enzymatic proteins. Serial rising titers of these antibodies over several weeks, followed by a slow fall in titers, are more supportive of the diagnosis of a previous streptococcal infection than is a single titer. The highest incidence of positive results is during the third week after the onset of acute symptoms of the poststreptococcal disease. By 6 months, only about 30% of patients have abnormal titers. By 12 months, levels return to normal.

One such extracellular enzyme produced by *streptococcus* is called *streptolysin O*, which has the ability to destroy (lyse) red blood corpuscles. The streptolysin O is antigenic stimulating the immunologic production of a neutralizing ASO antibody. ASO appears in the serum 1 week to 1 month after the onset of a streptococcal infection. A high ASO titer is not specific for a certain type of poststreptococcal disease (i.e., rheumatic fever versus glomerulonephritis), but merely indicates that a streptococcal infection is or has been present.

Like the ASO titer, *ADB* is used to detect previous streptococcal infections. Because a significant portion of individuals with normal antibody titers for one test will have elevated antibody titers for another test, one test is not used alone in the evaluation of streptococcal infections. The percentage of false-negatives can be reduced by performing two or more antibody tests. ADB is often run concurrently with the ASO titer and other serologic tests to provide more accurate results.

The *Streptozyme* assay detects antibodies to multiple extracellular antigens of group A *Streptococcus*, including antistreptolysin O, antistreptokinase, and antihyaluronidase. Approximately 80% of specimens positive by Streptozyme have antistreptolysin O, and 10% have antistreptokinase and/or antihyaluroni-dase. The remaining 10% of positive samples are apparently the result of ADB antibodies or other strep-tococcal extracellular antigens. Nephelometry is the laboratory method used to identify most of these antibodies.

Streptococcus Group B antigens accumulate in CSF, serum, or urine and provide a direct qualitative detection of bacterial antigens. These antigens indicate acute infection and are not related to post strep-tococcal sequelae as described. Confirmatory diagnosis of streptococcal infection is done by cultures (p. 761). Samples with extremely low levels of antigen may yield negative results.

Rapid antigen detection *(strept screen)* testing is another immunologic test in which the *Streptococcus* organism can be identified directly from the swab specimen. The rapid serologic tests can be performed in about 15 minutes in any lab or in most physicians' offices that treats children. This test is more thor-oughly discussed on p. 765.

INTERFERING FACTORS

- Increased beta-lipoprotein levels inhibit streptolysin O and give a falsely high ASO titer.
- Drugs that may cause *decreased* ASO levels include adrenocorticosteroids and antibiotics.

PROCEDURE AND PATIENT CARE

Before
- Explain the procedure to the patient.
- Tell the patient that no fasting is required.

During
- Collect a venous blood sample in a red-top tube.
- Avoid hemolysis of the blood specimen.
- Note on the laboratory slip any medications that may affect the test results.

After
- Apply pressure to the venipuncture site.
- Note that repeat testing may be done to determine the highest level of increase.

TEST RESULTS AND CLINICAL SIGNIFICANCE

▲ Increased Levels

Streptococcal infection,
Bacterial endocarditis,
Scarlet fever,
Streptococcal pyodermia:
> *These are acute streptococcal infections that will not immediately be associated with serologic changes because of the immunologic latency response.*

Acute rheumatic fever,
Acute glomerulonephritis:
> *Recent information suggests that rheumatic fever is associated with infection by rheumatogenic serotypes (M1, M3, M5, M6, M18, and M19), while glomerulonephritis follows infection by nephritogenic serotypes (M2, M12, M49, M57, M59, and M60). Streptococcal pyoderma is often associated with a reduced immunologic response as compared to throat infections.*

RELATED TEST

Throat culture (p. 765). The pharynx is a common anatomic site of streptococcal group A infection. Throat culture or rapid antigen testing are adequate to instigate antistreptococcal antibiotic therapy.

 Syphilis Detection (Serologic Test for Syphilis [STS], Venereal Disease Research Laboratory [VDRL], Rapid Plasma Reagin [RPR], Fluorescent Treponemal Antibody [FTA])

NORMAL FINDINGS

Negative or nonreactive

INDICATIONS

These serologic tests are used to diagnose and to document successful therapy of syphilis.

TEST EXPLANATION

Syphilis is caused by the spirochete *Treponema pallidum*. The disease is divided into four stages: acute, secondary, latent, and tertiary. The acute stage is marked by the development of a chancre on the skin near the infection (usually the genitalia). The chancre develops about 3 to 6 weeks after inoculation and lasts for about 4 to 6 weeks. The secondary stage is highlighted by a rash (often on the soles and palms) and generalized lymphadenopathy. This stage lasts for about 3 months. The latent stage represents a period of disease inactivity and can last for 5 years. Some patients are cured of the infection during this stage. Many go into the tertiary stage marked by central nervous system (CNS), cardiovascular, and ocular signs and symptoms.

The immunologic tests for syphilis detect antibodies to *T. pallidum*. There are two groups of antibodies. The first group of tests detects the presence of a nontreponemal antibody called reagin, which reacts to phospholipids in the body (which are probably similar to lipids in the membrane of *T. pallidum*). The second group of tests detects antibodies directed against the *Treponema* organism itself. The nontreponemal antibody tests are grouped as serologic screening tests for syphilis and are relatively nonspecific. These antibodies are most often detected by the Wassermann test or the Venereal Disease Research Laboratory (VDRL) test. A more sensitive nontreponemal test is the Rapid Plasma Reagin (RPR) test. The VDRL and RPR tests, by virtue of their testing for a nonspecific antibody, have a high false-positive (or cross-reactive) rate. The VDRL test becomes positive approximately 2 weeks after the patient's inoculation with *Treponema* and returns to normal after adequate treatment. The test is positive in nearly all primary and secondary stages of syphilis and in two thirds of patients with tertiary syphilis.

If the VDRL or RPR test is positive, the diagnosis must be confirmed by the more specific *Treponema* test, such as the *fluorescent treponemal antibody absorption test (FTA-ABS)*. The FTA test, which reacts to a specific treponemal antibody, is more accurate than the VDRL and RPR tests and becomes positive about 4 to 6 weeks after inoculation. To improve its specificity, non-*pallidum* antibodies are absorbed out of the patient's serum before the serum is added to the *T. pallidum*–impregnated slide. Anti–gamma globulin antibodies that are fluorescent are then added to the slide. If anti–*T. pallidum* antibodies exist in the patient's serum, they will react to the *T. pallidum* on the slide and the fluorescent anti–gamma globulin antibodies that were subsequently added will attach to the patient's serum

BOX 2-19	Diseases That Can Cause False-Positive Results on the VDRL and RPR Tests

- Malaria
- Typhus
- Leptospirosis
- Cat-scratch fever
- Leprosy
- Hepatitis
- Mononucleosis
- Periarteritis nodosa
- Systemic lupus erythematosus
- Acute viral or bacterial infections
- Lymphogranuloma venereum
- Hypersensitivity reactions
- Mycoplasmal pneumonia
- Recent vaccinations

RPR, Rapid plasma reagin; *VDRL,* Venereal Disease Research Laboratory.

antibody–*T. palladium* complex and make it visible under the fluorescent microscope. The FTA test is required before the diagnosis of syphilis can be made with certainty. A *microhemagglutination test (MHA-TP)* is also available and is comparable in accuracy to the "standard criterion" FTA-ABS test. Enzyme-linked immunosorbent assay (ELISA or EIA) methods are also available for detection of anti-treponemal/antibodies (IgG or IgM).

If the VDRL or RPR test is positive and the FTA-ABS is negative, other diseases that can cause positive results on screening serologic syphilis tests must be sought (Box 2-19).

Screening for syphilis is usually done during the first prenatal checkup of pregnant women using the VDRL or RPR test. Syphilis, if untreated, may cause abortion, stillbirth, or premature labor. The effect on the fetus can be CNS damage, hearing loss, or possible death. In patients who have symptoms compatible with primary syphilis, an FTA-ABS test is recommended. Congenital syphilis is difficult to distinguish from the passive immunity provided by a mother who has syphilis. However, in congenital syphilis the FTA-ABS result of the infant is usually much higher than the mother's. The term *TORCH* (toxoplasmosis, other, rubella, cytomegalovirus, herpes) has been applied to infections with recognized detrimental effects on the fetus. The effects on the fetus may be direct or indirect (e.g., precipitating abortion, premature labor). Included in the category of "other" are infections (e.g., syphilis). All of these tests are discussed separately.

During early primary syphilis, the first antibodies to appear are IgM, with IgG antibodies reaching significant titers later in the primary phase. As the disease progresses into the secondary phase, IgG *Treponema pallidum* antibodies reach peak titers. *Treponema pallidum* IgG antibodies persist indefinitely regardless of the course of the disease. If syphilis IgG and/or IgM is positive, results can be confirmed with FTA or MHA testing. The IgG- and IgM-specific antibodies assist in determining the etiology of neonatal syphilis. IgM does not pass through the placenta and if positive indicates active neonatal infection.

In general, serologic tests return to normal after successful treatment for syphilis. The earlier the disease is treated, the sooner the serologic tests return to normal. In the early primary stage the serologic tests may become negative in 2 to 4 months after successful antibiotic treatment. It may take longer than 1 year for the patient to convert to a seronegative result when treating later stages of the disease. In the tertiary stage the patient may never convert to negative. Testing should be routinely performed to document successful therapy.

INTERFERING FACTORS

- Excessive hemolysis and gross lipemia may cause false-positive STS test results.
- Excess chyle in the blood may cause false-positive STS test results. Testing should be performed after at least an 8-hour fast.
- Recent ingestion of alcohol may cause false-positive STS test results. Alcohol should be avoided for 24 hours before testing.
- Many conditions cause false-positive results when VDRL and RPR tests are used (see Box 2-19).
- If the patient is tested too soon after inoculation and before antibodies have developed, the tests may be falsely negative. The test should be repeated in 2 months or the patient should be treated despite the negative test results if clinical suspicion is high.

✔ Clinical Priorities

- If the patient is tested too soon after inoculation and before antibodies have developed, the tests may be falsely negative.
- Because the FTA tests for a specific treponemal antibody, it is more accurate than the VDRL and RPR tests. The FTA test becomes positive about 4 to 6 weeks after inoculation.
- Screening for syphilis is usually performed during the first prenatal checkup of pregnant women using the VDRL test.

PROCEDURE AND PATIENT CARE

Before

- Explain the procedure to the patient.
- Check with the laboratory regarding food and alcohol fasting requirements.

During

- Collect a venous blood sample in a red-top tube.

After

- Apply pressure or a pressure dressing to the venipuncture site.
- Check the venipuncture site for bleeding.
- If the test is positive, instruct the patient to inform recent sexual contacts so they can be evaluated.
- If the test is positive, be sure the patient receives the appropriate antibiotic therapy.
- If a screening serology test is positive, a more specific antitreponemal test is required to make the diagnosis.

TEST RESULTS AND CLINICAL SIGNIFICANCE

Positive Results

Syphilis

Testosterone (Total Testosterone Serum Level)

NORMAL FINDINGS

% Free Testosterone
Adult female: 0.1% - 0.3%
Adult male: 1.6% - 2.9%

FREE TESTOSTERONE, pg/mL

Female	Male
Tanner Stage I: <2.2 pg/mL	Tanner Stage I: ≤3.7 pg/mL
Tanner Stage II: 0.4-4.5 pg/mL	Tanner Stage II: 0.3-21 pg/mL
Tanner Stage III: 1.3-7.5 pg mL	Tanner Stage III: 1-98 pg mL
Tanner Stage IV: 1.1-15.5 pg/mL	Tanner Stage IV: 35-169 pg/mL
Tanner Stage V: 0.8-9.2 pg/mL	Tanner Stage V: 41-239 pg/mL
Postmenopausal: 0.6-3.8 pg/mL	

TOTAL TESTOSTERONE, ng/dL

Tanner Stage	Male	Female
7 months-9 years (Tanner Stage I)	<30	<30
10-13 years (Tanner Stage II)	<300	<40
14-15 years (Tanner Stage III)	170-540	<60
16-19 years (Tanner Stage IV, V)	250-910	<70
20 years and over	280-1080	<70

Dihydrotestosterone
Adult Male: 240-650 pg/mL
Adult Female: ≤300 pg/mL

INDICATIONS

Testosterone levels are used to evaluate ambiguous sex characteristics, precocious puberty, virilizing syndromes in the female, and infertility or impotency in the male. This test can also be used as a tumor marker for rare tumors of the ovary and testicle.

TEST EXPLANATION

Androgens include dehydroepiandrosterone (DHEA) (p. 29), androstenedione, and testosterone. In the adrenal glands, DHEA is produced in the process of making cortisol and aldosterone. DHEA is also produced de novo by the testes or the ovaries. DHEA is the precursor of androstenedione, which is the precursor of testosterone (and estrogen).

Testosterone levels vary by stage of maturity (indicated by Tanner Stage). Serum concentrations of testosterone in both sexes during the first week of life average about 25 ng/dL. In male infants, values increase sharply in the second week to a maximum (mean about 175 ng/dL) at about 2 months, which lasts until about 6 months of age. In female infants, values decrease in the first week and remain low throughout early childhood. Levels increase during puberty to adult values.

In the male most of the testosterone is made by the Leydig cells in the testicle; this accounts for 95% of the circulating testosterone in men. In the female about half of the testosterone is made by the conversion of DHEA to testosterone in the peripheral fat tissue. Another 30% is made by the same conversion of DHEA in the adrenal gland, and 20% is made directly by the ovaries.

Approximately 60% of circulating testosterone binds strongly to sex hormone–binding globulin (SHBG), which is also called testosterone-binding globulin. Most of the remaining testosterone is bound loosely to albumin, and approximately 2% is free or unbound. The unbound portion is the active component. Most assays for testosterone measure the total testosterone (i.e., bound and unbound portions). The free testosterone can be measured where the testosterone binding proteins may be altered (obesity, cirrhosis, thyroid disorders). Free testosterone is estimated in this panel by an indirect method, equilibrium ultrafiltration. It can be reported as a percentage of total testosterone, or as an absolute number.

In males a biofeedback mechanism exists that starts in the hypothalamus. Gonadotropin-releasing hormone (GnRH) induces the pituitary to produce luteinizing hormone (LH) (called interstitial cell–stimulating hormone in the male) and follicle-stimulating hormone (FSH). LH stimulates the Leydig cells to produce testosterone. FSH stimulates the Sertoli cells to produce sperm. Testosterone then acts to inhibit further secretion of GnRH.

Physiologically, testosterone stimulates spermatogenesis and influences the development of male secondary sexual characteristics. Overproduction of this hormone in the young male may cause precocious puberty. This can be caused by testicular, adrenal, or pituitary tumors. Overproduction of this hormone in females causes masculinization, which is manifested as amenorrhea and excessive growth of body hair (hirsutism). Ovarian and adrenal tumors/hyperplasia and medications (e.g., danazol) are all potential causes of masculinization in the female. Reduced levels of testosterone in the male suggest hypogonadism or Klinefelter syndrome.

Dihydrotestosterone (DHT) is the principal androgen made in body tissues, particularly the prostate. Levels of DHT remain normal with aging, despite a decrease in the plasma testosterone, and are not elevated in benign prostatic hyperplasia. Measurement of this hormone is useful in monitoring patients receiving 5 alpha-reductase inhibitor therapy such as finasteride or chemotherapy, which may affect prostate function. It is also useful in evaluating patients with possible 5 alpha-reductase deficiency.

There are several *testosterone stimulation tests* that can be performed to more accurately evaluate hypogonadism. Human chorionic gonadotropin, clomiphene, and GnRH can be used to stimulate testosterone secretion.

17-ketosteroids (17-KS) are metabolites of the testosterone and non-testosterone androgenic sex hormones that are excreted in the urine.

Methods used for the measurement of testosterone include radioimmunoassay and extraction chromatography. There is a slight diurnal variation in the secretion of testosterone. Levels are maximal around 7 AM and minimal around 8 PM.

INTERFERING FACTORS

▓ Drugs that may cause *increased* testosterone levels include anticonvulsants, barbiturates, estrogens, and oral contraceptives.

▓ Drugs that may cause *decreased* testosterone levels include alcohol, androgens, dexamethasone, diethylstilbestrol, digoxin, ketoconazole, phenothiazine, spironolactone, and steroids.

PROCEDURE AND PATIENT CARE

Before

☒ Explain the procedure to the patient.
☒ Tell the patient that no fasting is required.
- Because testosterone levels are highest in the early morning hours, blood should be drawn in the morning.

During

- Collect a venous blood sample in a red-top tube.

After

- Apply pressure or a pressure dressing to the venipuncture site.
- Assess the venipuncture site for bleeding.

TEST RESULTS AND CLINICAL SIGNIFICANCE

▲ Increased Levels (Male)

Idiopathic sexual precocity: *This is usually because of oversecretion of LH, which stimulates the testicles to produce testosterone.*

Pinealoma: *This is a hypothalamic tumor that produces an increased quantity of GnRH, which stimulates the pituitary to produce LH, which in turn stimulates the testicles to produce testosterone.*

Encephalitis: *This viral infection of the CNS can stimulate the hypothalamus to produce an increased quantity of GnRH, which stimulates the pituitary to produce LH, which in turn stimulates the testicles to produce testosterone.*

Congenital adrenal hyperplasia: *An enzyme deficiency in the production of cortisol causes an accumulation of large amounts of DHEA. DHEA is a precursor of androstenedione, which is a precursor of testosterone.*

Adrenocortical tumor: *Neoplasm involving the adrenal gland can produce large amounts of testosterone or DHEA. DHEA is a precursor of androstenedione, which is a precursor of testosterone.*

Testicular or extragonadal tumor: *Leydig cell tumors can produce testosterone, which can cause precocious puberty in males. However, no spermatogenesis occurs because gonadotropin hormones are not produced and are, in fact, inhibited.*

Hyperthyroidism: *These patients have elevated bound testosterone because of elevated SHBG proteins. This causes elevation of the total testosterone levels.*

Testosterone resistance syndromes: *These patients resist the effect of testosterone on tissue. In response, higher levels of testosterone are secreted.*

▼ Decreased Levels (Male)

Klinefelter syndrome: *These patients have an extra X chromosome (XXY). This syndrome is associated with primary testicular failure.*

Cryptorchidism: *These patients usually have normal testosterone levels, but occasionally testicles that fail to descend into the scrotum can be atrophic.*

Primary and secondary hypogonadism: *Infection, tumor, or congenital abnormalities are all possible causes of primary (testicular) or secondary (pituitary) failure.*

Trisomy 21: *The pathophysiology of this genetic defect is not defined.*

Orchiectomy: *The testicles must both be removed. Surgical removal of just one testicle does not cause deficient testosterone levels.*

Hepatic cirrhosis: *These patients have reduced proteins and therefore have reduced amounts of bound testosterone, which makes up most of the total testosterone that is measured.*

▲ Increased Levels (Female)

Ovarian tumor: *Arrhenoblastoma is an uncommon ovarian tumor that can produce testosterone.*

Adrenal tumor: *Neoplasms involving the adrenal gland can produce large amounts of testosterone or DHEA. DHEA is a precursor of androstenedione, which is a precursor of testosterone. Hirsutism in females is common with these tumors.*

Congenital adrenocortical hyperplasia: *An enzyme deficiency in the production of cortisol causes an accumulation of large amounts of DHEA. DHEA is a precursor of androstenedione, which is a precursor of testosterone. In females this can result in pseudohermaphroditism (ambiguous genitalia).*

Trophoblastic tumor: *These tumors (hydatidiform mole, choriocarcinoma) produce hCG, which can stimulate the production of testosterone.*

Polycystic ovaries: *This syndrome is associated with obesity, hirsutism, and amenorrhea. Patients have increased testosterone levels. The pathophysiology is not well defined.*

Idiopathic hirsutism: *The pathophysiology of this observation is not known.*

RELATED TEST

Adrenal Steroid Precursors (p. 29). Androstenedione is used in the diagnosis of virilizing syndromes, especially in the female.

Thromboelastography (Thromboelastometry)

NORMAL FINDINGS

5.3-12.4 dynes/cm^2

Critical Values

>12.4 dynes/cm^2

INDICATIONS

This test is performed to evaluate the coagulation system. It is used to:

- Identify potential hypercoagulable states
- Identify potential accelerated fibrinolysis
- Assess platelet and coagulating factor function

TEST EXPLANATION

Hemostasis is a well-regulated process in which the blood forms localized clots when the integrity of the vascular system is breeched. Trauma, infection, and inflammation all activate the blood's clotting system, which depends on the interaction of two separate systems: enzymatic proteins (clotting factors, intrinsic and extrinsic systems [Figure 2-29]) and platelets. The two systems work in concert to plug defects in the broken vessels. The clots that form in this process need to be of sufficient strength to resist dislodgement. If a particular clotting factor is dysfunctional or absent, as in hemophilia, an

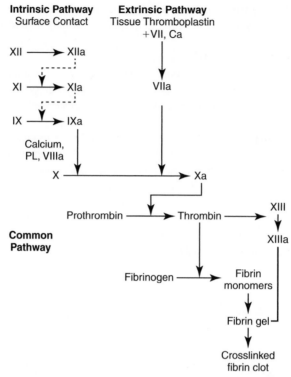

Figure 2-29 Simplified enzymatic cascade of fibrin clot formation.

insufficient amount of fibrin forms. Similarly, massive consumption of clotting factors in a trauma situation decreases the amount of fibrin formed. Inadequate numbers of platelets resulting from trauma, surgery, or chemotherapy also decrease platelet aggregation, as do genetic disorders, uremia, or medication therapy. Ultimately, reduced fibrin formation or platelet aggregation results in clots of inadequate tensile strength. This hypocoagulable state is associated with excessive bleeding. Conversely endothelial injury, stasis, cancer, genetic diseases, or other hypercoagulable states lead to thrombosis formation causing thromboembolic events.

In this test whole blood is rapidly transferred to a cuvette. Clot-activating catalysts may be added to speed up the process. The cuvette is rotated as a clot forms in a machine. The fibrin in the clot creates fluid resistance that is determined by a sensor transducer (also placed within the cuvette) that converts the tensile strength of the client to an electronic signal displayed on a graph. Thrombosis time and lysis time can be calculated and is reported as a coagulation index. This test is able to represent all global analysis of the hemostatic function from initial thrombin generation to clot lysis. When plotted on a graph, specific patterns can be identified, including normal, hemophilia, thrombocytopenia, decreased platelet function, increased fibrinolysis, and hypercoagulation.

This test is used to identify patients who are hypercoagulable and may experience a thromboembolic phenomenon when immobile (e.g., after surgery or trauma). It is particularly helpful in cardiac surgery and liver transplantation. It is also used to determine hyperfibrinolysis. Finally this shows the complete evaluation of platelet function. Usually three separate tracings using different reagents can determine the percent of platelet inhibition instigated by heparin, aspirin, and antiplatelet drugs (Plavix, Ticlid). This test correlates better with operative bleeding than does bleeding time, closure time (p. 404), or thromboxane levels. With the present instrumentation, point of service (e.g., in the operating room) testing can be performed.

INTERFERING FACTORS

Drugs that may cause *decreased* thromboelastography include antiplatelet drugs (e.g., ticlopidine), some antibiotics, aspirin, beta blockers, clofibrate, dextran, ethanol, heparin, nonsteroidal antiinflammatory drugs (NSAIDs), phenothiazines, tricyclics, theophylline, and warfarin sodium (Coumadin).

PROCEDURE AND PATIENT CARE

Before

Explain the procedure to the patient.

Tell the patient that no fasting is required.

During

- Collect a venous blood sample in a red-top tube.
- If the patient is receiving any drugs that may interfere with normal coagulation or has any diseases such as jaundice, hyperlipidemia, or hemolysis, this should be listed on the laboratory request slip.
- Immediately transfer the specimen to the laboratory.

After

- Apply pressure or a pressure dressing to the venipuncture site.
- Assess the venipuncture site for bleeding.
- Remember that abnormalities in platelet aggregation can prolong bleeding time, and a significant hematoma at the venipuncture site may occur.

TEST RESULTS AND CLINICAL SIGNIFICANCE

Hypocoagulability

Factor deficiency,
Anticoagulation,
Thrombocytopenia,
Platelet function abnormalities,
Increased fibrinolysis:

> *All associated with a fibrin clot with reduced tensile strength. Very succinct graph patterns can identify and differentiate these abnormalities.*

Hypercoagulability

Factor V-Leiden,
Protein S/C abnormality,
Genetic hypercoagulability,
Idiopathic hypercoagulability:

> *All are associated with an early fibrin clot. Again, very succinct graph patterns can be identified to differentiate these abnormalities.*

RELATED TESTS

Platelet Aggregation (p. 398). This is a measure of the abilities of the platelets to aggregate.
Platelet Function Assay (p. 404). This is a measure of platelet function.
Platelet Count (p. 401). This is an account of the number of thromboses.
Coagulating Factor Concentration (p. 163). These tests measure the quantity of each specific factor.
Factor V-Leiden (p. 231). This is an inherited abnormality affecting the coagulation cascade.
Protein C, Protein S (p. 432). These are important inhibitors of the coagulation system.
Plasminogen (p. 394). This protein is involved in the fibrinolytic process.

Thrombosis Indicators (Fibrin Monomers [Fibrin Degradation Products (FDPs)], Fibrin Split Products [FSPs], Fibrinopeptide A [FPA], Prothrombin Fragment [F1+2])

NORMAL FINDINGS

FDP: <10 mcg/mL or <10 mg/L (SI units)
FPA:
    Male: 0.4-2.6 mg/mL
    Female 0.7-3.1 mg/mL
F1+2: 7.4-103 mcg/L or 0.2-2.8 nmol/L

 Critical Values

FDP >40 mcg/mL

INDICATIONS

Identification of FDPs, FPA, and F1+2 is mostly used to document that fibrin clot formation and, therefore, thrombosis is occurring. These tests support the diagnosis of disseminated intravascular coagulation (DIC). They also provide an indication about the effectiveness of anticoagulation therapy. Finally, they are used to support the diagnosis and follow treatment for hypercoagulable states.

TEST EXPLANATION

F1+2 is liberated when prothrombin is converted to thrombin in reaction 4 of secondary hemostasis (see Figure 2-12, p. 167). These fragments are primarily used to indicate thrombosis. Significantly increased F1+2 levels are also noted in patients with leukemia, severe liver disease, and after myocardial infarction. Patients with elevated F1+2 concentration before the beginning of heparin therapy show decreases after 1 day of therapy. For patients in the stable phase of oral anticoagulant therapy decreasing F1+2 concentrations are noted with increasing INR values. Thus F1+2 determination is particularly helpful in monitoring anticoagulant therapy.

FPA is made up of two small peptide chains removed from the N-terminal segment of the alpha chains of fibrinogen during its conversion to fibrin. It is released into the bloodstream by that reaction during the blood coagulation process and is therefore a measure of thrombosis.

Measurement of *FDPs* provides a direct indication of the activity of the fibrinolytic system. The fibrinolytic system plays an important role in balancing clot formation and clot dissolution. Clot formation stimulates the activation of three major activators of the fibrinolytic system. These in turn act on plasminogen, which was previously absorbed into the clot, to form plasmin. Plasmin degenerates the fibrin polymer of the clot into fragments called FDPs (X, D, E, Y). These degradation products are usually cleared by macrophages. If present in increased quantities, they can have an anticoagulant effect by inhibiting fibrinogen conversion to fibrin and by interrupting fibrin polymerization to tighten the clot.

When present in large amounts, FDPs indicate increased fibrinolysis, as occurs in thrombotic states. The thrombosis stimulates the activation of the fibrinolytic system. Other diseases can secondarily activate the fibrinolytic system and elevate FDP levels. These may include extensive malignancy, tissue necrosis, and gram-negative sepsis. Thrombolytic therapy used in myocardial infarction (MI), for example, is associated with increased FDPs. Streptokinase or urokinase stimulates the conversion of plasminogen to plasmin. The plasmin splits the fibrinogen polymer into FDPs, as discussed above.

These products of hemostasis and fibrinolysis may also be elevated in patients with extensive malignancy, tissue necrosis, and gram-negative sepsis. For discussion of D-dimer fibrin degradation products, see p. 202.

INTERFERING FACTORS

- Traumatic venipunctures may increase FPA levels.
- Surgery or massive trauma is associated with increased levels of these indicators because of the thrombosis that is instigated by surgery.
- Menstruation may be associated with increased FDP levels.
- The presence of rheumatoid factor may give falsely high levels.
- Drugs that may cause *increased* levels include barbiturates, heparin, streptokinase, and urokinase.
- Drugs that may cause *decreased* indicator levels include warfarin and other oral anticoagulants.

PROCEDURE AND PATIENT CARE

Before
- Explain the procedure to the patient.
- Tell the patient that no fasting is required.
- Avoid prolonged use of a tourniquet.

During
- Draw the sample before initiating heparin therapy.
- Collect a venous blood sample in a small, blue-top tube or in the colored tube designated by the laboratory.
- Avoid excessive agitation of the blood sample.
- Note that it is best to place the blood on ice and take it immediately to the hematology laboratory.
- List on the laboratory slip any drugs that may cause elevated levels.

After
- Apply pressure to the venipuncture site.

TEST RESULTS AND CLINICAL SIGNIFICANCE

▲ Increased Levels
Disseminated intravascular coagulation (DIC),
Heart or vascular surgery,

Thromboembolism,
Thrombosis,
Advanced malignancy,
Severe inflammation,
Postoperative states,
Massive trauma:
   These diseases or states are all associated with increased thrombosis and/or fibrinolysis.
Deficiency in protein S and C: *The "protein C–protein S" system is an important inhibitor of coagulation. With deficiencies in these proteins, thrombosis proceeds without inhibition.*
Antithrombin III deficiency: *Antithrombin III complexes with activated coagulation proteins and blocks their biologic activity. Even mild reductions in this protein are therefore associated with marked increased thrombosis.*

▼   Decreased Levels

Anticoagulation therapy: *Reduction in thrombosis is associated with a reduction in all the proteins that are products of that biologic system.*

RELATED TEST

Disseminated Intravascular Coagulation (DIC) Screening (p. 210). This is a description of commonly used tests to diagnose DIC.

Thyroglobulin (Tg, Thyrogen-Stimulated Thyroglobulin)

NORMAL FINDINGS

Age	Male (ng/mL)	Female (ng/mL)
0-11 months	0.6-5.5	0.5-5.5
1-11 years	0.6-50.1	0.5-52.1
12 years and older	0.5-53.0	0.5-43.0

INDICATIONS

This test is primarily used as a tumor marker for well-differentiated thyroid cancer.

TEST EXPLANATION

Tg is the protein precursor of thyroid hormone and is made by normal well-differentiated benign thyroid cells or thyroid cancer cells. Because Tg is normally only made by thyroid cells, it serves a useful readout for the presence or absence of thyroid cells especially after thyroid cancer surgery. In the treatment of well-differentiated thyroid cancers, it is important to remove as much thyroid tissue as possible so that adjunctive radioactive iodine treatment will not go to residual thyroid gland tissue in the neck, but will go instead to any metastatic thyroid cells. If postoperative Tg levels are low, very little thyroid tissue remains.

Tg is also used as a "tumor marker" in these postoperative patients. Tg is a marker of disease activity and the volume of thyroid tumor. Ideally, the Tg levels will be low (<2 ng/mL) or undetectable after treatment (usually surgery followed by radioactive iodine). Rising levels herald tumor recurrence and progression. Although Tg levels may be elevated in patients with thyroid cancer, a large number of benign thyroid conditions may also be associated with elevated levels of Tg. Therefore an increased Tg alone in a patient is not a sensitive or specific test for the diagnosis of thyroid cancer. Simply examining the thyroid or carrying out a thyroid biopsy can produce significant elevations in the circulating blood level of Tg. Similarly, patients with thyroid inflammation can have very high levels of Tg. Some patients with antithyroglobulin antibodies (see p. 102) may have inaccurate Tg levels.

After thyroidectomy, thyroid hormone replacement is required for normal metabolic function. Because of thyroid hormone replacement therapy, thyroid-stimulating hormone (TSH) levels are usually very low and endogenous stimulation of any residual thyroid cells is minimal in these patients. As a result, Tg and thyroid endogenous thyroid hormones are low. Until recently, in order to stimulate Tg production in these patients for cancer surveillance testing, thyroid hormone was temporarily discontinued for as much as 6 weeks until the body was depleted of any thyroid hormone. TSH was then maximally stimulated and was able to stimulate the production of Tg from any thyroid cells. If there were any functioning thyroid cancer cells, Tg would be elevated. During the time of thyroid hormone withdrawal, the patient was very uncomfortable, lethargic, tired, and slow.

Thyrogen-stimulated testing has eliminated the need for withdrawal of thyroid hormone medications and provides a safe and effective method to elevate TSH levels so that even minimal levels of Tg can be detected. This allows patients to undergo periodic thyroid cancer follow-up evaluation while avoiding the often debilitating side effects of hypothyroidism caused by withdrawal of hormone medication. Thyrogen is a highly purified recombinant source of human thyroid-stimulating hormone. Thyrogen raises serum TSH levels and thereby stimulates Tg production. Normal thyroid remnant and well-differentiated thyroid tumors display a greater (>10-fold) serum Tg response to TSH stimulation. If Thyrogen-stimulated Tg levels are elevated after thyroid surgery, either a significant amount of normal thyroid gland was left in the neck or metastatic disease exists. If Thyrogen-stimulated Tg levels are elevated after postoperative therapeutic [131]I (given to destroy any residual thyroid tissue in the neck), metastatic disease certainly exists and will require treatment.

Thyrogen stimulation is also used for patients undergoing ^{131}I whole body scanning for metastatic thyroid cancer. Like Tg testing, in the past these patients had to withdraw from their thyroid hormone replacement medicine so that their endogenous TSH levels would rise, stimulate any metastatic thyroid cancer cells to pick up ^{131}I, and be detected on a nuclear scan of the body. Now with the use of Thyrogen, the ill effects of hormone withdrawal are not experienced.

INTERFERING FACTORS

- Tg levels are decreased in less well-differentiated thyroid cancers.
- Thyrogen stimulation of Tg levels is less in patients whose tumors do not have TSH receptors or whose tumors cannot make Tg.
- Tg autoantibodies cause either underestimation or overestimation of serum Tg measurements made by immunometric assay (IMA) and radioimmunoassay (RIA) methods, respectively.

 Clinical Priorities

- Thyroid cancer is the most common endocrine cancer and occurs in all age groups.
- Thyroid cancer is the cancer most increasing in incidence among women.
- Thyroid cancer may recur in up to 30% of patients, even decades after initial diagnosis.

Blood Studies

2

PROCEDURE AND PATIENT CARE

Before

Explain the procedure to the patient.

Tell the patient that no fasting is required.

- Determine if the patient is to have a whole body nuclear scan along with the Tg blood test.

During

- Collect a venous blood sample in a gold-top (serum separator) tube.
- If Thyrogen stimulation is to be used:
  1. Administer Thyrogen intramuscularly to the buttock every 24 hours for two or three doses.
  2. Collect blood in a gold-top (serum separator) tube in 3 days.
- For radioiodine imaging:
  1. The nuclear medicine technologist will administer radioiodine 24 hours following the final Thyrogen injection.
  2. Scanning is usually performed 48 hours after radioiodine administration. Whole-body images are acquired for a minimum of 30 minutes and/or should contain a minimum of 140,000 counts.
  3. Scanning times for single (spot) images of body regions may be obtained.

After

- Apply pressure or a pressure dressing to the venipuncture site.
- Assess the venipuncture site for bleeding.

TEST RESULTS AND CLINICAL SIGNIFICANCE

▲ Increased Levels

Residual thyroid tissue in the neck,

Metastatic thyroid cancer:

Normal thyroid cells and well-differentiated thyroid cancer cells make Tg as a precursor to thyroid hormone.

RELATED TEST

Antithyroglobulin Antibody (p. 102). Although used primarily to identify patients with thyroiditis, the presence of these antibodies can affect Tg test results.

Thyroid-Stimulating Hormone (TSH, Thyrotropin)

NORMAL FINDINGS

Adult: 0.3-5 μU/mL or 0.3-5 mU/L (SI units)

Newborn: 3-18 μU/mL or 3-18 mU/L

Cord: 3-12 μU/mL or 3-12 mU/L

Values vary among laboratories.

INDICATIONS

This test is used to diagnose primary hypothyroidism and to differentiate it from secondary (pituitary) and tertiary (hypothalamus) hypothyroidism.

TEST EXPLANATION

The TSH (also called thyrotropin) concentration aids in differentiating primary and secondary hypothyroidism. Pituitary TSH secretion is stimulated by hypothalamic thyroid-releasing hormone (TRH). Low levels of triiodothyronine (T_3) and thyroxine (T_4) are the underlying stimuli for TRH and TSH. Therefore a compensatory elevation of TRH and TSH occurs in patients with primary hypothyroid states, such as surgical or radioactive thyroid ablation; in patients with burned-out thyroiditis, thyroid agenesis, idiopathic hypothyroidism, or congenital cretinism; or in patients taking antithyroid medications.

In secondary or tertiary hypothyroidism the function of the pituitary or hypothalamus gland, respectively, is faulty as a result of tumor, trauma, or infarction. Therefore TRH and TSH cannot be secreted, and plasma levels of these hormones are near zero despite the stimulation that occurs with low T_3 and T_4 levels.

The *TRH Stimulation Test* is sometimes used to stimulate low levels of TSH to identify primary from secondary hypothyroidism in cases in which TSH is low. However, this test is not commonly used because extremely low levels of TSH can now be identified with the use of immunoassays.

The TSH test is used to monitor exogenous thyroid replacement or suppression as well. The goal of thyroid replacement therapy is to provide an adequate amount of thyroid medication so that TSH secretion is in the "low normal range," indicating a euthyroid state. The goal of thyroid suppression is to completely suppress the thyroid gland and TSH secretion by providing excessive thyroid medication. This treatment is used to diminish the size of a thyroid goiter. The dose of medication is given to keep the TSH level less than 2 for replacement. Even lower TSH levels are preferred if thyroid suppression is the clinical goal.

This test is also used to detect primary hypothyroidism in newborns with low screening T_4 levels. TSH and T_4 levels are frequently measured to differentiate pituitary and thyroid dysfunction. A decreased T_4 and normal or elevated TSH level can indicate a thyroid disorder. A decreased T_4 with a decreased TSH level can indicate a pituitary disorder.

INTERFERING FACTORS

- Recent radioisotope administration may affect test results.
- Severe illness may cause decreased TSH levels.
- There is a diurnal variation in TSH levels. Basal levels occur around 10 AM and highest levels (about two to three times basal levels) occur around 10 PM.
- Drugs that may cause *increased* levels include antithyroid medications, lithium, potassium iodide, and TSH injection.
- Drugs that may cause *decreased* levels include aspirin, heparin, nonsteroidal antiarthritics dopamine, steroids, and T_3.

✓ Clinical Priorities

- This test is useful for differentiating primary hypothyroidism and secondary (pituitary) and tertiary (hypothalamus) hypothyroidism. Elevations of TSH occur in patients with primary hypothyroid states. In contrast, plasma levels of TSH are near zero in patients with secondary and tertiary hypothyroidism.
- This test may be used to detect primary hypothyroidism in newborns with low screening T_4 levels.
- TSH levels are subject to a diurnal variation. Basal levels occur around 10 AM and highest levels occur around 10 PM.

PROCEDURE AND PATIENT CARE

Before

☒ Explain the procedure to the patient.
☒ Tell the patient that no food or drink restrictions are necessary.

During

- Collect a venous blood sample in a red-top tube.
- Use a heel stick to obtain blood from newborns.

After

- Apply pressure or a pressure dressing to the venipuncture site.
- Assess the venipuncture site for bleeding.

TEST RESULTS AND CLINICAL SIGNIFICANCE

▲ Increased Levels

Primary hypothyroidism (thyroid dysfunction),
Thyroiditis,
Thyroid agenesis,
Congenital cretinism,
Large doses of iodine,
Radioactive iodine injection,
Surgical ablation of thyroid,
Severe and chronic illnesses:
> *In these diseases, inadequate thyroid hormone levels act as a potent stimulant for the release of TSH from the anterior pituitary. TSH levels rise. In some cases, however, TSH may be diminished.*

Pituitary TSH-secreting tumor: *This is very rare, but when it occurs, TSH levels are increased.*

▼ Decreased Levels

Secondary hypothyroidism (pituitary or hypothalamus dysfunction): *Diseases of the hypothalamus diminish the capability of the hypothalamus to secrete TRH, which is the major factor that determines TSH production and secretion. Diseases of the pituitary diminish pituitary production of TSH.*

Hyperthyroidism: *Increased levels of thyroid hormones inhibit the release of TSH.*

Suppressive doses of thyroid medication: *When thyroid medication (e.g., Synthroid) is administered (usually to shrink a goiter), TSH levels fall because of inhibition by the thyroid medication.*

Factitious hyperthyroidism: *These patients take thyroid medication without prescription. These medications act to inhibit TSH production.*

RELATED TESTS

Thyroid-Stimulating Immunoglobulins (p. 491). LATS and other thyroid-stimulating immunoglobulins are used to support the diagnosis of Graves disease, especially when the diagnosis is complex.

Thyrotropin-Releasing Hormone Stimulation Test (p. 492). This test assists in the evaluation of patients with hyperthyroidism and hypothyroidism. It is especially helpful in the differential diagnosis of hypothyroidism.

Thyroid-Stimulating Hormone Stimulation (see following test). This test is also used to differentiate primary from secondary (and tertiary) hypothyroidism.

Thyroxine-Binding Globulin (p. 495). This is a measure of TBG, the major thyroid hormone protein carrier. It is used in the evaluation of patients who have abnormal total T_4 and T_3 levels. When performed concurrently with the T_4/T_3 test, T_4 and T_3 levels can more easily be interpreted.

Thyroxine, Total (p. 497). This is one of the first tests done for assessing thyroid function. It is used to diagnose thyroid function and to monitor replacement and suppressive therapy.

Triiodothyronine (p. 506). T_3 is used to evaluate thyroid function. It is mostly used to diagnose hyperthyroidism. It is also used to monitor thyroid replacement and suppressive therapy.

Thyroxine Index, Free. This test is used to evaluate thyroid function. It corrects for changes in thyroid hormone-binding serum proteins that can affect total T_4 levels. It is used to diagnose hyperthyroidism and hypothyroidism.

Thyroxine, Free (p. 497). The FT_4 is used to evaluate thyroid function in patients who may have protein abnormalities that could affect total T_4 levels. It is used to diagnose thyroid function and to monitor replacement and suppressive therapy.

Antithyroglobulin Antibody (p. 102). This test is used primarily in the differential diagnosis of thyroid diseases, such as Hashimoto thyroiditis and chronic lymphocytic thyroiditis (in children).

Thyroid-Stimulating Hormone Stimulation (TSH Stimulation)

NORMAL FINDINGS

Increased thyroid function with administration of exogenous TSH

INDICATIONS

This test is used to differentiate primary and secondary (and tertiary) hypothyroidism.

TEST EXPLANATION

The TSH stimulation test is used to differentiate primary (thyroid) hypothyroidism and secondary (hypothalamic-pituitary) hypothyroidism. Normal people and patients with hypothalamic-pituitary hypothyroidism are capable of increasing thyroid function when exogenous TSH is given. Patients with primary hypothyroidism because of disease in the thyroid, however, are not; their thyroid gland is inadequate and cannot function no matter how much stimulation it receives. Patients with less than a 10% increase in radioactive iodine uptake (RAIU) or less than a 1.5 mcg/dL rise in thyroxine (T_4) are considered to have primary hypothyroidism. If the hypothyroidism is caused by inadequate pituitary secretion of TSH or hypothalamic secretion of thyroid-releasing hormone (TRH), the RAIU should increase at least 10% and the T_4 level should rise 1.5 mcg/dL or more. This is characteristic of secondary hypothyroidism.

PROCEDURE AND PATIENT CARE

Before

 Explain the procedure to the patient.

- Obtain baseline levels of RAIU or T_4 as indicated.

Tell the patient that no fasting is required.

During

- Administer the prescribed dose of TSH intramuscularly for 3 days.
- Repeat the measurement of RAIU or T_4 as indicated.

After

- Apply pressure or a pressure dressing to the venipuncture site.
- Assess the venipuncture site for bleeding.

TEST RESULTS AND CLINICAL SIGNIFICANCE

▲ Increased Levels

Primary hypothyroidism (thyroid dysfunction),
Thyroiditis,
Thyroid agenesis,
Congenital cretinism,
Large doses of iodine,
Radioactive iodine injection,
Surgical ablation of thyroid,
Severe and chronic illnesses:
> In these diseases the thyroid is unable to increase T_4 levels or RAIU no matter how significant the stimulation, because the disease involves the thyroid itself.

Secondary hypothyroidism (pituitary or hypothalamus dysfunction): *The thyroid is capable of producing T_4 and RAIU, but the pituitary/hypothalamic stimulation is inadequate for appropriate stimulation of those functions. When TSH is administered, T_4 and RAIU increase significantly.*

RELATED TESTS

Long-Acting Thyroid Stimulator (p. 491). LATS and other thyroid-stimulating immunoglobulins are used to support the diagnosis of Graves disease, especially when the diagnosis is complex.

Thyrotropin-Releasing Hormone Stimulation Test (p. 492). This test assists in the evaluation of patients with hyperthyroidism and hypothyroidism. It is especially helpful in the differential diagnosis of hypothyroidism.

Thyroid-Stimulating Hormone (p. 486). This test is used to diagnose primary hypothyroidism and to differentiate it from secondary (pituitary) and tertiary (hypothalamus) hypothyroidism.

Thyroxine-Binding Globulin (p. 495). This is a measure of TBG, the major thyroid hormone protein carrier. It is used in the evaluation of patients who have abnormal total T_4 and T_3 levels. When performed concurrently with a T_4/T_3 test, the T_4 and T_3 levels can more easily be interpreted.

Thyroxine, Total (p. 497). This is one of the first tests done for assessing thyroid function. It is used to diagnose thyroid function and to monitor replacement and suppressive therapy.

Triiodothyronine (p. 506). T_3 is used to evaluate thyroid function. It is used primarily to diagnose hyperthyroidism. It is also used to monitor thyroid replacement and suppressive therapy.

Thyroxine Index, Free. This test is used to evaluate thyroid function. It corrects for changes in thyroid hormone-binding serum proteins that can affect total T_4 levels. It is used to diagnose hyperthyroidism and hypothyroidism.

Thyroxine, Free (p. 497). The FT_4 is used to evaluate thyroid function in patients who may have protein abnormalities that could affect total T_4 levels. It is used to diagnose thyroid function and to monitor replacement and suppressive therapy.

Antithyroglobulin Antibody (p. 102). This test is primarily used in the differential diagnosis of thyroid diseases, such as Hashimoto thyroiditis and chronic lymphocytic thyroiditis (in children).

Thyroid-Stimulating Immunoglobulins (TSI, Long-Acting Thyroid Stimulator [LATS], Thyroid-Binding Inhibitory Immunoglobulin [TBII], Thyrotropin Receptor Antibody)

NORMAL FINDINGS

TSI <130% of basal activity
TBII <10%

INDICATIONS

These are used to support the diagnosis of Graves disease, especially when the diagnosis is complex.

TEST EXPLANATION

Thyroid-stimulating immunoglobulins (TSI) represent a group of immunoglobulin-G (IgG) antibodies directed against the thyroid cell receptor for thyroid-stimulating hormone (TSH) and are associated with autoimmune thyroid disease states such as chronic thyroiditis and Graves disease. These autoantibodies bind and transactivate the TSH receptors (TSHRs). This instigates stimulation of the thyroid gland independent of the normal feedback–regulated thyroid-stimulating hormone (TSH) stimulation. This, in turn will stimulate the release of thyroid hormones from the thyroid cells. Some patients with Graves disease also have TSHR-blocking antibodies, which do not transactivate the TSHR. The balance between TSI and TSHR-blocking antibodies, as well as their individual titers, are felt to be determinants of Graves disease severity.

The use of these antibodies is helpful in the evaluation of patients for whom the diagnosis of Graves disease is confused by conflicting data (such as subclinical Graves hyperthyroidism or euthyroid patients with ophthalmopathy). In these cases, the antibodies help determine and support the diagnosis of Graves disease.

The effect of these antibodies on the thyroid may be long lasting, and titers do not decrease until nearly 1 year after successful treatment of the thyroid disease. However, measurement of these antibodies may be helpful in identifying remission or relapse of Graves disease after treatment. Because TSI can cross the placenta, they may be found in neonates whose mothers have Graves disease. These infants experience hyperthyroidism for as long as 4 to 8 months. This syndrome must be identified and treated early.

TSI and TSHR antibodies can be measured individually. Other antibodies associated with autoimmune thyroid diseases include thyroglobulin antibodies (p. 102) and antithyroid peroxidase antibodies (p. 104).

INTERFERING FACTORS

- Recent administration of radioactive iodine may affect test results.

PROCEDURE AND PATIENT CARE

Before

- Explain the procedure to the patient.
- Tell the patient that no fasting or special preparation is required.

During

- Collect a venous blood sample in a red-top or gold-top tube.

- Notify the laboratory if the patient has received radioactive iodine in the preceding 2 days.
- Handle the blood sample gently. Hemolysis may interfere with interpretation of test results.

After
- Apply pressure to the venipuncture site.

TEST RESULTS AND CLINICAL SIGNIFICANCE

▲ Increased Levels

Hyperthyroidism,
Neonatal thyrotoxicosis,
Malignant exophthalmos,
Graves disease,
Hashimoto thyroiditis:

> *These forms of hyperthyroidism have an autoimmune element to the disease process. IgG antibodies will be present in most cases. These antibodies can act to stimulate or inhibit thyroid function.*

RELATED TESTS

Thyrotropin-Releasing Hormone Stimulation Test (see following test). This test assists in the evaluation of patients with hyperthyroidism and hypothyroidism. It is especially helpful in the differential diagnosis of hypothyroidism.

Thyroid-Stimulating Hormone (p. 486). This test is used to diagnose primary hypothyroidism and to differentiate it from secondary (pituitary) and tertiary (hypothalamus) hypothyroidism.

Thyroid-Stimulating Hormone (TSH) Stimulation (p. 489). This test is also used to differentiate primary and secondary (and tertiary) hypothyroidism.

Thyroxine-Binding Globulin (p. 495). This is a measure of thyroxine-binding globulin (TBG), the major thyroid hormone protein carrier. It is used in the evaluation of patients who have abnormal total T_4 and T_3 levels. When done concurrently with a T_4/T_3 test, one can more easily interpret the T_4 and T_3 levels.

Thyroxine, Total (p. 497). This is one of the first tests done in assessing thyroid function. It is used to diagnose thyroid function and to monitor replacement and suppressive therapy.

Triiodothyronine (p. 506). T_3 is used to evaluate thyroid function. It is mostly used to diagnose hyperthyroidism. It is also used to monitor thyroid replacement and suppressive medical therapy.

Thyroxine, Free (p. 497). The FT_4 is used to evaluate thyroid function in patients who may have protein abnormalities that could affect total T_4 levels. It is used to diagnose thyroid function and to monitor replacement and suppressive therapy.

Antithyroglobulin Antibody (p. 102). This test is primarily used in the differential diagnosis of thyroid diseases such as Hashimoto thyroiditis and chronic lymphocytic thyroiditis (in children).

Thyrotropin-Releasing Hormone Stimulation Test (TRH Stimulation Test, Thyrotropin-Releasing Factor Stimulation Test [TRF Stimulation Test])

NORMAL FINDINGS

Prompt rise in serum thyroid-stimulating hormone (TSH) level to approximately twice the baseline value in 30 minutes after an intravenous (IV) bolus of TRH

Clinical Disease	Baseline Thyroid-Stimulating Hormone (μU/mL)	Stimulated TSH*
Euthyroid	<10	>2
Hyperthyroid	<10	<2
Primary hypothyroid (thyroid)	>10	>2
Secondary hypothyroid (pituitary)	<10	<2
Tertiary hypothyroid (hypothalamus)	<10	>2

*Stimulated TSH (times the baseline) is measured 30 minutes after the IV injection of thyrotropin-releasing hormone.

INDICATIONS

This test assists in the evaluation of patients with hyperthyroidism and hypothyroidism. It is especially helpful in the differential diagnosis of hypothyroidism.

TEST EXPLANATION

The TRH stimulation test assesses the anterior pituitary gland via its secretion of TSH in response to an IV injection of TRH. After the TRH injection the normally functioning pituitary gland should secrete TSH (and prolactin). In hyperthyroidism, either a slight increase or no increase in the TSH level is seen, because pituitary TSH production is suppressed by the inhibitory effect of excess circulating thyroxine (T_4) and triiodothyronine (T_3) on the pituitary gland. A normal result is considered reliable evidence for excluding the diagnosis of thyrotoxicosis. Since the development of a very sensitive radioimmunoassay for TSH, the TRH stimulation test is no longer required to diagnose hyperthyroidism. However, it still has a role in the evaluation of pituitary deficiency.

In addition to assessing the responsiveness of the anterior pituitary gland, this test aids in the detection of primary, secondary, and tertiary hypothyroidism. In primary hypothyroidism (thyroid gland failure) the increase in the TSH level is two or more times the normal result. With secondary hypothyroidism (anterior pituitary failure), no TSH response occurs. Tertiary hypothyroidism (hypothalamic failure) may be diagnosed by a delayed rise in the TSH level. Multiple injections of TRH may be needed to induce the appropriate TSH response in this case.

The TRH stimulation test also may be useful in differentiating primary depression, manic-depressive psychiatric illness, and secondary types of depression. In primary depression the TSH response is blunted in most patients, whereas patients with other types of depression have a normal TRH-induced TSH response.

INTERFERING FACTORS

- The normal response may be exaggerated in women.
- The normal response may be less than expected in the elderly.
- Pregnancy may increase the TSH response to TRH.
- Drugs that may modify the TSH response include antithyroid drugs, aspirin, corticosteroids, estrogens, levodopa, and T_4.

PROCEDURE AND PATIENT CARE

Before

Explain the procedure to the patient.

Instruct the patient to discontinue thyroid preparations for 3 to 4 weeks before the TRH test if indicated.

- Assess the patient for medications currently being taken.
- Tell the patient that no fasting or sedation is required.

During
- Administer an IV bolus of TRH.
- Obtain venous blood samples at intervals and measure TSH levels.

After
- Apply pressure or a pressure dressing to the venipuncture site.
- Assess the venipuncture site for bleeding.
- Indicate on the laboratory slip if the patient is pregnant.

TEST RESULTS AND CLINICAL SIGNIFICANCE

▲ Increased Levels

Hyperthyroidism: *Because the pituitary is already maximally suppressed by the high levels of T_3 and T_4, pituitary response to TRH will be blunted and baseline levels will be less than double.*

Primary hypothyroidism (thyroid disease): *Because the TSH is already stimulated by the lack of T_3 and T_4 stimulation will be maximized by the TRH and stimulated TSH will be more than double the baseline.*

Secondary hypothyroidism (pituitary disease): *Because the diseased pituitary is unable to produce TSH, no matter how significant the stimulation, TSH will not double after TRH stimulation.*

Tertiary hypothyroidism (hypothalamus): *The pituitary is functioning normally. If TRH is provided exogenously, the pituitary will respond normally and produce twice the TSH level.*

Psychiatric primary depression: *In primary depression the TSH response is blunted in most patients, whereas patients with other types of depression have a normal TRH-induced TSH response.*

RELATED TESTS

Thyroid-Stimulating Hormone (p. 486). This test is used to diagnose primary hypothyroidism and to differentiate it from secondary (pituitary) and tertiary (hypothalamus) hypothyroidism.

Thyroid-Stimulating Hormone Stimulation (p. 489). This test is also used to differentiate primary and secondary (and tertiary) hypothyroidism.

Thyroxine-Binding Globulin (p. 495). This is a measure of TBG, the major thyroid hormone protein carrier. It is used in the evaluation of patients who have abnormal total T_4 and T_3 levels. When performed concurrently with a T_4/T_3 test, the T_4 and T_3 levels can be more easily interpreted.

Thyroxine, Total (p. 497). This is one of the first tests done for assessing thyroid function. It is used to diagnose thyroid function and to monitor replacement and suppressive therapy.

Triiodothyronine (p. 506). T_3 is used to evaluate thyroid function. It is primarily used to diagnose hyperthyroidism. It is also used to monitor thyroid replacement and suppressive therapy.

Thyroxine Index, Free. This test is used to evaluate thyroid function. It corrects for changes in thyroid hormone-binding serum proteins that can affect total T_4 levels. It is used to diagnose hyperthyroidism and hypothyroidism.

Thyroxine, Free (p. 497). The FT_4 is used to evaluate thyroid function in patients who may have protein abnormalities that could affect total T_4 levels. It is used to diagnose thyroid function and to monitor replacement and suppressive therapy.

Long-Acting Thyroid Stimulator (p. 491). LATS and other thyroid-stimulating immunoglobulins are used to support the diagnosis of Graves disease, especially when the diagnosis is complex.

Antithyroglobulin Antibody (p. 102). This test is used primarily in the differential diagnosis of thyroid diseases, such as Hashimoto thyroiditis and chronic lymphocytic thyroiditis (in children).

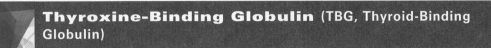

Thyroxine-Binding Globulin (TBG, Thyroid-Binding Globulin)

NORMAL FINDINGS

Age	Males (mg/dL)	Females (mg/dL)
1-5 days	2.2-4.2	2.2-4.2
1-11 months	1.6-3.6	1.7-3.7
1-9 years	1.2-2.8	1.5-2.7
10-19 years	1.4-2.6	1.4-3.0
>20 years	1.7-3.6	1.7-3.6
Oral contraceptives	—	1.5-5.5
Pregnancy (third trimester)	—	4.7-5.9

INDICATIONS

This is a measure of TBG, the major thyroid hormone protein carrier. It is used in the evaluation of patients who have abnormal total T_4 and T_3 levels. When performed concurrently with a T_4/T_3 test, the T_4 and T_3 levels can be more easily interpreted.

TEST EXPLANATION

Assays of T_4 and T_3 are a measure of total T_4/T_3 levels. That is, they are a measure of bound and unbound thyroid hormones. Most of these hormones are bound to TBG. The unbound or "free T_4/T_3" is the metabolically active hormone. Certain illnesses are associated with elevated or decreased TBG levels. With increased TBG levels, more T_4 and T_3 is bound to that protein. Less free, metabolically active T_4/T_3 is available. TSH is stimulated to produce higher levels of T_4 and T_3 to compensate. T_4 and T_3 levels increase but do not cause hyperthyroidism, because the increase is merely a compensation for the increased TBG. When total T_4 is elevated, one must ascertain whether that elevation is due to an elevation in TBG or a real elevation in T_4 alone associated with hyperthyroidism. There are other indirect measurements of TBG, including thyroid hormone-binding ratio (THBR).

The most common causes of elevated TBG are pregnancy, hormone replacement therapy, or use of oral contraceptives. Elevated TBG is also present in some cases of porphyria and in infectious hepatitis. Decreased TBG is commonly associated with other causes of hypoproteinemia (e.g., nephrotic syndrome, gastrointestinal [GI] malabsorption, malnutrition).

INTERFERING FACTORS

- Previous administration of diagnostic radioisotopes may confound test results, if TBG is measured by radioimmunoassay (RIA).
- Drugs that *increase* TBG include estrogens, methadone, oral contraceptives, and tamoxifen.
- Drugs that *decrease* TBG include androgens, danazol, phenytoin, propranolol, and steroids.

PROCEDURE AND PATIENT CARE

Before

☒ Explain the procedure to the patient.
☒ Tell the patient that no fasting is required.

During

- Collect a venous blood sample in a red-top tube.
- List on the laboratory slip any drugs that may affect test results.

After

- Apply pressure or a pressure dressing to the venipuncture site.
- Assess the venipuncture site for bleeding.

TEST RESULTS AND CLINICAL SIGNIFICANCE

▲ Increased Levels

Pregnancy (and estrogen-replacement therapy, estrogen-producing tumors): *All proteins, including TBG, are increased with increased estrogen levels.*
Infectious hepatitis: *The pathophysiology of this observation is not well known.*
Genetic increase of TBG: *Rarely a patient will have a genetic variation that causes elevated* TBG.
Acute intermittent porphyria: *The pathophysiology of this observation is not well known.*

▼ Decreased Levels

Protein-losing enteropathy,
Protein-losing nephropathy,
Malnutrition:
   Decreased protein levels include decreased TBG.
Testosterone-producing tumors: *Testosterone decreases TBG levels.*
Ovarian failure: *With reduced estrogens (e.g., menopause), TBG is reduced.*
Major stress: *Major stress is often associated with low proteins, including TBG.*

RELATED TESTS

Long-Acting Thyroid Stimulator (p. 491). LATS and other thyroid-stimulating immunoglobulins are used to support the diagnosis of Graves disease, especially when the diagnosis is complex.
Thyrotropin-Releasing Hormone (p. 492). This test assists in the evaluation of patients with hyperthyroidism and hypothyroidism. It is especially helpful in the differential diagnosis of hypothyroidism.
Thyroid-Stimulating Hormone (p. 486). This test is used to diagnose primary hypothyroidism and to differentiate it from secondary (pituitary) and tertiary (hypothalamus) hypothyroidism.
Thyroid-Stimulating Hormone Stimulation (p. 489). This test is also used to differentiate primary and secondary (and tertiary) hypothyroidism.
Thyroxine, Total (p. 497). This is one of the first tests done for assessing thyroid function. It is used to diagnose thyroid function and to monitor replacement and suppressive therapy.
Triiodothyronine (p. 506). T_3 is used to evaluate thyroid function. It is mostly used to diagnose hyperthyroidism. It is also used to monitor thyroid replacement and suppressive medical therapy.

Thyroxine, Free (see following test). The FT_4 is used to evaluate thyroid function in patients who may have protein abnormalities that could affect total T_4 levels. It is used to diagnose thyroid function and to monitor replacement and suppressive therapy.

Antithyroglobulin Antibody (p. 102). This test is used primarily in the differential diagnosis of thyroid diseases, such as Hashimoto thyroiditis and chronic lymphocytic thyroiditis (in children).

 Thyroxine, Total and Free (T$_4$, Thyroxine Screen, FT$_4$)

NORMAL FINDINGS

Free T_4
    0-4 days: 2-6 ng/dL or 26-77 pmol/L (SI units)
    2 weeks to 20 years: 0.8-2 ng/dL or 10-26 pmol/L (SI units)
    Adult: 0.8-2.8 ng/dL or 10-36 pmol/L (SI units)
Total T_4
    1-3 days: 11-22 mcg/dL
    1-2 weeks: 10-16 mcg/dL
    1-12 months: 8-16 mcg/dL
    1-5 years: 7-15 mcg/dL
    5-10 years: 6-13 mcg/dL
    10-15 years: 5-12 mcg/dL
    Adult male: 4-12 mcg/dL or 51-154 nmol/L (SI units)
    Adult female: 5-12 mcg/dL or 64-154 nmol/L (SI units)
    Adult >60 years: 5-11 mcg/dL or 64-142 nmol/L (SI units)

 Critical Values

Possible critical values of total T_4
    Newborn: <7 mcg/dL
    Adult: <2 mcg/dL if myxedema coma possible; >20 mcg/dL if thyroid storm possible

INDICATIONS

Thyroxine tests are used to determine thyroid function. Greater than normal levels indicate hyperthyroid states, and subnormal values are seen in hypothyroid states. T_4 and TSH are used to monitor thyroid replacement and suppressive therapy.

TEST EXPLANATION

Thyroid hormones are produced when tyrosine incorporates organic iodine to form monoiodotyrosine. This complex picks up iodine and becomes diiodotyrosine. Two diiodotyrosines combine to form tetraiodothyronine (also called T_4 thyroid hormone). If a diiodotyrosine combines with a monoiodotyrosine, triiodothyronine (p. 506) (also called T_3 thyroid hormone) is formed. T_4 makes up nearly 90% of what we call thyroid hormone. T_3 makes up less than 10% of thyroid hormone. Nearly all of T_4 and T_3 is bound to protein. Thyroxine-binding globulin (TBG) binds most of T_3 and T_4. Albumin and prealbumin bind the rest. Total T4 measurement consists of both the bound and unbound fractions. Free T4 is a measure of unbound metabolically active T4. Thyroid hormones regulate a number of developmental, metabolic, and neural activities throughout the body. Thyrotropin-releasing hormone (TRH) is secreted in the hypothalamus. This stimulates the anterior pituitary to secrete thyrotropin (thyroid-stimulating hormone [TSH]). TSH stimulates the thyroid to secrete thyroid hormone. The increased levels of T_3 and T_4 inhibit further production of TRH.

Abnormalities in protein levels can have a significant effect on the results of the total T_4. Pregnancy and hormone replacement therapy increase TBG and cause T_4 to be falsely elevated, suggesting that hyperthyroidism exists when in fact the patient is euthyroid. If the free T_4 is measured in these patients, it would be normal, indicating that free T_4 is a more accurate indicator of thyroid function than total T_4. In cases in which TBG is reduced (e.g., hypoproteinemia), the total T_4 is likewise reduced, suggesting hypothyroidism. Measurement of free T_4 would indicate normal levels and thereby discount the abnormal total T_4 as merely a result of the reduced TBG and not as a result of hypothyroidism.

Free thyroxine (FT4) is measured using an automated, competitive, chemiluminescent immunoassay. Total thyroxine is measured by immunoenzymatic assay.

Clinical Priorities

- This test is used to diagnose thyroid function and monitor replacement or suppressive therapy.
- High levels of thyroid hormones indicate hyperthyroidism and low levels indicate hypothyroidism.
- Newborns are screened using total T_4 tests to detect hypothyroidism. A heel stick is used to collect the blood. Mental retardation can be prevented with early diagnosis.

INTERFERING FACTORS

- Neonates have higher free T_4 levels than older children and adults.
- Prior use of iodinated radioisotopes or iodinated contrast can alter test results.
- Pregnancy causes increased total T4 levels.
- Drugs that *increase* free T_4 levels include aspirin, danazol, heparin, and propranolol.
- Drugs that *decrease* free T_4 levels include furosemide, methadone, phenytoins, and rifampicin.
- Exogenously administered thyroxine causes *increased* free T_4 results.
- Drugs that may cause *increased* total T_4 levels include clofibrate, estrogens, heroin, methadone, and oral contraceptives.
- Drugs that may cause *decreased* T_4 levels include anabolic steroids, androgens, antithyroid drugs (e.g., propylthiouracil), lithium, phenytoin, and propranolol.

PROCEDURE AND PATIENT CARE

Before

 Explain the procedure to the patient.
Evaluate the patient's medication history.
If indicated, instruct the patient to stop exogenous T_4 medication 1 month before testing.
Tell the patient that no fasting is required.

🖎 Explain to parents that newborns should be screened before discharge (regardless of age), because of the consequences of delayed diagnosis.
- Note that the optimal collection time is 2 to 4 days after birth.

During
- Collect a venous blood specimen in a red-top tube.
- Follow the following steps for newborns:
  1. Perform a heel stick to obtain blood.
  2. Thoroughly saturate the circles on the filter paper with blood.
- Note that prompt collection and processing are crucial to the early detection of hypothyroidism.

After
- Apply pressure to the venipuncture site.

TEST RESULTS AND CLINICAL SIGNIFICANCE

▲ Increased Levels

Primary hyperthyroid states (e.g., Graves disease, Plummer disease, toxic thyroid adenoma): *The thyroid produces increased T_4 despite lack of TSH stimulation.*

Acute thyroiditis: *The thyroid secretes increased T_4 during the acute inflammatory stages of thyroiditis (e.g., Hashimoto thyroiditis). However, in the latter stages the thyroid may become burned out and the patient may develop hypothyroidism.*

Familial dysalbuminemic hyperthyroxinemia: *These patients have a genetically defective form of albumin that binds T_4 unusually tightly. As a result, the bound portion of T_4 increases. The patient is not hyperthyroid because the protein-bound T_4 is not metabolically active.*

Factitious hyperthyroidism: *Patients who self-administer T_4 will have elevated levels. Many patients believe they will feel more energetic or will lose weight faster if they take T_4.*

Struma ovarii: *Ectopic thyroid tissue in the ovary or anywhere can produce excess T_4.*

TBG increase (e.g., as occurs in pregnancy, hepatitis, congenital hyperproteinemia): *Because the T_4 assay measures total bound and unbound T_4 any condition associated with elevated TBG will cause an elevation of T_4.*

▼ Decreased Levels

Hypothyroid states (e.g., cretinism, surgical ablation, myxedema): *The thyroid in these diseases cannot produce an adequate amount of T_4 despite the stimulation provided.*

Pituitary insufficiency: *The pituitary produces an insufficient amount of thyrotropin. As a result, the thyroid is not stimulated to produce T_4.*

Hypothalamic failure: *The hypothalamus produces an insufficient amount of TRH. As a result, the pituitary does not produce thyrotropin, and the thyroid is not stimulated to produce T_4.*

Protein malnutrition and other protein-depleted states (e.g., nephrotic syndrome): *With a reduced protein source, TBG and albumin decrease. Because T_4 assay measures hormone bound to these proteins, T_4 can be expected to be reduced.*

Iodine insufficiency: *Iodine is the basic raw material for T_4. Without iodine, T_4 cannot be produced. With the introduction of iodide in most table salts, iodine insufficiency is rare in the United States.*

Nonthyroid illnesses (e.g., renal failure, Cushing disease, cirrhosis, surgery, advanced cancer): *The pathophysiology of these observations is not well known. It may be in part because of a depletion of thyroid-binding proteins associated with severe medical illnesses.*

RELATED TESTS

Thyroid-Stimulating Immunoglobulins (p. 491). This and other thyroid-stimulating immunoglobulins are used to support the diagnosis of Graves disease, especially when the diagnosis is complex.

Thyrotropin-Releasing Hormone (p. 492). This test assists in the evaluation of patients with hyperthyroidism and hypothyroidism. It is especially helpful in the differential diagnosis of hypothyroidism.

Thyroid-Stimulating Hormone (p. 486). This test is used to diagnose primary hypothyroidism and to differentiate it from secondary (pituitary) and tertiary (hypothalamus) hypothyroidism. The free thyroxine value, combined with the TSH value, gives a more accurate picture of the thyroid status in patients with abnormal thyroid-binding globulin levels.

Thyroid-Stimulating Hormone Stimulation (p. 489). This test is also used to differentiate primary and secondary (and tertiary) hypothyroidism.

Thyroxine-Binding Globulin (p. 495). This is a measure of TBG, the major thyroid hormone protein carrier. It is used in the evaluation of patients who have abnormal total T_4 and T_3 levels. When performed concurrently with a T_4/T_3 test, the T_4 and T_3 levels can be more easily interpreted.

Triiodothyronine (p. 506). T_3 is used to evaluate thyroid function. It is primarily used to diagnose hyperthyroidism. It is also used to monitor thyroid replacement and suppressive therapy.

Antithyroglobulin Antibody (p. 102). This test is primarily used in the differential diagnosis of thyroid diseases, such as Hashimoto thyroiditis and chronic lymphocytic thyroiditis (in children).

Toxoplasmosis Antibody Titer

NORMAL FINDINGS

IgG titers: <1:16 indicate no previous infection.
IgG titers: 1:16-1:256 are usually prevalent in the general population.
IgG titers: >1:256 suggest recent infection.
IgM titers: >1:256 indicate acute infection.

INDICATIONS

These serologic tests are used to diagnose acute toxoplasmosis in immunosuppressed patients, pregnant women, and newborn infants. Immunity obtained from prior infection (e.g., fetal infection) is also determined by this test.

TEST EXPLANATION

Toxoplasmosis is a protozoan disease caused by *Toxoplasma gondii,* which is found in humans and many animals (especially cats). Humans become infected by eating poorly cooked or raw meat. Exposure to feces of cats or other infected material can cause infection. Infected humans are most often asymptomatic. When symptoms occur, this disease is characterized by CNS lesions, which may lead to blindness, brain damage, and death. The condition may occur congenitally or some time after birth. Because approximately 25% to 70% of the adult population have been exposed to toxoplasmosis as determined by positive antibody titers, the Centers for Disease Control and Prevention (CDC) recommends that pregnant women be serologically tested for this disease. Again, most acutely infected pregnant women are asymptomatic, and the best way to diagnose infection is by antibody testing.

The presence of antibodies before pregnancy indicates prior exposure and chronic asymptomatic infection. The presence of these antibodies probably ensures protection against congenital toxoplasmosis in the child. Fetal infection occurs if the mother acquires toxoplasmosis after conception and passes it to the fetus through the placenta. Repeat testing of pregnant patients with low or negative titers may be done before the twentieth week and before delivery to identify antibody converters and determine appropriate therapy (e.g., therapeutic abortion at 20 weeks, treatment during the remainder of the pregnancy, or treatment of the newborn).

Hydrocephaly, microcephaly, chronic retinitis, and convulsions are complications of congenital toxoplasmosis. Congenital toxoplasmosis is diagnosed when the antibody levels are persistently elevated or a rising titer is found in the infant 2 to 3 months after birth.

The term TORCH (toxoplasmosis, other, rubella, cytomegalovirus, herpes) has been applied to maternal infections with recognized detrimental effects on the fetus. TORCH testing refers to the testing for IgG (indicating past infection) and IgM (indicating recent infection) antibodies to the particular infectious agents as described. Included in the category of *other* are infections such as syphilis. All of these tests are discussed separately:

Toxoplasmosis, p. 500
Rubella, p. 457
Cytomegalovirus, p. 200
Herpesvirus, p. 731

Because of the difficulty in growing *Toxoplasma* in culture, the best way to diagnose this disease is by serologic testing. A commonly used test is the indirect fluorescent antibody test. With this technique, immunoglobulin (Ig)M and IgG can be detected in sum or separately. IgM rises about 1 week after inoculation, peaks in about 2 to 3 months, and declines to undetectable levels in about 1 year. IgG begins to rise about 2 weeks after inoculation, peaks in about 2 to 3 months, and declines to low but persistent levels in about 6 months. Low titers of IgG especially indicate past infections and protection from passing acute infection to an unborn child. High or rapidly rising titers of either IgM or IgG indicate acute infection in the adult or newborn infant. Hemagglutination is another more easily performed method of detecting IgG antibodies to toxoplasmosis. This is often used to screen new mothers. Enzyme-linked immunosorbent assay (ELISA) and radioimmunoassay (RIA) are other techniques to identify antibodies.

Elevated IgM antibodies, IgG titers greater than 1:1000, or a fourfold rise in IgG antibodies indicates an acute *Toxoplasma* infection. Low but significant titers of IgG indicate past infection. High, nonrising titers indicate acute infection more than 3 to 12 months before testing.

INTERFERING FACTORS

- Rheumatoid factor or antinuclear antibodies can cause false-positive results.
- Other active congenital infections can cause false-positive results.

PROCEDURE AND PATIENT CARE

Before

Explain the procedure to the patient.
Tell the patient that no fasting is required.

During

- Collect a venous blood sample in a red- or green-top tube, depending on laboratory protocol.
- Indicate on the laboratory slip if the patient is pregnant or has been exposed to cats.

After

- Apply pressure or a pressure dressing to the venipuncture site.
- Assess the venipuncture site for bleeding.

TEST RESULTS AND CLINICAL SIGNIFICANCE

▲ **Increased Levels**

Toxoplasmosis

Transferrin Receptor Assay (TfR)

NORMAL FINDINGS

Men: 2-5.0 mg/L
Women: 1.9-4.4 mg/L
(Results vary depending on the testing method.)

INDICATIONS

Serum transferrin receptor (TfR) concentration is used to differentiate iron deficiency anemia from the anemia of chronic disease (ACD) or other "iron low" anemias—particularly in children.

TEST EXPLANATION

Both iron metabolism and transport are altered in chronic and critical illness. Differentiation of the ACD (also called anemia of inflammation or anemia of aging) from iron deficiency anemia may be difficult, and the results of conventional laboratory assessment of iron stores may not be definitive. The most valuable iron store marker in distinguishing these two entities is the TfR concentration.

TfR is a cell surface protein found on most cells and especially those with a high requirement for iron, such as immature erythroid and malignant cells. Its function is to internalize absorbed iron into target cells. TfR is increased when erythropoiesis is enhanced (such as often occurs in iron deficiency). The concentration of cell surface–transferrin receptor is carefully regulated by transferrin receptor mRNA, according to the internal iron content of the cell and its individual iron requirements. Iron-deficient cells contain increased numbers of receptors, while receptor numbers are downregulated in iron-replete cells.

An increased mean TfR concentration is noted in patients with iron deficiency anemia as compared with patients with anemia secondary to chronic critical illnesses. TfR is also useful in distinguishing iron deficiency anemia from situations that are commonly encountered in childhood, adolescence, and during pregnancy when iron stores are uniformly low to absent. In these situations, iron-deficient erythropoiesis is not necessarily present, and TfR levels are not elevated. Finally, in situations in which iron deficiency anemia coexists with anemia of chronic disease, transferrin receptor concentrations increase secondary to the underlying iron deficiency, thus avoiding the need for a bone marrow examination.

In general, to increase sensitivity and specificity, the measurement of serum soluble transferrin receptor should be performed in combination with other tests of iron status, including ferritin, TIBC, and serum iron (Table 2-46). Calculation of the ratio of transferrin receptor to log ferritin concentration provides an even higher sensitivity and specificity for the detection of Fe deficiency.

TABLE 2-46	Tests Used to Evaluate Iron Status			
	Tests for Changes in:	Iron Deficiency Anemia	Anemia of Chronic Disease	Iron Deficiency and Anemia of Chronic Disease
Ferritin	Iron stores	Low	High	Normal or high
TIBC	Iron status	High	Low	Normal or high
Serum Iron	Iron status	Low	Low	Low
TfR	Iron status	High	Normal	High

The principal method for measurement of soluble transferrin receptor (TfR) is immunoturbidimetry using a commercially available clinical analyzer. Latex-bound anti-TfR antibodies react with the antigen in the sample to form an antigen-antibody complex. Following agglutination, this is measured turbidimetrically.

INTERFERING FACTORS

- Individuals who live at high altitudes have a reference range that extends 6% higher than the upper level of this reference interval.
- Results are related to ethnicity. Individuals of African descent can be expected to have higher levels.
- Drugs that may cause *increased* TfR levels include recombinant human erythropoietins.

PROCEDURE AND PATIENT CARE

Before
- Explain the procedure to the patient.
- Tell the patient that no fasting is required.

During
- Collect a venous blood in a red-top or green-top tube (depending on laboratory preferences/techniques).

After
- Apply pressure to the venipuncture site.
- Assess the venipuncture site for bleeding.

TEST RESULTS AND CLINICAL SIGNIFICANCE

▲ Increased Plasma TfR

Iron deficiency anemia: *TfR receptors are affected by intracellular stores of iron. Low intracellular iron will instigate (through mRNA stimulus) TfR proliferation.*

▼ Decreased Plasma TfR

Hemochromatosis: *Elevated iron stores will diminish TfR.*

RELATED TESTS

Ferritin (p. 234). This is the most sensitive test to determine iron-deficiency anemia.
Serum Iron and Total Iron-Binding Capacity (p. 322). These tests of iron status and storage are critical in the diagnosis of iron deficiency anemia.

Blood Studies

2

Triglycerides (TGs)

NORMAL FINDINGS

Adult/elderly
    Male: 40-160 mg/dL or 0.45-1.81 mmol/L (SI units)
    Female: 35-135 mg/dL or 0.40-1.52 mmol/L (SI units)

Children (yr)	Male (mg/dL)	Female (mg/dL)
0-5	30-86	32-99
6-11	31-108	35-114
12-15	36-138	41-138
16-19	40-163	40-128

 Critical Values

>400 mg/dL

INDICATIONS

TGs identify the risk of developing coronary heart disease (CHD). This test is part of a lipid profile that includes the measurement of cholesterol and lipoproteins. This test is also performed on patients with suspected fat metabolism disorders.

TEST EXPLANATION

TGs are a form of fat in the bloodstream. They are transported by very-low-density lipoproteins (VLDLs) and low-density lipoproteins (LDLs). TGs are produced in the liver using glycerol and other fatty acids as building blocks. TGs act as a storage source for energy. When TG levels in the blood are high, TGs are deposited in the fatty tissues. TGs constitute most of the fat in the body and are a part of a lipid profile that also evaluates cholesterol and lipoprotein. A lipid profile is performed to assess the risk of coronary and vascular disease.

INTERFERING FACTORS

- Ingestion of fatty meals may cause elevated TG levels.
- Ingestion of alcohol may cause elevated levels of TG by increasing the production of VLDL.
- Pregnancy may cause increased levels.
- Drugs that may cause *increased* TG levels include cholestyramine, estrogens, and oral contraceptives.
- Drugs that may cause *decreased* levels include ascorbic acid, asparaginase, clofibrate, colestipol, fibrates, and statins.

PROCEDURE AND PATIENT CARE

Before

- Explain the procedure to the patient.
- Instruct the patient to fast for 12 to 14 hours before the test. Only water is permitted.

Tell the patient not to drink alcohol for 24 hours before the test.
Inform the patient that dietary indiscretion for as much as 2 weeks before this test will influence results.

During

- Collect a venous blood sample in a red-top tube.

After

- Apply pressure or a pressure dressing to the venipuncture site.
- Assess the venipuncture site for bleeding.
- Mark the patient's age and gender on the laboratory slip.
- Instruct patients with increased TG levels regarding diet, exercise, and appropriate weight.

TEST RESULTS AND CLINICAL SIGNIFICANCE

▲ Increased Levels

Glycogen storage disease (von Gierke disease): *VLDL (TG-carrying proteins) synthesis is increased, whereas catabolism is decreased. TG levels in the blood increase.*

Familial hypertriglyceridemia: *This is a genetic predisposition to elevated TGs.*

Apoprotein C-II deficiency: *This congenital disease is associated with lipoprotein lipase deficiency. TGs accumulate.*

Hyperlipidemias: *As lipids in the blood increase, so does TG, the major blood lipid.*

Hypothyroidism: *Catabolism of TG is diminished.*

High-carbohydrate diet: *Excess carbohydrates are converted into TG and blood levels of TG rise.*

Poorly controlled diabetes: *Diabetics have an increased synthesis of TG-carrying VLDL and a decreased catabolism of the same. Therefore TG blood levels increase.*

Nephrotic syndrome: *The loss of proteins diminishes the plasma oncotic pressures. This appears to stimulate hepatic lipoprotein synthesis of VLDL and LDL. Also, lipoprotein disposal is possibly diminished.*

Chronic renal failure: *Insulin levels are high in these patients, because insulin is excreted by the kidney. Insulin increases lipogenesis and causes TG levels to increase. Also, these patients have a deficiency in lipoprotein lipase that clears the blood of TG.*

▼ Decreased Levels

Malabsorption syndrome: *These patients have a malabsorption of fat from the diet. As TG is the major component of dietary fat, TG levels can be expected to fall in light of poor gastrointestinal (GI) absorption.*

Abetalipoproteinemia: *Not only do these patients have a malabsorption of fat, but they also have a defective synthesis of apoprotein B (TG-carrying lipoproteins). TG blood levels are low.*

Malnutrition: *These patients have diminished fat in the diet. As TG is the major component of dietary fat, TG levels can be expected to fall.*

Hyperthyroidism: *The catabolism of VLDL, the main TG-carrying lipoprotein, is increased. Therefore, TG blood levels diminish.*

RELATED TESTS

Cholesterol (p. 154). This is a measure of total cholesterol in the blood. It is a part of the lipid profile.

Lipoprotein (HDL, VLDL, and LDL) (p. 342). These proteins play an important role in the transport of lipids in the bloodstream. They, too, have been used in the assessment of risk for coronary heart disease.

Triiodothyronine (Total T_3 Radioimmunoassay [T_3 by RIA], Free T_3)

NORMAL FINDINGS

1-3 days	100-740 ng/dL
1-11 months	105-245 ng/dL
1-5 years	105-270 ng/dL
6-10 years	95-240 ng/dL
11-15 years	80-215 ng/dL
16-20 years	80-210 ng/dL
20-50 years	70-205 ng/dL or 1.2-3.4 nmol/L (SI units)
>50 years	40-180 ng/dL or 0.6-2.8 nmol/L (SI units)

INDICATIONS

T_3 is used to evaluate thyroid function. It is used primarily to diagnose hyperthyroidism. It is also used to monitor thyroid replacement and suppressive therapy.

TEST EXPLANATION

Thyroid hormones are produced when tyrosine incorporates organic iodine to form a monoiodotyrosine. This complex picks up another iodine and becomes diiodotyrosine. Two diiodotyrosines combine to form tetraiodothyronine (also called T_4 thyroid hormone). If a diiodotyrosine combines with a monoiodotyrosine, triiodothyronine (also called T_3 thyroid hormone) is formed. A large proportion of T_3 is formed in the liver by conversion of T_4 to T_3. As with the T_4 test, the serum T_3 test is an accurate indicator of thyroid function. T_3 is less stable than T_4 because it is much less tightly bound to serum proteins than T_4. Only about 7% to 10% of thyroid hormone is composed of T_3. And 70% of that T_3 is bound to proteins (thyroxine-binding globulin [TBG] and albumin). Only minute quantities are unbound or "free." It is the *free T3* that is metabolically active. Furthermore, measurement of free T_3 is not subject to the effects that alterations of serum proteins have on the total T_3, which is described in this test. This test measures the total bound and unbound (free) T_3. Generally, when the T_3 level is below normal, the patient is in a hypothyroid state.

Other severe non-thyroid diseases can decrease T_3 levels by diminishing the conversion of T_4 to T_3 in the liver. This makes T_3 levels less useful in indicating hypothyroid states. Furthermore, there is considerable overlap between hypothyroid states and normal thyroid function. Because of this, T_3 levels are used primarily to assist in the diagnosis of hyperthyroid states. An elevated T_3 indicates hyperthyroidism, especially when T_4 is also elevated. In a rare form of hyperthyroidism called "T_3 toxicosis," T_4 is normal and T_3 is elevated.

In the hypothalamus, thyrotropin-releasing hormone (TRH) is secreted. This stimulates the anterior pituitary to secrete thyrotropin (thyroid-stimulating hormone [TSH]). TSH stimulates the thyroid to secrete thyroid hormone. The increased levels of T_3 and T_4 inhibit further production of TRH.

This test is performed by direct dialysis extraction of both bound T_3 and free T_3 and is measured by RIA. This test is not the same as the T_3 uptake test and should not be confused with it.

INTERFERING FACTORS

- Radioisotope administration before the test may alter the results, if this test is performed by RIA methods.

- Total T_3 values are increased in pregnancy, because serum proteins are increased at that time. Free T_3, however, is not affected by protein levels.
- Drugs that may cause *increased* levels include estrogen, methadone, and oral contraceptives.
- Drugs that may cause *decreased* levels include anabolic steroids, androgens, phenytoin (Dilantin), propranolol (Inderal), reserpine, and salicylates (high dose).

Clinical Priorities

- The T_3 test is used primarily to diagnose hyperthyroidism.
- T_3 is less useful in the diagnosis of hypothyroidism because other nonthyroid diseases can decrease T_3 levels by decreasing the conversion of T_4 to T_3 in the liver.
- This test is not the same as the T_3 resin uptake test, which is rarely done today.

PROCEDURE AND PATIENT CARE

Before
- Explain the procedure to the patient.
- Determine whether the patient is taking any exogenous T_3 medication, because this will affect test results.
- Withhold drugs that may affect results (with physician's approval).
- Tell the patient that no fasting is required.

During
- Collect a venous blood sample in a red-top tube.

After
- Apply pressure or a pressure dressing to the venipuncture site.
- Observe the venipuncture site for bleeding.

TEST RESULTS AND CLINICAL SIGNIFICANCE

▲ Increased Levels

Primary hyperthyroid states (e.g., Graves disease, Plummer disease, toxic thyroid adenoma): *The thyroid produces increased T_3 despite lack of TSH stimulation.*

Acute thyroiditis: *The thyroid secretes increased T_3 during the acute inflammatory stages of thyroiditis (e.g., Hashimoto thyroiditis). However, in the latter stages the thyroid may become burned out and the patient may develop hypothyroidism.*

Factitious hyperthyroidism: *Patients who self-administer T_3 will have elevated levels. Many patients believe they will feel more energetic or will lose weight faster if they take T_3.*

Struma ovarii: *Ectopic thyroid tissue in the ovary or anywhere can produce excess T_3.*

TBG increase (e.g., as occurs in pregnancy, hepatitis, congenital hyperproteinemia): *Because T_3 assay measures total bound and unbound T_3, any condition associated with elevated TBG will cause elevation of T_3. Free T_3 will not be elevated, however.*

▼ Decreased Levels

Hypothyroid states (e.g., cretinism, surgical ablation, myxedema): *The thyroid in these diseases cannot produce an adequate amount of T_3 despite the stimulation provided.*

Pituitary insufficiency: *The pituitary produces an insufficient amount of thyrotropin. As a result, the thyroid is not stimulated to produce T_3.*

Hypothalamic failure: *The hypothalamus produces an insufficient amount of TRH. As a result, the pituitary does not produce thyrotropin, and the thyroid is not stimulated to produce T_3.*

Protein malnutrition and other protein-depleted states (e.g., nephrotic syndrome): *With a reduced protein source, TBG and albumin decrease. Because the T_3 assay measures hormones bound to these proteins, T_3 can be expected to be reduced. Free T_3 levels will be unaffected by serum protein changes.*

Iodine insufficiency: *Iodine is the basic raw material for T_3. Without iodine, T_4 cannot be produced. With the introduction of iodide in most table salts, iodine insufficiency has become rare in the United States.*

Nonthyroid illnesses (e.g., renal failure, Cushing disease, cirrhosis, surgery, advanced cancer): *The pathophysiology of these observations is not well known. It may be, in part, because of a depletion of thyroxine-binding proteins, which is associated with severe medical illnesses. T_3 is more significantly affected by these diseases than is T_4.*

Hepatic diseases: *Because a large proportion of T_3 is made by conversion of T_4 in the liver, severe liver dysfunction may affect T_3 levels. Often, however, other peripheral tissues take over T_3 synthesis by T_4 conversion.*

RELATED TESTS

Long-Acting Thyroid Stimulator (LATS) (p. 491). This and other thyroid-stimulating immunoglobulins are used to support the diagnosis of Graves disease, especially when the diagnosis is complex.

Thyrotropin-Releasing Hormone Stimulation Test (p. 492). This test assists in the evaluation of patients with hyperthyroidism and hypothyroidism. It is especially helpful in the differential diagnosis of hypothyroidism.

Thyroid-Stimulating Hormone (p. 486). This test is used to diagnose primary hypothyroidism and to differentiate it from secondary (pituitary) and tertiary (hypothalamus) hypothyroidism.

Thyroid-Stimulating Hormone (TSH) Stimulation (p. 489). This test is also used to differentiate primary and secondary (and tertiary) hypothyroidism.

Thyroxine-Binding Globulin (p. 495). This is a measure of TBG, the major thyroid hormone protein carrier. It is used in the evaluation of patients who have abnormal total T_4 and T_3 levels. When performed concurrently with a T_4/T_3 test, the T_4 and T_3 levels can be more easily interpreted.

Thyroxine, Total (p. 497). This is one of the first tests done for assessing thyroid function. It is used to diagnose thyroid function and to monitor replacement and suppressive therapy.

Thyroxine, Free (p. 497). The FT_4 is used to evaluate thyroid function in patients who may have protein abnormalities that could affect total T_4 levels. It is used to diagnose thyroid function and to monitor replacement and suppressive therapy.

Antithyroglobulin Antibody (p. 102). This test is primarily used for the differential diagnosis of thyroid diseases, such as Hashimoto thyroiditis and chronic lymphocytic thyroiditis (in children).

Troponins (Cardiac-Specific Troponin T [cTnT], Cardiac-Specific Troponin I [cTnI])

NORMAL FINDINGS

Cardiac troponin T: <0.1 ng/mL
Cardiac troponin I: <0.03 ng/mL

INDICATIONS

This test is performed on patients with chest pain to determine if the pain is caused by cardiac ischemia. It is a specific indicator of cardiac muscle injury. It is also helpful in predicting the possibility of future cardiac events.

TEST EXPLANATION

Cardiac troponins are biochemical markers for cardiac disease. This test is used to assist in the evaluation of patients with suspected acute coronary ischemic syndromes. In addition to improving the diagnosis of acute ischemic disorders, troponins are also valuable for early risk stratification in patients with unstable angina. They can be used to predict the likelihood of future cardiac events.

Troponins are proteins that exist in skeletal and cardiac muscle that regulate the calcium-dependent interaction of myosin with actin for the muscle contractile apparatus. Cardiac troponins can be separated from skeletal troponins by the use of monoclonal antibodies or enzyme-linked immunosorbent assay (ELISA). There are two cardiac-specific troponins: cardiac troponin T (cTnT), and cardiac troponin I (cTnI).

Because of their extraordinarily high specificity for myocardial cell injury, cardiac troponins are very helpful in the evaluation of patients with chest pain. Their use is similar to that of creatine phosphokinase MB (CPK-MB) (see p. 186). However, there are several advantages that cardiac troponins have over CPK-MB. Cardiac troponins are more specific for cardiac muscle injury. CPK-MB can be elevated with severe skeletal muscle injury, with brain or lung injury, or in renal failure. Cardiac troponins will nearly always be normal in noncardiac muscle diseases. Cardiac troponins become elevated sooner and remain elevated longer than CPK-MB. This expands the time window of opportunity for diagnosis and thrombolytic treatment of myocardial injury. Finally, cTnT and cTnI are more sensitive to muscle injury than CPK-MB. That is most important in evaluating patients with chest pain.

Cardiac troponins become elevated as early as 2-3 hours after myocardial injury. Typically 2-3 sets of troponins over the course of a day are required to indicate myocardial infarction. Levels of cTnI may remain elevated for 7 to 10 days after myocardial infarction, and cTnT levels may remain elevated for up to 10 to 14 days. Measurement of these troponins is preferable to measurement of LDH (see p. 329) and its isoenzymes in patients who seek medical attention more than 24 to 48 hours after the onset of symptoms. However, if reinfarction is considered, troponins are not helpful because they could be elevated just from the first ischemic event. Each cardiac monitor has its specific use depending on the time from onset of chest pain to the time of presentation to the hospital.

Troponins can be detected by monoclonal antibody immunoassay; by ELISA; and most recently, by monoclonal "sandwich" antibody qualitative testing. The test results using the first two laboratory techniques listed are available after about 2 hours. The "sandwich" technique is performed at the bedside in about 20 minutes and is read visually much like a glucometer. This fast turnaround time for this blood test is extremely useful. The earlier myocardial injury is detected, the more rapidly treatment directed toward revascularization can begin. The earlier revascularization occurs, the less myocardial muscle is injured.

Cardiac troponins are used in the following cardiac clinical situations:

1. Evaluation of patient with unstable angina. These patients can be separated into two groups based on cardiac troponins. If cardiac troponin levels are normal, no myocardial injury has occurred, and there will be no lasting cardiac dysfunction. If cardiac troponin levels are elevated, muscle injury has occurred. Thrombolytic therapy may be indicated because this latter group is at great risk for a subsequent cardiac event (infarction or sudden death).

2. Detection of reperfusion associated with coronary recanalization. A "washout" or second peak of cardiac troponin levels accurately indicates reperfusion by way of recanalization or coronary angioplasty.

3. Estimation of MI size. Late (4 weeks) cardiac troponin levels are inversely related to left ventricular ejection fraction. These late elevations in cardiac troponins are related to degradation of the contractile apparatus.
4. Detection of perioperative MI. The use of CPK-MB determinations in the diagnosis of MI after surgery is difficult because of the frequent increase of this enzyme associated with skeletal muscle injury during surgery. Cardiac troponins are not affected by skeletal muscle injury.
5. Evaluation of the severity of pulmonary emboli. Elevated levels may indicate more severe disease and the need for thrombolytic therapy.
6. Congestive heart failure—persistently elevated tropinins indicate continued ventricular strain.

Elevations of troponin T do not in and of themselves indicate the presence of an ischemic mechanism. Many other disease states are associated with elevations of troponin T via mechanisms different from those that cause injury in patients with acute coronary syndromes. These include cardiac trauma (e.g., contusion ablation or pacing), congestive heart failure, hypertension, hypotension (often with arrhythmias), pulmonary embolism, renal failure, and myocarditis.

INTERFERING FACTORS

• Troponin T levels are falsely *elevated* in patients on dialysis.

PROCEDURE AND PATIENT CARE

Before

☒ Explain the procedure to the patient.
☒ Discuss with the patient the need and reason for frequent venipuncture in diagnosing MI.
☒ Tell the patient that no food or fluid restrictions are necessary.

During

• Collect a venous blood sample in a yellow-top (serum separator) tube. This is usually done initially and 12 hours later followed by daily testing for 3 to 5 days and possibly weekly for 5 to 6 weeks.
• Rotate the venipuncture sites.
• Record the exact time and date of venipuncture on each laboratory slip. This aids in the interpretation of the temporal pattern of enzyme elevations.
• If a qualitative immunoassay is to be done at the bedside, whole blood is obtained in a micropipette and placed in the sample well of the testing device. A red or purple color in the "read" zone indicates that 0.2 ng/mL or more cardiac troponin is present in the patient's blood.

After

• Apply pressure or a pressure dressing to the venipuncture site.
• Observe the venipuncture site for bleeding.

TEST RESULTS AND CLINICAL SIGNIFICANCE

▲ Increased Levels

Myocardial injury,
Myocardial infarction:
  This myocardial intracellular protein becomes available to the bloodstream after myocardial cell death because of ischemia. Blood levels therefore rise. Normally, no troponins can be detected in the blood.

RELATED TESTS

Creatine Phosphokinase MB (p. 186). Elevation of CPK-MB on this blood test is closely linked to myocardial muscle. It is elevated early in myocardial injury. Its usefulness is limited in patients who have had chest pain for more than 24 hours.

Myoglobin (p. 365). This protein is a nonspecific indicator of cardiac disease. However, it is also elevated with skeletal muscle disease or trauma.

Electrocardiography (p. 544). This is the electrodiagnostic test most commonly used to detect myocardial injury and infarction.

Urea Nitrogen, Blood (Blood Urea Nitrogen [BUN], Serum Urea Nitrogen)

NORMAL FINDINGS

Adult: 10-20 mg/dL or 3.6-7.1 mmol/L (SI units)
Elderly: may be slightly higher than adult
Child: 5-18 mg/dL
Infant: 5-18 mg/dL
Newborn: 3-12 mg/dL
Cord: 21-40 mg/dL

 Critical Values

>100 mg/dL (indicates serious impairment of renal function)

INDICATIONS

BUN is an indirect and rough measurement of renal function and glomerular filtration rate (if normal liver function exists). It is also a measurement of liver function. It is performed on patients undergoing routine laboratory testing. It is usually performed as a part of a multiphasic automated testing process.

TEST EXPLANATION

The BUN measures the amount of urea nitrogen in the blood. Urea is formed in the liver as the end product of protein metabolism and digestion. During ingestion, protein is broken down into amino acids. In the liver these amino acids are catabolized and free ammonia is formed. The ammonia molecules are combined to form urea, which is then deposited in the blood and transported to the kidneys for excretion. Therefore the BUN is directly related to the metabolic function of the liver and the excretory function of the kidney. It serves as an index of the function of these organs. Patients who have elevated BUN levels are said to have azotemia or be azotemic.

Nearly all renal diseases cause an inadequate excretion of urea, which causes the blood concentration to rise above normal. If the disease is unilateral, however, the unaffected kidney can compensate for the diseased kidney and the BUN may not become elevated. The BUN also increases in conditions other than primary renal disease. Prerenal azotemia refers to elevation of the BUN as a result of pathologic conditions that affect urea nitrogen accumulation before it gets to the kidney. Examples of prerenal azotemia include shock, dehydration, congestive heart failure, and excessive protein catabolism.

Another example of prerenal azotemia is gastrointestinal bleeding that causes variable and sometimes significant blood in the intestinal tract. The proteins in the blood and blood cells are digested to urea. As the marked increase in intestinal urea is absorbed, the BUN can be expected to increase, sometimes significantly. Postrenal azotemia refers to pathologic conditions that affect urea nitrogen accumulation after it gets to the kidney. Examples of this include ureteral and urethral obstruction.

Finally, the synthesis of urea depends on the liver. Patients with severe primary liver disease will have a decreased BUN. With combined liver and renal disease (as in hepatorenal syndrome), the BUN can be normal because poor hepatic functioning results in decreased formation of urea and is not an indicator that renal excretory function is adequate.

The BUN is interpreted in conjunction with the creatinine test. These tests are referred to as "renal function studies." The BUN/creatinine ratio is a good measurement of kidney and liver function. The normal adult range is 6 to 25, with 15.5 being the optimal value.

INTERFERING FACTORS

- Changes in protein intake may affect BUN levels. Low-protein diets will decrease BUN if caloric intake is maintained with carbohydrates. High-protein diets or alimentary tube feeding is associated with elevated BUN levels.
- To some degree, muscle mass determines BUN levels. Women and children tend to have lower BUN levels than men.
- Advanced pregnancy may cause increased levels as a result of high protein metabolism.
- Gastrointestinal bleeding can cause increased BUN levels.
- Overhydration and underhydration will affect levels. Overhydrated patients tend to dilute the BUN and have lower levels. Dehydrated patients tend to concentrate BUN and have higher levels.
- Drugs that may cause *increased* BUN levels include allopurinol, aminoglycosides, cephalosporins, chloral hydrate, cisplatin, furosemide, guanethidine, indomethacin, methotrexate, methyldopa, nephrotoxic drugs (e.g., aspirin, amphotericin B, bacitracin, carbamazepine, colistin, gentamicin, methicillin, neomycin, penicillamine, polymyxin B, probenecid, vancomycin), propranolol, rifampin, spironolactone, tetracyclines, thiazide diuretics, and triamterene.
- Drugs that may cause *decreased* levels include chloramphenicol and streptomycin.

✔ Clinical Priorities

- Almost all renal diseases cause an inadequate excretion of urea, which causes the BUN to rise. Since the synthesis of urea depends on the liver, severe liver disease can cause a decreased BUN. Therefore the BUN is directly related to the metabolic function of the liver and the excretory function of the kidney.
- Changes in protein intake can affect BUN levels. Low-protein diets can decrease the BUN and high-protein diets can increase BUN levels.
- Hydration status can also affect levels. Overhydration will dilute the BUN and cause lower levels. Dehydration tends to concentrate the BUN and cause higher levels.

PROCEDURE AND PATIENT CARE

Before
- Explain the procedure to the patient.
- Tell the patient that no fasting is required.

During
- Collect a venous blood sample in a red-top tube.
- Avoid hemolysis.

After
- Apply pressure or a pressure dressing to the venipuncture site.
- Observe the venipuncture site for bleeding.

TEST RESULTS AND CLINICAL SIGNIFICANCE

▲ Increased Levels

Prerenal Causes
Hypovolemia,

Shock,

Burns,

Dehydration:
> With reduced blood volume, renal blood flow is diminished. Therefore renal excretion of BUN is decreased and BUN levels rise.

Congestive heart failure,

Myocardial infarction:
> With reduced cardiac function, renal blood flow is diminished. Therefore renal excretion of BUN is decreased and BUN levels rise.

GI bleeding,

Excessive protein ingestion (alimentary tube feeding):
> Blood or feeding supplements overload the gut with protein. Urea is formed at a higher rate and BUN accumulates.

Excessive protein catabolism,

Starvation:
> As protein is broken down to amino acids at an accelerated rate, urea is formed at a higher rate and BUN accumulates.

Sepsis: *For a host of reasons, renal blood flow and primary renal function are reduced. BUN levels rise.*

Renal Causes
Renal disease (e.g., glomerulonephritis, pyelonephritis, acute tubular necrosis),

Renal failure,

Nephrotoxic drugs:
> Primary renal diseases are all associated with reduced excretion of BUN.

Postrenal Azotemia
Ureteral obstruction from stones, tumor, or congenital anomalies,

Bladder outlet obstruction from prostatic hypertrophy or cancer or bladder/urethral congenital anomalies:
> Obstruction of the flow of urine causes reduced excretion and BUN levels rise.

▼ Decreased Levels

Liver failure: *BUN is made in the liver from urea. Reduced liver function is associated with reduced BUN levels.*

Overhydration because of fluid overload syndrome of inappropriate antidiuretic hormone secretion (SIADH): *BUN is diluted by fluid overload.*

Negative nitrogen balance (e.g., malnutrition, malabsorption): *With protein depletion, urea production is reduced and therefore BUN is reduced.*

Pregnancy: *Early pregnancy is associated with increased water retention and BUN dilution.*

Nephrotic syndrome: *This syndrome is associated with protein loss in the urine. With protein depletion, BUN is reduced.*

RELATED TESTS

Creatinine, Blood (p. 190). This is a more accurate test of renal function that is not dependent on liver function.

Creatinine Clearance (p. 193). Like creatinine, this is a more accurate test of renal function.

Uric Acid, Blood

NORMAL FINDINGS

Adult
  Male: 4.0-8.5 mg/dL or 0.24-0.51 mmol/L
  Female: 2.7-7.3 mg/dL or 0.16-0.43 mmol/L
Elderly: Values may be slightly increased
Child: 2.5-5.5 mg/dL or 0.12-0.32 mmol/L
Newborn: 2.0-6.2 mg/dL
Physiologic saturation threshold: >6 mg/dL or >0.357 mmol/L
Therapeutic target for gout: <6 mg/dL or <0.357 mmol/L

 Critical Values

>12 mg/dL

TEST EXPLANATION

Uric acid is a nitrogenous compound that is a product of purine (a deoxyribonucleic acid [DNA] building block) catabolism. Uric acid is excreted to a large degree by the kidney and to a smaller degree by the intestinal tract. When uric acid levels are elevated (hyperuricemia), the patient may have gout. Gout is a common metabolic disorder characterized by chronic hyperuricemia, defined as serum urate greater than 6.8 mg/dL (>0.360 mmol/L). At this level, uric acid concentrations exceed the physiologic saturation threshold and monosodium urate crystals may be deposited in the joints and soft tissues. Gout may be managed through urate-lowering therapy with the goal of treatment being uric acid less than 6 mg/dL or less than 0.357 mmol/L.

Causes of hyperuricemia can be overproduction or decreased excretion of uric acid (e.g., kidney failure). Overproduction of uric acid may occur in patients with a catabolic enzyme deficiency that stimulates purine metabolism or in patients with cancer in whom purine and DNA turnover is great. Other causes of hyperuricemia may include alcoholism, leukemia, metastatic cancer, multiple myeloma, hyperlipoproteinemia, diabetes mellitus, renal failure, stress, lead poisoning, and dehydration caused by diuretic therapy. Ketoacids (as occur in diabetic or alcoholic ketoacidosis) may compete with uric acid for tubular excretion and may cause decreased uric acid excretion. Many causes of hyperuricemia are undefined and therefore labeled as *idiopathic*.

INTERFERING FACTORS

- Stress may cause increased uric acid levels.
- X-ray contrast agents increase uric acid excretion and may cause decreased levels.
- High-protein infusion (especially glycine), as in total parental nutrition, may cause increased uric acid, which is a breakdown product of glycine.
- ⚖ Drugs that may cause *increased* levels include alcohol, ascorbic acid, aspirin (low dose), caffeine, cisplatin, diazoxide, epinephrine, ethambutol, levodopa, methyldopa (Aldomet), nicotinic acid, phenothiazines, and theophylline.
- ⚖ Drugs that may cause *decreased* levels include allopurinol, aspirin (high dose), azathioprine (Imuran), clofibrate, corticosteroids, diuretics, estrogens, glucose infusions, guaifenesin, mannitol, probenecid, and warfarin.

PROCEDURE AND PATIENT CARE

Before

- ✍ Explain the procedure to the patient.
- Follow the institution's requirements regarding fasting. (Some recommend that the patient fast.)

During

- Collect a venous blood sample in a red-top tube.

After

- Apply pressure or a pressure dressing to the venipuncture site.
- Assess the venipuncture site for bleeding.

TEST RESULTS AND CLINICAL SIGNIFICANCE

▲ Increased Levels (Hyperuricemia)

Increased Production of Uric Acid

Increased ingestion of purines: *Nucleic acid content is high in such foods as liver, sweetbreads, kidney, and anchovies.*

Genetic inborn error in purine metabolism: *The most common is an X-linked disorder that causes an increase in an enzyme that produces increased synthesis of purines and therefore an increased amount of purine breakdown products, including uric acid. A second type of genetic error is a deficiency of an enzyme that produces ribonucleic acid (RNA) and DNA from building blocks of those substances. With a deficiency of these enzymes, these building blocks accumulate and are broken down to uric acid, which is then present in high levels in the blood.*

Metastatic cancer,

Multiple myeloma,

Leukemia,

Lymphoma,

Cancer chemotherapy:

Rapid cell destruction associated with rapidly growing cancers (with high cell turnover) and especially after chemotherapy for rapidly growing tumors causes the cells to lyse and spill their nucleic acids into the bloodstream. These free nucleic acids are converted to uric acid in the liver. Levels of uric acid increase.

Hemolysis: *The nucleic acid in the RBC and adenosine triphosphate (ATP) in the RBC are spilled into the bloodstream when hemolysis occurs. These free nucleic acids are converted to uric acid in the liver. Levels of uric acid increase.*

Rhabdomyolysis (e.g., heavy exercise, burns, crush injury, epileptic seizure, myocardial infarction): *Muscle cell lysis leads to excessive muscle ATP (uric acid is a breakdown product of adenosine) in the blood. Uric acid levels increase.*

Decreased Excretion of Uric Acid

Idiopathic: *This is the most common cause of hyperuricemia. For unknown reasons, these patients have reduced uric acid clearance in the kidney. As a result, uric acid accumulates in the blood. Patients with gout excrete less than half the uric acid in their urine as normal persons.*

Chronic renal disease: *The pathophysiology regarding why these individuals cannot excrete uric acid in appropriate quantities is not known for sure. It may be because of decreased glomerular filtration only, but other mechanisms seem to be at work here.*

Acidosis (ketotic [diabetic or starvation] or lactic): *Decreased renal tubular secretion of uric acid in the urine causes reduced excretion of uric acid. Furthermore, ketoacids (as occur in diabetic or alcoholic ketoacidosis) may compete with uric acid for tubular excretion and may cause decreased uric acid excretion. Uric acid levels increase in the blood.*

Hypothyroidism,

Toxemia of pregnancy,

Hyperlipoproteinemia: *The pathophysiology of these observations is not well defined.*

Alcoholism: *Alcohol consumption causes accelerated breakdown of ATP in the liver, which increases uric acid production. The chronic acidosis from excessive alcohol ingestion decreases renal tubular secretion of uric acid into the urine. Both lead to hyperuricemia.*

Shock or chronic blood volume depletion states: *The increased tubular reabsorption of water and electrolytes causes increased tubular reabsorption of uric acid.*

▼ Decreased Levels

Wilson disease,

Fanconi syndrome,

Lead poisoning: *Wilson disease and accompanying Fanconi syndrome are associated with increased uric acid renal excretion. Heavy metal poisoning is also associated with this observation.*

Yellow atrophy of liver: *With severe liver dysfunction, uric acid will not be made and levels in the blood will be low.*

RELATED TEST

Uric Acid, Urine (p. 954). This test is used to evaluate uric acid levels in the urine and is used in the evaluation of patients with nephrolithiasis.

Uroporphyrinogen-1-Synthase

NORMAL FINDINGS

1.27-2.00 mU/g of hemoglobin or 81.9-129.6 units/mol Hgb (SI units)

BOX 2-20	Drugs That Precipitate Acute Porphyrias

- Barbiturates
- Sulfonamides
- Succinimides
- Carbamazepine
- Methyprylon
- Phenytoins
- Ergots
- Estrogens/progestins
- Valproic acid
- Griseofulvin
- Methyldopa
- Theophylline
- Danazol
- Alcohol
- Chlordiazepoxide
- Phenylbutazone
- Amphetamines
- Meprobamate
- Glutethimide
- Arsenic

INDICATIONS

This test is used to identify persons at risk for porphyria. It is also used to diagnose porphyria in the acute and latent stages.

TEST EXPLANATION

Porphyria is a group of genetic disorders characterized by an accumulation of porphyrin products in the liver or RBC. Liver porphyrias are much more common. Symptoms of liver porphyrias include abdominal pain, neuromuscular signs and symptoms, constipation, and occasionally psychotic behavior. This group of disorders results from enzymatic deficiencies in the synthesis of heme (a portion of hemoglobin). Acute intermittent porphyria (AIP) is the most common form of liver porphyria; this is caused by a deficiency in uroporphyrinogen-1-synthase (also called porphobilinogen deaminase). This enzyme is necessary for erythroid cells to make heme.

Most patients with AIP have no symptoms (latent phase) until the acute phase is precipitated by surgery, infection, a low-calorie diet, or certain drugs (Box 2-20). The acute phase is highlighted by symptoms of abdominal and muscular pain, nausea, vomiting, hypertension, mental symptoms (anxiety, insomnia, hallucinations, paranoia), sensory loss, and urinary retention. Hemolytic anemia also may occur with these acute attacks. These acute symptoms are associated with increased serum and urine levels of porphyrin precursors (see urine tests for aminolevulinic acid, porphyrins, and porphobilinogens).

This enzyme is significantly reduced during the acute and latent phases of this disorder. It is important to identify this disease process, because acute bouts of porphyria occasionally may be fatal. The acute phase can be avoided by controlling factors that can precipitate the acute symptoms.

PROCEDURE AND PATIENT CARE

Before
☒ Explain the procedure to the patient.
☒ Tell the patient that no fasting is required.

During
- Collect a peripheral venous blood sample in a lavender-top tube.
- Because this test is based on the hemoglobin measurement, measure the patient's hemoglobin level at the same time.

After
- Blood samples should be stored frozen during laboratory transfer to avoid a false decrease in enzyme level.

- Indicate on the laboratory slip if the patient is having symptoms of acute porphyria.
- Apply pressure or a pressure dressing to the venipuncture site.
- Assess the venipuncture site for bleeding.

TEST RESULTS AND CLINICAL SIGNIFICANCE

▼ Decreased Levels

Acute intermittent porphyria

RELATED TESTS

Delta-Aminolevulinic Acid, Urine (p. 922). This test is used to diagnose porphyria. It is also used in the evaluation of children with subclinical lead poisoning.

Porphyrins and Porphobilinogens, Urine (p. 940). This is a quantitative measurement of porphyrins and porphobilinogen in the urine. This test helps define the porphyrin pattern that can classify the type of porphyria.

Vitamin B$_{12}$ and Methylmalonic Acid (MMA)

NORMAL FINDINGS

Vitamin B$_{12}$: 160-950 pg/mL or 118-701 pmol/L (SI units)
MMA: <3.6 μmol/mmol creatinine

INDICATIONS

This test measures the amount of vitamin B$_{12}$ (Cyanocobalamin) in the blood. It is used to identify the cause of megaloblastic anemia and to evaluate malnourished patients.

TEST EXPLANATION

Vitamin B$_{12}$ is necessary for conversion of the inactive form of folate to the active form. This reaction is vital for the synthesis of nucleic acids and amino acids. This is most notable in the formation and function of red blood cells (RBCs). Vitamin B$_{12}$ deficiency, like folic acid deficiency, causes anemia. The RBCs formed in light of these deficiencies become large megaloblastic RBCs. These RBCs cannot conform to the size of small capillaries. Instead they fracture and hemolyze. The shortened life span ultimately leads to anemia. RBCs are not the only blood cells affected. Other marrow cells are also affected—causing, for example, giant segmented neutrophils and large nucleated platelets. It may take 6 to 18 months of vitamin B$_{12}$ depletion before anemia develops.

Meats, eggs, and dairy products are the main source of vitamin B$_{12}$. In the stomach, gastric acid detaches vitamin B$_{12}$ from its binding proteins. Intrinsic factor (IF), necessary for vitamin B$_{12}$ absorption in the small intestine, is made in the stomach mucosa. Without IF, vitamin B$_{12}$ cannot be absorbed. Deficiency of IF is the most common cause of vitamin B$_{12}$ deficiency (pernicious anemia [PA]). The next most common cause of vitamin B$_{12}$ deficiency is lack of gastric acid to separate the ingested vitamin B$_{12}$ from its binding proteins. A third cause of vitamin B$_{12}$ deficiency is malabsorption caused by diseases of the small terminal ileum.

BOX 2-21   Other Vitamin Testing

- Vitamin B$_1$ (Thiamine)
- Vitamin B$_2$ (Riboflavin)
- Vitamin B$_3$ (Niacin)
- Vitamin B$_5$ (Pantothenic acid)
- Vitamin B$_6$ (Pyridoxine)
- Vitamin B$_7$ (Biotin)
- Vitamin B$_9$ (Folate)
- Vitamin B$_{12}$ (Cyanocobalamin)
- Vitamin C (Ascorbic acid)
- Vitamin A (Retinol)
- Vitamin D (25-Hydroxy vitamin D)
- Vitamin E (Alpha-tocopherol)
- Vitamin K$_1$ (Aqua-Mephyton)

Serum B$_{12}$ is a measurement of recent B$_{12}$ ingestion. More prolonged B$_{12}$ deficiency is better and more easily measured by urinary *methylmalonic acid (MMA)* measurement. Elevated serum MMA levels and urinary excretion of MMA are direct measures of tissue vitamin B$_{12}$ activity. The active form of B$_{12}$ is essential in the intracellular conversion of L-methylmalonyl coenzyme A (MMA CoA) to succinyl CoA. Without B$_{12}$, MMA CoA metabolism is diverted to make large quantities of MMA. MMA is then excreted by the kidneys. MMA testing is the most sensitive test for vitamin B$_{12}$ deficiency.

With the exception of vitamin D, most other vitamins are not commonly measured (Box 2-21).

INTERFERING FACTORS

▤ Chloral hydrate is known to *increase* vitamin B$_{12}$ levels.

▤ Drugs known to *decrease* vitamin B$_{12}$ levels include alcohol, aminoglycosides, aminosalicylic acid, anticonvulsants, colchicine, and oral contraceptives.

PROCEDURE AND PATIENT CARE

Before

🖉 Explain the procedure to the patient.

🖉 Tell the patient that no fasting is usually required. (However, some laboratories prefer an 8-hour fast.)

🖉 Instruct the patient not to consume alcoholic beverages before the test.

- Draw the specimen before starting vitamin B$_{12}$ therapy.

During

- Collect a venous blood sample in a red-top tube.

After

- Apply pressure or a pressure dressing to the venipuncture site.
- Assess the venipuncture site for bleeding.
- Transport the blood immediately to the laboratory after collection.

TEST RESULTS AND CLINICAL SIGNIFICANCE

▲   Increased Levels

Leukemia,
Polycythemia vera:
  The pathophysiology of these observations is not well known.
Severe liver dysfunction,
Myeloproliferative disease:
  In the above-noted illnesses, transcobalamin (a vitamin B_{12} carrier protein) is increased, giving a falsely high vitamin B_{12} level.

▼   Decreased Levels

Pernicious anemia: *Intrinsic factor, necessary for vitamin B_{12} absorption, is deficient.*
Malabsorption syndromes (e.g., inflammatory bowel disease, sprue, Crohn disease): *Absorption of vitamin B_{12} is inadequate.*
Intestinal worm infestation: *Competition for vitamin B_{12} in the gut leaves very little vitamin B_{12} for absorption.*
Atrophic gastritis,
Zollinger-Ellison syndrome,
Large proximal gastrectomy:
  Intrinsic factor, necessary for vitamin B_{12} absorption, is deficient, because the mucosal gastric cells necessary for production of IF are absent.
Resection of terminal ileum: *Vitamin B_{12} is absorbed at the terminal portion of the ileum. Without that piece of intestine, vitamin B_{12} cannot be absorbed.*
Achlorhydria: *Gastric acid is necessary to separate vitamin B_{12} from binding proteins. Without gastric acid, vitamin B_{12} stays bound and cannot be absorbed from the intestine.*
Pregnancy: *Vitamin B_{12} deficiency in pregnancy is probably caused by a combination of inadequate intake and increased demand placed by the fetus on the maternal source of folic acid.*
Vitamin C deficiency,
Folic acid deficiency:
  The pathophysiology of these observations is not clear.

RELATED TESTS

Folic Acid (p. 242). This is a measurement of serum folic acid level. Folic acid should always be determined when vitamin B_{12} levels are measured. The clinical symptoms of either deficiency are the same.
Complete Blood Cell Count (CBC) (p. 174). This is performed routinely and can identify megaloblastic anemia.

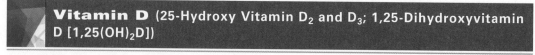

Vitamin D (25-Hydroxy Vitamin D_2 and D_3; 1,25-Dihydroxyvitamin D [1,25$(OH)_2$D])

NORMAL FINDINGS

Total 25-hydroxy D ($D_2 + D_3$): 25-80 ng/mL
1,25 $(OH)_2$D
  Males: 18-64 pg/mL
  Females: 18-78 pg/mL

INDICATIONS

Vitamin D levels are used to ensure that postmenopausal women have adequate vitamin D levels to absorb dietary calcium. Because of the increased number of research studies investigating the role of vitamin D in osteoporosis and cancer prevention, more and more patients are having this blood test.

TEST EXPLANATION

Vitamin D is a fat-soluble vitamin. The two major forms of vitamin D are vitamin D_2 (or ergocalciferol) and vitamin D_3 (or cholecalciferol). The term vitamin D also refers to the "hydroxy-" metabolites of these substances. Vitamin D_2 is provided by dietary sources. Because only fish is naturally rich in vitamin D, most of the vitamin D_2 intake in the industrialized world is from fortified products including milk, soy milk, and breakfast cereals or supplements.

Vitamin D_3 is produced in skin exposed to sunlight, specifically ultraviolet B (UVB) radiation. In this scenario, 7-dehydrocholesterol reacts with UVB ultraviolet light at wavelengths between 270 to 300 nm to produce vitamin D_3. These wavelengths are present in sunlight at sea level when the UV index is greater than 3. These wavelengths occur on a daily basis within the tropics, daily during the spring and summer seasons in temperate regions, and almost never within the arctic circles. Adequate amounts of vitamin D_3 can be made in the skin after only 10 to 15 minutes of sun exposure at least 2 times per week to the face, arms, hands, or back without sunscreen. Melanin functions as a light filter in the skin. Individuals with higher skin melanin content require more time in sunlight to produce the same amount of vitamin D as individuals with lower melanin content.

Once vitamin D is produced in the skin or consumed in food, it is converted in the liver and kidney to form 1,25-dihydroxyvitamin D (1,25[OH]$_2$D), the physiologically active form of vitamin D. Following this conversion, the hormonally active form of vitamin D is released into the circulation. After binding to a carrier protein in the plasma, vitamin D–binding protein (VDBP), it is transported to various target organs. The hormonally active form of vitamin D mediates its biologic effects by binding to the vitamin D receptor (VDR), which is principally located in the nuclei of target cells. The binding of D_3 to the VDR allows the VDR to act as a transcription factor that modulates the gene expression of transport proteins (such as TRPV6 and calbindin), which encourage calcium absorption in the intestine. VDR activation in the intestine, bone, kidney, and parathyroid gland cells leads to the maintenance of calcium and phosphorus levels in the blood.

Vitamin D regulates the calcium and phosphorus levels in the blood by promoting their absorption from food in the intestines, and by promoting reabsorption of calcium in the kidneys. This enables normal mineralization of bone needed for bone growth and bone remodeling.

Vitamin D inhibits parathyroid hormone secretion from the parathyroid gland. Vitamin D promotes the immune system by increasing phagocytosis, antitumor activity, and other immunomodulatory functions.

Vitamin D deficiency can result from inadequate dietary intake, inadequate sunlight exposure, malabsorption syndromes, liver or kidney disorders, or by a number of metabolic hereditary disorders. Deficiency results in impaired bone mineralization and leads to bone softening diseases (rickets in children and osteomalacia in adults). Vitamin D deficiency may also contribute to the development of osteoporosis.

VDR is thought to be involved in cell proliferation/apoptosis and cell differentiation. This may have some influence on the recent observations that vitamin D deficiencies are associated with cancers in the colon, breast, and pancreas. Several recent reports indicate a beneficial correlation between vitamin D intake and prevention of cancer. Vitamin D deficiency is associated with an increase in high blood

TABLE 2-47	Clinical Features and Associated Vitamin D Blood Levels
ng/mL	**Clinical Features**
<11	Associated with vitamin D deficiency and rickets in infants and young children
<10-15	Generally considered inadequate for bone and overall health in healthy individuals
≥30	Proposed by some as desirable for overall health and disease prevention, although a recent government-sponsored expert panel concluded that insufficient data are available to support these higher levels.
Consistently >200	Considered potentially toxic, leading to hypercalcemia and hyperphosphatemia, although human data are limited. In an animal model, concentrations ≤400 ng/mL (≤1000 nmol/L) demonstrated no toxicity.

TABLE 2-48	Adequate Intakes for Vitamin D		
Age	**Children**	**Men**	**Women**
Birth to 13 years	5 mcg (200 international units)		
14-18 years		5 mcg (200 international units)	5 mcg (200 international units)
19-50 years		5 mcg (200 international units)	5 mcg (200 international units)
51-70 years		10 mcg (400 international units)	10 mcg (400 international units)
71+ years		15 mcg (600 international units)	15 mcg (600 international units)

pressure and cardiovascular risk. Vitamin D also affects the immune system through VDR expressed in monocytes and activated T and B cells.

Vitamin D levels can be measured in the blood. Usually 25 hydroxy D_2 and D_3 are measured and added to obtain the total 25 hydroxy D level. Therapy is based on the measurement of total hydroxy D levels. Levels below 20 ng/mL indicate a vitamin D deficiency. D levels between 20 and 30 ng/mL suggest insufficiency. Optimal levels are greater than 30 ng/mL (Table 2-47). Dietary Guidelines for Americans recommend that older adults, people with dark skin, and those exposed to insufficient ultraviolet radiation (i.e., sunlight) consume extra vitamin D from vitamin D–fortified foods (such as milk) and/or supplements. Fish liver oils and eggs are naturally high in vitamin D.

Vitamin D requirements increase with age, while the ability of skin to convert 7-dehydrocholesterol to D_3 decreases. At the same time, the ability of the kidneys to convert D_2 to its active form also decreases with age, prompting the need for increased D supplementation in elderly individuals (Table 2-48). Others particularly at risk for D deficiency include:

- Breastfed infants because human milk alone does not have adequate D levels
- People with limited sun exposure, such as homebound individuals and people living in northern latitudes (such as New England and Alaska)
- Women who wear long robes and head coverings for religious reasons
- People with occupations that prevent sun exposure

- Individuals with a body mass index (BMI) ≥30 because D_2 is trapped in the subcutaneous fat and cannot get into the bloodstream
- Individuals who have a reduced ability to absorb dietary fat because, as a fat-soluble vitamin, vitamin D requires some dietary fat in the gut for absorption
- Patients with liver or renal disease because they cannot convert vitamin D to its active metabolic forms

Vitamin D toxicity can cause nonspecific symptoms such as nausea, vomiting, poor appetite, constipation, weakness, weight loss, confusion, and heart rhythm abnormalities (associated with hypercalcemia). The use of the supplements calcium and vitamin D by postmenopausal women to decrease the risk of osteoporosis has been associated with a 17% increase in the risk of kidney stones.

INTERFERING FACTORS

- Corticosteroid drugs can *decrease* vitamin D levels by reducing calcium absorption.
- The weight-loss drug, orlistat, and the cholesterol-lowering drug, cholestyramine, can *decrease* vitamin D levels by reducing the absorption of vitamin D and other fat-soluble vitamins.
- Barbiturates and phenytoin *decrease* vitamin D levels by increasing hepatic metabolism of vitamin D to inactive compounds.

PROCEDURE AND PATIENT CARE

Before

- Explain the test to the patient. Tell the patient that fasting is not necessary.
- Obtain a list of medications the patient is taking, including supplements and OTC preparations.

During

- Collect a venous blood sample in a red- or green-top tube.

After

- Apply pressure or a pressure dressing to the venipuncture site.
- Assess the site for bleeding.
- If the patient has a vitamin D deficiency, educate him or her about dietary food sources and about the importance of sunlight.

TEST RESULTS AND CLINICAL SIGNIFICANCE

▲ Increased Levels

Williams syndrome (WS): *This is a rare genetic disorder characterized by mild to moderate mental retardation or learning difficulties, a distinctive facial appearance, and a unique personality that combines over-friendliness and high levels of empathy with anxiety. The most significant medical problem associated with WS is cardiovascular disease caused by narrowed arteries. WS is also associated with elevated blood calcium and vitamin D levels in infancy.*

Excess dietary supplements: *With increased oral ingestion of vitamin D, blood levels can rise to toxic levels.*

▲ Decreased Levels

Rickets,
Osteomalacia,

Osteoporosis:

Vitamin D encourages the absorption of calcium from the intestines. Bone matrix formation depends on adequate levels of calcium.

Gastrointestinal malabsorption syndromes: *Vitamin D is a fat-soluble vitamin that will not be absorbed in diseases of maldigestion or malabsorption.*

Renal disease,

Liver disease:

Diseases affecting the metabolic function of these organs will inhibit the conversion of vitamin D to its active form, 1,25 dihydroxyvitamin D.

Familial hypophosphatemic rickets (X-linked hypophosphatemic rickets): *This is a disease caused by a mutation in the PHEX gene on the X chromosome. These patients experience high levels of phosphaturia that is resistant to vitamin D therapy.*

Acute inflammatory disease: *Because inflammation leads to the increased conversion of 25 hydroxy D into 1,25 hydroxy D, 25 hydroxy D (total) will be decreased.*

Inadequate dietary intake: *With decreased oral ingestion of vitamin D, blood levels can fall to insufficient or deficient levels.*

Inadequate exposure to sunlight: *With decreased exposure to adequate sunlight, endogenous production of vitamin D levels can fall to insufficient or deficient levels.*

RELATED TESTS

Calcium (p. 138). This test is used to evaluate parathyroid function and calcium metabolism by measuring the calcium in the blood.

Bone Mineral Density (p. 1002). This test determines bone mineral content and density to diagnosis osteoporosis.

Phosphorus (p. 391). This test assists in the interpretation of studies investigating parathyroid and calcium abnormalities.

West Nile Virus Testing

NORMAL FINDINGS

Negative for West Nile antibody

INDICATIONS

Testing for West Nile virus is indicated when the flu like symptoms occur in an area in which the virus exists. In other areas, testing is only performed when the disease has progressed to one of the more complicated syndromes as discussed below.

TEST EXPLANATION

West Nile virus (WNV) is a RNA virus of the Flavivirus family. Reservoir hosts include birds (especially crows and jays) and farm animals (particularly horses). The vector is the common household mosquito, which carries the virus from the hosts to humans. WNV is not transmitted from human to human. Before 1999, this disease was mostly limited to the African continent. Now, every state in America has reported cases of the disease. It is most common during peak mosquito season (July through October).

Common symptoms of this infection are flu like and include fever, lethargy, headache, neck/body aches, and a skin rash. This disease can progress to encephalitis, aseptic meningitis, and an atypical form of Guillain Barré acute flaccid paralysis.

Front-line testing measures IgM antibodies to flaviviruses and is not specific to WNV. This antibody is measurable by enzyme-linked immunosorbent assay (ELISA) or indirect immunofluorescent antibody assay about 10 days after symptoms start in nearly all patients. If the front-line test for IgM is positive and the symptoms fulfill the Centers for Disease Control and prevention (CDC) criteria, the diagnosis of WNV can be made and treatment altered. This is especially true if the person lives or has traveled to an area that is known to harbor WNV.

If the rapid front-line testing is positive, confirmatory tests may be carried out (especially in areas in which WNV has not been previously known to exist). This testing is more important for public health officials and researchers. Confirmatory tests may include:

- A second IgM serology on convalescing serum 3 to 4 weeks later. A fourfold rise would be confirmatory.
- Direct detection of WNV RNA by nucleic acid amplification testing (NAT) (Plague Reduction Neutralization test performed by the CDC)
- Detection of IgM West Nile virus antibodies in the cerebrospinal fluid

Unfortunately, the sensitivity of the PCR testing is low; therefore negative PCR testing does not exclude West Nile virus infection. WNV can be transmitted through donated blood or blood components. For that reason, in some centers WNV testing kits for WNV antibodies are routinely performed on all donated blood.

Because arboviruses (viruses transmitted by mosquitoes and ticks) are closely related and exhibit serologic cross-reactivity, sometimes it may be epidemiologically important to attempt to pinpoint the infecting virus by conducting cross-neutralization tests using an appropriate battery of closely related viruses (e.g., California, St. Louis, Eastern equine, and Western equine). WNV diseases can be prevented by applying insect repellent containing DEET to exposed skin and clothing.

INTERFERING FACTORS

- Other flavivirus infections, such as St. Louis encephalitis virus, will cause elevations of serologic testing—especially when combined total immunoglobulin (Ig) M and IgG are tested.

PROCEDURE AND PATIENT CARE

Before
✗ Explain the procedure to the patient and family.

During
- Blood: Obtain a venous blood sample in a red-top tube.
- CSF: During lumbar puncture (see p. 651), 1 to 2 mL is reserved in a sterile tube until bacteriologic specimens are found to be negative. Then, the reserved specimen is sent out for testing.

After
- Although there is no treatment specific for WNV, these patients may need acute medical/nursing support for neurologic and respiratory sequelae.
✗ Explain to patient and family that testing is only carried out at a few centers and the specimen must be sent out.
✗ Explain that results may not be available for 2 weeks.

TEST RESULTS AND CLINICAL SIGNIFICANCE

West Nile virus infections: *Most infected people have no symptoms. About 25% may develop a mild fever; head and body aches occur about 3 to 15 days after a mosquito bite. Some may even have a rash or enlarged lymph nodes.*

White Blood Cell Count and Differential Count
(WBC and Differential, Leukocyte Count, Neutrophil Count, Lymphocyte Count, Monocyte Count, Eosinophil Count, Basophil Count)

NORMAL FINDINGS
Total WBCs

Adult/child >2 years: 5000-10,000/mm^3 or 5-10 × 10^9/L (SI units)
Child ≤2 years: 6200-17,000/mm^3
Newborn: 9000-30,000/mm^3

Differential Count

	Percentage (%)	Absolute (per mm^3)
Neutrophils	55-70	2500-8000
Lymphocytes	20-40	1000-4000
Monocytes	2-8	100-700
Eosinophils	1-4	50-500
Basophils	0.5-1.0	25-100

 Critical Values

WBCs <2000 or >40,000/mm^3

INDICATIONS

The measurement of the total and differential WBC count is a part of all routine laboratory diagnostic evaluations. It is especially helpful in the evaluation of the patient with infection, neoplasm, allergy, or immunosuppression (Box 2-22).

 Age-Related Concerns

- The WBC values tend to be age related.
- Normal newborns and infants tend to have higher WBC values than adults.
- It is not uncommon for the elderly to fail to respond to infection by the absence of leukocytosis. The elderly may not develop an increased WBC count even in the presence of a severe bacterial infection.

| BOX 2-22 | Precautions for Immunocompromised Patients |

- Observe protective isolation:
  - Wash hands before entering room.
  - Restrict visitors, per institution policy.
  - Prohibit visitation by people with infections (viral, fungal, bacterial).
- Avoid bacteremia from patient's own bacterial flora:
  - Do not take rectal temperatures.
  - Do not perform rectal examinations or administer enemas.
  - Do not allow patient to floss teeth.
  - Encourage frequent gentle oral hygiene.
  - Encourage daily hygienic skin care.
- Avoid bacterial contamination from foods:
  - Serve only foods from newly opened packages.
  - Avoid fresh fruits and vegetables, per institution policy.
  - Avoid cheese with active mold growth.
- Avoid infection by administration of intramuscular (IM) injections, if possible.
- Administer antibiotics within 1 hour after being ordered.
- Observe closely for infections or fever.

TEST EXPLANATION

The WBC count has two components. The first is a count of the *total number of WBCs* (leukocytes) in 1 mm^3 of peripheral venous blood. The other component, the *differential count,* measures the percentage of each type of leukocyte present in the same specimen. An increase in the percentage of one type of leukocyte means a decrease in the percentage of another. Neutrophils and lymphocytes make up 75% to 90% of the total leukocytes. These leukocyte types can be identified easily by their morphology on a peripheral blood smear (see p. 710) or by automated counters. The total leukocyte count has a wide range of normal values, but many diseases may induce abnormal values.

An increased total WBC count (leukocytosis, WBC count >10,000) usually indicates infection, inflammation, tissue necrosis, or leukemic neoplasia. Trauma or stress, either emotional or physical, may increase the WBC count. In some infections, especially sepsis, the WBC count may be extremely high and reach levels associated with leukemia. This is called a "leukemoid" reaction and quickly resolves as the infection is successfully treated.

A decreased total WBC count (leukopenia; WBC count <4000) occurs in many forms of bone marrow failure (e.g., following antineoplastic chemotherapy or radiation therapy, marrow infiltrative diseases, overwhelming infections, dietary deficiencies, autoimmune diseases).

The major function of WBCs is to fight infection and react against foreign bodies or tissues. Five types of WBCs may easily be identified on a routine blood smear. These cells, in order of frequency, include neutrophils, lymphocytes, monocytes, eosinophils, and basophils. All of these WBCs arise from the same "pluripotent" stem cell within the bone marrow as the RBC (Figure 2-30). Beyond this origin, however, each cell line differentiates separately. Most mature WBCs are then deposited into the circulating blood.

White blood cells are divided into granulocytes and nongranulocytes. Granulocytes include neutrophils, basophils, and eosinophils. Because of their multilobed nuclei neutrophils are sometimes referred to as polymorphonuclear leukocytes (PMNs or "polys"). The normal ranges for absolute counts depend on age, sex, and ethnicity. For example, normal range for absolute neutrophils for adult African American males is 1400 to 7000 cells/microliter.

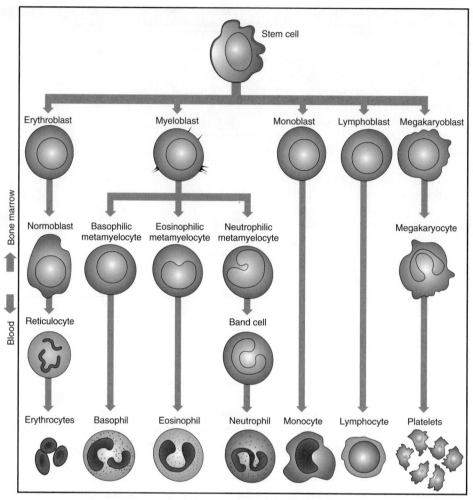

Figure 2-30 Development of blood cells.

The most common granulocyte, *neutrophils,* are produced in 7 to 14 days, and exist in the circulation for only 6 hours. The primary function of the neutrophil is phagocytosis (killing and digestion of bacterial microorganisms). Acute bacterial infections and trauma stimulate neutrophil production, resulting in an increased WBC count. When neutrophil production is significantly stimulated, early immature forms of neutrophils often enter the circulation. These immature forms are called *band* or *stab cells.* This occurrence, referred to as a "shift to the left" in WBC production, is indicative of an ongoing acute bacterial infection.

Basophils (also called *mast cells*) and especially *eosinophils* are involved in the allergic reaction. They are capable of phagocytosis of antigen-antibody complexes. As the allergic response diminishes, the eosinophil count decreases. Eosinophils and basophils do not respond to bacterial or viral infections. The cytoplasm of basophils contains heparin, histamine, and serotonin. These cells infiltrate the tissue (e.g., hive in the skin) involved in the allergic reaction and serve to further the inflammatory reaction. Parasitic infestations also are capable of stimulating the production of these cells.

Nongranulocytes (mononuclear cells) include lymphocytes and monocytes (the count also includes histiocytes). They have no cytoplasmic granules and have a small, single, rounded nuclei. *Lymphocytes*

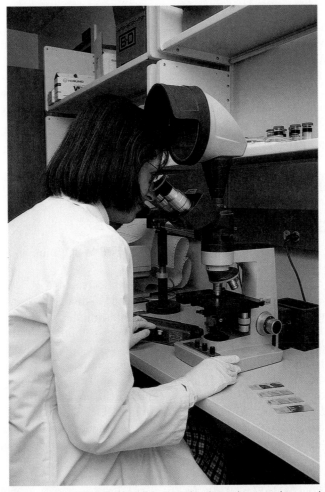

Figure 2-31 Medical technologist conducting microscopic examination of a blood smear after the automated Beckman-Coulter CBC analyzer indicated a population of abnormal white blood cells.

are divided into two types: T cells (mature in the thymus) and B cells (mature in the bone marrow). T cells are involved primarily with cellular-type immune reactions, whereas B cells participate in humoral immunity (antibody production). T cells are the killer cells, suppressor cells, and the T4 helper cells (see lymphocyte immunophenotyping on p. 147). The primary function of lymphocytes is to fight chronic bacterial infection and acute viral infections. The differential count does not separate the T and B cells but rather counts the combination of the two.

Monocytes are phagocytic cells capable of fighting bacteria similar to the way neutrophils do. Through phagocytosis, they remove necrotic debris and microorganisms from the blood. The monocytes produce interferon, which is the body's endogenous immunostimulant. Monocytes can be produced more rapidly, however, and can spend a longer time in the circulation than the neutrophils.

The WBC and differential count are routinely measured as part of the complete blood cell count (see p. 174) (Figure 2-31). Serial WBC counts and differential counts have both diagnostic and prognostic value. For example, a persistent increase in the WBC count (and particularly the neutrophils) may indicate worsening of an infectious process (e.g., appendicitis). A reduction in WBC count to the normal range from a previously elevated range indicates resolution of an infection. A dramatic decrease in the WBC count below the normal range may indicate marrow failure. In patients receiving chemotherapy, a reduced WBC count may contraindicate further chemotherapy.

The absolute count is calculated by multiplying the differential count (%) by the total WBC count. For example, the *absolute neutrophil count* (ANC) is helpful in determining the patient's real risk for infection. It is calculated by multiplying the WBC count by the percent of neutrophils and percent of bands, that is:

$$ANC = WBC \times (\% \text{ Neutrophils} + \% \text{ Bands})$$

If the ANC is below 1000, the patient may need to be placed in protective isolation as he or she could be severely immunocompromised (see Box 2-22, p. 527) and is at great risk for infection.

INTERFERING FACTORS

- Eating, physical activity, and stress may cause an increased WBC count and alter the differential values.
- Pregnancy (final month) and labor may be associated with increased WBC levels.
- Patients who have had a splenectomy have a persistent mild to moderate elevation of WBC counts.
- The WBC count tends to be lower in the morning and higher in the late afternoon.
- The WBC count tends to be age related. Normal newborns and infants tend to have higher WBC counts than adults. It is not uncommon for the elderly to fail to respond to infection by the absence of leukocytosis. In fact, the elderly may not develop an increased WBC count even in the face of a severe bacterial infection.

 Drugs that may cause *increased* WBC levels include adrenaline, allopurinol, aspirin, chloroform, epinephrine, heparin, quinine, steroids, and triamterene (Dyrenium).

 Drugs that may cause *decreased* WBC levels include antibiotics, anticonvulsants, antihistamines, antimetabolites, antithyroid drugs, arsenicals, barbiturates, chemotherapeutic agents, diuretics, and sulfonamides.

✓ Clinical Priorities

- An increased WBC count (leukocytosis) usually indicates infection, inflammation, tissue necrosis, or leukemic neoplasia.
- Serial WBC and differential counts have both diagnostic and prognostic value. For example, a persistent increase in the WBC count may indicate a worsening of an infectious process (e.g., appendicitis).
- A drastic decrease in WBCs below the normal range may indicate bone marrow failure and subsequent high risk of septicemia and death.

PROCEDURE AND PATIENT CARE

Before
- Explain the procedure to the patient.
- Tell the patient that no fasting is required.

During
- Collect a venous blood sample in a lavender-top tube.

After

- Apply pressure or a pressure dressing to the venipuncture site.
- Check the venipuncture site for bleeding.

TEST RESULTS AND CLINICAL SIGNIFICANCE

▲ Increased WBC Count (Leukocytosis)

Infection: *WBCs are integral to initiating and maintaining the body's defense mechanism against infection.*

Leukemic neoplasia or other myeloproliferative disorders: *These neoplastic cells are produced by the marrow and are released into the bloodstream.*

Other malignancy: *Advanced non-marrow cancers (e.g., lung) are associated with leukocytosis. The pathophysiology of this observation is not defined.*

Trauma, stress, or hemorrhage: *The WBC count is probably under hormonal influence (e.g., epinephrine). However, the pathophysiology of this observation is not defined.*

Tissue necrosis,

Inflammation:

The pathophysiology of these observations is complex, including the recognition of necrotic or normal tissue as "foreign" so that a WBC response is instituted.

Dehydration: *Not only is dehydration a stress that, by itself, increases the WBC count, but also by virtue of hemoconcentration, the WBC count increases.*

Thyroid storm: *The WBC count is probably influenced by thyroid hormones. Marked increases in these hormones could be associated with an increased WBC count.*

Steroid use: *Glucocorticosteroids stimulate WBC production.*

▼ Decreased WBC Count (Leukopenia)

Drug toxicity (e.g., cytotoxic chemotherapy; see also drugs that decrease the WBC count),

Bone marrow failure,

Overwhelming infections,

Dietary deficiency (e.g., vitamin B_{12}, iron deficiency),

Congenital marrow aplasia,

Bone marrow infiltration (e.g., myelofibrosis):

The above are associated with all different forms of bone marrow failure whereby WBC production is reduced.

Autoimmune disease: *The pathophysiology of this observation is not known.*

Hypersplenism: *The spleen more aggressively extracts WBCs from the bloodstream.*

▲ Increased/▼ Decreased Differential Results

See Table 2-49.

RELATED TESTS

Lymphocyte Immunophenotyping (p. 147). This test is used to detect the progressive depletion of CD4 T lymphocytes, which is associated with an increased likelihood of clinical complications from acquired immunodeficiency syndrome (AIDS). Test results can indicate if an AIDS patient is at risk for developing opportunistic infections.

Peripheral Blood Smear (p. 710). This is a direct microscopic analysis of the cellular components of the blood.

TABLE 2-49	Causes of Abnormalities in the White Blood Cell Differential Count	

Type of White Blood Cell	Elevated	Decreased
Neutrophils	"Neutrophilia" Physical or emotional stress Acute suppurative infection Myelocytic leukemia Trauma Cushing syndrome Inflammatory disorders (e.g., rheumatic fever, thyroiditis, rheumatoid arthritis) Metabolic disorders (e.g., ketoacidosis, gout, eclampsia)	"Neutropenia" Aplastic anemia Dietary deficiency Overwhelming bacterial infection (especially in the elderly) Viral infections (e.g., hepatitis, influenza, measles) Radiation therapy Addison disease Drug therapy: myelotoxic drugs (as in chemotherapy)
Lymphocytes	"Lymphocytosis" Chronic bacterial infection Viral infection (e.g., mumps, rubella) Lymphocytic leukemia Multiple myeloma Infectious mononucleosis Radiation Infectious hepatitis	"Lymphocytopenia" Leukemia Sepsis Immunodeficiency diseases Lupus erythematosus Later stages of human immunodeficiency virus infection Drug therapy: adrenocorticosteroids, antineoplastics Radiation therapy
Monocytes	"Monocytosis" Chronic inflammatory disorders Viral infections (e.g., infectious mononucleosis) Tuberculosis Chronic ulcerative colitis Parasites (e.g., malaria)	"Monocytopenia" Aplastic anemia Hairy cell leukemia Drug therapy: prednisone
Eosinophils	"Eosinophilia" Parasitic infections Allergic reactions Eczema Leukemia Autoimmune diseases	"Eosinopenia" Increased adrenosteroid production
Basophils	"Basophilia" Myeloproliferative disease (e.g., myelofibrosis, polycythemia rubra vera) Leukemia	"Basopenia" Acute allergic reactions Hyperthyroidism Stress reactions

D-Xylose Absorption (Xylose Tolerance)

NORMAL FINDINGS

Age	60-min Plasma (mg/dL)	120-min Plasma (mg/dL)	Urine (g/5 hr)
Child	>15-20	>20	>4 (16%-32%)
Adult	20-57	30-58	>3.5-4 (>14%)

INDICATIONS

This test is used to evaluate the absorptive capability of the intestines. It is used in the evaluation of patients with suspected malabsorption.

TEST EXPLANATION

D-Xylose is a monosaccharide that is easily absorbed by the normal intestine. In patients with malabsorption, intestinal D-xylose absorption is diminished, and as a result, blood levels and urine excretion will be reduced. D-Xylose is the monosaccharide chosen for the test because it is not metabolized by the body. Serum levels directly reflect intestinal absorption.

This monosaccharide is also used because absorption does not require pancreatic or biliary exocrine function. Its absorption is directly determined by the absorptive function of the small intestine. This test is used to differentiate diarrhea caused by maldigestion (pancreatic/biliary dysfunction) and diarrhea caused by malabsorption (sprue, Whipple disease, Crohn disease). It is also used to quantitate the degree of malabsorption to monitor therapy.

In this test the patient is asked to drink a fluid containing a prescribed amount of D-xylose. Blood and urine levels are subsequently evaluated. Excellent gastrointestinal (GI) absorption is documented by high blood levels and good urine excretion of D-xylose. Poor intestinal absorption is marked by low blood levels and urine excretion.

CONTRAINDICATIONS

- Patients who are dehydrated, because the dose of D-xylose can cause diarrhea and may precipitate hypovolemia in these patients

INTERFERING FACTORS

- Patients with abnormal kidney function, because they may not be able to excrete the xylose. The urine measurement for D-xylose should not be performed, and the interpretation should be based on the blood test results only.
- Drugs that may affect test results include aspirin, atropine, and indomethacin.

PROCEDURE AND PATIENT CARE

Before

- Explain the procedure to the patient.
- Instruct the adult patient to fast for 8 hours before testing. Water should be encouraged, however.
- Tell the pediatric patient or the parents that the patient should fast for at least 4 hours before testing.

During

- Collect a venous blood sample in a red-top tube before the patient ingests the D-xylose.
- Collect a first-voided morning urine specimen and send it to the laboratory.
- Ask the patient to take the prescribed dose of D-xylose dissolved in 8 ounces of water. Record the time of ingestion.
- Calibrate pediatric doses according to the patient's body weight.
- Repeat venipunctures to obtain blood in exactly 2 hours for an adult and 1 hour for a child.
- Collect urine for a designated time, usually 5 hours, in a dark bottle. Refrigerate the urine during the collection period.
- Observe the patient for nausea, vomiting, and diarrhea, which may occur as side effects of D-xylose ingestion.
- Instruct the patient to remain in a restful position. Intense physical activity may alter the digestive process and affect the test results.

After

- Apply pressure or a pressure dressing to the venipuncture site.
- Observe the venipuncture site for bleeding.
- Provide the patient with food or drink and inform the patient that normal activity may be resumed after completion of the study.

TEST RESULTS AND CLINICAL SIGNIFICANCE

▼ Decreased Levels

Malabsorption caused by sprue, lymphatic obstruction, enteropathy (e.g., radiation), Crohn disease, or Whipple disease: *The D-xylose is not absorbed in these patients; therefore blood and urine levels are not as normally expected.*

Short-bowel syndrome: *Because of the lack of absorptive surface, absorption of D-xylose does not occur. Therefore blood and urine levels are not as normally expected.*

RELATED TEST

Small Bowel Follow-Through (p. 1064). This is an x-ray test that visualizes the mucosa of the small intestine. Patients with Crohn disease and other malabsorption syndromes may have obvious abnormal findings.

Zinc Protoporphyrin (ZPP)

NORMAL FINDINGS

0-69 μmol ZPP/mol heme

INDICATIONS

ZPP is a screening test for lead poisoning and iron deficiency anemia.

TEST EXPLANATION

ZPP is used in screening for iron deficiency anemia or lead poisoning. It is also used in monitoring the treatment/interventions of chronic lead poisoning. ZPP is found in red blood cells when heme production is inhibited by lead toxicity. Lead prevents iron, but not zinc, from attaching to the protoporphyrin. Or, if there is iron deficiency, instead of incorporating a ferrous ion to form heme, protoporphyrin (the immediate precursor of heme) incorporates a zinc ion, forming ZPP. In addition to lead poisoning and iron deficiency, zinc protoporphyrin levels can be elevated as the result of a number of other conditions (e.g., sickle cell anemia). Because of this lack of specificity, ZPP is not commonly used as a screening test for lead poisoning.

The fluorescent properties of ZPP in intact red cells allow the ZPP/heme molar ratio to be measured quickly, at low cost, and in a small sample volume. However, it is more commonly measured using a hematofluorometer, which is able to measure the ZPP/heme ratio.

PROCEDURE AND PATIENT CARE

Before
🖉 Instruct the patient to fast for 12 hours before the blood test. Water is permitted.

During
- Collect a venous blood sample in a royal blue-, tan-, lavender-, or pink-top tube.
- Indicate on the laboratory slip any drugs that may affect test results.

After
- Apply pressure to the venipuncture site.

TEST RESULTS AND CLINICAL SIGNIFICANCE

▲ Increased Levels

Lead poisoning,
Vanadium exposure:
> Lead and a few other heavy metals inhibit the action of the enzyme ferrochelatase, which facilitates the uptake of iron into protoporphyrin IX in the production of hemoglobin. As a result, zinc is taken up by the protoporphyrin and incorporated into ZPP. Increased ZPP is noted.

Iron deficiency,
Anemia of chronic illness,
Sickle cell anemia,
Sideroblastic anemia:
> When iron is deficient or hemoglobin synthesis outstrips iron availability, zinc is preferentially taken up by protoporphyrin IX in the production of hemoglobin. As a result, zinc is taken up by the protoporphyrin and incorporated into ZPP. Increased ZPP is noted.

RELATED TESTS

Lead (p. 334). This is a measure of lead in the blood.
Iron Level and Total Iron Binding Capacity (p. 322). This is a measure of iron in the blood.
Transferrin Receptor Assay (p. 502). This test is used to help differentiate the various causes of iron deficiency anemia.

3

Electrodiagnostic Tests

OVERVIEW

TESTS

Overview

REASONS FOR PERFORMING ELECTRODIAGNOSTIC STUDIES

Most electrodiagnostic studies use electrical activity and electronic devices to evaluate disease or injury to a specified area of the body. The electrical impulses can be generated spontaneously or can be stimulated. For example, electrocardiography records spontaneous electrical impulses generated by the heart during the cardiac cycle. In electromyography, the electrical impulses are stimulated by an electrical shock applied to the body. For the caloric study, nystagmus is induced by irrigating the ear canal with water. The electrical activity is usually detected by electrodes placed on the body. The electrodes are attached to instruments for receiving and recording electrical impulses. Table 3-1 lists the various areas of the body that can be evaluated by electrodiagnostic studies.

PROCEDURAL CARE FOR ELECTRODIAGNOSTIC STUDIES

Before

🖉 Explain the procedure to the patient.

- Obtain baseline values for comparison during and after the test.

TABLE 3-1	Body Areas Evaluated by Electrodiagnostic Studies
Name of Test	**Evaluation**
Caloric study	Cranial nerve VIII
Cardiac stress	Cardiac muscle
Electrocardiography	Cardiac muscle and conduction system
Electroencephalography	Brain
Electromyography	Neuromuscular system
Electroneurography	Peripheral nerves
Electronystagmography	Oculovestibular reflex pathway
Electrophysiologic studies	Cardiac conduction system
Evoked potential studies	Sensory pathways of the eyes, ears, and peripheral nerves
Contraction stress (fetal)	Fetal viability
Nonstress (fetal)	Fetal viability
Holter monitoring	Cardiac rhythm
Pelvic floor sphincter electromyography	Urinary or fecal continence

Explain food restrictions, if indicated. For example, caloric studies require fasting to reduce the possibility of nausea and vomiting. On the other hand, fasting would affect electroencephalography results by causing hypoglycemia.
- Determine if there are any drug restrictions. Sedatives may adversely affect most test results.
- Because of its stimulating effect, caffeine is restricted before most studies.
- Most of these studies are considered noninvasive and do not require a consent form.

During
- For most tests, some type of electrode is applied to the patient to record electrical activity.
- Some tests (such as electromyography) require some type of stimulation. Slight discomfort may be felt if electrical stimulation is applied.
- The patient needs to remain still during testing. Any movement can alter test results.

After
- Monitor the patient for a return to pretest baseline activity.
- Some studies may cause nausea and vomiting. The patient should rest until these symptoms subside.
- If any sedation was given, safety precautions should be in effect.

POTENTIAL COMPLICATIONS OF ELECTRODIAGNOSTIC STUDIES

Most tests in this category have few potential complications. Those mentioned below apply to specific tests and are grouped accordingly.

Cardiac Stress Testing
Cardiac arrhythmias
Severe angina
Fainting
Myocardial infarction

Contraction Stress Test

Premature labor

REPORTING OF RESULTS

Many of these tests are performed by technicians. Test results are available after interpretation by a physician.

Caloric Study (Oculovestibular Reflex Study)

NORMAL FINDINGS

Nystagmus with irrigation

INDICATIONS

This test is used to evaluate the function of cranial nerve VIII. It also can indicate disease in the temporal portion of the cerebrum.

TEST EXPLANATION

Caloric studies are used to evaluate the vestibular portion of the eighth cranial nerve (CN VIII) by irrigating the external auditory canal with hot or cold water. This is usually part of a complete neurologic examination. Stimulation with cold water normally causes rotary nystagmus (involuntary rapid eye movement) away from the ear being irrigated; hot water induces nystagmus toward the side of the ear being irrigated. If the labyrinth is diseased or CN VIII is not functioning (e.g., from tumor compression), no nystagmus is induced. This study aids in the differential diagnosis of abnormalities that may occur in the vestibular system, brainstem, or cerebellum. When results are inconclusive, electronystagmography (p. 557) may be performed.

CONTRAINDICATIONS

- Patients with a perforated eardrum. Cold air may be substituted for the fluid, although this method is less reliable.
- Patients with an acute disease of the labyrinth (e.g., Ménière syndrome). The test can be performed when the acute attack subsides.

INTERFERING FACTORS

 Drugs such as sedatives and antivertigo agents can alter test results.

Clinical Priorities

- This study aids in evaluating the vestibular portion of the eighth cranial nerve.
- During this test, the external auditory canal is irrigated with hot or cold water to induce nystagmus.
- Most patients experience nausea and dizziness during this test. Patients with a decreased level of consciousness should be safely positioned to avoid potential aspiration from vomiting.

PROCEDURE AND PATIENT CARE

Before

📵 Explain the procedure to the patient.
- Hold solid foods before the test to reduce the incidence of vomiting.

During

- Although the exact procedures for caloric studies vary, note the following steps in a typical test:
  1. Before the test, the patient is examined for the presence of nystagmus, postural deviation (Romberg sign), and past-pointing. This examination provides the baseline values for comparison during the test.
  2. The ear canal should be examined and cleaned before testing to ensure that the water will flow freely to the middle ear area.
  3. The ear on the suspected side is irrigated first because the patient's response may be minimal.
  4. After an emesis basin is placed under the ear, the irrigation solution is directed into the external auditory canal until the patient complains of nausea and dizziness, or nystagmus is observed. This usually occurs in 20 to 30 seconds.
  5. If after 3 minutes no symptoms occur, the irrigation is stopped.
  6. The patient is tested again for nystagmus, past-pointing, and Romberg sign.
  7. After approximately 5 minutes, the procedure is repeated on the other side.
- Note that this procedure is usually performed by a physician or technician in approximately 15 minutes.

📵 Tell the patient that he or she will probably experience nausea and dizziness during the test. If the patient has a decreased level of consciousness, position safely to avoid potential aspiration from vomiting.

After

- Usually, place the patient on bed rest for approximately 30 to 60 minutes until nausea or vomiting subsides.
- Ensure patient safety related to dizziness.

TEST RESULTS AND CLINICAL SIGNIFICANCE

Brainstem inflammation, infarction, or tumor,
Cerebellar inflammation, infarction, or tumor,
Vestibular or cochlear inflammation or tumor,
Acoustic neuroma,
Eighth nerve neuritis or neuropathy:
  The above-noted diseases involve the central nervous system (CNS) from the vestibular/cochlear end organ to the temporal area of the cerebrum.

RELATED TEST

Electronystagmography (p. 557). During this test, nystagmus is stimulated in a manner similar to that described for caloric studies. The direction, velocity, and amplitude of the nystagmus are recorded through the use of electrodes.

Cardiac Stress Testing (Stress Testing, Exercise Testing, Electrocardiograph [EKG] Stress Testing, Nuclear Stress Testing, Echo Stress Testing)

NORMAL FINDINGS

Patient able to obtain and maintain maximal heart rate of 85% for predicted age and gender with no cardiac symptoms or EKG change
No cardiac muscle wall dysfunction

INDICATIONS

Stress testing is used in the following situations:

1. To evaluate chest pain in a patient with suspected coronary disease (Occasionally a person may have significant coronary stenosis that is not apparent during normal physical activity. If, however, the pain can be reproduced with exercise, coronary occlusion may be present.)
2. To determine the limits of safe exercise during a cardiac rehabilitation program or to assist patients with cardiac disease in maintaining good physical fitness
3. To detect labile or exercise-related hypertension
4. To detect intermittent claudication in patients with suspected vascular occlusive disease in the extremities (In this situation, the patient may experience leg muscle cramping while performing the exercise.)
5. To evaluate the effectiveness of treatment in patients who take antianginal or antiarrhythmic medications
6. To evaluate the effectiveness of cardiac intervention (such as bypass grafting or angioplasty)

TEST EXPLANATION

Stress testing is a noninvasive study that provides information about the patient's cardiac function. In stress testing the heart is stressed in some way. The heart is then evaluated during the stress. Changes indicating ischemia point to coronary occlusive disease. By far the most commonly used method of stress is exercise (usually treadmill). Chemical stress methods are becoming more common because of their safety and increased accuracy. A third method, less frequently used, is pacer stress (Box 3-1).

During *exercise stress testing*, the EKG, heart rate, and blood pressure are monitored while the patient engages in some type of physical activity (stress). Two methods of stress testing are pedaling a stationary

BOX 3-1	Commonly Used Methods of Stressing the Heart	
Exercise	**Chemical**	**Pacing**
• Bicycle	• Adenosine	• Cardiac pacemaker
• Treadmill	• Dipyridamole	
	• Dobutamine	
	• Stimulatory drugs	
	• Vascular dilation drugs	

bike and walking on a treadmill. With the stationary bicycle the pedaling tension is slowly increased to increase the heart rate. With the treadmill test the speed and grade of incline are increased. The treadmill test is the most frequently used because it is the most easily standardized and reproducible (Figure 3-1). The various grades of exercise are determined by the cardiologist in attendance based on estimation of cardiac function capabilities.

The usual goal of the exercise stress testing is to increase the heart rate to just below maximal levels or to the "target heart rate." This target heart rate is usually 80% to 90% of the maximal heart rate. The test is usually discontinued if the patient reaches that target heart rate or develops any symptoms or EKG changes. The maximal heart rate is determined by a chart that takes into account the patient's age (about 220 minus the patient's age) and gender. The normal maximal heart rate for adults varies from 150 to 200 beats/min; patients taking calcium channel blockers and sympathetic blockers have a lower-than-expected maximal heart rate.

Exercise stress testing is based on the principle that occluded arteries will be unable to meet the heart's increased demand for blood during the testing. This may become obvious with symptoms (e.g., chest pain, fatigue, dyspnea, tachycardia, cardiac arrhythmias [dysrhythmias], fall in blood pressure) or EKG changes (e.g., ST-segment variance >1 mm, increasing premature ventricular contractions, other rhythm disturbances). An advantage of stress testing is that these symptoms can be stimulated and identified in a safe environment. Besides the electrodiagnostic method of cardiac evaluation, the stressed heart also can be evaluated by nuclear scanning or echocardiography, which are more sensitive and accurate. Findings of ischemia are discussed in "Test Results and Clinical Significance."

When exercise testing is not advisable or the patient is unable to exercise to a level adequate to stress the heart (patients with an orthopedic, arthritic, neurologic, or pulmonary limitation), *chemical stress testing* is recommended. Chemical stress testing is being increasingly used because of its accuracy and ease of performance. Although chemical stress testing is less physiologic than exercise testing, it is safer and more controllable. *Dipyridamole (Persantine)* is a coronary vasodilator. If one coronary artery is significantly occluded, the coronary blood flow is diverted to the opened vessels. This causes a "steal syndrome" away from the stenotic or occluded coronary vessel. That is, the dipyridamole-induced vascular dilation "steals" the blood from the ischemic areas and diverts it to the open, dilated coronary vessels. Caution must be taken, however, because this can precipitate angina or myocardial infarction (MI). This test should be performed only with a cardiologist in attendance. Intravenous (IV) aminophylline can reverse the effect of dipyridamole. *Adenosine* works similarly to dipyridamole.

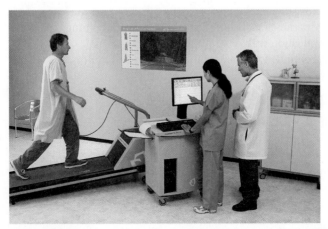

Figure 3-1 Patient taking exercise stress test while nurse monitors the EKG response.

BOX 3-2	Commonly Used Methods of Cardiac Evaluation During Stress Testing

- Cardiac nuclear scanning (p. 791)
- Echocardiography (p. 877)
- Electrophysiologic parameters: EKG, blood pressure, and heart rate

BOX 3-3	Criteria for Discontinuation of an Exercise Stress Test

- Abnormal EKG changes
  - Ectopy
  - Flipped T waves
  - ST changes
- Attainment of maximal performance
- Chest pain
- Cyanosis
- Excessive heart rate changes: tachycardia or bradycardia
- Excessive hypertension or hypotension
- Leg claudication
- Severe shortness of breath
- Syncope

Dobutamine is another chemical that can stress the heart. Dobutamine stimulates heart muscle function. This entails administration of progressively greater amounts of dobutamine over 3-minute intervals. The normal heart muscle increases its contractility (wall motion). Ischemic muscle has no augmentation. In fact, in time the ischemic area becomes hypokinetic. Infarcted tissue is akinetic. In chemical stress testing the stressed heart is evaluated by nuclear scanning or echocardiography.

Pacing is another method of stress testing. In patients with permanent pacemakers, the rate of capture can be increased to a rate that would be considered a cardiac stress. The heart is then evaluated electrodiagnostically or with nuclear scanning or echocardiography.

As indicated in Box 3-2, the methods of evaluating the heart are nuclear scanning, echocardiography, and electrophysiologic parameters. Echocardiography is fast becoming the method of choice for urgent and elective cardiac evaluation with or without stress testing.

Stress testing is discontinued with any of the criteria noted in Box 3-3.

CONTRAINDICATIONS

- Patients with unstable angina, because stress may induce an infarction.
- Patients with severe aortic valvular heart disease (especially stenotic lesions), because their stress tolerance is easily reached and is quite low.
- Patients who cannot participate in an exercise program because of their impaired lung or motor function. However, they can be stressed chemically.
- Patients who have recently had a myocardial infarction (MI). However, limited stress testing may be done.
- Patients with severe congestive heart failure.

- Patients who have severe claudication and cannot walk adequately to stress their hearts. However, they can be stressed chemically.
- Patients with known severe left main coronary artery disease.

POTENTIAL COMPLICATIONS

- Fatal cardiac arrhythmias
- Severe angina
- MI
- Fainting

INTERFERING FACTORS

- Heavy meals before testing can divert blood to the gastrointestinal tract.
- Nicotine from smoking can cause coronary artery spasm.
- Caffeine blocks the effect of dipyridamole.
- Medical problems such as hypertension, valvular heart disease (especially of the aortic valve), severe anemia, hypoxemia, and chronic pulmonary disease can affect results.
- Left ventricular hypertrophy may affect test results.
- The EKG is not a reliable indicator of ischemia in patients with left bundle branch block.
- Drugs that can affect test results include beta blockers (e.g., propranolol [Inderal]), calcium channel blockers, digoxin, and nitroglycerin.

PROCEDURE AND PATIENT CARE

Before

- Explain the procedure to the patient.
- Instruct the patient to abstain from eating, drinking, and smoking for 4 hours.
- Inform the patient about the risks of the test and obtain informed consent.
- Instruct the patient to bring comfortable clothing and athletic shoes for exercise. Slippers are not acceptable.
- Inform the patient if any medications should be discontinued before testing.
- Obtain a pretest EKG.
- Record the patient's vital signs for baseline values. Monitor the blood pressure during the testing.
- Apply and secure appropriate EKG electrodes.

During

- Note that a physician usually is present during stress testing.
- After the patient begins to exercise, adjust the treadmill machine settings to apply increasing levels of stress at specific intervals. Encourage and support the patient at each level of increased stress.
- Encourage patients to verbalize any symptoms.
- Note that during the test the EKG tracing and vital signs are monitored continuously.
- Terminate the test if the patient complains of chest pain, exhaustion, dyspnea, fatigue, or dizziness.
- Note that testing usually takes approximately 45 minutes.
- Inform the patient that the physician in attendance usually interprets the results and explains them to the patient.

After

- Place the patient in the supine position to rest after the test.
- Monitor the EKG tracing and record vital signs at poststress intervals until recordings and values return to pretest levels.
- Remove electrodes and paste.

TEST RESULTS AND CLINICAL SIGNIFICANCE

Coronary artery occlusive disease: *Subclinical coronary artery occlusive disease often becomes evident with stress testing.*

Exercise-related hypertension or hypotension: *The blood pressure is higher or lower than what is considered normal for the level of exercise.*

Intermittent claudication: *As with the coronary system, peripheral vascular stenosis or occlusion may not become evident until the legs are stressed as in an exercise stress test.*

Abnormal cardiac rhythms such as ventricular tachycardia or supraventricular tachycardia: *Ectopy may not occur or become symptomatic until the person is stressed.*

RELATED TESTS

Cardiac Nuclear Scan (p. 791). This test is used to evaluate the heart during stress testing.
Echocardiography (p. 877). This test is also used to evaluate the heart during stress testing.

Electrocardiography (Electrocardiogram [ECG, EKG])

NORMAL FINDINGS

Normal heart rate (60-100 beats/min), rhythm, and wave deflections

INDICATIONS

This electrodiagnostic test records the electrical impulses that stimulate the heart to contract. It is used to evaluate arrhythmias, conduction defects, myocardial injury and damage, hypertrophy—both left and right, and pericardial diseases. It is also used to assist in the diagnosis of other noncardiac conditions such as electrolyte abnormalities, drug level abnormalities, and pulmonary diseases.

TEST EXPLANATION

The EKG is a graphic representation of the electrical impulses that the heart generates during the cardiac cycle. These electrical impulses are conducted to the body's surface, where they are detected by electrodes placed on the patient's limbs and chest. The monitoring electrodes detect the electrical activity of the heart from a variety of spatial perspectives. The EKG lead system is composed of several electrodes that are placed on each of the four extremities and at varying sites on the chest. Each combination of electrodes is called a *lead*.

A 12-lead EKG provides a comprehensive view of the flow of the heart's electrical currents in two different planes. There are six limb leads (combination of electrodes on the extremities) and six chest leads (corresponding to six sites on the chest).

The limb leads provide a *frontal* plane view that bisects the body, separating it front to back. The chest leads provide a *horizontal* plane view that bisects the body, separating it top to bottom (Figure 3-2). Leads I, II, and III are considered the *standard limb leads*. Lead I records the difference in electrical potential between the left arm (LA) and the right arm (RA). Lead II records the electrical potential between the RA and the left leg (LL). Lead III reflects the difference between the LA and the LL. The right leg (RL) electrode is an inactive ground in all leads. There are three *augmented limb leads:* aV_R, aV_L, and aV_F (*a*, augmented; *V*, vector [unipolar]; *R*, right arm; *L*, left arm; *F*, left foot or leg). The augmented leads measure the electrical potential between the center of the heart and the right arm (aV_R), the left arm (aV_L), and the left leg (aV_F). The six standard *chest*, or *precordial*, *leads* (V_1, V_2, V_3, V_4, V_5, V_6) are recorded by placing electrodes at six different positions on the chest, surrounding the heart. (The exact locations of the leads are indicated in "Procedure and Patient Care.")

In general, leads II, III, and aVF look at the inferior portion of the heart. Leads aVL and I look at the lateral portion of the heart. Leads V2 to V4 look at the anterior portion of the heart.

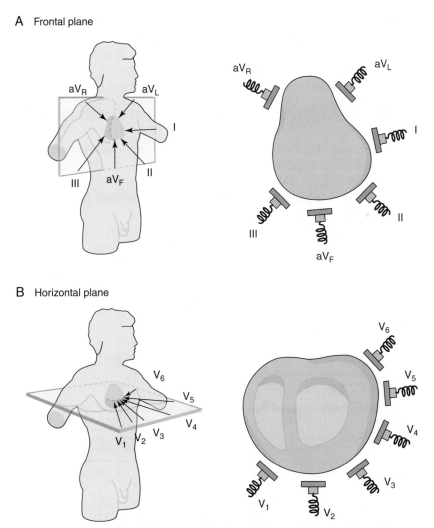

Figure 3-2 Planes of reference. **A,** The frontal plane. **B,** The horizontal plane.

The EKG is recorded on special paper with a graphic background of horizontal and vertical lines for rapid measurement of time intervals (X coordinate) and voltages (Y coordinate). Time duration is measured by vertical lines 1 mm apart, each representing 0.04 second. Voltage is measured by horizontal lines 1 mm apart. Five 1-mm squares equal 0.5 mV.

The normal EKG pattern is composed of waves arbitrarily designated by the letters P, Q, R, S, and T. The Q, R, and S waves are grouped together and described as the QRS complex. The significance of the waves and the time intervals are as follows (Figure 3-3):

- *P wave.* This represents atrial electrical depolarization associated with atrial contraction. It represents electrical activity associated with the spread of the original impulse from the sinoatrial (SA) node through the atria. If the P waves are absent or altered, the cardiac impulse originates outside the SA node.
- *PR interval.* This represents the time required for the impulse to travel from the SA node to the atrioventricular node. If this interval is prolonged, a conduction delay exists in the atrioventricular node (e.g., a first-degree heart block). If the PR interval is shortened, the impulse must have reached the ventricle through a "shortcut" (as in Wolff-Parkinson-White syndrome).
- *QRS complex.* This represents ventricular electrical depolarization associated with ventricular contraction. This complex consists of an initial downward (negative) deflection (Q wave), a large upward (positive) deflection (R wave), and a small downward deflection (S wave). A widened QRS complex indicates abnormal or prolonged ventricular depolarization time (as in a bundle branch block).
- *ST segment.* This represents the period between the completion of depolarization and the beginning of repolarization of the ventricular muscle. This segment may be elevated or depressed in transient muscle ischemia (e.g., angina) or in muscle injury (as in the early stages of myocardial infarction [MI]).
- *T wave.* This represents ventricular repolarization (i.e., return to neutral electrical activity).
- *QT interval.* This represents the time between the onset of ventricular depolarization and the end of ventricular depolarization. This interval varies with age, sex, heart rate, and medications.
- *U wave.* This deflection follows the T wave and is usually quite small. It represents repolarization of the Purkinje fibers within the ventricles.

Through the analysis of these wave forms and time intervals, valuable information about the heart may be obtained. The EKG is used primarily to identify abnormal heart rhythms (arrhythmias, or dysrhythmias) and to diagnose acute MI, conduction defects, and ventricular hypertrophy. It is important to note that the EKG may be normal, even in the presence of heart disease, if the heart disorder does not affect the electrical activity of the heart.

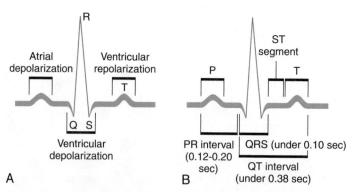

Figure 3-3 A, Normal EKG deflections during depolarization and repolarization of the atria and ventricles. **B,** Principal EKG intervals between P, QRS, and T waves.

For some patients at high risk for malignant ventricular dysrhythmias, a *signal-averaged EKG* (SAEKG) can be performed. This test averages several hundred QRS waveforms to detect late potentials that are likely to lead to ventricular dysrhythmias. SAEKG has been a useful precursor to electrophysiologic studies (EPS) (p. 559) because it can identify ventricular tachycardia in patients with unexplained syncope. The SAEKG can be performed at the bedside in 15 to 20 minutes and must be ordered separately from a standard EKG.

Microvolt T-wave alternans (MTWA) detects T-wave alternans (variations in the *vector* and *amplitude* of the *T waves*) on EKG signals as small as one-millionth of a volt. Microvolt T-wave alternans is defined as an alternation in the morphology of the T-wave in an every-other-beat pattern. It has long been associated with ventricular arrhythmias and sudden death. T-wave alternans is linked to the rapid onset of ventricular tachyarrhythmias.

MTWA is significant in the clinical context because it acts as a risk stratifier between patients who need implantable cardiac defibrillators (ICDs) and those who do not. Patients who test negative for MTWA have a very low risk for sudden cardiac death and are less likely to require implantable cardiac defibrillators than those who test positive.

In this test, high-fidelity EKG leads are placed on the patient's chest during an exercise test. The goal is to get the patient walking fast enough to get the heart rate in the range of 105 to 110 beats/min, but no higher. Minute changes in T waves are measured and recorded via computer analysis.

INTERFERING FACTORS

- Inaccurate placement of the electrodes
- Electrolyte imbalances
- Poor contact between the skin and the electrodes
- Movement or muscle tremors (twitching) during the test
- Drugs that can affect results include barbiturates, digitalis, and quinidine.

PROCEDURE AND PATIENT CARE

Before

- Explain the procedure to the patient.
- Tell the patient that no food or fluid restriction is necessary.
- Assure the patient that the flow of electric current is from the patient. He or she will feel nothing during this procedure.
- Expose only the patient's chest, arms, and lower legs. Keep the abdomen and thighs adequately covered.

During

- Note the following procedural steps:
  1. The skin areas designated for electrode placement are prepared by using alcohol swabs or sandpaper to remove skin oil or debris. Sometimes the skin is shaved if the patient has a large amount of hair.
  2. Prelubricated leads are applied to ensure electrical conduction between the skin and the electrodes.
  3. The four limb leads are usually held in place by clamps that can easily be opened and applied to the extremity.
  4. Many cardiologists recommend that arm electrodes be placed on the upper arm, because fewer muscle tremors are detected there.

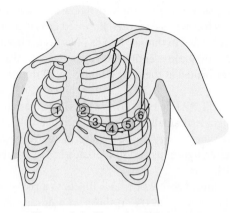

Figure 3-4 Chest lead placement.

5. The chest leads are applied one at a time, three at a time, or six at a time, depending on the type of EKG machine used. These leads are positioned (Figure 3-4) as follows:

V_1: in the fourth intercostal space (4 ICS) at the right sternal border

V_2: in 4 ICS at the left sternal border

V_3: midway between V_2 and V_4

V_4: in 5 ICS at the midclavicular line

V_5: at the left anterior axillary line at the level of V_4 horizontally

V_6: at the left midaxillary line at the level of V_4 horizontally

- Note that cardiac technicians, nurses, or physicians perform this procedure in less than 5 minutes at the bedside or in the cardiology clinic.
- Tell the patient that although this procedure causes no discomfort, he or she must lie still in the supine position without talking while the EKG is recorded.

After

- Remove the electrodes from the patient's skin and wipe off the electrode gel.
- Indicate on the EKG strip or request slip if the patient was experiencing chest pain during the study. The pain may be correlated to an arrhythmia on the EKG.

TEST RESULTS AND CLINICAL SIGNIFICANCE

Arrhythmia (dysrhythmia): *Arrhythmias can start in the atrium or the ventricle. They can cause the heart to speed up (tachyarrhythmias) or to slow down (bradyarrhythmias). With serious arrhythmias, cardiac output can fall significantly, causing the patient to lose consciousness (syncope). Often the patient may experience palpitations during some arrhythmias. Most arrhythmias are asymptomatic, however.*

Acute MI,

Myocardial ischemia,

Old MI:

    Acute myocardial muscle damage is often seen as elevations in the ST segment or as inverted T waves. Old MIs (or areas of dead muscle tissue) appear as deep Q waves on the EKG. The EKG should be one of the first tests to be performed on an adult patient who complains of chest pain.

Conduction defects,

Conduction system disease,

TABLE 3-2	Electrolyte Abnormalities and Associated EKG Abnormalities
Electrolyte Abnormality	**EKG Abnormality**
Increased calcium	Prolonged PR interval Shortened QT interval
Decreased calcium	Prolonged QT interval
Increased potassium	Narrowed, elevated T waves AV conduction changes Widened QRS complex
Decreased potassium	Prolonged U wave Prolonged QT interval

Wolff-Parkinson-White syndrome:
> *The number and type of conduction defects are too great to discuss within the scope of this book. Some conduction defects slow the normal conduction of electrical voltage through the heart (e.g., bundle branch block). Some (e.g., Wolff-Parkinson-White syndrome) speed up the electrical conduction.*

Ventricular hypertrophy: *As a result of prolonged strain on the left ventricle (e.g., aortic stenosis), the thickened myocardium produces large R waves in V5 and V6 and large S waves in V1.*

Cor pulmonale,

Pulmonary embolus:
> *The right heart strain associated with acute pulmonary diseases (e.g., embolism) is called acute cor pulmonale. The classic EKG findings are "S1 Q3 T3," which means the presence of an S wave in lead I, a Q wave in lead III, and T wave inversion in lead III. Many times, however, there may be no changes other than tachycardia associated with pulmonary emboli.*

Electrolyte imbalance: *Each electrolyte abnormality is associated with different EKG changes (Table 3-2).*

Pericarditis: *The EKG findings of pericarditis are classic for that disease. There are widespread elevations of the ST segments involving most of the leads (except aVR). The QRS complexes are normal. When effusion is associated with the pericarditis, the voltages are diminished throughout.*

RELATED TESTS

Echocardiography (p. 877). This is another method of imaging the heart with the use of ultrasound.
Cardiac Nuclear Scan (p. 791). This is a nuclear method of cardiac imaging.

Electroencephalography (Electroencephalogram [EEG])

NORMAL FINDINGS

Normal frequency, amplitude, and characteristics of brain waves

INDICATIONS

This electrodiagnostic test is performed to identify and evaluate patients with seizures. Pathologic conditions involving the brain cortex (such as tumors, infarction) can also be detected. The EEG is also a confirmatory test for determination of brain death.

TEST EXPLANATION

The EEG is a graphic recording of the electrical activity of the brain. EEG electrodes are placed on the scalp overlying multiple areas of the brain to detect and record electrical impulses within the brain. This study is invaluable in the investigation of epileptic states, in which the focus of seizure activity is characterized by rapid, spiking waves seen on the graph. Patients with cerebral lesions (e.g., tumors, infarctions) will have abnormally slow EEG waves, depending on the size and location of the lesion. Because this study determines the overall electrical activity of the brain, it can be used to evaluate trauma and drug intoxication and also to determine cerebral death in comatose patients.

The EEG also can be used to monitor the electrophysiologic effects of cerebral blood flow during surgical procedures. For example, during carotid endarterectomy, the carotid vessel must be temporarily occluded. When this surgery is performed with the patient under general anesthesia, the EEG can be used for the early detection of cerebral tissue ischemia, which would indicate that continued carotid occlusion will result in a cerebrovascular accident (stroke) syndrome. Temporary shunting of the blood during the surgery is then required.

Electrocorticography (ECoG) is a form of EEG performed during craniotomy in which electrodes are placed directly on the exposed surface of the brain to record electrical activity from the cerebral cortex. ECoG is currently considered to be the "gold standard" for defining epileptogenic zones before attempts at surgical interruption are carried out. This procedure is invasive. The same information can be obtained by a noninvasive brain imaging technique called *magnetoencephalography (MEG)*.

MEG measures the magnetic fields produced by electrical activity in the brain with an extremely sensitive device called a superconducting quantum interference device (SQID). The data obtained by MEG are commonly used to assist neurosurgeons in localizing pathology or defining sites of origin for epileptic seizures. MEG is also used in localizing important adjacent cortical areas for surgical planning in patients with brain tumors or intractable epilepsy. This allows the surgeon to identify and avoid injury of important nearby cortical tissue that, if injured, would cause grave neurologic defects (such as blindness, aphasia, or loss of sensation).

INTERFERING FACTORS

- Fasting may cause hypoglycemia, which could modify the EEG pattern.
- Drinks containing caffeine (e.g., coffee, tea, cocoa, cola) interfere with the test results.
- Body and eye movements during the test can cause changes in the brain wave patterns.
- Lights (especially bright or flashing) can alter test results.
- Drugs that may affect test results include sedatives.

✓ Clinical Priorities

- The patient should not be in the fasting state during this test. Hypoglycemia could modify the EEG pattern.
- Stimulants (such as coffee, tea, cola) should not be taken before testing because of their stimulating effects.
- Sleep may need to be shortened if a sleep EEG will be attempted.

PROCEDURE AND PATIENT CARE

Before

- Explain the procedure to the patient.
- Assure the patient that this test cannot "read the mind" or detect senility.
- Assure the patient that the flow of electrical activity is *from* the patient. He or she will not feel anything during the test.
- Instruct the patient to wash his or her hair the night before the test. No oils, sprays, or lotion should be used.
- Check if the physician wants the patient to discontinue any medications before the study. (Anticonvulsants should be taken unless contraindicated by the physician.)
- Instruct the patient if sleeping time should be shortened the night before the test. Adults may not be allowed to sleep more than 4 or 5 hours, and children not more than 5 to 7 hours, if a sleep EEG will be attempted at the time of testing.
- Do not administer any sedatives or hypnotics before the test because they will cause abnormal waves on the EEG.
- Tell the patient not to fast before the study. Fasting may cause hypoglycemia, which could alter test results.
- Instruct the patient not to drink any coffee, tea, cocoa, or cola on the morning of the test because of their stimulating effect.
- Tell the patient that he or she needs to remain still during the test. Any movement, including opening the eyes, will create interference and alter the EEG recording.

During

- Note the following procedural steps:
  1. The EEG is usually performed in a specially constructed room that is shielded from outside disturbances.
  2. The patient is placed in a supine position on a bed or reclining on a chair.
  3. Sixteen or more electrodes are applied to the scalp with electrode paste in a specified pattern (as determined by the *10-20 system*) over both sides of the head, covering the prefrontal, frontal, temporal, parietal, and occipital areas (Figures 3-5 and 3-6). In some laboratories the electrodes are tiny needles superficially placed in the skin of the scalp.
  4. One electrode may be applied to each earlobe for grounding.
  5. After the electrodes are applied, the patient is instructed to lie still with his or her eyes closed.
  6. The technician continuously observes the patient during the EEG recording for any movements that could alter results.
  7. Approximately every 5 minutes the recording is interrupted to permit the patient to move if desired.
- In addition to the resting EEG, note that the following *activating procedures* can be performed:
  1. The patient is *hyperventilated* (asked to breathe deeply 20 times a minute for 3 minutes) to induce alkalosis and cerebral vasoconstriction, which can activate otherwise hidden abnormalities.
  2. *Photostimulation* is performed by flashing a light at variable speeds over the patient's face with the eyes opened or closed. Photostimulated seizure activity may be seen on the EEG.
  3. A *sleep* EEG may be performed to aid in the detection of some abnormal brain waves that are seen only if the patient is sleeping (e.g., frontal lobe epilepsy). The sleep EEG is performed after orally administering a sedative or hypnotic. A recording is performed while the patient is falling asleep, while the patient is asleep, and while the patient is waking.

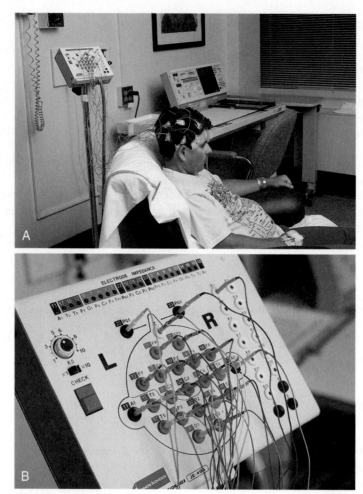

Figure 3-5 Electroencephalography (EEG). A routine EEG takes approximately 1¼ hours. The actual test lasts approximately 30 minutes. Electrodes are attached to the patient's head (**A**) with the wires leading to corresponding areas on the equipment (**B**) for recording brain wave activity.

• Note that this study is performed by an EEG technician in approximately 45 minutes to 2 hours.

🖎 Tell the patient that no discomfort is associated with this study, other than possibly missing sleep.

After

• Help the patient to remove the electrode paste. The paste may be removed with acetone or witch hazel.

🖎 Instruct the patient to shampoo the hair.

• Ensure safety precautions until the effects of any sedatives have worn off. Keep the bed's side rails up.

🖎 Tell the patient who has had a sleep EEG not to drive home alone.

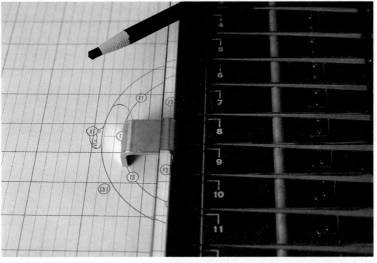

Figure 3-6 Equipment used to record brain waves during EEG.

BOX 3-4	**Criteria for Brain Death**

- Absence of hypothermia (temperature greater than 32.2° C)
- Absence of neuromuscular blockade administration
- Absence of possibility of drug- or metabolic-induced coma
- Absence of response to painful or other noxious stimuli
- Confirmatory tests (not necessary, but helpful)
  - Cerebral flow study indicating no blood flow to the brain
  - Isoelectric EEG (may be repeated in 6 hours)
- No attempt at respiration with a Pco_2 of >50 mm Hg
- No brainstem reflexes
  - Fixed pupils
  - No corneal reflexes

TEST RESULTS AND CLINICAL SIGNIFICANCE

Seizure disorders (e.g., epilepsy): *Major, minor, and focal motor seizures can be detected by the EEG only when they are occurring. Between seizures the EEG may be normal.*

Brain tumor,

Brain abscess,

Intracranial hemorrhage,

Cerebral infarct:
   Most pathologic areas of the brain exhibit localized slowing of brain waves.

Cerebral death: *Cerebral death is total cessation of brain blood flow and function while the patient is being ventilated. The EEG is flat, that is, there is no electrical activity. Box 3-4 lists the criteria for brain death.*

Encephalitis: *Diffuse global slowing of the EEG waves may be noted.*

Narcolepsy: *Sleep waves are noted during what are normally waking hours.*

Metabolic encephalopathy: *This may be drug induced or may occur with hypoxia (e.g., after a cardiac arrest), hypoglycemia, etc. The EEG usually shows diffuse slowing of electrical activity.*

RELATED TEST

Evoked Potential Studies (p. 562). These tests are used to evaluate specific areas of the cortex that receive incoming stimulus from the eyes, ears, and lower- or upper-extremity sensory nerves.

Electromyography (EMG)

NORMAL FINDINGS

No evidence of neuromuscular abnormalities

INDICATIONS

This test is used in the evaluation of patients with diffuse or localized muscle weakness/atrophy. Combined with electroneurography, EMG can identify primary muscle diseases and differentiate them from primary neurologic pathologic conditions.

This test is also used to evaluate the peripheral nervous system in patients with paresthesias and neurogenic pain.

TEST EXPLANATION

By placing a recording electrode into a skeletal muscle, one can monitor the electrical activity of a skeletal muscle in a way very similar to electrocardiography. The electrical activity is displayed on an oscilloscope as an electrical waveform. An audio electrical amplifier can be added to the system so that both the appearance and sound of the electrical potentials can be analyzed and compared simultaneously. EMG is used to detect primary muscular disorders as well as muscular abnormalities caused by other system diseases (e.g., nerve dysfunction, sarcoidosis, paraneoplastic syndrome).

Spontaneous muscle movement, such as fibrillation and fasciculation, can be detected during EMG. When evident, these waveforms indicate injury or disease of the nerve or muscle being evaluated. A decrease in the number of muscle fibers able to contract is typically observed with peripheral nerve damage. This study is usually done in conjunction with nerve conduction studies (p. 574) and also may be called electromyoneurography.

The EMG is performed by a physiatrist, musculoskeletal physician, or neurologist in approximately 30 to 60 minutes. The small needle size helps reduce discomfort.

CONTRAINDICATIONS

- Some patients who are receiving aggressive anticoagulant therapy, because the electrodes may induce intramuscular bleeding
- Patients with skin infection, because the electrodes may penetrate the infected skin and spread the infection to the muscle

POTENTIAL COMPLICATIONS

- Rarely, hematoma at the needle insertion site

INTERFERING FACTORS

- Edema, hemorrhage, or thick subcutaneous fat can interfere with the transmission of electrical waves to the electrodes and alter test results.
- Patients with excessive pain that precludes the patient's ability to relax

Clinical Priorities

- This test cannot be done on patients receiving anticoagulation therapy because the electrodes may induce bleeding.
- Slight discomfort may occur with insertion of the needle electrodes into the muscle.
- If ordered, serum enzyme tests (e.g., aspartate aminotransferase [AST], lactic dehydrogenase [LDH], creatine phosphokinase [CPK]) should be done 5 to 10 days after EMG because penetration of the muscle may cause misleading elevations of the enzymes.

PROCEDURE AND PATIENT CARE

Before

- Explain the procedure to the patient. Allay any fears and allow the patient to express concerns.
- Obtain informed consent if required by the institution.
- Tell the patient that fasting is not usually required; however, some facilities may restrict stimulants (coffee, tea, cocoa, cola, cigarettes) for 2 to 3 hours before the test.
- If serum enzyme tests (e.g., aspartate aminotransferase [AST], creatine phosphokinase [CPK], lactic dehydrogenase [LDH]) are ordered, the specimen should be drawn before EMG or 5 to 10 days afterward because the penetration of the muscle by the electrodes may cause misleading elevations of these enzymes, which can be produced by the muscle tissue.
- Premedication or sedation is usually avoided because of the need for patient cooperation. The small needle size makes the test nearly painless.

During

- Note the following procedural steps:
  1. This study is usually done in an EMG laboratory. This may be specially designed (with copper-lined walls) to minimize extraneous electrical activity.
  2. The patient's position and the position of the electrode depend on the muscle being studied.
  3. A tiny needle that acts as a reference electrode is inserted into the muscle being examined (Figure 3-7) or overlying the nerve itself. In most circumstances, however, that reference electrode is in the needle itself.
  4. A reference electrode is placed nearby on the skin surface.
  5. The patient is asked to keep the muscle at rest.
  6. The oscilloscope display is viewed for any evidence of spontaneous electrical activity, such as fasciculation or fibrillation.
  7. The patient is asked to contract the muscle slowly and progressively.
  8. The electrical waves produced are examined for their number, form, and amplitude. This evaluates the muscular component of the test.
  9. Next, a nerve innervating a particular muscle group is stimulated, and the resulting muscle contraction is evaluated as described if nerve conduction studies are performed concomitantly.

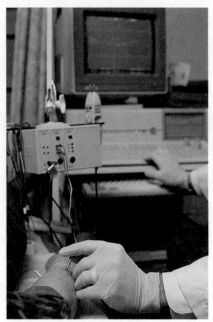

Figure 3-7 Patient having electromyogram (EMG) of forearm. Tiny needle size makes procedure nearly painless.

After

- Observe the needle site for hematoma or inflammation.
- Postprocedure pain medications are rarely needed.

TEST RESULTS AND CLINICAL SIGNIFICANCE

Polymyositis: *This disease is evidenced by early to recruit, small, spontaneous waveforms (myotonia), caused by hyperirritability of the muscle membrane.*

Muscular dystrophy,

Myopathy,

Traumatic injury:

   These primary muscle diseases are denoted by decreased electrical activity and amplitude. Even with nerve stimulation, little or no activity is seen. This indicates weakened muscle tissue.

Hyperadrenalism,

Hypothyroidism:

   These endocrine diseases are marked by decreased electrical activity in both amplitude and frequency. This indicates weakened muscle tissue.

Paraneoplastic syndrome (e.g., lung cancer),

Sarcoidosis:

   These two diseases can be associated with ectopic production of adrenocorticotropic hormone. As in hyperadrenalism, decreased electrical activity in both amplitude and frequency are noted. This indicates weakened muscle tissue.

Guillain-Barré syndrome,

Myasthenia gravis,

Peripheral nerve injury, entrapment, or compression,
Acetylcholine blockers (e.g., curare, snake venom),
Diabetic neuropathy,
Anterior poliomyelitis,
Muscle denervation,
Amyotrophic lateral sclerosis:

> *These neurologic diseases and injuries are indicated by reduced muscle electrical activity with spontaneous contraction. With electrical stimulation, the electrical activity within the muscle is more normal.*

RELATED TEST

Nerve Conduction Studies (p. 574). This is similar to EMG except that it evaluates the integrity of the peripheral nerves. This test is often performed with EMG.

Electronystagmography (ENG, Electrooculography)

NORMAL FINDINGS

Normal nystagmus response
Normal oculovestibular reflex

INDICATIONS

This electrodiagnostic test is used to evaluate patients with vertigo and to differentiate organic from psychogenic vertigo. With this test, central (cerebellum, brainstem, eighth cranial nerve) pathologic conditions can be differentiated from peripheral (vestibular-cochlear) pathologic conditions. If a known lesion exists, ENG can identify the site of the lesion. This test is also used to evaluate unilateral deafness.

TEST EXPLANATION

ENG is used to evaluate nystagmus (involuntary rapid eye movement) and the muscles controlling eye movement. By measuring changes in the electrical field around the eye, this study can make a permanent recording of eye movement at rest, with a change in head position, and in response to various stimuli. The test delineates the presence or absence of nystagmus, which is caused by the initiation of the oculovestibular reflex. Nystagmus should occur when initiated by positional, visual, or caloric (p. 557) stimuli. Unlike caloric studies, in which nystagmus is usually determined visually, with ENG, the direction, velocity, and degree of nystagmus can be recorded. If nystagmus does not occur with stimulation, the vestibular-cochlear apparatus, cerebral cortex (temporal lobe), auditory nerve, or brainstem is abnormal. Tumors, infection, ischemia, and degeneration can cause such abnormalities. The pattern of nystagmus when put together with the entire clinical picture helps in the differentiation between central and peripheral vertigo. This test is used in the differential diagnosis of lesions in the vestibular system, brainstem, and cerebellum.

It also may help evaluate unilateral hearing loss and vertigo. Unilateral hearing loss may be related to middle ear problems or nerve injury. If the patient experiences nystagmus with stimulation, the auditory nerve is working and hearing loss can be blamed on the middle ear.

CONTRAINDICATIONS

- Patients with perforated eardrums, who should not have water irrigation
- Patients with pacemakers

INTERFERING FACTORS

- Blinking of the eyes can alter test results.
- Drugs that can alter results include antivertigo agents, sedatives, and stimulants.

✓ Clinical Priorities

- Various procedures are used to stimulate nystagmus, such as pendulum tracking, changing head position, and changing gaze position.
- Sedatives, stimulants, and antivertigo drugs can alter test results.
- Food should not be eaten before this test to reduce the possibility of vomiting.

PROCEDURE AND PATIENT CARE

Before

- Explain the procedure to the patient.
- Instruct the patient not to apply facial makeup before the test because electrodes will be taped to the skin around the eyes.
- Instruct the patient not to eat solid food before the test to reduce the likelihood of vomiting.
- Instruct the patient not to drink caffeine or alcoholic beverages for approximately 24 to 48 hours (as ordered) before the test.
- Check with the physician regarding withholding any medications that could interfere with the test results.

During

- Note the following procedural steps:
  1. This procedure is usually performed in a darkened room with the patient seated or lying down on an examining table.
  2. If there is any wax in the ear, it is removed.
  3. Electrodes are taped to the skin around the eyes (Figure 3-8).
  4. Various procedures are used to stimulate nystagmus, such as pendulum tracking, changing head position, changing gaze position, and caloric studies (p. 538).
  5. Several recordings are made with the patient at rest and demonstrating patient response to various procedures (e.g., blowing air into the ear, irrigating the ear with water).
  6. Nystagmus response is compared with the expected ranges, and the results are recorded as "normal," "borderline," or "abnormal."
- Note that this procedure is performed by a physician or audiologist in approximately 1 hour.
- Tell the patient that nausea and vomiting may occur during the test.

After

- Consider prescribing bed rest until nausea, vertigo, or weakness subsides.

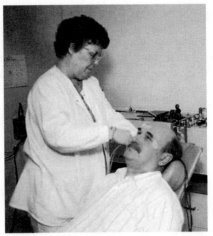

Figure 3-8 Electrodes are applied to a patient in preparation for ENG.

TEST RESULTS AND CLINICAL SIGNIFICANCE

Brainstem lesions,

Cerebellum lesions,

Eighth cranial nerve injury:

Tumors, infection, or degeneration of the central nervous system can be diagnosed, localized, and differentiated from peripheral vestibular diseases.

Vestibular system lesions: *Infection is the most common pathologic condition affecting the peripheral vestibular system.*

Congenital disorder,

Demyelinating disease:

The demyelinating disorders (such as multiple sclerosis) are usually central, whereas the congenital disorders are usually peripheral.

RELATED TEST

Caloric Study (p. 538). This is a test in which nystagmus is stimulated by warm or cold water (or air) and the presence or absence of nystagmus is observed.

Electrophysiologic Study (EPS, Cardiac Mapping)

NORMAL FINDINGS

Normal conduction intervals, refractive periods, and recovery times

INDICATIONS

EPS is a method of studying evoked potentials within the heart. It is used to evaluate patients with syncope, palpitations, or arrhythmias. It is used to identify the location of conduction defects that cause abnormal electroconduction and arrhythmias. It can also be used to monitor antiarrhythmic therapy. Through EPS the area known to induce arrhythmias can be obliterated by radiofrequency waves.

TEST EXPLANATION

In this invasive procedure, fluoroscopic guidance is used to place multiple-electrode catheters through a peripheral vein and into the right atrium and/or ventricle or, less often, through an artery into the left atrium and/or ventricle. With close cardiac monitoring the electrode catheters are used to pace the heart and potentially induce arrhythmias (dysrhythmias). Defects in the heart conduction system can then be identified; arrhythmias that are otherwise not apparent also can be induced, identified, and treated. The effectiveness of antiarrhythmic drugs (e.g., lidocaine, phenytoin, quinidine) can be assessed by determining the electrical threshold required to induce arrhythmias.

EPS can also be therapeutic. With the use of radiofrequency waves, sites with documented low thresholds for inducing arrhythmias can be obliterated to stop the arrhythmias.

CONTRAINDICATIONS

- Patients who are uncooperative
- Patients with acute myocardial infarction

POTENTIAL COMPLICATIONS

- Cardiac arrhythmias leading to ventricular tachycardia or fibrillation
- Perforation of the myocardium
- Catheter-induced embolic cerebrovascular accident (stroke) or myocardial infarction
- Peripheral vascular problems
- Hemorrhage
- Phlebitis at the venipuncture site

INTERFERING FACTORS

Drugs that may interfere with test results include analgesics, sedatives, and tranquilizers.

✓ Clinical Priorities

- In this procedure, fluoroscopic guidance is used to place electrode catheters into the heart to pace the heart and to induce arrhythmias. The effectiveness of antiarrhythmic drugs can be evaluated.
- After this procedure, the patient is kept on bed rest for about 6 to 8 hours to allow the blood vessel access site to seal.
- After this test the patient is carefully monitored for arrhythmias and hypotension.

PROCEDURE AND PATIENT CARE

Before

Instruct the patient to fast for 6 to 8 hours before the procedure. Fluids are usually permitted until 3 hours before the test.

- Obtain an informed consent from the patient.
- Encourage the patient to verbalize any fears regarding this test.
- Prepare the catheter insertion site as directed.

- Collect a blood sample for potassium or drug levels, if indicated.
- Obtain peripheral intravenous (IV) access for the administration of drugs.

During

- Note the following procedural steps:
    1. After being transported to the cardiac catheterization laboratory, the patient has electrocardiographic (EKG) leads attached.
    2. The catheter insertion site, usually the femoral artery or vein, is prepared and draped in a sterile manner.
    3. Under fluoroscopic guidance the catheter is passed to the atrium and ventricle.
    4. Baseline surface intracardiac EKGs are recorded.
    5. Various parts of the cardiac electroconduction system are stimulated by atrial or ventricular pacing.
    6. Mapping of the electroconduction system and its defects is performed by measuring evoked potentials.
    7. Arrhythmias (dysrhythmias) are identified.
    8. Drugs may be administered to assess their efficacy in preventing EPS-induced arrhythmias.
    9. Because dangerous arrhythmias can be prolonged, cardioversion must be immediately available.
    10. Not only are vital signs and the heart monitored, but also the patient is constantly engaged in light conversation to assess mental status and consciousness.
- Note that this procedure is performed by a cardiologist within a darkened cardiac catheterization laboratory in approximately 1 to 4 hours.
- 🖊 Tell the patient that he or she may experience palpitations, light-headedness, or dizziness when arrhythmias are induced. The patient should report these sensations to the physician. For most patients, this is an anxiety-producing experience.
- 🖊 Inform the patient that discomfort from catheter insertion is minimal.

After

- Keep the patient on bed rest for approximately 6 to 8 hours.
- Apply pressure to the catheter insertion site. Evaluate the venous access site for swelling and bleeding.
- Monitor the patient's vital signs for at least 2 to 4 hours for hypotension and arrhythmias (dysrhythmias). Additional monitoring is especially important for certain medications that the patient received during the test. For example, if the patient received quinidine, he or she should be monitored for hypotension and abdominal cramping.
- Continue cardiac monitoring to identify arrhythmias. Transfer arrangements to a monitored unit may be necessary.
- Cover the area with sterile dressings if the electrical catheter is left in place for subsequent studies.

TEST RESULTS AND CLINICAL SIGNIFICANCE

Electroconduction defects,
Cardiac arrhythmia,
Sinoatrial node defects (e.g., sick sinus syndrome),
Atrioventricular node defects and heart blocks,
Inducible arrhythmias (e.g., ventricular tachycardia and Wolff-Parkinson-White):

These arrhythmias and others can be determined by EPS. The site and actual presence could only be guessed before EPS. Furthermore, areas of arrhythmia inducement can be obliterated by burning the tissue with radiofrequency waves.

Vasomotor syncope syndrome

3 Electrodiagnostic Tests

RELATED TEST

Electrocardiography (EKG) (p. 544). This is the only other mechanism available to identify and locate the source of arrhythmia.

Evoked Potential Studies (EP Studies, Evoked Brain Potentials, Evoked Responses, Visual-Evoked Responses [VERs], Auditory Brainstem-Evoked Potentials [ABEPs], Somatosensory-Evoked Responses [SERs])

NORMAL FINDINGS

No neural conduction delay

INDICATIONS

EP studies are indicated for patients who have a suspected sensory deficit but are unable to indicate or are unreliable in indicating recognition of a stimulus. These may include infants, comatose patients, or patients who are unable to communicate. These tests are used to evaluate specific areas of the cortex that receive incoming stimulus from the eyes, ears, and lower or upper extremities' sensory nerves. They are used to monitor natural progression or treatment of deteriorating neurologic diseases (e.g., multiple sclerosis). Finally, they are also used to identify histrionic or malingering patients who have sensory deficit complaints.

TEST EXPLANATION

EP studies focus on changes and responses in brain waves that are evoked from stimulation of a sensory pathway. The study of EPs grew out of early work with the electroencephalogram (EEG) (p. 549). Although the EEG measures "spontaneous" brain electrical activity, the sensory EP study measures minute voltage changes produced in response to a specific stimulus, such as a light pattern, an audible click, or a shock. In contrast to the EEG, which records signals that reach amplitudes of up to 50 to 100 mV, EP signals are usually less than 5 mV. Because of this, they can be detected only with an averaging computer. The computer averages out (or cancels) unwanted random waves to sum the evoked response that occurs at a specific time after a given stimulus.

EP studies allow one to measure and assess the entire sensory pathway from the peripheral sensory organ all the way to the brain cortex (recognition of the stimulus). Clinical abnormalities are usually detected by an increase in latency, which refers to the delay between the stimulus and the wave response. Normal latency times are calculated depending on body size, position of the body where the stimulus is applied, conduction velocity of axons in the neural pathways, number of synapses in the system, location of nerve generators of EP components (brainstem or cortex), and presence of central nervous system (CNS) pathologic conditions. Conduction delays indicate damage or disease anywhere along the neural pathway from the sensory organ to the cortex.

Sensory stimuli used for the EP study can be visual, auditory, or somatosensory. The sensory stimulus chosen depends on what sensory system is suspected to be pathologic (e.g., questionable blindness, deafness, or numbness). Also, the sensory stimulus chosen may depend on the area of brain in which abnormality is suspected. (Auditory stimuli check the brainstem and temporal lobes of the brain; visual stimuli test the optic nerve, central neural visual pathway, and occipital portions of the brain;

TABLE 3-3   Overview of Evoked Potential Studies

Type of Evoked Potential	Targeted Area of Brain/Nervous System	Stimulus	Examples of Clinical Applications
Visual-evoked response (VER)	Optic nerve Central neural visual pathway Occipital area	Strobe light flash Reversible checkerboard Retinal stimuli	Muscular sclerosis Parkinson disease Optic nerve lesions Blindness Gross visual acuity in infants
Auditory brainstem-evoked potentials (ABEP)	Brainstem Temporal lobe	Clicking sounds	Brainstem lesions Hearing disorder in infants Brain tumors
Somatosensory-evoked responses (SER)	Peripheral nerves Spinal cord Parietal lobe	Sensory stimulus to an area of the body	Spinal cord injuries Head injury Malingering Monitor multiple sclerosis treatment

somatosensory stimuli check the peripheral nerves, spinal cord, and parietal lobe of the brain.) Increased latency (i.e., abnormally prolonged period from the time of stimulus to the time of brain EEG recognition) indicates a pathologic condition of the sensory organ or the specific neural pathway as described previously. See Table 3-3.

Visual-evoked responses (VERs) are usually stimulated by a strobe light flash, reversible checkerboard pattern, or retinal stimuli (Figure 3-9). A visual stimulus to the eye causes an electrical response in the occipital area that can be recorded with "EEG-like" electrodes placed on the scalp overlying the vertex and on the occipital lobes. Ninety percent of patients with multiple sclerosis show abnormal latencies in VERs, a phenomenon attributed to demyelination of nerve fibers. In addition, patients with other neurologic disorders (e.g., Parkinson disease) show an abnormal latency with VERs. The degree of latency seems to correlate with the disease severity. Abnormal results also may be seen in patients with lesions of the optic nerve, optic tract, visual center, and the eye itself. Absence of binocularity, which is a neurologic developmental disorder in infants, can be detected and evaluated by VERs. Eyesight problems or blindness can be detected in infants through VERs or *electroretinography*. This test also can be used during eye surgery to provide a warning of possible damage to the optic nerve. Infants' gross visual acuity can even be checked using VERs.

Auditory brainstem-evoked potentials (ABEPs) are usually stimulated by clicking sounds to evaluate the central auditory pathways of the brainstem (Figure 3-10). Either ear can be evoked to detect lesions in the brainstem that involve the auditory pathway without affecting hearing. One of the most successful applications of ABEPs has been screening low-birth-weight (LBW) newborns and other infants for hearing disorders. Recognition of deafness enables infants to be fitted with corrective devices as early as possible. Use of these devices before affected children learn to speak helps prevent speech abnormalities. ABEPs also have great therapeutic implications in the early detection of posterior fossa brain tumors.

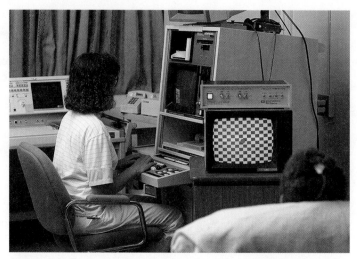

Figure 3-9 Patient undergoing test for visual-evoked responses. The patient is asked to concentrate on the yellow dot in the middle of the screen while the checkerboard pattern moves. Usually a patch is placed over one eye at a time. The room is darkened for the actual procedure.

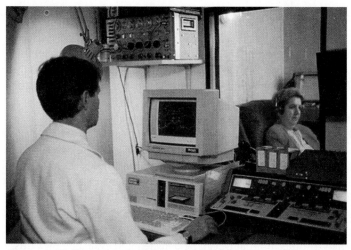

Figure 3-10 Patient undergoing test for auditory brainstem-evoked potentials (ABEPs).

Somatosensory-evoked responses (SERs) are usually initiated by sensory stimulus to an area of the body. The time is then measured for the current of the stimulus to travel along the nerve to the cortex of the brain. SERs are used to evaluate patients with spinal cord injuries and to monitor spinal cord functioning during spinal surgery. They are also used to monitor treatment of diseases (e.g., multiple sclerosis), to evaluate the location and extent of areas of brain dysfunction after head injury, and to pinpoint tumors at an early stage. These tests can also be used to identify malingering or hysterical numbness. The latency is normal in these patients despite the fact that they indicated numbness.

One of the main benefits of EPs is their objectivity, because voluntary patient response is not needed. This makes EPs useful with nonverbal and uncooperative patients. This objectivity permits the distinction of organic from psychogenic problems. This is invaluable in settling lawsuits concerning workers' compensation insurance. The projected future of EPs is that they will aid in diagnosing and monitoring mental disorders and learning disabilities.

PROCEDURE AND PATIENT CARE

Before

🖉 Explain the procedure to the patient.
🖉 Instruct the patient to shampoo his or her hair before the test.
🖉 Tell the patient that no fasting or sedation is required.

During

- Note that the position of the electrode depends on the type of EP study to be done:
  1. For VERs, electrodes are placed on the scalp along the vertex and the cortex lobes. Stimulation occurs by using a strobe light, checkerboard pattern, or retinal stimuli.
  2. ABEPs are stimulated with clicking noises or tone bursts delivered via earphones. The responses are detected by scalp electrodes placed along the vertex and on each earlobe.
  3. SERs are stimulated using electrical stimuli applied to nerves at the wrist (medial nerve) or the knee (peroneal nerve). The response is detected by electrodes placed over the sensory cortex of the opposite hemisphere on the scalp.
- Note that this study is performed by a physician or technician in less than 30 minutes.
🖉 Tell the patient that little or no discomfort is associated with this study.

After

- Remove the gel used for the adherence of the electrodes.

TEST RESULTS AND CLINICAL SIGNIFICANCE

Prolonged Latency for VERs

Parkinson disease,
Demyelinating diseases (e.g., multiple sclerosis):
   Diseases affecting the peripheral and CNS prolong VER latency.
Optic nerve damage: *In the absence of a functioning optic nerve, the stimulus cannot reach the cortex. VER latency will be prolonged or absent.*
Ocular disease or injury,
Blindness:
   Without visual sensory functioning, the stimulus cannot reach the cortex, so stimulus recognition will not occur.
Optic tract disease,
Occipital lobe tumor or cerebrovascular accident (CVA):
   Unilateral or bilateral latency may be noted in diseases that compress or destroy occipital cortical tissue.
Absence of binocularity,
Visual field defects:
   These defects are caused by congenital or acquired diseases, infections, tumors, etc.

Prolonged Latency for ABEPs

Demyelinating diseases (e.g., multiple sclerosis): *Demyelinating diseases destroy the function and integrity of the peripheral and central nervous system. Latency is prolonged.*

Tumor—acoustic neuroma: *These tumors grow where the eighth cranial nerve passes under the temporal lobe. Destruction by compression prolongs latency.*

CVA (stroke),

Temporal lobe cortex,

Brainstem:

    Infarctions of either portion of the brain will prolong ABEP latency. The brainstem is an important part of the reflex auditory mechanism.

Auditory nerve damage: *If the auditory nerve is not functioning, the stimulus cannot reach the cortex. ABEP latency will be prolonged or absent.*

Deafness: *Without auditory sensory functioning, the stimulus cannot reach the cortex. Stimulus recognition will not occur. The test can be performed with vibratory stimuli, however. This bypasses the function of the inner ear.*

Abnormal Latency for SERs

Spinal cord injury,

Cervical disk disease,

Spinal cord demyelinating diseases:

    Because the spinal cord is the path by which the stimulus reaches the cortex, diseases affecting the spinal cord will prolong latency.

Peripheral nerve injury, transection, or disease: *The somatic stimulus must travel by way of sensory peripheral nerves to the spinal cord. Diseases that affect the function of these nerves will prolong latency.*

Parietal cortical tumor or CVA: *Unilateral or bilateral latency may be noted in diseases that compress or destroy parietal cortical tissue.*

RELATED TEST

Electroencephalography (EEG) (p. 549). This electrodiagnostic test is used to detect large electrical waves generated by the cortical structures of the brain and to identify areas of seizure activity or wave slowing compatible with specific pathologic conditions.

Fetal Contraction Stress Test (CST, Oxytocin Challenge Test [OCT])

NORMAL FINDINGS

Negative

INDICATIONS

The fetal CST is a method to evaluate the viability of a fetus. It documents the ability of the placenta to provide an adequate blood supply to the fetus. The CST can be used to evaluate any high-risk pregnancy in which fetal well-being may be threatened. These pregnancies include those marked by diabetes, hypertensive disease of pregnancy (toxemia), intrauterine growth restriction, Rh-factor sensitization, history of stillbirth, postmaturity, or low estriol levels.

TEST EXPLANATION

The CST, frequently called the oxytocin challenge test (OCT), is a relatively noninvasive test of fetoplacental adequacy used in the assessment of high-risk pregnancy. (Other tests used to evaluate the fetoplacental unit are listed in Box 3-5.) For this study, a temporary stress in the form of uterine contractions is applied to the fetus after the intravenous (IV) administration of oxytocin. The reaction of the fetus to the contractions is assessed by an external fetal heart monitor. Uterine contractions cause transient impediment of placental blood flow. If the placental reserve is adequate, the maternal-fetal oxygen transfer is not significantly compromised during the contractions and the fetal heart rate (FHR) remains normal (a *negative* test). The fetoplacental unit can then be considered adequate for the next 7 days.

If the placental reserve is inadequate, the fetus does not receive enough oxygen during the contraction. This results in intrauterine hypoxia and late deceleration of the FHR. The test is considered to be *positive* if consistent, persistent, late decelerations of the FHR occur with two or more uterine contractions. False-positive results caused by uterine hyperstimulation can occur in 10% to 30% of patients. Thus, positive test results warrant a complete review of other studies (e.g., amniocentesis) before the pregnancy is terminated by delivery.

The test is considered to be *unsatisfactory* if the results cannot be interpreted (e.g., because of hyperstimulation of the uterus, excessive movement of the mother, or deceleration of unknown meaning [not associated with contractions]). In the case of unsatisfactory results, other means of evaluation should be considered (ultrasound or amniocentesis).

Although this test can be performed reliably at 32 weeks of gestation, it usually is done after 34 weeks. The CST can induce labor, and a fetus at 34 weeks is more likely to survive an unexpectedly induced delivery than a fetus at 32 weeks. The Fetal Nonstress Test (p. 569) is the preferred test in almost every instance and can be performed more safely at 32 weeks; it can then be followed 2 weeks later by the CST if necessary. The CST may be performed weekly until delivery terminates pregnancy.

Although rarely done, there is a noninvasive, alternative method of performing the CST called the *breast stimulation* or *nipple stimulation technique*. Stimulation of the nipple causes nerve impulses to the hypothalamus that trigger the release of oxytocin into the mother's bloodstream. This causes uterine contractions and may eliminate the need for IV administration of oxytocin. Uterine contractions are usually satisfactory after 15 minutes of nipple stimulation (gentle twisting of the nipples). Advantages of this technique include the ease of performing the test, shorter duration of the study, and elimination of the need to start, monitor, and stop IV infusions. If sufficient contractions do not result from nipple stimulation, the standard CST procedure is followed.

The CST is performed safely on an outpatient basis in the labor and delivery unit, where qualified nurses and necessary equipment are available. The test is performed by a nurse with a physician available. The duration of this study is approximately 2 hours. The discomfort associated with the CST may consist of mild labor contractions. Breathing exercises are usually sufficient to control any discomfort.

BOX 3-5	Tests Used in the Evaluation of the Fetoplacental Unit	
• Alpha-fetoprotein	• Contraction stress test	• Nonstress test
• Amniocentesis	• Estriol excretion	• Obstetric ultrasound
• Biophysical profile	• Fetoscopy	• Pregnanediol

CONTRAINDICATIONS

- Patients pregnant with multiple fetuses, because the myometrium is under greater tension and is more likely to be stimulated to premature labor
- Patients with a prematurely ruptured membrane, because labor may be stimulated by the CST
- Patients with placenta previa, because vaginal delivery may be induced
- Patients with abruptio placentae, because the placenta may separate from the uterus as a result of the oxytocin-induced uterine contractions
- Patients with a previous hysterotomy, because the strong uterine contractions may cause uterine rupture
- Patients with a previous vertical or classic cesarean section, because the strong uterine contractions may cause uterine rupture. (The test can be performed, however, if it is carefully monitored and controlled.)
- Patients with pregnancies of less than 32 weeks, because early delivery may be induced by the procedure

POTENTIAL COMPLICATIONS

- Premature labor

INTERFERING FACTORS

- Hypotension may cause false-positive results.

Clinical Priorities

- The blood pressure needs to be carefully monitored during this test to avoid hypotension, which may cause diminished fetal blood flow and a false-positive test result.
- This test is usually performed after 34 weeks' gestation because it could induce labor.
- The breast stimulation technique is an alternative method of performing the CST that eliminates the need for IV administration of oxytocin.

PROCEDURE AND PATIENT CARE

Before

 Explain the procedure to the patient.
- Obtain informed consent for the procedure.

Teach the patient breathing and relaxation techniques.
- Record the patient's blood pressure and the FHR before the test as baseline values.
- If the CST is performed on an elective basis, the patient may be kept on nothing by mouth (NPO) status in case labor occurs.

During

- Note the following procedural steps:
  1. After the patient empties her bladder, place her in a semi-Fowler's position and tilted slightly to one side to avoid vena caval compression by the enlarged uterus.
  2. Check her blood pressure every 10 minutes to avoid hypotension, which may cause diminished placental blood flow and a false-positive test result.
  3. Place an external fetal monitor over the patient's abdomen to record the fetal heart tones. Attach an external tocodynamometer to the abdomen at the fundal region to monitor uterine contractions.

4. Record the output of the fetal heart tones and uterine contractions on a two-channel strip recorder.
5. Monitor baseline FHR and uterine activity for 20 minutes.
6. If uterine contractions are detected during this pretest period, withhold oxytocin and monitor the response of the fetal heart tone to spontaneous uterine contractions.
7. If no spontaneous uterine contractions occur, administer oxytocin (Pitocin) by IV infusion pump.
8. Increase the rate of oxytocin infusion until the patient is having moderate contractions, then record the FHR pattern.
9. After the oxytocin infusion is discontinued, continue FHR monitoring for another 30 minutes until the uterine activity has returned to its preoxytocin state. The body metabolizes oxytocin in approximately 20 to 25 minutes.

After

- Monitor the patient's blood pressure and the FHR.
- Discontinue the IV line and assess the site for bleeding.

TEST RESULTS AND CLINICAL SIGNIFICANCE

Fetoplacental inadequacy: *Any disease, trauma, or alteration in the fetoplacental unit will cause deceleration of the FHR. This would include maternal causes, placental causes, or fetal diseases (or severe genetic defects).*

RELATED TEST

Fetal Nonstress Test (see following test). This is a preferred method to evaluate the fetoplacental unit. This test is performed in a manner similar to that described for the CST except that oxytocin is not used.

Fetal Nonstress Test (NST, Fetal Activity Determination)

NORMAL FINDINGS

"Reactive" fetus (heart rate acceleration associated with fetal movement)

INDICATIONS

The NST is a method to evaluate the viability of a fetus. It documents the placenta's ability to provide an adequate blood supply to the fetus. The NST can be used to evaluate any high-risk pregnancy in which fetal well-being may be threatened. These pregnancies include those marked by diabetes, hypertensive disease of pregnancy (toxemia), intrauterine growth restriction, Rh-factor sensitization, history of stillbirth, postmaturity, or low estriol levels.

TEST EXPLANATION

The NST is a noninvasive study that monitors acceleration of the fetal heart rate (FHR) in response to fetal movement. This FHR acceleration reflects the integrity of the central nervous system (CNS) and fetal well-being. Fetal activity may be spontaneous, induced by uterine contraction, or induced by external manipulation. Oxytocin stimulation is not used. Fetal response is characterized as "reactive" or "nonreactive." The NST indicates a reactive fetus when, with fetal movement, two or more FHR accelerations are detected, each of which must be at least 15 beats/min for 15 seconds or more within any 10-minute period. The test is 99% reliable in indicating fetal viability and negates the need for the fetal contraction stress test (CST, p. 566). If the test detects a nonreactive fetus (i.e., no FHR acceleration with fetal movement) within 40 minutes, the patient is a candidate for the CST. A 40-minute test period is used because this is the average duration of the sleep-wake cycle of the fetus. The cycle may vary considerably, however.

The NST is useful in screening high-risk pregnancies and in selecting those patients who may require the CST. The NST is how routinely performed before the CST to avoid the complications associated with oxytocin administration. No complications are associated with the NST.

Clinical Priorities

- An NST is routinely performed before the CST to avoid the complications associated with oxytocin administration.
- Fetal activity is enhanced by a high maternal serum glucose level. Therefore the mother should eat before this study.
- If this test indicates a nonreactive fetus, further testing (such as the CST) is indicated to evaluate fetal health.

PROCEDURE AND PATIENT CARE

Before

 Explain the procedure to the patient.

Encourage verbalization of the patient's fears. The necessity for the study usually raises realistic fears in the expectant mother.

If the patient is hungry, instruct her to eat before the NST is begun. Fetal activity is enhanced with a high maternal serum glucose level.

During

- After the patient empties her bladder, place her in the Sims' position.
- Place an external fetal monitor on the patient's abdomen to record the FHR. The mother can indicate fetal movement by pressing a button on the fetal monitor whenever she feels the fetus move. The FHR and fetal movement are concomitantly recorded on a two-channel strip graph.
- Observe the fetal monitor for FHR accelerations associated with fetal movement.
- If the fetus is quiet for 20 minutes, stimulate fetal activity by external methods, such as rubbing or compressing the mother's abdomen, ringing a bell near the abdomen, or placing a pan on the abdomen and hitting the pan.
- Note that a nurse performs the NST in approximately 20 to 40 minutes in the physician's office or a hospital unit.

Tell the patient that no discomfort is associated with the NST.

After

If the results detect a nonreactive fetus, calmly inform the patient that she is a candidate for the CST. Provide appropriate education.

TEST RESULTS AND CLINICAL SIGNIFICANCE

Nonreactive fetus: *This result alone does not indicate fetal distress, but when it is combined with other noninvasive tests such as CST, biophysical profile, alpha-fetoprotein, pregnanediol, and obstetric ultrasound, fetal health can be accurately determined.*

RELATED TEST

Fetal Contraction Stress Test (p. 566). This test is frequently called the oxytocin challenge test. It is a relatively noninvasive test of fetoplacental adequacy used in the assessment of high-risk pregnancy.

Holter Monitoring (Ambulatory Monitoring, Ambulatory Electrocardiography, Event Recorder)

3 Electrodiagnostic Tests

NORMAL FINDINGS

Normal sinus rhythm

INDICATIONS

Holter monitoring is used to record a patient's heart rate and rhythm for one or more days. It is indicated in patients who experience syncope, palpitations, atypical chest pains, or unexplained dyspnea.

TEST EXPLANATION

Holter monitoring is a continuous recording of the electrical activity of the heart. This can be performed for periods up to 72 hours. With this technique, an electrocardiogram (EKG) is recorded continuously on magnetic tape during unrestricted activity, rest, and sleep. The Holter monitor is equipped with a clock that permits accurate time monitoring on the EKG tape. The patient is asked to carry a diary and record daily activities, as well as any cardiac symptoms that may develop during the period of monitoring (Figure 3-11).

Most units are equipped with an "event marker." This is a button the patient can push when symptoms such as chest pain, syncope, or palpitations are experienced. This type of monitor is referred to as an event recorder. Many recorders store the rhythm immediately preceding activation of the recorder. Stored information can be transmitted by telephone to a recording station.

The Holter monitor is used primarily to identify suspected cardiac rhythm disturbances and to correlate these disturbances with symptoms such as dizziness, syncope, palpitations, or chest pain. The monitor is also used to assess pacemaker function and the effectiveness of antiarrhythmic medications.

After completion of the determined time period, usually 24 to 72 hours, the Holter monitor is removed from the patient and the record tape is played back at high speed. The EKG tracing is usually interpreted by computer, which can detect any significant abnormal waveform patterns that occurred during the testing. Two different computer printouts can be generated. The first is generated from an "event recording," in which representative tracings during noted events are printed out. Tracings demonstrating maximum and minimum heart rates are also printed. A report then can be generated regarding the frequency and severity of abnormal cardiac events, especially in relation to the patient's symptoms. The second type of report is generated from a "full disclosure recording," in which all the beats are printed out and are scanned by a technologist, who looks for aberrant waveforms. These aberrations are then provided to the cardiologist for review.

Implantable loop recorders (ILRs) are used when long-term monitoring is required. These recorders are implanted subcutaneously via a small incision. They record electrocardiographic tracings continuously or only when purposefully activated by the patient. The recording device can be automatically activated by a predefined arrhythmia that will trigger device recording. If nothing irregular happens, the information is subsequently erased. But if an arrhythmia does occur, the device locks it in and saves it to memory. ILRs can provide a diagnosis in many patients with unexplained syncope or presyncope.

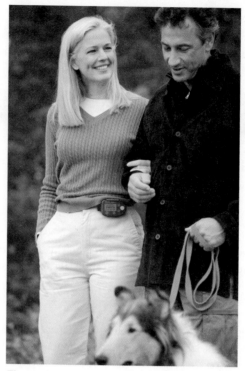

Figure 3-11 Patient wearing Holter monitor.

CONTRAINDICATIONS

- Patients who are unable to cooperate with maintaining the lead placement
- Patients who are unable to maintain an accurate diary of significant activities or events

INTERFERING FACTORS

- Interruption in the electrode contact with the skin

PROCEDURE AND PATIENT CARE

Before

- Explain the procedure to the patient.
- Instruct the patient about care of the Holter monitor (Figure 3-12).
- Inform the patient about the necessity of ensuring good contact between the electrodes and the skin.
- Teach the patient how to maintain an accurate diary. Stress the need to record activities and significant symptoms.
- Instruct the patient to note in the diary if any interruption in Holter monitoring occurs.
- Assure the patient that the electrical flow is coming *from* the patient and that he or she will not experience any electrical stimulation from the machine.
- Instruct the patient not to bathe during the period of cardiac monitoring.
- Tell the patient to minimize the use of electrical devices (e.g., electric toothbrushes, shavers), which may cause artificial changes in the EKG tracing.

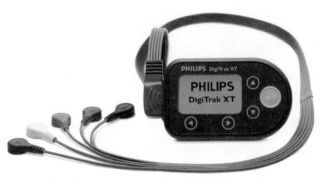

Figure 3-12 Holter monitor.

During

- Prepare the sites for electrode placement with alcohol (this is usually done in the cardiology department by a technologist). (See equipment in Figure 3-12.)
- Securely place the gel and electrodes at the appropriate sites. The chest and abdomen are usually the most appropriate locations for limb-lead electrode placement. The precordial leads also may be placed.
- Usually, do not use the extremities for electrode placement to minimize alterations in tracing that occur with normal physical activity.

 Encourage the patient to call if he or she has any difficulties.

- Use a tight undershirt or netlike dressing to hold the leads in place.

After

- Gently remove the tape and other paraphernalia securing the electrodes.
- Wipe the patient clean of electrode gel.

 Inform the patient when the Holter monitoring interpretation will be available.

TEST RESULTS AND CLINICAL SIGNIFICANCE

Cardiac arrhythmia (dysrhythmia): *Tachycardia or bradycardia may be noted and may be a cause of syncope. Frequent premature beats may be identified.*

Ischemic changes: *If a patient experiences unusual pain symptoms during a particular exercise, a monitor can be applied and that particular exercise performed. If the pain occurs and associated EKG ischemic changes are noted on the monitor, the diagnosis of angina can be made even though the pain is atypical.*

RELATED TEST

Electrocardiography (EKG) (p. 544). This is an electrodiagnostic test of the heart taken at one point in time, whereas Holter monitoring continually records EKG data during the entire monitoring period.

Nerve Conduction Studies (NCS, Electroneurography)

NORMAL FINDINGS

No evidence of peripheral nerve injury or disease (Conduction velocity is usually decreased in elderly people.)

INDICATIONS

This test is performed to identify peripheral nerve injury in patients with localized or diffuse weakness, muscle atrophy, dysesthesia, paresthesia, and neurogenic pain to differentiate primary peripheral nerve disease from muscular injury. NCS can document the severity of injury. It also is used to monitor the nerve injury and response to treatment.

TEST EXPLANATION

Nerve conduction studies evaluate the integrity of the nerves and allow the detection and location of peripheral nerve injury or disease. By initiating an electrical impulse at one site (proximal, when evaluating motor nerves or distal when evaluating sensory nerves) of a nerve and recording the time required for that impulse to travel to a second site (opposite above) of the same nerve, the conduction velocity of an impulse in that nerve can be determined. This study is usually done in conjunction with EMG (p. 554) and also may be called *electromyoneurography.*

The normal value for conduction velocity may only slightly vary. It is always best to compare the conduction velocity of the suspected side with the contralateral nerve conduction velocity. In general, a range of normal conduction velocity for the upper extremities will be approximately 50 to 60 m/sec. For the lower extremities, normal conduction velocity is 40 to 50 m/sec.

Trauma to or contusion of a nerve usually cause slowing of conduction velocity in the affected side compared with the normal side. Neuropathies, both local and generalized, also cause a slowing of conduction velocity. A velocity greater than normal does not indicate a pathologic condition. With complete nerve transection, no nerve conduction is noted.

Because conduction velocity may require contraction of a muscle as an indication of an impulse arriving at the recording electrode, significant primary muscular disorders may cause a falsely slow nerve conduction velocity. This "muscular" variable is eliminated if one evaluates the suspected pathologic muscle group before performing nerve conduction studies. This muscular factor is evaluated by measuring distal latency (i.e., the time required for stimulation of the nerve to cause muscular contraction). As the distal latency is calculated, the motor nerve conduction study is performed normally by stimulating the nerve bundle. Conduction velocity can then be determined by the following equation:

$$\text{Conduction velocity (in meters per second)} = \frac{\text{Distance (in meters)}}{\text{Total latency} - \text{Distal latency}}$$

NCS can also indicate diseases affecting either the motor or sensory nerves. Diseases affecting the neuromuscular junction, nerve axon loss, and variations in nerve recovery time can be evaluated.

NCS takes about 15 minutes and is performed by a physiatrist, neurologist, or trained technologist. It may be uncomfortable because a mild shock is required for nerve impulse stimulation.

INTERFERING FACTOR

- Patients in severe pain may have false results.

PROCEDURE AND PATIENT CARE

Before

- Explain the procedure to the patient. Allay any fears and allow the patient to express concerns.
- Obtain informed consent if required by the institution.
- Tell the patient that no fasting or sedation is usually required.

During

- Note the following procedural steps:
  1. This test can be performed in a nerve conduction laboratory, office setting, or at the patient's bedside.
  2. The patient's position depends on the area of suspected peripheral nerve injury or disease.
  3. A recording electrode is placed on the skin overlying a muscle innervated solely by the relevant nerve.
  4. A reference electrode is placed nearby.
  5. All skin-to-electrode connections are ensured by using electrical paste.
  6. The nerve is stimulated by a shock-emitting device at an adjacent location.
  7. For the evaluation of a motor nerve, the time between nerve impulse and muscular contraction (distal latency) is measured in milliseconds on an EMG machine.
  8. The nerve is similarly stimulated at a location proximal to the area of suspected injury or disease.
  9. The time required for the impulse to travel from the site of initiation to muscle contraction (total latency) is recorded in milliseconds.
  10. The distance between the site of stimulation and the recording electrode is measured in centimeters.
  11. Conduction velocity is converted to meters per second and is computed as in the previous equation.
- Note that this test takes approximately 40 minutes and is performed by a physiatrist, neurologist, or trained technologist.
- This test may be uncomfortable because a mild shock is required for nerve impulse stimulation.

After

- Remove the electrodes and gel from the patient's skin.

TEST RESULTS AND CLINICAL SIGNIFICANCE

Peripheral nerve injury or disease,
Carpal tunnel syndrome,
Poliomyelitis,
Diabetic neuropathy:

With peripheral nerve injury, nerve conduction is reduced. Treatment of the nerve entrapment can improve the nerve function and conduction.

Myasthenia gravis,
Guillain-Barré syndrome:

The extent to which the peripheral nerve is diseased will determine the extent of abnormality of the nerve conduction velocity.

RELATED TEST

Electromyography (EMG) (p. 554). This test is often performed simultaneously with electroneurography to determine distal latency (muscular contraction) and identify muscular disorder as a contributing cause of weakness.

Pelvic Floor Sphincter Electromyography (Pelvic Floor Sphincter EMG, Rectal EMG Procedure)

NORMAL FINDINGS

Increased EMG signal during bladder filling
Silent EMG signal on voluntary micturition
Increased EMG signal at the end of voiding
Increased EMG signal with voluntary contraction of the anal sphincter

INDICATIONS

This test is used to document pelvic diaphragm muscle weakness or paralysis. It is performed most often in patients who have urinary or fecal incontinence. The pathologic condition causing the muscle weakness can be muscular or neurologic.

TEST EXPLANATION

This urodynamic test uses the placement of electrodes on or in the pelvic floor musculature to evaluate the neuromuscular function of the urinary or anal sphincter. The main benefit of this study is to evaluate the external sphincter (skeletal muscle) activity during voiding. This test is also used to evaluate the bulbocavernosus reflex and voluntary control of external sphincter or pelvic floor muscles. The pelvic floor sphincter EMG also aids in the investigation of "functional" or "psychologic" disturbances of voiding. Fecal incontinence caused by muscular dysfunction can also be identified by rectal sphincter EMG.

Three electrodes are used for this procedure. Recordings may be made from surface electrodes or needle electrodes within the muscle; surface electrodes are most often used. These electrodes allow for observation of and change in the muscle activity before and during voiding.

Patient cooperation is essential. If the patient does not cooperate, the interpretation of the test results will be difficult. This test is performed by a urologist, physiatrist, or neurologist in less than 30 minutes. This study is slightly more uncomfortable than urethral catheterization.

CONTRAINDICATIONS

- Patients who cannot cooperate during the procedure

PROCEDURE AND PATIENT CARE

Before

 Explain the procedure to the patient.
 Inform the patient that cooperation is essential.

During

- Note the following procedural steps:
  1. Two electrodes are placed at the 2 o'clock and 10 o'clock positions on the perianal skin to monitor the pelvic floor musculature during voiding.
  2. The third electrode is usually placed on the thigh and serves as a ground.

3. Electrical activity is recorded with the bladder empty and the patient relaxed.
4. Reflex activity is evaluated by asking the patient to cough and by stimulating the urethra and trigone by gently tugging on an inserted Foley catheter (bulbocavernosus reflex).
5. Voluntary activity is evaluated by asking the patient to contract and relax the sphincter muscle.
6. The bladder is filled with sterile water at room temperature at a rate of 100 mL/min.
7. The EMG responses to filling and detrusor hyperreflexia (if present) are recorded.
8. Finally, when the bladder is full and with the patient in a voiding position, the filling catheter is removed and the patient is asked to urinate. In the normal patient, the EMG signals build during bladder filling and cease promptly on voluntary micturition, remaining silent until the pelvic floor contracts at the end of voiding.
9. The electrical waves produced are examined for their number, amplitude, and form.
10. The patient may be asked when there is the first urge to void and when there is a strong urge to void. This is recorded.

After

- If needle electrodes were used, observe the needle site for hematoma or inflammation.

TEST RESULTS AND CLINICAL SIGNIFICANCE

Neuromuscular dysfunction of the lower urinary sphincter,
Pelvic floor muscle dysfunction of the anal sphincter:

> *With overly relaxed pelvic musculature, the frequency and amplitude of the electrical waveform are diminished. This is most commonly seen in older adult women who have had significant muscle stretching during childbirth. It is also seen in patients who have neurologic injury to the nerves innervating the pelvic muscles. The resultant weakness can affect the posterior portion of the pelvic sling and cause anal incontinence. It can affect the anterior portion of the pelvic muscle and cause cystocele, uterine prolapse, and/or urinary incontinence.*

RELATED TESTS

Electromyography (EMG) (p. 554). This test is used to diagnose peripheral muscle pathologic conditions. Theoretically these two studies are similar.

Urine Flow Studies (p. 701). This test is often performed at the same time to evaluate incontinent patients.

CHAPTER

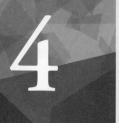

Endoscopic Studies

OVERVIEW

TESTS

 Overview

INDICATIONS FOR ENDOSCOPY

Endoscopy is a general term referring to the inspection of the internal body organs and cavities by using an instrument called an endoscope. Endoscopic procedures are named for the organ or body area to be visualized and/or treated. Table 4-1 provides an overview of body areas viewed by endoscopy.

In addition to direct observation, endoscopy permits biopsy of suspicious tissue, removal of polyps, injection of variceal blood vessels, and the performance of many surgical procedures as indicated in Box 4-1. Furthermore, areas of stricture within a lumen of a hollow viscus can be dilated and stented during endoscopy.

TABLE 4-1	Types of Endoscopies and Areas of Visualization
Type	**Area of Visualization**
Arthroscopy	Joints
Bronchoscopy	Larynx, trachea, bronchi, and alveoli
Colonoscopy	Rectum and colon
Colposcopy	Vagina and cervix
Cystoscopy	Urethra, bladder, ureters, and prostate
Enteroscopy	Upper colon and small intestines
Endoscopic retrograde cholangiopancreatography (ERCP)	Pancreatic and biliary ducts
Esophagogastroduodenoscopy (EGD)	Esophagus, stomach, duodenum
Fetoscopy	Fetus
Gastroscopy (part of EGD)	Stomach
Hysteroscopy	Uterus
Laparoscopy	Abdominal cavity
Mediastinoscopy	Mediastinal lymph nodes
Sigmoidoscopy	Anus, rectum, sigmoid colon
Sinus endoscopy	Sinus cavities
Thoracoscopy	Pleura and lung
Transesophageal echocardiography (TEE)	Heart
Urologic endoscopy (endourology)	Bladder and urethra

Endoscopic Studies

4

BOX 4-1	Endoscopic Surgical Procedures

Laparoscopy
- Cholecystectomy
- Hiatal hernia repair
- Inguinal hernia repair
- Video-assisted colectomy

Pelviscopy
- Oophorectomy
- Video-assisted hysterectomy
- Tubal ligation
- Oophoropexy
- Ovarian cystectomy

Thoracoscopy
- Wedge lung resection
- Video-assisted lung resection

Arthroscopy
- Meniscus removal or repair
- Ligamentous repair
- Tendon repair
- Tendon release (carpal tunnel)

Sinus endoscopy
- Drainage of sinuses

Cystoscopy
- Transurethral resection of prostate (TURP)
- Transurethral resection of superficial bladder tumors
- Removal of ureteral and bladder calculi
- Retrograde cystoscopy
- Ureteral stent placement

Esophagogastroduodenoscopy (EGD)
- Dilation of lumen strictures
- Placement of esophageal stents

Endoscopic Retrograde Cholangio-pancreatography (ERCP)
- Stent placement in the pancreatobiliary tree

Fetoscopy
- Placement of central nervous system (CNS) shunts

INSTRUMENTATION

Endoscopes are tubular instruments with a light source and a viewing lens for observation. The endoscope can be inserted through a body orifice (e.g., rectum) or through a small incision (e.g., arthroscopy). There are two basic types of endoscopes: rigid and flexible. *Rigid metal scopes* were the first type available and are still used in operative endoscopy (e.g., arthroscopy). *Flexible fiberoptic scopes* are most often used in pulmonary and gastrointestinal (GI) endoscopy. An example of a flexible fiberoptic endoscope used in esophagogastroduodenoscopy (EGD) is shown in Figure 4-1. These scopes allow the transmission of images over flexible, light-carrying bundles of glass wires. The scopes contain an accessory lumen(s) for the insertion of water or medication or the suctioning of debris. Also, instruments can be inserted through these lumens to do the following:

- Obtain biopsy specimens (with forceps or brushes)
- Coagulate blood vessels
- Provide laser beams to coagulate vessels or remove tissue

Most often endoscopic procedures are performed via a video chip in the tip of a camera that is placed over the viewing lens. The image is then transmitted in color to a nearby television monitor (Figure 4-2) where body cavities or organs are viewed. This permits others in the room to observe the procedure and more actively provide assistance. In many situations, endoscopy eliminates the need for open surgery.

PROCEDURAL CARE FOR THE ENDOSCOPY PATIENT
PULMONARY AND GASTROINTESTINAL ENDOSCOPY

Endoscopic procedures are generally considered invasive. Client preparation and care are similar to those for most minor surgical procedures. General principles are described in this section. Detailed descriptions are included in this chapter with each individual test.

Before

🖉 Explain the test preparation.

- Ensure that written and informed consent is obtained from the patient.
- Preparation varies with the type of endoscopy to be performed. For example, gastroscopy requires that the patient be kept on nothing by mouth (NPO) status for 8 to 12 hours before the procedure to prevent vomiting and aspiration.

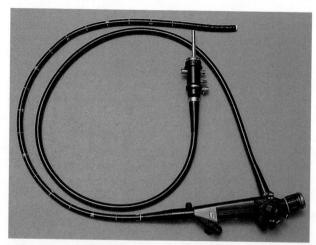

Figure 4-1 Endoscope used to perform esophagogastroduodenoscopy (EGD).

- Dentures should be removed, and loose teeth should be noted and recorded.
- For colonoscopy the bowel must be cleansed and free of fecal material to allow adequate visualization of the mucosa.
- GI endoscopy should precede barium contrast studies. Barium can coat the GI mucosa and preclude adequate visualization of the mucosa.
- Baseline laboratory tests (e.g., measurement of hemoglobin, hematocrit, electrolyte levels) should be performed, especially if a surgical procedure or biopsy is possible.
- A history concerning bleeding tendencies and allergies should be obtained before the procedure.
- Because GI endoscopy is considered clean (not sterile), intravenous (IV) antibiotics are recommended for patients who have cardiac valvular disease (to prevent endocarditis) or patients who have prosthetic joints (to prevent seeding of the joint).

During

- Endoscopic procedures are preferably performed in a specially equipped endoscopy room or in the operating room. However, in cases of emergency, endoscopy can be performed at the bedside.

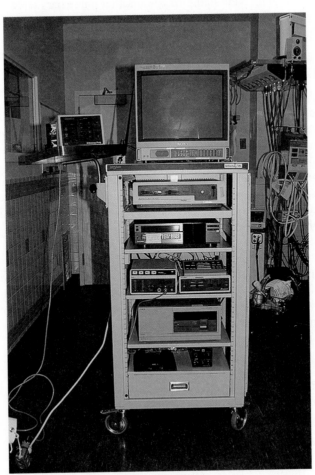

Figure 4-2 Video endoscopy equipment.

- Because sedation is provided, resuscitative equipment should be available.
- Air or CO_2 is instilled into the bowel during GI endoscopy to maintain patency of the bowel lumen and to allow better visualization of the mucosa. If cautery is to be used, the air is exchanged for carbon dioxide to prevent ignition of oxygen or methane inside the bowel.
- Because air or CO_2 insufflation is used, the patient may experience gas pains during the procedure and after the procedure.
- Any surgical or biopsy procedures can be performed.

After

- Specific postprocedure interventions are determined by the type of endoscopic examination performed. All GI procedures have the potential complication of perforation and bleeding. See the discussion of potential complications.
- These procedures use sedation. Safety precautions (such as someone staying with the patient) should be observed until the effects of the sedatives have worn off.
- A family member or friend should drive the patient home after the test.
- After lower GI tract endoscopy, the patient may complain of rectal discomfort. A warm tub bath may be soothing.
- Usually the patient is kept on NPO status for 2 hours after pulmonary endoscopy or upper GI tract endoscopy. Be certain that the swallowing mechanism and cough reflex have returned to normal before allowing fluids or food.

OPERATIVE ENDOSCOPY AND ENDOUROLOGY
Before

- These procedures usually require general anesthesia. Furthermore, complications of operative endoscopy may require open surgical treatment. Therefore the patient must be prepared for general anesthesia and the possibility of open surgery. Routine preoperative care and teaching must be performed.
- The area to be examined should be shaved to remove hair if preferred by the surgeon.
- Because genitourinary (GU) endoscopy is considered clean (not sterile), IV antibiotics are recommended for patients who have cardiac valvular disease (to prevent endocarditis) or patients who have prosthetic joints (to prevent seeding of the joint).

During

- During laparoscopy, CO_2 is instilled into the peritoneal cavity. This may cause significant gas pains and referred shoulder pain postoperatively if not all the CO_2 is allowed to escape.
- During cystoscopy, water is used to distend the bladder to allow visualization of the bladder mucosa. Accurate measurement of intake and output is difficult.
- The appropriate surgical procedure is performed as indicated in each test.

After

- Patients undergoing endoscopic surgical procedures should be monitored in the same way as any postsurgical patient.

POTENTIAL COMPLICATIONS OF ENDOSCOPY

Specific complications depend on the type of endoscopic procedure performed. The following guidelines apply to most types of endoscopies.

Perforation of Organ or Cavity

Examine the abdomen for evidence of organ perforation. Assess for abdominal distention, tenderness, and pain.

Persistent Bleeding from a Biopsy Site

Assess the vital signs. Watch for a decrease in blood pressure and an increase in pulse rate. Inspect body secretions (such as stool, urine, sputum) for blood.

Respiratory Depression as a Result of Oversedation

Carefully assess the patient for respiratory depression. Naloxone (Narcan) may be used to reverse opiates, such as fentanyl or morphine. Flumazenil (Romazicon) may be used to reverse the effects of benzodiazepines, such as diazepam (Valium) and midazolam (Versed).

Infections and Transient Bacteremia

This is a special concern with cystoscopy. Patients need to be encouraged to drink a lot of fluids to maintain a constant flow of urine to prevent stasis and accumulation of bacteria in the bladder. Observe also for signs and symptoms of sepsis, which include elevated temperature, flushing, chills, hypotension, and tachycardia.

Aspiration When Upper Airway or Upper GI Tract Was Evaluated

Instruct the patient not to eat or drink anything until tracheal anesthesia has worn off and the gag reflex has returned.

Cardiovascular Problems

Arrhythmias and even myocardial infarction can result. Vasovagal-induced bradycardia can be treated with atropine.

REPORTING OF RESULTS

Most results are directly observed by the physician performing the procedure. Tissues for biopsy or culture need to be sent to the laboratory for evaluation. Results are discussed with the patient as soon as the effect of any sedation has worn off. However, because the sedation has an amnesic effect, the patient may not recall the results of the test. If possible a written reminder of the physician's findings and instructions should be provided to the patient.

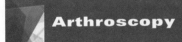

Arthroscopy

NORMAL FINDINGS

Normal ligaments, menisci, and articular surfaces of the joint

INDICATIONS

Arthroscopy is an endoscopic procedure that allows examination of a joint interior with a specially designed endoscope.

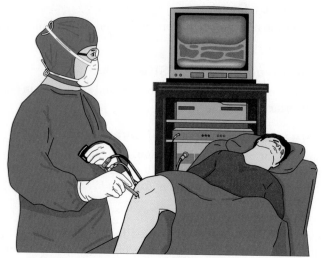

Figure 4-3 Arthroscopy. The arthroscope is placed within the joint space of the knee. Video arthroscopy requires the availability of a water source to distend the joint space, a light source to see the contents of the joint, and a TV monitor to project the image. Other trocars are used for access of the joint space for other operative instruments.

TEST EXPLANATION

Arthroscopy is a highly accurate test because it allows direct visualization of an anatomic site (Figure 4-3). Although this technique can visualize many joints of the body, it is most often used to evaluate the knee for meniscus cartilage or ligament injury. It is also used in the differential diagnosis of acute and chronic disorders of the knee (e.g., arthritic inflammation versus injury).

Physicians can now perform corrective surgery on the knee through the endoscope. Meniscus removal, spur removal, ligamentous repair, and biopsy are but a few of the procedures that are done through the arthroscope. Arthroscopy provides a safe, convenient alternative to open surgery (arthrotomy) because surgery is done through small trocars that are placed into the joint. Surgical maneuvers are carried out under direct vision of the camera that is attached to the arthroscope. Because a large incision is avoided, recovery is faster and more comfortable.

Arthroscopy is also used to monitor the progression of disease and the effectiveness of therapy. Visual findings may be recorded by attaching a video camera to the arthroscope. Joints that can be evaluated by the arthroscope include the tarsal, ankle, knee, hip, carpal, wrist, shoulder, and temporomandibular joints. Synovial fluid can be obtained for fluid analysis (see Arthrocentesis, p. 640).

This procedure is performed in the operating room by an orthopedic surgeon in approximately 30 minutes to 2 hours. Patients receiving local anesthesia have transient discomfort from the injection of the local anesthetic and the pressure of the tourniquet. A thumping sensation may be felt as the arthroscope is inserted into the joint. The joint may be painful and slightly swollen for several days or weeks, depending on the extent of surgery performed.

CONTRAINDICATIONS

• Patients with ankylosis, because it is almost impossible to maneuver the instrument into a joint stiffened by adhesions

- Patients with local skin or wound infections, because of the risk of sepsis
- Patients who have recently had an arthrogram, because they will have some residual inflammation subsequent to the injection of the contrast dye

POTENTIAL COMPLICATIONS

- Infection
- Hemarthrosis
- Swelling
- Thrombophlebitis
- Joint injury
- Synovial rupture

PROCEDURE AND PATIENT CARE

Before

- Explain the procedure to the patient.
- Ensure that the physician has obtained written consent for this procedure.
- Follow the routine preoperative procedure of the institution.
- Keep the patient on nothing by mouth (NPO) status after midnight on the day of the test because general anesthesia is usually required.
- Tell the patient to use crutches after arthroscopy until he or she can walk without limping. Instruct the patient regarding the appropriate crutch gait.
- Shave the hair in the area 6 inches above and below the joint before the test (as ordered).

During

- Place the patient on his or her back on an operating room table.
- Note the following procedural steps:
  1. General anesthesia is usually used to diminish pain and to allow for complete relaxation of the muscles around the knee.
  2. The leg is carefully scrubbed, elevated, and wrapped with an elastic bandage from the toes to the lower thigh to drain as much blood from the leg as possible.
  3. A tourniquet is placed on the patient's leg. If the tourniquet is not used, a fluid solution (usually saline) is instilled into the patient's knee immediately before insertion of the arthroscope to distend the knee and to help reduce bleeding.
  4. The foot of the table is lowered so that the patient's knee can be bent between a 45- and a 90-degree angle.
  5. A small incision is made in the skin around the knee.
  6. The arthroscope (a lighted instrument) is inserted into the joint space to visualize the inside of the knee joint.
  7. Although the entire joint can be viewed from one puncture site, additional punctures for better visualization and surgical maneuvers are often necessary.
  8. After the area is examined, biopsy or appropriate surgery can be performed.
  9. Before removal of the arthroscope, the joint is irrigated. Steroids are sometimes injected to decrease inflammation. Pressure is then applied to the knee to remove the irrigating solution.
  10. After a few stitches are placed into the skin, a pressure dressing is applied over the incision site.

After

- Assess the patient's neurologic and circulatory status.
- Assess vital signs and observe the patient for signs of bleeding or infection.
- Instruct the patient to elevate the knee when sitting and to avoid overbending the knee so that swelling is minimized.
- Inform the patient that he or she can usually walk with the assistance of crutches; however, this depends on the extent of the procedure and the physician's protocol. A referral may be made for physical therapy.
- Tell the patient to minimize use of the joint for several days.
- Examine the incision site for bleeding.
- Apply ice to reduce pain and swelling.
- Inform the patient that the sutures will be removed in approximately 7 to 10 days.

Home Care Responsibilities

- Teach the patient to walk on crutches.
- Educate the patient to observe for signs of bleeding into the joint (significant swelling, increasing pain, or joint weakness).
- Teach the patient to observe for signs of infection of the joint (fever, swelling, drainage, redness about the joint, and increasing pain).
- Educate the patient to observe for signs of phlebitis. This is not uncommon in a person immobilized by joint pain. The involved leg may become swollen, painful, and edematous.
- Instruct the patient not to drive until approved by the physician.
- Ice should be applied at home to minimize the normal swelling that may occur around the involved joint.

TEST RESULTS AND CLINICAL SIGNIFICANCE

Torn cartilage: *Either meniscus (in the knee) is fractured. It may further injure the underlying joint surface.*

Torn ligament: *Ligaments support the joint. Injury to this structure weakens joint stability.*

Patellar disease,

Patellar fracture:

Fracture, inflammation, and malformation can be seen with knee arthroscopy.

Chondromalacia: *Disease or structural damage to the cartilaginous joint surfaces can cause joint pain and dysfunction.*

Osteochondritis dissecans: *Injury to the joint surfaces can occur as a result of joint fragments in the joint space.*

Cyst (e.g., Baker): *This is a synovial cyst behind the knee as a result of synovial fluid herniating into the soft tissue surrounding the knee.*

Synovitis: *This is an inflammation of the lining of the joint.*

Rheumatoid arthritis,

Degenerative arthritis:

Destruction of the articular surfaces causes inflammation in the joint.

Trapped synovium: *Synovial tissue can become trapped between two bones of the joint, causing pain and inflammation.*

RELATED TESTS

Arthrocentesis (p. 640). This procedure is performed by inserting a needle into the joint space to obtain synovial fluid for analysis.

Arthrography. This x-ray test of the joint space provides information about anatomic and disease abnormalities affecting the joint.

Magnetic Resonance Imaging (MRI) of the Knee (p. 1106). This scanning technique provides valuable information by placing the patient in a magnetic field.

Bronchoscopy

NORMAL FINDINGS

Normal larynx, trachea, bronchi, and alveoli

INDICATIONS

Bronchoscopy permits endoscopic visualization of the larynx, trachea, and bronchi by either a flexible fiberoptic bronchoscope or a rigid bronchoscope. Reasons for these procedures are described below.

TEST EXPLANATION

There are many diagnostic and therapeutic uses for bronchoscopy. *Diagnostic* uses of bronchoscopy include the following:

1. Direct visualization of the tracheobronchial tree for abnormalities (e.g., tumors, inflammation, strictures)
2. Biopsy of tissue from observed lesions
3. Aspiration of "deep" sputum for culture and sensitivity and for cytologic determinations
4. Direct visualization of the larynx for identification of vocal cord paralysis, if present. With pronunciation of "eeee" the cords should move toward the midline.

Therapeutic uses of bronchoscopy include the following:

1. Aspiration of retained secretions in patients with airway obstruction or postoperative atelectasis
2. Control of bleeding within the bronchus
3. Removal of foreign bodies that have been aspirated
4. Brachytherapy, which is endobronchial radiation therapy using an iridium wire placed via the bronchoscope
5. Palliative laser obliteration of bronchial neoplastic obstruction

The rigid bronchoscope is a wide-bore metal tube that permits visualization of only the larger airways. It is used mainly for the removal of large foreign bodies. Its use has radically diminished since the advent of the newer flexible fiberoptic bronchoscope.

Because of its smaller size and its flexibility, the flexible fiberoptic bronchoscope has increased the diagnostic reach to the smaller bronchi. It also has accessory lumens through which cable-activated instruments can be used for removing biopsy specimens of pathologic lesions (Figure 4-4). In addition, the collection of bronchial washings (obtained by flushing the airways with saline solution), respiratory hygiene, and the instillation of anesthetic agents can be carried out through these extra lumens. Double-sheathed, plugged protected brushes also can be passed through this accessory lumen. Specimens for cytologic and bacteriologic study can be obtained with these brushes. This allows more

4

Endoscopic Studies

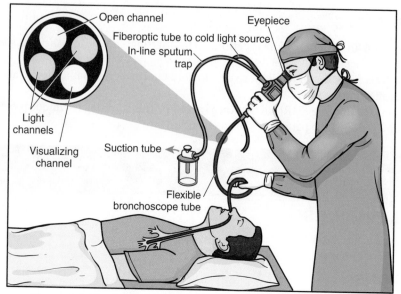

Figure 4-4 Flexible fiberoptic bronchoscope. The four channels consist of two that provide a light source, one vision channel, and one open channel that accommodates instruments or allows administration of an anesthetic or oxygen.

accurate determination of pulmonary infectious agents. Needles or biopsy forceps can be placed through the scope to obtain biopsy specimens from tissue immediately adjacent to the bronchi. Laser therapy can now be performed through the bronchoscope to burn out endotracheal lesions.

This procedure is performed by a physician, usually a pulmonary specialist or a surgeon, in approximately 30 to 45 minutes. No discomfort is usually felt. This test is performed at the bedside or in an appropriately equipped endoscopy room.

Laryngoscopy is often performed through a short bronchoscope to allow inspection of the larynx and perilaryngeal structures. This is most commonly performed by an ENT surgeon. Cancers, polyps, inflammation, and infections of those structures can be identified. The vocal cord motion can be evaluated also. Anesthesiologists use laryngoscopy to visualize the vocal cord structures on patients who are difficult to intubate for general anesthesia. In this instance, the laryngoscope is shaped very much like a rigid scope routinely used to see the vocal cords under direct visualization using retraction of the anterior neck during intubation. This endoscopic laryngoscope, however, is attached to a camera that projects the image of the vocal cords onto a monitor.

CONTRAINDICATIONS

- Patients with hypercapnia and severe shortness of breath who cannot tolerate interruption of high-flow oxygen (Bronchoscopy, however, can be performed through a special oxygen mask or an endotracheal tube so that the patient can receive oxygen if required.)
- Patients with severe tracheal stenosis, which may make it difficult to pass the scope

POTENTIAL COMPLICATIONS

- Fever
- Bronchospasm

- Hemorrhage (after biopsy)
- Hypoxemia
- Pneumothorax
- Infection
- Laryngospasm
- Aspiration
- Cardiac arrest

 Age-Related Concerns

- Children have a smaller bronchus. The bronchoscope can significantly decrease the available space for them to breathe. They are at higher risk of hypoxemia than adults.

PROCEDURE AND PATIENT CARE

Before

- Explain the procedure to the patient. Allay any fears and allow the patient to verbalize any concerns.
- Obtain informed consent for this procedure.
- Keep the patient on nothing by mouth (NPO) status for 4 to 8 hours before the test to reduce the risk of aspiration.
- Instruct the patient to perform thorough mouth care to minimize the risk of introducing bacteria into the lungs during the procedure. Assist if needed.
- Remove and safely store the patient's dentures, glasses, or contact lenses before administering the preprocedural medications.
- Administer the preprocedural medications as ordered. Atropine may be used to prevent vagal-induced bradycardia and to minimize secretions. Fentanyl or versed may be used to sedate the patient and relieve anxiety.
- Reassure the patient that he or she will be able to breathe during this procedure.
- Instruct the patient not to swallow the local anesthetic sprayed into the throat.
- Provide a basin for expectoration of the anesthetic.

During

- Note the following procedural steps for *fiberoptic bronchoscopy*:
  1. The patient's nasopharynx and oropharynx are anesthetized topically with lidocaine spray before the insertion of the bronchoscope. A bite block may be used.
  2. The patient is placed in the sitting or supine position, and the scope is inserted through the nose or mouth and into the pharynx (Figure 4-5).
  3. After the scope passes into the larynx and through the glottis, more lidocaine is sprayed into the trachea to prevent the cough reflex.
  4. The scope is passed farther, well into the trachea, bronchi, and the first- and second-generation bronchioles, for systematic examination of the bronchial tree.
  5. Biopsy specimens and washings are taken if a pathologic condition is suspected.
  6. If bronchoscopy is performed for pulmonary hygiene (removal of mucus), each bronchus is aspirated until clear.

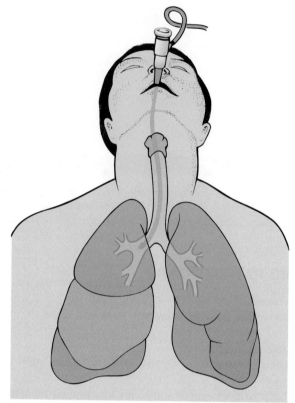

Figure 4-5 Bronchoscopy. A bronchoscope is inserted through the trachea and into the bronchus.

7. Monitor the patient's oxygen saturation to be sure that the patient is well oxygenated. These patients often have pulmonary diseases that already compromise their oxygenation. When a scope is placed, breathing may be further impaired.

After

⬨ Instruct the patient not to eat or drink anything until the tracheobronchial anesthesia has worn off and the gag reflex has returned.

• Observe the patient's sputum for hemorrhage if biopsy specimens were removed. A small amount of blood streaking may be expected and is normal for several hours. Large amounts of bleeding can cause a chemical pneumonitis.

• Observe the patient closely for evidence of impaired respiration or laryngospasm. The vocal cords may go into spasms after intubation. Emergency resuscitation equipment should be readily available.

⬨ Inform the patient that postbronchoscopy fever often develops within the first 24 hours. A low-grade temperature is normal.

• If a tumor is suspected, collect a postbronchoscopy sputum sample for a cytologic determination.

⬨ Inform the patient that warm saline gargles and lozenges may be helpful if a sore throat develops.

• Note that a chest x-ray film may be ordered to identify a pneumothorax if a deep biopsy was obtained.

Home Care Responsibilities

- Suggest that the patient gargle with saline or soothing mouthwash to minimize a sore throat.
- Fever is not uncommon after bronchoscopy. High persistent fever should be reported immediately.
- Bronchospasm or laryngospasm should be reported immediately to emergency personnel.
- Inform the patient that biopsy or culture reports will be available in 2 to 7 days.

TEST RESULTS AND CLINICAL SIGNIFICANCE

Inflammation: *Bronchitis is readily obvious with this method. Cultures can be obtained to identify infections.*

Strictures: *Strictures can be identified and sometimes dilated with this technique.*

Cancer: *Neoplasm of the larynx, bronchus, or lung can be identified, and a biopsy can be performed. The extent of the tumor and its resectability can sometimes be determined. The amount of lung that is required to be removed can be estimated at bronchoscopy. Laser energy can be delivered to diminish the intraluminal size of the tumor. Iridium radiation strips can be positioned accurately at bronchoscopy.*

Hemorrhage: *Hemorrhage can be identified and sometimes controlled by this technique. The source of the hemorrhage can be determined.*

Foreign body: *Often foreign bodies can be removed by fiberoptic flexible bronchoscopy. Large-bore rigid bronchoscopy may be required.*

Abscess: *Pockets of infection can be diagnosed and drained by bronchoscopy. Valuable cultures can be obtained.*

Infection: *Infections can be identified and cultures can be obtained to provide information for treatment. Difficult-to-grow organisms can be better cultured by this technique. This is especially helpful for tuberculosis, fungal infections, and* Pneumocystis jiroveci.

RELATED TESTS

Computed Tomography (CT) of the Chest (p. 1029). This test can visualize the pulmonary, bronchial, and mediastinal structure but cannot be specific about a disease process.

Chest X-Ray (p. 1014). This test is important in the complete evaluation of the pulmonary and cardiac systems.

Colonoscopy

NORMAL FINDINGS

Normal rectum, colon, and distal small bowel

INDICATIONS

This test allows for direct visualization of the rectum, colon, and small bowel. It is used to diagnose suspected pathologic conditions of these organs. It is recommended for patients who have had a change in bowel habits or obvious or occult blood in the stool or who have abdominal pain. It is also used as a surveillance tool for patients who have had colorectal cancer, inflammatory bowel disease, or polyposis.

TEST EXPLANATION

With fiberoptic colonoscopy the entire colon from anus to cecum (and often a portion of terminal ileum) can be examined in most patients. (Table 4-2 lists types of gastrointestinal [GI] endoscopies.) As with sigmoidoscopy (p. 623), benign and malignant neoplasms, polyps, mucosal inflammation, ulceration, and sites of active hemorrhage can be visualized. Diseases such as cancer, polyps, ulcers, and arteriovenous (AV) malformations also can be visualized. Biopsy specimens of cancers, polyps, and inflammatory bowel diseases can be taken through the colonoscope with cable-activated instruments. Sites of active bleeding can be coagulated with the use of laser, electrocoagulation, and injection of sclerosing agents.

This test is recommended for patients who have Hemoccult-positive stools, abnormal sigmoidoscopy, lower GI tract bleeding, or a change in bowel habits. This test is also recommended for patients who are at high risk for colon cancer. They include patients with a strong personal or family history of colon cancer, polyps, or ulcerative colitis. Colonoscopy is also used for colorectal screening in asymptomatic patients without increased risks for cancer. This screening for colorectal cancer has been well defined by several professional organizations such as The U.S. Preventive Services Task Force on Screening for Colorectal Cancer and the American Cancer Society. The recommendations vary slightly, but are summarized in Table 4-3. Virtual colonoscopy (see p. 1020) is now an option.

The test is performed by a physician trained in GI endoscopy in approximately 30 to 60 minutes. It is usually performed in an endoscopy suite or the operating room. Because the patient is heavily sedated, he or she experiences very little discomfort and may not have recall of the procedure.

See p. 1020 for a discussion of a virtual colonoscopy.

CONTRAINDICATIONS

- Patients who are uncooperative: As in all studies that require technical finesse, patient cooperation is essential to successful completion of the test.
- Patients whose medical conditions are not stable: This test requires sedation, which may induce hypotension in medically unstable patients.
- Patients who are bleeding profusely from the rectum: The viewing lens will become covered with blood clots, preventing visualization of the lower intestinal tract.
- Patients with a suspected perforation of the colon: The air insufflated during colonoscopy may worsen the fecal peritoneal soilage.
- Patients with toxic megacolon: The condition may worsen with the test preparation.
- Patients with a recent colon anastomosis (within the past 14 to 21 days): The anastomosis may break down with significant insufflation of carbon dioxide.

TABLE 4-2	Types of GI Endoscopies
Endoscopy	**Portion of Bowel Examined**
Anoscopy	Anus and distal rectum
Proctoscopy	Rectum
Sigmoidoscopy	
Rigid	Anus, rectum, and sigmoid colon to 25 cm
Flexible	Anus, rectum, and sigmoid colon to 60 cm
Colonoscopy	Anus, rectum, and entire colon

TABLE 4-3	Summary of Recommendations for Colorectal Cancer Screening		
Population	**<50 years**	**Ages 50-75**	**Ages 76-85**
Recommendations	Screen only if high risk	Screen routinely	Screen only if high risk and no comorbidity
Testing	Fecal occult blood testing (FOBT) (see p. 857)		
	Fecal immunochemical Testing (FIT) (see p. 857)		
	Sigmoidoscopy		
	Colonoscopy		
	Double contrast barium enema (DCBE)		
	Virtual colonoscopy with computerized tomography (VC with CT)		
Screening Intervals	FOBT annually		
	FIT annually		
	Sigmoidoscopy every 5 years with FOBT every 3 years		
	Colonoscopy every 10 years		
	DCBE every 5 years		
	VC with CT every 5 years		

 Age-Related Concerns

- The elderly should be cautious because of the dehydration and exhaustion that may result from the test preparation. It may be helpful for someone to stay with the older adult patient if this is done on an outpatient basis.
- The elderly may have longer-lasting effects from the sedatives.

POTENTIAL COMPLICATIONS

- Bowel perforation
- Persistent bleeding from a biopsy site
- Respiratory depression as a result of oversedation

INTERFERING FACTORS

- Poor bowel preparation may result in the stool immediately obstructing the lens and precluding adequate visualization of the colon.
- Active bleeding may obstruct the lens system and preclude adequate visualization of the colon.

✓ **Clinical Priorities**

- Patients need to drink large amounts of fluids to preclude dehydration from the test preparation.
- It is recommended that the patient drink the entire gallon of the glycol preparation within 4 hours.
- Nausea and vomiting should indicate immediate cessation of the preparation procedure.
- Patients with valvular heart disease should receive prophylactic antibiotics before the test.

Endoscopic Studies

4

PROCEDURE AND PATIENT CARE

Before

- Explain the procedure to the patient.
- Fully inform the patient about the risks of the procedure and obtain an informed consent.
- Instruct the patient in the appropriate bowel preparation. One type is *the 2-day bowel preparation,* which uses clear liquids for 2 days, along with a strong cathartic such as magnesium citrate and bisacodyl (Dulcolax). On the day of examination, an enema is given. A *1-day preparation* involving a clear liquid diet and using a glycol bowel preparation (Colyte or GoLYTELY) is more widely used. Flavor packets from the manufacturer may improve the flavor. After the patient ingests the glycol solution, enemas are not usually needed.
- The gallon should be consumed within 4 hours if possible.
- Lemonade powder may be added to the glycol cathartic to improve its flavor.
- Avoid an oral bowel preparation in patients with upper GI tract obstruction, suspected acute diverticulitis, or recent bowel resection surgery.
- Assure patients that they will be appropriately draped to avoid unnecessary embarrassment.
- Administer appropriate preendoscopy sedation, usually Fentanyl and midazolam (Versed). Atropine is often ordered to minimize patient secretions.

During

- Note the following procedural steps:
  1. Intravenous (IV) access is obtained for sedation and analgesia.
  2. After a rectal examination indicates adequate bowel preparation, the patient is sedated.
  3. The patient is placed in the lateral decubitus position, and the colonoscope is placed into the rectum.
  4. Under direct visualization, the colonoscope is directed to the cecum. Often a significant amount of manipulation is required to obtain this position.
  5. As in all endoscopy, air is insufflated to distend the bowel for better visualization.
  6. Complete examination of the large bowel is carried out.
  7. Polypectomy, biopsy, and other endoscopic surgery is performed after appropriate visualization.
  8. When the laser or coagulator is used, the air is removed and carbon dioxide is used as an insufflating agent to avoid explosion.

After

- Explain to the patient that air has been insufflated into the bowel. The patient may experience flatulence or gas pains.
- Examine the abdomen for evidence of colon perforation (abdominal distention and tenderness).
- Monitor the patient's vital signs for a decrease in blood pressure and an increase in pulse rate as an indication of hemorrhage.
- Inspect the stools for gross blood.
- Notify the physician if the patient develops increased pain or significant GI bleeding.
- Allow the patient to eat when fully alert if no evidence of bowel perforation exists.
- Encourage the patient to drink large amounts of fluids when intake is allowed. This will make up for the dehydration associated with the bowel preparation.

TEST RESULTS AND CLINICAL SIGNIFICANCE

Colon cancer: *This is seen as a red, friable, fleshy tumor concentrically involving the mucosa of the bowel.*
Colon polyp: *This is a tumor that protrudes from only one part of the mucosa of the bowel. Some cancers and most polyps can be removed with the colonoscope. A biopsy specimen can be obtained from neoplasms.*

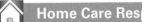

Home Care Responsibilities

- Observe for increasing abdominal pain, which may indicate bowel perforation.
- Inform the patient that frequent, bloody bowel movements may indicate poor hemostasis if biopsy or polypectomy was performed.
- Observe for abdominal bloating and inability to pass flatus, which may indicate colon obstruction if a neoplasm was identified.
- Assess for weakness and dizziness, which may indicate orthostasis and hypovolemia because of dehydration.
- Evaluate for fever and chills, which may indicate a bowel perforation.

Inflammatory bowel disease (e.g., ulcerative or Crohn colitis): *The mucosa of the bowel is red, friable, and thickened. Patients with ulcerative colitis are at great risk for the development of cancer over time. These patients should frequently undergo colonoscopy to identify any cancer or precancerous conditions.*

AV malformations: *These are small red dots on the mucosa of the bowel. They are a common form of bleeding in the adult, especially those with aortic sclerosis and valvular disease. These lesions can be fulgurated by electrocautery through the colonoscope.*

Hemorrhoids: *These are excess fleshy tissue immediately inside the anus.*

Diverticulosis: *This is the presence of diverticula, which are outpouchings in the wall of the colon. Recognition of these abnormalities is important but usually does not require surgical therapy.*

Ischemic or postinflammatory stricture: *This is a fibrotic narrowing of the bowel lumen. Stricture may follow any injury to the bowel. It is a result of fibrosis and scarring that follows an acute insult to the bowel.*

RELATED TESTS

Barium Enema (p. 994). This is another form of visualization of the bowel. It is not as accurate as colonoscopy.

Virtual Colonoscopy (p. 1020). This is a noninterventional method of examining the entire colon by using computerized tomography. Positron Emission Tomography (PET) scan (p. 821) may be added to the CT scan and will add accuracy to this form of colon examination.

Septin 9 DNA Methylation Assay (p. 460). This blood test is used to screen asymptomatic patients for colorectal cancer.

Colposcopy

NORMAL FINDINGS

Normal vagina and cervix

INDICATIONS

Colposcopy is used to identify malignant and premalignant lesions of the vagina and cervix. It is helpful in the more thorough evaluation of abnormal Papanicolaou (Pap) tests.

TEST EXPLANATION

Colposcopy provides an in situ macroscopic examination of the vagina and the cervix with a colposcope, which is a macroscope with a light source and a magnifying lens (Figure 4-6). With this procedure, tiny areas of dysplasia, carcinoma in situ, and invasive cancer that would be missed by the naked eye can be visualized, and biopsy specimens can be obtained. The study is performed on patients with abnormal vaginal epithelial patterns, cervical lesions, or suspicious Pap test results and on those women who were exposed to diethylstilbestrol in utero. It may be a sufficient substitute for cone biopsy (removal and examination of a cone of tissue from the cervix) in evaluating the cause of abnormal cervical cytologic findings (Table 4-4).

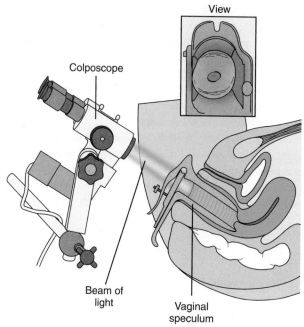

Figure 4-6 Colposcopy. A colposcope is used to evaluate patients with an abnormal Pap test and a grossly normal cervix.

TABLE 4-4	Gynecologic Procedures	
Test	**Advantage**	**Disadvantage(s)**
Colposcopy	Evaluates the vagina and cervix	Cannot evaluate the endocervix
		High false-positive rate
Hysteroscopy	Evaluates the endometrium	Cannot evaluate the cervix and endocervix
Cone biopsy of the cervix	Evaluates the cervix and endocervix	Cannot evaluate the endometrium
Pap test	Evaluates the cervix, endocervix, and endometrium	Misses important pathologic conditions of those tissues and may overread inflammation
		Cannot localize the lesion

It is important to realize that colposcopy is useful only in identifying a suspicious lesion. Definitive diagnosis requires biopsy of the tissue. One of the major advantages of this procedure is that of directing the biopsy to the area most likely to be truly representative of the lesion. A biopsy performed without colposcopy may not necessarily be representative of the lesion's true pathologic condition, resulting in a significant risk of missing a serious lesion.

The patient will need to have diagnostic conization in the following instances:

1. Colposcopy and endocervical curettage do not explain the problem or match the cytologic findings of the Pap test within one grade.
2. The entire transformation zone (between squamous and columnar epithelium) is not seen. This area is also called the endocervix, in which many cancers can initiate.
3. The lesion extends up the cervical canal beyond the vision of the colposcope.

The need for up to 90% of cone biopsies is eliminated with examination by an experienced colposcopist. Endocervical curettage may accompany colposcopy to detect unseen lesions in the endocervical canal.

Colposcopy is performed by a physician, nurse practitioner, or physician's assistant in approximately 5 to 10 minutes. Some women complain of pressure pains from the vaginal speculum, and momentary discomfort may be felt if biopsy specimens are obtained. If the discomfort exceeds that which mild sedation treats, a paracervical block can be performed.

CONTRAINDICATIONS

- Patients with heavy menstrual flow

POTENTIAL COMPLICATIONS

- Infectious cervicitis
- Hemorrhage
- Vasovagal reaction

INTERFERING FACTORS

- Failure to cleanse the cervix of foreign materials (e.g., creams, medications) may impair visualization.

PROCEDURE AND PATIENT CARE

Before

- Explain the procedure to the patient.
- Obtain informed consent if required by the institution.

During

- Note the following procedural steps:
  1. The patient is placed in the lithotomy position, and a vaginal speculum is used to expose the vagina and cervix. An endocervical curettage is performed to minimize any dropping of endocervical cells onto the external surface of the cervix.
  2. After the cervix is sampled for cytologic findings, it is cleansed with a 3% acetic acid solution to remove excess mucus and cellular debris. The acetic acid also accentuates the difference between normal and abnormal epithelial tissues.

3. The colposcope is focused on the cervix, which is then carefully examined. Photographs and rough sketches of the cervix may be created.

4. Usually the entire lesion can be outlined, and the most atypical areas can be selected for biopsy specimen removal.

5. A biopsy can be performed at this time on any abnormality.

After

• The cervix is cleaned with normal saline solution, and hemostasis is ensured.

 Inform the patient that she may have vaginal bleeding if biopsy specimens were taken. Suggest that she wear a sanitary pad.

 Instruct the patient to abstain from intercourse and not to insert anything (except a tampon) into the vagina until healing of the biopsy is confirmed.

 Inform the patient when and how to obtain the results of this study.

TEST RESULTS AND CLINICAL SIGNIFICANCE

Dysplasia: This is visible as a white, sharply bordered lesion after acetic acid is applied.

Carcinoma in situ: This is visible as a pink or reddened well-circumscribed punctate lesion.

Invasive cancer: This lesion is noted by its disarray of blood vessels and a mass effect in the cervix.

RELATED TESTS

Cervical Biopsy (p. 720). A biopsy of the cervix is performed to more accurately identify and treat premalignant and superficial malignant lesions of the cervix.

Papanicolaou (Pap) Test (p. 743). This is a test of the cells that have been shed by the cervix and uterus. Early detection of cancer of the uterus and cervix can be accomplished by routine use of this test.

Conization/Cytology (p. 720). A concentric piece of cervix and endocervix is obtained for microscopic evaluation.

Cystoscopy (Endourology)

NORMAL FINDINGS

Normal structure and function of the urethra, bladder, ureters, and prostate (in males)

INDICATIONS

This endoscopic test is used to evaluate patients with suspected pathologic conditions involving the urethra, bladder, and lower ureters. It is also used to perform a biopsy on and to treat pathologic conditions related to those structures. This procedure is commonly performed for patients with the following problems:

• Hematuria
• Recurrent or resistant urinary tract infections
• Urinary symptoms of dysuria, frequency, urinary retention, inadequate urinary stream, urgency, and incontinence

TEST EXPLANATION

Cystoscopy provides direct visualization of the urethra and bladder through the transurethral insertion of a cystoscope into the bladder (Figure 4-7). Cystoscopy is used *diagnostically* to allow the following:

1. Direct inspection and biopsy of the prostate, bladder, and urethra
2. Collection of a separate urine specimen directly from each ureter by the placement of ureteral catheters
3. Measurement of bladder capacity and determination of ureteral reflux
4. Identification of bladder and ureteral calculi
5. Placement of ureteral catheters (Figure 4-8) for retrograde pyelography (p. 1056)
6. Identification of the source of hematuria

Cystoscopy is used *therapeutically* to provide the following:

1. Resection of small, superficial bladder tumors (transurethral resection of the bladder)
2. Removal of foreign bodies and stones
3. Dilation of the urethra and ureters
4. Placement of stents to drain urine from the renal pelvis
5. Coagulation of bleeding areas
6. Implantation of radium seeds into a tumor
7. Resection of hypertrophied or malignant prostate gland overgrowth (transurethral resection of the prostate [TURP])
8. Placement of ureteral stents for identification of ureters during pelvic surgery

The cystoscope consists primarily of an obturator and a telescope. The obturator is used to insert the cystoscope atraumatically. After the cystoscope is within the bladder, the obturator is removed and the telescope is passed through the cystoscope. The lens and lighting system of the telescope permit adequate visualization of the lower genitourinary (GU) tract. Transendoscopic instruments, such as forceps, scissors, needles, and electrodes, are used when needed.

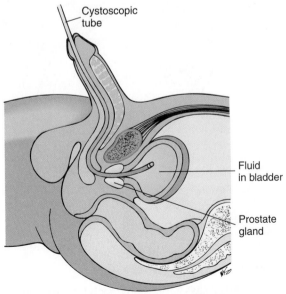

Figure 4-7 Cystoscopic examination of the male bladder.

Endoscopic Studies

4

Endourology is an endoscopic procedure that visualizes the bladder and urethra. It is more comprehensive than cystoscopy because it includes a detailed visualization of the urethra. This test is important in the evaluation of hematuria, chronic infection, suspected stones, and radiographic filling defects. On inspection the urethra may show inflammation or structural causes of obstruction (e.g., stricture, neoplasia, prostatic hypertrophy). If the obstruction is functional rather than structural (e.g., detrusor–bladder neck dyssynergia), no site of obstruction will be demonstrated by endoscopy.

Although usually performed in the operating room using general anesthesia, diagnostic cystoscopy can be done in the urologist's office in about 10 minutes. A flexible scope is used for this. The urethra is anesthetized with an anesthetic gel. The only discomfort felt is when the scope passes through the sphincter. When a rigid scope is to be used for diagnostic or therapeutic cystoscopy, general or spinal anesthesia is used.

POTENTIAL COMPLICATIONS

- Perforation of the bladder or ureters
- Sepsis by seeding the bloodstream with bacteria from infected urine
- Hematuria
- Urinary retention

PROCEDURE AND PATIENT CARE

Before

- Explain the procedure to the patient.
- Ensure that an informed consent is obtained.

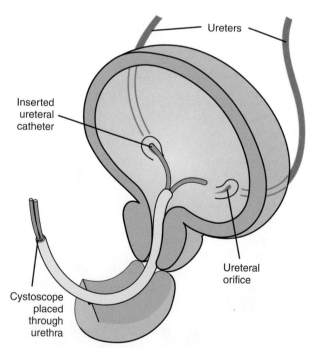

Figure 4-8 Ureteral catheterization through the cystoscope. Note the ureteral catheter inserted into the right orifice. The left ureteral catheter is ready to be inserted.

🖉 If enemas are ordered to clear the bowel, assist the patient as needed and record the results.

🖉 Encourage the patient to drink fluids the night before the procedure to maintain a continuous flow of urine for collection and to prevent multiplication of bacteria that may be introduced during this technique.

• If the procedure will be done using local anesthesia, small volumes of liquids may be acceptable. Verify this with the doctor.

🖉 When local anesthesia will be used, inform the patient of the associated discomfort (much more than with urethral catheterization).

🖉 If the procedure will be performed with the patient under general anesthesia, follow routine precautions. Keep the patient on nothing by mouth (NPO) status after midnight on the day of the test. Intravenous fluids may be given.

• Administer the preprocedural medications as ordered 1 hour before the study. Sedatives decrease the spasm of the bladder sphincter, decreasing the patient's discomfort.

During

• Note the following procedural steps:
  1. Cystoscopy is performed in the operating room or in the urologist's office.
  2. The patient is placed in the lithotomy position with his or her feet in stirrups.
  3. The external genitalia are cleansed with an antiseptic solution such as povidone-iodine (Betadine).
  4. A local anesthetic gel is instilled into the urethra if the patient is not under general anesthesia.
  5. The cystoscope is inserted, and the bladder is distended with saline.
  6. The desired diagnostic or therapeutic studies are performed.

🖉 Instruct the patient to lie very still during the entire procedure to prevent trauma to the urinary tract.

🖉 Tell the patient that he or she will have the desire to void as the cystoscope passes the bladder neck and with bladder distention.

• When the procedure is completed, bed rest should be prescribed for a short time if biopsies were performed.

• Note that this procedure is performed by a urologist in approximately 25 minutes.

After

🖉 Instruct the patient not to walk or stand alone immediately after the legs have been removed from the stirrups. The orthostasis that may result from standing erect may cause dizziness and fainting.

• Assess the patient's ability to void for at least 24 hours after the procedure if the patient is hospitalized. Urinary retention may be secondary to edema caused by instrumentation.

• Note the urine color. Pink-tinged urine is common. The presence of bright-red blood or clots should be reported to the physician.

• Monitor the patient for complaints of back pain, bladder spasms, urinary frequency, and burning on urination. Warm sitz baths and mild analgesics may be ordered and given. Sometimes belladonna and opium (B&O) suppositories are given to relieve bladder spasms. Warm, moist heat to the lower abdomen may help to relieve pain and to promote muscle relaxation.

• The first few times the patient voids after cystoscopy, burning will be felt in the urethra. This may be intense. Encourage men to urinate while sitting to avoid a vagal reaction related to severe dysuria.

🖉 Encourage increased intake of fluids. A dilute urine decreases dysuria. Fluids also maintain a constant flow of urine to prevent stasis and the accumulation of bacteria in the bladder.

- Monitor and record the patient's vital signs. Watch for a decrease in blood pressure and an increase in pulse rate as an indication of hemorrhage.
- Observe for signs and symptoms of sepsis (elevated temperature, flushing, chills, decreased blood pressure, increased pulse rate).
- Note that antibiotics are occasionally ordered 1 day before and continuing through 3 days following the procedure to reduce the incidence of bacteremia that may occur with instrumentation of the urethra and bladder.
- Encourage the patient to use cathartics, especially after cystoscopic surgery. Increases in intraabdominal pressure caused by constipation may initiate urologic bleeding.
- If postprocedure irrigation is ordered, use an isotonic solution containing mannitol, glycine, or sorbitol to prevent fluid overhydration in the event any of the irrigation is absorbed through opened venous sinuses in the bladder.
- If a catheter is left in after the procedure, provide catheter care instructions.

Home Care Responsibilities

- Watch for signs of urinary retention for 24 to 48 hours.
- Watch for signs of bleeding. Pink urine is normal; clots are not.
- Report symptoms of increasing lower abdominal pain immediately.
- Use warm sitz baths or B&O suppositories to reduce bladder spasms.
- Encourage the patient to drink large amounts of fluids.
- Watch for fever, shaking chills, or prolonged dysuria as possible signs of urinary tract infection.
- Stress the importance of taking postprocedure antibiotics if ordered.

TEST RESULTS AND CLINICAL SIGNIFICANCE

Lower urologic tract tumor: *Bladder cancers or polyps are seen as red friable tumors arising from the mucosa. Sometimes noninvasive tumors can be completely removed with the cystoscope.*

Stones in the ureter or bladder: *These can be retrieved through endourologic surgery. If the stones are too large for retrieval, they can be fractured mechanically or with laser or ultrasound.*

Prostatic hypertrophy: *This is a benign lesion that occludes the urethra. Removal of the portion of the prostate blocking the urethra (by TURP) resolves the obstruction.*

Prostate cancer: *This malignant lesion can obstruct the urethra. Removal of the portion of the prostate cancer that is blocking the urethra (by TURP) resolves the obstruction. In the elderly, this is not an aggressive tumor.*

Inflammation of the bladder and urethra: *A red thickened bladder mucosa indicates chronic infection. This may be because of urethral stricture, bladder diverticula, or inadequate bladder function.*

Urethral, ureteral, or vesical stricture: *A fibrous obstruction of the urethra or ureteral opening into the bladder indicates stricture, which is usually benign.*

RELATED TESTS

Cystometry (p. 688). This is a test of bladder function and capacity.

Cystography (p. 1036). This is an x-ray study of the bladder. It is used to identify bladder tumors, leaks, or fistulas.

Ductoscopy (Mammary Ductoscopy)

NORMAL FINDINGS

No tumor or premalignant changes

INDICATIONS

Ductoscopy is used to visualize the breast ducts in women who have nipple discharge. Its accuracy and diagnostic potential depend on the experience of the surgeon and the patient's anatomy.

TEST EXPLANATION

Most breast cancers start in the cells that line the milk ducts within the breast ducts. Mammary ductoscopy refers to a procedure in which a "miniaturized endoscope" is used to get a closer look at the lining of milk ducts of the breast and provide access for biopsy or retrieval of cells lining the ducts.

The mammary ductoscopy consists of a tiny outer sheath with an external diameter only barely larger than a piece of thread. The sheath has two channels. In one channel, the camera light source is inserted. In the other channel, water is injected to dilate the ducts for better visibility. A video/endoscopic camera is attached and the images are projected on a TV monitor through a video system (Figure 4-9). The scope is then advanced to the smallest branches of the milk ducts.

With the use of this technique, breast diseases, including cancers, can be found at their very earliest stages. Ductoscopy can identify cancers so small that mammography, ultrasound, or even magnetic resonance imaging (MRI) cannot see them. With this technique, premalignant changes can be identified and treated in an attempt to prevent breast cancer. Mammary ductoscopy is used as a diagnostic technique in women with nipple discharge.

Ductal lavage (p. 645) is a technique used to obtain and identify premalignant atypical cells from breast ducts in patients who are considered high risk for cancer and who have no evidence of breast

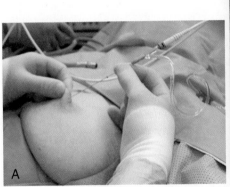
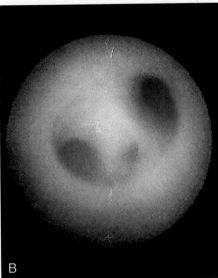

Figure 4-9 **A,** Ductoscope is passed into the breast nipple. **B,** Image of normal ducts in the breast.

malignancy on mammogram or ultrasound. Ductoscopy is used to look into these ducts in the hopes of identifying the causes of those changes (e.g., intraductal papillomas or early cancers) in these ducts and possibly delivering ablative therapies to eradicate them.

INTERFERING FACTORS

- The inability to access the duct (e.g., narrowed or convoluted) precludes performance of this endoscopic procedure.

PROCEDURE AND PATIENT CARE

Before

- Explain the procedure to the patient.
- Be sure the breast exam and mammogram are normal.
- Obtain informed consent.
- If the procedure is to be performed under general anesthesia, keep the patient on nothing by mouth (NPO) status for at least 8 hours.
- If the procedure is to be performed under local anesthesia, apply a topical anesthetic to the nipple area for about 30 to 60 minutes before the test.

During

- Note the following procedural steps:
  1. The breast is massaged to promote the discharge of nipple fluid. This helps to visually identify the ductal orifice in the nipple for endoscopy.
  2. The ductal opening in the nipple is gently dilated with increasing sized tiny dilators, and the mammary sheath containing the ductoscope is inserted and advanced under direct visualization as saline is injected to dilate the branches of the duct for visualization.
  3. The ductoscopy findings can be recorded by videotape.
  4. If any disease is identified, the scope can lead the surgeon directly to the area for directed surgical removal.
  5. Ductal washings can also be obtained by aspiring some of the fluid for microscopic analysis.
- This procedure is usually performed by a surgeon in the office in approximately 30 minutes.

After

- Inform the patient to contact the physician is she develops any redness, breast pain, or elevated temperature that may indicate mastitis.

TEST RESULTS AND CLINICAL SIGNIFICANCE

Invasive ductal cancer: *This is usually only evident by complete obstruction of the breast ducts.*
Noninvasive ductal cancer,
Atypical ductal hyperplasia:
   These diseases are evident by changes in the epithelial lining of the breast ducts.
Papilloma: *This is a small polypoid tumor projecting into the breast duct lumen.*

RELATED TEST

Breast Ductal Lavage (p. 645). With this procedure the breast ducts are flushed. Cells are obtained for cytology to identify malignant or premalignant cells.

Endoscopic Retrograde Cholangiopancreatography (ERCP, ERCP of the Biliary and Pancreatic Ducts)

NORMAL FINDINGS

Normal size of biliary and pancreatic ducts
No obstruction or filling defects within the biliary or pancreatic ducts

INDICATIONS

This test is used in the evaluation of the jaundiced patient. It is also used to evaluate patients with unexplained upper abdominal pain or pancreatitis.

TEST EXPLANATION

With the use of a fiberoptic endoscope, ERCP provides radiographic visualization of the bile and pancreatic ducts. This is especially useful in patients with jaundice. If a partial or total obstruction of those ducts exists, characteristics of the obstructing lesion can be demonstrated. Stones, benign strictures, cysts, ampullary stenosis, anatomic variations, and malignant tumors can be identified. Only ERCP and percutaneous transhepatic cholangiography (PTHC) can provide direct radiographic visualization of the biliary and pancreatic ducts. PTHC (p. 1053) is an invasive procedure with significant morbidity; ERCP is associated with much less morbidity but must be performed by an experienced endoscopist.

Incision of the papillary muscle in the ampulla of Vater can be performed through the scope at the time of ERCP. This incision widens the distal common duct so that common bile duct gallstones can be removed. Stents can be placed through strictured bile ducts during ERCP, allowing the bile of jaundiced patients to be internally drained. Pieces of tissue and brushings of the common bile duct can be obtained by ERCP for pathologic review.

Manometric studies of the sphincter of Oddi and pancreatobiliary ducts can be performed at the time of ERCP. These are used to investigate unusual functional abnormalities of these structures.

CONTRAINDICATIONS

- Patients who are uncooperative: Cannulation of the ampulla of Vater requires that the patient lie very still
- Patients whose ampulla of Vater is not accessible endoscopically because of previous upper gastrointestinal (GI) tract surgery (e.g., gastrectomy patients whose duodenum containing the ampulla is surgically separated from the stomach)
- Patients with esophageal diverticula: The scope can fall into a diverticulum and perforate its wall
- Patients with known acute pancreatitis, because ERCP can worsen this inflammation

POTENTIAL COMPLICATIONS

- Perforation of the esophagus, stomach, or duodenum
- Gram-negative sepsis: This results from introducing bacteria through the biliary system and into the blood. Usually this occurs in patients who have obstructive jaundice
- Pancreatitis: This results from pressure of the dye injection

- Aspiration of gastric contents into the lungs
- Respiratory arrest as a result of oversedation

INTERFERING FACTORS

- Barium within the abdomen as a result of a previous upper GI series or barium enema x-ray studies precludes adequate visualization of the biliary and pancreatic ducts.

PROCEDURE AND PATIENT CARE

Before

⊗ Explain the procedure to the patient.
- Obtain informed consent from the patient.
⊗ Inform the patient that breathing will not be compromised by the insertion of the endoscope.
⊗ Keep the patient on nothing by mouth (NPO) status as of midnight on the day of the test.
⊗ Tell the patient that no discomfort is associated with the dye injection but that minimal gagging may occur during the initial introduction of the scope into the oral pharynx.
- Administer appropriate premedication (e.g., midazolam [Versed] and atropine), if ordered.

During

- Note the following procedural steps:
  1. A flat plate of the abdomen (see p. 1040) is taken to ensure that any barium from previous studies will not obscure visualization of the bile duct.
  2. The patient is placed in the supine position or on the left side.
  3. The patient is usually sedated with a narcotic and a sedative/hypnotic.
  4. The pharynx is sprayed with a local anesthetic (lidocaine) to inactivate the gag reflex and to lessen the discomfort caused by the passage of the scope.
  5. A side-viewing fiberoptic duodenoscope is inserted through the oral pharynx and passed through the esophagus and stomach and into the duodenum (Figure 4-10). A bite block may be used.

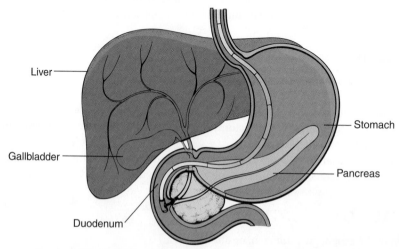

Figure 4-10 Endoscopic retrograde cholangiopancreatography (ERCP). The fiberoptic scope is passed into the duodenum. Note the small catheter being advanced into the biliary duct.

6. Glucagon is often administered intravenously to minimize the spasm of the duodenum and to improve visualization of the ampulla of Vater. Simethicone may be instilled to diminish any bubbles present that may inhibit visualization of the ampulla.

7. Through the accessory lumen within the scope, a small catheter is passed through the ampulla and into the common bile or pancreatic ducts.

8. Radiographic dye is injected, and x-ray images are taken.

- Note that the test usually takes approximately 1 hour and is performed by a physician trained in endoscopy. The x-ray images are interpreted by the radiologist.

After

 Do not allow the patient to eat or drink until the gag reflex returns to prevent aspiration.

- Observe the patient closely for development of abdominal pain, nausea, and vomiting. This may herald the onset of ERCP-induced pancreatitis.
- Observe safety precautions until the effects of the sedatives have worn off.
- Monitor the patient for signs of respiratory depression. Medication (e.g., naloxone) should be available to counteract serious respiratory depression. Resuscitative equipment should also be present.
- Assess the patient for signs and symptoms of septicemia, which may indicate the onset of ERCP-induced cholangitis.

Inform the patient that he or she may be hoarse and have a sore throat for several days. Drinking cool fluids and gargling will help to relieve some of this soreness.

> ### 🏠 Home Care Responsibilities
>
> - A sore throat is expected. A soothing mouthwash gargle may help.
> - Notify the doctor immediately if increasing abdominal pain, nausea, or vomiting occurs. These may be the early signs of pancreatitis or gastroduodenal perforation.
> - Notify the physician immediately of fever or shaking chills. These may indicate possible cholangitis.
> - Encourage the patient to eat lightly for the next 12 to 24 hours.

TEST RESULTS AND CLINICAL SIGNIFICANCE

Tumor, strictures, or gallstones of the common bile duct: *This is obvious in the presence and character of the filling defect noted in the dye-filled duct.*

Sclerosing cholangitis,

Biliary sclerosis:
  These are apparent as a long area of strictures involving, but not limited to, the extrahepatic ducts.

Cysts of the common bile duct: *These congenital cysts are seen as large balloon-like dilations of any portion of the extrahepatic ducts.*

Tumor, strictures, or inflammation of the pancreatic duct: *Some tumors of the pancreas present as large cystic structures involving and leading from the pancreatic duct. Most pancreatic tumors, however, appear as a localized narrowing of the pancreatic duct with a dilated duct distal to the narrowing. Strictures and inflammation usually involve the entire duct with very little duct dilation beyond the narrowing.*

Pseudocyst of the pancreatic duct: *This results from pancreatic duct injury (usually following severe pancreatitis). The pancreatic juices leak out of the duct and into the peripancreatic tissue. A cyst is formed that communicates with the main pancreatic duct.*

Chronic pancreatitis: *This may be seen as multiple small partial strictures involving multiple short segments of the pancreatic duct with dilation of the duct in between the strictures. This gives the appearance of "beading" along the duct.*

Anatomic biliary or pancreatic duct variations: *Variable pathologic and nonpathologic anomalies can occur. Usually no symptoms are caused by these abnormalities.*

Cancer of the duodenum or ampulla: *These cancers are quite obvious as friable tumor masses emanating from the mucosa of those regions.*

RELATED TEST

Percutaneous Transhepatic Cholangiography (p. 1053). The liver is percutaneously punctured with a needle, and a catheter is threaded into the biliary duct radical. Dye is injected, and the biliary tree can be visualized radiographically.

Esophagogastroduodenoscopy (EGD, Upper Gastrointestinal [UGI] Endoscopy, Gastroscopy)

NORMAL FINDINGS

Normal esophagus, stomach, and duodenum

INDICATIONS

This test is used to visualize the lumen of the esophagus, stomach, and duodenum. It is used to evaluate patients with the following:

- Dysphagia
- Weight loss
- Early satiety
- Upper abdominal pain
- "Ulcer symptoms" or dyspepsia
- Alcoholism and suspected varices
- Results of barium swallow or upper gastrointestinal (GI) x-ray study that are suggestive of a pathologic condition

TEST EXPLANATION

Endoscopy enables direct visualization of the upper GI tract by means of a long, flexible, fiberoptic-lighted scope. The lumen of the esophagus, stomach, and duodenum are examined for tumors, varices, mucosal inflammations, hiatal hernias, polyps, ulcers, and obstructions. The endoscope has one to three channels. The first channel is used for viewing, the second for insufflation of air and aspiration of fluid, and the third for passing cable-activated instruments to perform a biopsy of suspected pathologic tissue. Probes also can be passed through the third channel to allow coagulation or injection of sclerosing agents to areas of active GI bleeding. A laser beam can pass through the endoscope to perform endoscopic surgery (e.g., obliteration of tumors or polyps, control of bleeding), and the fiberoptics of endoscopy are so refined that video images and "still pictures" can be taken.

    With endoscopy, one can not only evaluate the esophagus, stomach, and duodenum, but with the use of an extra-long fiberoptic endoscope, one can also visualize and perform a biopsy of tissue in the upper

TABLE 4-5   Gastrointestinal Tract Endoscopy

Endoscopy	Area Evaluated
Esophagoscopy	Esophagus
Gastroscopy	Esophagus and stomach
Esophagogastroduodenoscopy (EGD)	Esophagus, stomach, and duodenum
Enteroscopy	Esophagus, stomach, duodenum, and upper jejunum
Panendoscopy	Esophagus, stomach, duodenum, upper jejunum and colon (per colonoscopy)
Endoscopic retrograde cholangiopancreatography (ERCP)	Duodenum, ampulla, and pancreatobiliary ducts

small intestinal tract. This procedure is referred to as *enteroscopy* (Table 4-5). Abnormalities of the small intestine, such as arteriovenous (AV) malformations, tumors, enteropathies (e.g., celiac disease), and ulcerations, can be diagnosed with enteroscopy.

Until recently, there was no good way to directly visualize the mid and distal small bowel. *Capsule endoscopy* (or *wireless capsule endoscopy*) uses a capsule containing a miniature camera that records images of the entire digestive tract, particularly the small intestine. This capsule is about the size of a large vitamin and contains a color video camera, a radiofrequency transmitter, four LED lights, and enough battery power to take 50,000 color images during an 8-hour journey through the digestive tract. It moves through the digestive track naturally with the aid of peristaltic activity. During the 6- to 10-hour examination, the images are continuously transmitted to special antenna pads placed on the body and captured on a recording device about the size of a portable radio that is worn around the patient's waist. After the examination, the patient returns to the doctor's office and the recording device is removed. The stored images are transferred to a computer workstation, where they are transformed into a digital movie that the doctor can later examine on the computer monitor.

Patients are not required to retrieve and return the video capsule to the physician. It is disposable and expelled normally and effortlessly with the next bowel movement. The most common reason for doing capsule endoscopy is to search for a cause of bleeding from the small intestine. It may also be useful for detecting polyps, inflammatory bowel disease (Crohn disease), ulcers, and tumors of the small intestine. Capsule endoscopy is not accurate for the detection of colon neoplasia.

Besides being much more sensitive and specific than an upper GI x-ray series in diagnosing diseases of the esophagus, stomach, and duodenum, EGD also can be used therapeutically. An experienced endoscopist often can control active GI tract bleeding by electrocoagulation, laser coagulation, or the injection of sclerosing agents, such as alcohol. Also, with the endoscope, benign and malignant strictures can be dilated to reestablish patency of the upper GI tract. Biliary stents and a percutaneous gastrostomy tube can be placed with the use of EGD. The role of endoscopic surgery is expanding in light of its dramatic success and minimal morbidity.

CONTRAINDICATIONS

- Patients who cannot cooperate fully: As in all studies that require technical finesse, patient cooperation is essential for successful, safe, and accurate test completion.
- Patients with severe upper GI tract bleeding: The viewing lens will become covered with blood clots, preventing adequate visualization. However, if the stomach can be lavaged and aspirated to clear the blood clots, EGD can be performed.

- Patients with esophageal diverticula: The scope can easily fall into the diverticulum and perforate the wall of the esophagus.
- Patients with suspected perforation: The perforation can be worsened by the insufflation of pressurized air into the GI tract.
- Patients who have had recent upper GI tract surgery: The anastomosis may not be able to withstand the pressure of the required air insufflation. This may lead to anastomotic disruption.

POTENTIAL COMPLICATIONS

- Perforation of the esophagus, stomach, and duodenum
- Bleeding from a biopsy site
- Pulmonary aspiration of gastric contents
- Oversedation from the medication administered during the test
- Hypotension induced by the sedative medication: Usually the patient already has some significant element of hypovolemia or dehydration.
- Local intravenous (IV) phlebitic reaction to the injection of sclerosing sedative medication

INTERFERING FACTORS

- Food in the stomach
- Excessive GI tract bleeding

PROCEDURE AND PATIENT CARE

Before

- Explain the procedure to the patient.
- Obtain informed consent.
- Instruct the patient to abstain from eating as of midnight the day of the test.
- Inform the patient that this test is mildly uncomfortable. Tell the patient that the throat will be anesthetized with a spray to depress the gag reflex.
- Encourage the patient to verbalize concerns. Provide support.
- Inform the patient that dentures and eyewear will need to be removed before the procedure starts.
- Remind the patient that he or she will not be able to speak during the test but that respiration will not be affected.
- Instruct the patient not to bite down on the endoscope.
- Instruct the patient to perform thorough oral hygiene because the tube will be passed through the mouth.

During

- Note the following procedural steps:
  1. The patient is placed on the endoscopy table in the left lateral decubitus position.
  2. The throat is topically anesthetized with viscous lidocaine or another anesthetic spray. This is to decrease the gag reflex caused by passage of the endoscope.
  3. The patient is usually sedated. This minimizes anxiety and allows the patient to experience a "light" sleep.
  4. The endoscope is gently passed through the mouth and finally into the esophagus; once in the esophagus, visualization can be performed. A bite block may be used.

5. Air is insufflated to distend the upper GI tract for adequate visualization.
6. The esophagus, stomach, and duodenum are evaluated.
7. During enteroscopy, the upper small bowel is visualized and a biopsy is performed if needed.
8. Biopsy or any endoscopic surgery is performed with direct visualization.
9. At the completion of direct inspection and surgery, the excess air and GI tract secretions are aspirated through the scope.
- Note that the test is performed in the endoscopy laboratory by a physician trained in GI endoscopy and takes approximately 20 to 30 minutes.

After

- Inform the patient that he or she may have hoarseness or a sore throat after the test.
- Withhold any fluids until the patient is completely alert and the swallowing reflex returns to normal, usually 2 to 4 hours.
- Observe the patient's vital signs. Evaluate the patient for bleeding, fever, abdominal pain, dyspnea, or dysphagia.
- Inform the patient that he or she may experience some postendoscopic bloating, belching, and flatulence.
- Observe safety precautions until the effects of the sedatives have worn off.
- Inform the patient that the sedation may cause some retrograde and antegrade amnesia for a few hours.

Home Care Responsibilities

- A sore throat is expected after EGD. A soothing mouthwash may help.
- Notify the doctor immediately if bleeding, fever, abdominal pain, dyspnea, or dysphagia occurs.
- Inform the patient that it is normal to have some bloating, belching, and flatulence after the procedure.

TEST RESULTS AND CLINICAL SIGNIFICANCE

Tumors (benign or malignant) of the esophagus, stomach, or duodenum: *These appear as red, friable ulcers or masses in the mucosa of the respective organ. These tumors can obstruct, bleed, or perforate.*

Esophageal diverticula: *These are outpouchings of the esophagus at the level of the cricopharyngeal muscle or the diaphragm.*

Hiatal hernia: *A hiatal hernia exists when a portion of the stomach is above the diaphragm (seen as an extrinsic compression of the lower esophagus).*

Esophagitis, gastritis, duodenitis: *A reddened friable mucosa without ulcer or mass is classic for inflammation.*

Gastroesophageal varices: *Submucosal vessels that protrude into the lumen of the distal esophagus and stomach are called varices and indicate a reversal of portal blood flow because of hepatic cirrhosis.*

Peptic ulcer: *This benign, acid-induced ulcer usually occurs in the duodenum but may occur in the distal stomach. It is a small to moderate-sized ulcer seen in the mucosa of the organ.*

Peptic stricture and subsequent scarring: *Following healing of an ulcer or inflammation, scarring and stricture can form and partially obstruct the lumen of the organ involved (usually the esophagus).*

Extrinsic compression by a cyst or tumor outside the upper GI tract: *Tumors, cysts, or enlarged organs can compress the upper GI tract. This is noted by a convex narrowing involving the organ being evaluated.*

Source of upper GI tract bleeding: *Ulcers, tumors, varices, AV malformations, inflammation, and bleeding can be identified and often treated by EGD.*

RELATED TESTS

Barium Swallow and Upper Gastrointestinal Tract Series (pp. 999 and 1072). These x-ray contrast studies also evaluate the upper GI tract. They are not as accurate as EGD. Furthermore, biopsy and therapy cannot be performed using the x-ray studies, but they can be performed with EGD.

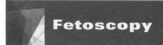

Fetoscopy

NORMAL FINDINGS

No fetal distress or diseases seen
No hematologic abnormalities noted

INDICATIONS

Fetoscopy is indicated for any woman who is at risk for delivery of a baby with a significant birth defect. It is used also to perform corrective surgery on the fetus when possible.

TEST EXPLANATION

Fetoscopy is an endoscopic procedure that allows direct visualization of the fetus via the insertion of a tiny, telescope-like instrument through the abdominal wall and into the uterine cavity (Figure 4-11). Direct visualization may lead to diagnosis of a severe malformation, such as a neural tube defect. During the procedure, fetal blood samples to detect congenital blood disorders (e.g., hemophilia, sickle cell anemia) can be drawn from a blood vessel in the umbilical cord for biochemical analysis. Fetal skin biopsies also can be done to detect primary skin disorders. Fetoscopic surgery (placement of central nervous system [CNS] shunts, etc.) is becoming more and more a reality.

Fetoscopy is performed at approximately 18 weeks' gestation. At this time the vessels of the placental surface are of adequate size and the fetal parts are readily identifiable. A therapeutic abortion would not be as hazardous at this time as it would be if it were done later in the pregnancy. An ultrasound examination is usually performed the day after the procedure to confirm the adequacy of the amniotic fluid and fetal viability.

POTENTIAL COMPLICATIONS

- Spontaneous abortion
- Premature delivery
- Amniotic fluid leak
- Intrauterine fetal death
- Amnionitis

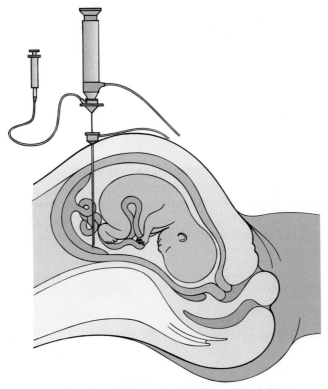

Figure 4-11 Fetoscopy for fetal blood sampling.

✓ Clinical Priorities

- Ultrasound examination is performed before the procedure to identify a safe area to enter the uterine cavity.
- After the test, mothers who are Rh negative should receive RhoGAM unless the fetal blood is also Rh negative.
- Ultrasound examination is usually performed the day after the procedure to confirm the adequacy of the amniotic fluid and to assess fetal viability.

PROCEDURE AND PATIENT CARE

Before

 Explain the procedure to the patient.
- Obtain informed consent for this procedure.
- Assess the fetal heart rate (FHR) before the test to serve as a baseline value.
- Administer fentanyl, if ordered, before the test because it crosses the placenta and quiets the fetus. This prevents excessive fetal movement, which would make the procedure more difficult.
- Tell the patient that the only discomfort associated with this study is the injection of the local anesthetic.

During

- Note the following procedural steps:
  1. The woman is placed in the supine position on an examining table.

2. The abdominal wall is anesthetized locally.
3. Ultrasonography is performed to locate the fetus and the placenta and to identify a safe area to penetrate the uterus.
4. The endoscope is inserted.
5. Biopsy specimens and blood samples may be obtained.
• Note that this procedure is performed by a physician in 1 to 2 hours.

After

• Assess the FHR and compare with the baseline value to detect any side effects related to the procedure.
• Monitor the mother and fetus carefully for alterations in blood pressure, pulse rate, uterine activity, and fetal activity; vaginal bleeding; and loss of amniotic fluid.
• Administer RhoGAM to mothers who are Rh negative unless the fetal blood is found to be Rh negative.
• If ordered, administer antibiotics prophylactically after the test to prevent amnionitis.

Home Care Responsibilities

• Instruct the mother to avoid strenuous activity for 1 to 2 weeks following the procedure.
• Advise the mother to report any pain, bleeding, amniotic fluid loss, or fever.

TEST RESULTS AND CLINICAL SIGNIFICANCE

Developmental defects (e.g., neural tube defects): *These defects are visible on a fetus exceeding 20 weeks in age.*
Congenital blood disorders (e.g., hemophilia, sickle cell anemia): *These congenital abnormalities are identified by evaluation of the fetal blood.*
Primary skin disorders: *These may be obvious at the time of fetoscopy. Skin biopsies can be performed.*

RELATED TESTS

Amniocentesis (p. 632). This procedure involves placing a needle through the abdominal and uterine walls into the amniotic cavity to withdraw fluid for analysis. Valuable information about fetal status is obtained.
Chorionic Villus Sampling (p. 1088). This is a test whereby the chorionic placental tissue (which has the same genetic material as the fetus) is tested for genetic analysis and karyotyping. This is a rapid and accurate method of determining genetic defects. CVS can be performed earlier in pregnancy than can amniocentesis.

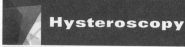
Hysteroscopy

NORMAL FINDINGS

Normal structure and function of the uterus

INDICATIONS

This test allows direct visualization of the endometrial cavity. It is indicated for women with an abnormal Papanicolaou (Pap) test, dysfunctional uterine bleeding, or postmenopausal bleeding.

TEST EXPLANATION

Hysteroscopy is an endoscopic procedure that provides direct visualization of the uterine cavity by inserting a hysteroscope (a thin, telescope-like instrument) through the vagina and cervix and into the uterus (Figure 4-12). Hysteroscopy can be used to identify the cause of abnormal uterine bleeding, infertility, and repeated miscarriages. It is also used to evaluate and diagnose uterine adhesions (Asherman syndrome), polyps, and fibroids and to detect displaced intrauterine devices (IUDs).

In addition to diagnosing and evaluating uterine problems, hysteroscopy can also correct uterine problems. For example, uterine adhesions and small fibroids can be removed through the hysteroscope, thus avoiding open abdominal surgery. Hysteroscopy can also be used to perform endometrial ablation, which destroys the uterine lining to treat some cases of heavy uterine bleeding.

Hysteroscopy may confirm the results of other tests, such as hysterosalpingography (p. 1038). Depending on the amount of surgery and time associated with hysteroscopy, general, spinal, or light sedative anesthesia is used. It takes only about 30 minutes for simple hysteroscopy. This test is usually performed by a gynecologist in the operating room. The patient receiving local anesthesia

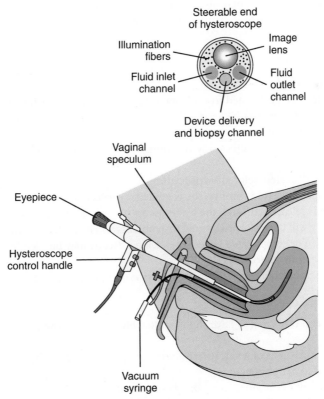

Figure 4-12 Hysteroscopy.

or only light sedation may feel some cramping during the procedure. In general, it is not a painful procedure.

CONTRAINDICATIONS

- Patients with pelvic inflammatory disease
- Patients with vaginal discharge

POTENTIAL COMPLICATIONS

- Uterine perforation
- Infection

PROCEDURE AND PATIENT CARE

Before

- Explain the procedure to the patient.
- Obtain informed consent for this procedure.
- Schedule the procedure after menstrual bleeding has ceased and before ovulation. This allows better visualization of the inside of the uterus and avoids damage to a newly formed pregnancy.
- Inform the patient that hysteroscopy may be performed with local, regional, or general anesthesia. If general anesthesia will be given, the patient should be on nothing by mouth (NPO) status for at least 8 hours before the test. This test may also be performed without anesthesia.
- Tell the patient to void before the procedure because a distended bladder can be more easily perforated.

During

- Note the following procedural steps:
  1. Hysteroscopy may be performed in the operating room or in the doctor's office. Local, regional, general, or no anesthesia may be used. (The type of anesthesia depends on other procedures that may be done at the same time.)
  2. The patient is placed in the lithotomy position. The vaginal area is cleansed with an antiseptic solution.
  3. The cervix may be dilated before this procedure.
  4. The hysteroscope is inserted through the vagina and cervix and into the uterus.
  5. A liquid or gas is released through the hysteroscope to expand the uterus for better visualization.
  6. If minor surgery will be performed, small instruments will be inserted through the hysteroscope.
  7. For more detailed or complicated procedures, a laparoscope may be used (p. 617) to concurrently view the outside of the uterus.
  8. After the desired procedure is performed, the hysteroscope is removed.

After

- Tell the patient that it is normal to have slight vaginal bleeding and cramps for a day or two after the procedure.
- Inform the patient that signs of fever, severe abdominal pain, or heavy vaginal discharge or bleeding should be reported to her physician.
- If the patient has any discomfort from the gas inserted during the hysteroscopy or laparoscopy, assure her that this usually lasts less than 24 hours.

TEST RESULTS AND CLINICAL SIGNIFICANCE

Endometrial cancer, polyps, or hyperplasia: *Cancer appears as thickened endometrium in one or multiple portions of the uterus. Hyperplasia looks similar but is not as isolated and seems more diffuse. Polyps appear as pedunculated mucosal tissue protruding from the endometrium.*

Uterine fibroids: *Small fibroids are easily seen because they distort the endometrium.*

Asherman syndrome: *Intrauterine adhesions may be associated with previous uterine infections and can be lysed through hysteroscopy.*

Septate uterus: *This and other developmental abnormalities can be visualized by hysteroscopy.*

Displaced IUD: *The location of a displaced IUD is easily seen.*

RELATED TEST

Dilation and Curettage (D&C) (p. 726). This is another procedure that allows one to examine scrapings of the endometrium under a microscope. This test has nearly the same indications as hysteroscopy. However, sampling is random, and serious lesions may be missed.

Laparoscopy (Pelvic Endoscopy, Gynecologic Video Laparoscopy, Peritoneoscopy)

NORMAL FINDINGS

Normal-appearing female reproductive organs
Normal-appearing abdominal and pelvic organs (male and female)

INDICATIONS

Laparoscopy is used to directly visualize the abdominal and pelvic organs when a pathologic condition is suspected. It is used to evaluate patients with the following:

- Acute abdominal or pelvic pain
- Chronic abdominal or pelvic pain
- Suspected advanced cancer
- Abdominal mass of uncertain cause
- Unexplained infertility

Operative procedures that can be performed with laparoscopic surgery include oophorectomy, appendectomy, cholecystectomy, colectomy, hernia repair, liver biopsy, nephrectomy, tubal ligation, and gastrectomy.

TEST EXPLANATION

During laparoscopy the abdominal organs can be visualized by inserting a scope through the abdominal wall and into the peritoneum (Figure 4-13). An attached camera is applied to the scope, and the scope's view is seen on color monitors. This is particularly helpful in diagnosing abdominal and pelvic adhesions, tumors and cysts affecting any abdominal organ, and tubal and uterine causes of infertility. In addition, endometriosis, ectopic pregnancy, ruptured ovarian cyst, and salpingitis can be detected during an evaluation for pelvic pain. This procedure is also used to stage cancers and determine their resectability. Surgical procedures, as described above, can be performed with the laparoscope.

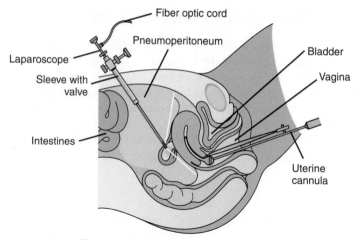

Figure 4-13 Gynecologic laparoscopy.

	Laparotomy	Laparoscopy
Difficulty in technique	Moderate	High
Size of incision	One large	Multiple and small
Expense of equipment in the operating room	Moderate	High
Expense of postoperative care	High	Low
Postoperative mobility	Low	High
Postoperative pain	High	Minimal to moderate
Postoperative hospitalization	4-10 days	1-2 days
Duration of postoperative recovery	Weeks	Days
Return to work	6 weeks	1 week

TABLE 4-6   Differences Between Laparotomy and Laparoscopy

As noted in Table 4-6, laparoscopy affords many advantages to the patient in comparison with an open laparotomy.

Laparoscopy is performed by a surgeon. The patient is under general anesthesia so that no pain or discomfort is experienced during the procedure. Most patients have mild to moderate incisional pain. However, the patient may complain of shoulder or subcostal discomfort from diaphragmatic irritation caused by pneumoperitoneum.

CONTRAINDICATIONS

- Patients who have had multiple abdominal surgical procedures, because adhesions may have formed between the viscera and the abdominal wall, making safe access to the abdomen impossible: There are techniques that allow limited laparoscopy in these situations.

- Patients with suspected intraabdominal hemorrhage, because visualization through the scope will be obscured by the blood

POTENTIAL COMPLICATIONS

- Perforation of the bowel, with spilling of intestinal contents into the peritoneum
- Hemorrhage from the trocar site or surgical site
- Umbilical hernia resulting from inadequate repair of the hole in the fascia used to insert the laparoscope
- Incisional hernias

INTERFERING FACTORS

- Adhesions may obstruct the field of vision.

✓ Clinical Priorities

- During the procedure the peritoneal cavity is filled with 3 to 4 L of CO_2 to separate the abdominal wall from the intraabdominal viscera.
- After the procedure, patients may have shoulder or subcostal discomfort from pneumoperitoneum. This usually lasts only 24 hours.
- After the procedure, patients should be assessed for bleeding (increased pulse rate, decreased blood pressure) and perforated viscus (abdominal tenderness, guarding, decreased bowel sounds).

PROCEDURE AND PATIENT CARE

Before

 Explain the procedure to the patient.

 Ensure that an informed consent for this procedure is obtained. Because of the possibility of intraabdominal injury, an open laparotomy may be required. Be sure the patient is aware of that.

 If enemas are ordered to clear the bowel, assist the patient as needed and record the results.

- Because the procedure is usually performed with the patient under general anesthesia, follow the routine general anesthesia precautions.
- Shave and prepare the patient's abdomen as ordered.

 Keep the patient on nothing by mouth (NPO) status after midnight on the day of the test. Intravenous (IV) fluids may be given.

 Instruct the patient to void before going to the operating room because a distended bladder can be easily penetrated.

During

- After general anesthesia is induced, a catheter and nasogastric tube are inserted to minimize the risk of penetrating a distended stomach or bladder with the initial needle placement.
- Note the following procedural steps:
  1. Laparoscopy is performed in the operating room. The patient is initially placed in supine position. Other positions may be assumed to maximize visibility.
  2. After the abdominal skin is cleansed, a blunt-tipped (Verres) needle is inserted through a small incision in the periumbilical area and into the peritoneal cavity. Alternatively, a slightly larger

incision is placed in the skin and the abdominal wall is separated under direct vision. The peritoneal cavity is entered directly. Adhesions can be lysed under direct vision.

3. The peritoneal cavity is filled with approximately 2 to 3 L of CO_2 to separate the abdominal wall from the intraabdominal viscera, enhancing visualization of pelvic and abdominal structures.

4. A laparoscope is inserted through a trocar to examine the abdomen (see Figure 4-13). Other trocars can be placed as conduits for other instrumentation.

5. After the desired procedure is completed, the laparoscope is removed and the CO_2 is allowed to escape.

6. The incision(s) is closed with a few skin stitches and covered with an adhesive bandage.

After

- Assess the patient frequently for signs of bleeding (increased pulse rate, decreased blood pressure) and perforated viscus (abdominal tenderness, guarding, decreased bowel sounds). Report any significant findings to the physician.

 If patients have shoulder or subcostal discomfort from pneumoperitoneum, assure them that this usually lasts only 24 hours. Minor analgesics usually relieve this discomfort.

- If a surgical procedure has been performed laparoscopically, provide appropriate specific postsurgical care.

Home Care Responsibilities

- Observe for increasing abdominal pain, which may indicate bowel perforation.
- Note that fever and chills may indicate a bowel perforation.
- Inform the patient that discomfort in the shoulder area or under the ribs may result from the carbon dioxide inserted into the peritoneal cavity during the procedure.

TEST RESULTS AND CLINICAL SIGNIFICANCE

Abdominal adhesions: *Occasionally these can be the source of chronic abdominal pain.*

Ovarian tumor or cyst: *These are obvious as masses affecting the ovaries.*

Endometriosis: *Endometriosis varies from small white wispy scars on the peritoneal surface to large inflammatory masses distorting normal anatomy.*

Ectopic pregnancy: *This usually appears to be a large mass with or without a surrounding inflammation involving just one fallopian tube.*

Pelvic inflammatory disease (salpingitis): *The pelvic structures are red and inflamed.*

Uterine fibroids: *Large soft masses are seen on and in the uterus.*

Abscess or infection: *This can come from any number of abdominal or pelvic causes, including appendicitis, infection of fallopian tubes, diverticulitis, or acute cholecystitis.*

Cancer: *A large primary or metastatic cancer in the abdomen is usually obvious. The extent of tumor spread can be assessed.*

Ascites: *Fluid within the abdomen can be aspirated and tested to indicate its source if not apparent at laparoscopy.*

Other abdominal pathologic conditions: *Every abdominal abnormality cannot be mentioned here. Suffice it to say that nearly every significant abdominal pathologic process that affects the visceral or parietal peritoneal surface can usually be seen.*

Mediastinoscopy

NORMAL FINDINGS

No mediastinal tumors or abnormal lymph nodes

INDICATIONS

This procedure provides direct visualization of the mediastinum and the lymph nodes contained within. It is used most commonly to determine the cancer stage of a person with known lung cancer. It is also used to evaluate patients with mediastinal masses of uncertain causes.

TEST EXPLANATION

Mediastinoscopy is a surgical procedure in which a rigid mediastinoscope (a lighted instrument scope) is inserted through a small incision made at the suprasternal notch. The scope is passed into the superior mediastinum to inspect the mediastinal lymph nodes and to remove biopsy specimens. Because these lymph nodes receive lymphatic drainage from the lungs, assessment of them can provide information on intrathoracic diseases such as carcinoma, granulomatous infections, and sarcoidosis; therefore mediastinoscopy is used in establishing the diagnosis of various intrathoracic diseases. This procedure is also employed to "stage" patients with lung cancer and to assess whether they are candidates for surgery. Evidence of metastasis to the mediastinal lymph nodes is usually a contraindication to thoracotomy because the tumor is considered inoperable. Biopsies of tumors occurring in the mediastinum (e.g., thymoma or lymphoma) can also be performed through the mediastinoscope.

CONTRAINDICATIONS

- Patients who have superior vena cava obstruction: These patients have tremendous venous collateralization in the mediastinum. Mediastinoscopy in this group of patients is fraught with danger from hemorrhage.

POTENTIAL COMPLICATIONS

- Puncture of the esophagus, trachea, or great blood vessels
- Pneumothorax
- Infection
- Hemorrhage
- Chylothorax

PROCEDURE AND PATIENT CARE

Before

- Explain the procedure to the patient.
- Ensure that the physician has obtained an informed consent for this procedure.
- Check whether the patient's blood needs to be typed and crossmatched.
- Provide preoperative care as with any other surgical procedure.

Keep the patient on nothing by mouth (NPO) status after midnight on the day of the test.

Inform the patient that he or she will be asleep during the procedure.

- Administer preprocedural medication approximately 1 hour before the test, as ordered.

During

- Note the following procedural steps:
  1. The patient is taken to the operating room for this surgical procedure.
  2. The patient is placed under general anesthesia.
  3. An incision is made in the suprasternal notch.
  4. The mediastinoscope is passed through this neck incision and into the superior mediastinum.
  5. Biopsies of the lymph nodes are performed.
  6. The scope is withdrawn, and the incision is sutured closed.
- Note that this procedure is performed by a surgeon in approximately 1 hour.

After

- Provide postoperative care as with any other surgical procedure.

 Home Care Responsibilities

- Assess for cough or shortness of breath, which may indicate a pneumothorax.
- Note that subcutaneous emphysema may indicate a pneumothorax.
- Assess for mediastinal crepitus on auscultation, which may indicate mediastinal air from a pneumothorax or the bronchus or esophagus.
- Note that distended neck veins and pulsus paradoxus (abnormal decrease in systolic blood pressure and pulse wave amplitude during inspiration) may indicate lack of cardiac filling because of a large mediastinal hematoma.
- Observe for hypotension and tachycardia, which may indicate bleeding from the biopsy site or the great vessels.
- Evaluate for hoarseness, which may indicate injury to the recurrent laryngeal nerve.
- Assess for fever, chills, and sepsis, which may indicate mediastinitis from infection.

TEST RESULTS AND CLINICAL SIGNIFICANCE

Lung cancer—primary into the mediastinum or metastatic to the lymph nodes: *It is routine to stage lung cancers with mediastinoscopy prior to thoracotomy.*

Thymoma: *These tumors of the anterior superior mediastinum can be easily seen by this technique.*

Tuberculosis or sarcoidosis: *Granulomatous inflammations can involve the mediastinal lymph nodes.*

Lymphoma or Hodgkin disease: *Lymphomas routinely involve the mediastinum. In a patient with previously established lymphoma, this procedure is not needed. However, mediastinoscopy may be the least invasive method of diagnosis if lymphoma has not yet been diagnosed.*

Infection (fungal, mycoplasma, etc.): *Coccidioidomycosis, histoplasmosis, and* Pneumocystis jiroveci *can be diagnosed by this technique if the mediastinum is involved.*

RELATED TEST

Computed Tomography (CT) of the Chest (p. 1029). This test can visualize the mediastinal structure but cannot be specific about a disease process.

Sigmoidoscopy (Proctoscopy, Anoscopy)

NORMAL FINDINGS

Normal anus, rectum, and sigmoid colon

INDICATIONS

This test allows for direct visualization of the rectum and sigmoid colon. It is used to diagnose suspected pathologic conditions of these organs. It is recommended for patients who have had a change in bowel habits or obvious or occult blood in the stool or who have abdominal pain. It is part of routine screening for colorectal cancer in people over age 50 years.

TEST EXPLANATION

Endoscopy of the lower gastrointestinal (GI) tract allows one to visualize and perform biopsies of tumors, polyps, hemorrhoids, or ulcers of the anus, rectum, and sigmoid colon. *Anoscopy* refers to examination of the anus; *proctoscopy* to examination of the anus and rectum; and *sigmoidoscopy* (the most frequent procedure) to examination of the anus, rectum, and sigmoid colon. This test can be performed with a rigid (to 25 cm from the anus) or flexible (to 60 cm from the anus) sigmoidoscope. Because the lower GI tract is difficult to visualize radiographically, direct visualization by sigmoidoscopy is diagnostically helpful.

Furthermore, sigmoidoscopy, like colonoscopy, can be therapeutic. Reduction of sigmoid volvulus, removal of polyps, and obliteration of hemorrhoids can be performed through the sigmoidoscope. For those having no colorectal cancer risk, the American Cancer Society recommends a sigmoidoscopy every 3 to 5 years after age 50 years. If a neoplastic abnormality (benign or malignant) is found, a total colonoscopy (p. 591) should be performed.

Note that a physician trained in GI endoscopy usually performs this procedure in the GI laboratory, operating room, or outpatient clinic or at the patient's bedside in approximately 15 to 20 minutes. Very little discomfort is associated with the test. A sense of having to defecate during the procedure is uncomfortable. It is caused by the scope within the rectum.

CONTRAINDICATIONS

- Patients who are uncooperative
- Patients with diverticulitis: The insufflation of air needed to distend the rectum and colon for passage of the scope may cause a perforation of the diverticulitis.
- Patients with painful anorectal conditions (e.g., fissures, fistulas, hemorrhoids), because of the anal pain associated with passage of the scope
- Patients with severe bleeding: Blood clots obstruct the view of the scope.
- Patients suspected of having perforated colon lesions

POTENTIAL COMPLICATIONS

- Perforation of the colon
- Bleeding from biopsy sites

INTERFERING FACTORS

- Poor bowel preparation may obscure visualization of the bowel mucosa.
- Rectal bleeding may obstruct the lens system and preclude adequate visualization.

PROCEDURE AND PATIENT CARE

Before

- Explain the procedure to the patient.
- Obtain informed consent for this procedure.
- Assist the patient with the bowel preparation. In most cases, two Fleet enemas are sufficient for examining the lower sigmoid colon and rectum. An oral cathartic is usually required to examine as far as 60 cm.
- Instruct the patient to ingest only a light breakfast on the morning of the endoscopy.
- Assure patients that they will be properly draped to avoid unnecessary embarrassment.

During

- Note the following procedural steps:
  1. The patient is placed on the endoscopy table or bed in the left lateral decubitus position. Some physicians prefer the knee-chest position; many operating and examining tables are easily converted to make the knee-chest position more comfortable. This procedure also can be performed with the patient in the lithotomy position.
  2. Usually no sedation is required.
  3. The anus is mildly dilated with a well-lubricated finger.
  4. The rigid or flexible sigmoidoscope is placed into the rectum and advanced to its point of maximal penetration.
  5. Air is insufflated during the procedure to more fully distend the lower intestinal tract.
  6. The sigmoid, rectum, and anus are visualized.
  7. Biopsy specimens can be obtained and polypectomy can be performed at the time of sigmoidoscopy.

After

- Inform the patient that because air has been insufflated into the bowel during the procedure, he or she may have flatulence or gas pains. Ambulation may help.
- Observe the patient for signs of abdominal distention, increased tenderness, or rectal bleeding.
- Tell the patient that slight rectal bleeding may occur if biopsy specimens have been taken.

Home Care Responsibilities

- Observe for increasing abdominal pain, which may indicate bowel perforation.
- Note that fever and chills may indicate a bowel perforation.
- Inform the patient that frequent bloody bowel movements may indicate poor hemostasis if biopsy or polypectomy was performed.
- Observe for abdominal bloating and inability to pass flatus, which may indicate colon obstruction if a neoplasm was identified.

TEST RESULTS AND CLINICAL SIGNIFICANCE

Colorectal cancer: *This is seen as a red friable fleshy tumor concentrically involving the mucosa of the bowel.*

Colorectal polyp: *This is a tumor that protrudes from only one part of the mucosa of the bowel. Some cancers and most polyps can be removed with the sigmoidoscope. Biopsy specimens can be obtained from neoplasms.*

Ulcerative proctitis: *Ulcerative colitis frequently involves the rectum. That is one characteristic that separates ulcerative colitis from Crohn disease.*

Pseudomembranous colitis: *The rectum is the best location to most easily make the diagnosis of this disease. Usually this inflammation is the result of* Clostridium *overgrowth caused by prolonged use of clindamycin.*

Intestinal ischemia: *This usually is apparent as dark mucosa in the sigmoid colon. The sigmoid colon is the portion of colon most vulnerable if ischemia occurs. Ischemia always shows up in the mucosa first.*

RELATED TESTS

Barium Enema (p. 994). This is an x-ray contrast study of the colon and rectum. The rectum, however, is not well evaluated by this study.

Colonoscopy (p. 591). This is a direct visualization of the entire colon and rectum. It is more extensive and invasive than sigmoidoscopy. The required preparation is more complete.

Sinus Endoscopy

NORMAL FINDINGS

Normal sinuses

INDICATIONS

This procedure is used to evaluate and treat patients with recurrent or resistant sinus infections.

TEST EXPLANATION

Patients with recurrent or resistant sinus infections often require surgical drainage. However, with the advent of sinus endoscopy (Figure 4-14), the sinus cavities can be accessed and drained without surgery. Cultures can be obtained, and antibiotic therapy can be more appropriately provided. The treatment of sinusitis is important to prevent the development of complications, such as mucoceles, cysts, or sinus bone destruction. The most accessible sinuses include the anterior ethmoid, middle turbinate, and middle meatus areas.

This procedure can also be used to visualize suspected neoplasms involving the sinuses. The test is usually performed by a surgeon trained in ear, nose, and throat (ENT) diseases. There is usually little postoperative pain associated with this procedure.

4 Endoscopic Studies

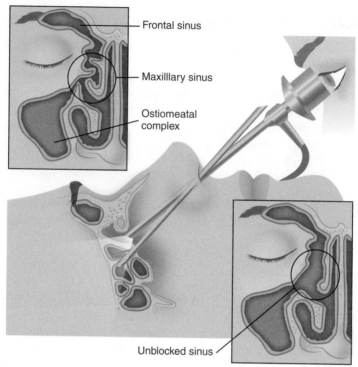

Frontal sinus

Maxilllary sinus

Ostiomeatal complex

Unblocked sinus

Figure 4-14 With sinus endoscopy, the sinus cavities can be examined and drained without surgery.

POTENTIAL COMPLICATIONS

- Bleeding
- Cerebrospinal fluid (CSF) leak (occurs only with ethmoid sinus endoscopy)

PROCEDURE AND PATIENT CARE

Before

- Explain the procedure to the patient.
- Ensure that an informed consent for this procedure is obtained.
- If the procedure is to be performed under general anesthesia, keep the patient on nothing by mouth (NPO) status after midnight on the day of the test. Intravenous (IV) fluids may be given. This procedure can also be done using local anesthesia, depending on the amount of endoscopic surgery that will be required.

During

- Note the following procedural steps:
  1. Sinus endoscopy is performed in the operating room if general anesthesia is required; otherwise it can be done in the office. The patient is initially placed in the supine position.
  2. After the skin near the nose and mouth is cleansed, the nose is sprayed with a Xylocaine/epinephrine solution to diminish any bleeding.
  3. The sinuses are viewed with an endoscope preformed at various angles to permit optimal viewing.
  4. Sinus contents are examined and aspirated for culture testing.

After

- Place a 4 × 4 gauze pad under the nose to collect any fluid or blood that may further drain from the nose.
- If a cerebral spinal fluid leak is suspected, the fluid can be checked for sugar with a Dextrostix. Spinal fluid contains glucose.
- Assess the patient frequently for signs of bleeding. Report any significant findings to the physician.
- Allow the patient to have oral fluids.

TEST RESULTS AND CLINICAL SIGNIFICANCE

Chronic or resistant sinusitis: *These diseases usually come from inadequate drainage of the sinuses. Endoscopy should hasten cure.*
Sinus tumors: *These can be visualized and cells obtained to assist in the diagnosis of these tumors.*
Sinus cysts,
Sinus mucoceles:
  These usually occur after years of chronic sinus infections.

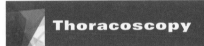

Thoracoscopy

NORMAL FINDINGS

Normal pleura and lung

INDICATIONS

This procedure is used to directly visualize the pleura, lung, and mediastinum. Tissue can be obtained for testing. It is also helpful in assisting in the staging and dissection of lung cancers.

TEST EXPLANATION

Thoracoscopy is experiencing a renewal as a result of the development of instrumentation for operative laparoscopy. With this technique the parietal pleura, visceral pleura, and mediastinum can be directly visualized. Tumors involving the chest cavity can be staged by direct visualization. A biopsy of any abnormality can be performed. Collections of fluid can be drained and aspirated for testing. Dissection for lung resection can be carried out with the thoracoscope (*video-assisted thoracotomy* [VAT]), thereby minimizing the extent of a thoracotomy incision. VAT is especially helpful for lung biopsy in patients with pulmonary nodules of uncertain cause or for suspected *Pneumocystis* infections in immunocompromised patients.

The patient must be aware of the possibility of requiring an open thoracotomy if the procedure cannot be performed thoracoscopically or if bleeding occurs that cannot be controlled any other way. Any patient who can have an open thoracotomy can have a thoracoscopy.

CONTRAINDICATIONS

- Patients with previous lung surgery, because it is difficult to obtain access to the free pleural space

POTENTIAL COMPLICATIONS

- Bleeding
- Infection or empyema
- Prolonged pneumothorax

PROCEDURE AND PATIENT CARE

Before

✗ Explain the procedure to the patient.

✗ Ensure that an informed consent for this procedure is obtained. Because of the possibility of intra-thoracic injury, an open thoracotomy may be required. Inform the patient of this possibility.

- Because the procedure is usually performed with the patient under general anesthesia, follow the routine general anesthesia precautions.
- Shave and prepare the patient's chest as ordered.

✗ Keep the patient on nothing by mouth (NPO) status after midnight on the day of the test. Intravenous (IV) fluids may be given.

During

- Note the following procedural steps:
  1. Thoracoscopy is performed in the operating room. The patient is initially placed in the lateral decubitus position.
  2. After the thorax is cleansed, a blunt-tipped (Verres) needle is inserted through a small incision and the lung is collapsed.
  3. A thoracoscope is inserted through a trocar to examine the chest cavity. Other trocars can be placed as conduits for other instrumentation.
  4. After the desired procedure is completed, the scope and trocars are removed.
  5. Usually a small chest tube is placed to ensure full reexpansion of the lung.
  6. The incision(s) is closed with a few skin stitches and covered with an adhesive bandage.

After

- Assess the patient frequently for signs of bleeding (increased pulse rate, decreased blood pressure). Report any significant findings to the physician.
- Provide analgesics to relieve the minor to moderate pain that may be experienced.
- If a surgical procedure has been performed thoracoscopically, provide appropriate specific postsurgical care.
- Note that a chest x-ray examination is performed after the procedure to ensure complete reexpansion of the lung.
- If a chest tube is left in place, provide assessment and care.

TEST RESULTS AND CLINICAL SIGNIFICANCE

Primary lung cancer,

Metastatic cancer to the lung or pleura:

   Often these tumors can be easily seen and biopsies performed, or the tumors can be removed through or with the help of thoracoscopy.

Empyema: *The infected fluid can be drained directly and valuable specimens obtained for cultures.*

Pleural diseases such as tumor, infection, or inflammation: *Biopsies of either the parietal or visceral pleura can be performed during this procedure.*

Pulmonary infection: *Thoracoscopy is particularly helpful in obtaining lung tissue for suspected infections such as tuberculosis,* Pneumocystis jiroveci, *coccidioidomycosis, or histoplasmosis.*

RELATED TEST

Laparoscopy (p. 617). This test is to the abdomen as thoracoscopy is to the chest. Most of the instruments are the same.

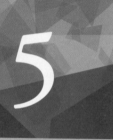

Fluid Analysis Studies

OVERVIEW

TESTS

 Overview

REASONS FOR PERFORMING FLUID ANALYSIS

Body fluid analysis can provide a significant amount of information concerning diseases that affect a patient. Normal body fluids can provide information concerning the body's hormonal status (cervical mucus test) and fertility (semen analysis, Sims-Huhner test). Cerebrospinal fluid (CSF) analysis (obtained by lumbar puncture) can provide significant data concerning diseases involving the CNS (brain and spinal cord). The normal collection of fluid that surrounds a fetus during pregnancy can be aspirated to gain information about the present and future health of the child and mother.

Abnormal accumulations of fluid *(effusions)* can be aspirated from the body to gain information about the disease process that caused the fluid to develop. Effusions can occur nearly anywhere in the body. Their presence is abnormal. In this chapter we discuss effusions within the pericardium, pleura, peritoneum, and joints. Effusions are classified as a transudate or an exudate. The purpose of this classification is to categorize possible diagnoses. In general, exudates are caused by inflammatory, infectious, or neoplastic diseases. Transudates are generally caused by venous engorgement, hypoproteinemia, or fluid overload.

Other body fluids are analyzed to indicate specific disease such as cystic fibrosis (sweat electrolytes or pancreatic enzymes). The secretion of these body fluids is stimulated to obtain enough fluid for analysis.

Most body fluids are not easily obtained. Usually a cavity of the body must be invaded to obtain the fluids for analysis. A needle is used for aspiration of fluid from the subarachnoid space of the central nervous system (CNS) (lumbar puncture), uterus (amniocentesis), pericardium (pericardiocentesis), pleura (thoracentesis), peritoneum (paracentesis), or joint (arthrocentesis). This aspiration must be done under complete and ensured sterile technique to avoid the introduction of infection to the body cavity. The quantity aspirated can vary from 20 mL to 5 L, depending on the location and original volume of the fluid. Testing of the fluid should be performed immediately to prevent inaccurate results caused by cellular or chemical deterioration. If testing cannot be done immediately, guidelines for preservation should be closely followed. Usually the fluid is evaluated for gross appearance, color, odor, red and white cell counts and differential, albumen and protein content, glucose and lactic dehydrogenase (LDH) levels, cytology, fungi, tuberculosis, and bacteria (culture or Gram stain). Other tests may be performed, depending on the specifics of the fluid or the suspected disease.

Not only is the aspiration of fluid helpful diagnostically, but it is often helpful therapeutically. The aspiration of fluid from the pleura often improves ventilation and oxygenation. Aspiration of fluid from the peritoneum often relieves pressure and allows the patient to breathe more easily and eat more comfortably. Joint fluid aspiration may improve joint function. Pericardial fluid aspiration improves diastolic filling and cardiac output. Furthermore, therapeutic drugs (steroids or antibiotics) or diagnostic contrast materials (for x-ray evaluation) can be injected through the aspirating needle.

Although some other body fluids do not require aspiration, care must still be applied to obtaining and transporting the fluid properly (semen analysis, cervical mucus, sweat electrolytes, and pancreatic enzymes). One must be aware that the evaluation of some body fluids may be very important as criminal legal evidence (Sims-Huhner test in rape cases). It is extremely important that cross-contamination of fluid samples be prevented. It is possible to cross-contaminate specimens merely by failing to change gloves or by labeling specimens improperly.

PROCEDURAL CARE FOR FLUID ANALYSIS

Before

- Explain the procedure to the patient.
- Obtain informed consent for this procedure.
- Tell the patient that no fasting is necessary unless heavy sedation or an operative procedure is used to obtain the fluid.
- Have the patient urinate or empty the bladder before the test to avoid inadvertent puncture of the bladder during paracentesis or hip joint aspiration.
- Obtain the patient's weight.
- Obtain baseline vital signs.

During

- The patient is positioned in a manner designed to make the fluid most accessible to the aspirating needle.
- Aspirating techniques are always performed under sterile conditions.
- When obtaining semen or cervical mucus, penile or vaginal preparation is contraindicated.
- With aspiration techniques a variable amount of fluid is aspirated. Small volumes are aspirated into a syringe. For larger volumes the aspirating needle is attached to a plastic tubing. The other end of the tubing is placed in the collection receptacle (usually a container with a pressurized vacuum).

- If medications are to be administered, a syringe containing the preparation is attached to the needle and the drug is injected.
- To compare fluid levels to blood level and to calculate ratios, blood is simultaneously drawn for glucose, albumin, total protein, LDH, and so on.

After

- All tests performed on fluid should be performed immediately to avoid false results because of chemical or cellular deterioration.
- Place a small bandage over the needle site after aspiration is performed.
- Label the specimen with the patient's name, date, source of fluid, and diagnosis.
- Send the specimen promptly to the laboratory.
- Observe the puncture site for bleeding, continued drainage, or signs of infection if aspiration is performed.
- Monitor vital signs for evidence of hemodynamic changes if large volumes of fluid are withdrawn.
- Write any recent antibiotic therapy on the microbiology laboratory requisition slip.
- Place the patient is a position designed to minimize further leakage of fluid from an aspiration site.
- Monitor the patient and educate the patient about signs of potential complications.

POTENTIAL COMPLICATIONS OF FLUID ANALYSIS TESTING

The complications associated with fluid analysis are those of aspirating fluid for analysis. In general, they include the following:

- Injury to an organ by penetration with the aspirating needle
- Bleeding into the fluid space as a result of blood vessel penetration during aspiration
- Reflex bradycardia and hypotension because of the patient's anxiety about the procedure
- Infection of the soft tissue around the needle aspiration site
- Infection of the remaining fluid within the fluid space
- Seeding of the aspirating needle tract with tumor when malignant effusion exists
- Persistent leakage of effusion fluid after withdrawal of the aspirating needle

Other specific complications are discussed with each test.

REPORTING RESULTS

In most instances, fluid is obtained by a physician. The laboratory tests are performed by technologists and are usually reported the same day. Cytologic study results are interpreted by a pathologist and are reported after several days. Culture and sensitivity reports also take several days.

 Amniocentesis (Amniotic Fluid Analysis)

NORMAL FINDINGS

Weeks' Gestation	Amniotic Fluid Volume (mL)
15	450
25	750
30-35	1500
Full term	>1500

Amniotic fluid appearance: clear; pale to straw yellow

Lecithin/sphingomyelin (L/S) ratio: ≥2:1

Bilirubin: <0.2 mg/dL

No chromosomal or genetic abnormalities

Phosphatidylglycerol (PG): positive for PG

Lamellar body count: >30,000

Alpha-fetoprotein: dependent on gestational age and laboratory technique

Fetal lung maturity (FLM)

    Mature: <260 mPOL

    Transitional: 260-290 mPOL

    Immature: >290 mPOL

INDICATIONS

Amniocentesis is performed on women to gather information about the fetus. Fetal maturity, fetal distress, and risk for respiratory distress syndrome can be assessed. Genetic and chromosomal abnormalities can be identified. Maternal-fetal Rh incompatibility can be diagnosed. The sex of the child can be ascertained. This is important for a mother carrying a sex-linked gene. Neural tube defects can also be recognized. The test is performed on mothers whose pregnancies are considered to be high risk. These may include diabetic mothers, very obese mothers, older mothers (over 35 to 40 years) especially if there is a family history of trisomy 21, mothers with repeated spontaneous abortions, mothers whose prior children have genetic defects, and mothers in a couple in which either the mother or the father is a carrier for genetic defects. This test is also done on women who have an abnormal obstetric ultrasound.

TEST EXPLANATION

Amniocentesis involves the placement of a needle through the patient's abdominal and uterine walls into the amniotic cavity to withdraw fluid for analysis. Studying amniotic fluid is vitally important in assessing the following:

1. **Fetal maturity status,** especially pulmonary maturity (when early delivery is preferred). Fetal maturity is determined by analysis of the amniotic fluid in the following manner:

    a. *Lecithin and sphingomyelin (L/S ratio).* The measurement of the ratio of the lipids L/S ratio has emerged as the standard criterion test to evaluate fetal lung maturity. Lecithin is the major constituent of surfactant, an important substance required for alveolar ventilation. If surfactant is insufficient, the alveoli collapse during expiration. This results in atelectasis and respiratory distress syndrome (RDS), which is a major cause of death in immature babies. In the immature fetal lung, the sphingomyelin concentration in amniotic fluid is higher than the lecithin concentration. At 35 weeks of gestation, the concentration of lecithin rapidly increases, whereas the sphingomyelin concentration decreases. An L/S ratio of 2:1 (3:1 in mothers with diabetes) or greater is a highly reliable indication that the fetal lung, and therefore the fetus, is mature. In such a case the infant would be unlikely to develop RDS after birth. As the L/S ratio decreases, the risk of RDS increases.

    Unfortunately, the L/S ratio assay involves a long and labor-intensive thin layer chromatography separation of the lipids. An alternative test is an assay based on fluorescence depolarization, implemented on the TDx fluorescence polarimeter and is called TDx *Fetal Lung Maturity (FLM)* test. This test, which yields the ratio of surfactant to albumin (S/A ratio), is quite sensitive.

FLM results are less affected by other factors such as contaminated blood or meconium. A fluorescent phospholipid analogue (C6-NBD-PC) is added to amniotic fluid and its fluorescence polarization is measured with a TDx fluorescence polarimeter. Polarization values decrease during gestation in parallel with maturation of the pulmonary surfactant system. Polarization value can be used to predict the probability that a fetus will develop respiratory distress syndrome following birth. Infrared (IR) spectroscopy offers an alternative method to detect and quantitate the key surfactants. The infrared spectrum of amniotic fluid shows strong absorptions from protein such as albumin when compared with the surfactant lipids contributing subtle absorption differences to the overall profile.

b. *Phosphatidylglycerol (PG)*. This is a minor component (about 10%) of lung surfactant phospholipids. However, because PG is synthesized almost entirely by mature lung alveolar cells, it is a good indicator of lung maturity. Because PG appears late in gestation, this test indicates a more mature surfactant than that found in the L/S ratio described previously. In healthy pregnant women, PG appears in amniotic fluid after 35 weeks of gestation, and levels gradually increase until term. An advantage of the PG assay is that it is not affected by contamination of amniotic fluid by blood or meconium. These two contaminants cause false-positive and false-negative results for the L/S ratio evaluation. In addition, the presence of PG in the amniotic fluid in the vagina after the membranes are ruptured indicates a low risk for RDS of the newborn. The simultaneous determination of the L/S ratio and the presence of PG is an excellent method of assessing fetal maturity based on pulmonary surfactant.

c. *Lamellar body count*. This newer test to determine fetal maturity is also based on the presence of surfactant. Lamellar bodies are concentrically layered structures produced by type II pneumocytes. On cross section, these small (about 3 μm) structures look like an onion. These lamellar bodies represent the storage form of pulmonary surfactant. Because lamellar bodies and platelets are indistinguishable to cell counters, the lamellar body count is obtained by analyzing the amniotic fluid with a cell counter and recording the platelet count. Lamellar body results are calculated in units of particle density per microliter of amniotic fluid. Some researchers have recommended cutoffs of 30,000/μL and 10,000/μL to predict low and high risk for RDS, respectively. If the count is greater than 30,000/μL, the negative predictive value for RDS is 100% (i.e., there is a 100% chance that the infant's lungs are mature enough to not experience RDS). If the lamellar body count is less than 10,000/μL, the probability of RDS is high (67%). Values between 10,000/μL and 30,000/mcL represent intermediate risk for RDS. At this time, not enough information is available on lamellar body count in diabetics to advocate its use in this high-risk group. There are several advantages of lamellar body counts. First, they are faster, more precise, and more objective, and they require less amniotic fluid than phospholipid analysis. Second, test results are not invalidated by the presence of blood or meconium. Third, the instrumentation required for this test is readily available, thus allowing it to be performed in all laboratories.

d. *Microviscosity*. Microvisocity in lipid aggregates is dependent on the L/S ratio and the degree of saturation of fatty acid side chains. The pattern of change of amniotic fluid microviscosity during gestation parallels the expected development of the surfactant system. Amniotic fluid microviscosity is high during early gestation and abruptly and sequentially decreases between the 28th and 36th week of gestation. The measurements are an accurate reflection of the development of the surfactant system and thereby fetal lung maturity. With the development of more accurate testing such as FLM as described above, this testing is no longer routinely performed and is included here more for recent historical value.

2. **Sex of the fetus.** Sons of mothers who are known to be carriers of X-linked recessive traits have a 50:50 risk of inheritance. It is important to note that amniocentesis is not done to determine the sex of the child just out of interest.

3. **Genetic and chromosomal aberrations,** such as hemophilia, Down syndrome, and galactosemia. Genetic and chromosomal studies performed on cells aspirated within the amniotic fluid can indicate the gender of the fetus (important in sex-linked diseases such as hemophilia) or many genetic and chromosomal aberrations (e.g., trisomy 21). (See Laboratory Genetics, p. 1104).

4. **Fetal status affected by Rh isoimmunization.** Mothers with Rh isoimmunization have a series of amniocentesis procedures during the second half of pregnancy to assess the level of bilirubin pigment in the amniotic fluid. The quantity of bilirubin is used to assess the severity of hemolytic anemia in Rh-sensitized pregnancy. The higher the amount of bilirubin, the lower is the amount of fetal hemoglobin. Amniocentesis is usually initiated at 24 to 25 weeks. This allows assessment of the severity of the disease and the status of the fetus. Early delivery or blood transfusion may be indicated. It is important to take into consideration the volume of amniotic fluid because bilirubin concentration will be affected by total fluid volume.

5. **Hereditary metabolic disorders,** such as cystic fibrosis.

6. **Anatomic abnormalities,** such as neural tube closure defects (myelomeningocele, anencephaly, spina bifida). Increased levels of alpha-fetoprotein (AFP) in the amniotic fluid may indicate a neural crest abnormality (p. 54). Decreased levels of AFP may be associated with increased risk of trisomy 21.

7. **Fetal distress,** detected by meconium staining of the amniotic fluid. This is caused by relaxation of the anal sphincter. In this case the normally colorless and pale, straw-colored amniotic fluid may be tinged with green. Other color changes may also indicate fetal distress. For example, a yellow discoloration may indicate a blood incompatibility. A yellow-brown opaque appearance may indicate intrauterine death. A red color indicates blood contamination from either the mother or the fetus.

Amniocentesis may be done on the premise that elective abortion could be performed if the fetus is severely defective. Chorionic villus sampling (CVS) may be even better than amniocentesis for karyotyping and genetic analysis. CVS can be performed earlier in the pregnancy than can amniocentesis. (The earliest one can obtain amniotic fluid is at about 12 to 14 weeks.) Thus with CVS a decision can be made concerning abortion much earlier in the pregnancy than with amniocentesis.

The timing of the amniocentesis varies according to the clinical circumstances. With advanced maternal age and if chromosomal or genetic aberrations are suspected, the test should be done early enough to allow a safe abortion. If information on fetal maturity is sought, performing the study during or after the thirty-fifth week of gestation is best. Placental localization by ultrasonography (see p. 887) should be done before amniocentesis to avoid the needle passing into the placenta, possibly interrupting the placenta, and inducing bleeding or abortion.

CONTRAINDICATIONS

- Patients with abruptio placentae
- Patients with placenta previa
- Patients with a history of premature labor (before 34 weeks of gestation, unless the patient is receiving anti-labor medication)
- Patients with an incompetent cervix

POTENTIAL COMPLICATIONS

- Miscarriage
- Fetal injury

Fluid Analysis Studies

5

- Leak of amniotic fluid
- Infection (amnionitis)
- Abortion
- Premature labor
- Maternal hemorrhage with possible maternal Rh isoimmunization
- Amniotic fluid embolism
- Abruptio placentae
- Inadvertent damage to the bladder or intestines

INTERFERING FACTORS

- Fetal blood contamination can cause falsely elevated AFP levels.
- Hemolysis of the specimen can alter results.
- Contamination of the specimen with meconium or blood may result in inaccurate L/S ratios.

Clinical Priorities

- Instructions regarding emptying the bladder vary according to gestational age. Before 20 weeks, the bladder should be kept full to support the uterus. After 20 weeks, the bladder must be emptied to minimize the chance of puncture.
- Before this procedure the placenta should be localized by ultrasonography to select a site to avoid placental puncture.
- Women who have Rh-negative blood should receive RhoGAM because of the risk of immunization from fetal blood.

PROCEDURE AND PATIENT CARE

Before

 Explain the procedure to the patient. Allay any fears and allow the patient to verbalize her concerns.
- Obtain an informed consent from the patient and her partner.
 Tell the patient that no food or fluid is restricted.
- Evaluate the mother's blood pressure and the fetal heart rate.
- Follow instructions regarding emptying the bladder, which depend on gestational age. Before 20 weeks of gestation, the bladder may be kept full to support the uterus. After 20 weeks, the bladder may be emptied to minimize the chance of puncture.
- Localize the placenta by ultrasound examination before the study to permit selection of a site that will avoid placental puncture.

During

- Place the patient in the supine position.
- Note the following procedural steps:
  1. The skin overlying the chosen site (often determined by obstetric ultrasonography) is prepared and usually anesthetized locally.
  2. A needle with a stylet is inserted through the midabdominal wall and directed at an angle toward the middle of the uterine cavity (Figure 5-1).

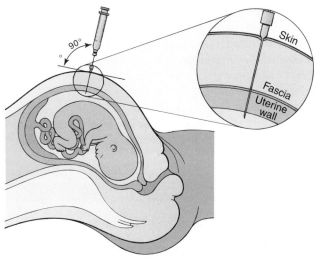

Figure 5-1 Amniocentesis. Ultrasound scanning is usually used to determine the placental site and to locate a pocket of amniotic fluid. The needle is then inserted. Three levels of resistance are felt as the needle penetrates the skin, fascia, and uterine wall. When the needle is placed within the uterine cavity, amniotic fluid is withdrawn.

Fluid Analysis Studies

5

3. The stylet is then removed and a sterile plastic syringe attached.
4. After 5 to 10 mL of amniotic fluid is withdrawn, the needle is removed. (This fluid volume is replaced by newly formed amniotic fluid within 3 to 4 hours after the procedure.)
5. The specimen is placed in a light-resistant container to prevent breakdown of bilirubin.
6. The site is covered with an adhesive bandage.
7. If the amniotic fluid is bloody, the physician must determine whether the blood is maternal or fetal in origin. Kleihauer-Böetke stain will stain fetal cells pink. Meconium in the fluid is usually associated with a compromised fetus.

- Amniotic fluid volume is calculated by injecting a known concentration of solute (such as para-aminohippuric acid [PAH]) into the amniotic fluid to distribute throughout the amniotic fluid. Amniotic fluid is then withdrawn, and the PAH concentration is determined.
- Note that this procedure is performed by a physician and takes approximately 20 to 30 minutes.
- Tell the patient that the discomfort associated with amniocentesis is usually described as a mild uterine cramping that occurs when the needle contacts the uterus. Some women may complain of a "pulling" sensation as the amniotic fluid is withdrawn.
- Remember that many women are extremely anxious during this procedure.

After

- Place amniotic fluid in a sterile, siliconized glass container and transport it to a special chemistry laboratory for analysis. Sometimes the specimen may be sent by air mail to another commercial laboratory for genetic and other testing.
- Inform the patient that the results of this study are usually not available for over 1 week.

- For women who have Rh-negative blood, administer RhoGAM because of the risk of immunization from the fetal blood.
- Assess the fetal heart rate after the test to detect any ill effects related to the procedure. Compare this value with the preprocedural baseline value.
- If the patient felt dizzy or nauseated during the procedure, instruct her to lie on her left side for several minutes before leaving the examining room.
- Observe the puncture site for bleeding or other drainage.
- Instruct the patient to call her physician if she has any amniotic fluid loss, bleeding, temperature elevation, abdominal pain or cramping, fetal hyperactivity, or unusual fetal lethargy.

🏠 Home Care Responsibilities

- Inform the patient that the puncture site should be checked for bleeding and amniotic fluid loss.
- Instruct the patient to call her physician if she has any fluid loss, bleeding, chills, temperature elevation, abdominal cramping, or unusual fetal movement.

TEST RESULTS AND CLINICAL SIGNIFICANCE

Hemolytic disease of the newborn: *This may be apparent as increased bilirubin in the amniotic fluid. The fetal hemolysis causes free heme to form. This is then catabolized to bilirubin.*

Rh isoimmunization: *A rising anti-Rh antibody titer in an Rh-negative woman would indicate potential for erythroblastosis fetalis (Rh-positive fetus). The higher the bilirubin in the amniotic fluid, the greater is the risk to the fetus.*

Neural tube closure defects (e.g., myelomeningocele, anencephaly, spina bifida),
Abdominal wall closure defects (e.g., gastroschisis, omphalocele),
Sacrococcygeal teratoma:
   An elevated AFP level most commonly indicates neural tube defects. However, other closing defects (e.g., abdominal wall) can occur. Neoplasms associated with neural tube defects may also be associated with increased AFP levels. Blood levels of AFP are also increased with these abnormalities.

Meconium staining: *This is evidence of fetal distress and is noted as greenish staining of the amniotic fluid.*

Immature fetal lungs: *This may occur with premature labor, maternal hypertension, or placental injuries. The risk of RDS increases as evidence of fetal lung immaturity increases. Fetal lung maturity is diminished in diabetic mothers. This is also noted in hydrops fetalis.*

Hereditary metabolic disorders (e.g., cystic fibrosis, Tay-Sachs disease, galactosemia),
Genetic or chromosomal aberrations (e.g., sickle cell anemia, thalassemia, Down syndrome),
Sex-linked disorders (e.g., hemophilia):
   The genetic defects of many diseases can be recognized through gene recognition and karyotyping. Other genetic defects causing metabolic disorders can be recognized by the results of protein analysis of the amniotic fluid.

Polyhydramnios: *This occurs in patients who have diabetes. When polyhydramnios (>2000 mL) is present, the risk of congenital aberrations increases significantly.*

Oligohydramnios: *This is recognized as less than 300 mL of amniotic fluid at 25 weeks' gestation. It is associated with fetal renal diseases. Near term, it is associated with early membrane rupture, intrauterine growth restriction, or significant postterm pregnancy.*

RELATED TESTS

Chorionic Villus Sampling (CVS) (p. 1088). This is a test whereby the chorionic placental tissue (which has the same genetic material as the fetus) is tested for genetic analysis and karyotyping. This is a rapid and accurate method of determining genetic defects. CVS can be performed earlier in pregnancy than can amniocentesis.

Maternal Screen Testing, (p. 354). This is a series of screening tests that can identify fetal distress and chromosomal abnormalities.

Fetoscopy (p. 612). This is another method of obtaining fetal tissue for genetic and maturity testing.

Obstetric Ultrasound (p. 887). Significant fetal disease and evidence of fetal distress can be detected on ultrasound examination. If findings are abnormal, amniocentesis is indicated.

Amyloid Beta Protein Precursor, Soluble (sBPP)

NORMAL FINDINGS

>450 units/L

INDICATIONS

This test is performed on patients who become increasingly demented and confused. It is a test used to help diagnose Alzheimer disease (AD) and other forms of senile dementia.

TEST EXPLANATION

Amyloid protein is a 42-amino-acid peptide that is broken off of a larger amyloid pre-cursor protein (beta APP). These beta amyloid proteins have been shown to be neurotrophic and neuroprotective. Beta amyloid is deposited on the brain in the form of plaques in patients with AD. It has been discovered that these plaques contain damaged nerve cells in a compacted core of beta amyloid protein. As a result of this deposition, levels of beta amyloid are decreased in the cerebrospinal fluid of patients with AD and other forms of dementia. Research has demonstrated the diagnostic potential of this biochemical marker for AD.

Ongoing research has also focused on using cerebrospinal fluid (CSF) levels of *tau protein* as another biochemical marker for AD. Neurofibrillary tangles, also noted in the brains of patients with AD, are composed primarily of hyperphosphorylated tau. There is a general consensus that CSF levels of tau are significantly increased in patients with AD as compared with healthy control subjects and patients with non-AD neurologic disease. These tests require a CSF sample obtained by lumbar puncture (p. 651).

At this time, there is little or no consensus on the use of screening tests for diagnosing early AD. This is due to lack of sensitivity and specificity and sufficient normative data. However, there is consensus that using a combination of early neuropsychologic changes and biomarkers will facilitate making the diagnosis of prodromal AD earlier than current criteria for probable AD allow.

Recently, PET scanning with amyloid imaging (p. 823) has shown promise for the diagnosis of AD. Pittsburgh Agent B (PIB) appears to reliably detect brain amyloid due to the accumulation of A beta 42 within plaques. Studies so far have revealed high levels of amyloid retention in the brain at prodromal stages of AD and the possibility of discriminating AD from other dementia disorders by scanning with PIB. The PET scans using PIB as the imaging agent have shown a dramatically different amyloid deposition pattern in AD versus normal brains. Since amyloid accumulation is one of the earliest signs of AD, early diagnosis may be facilitated by identifying amyloid early in the disease progression, perhaps before symptoms emerge.

Anti-amyloid beta precursor protein antibody can be identified in brain tissue by immunohisto-chemistry and is diagnostic for AD.

PROCEDURE AND PATIENT CARE

Before

⚕ Explain the procedure to the patient.
- Refer to the instructions for a lumbar puncture and CSF examination (p. 651).

During

- Collect a CSF specimen as indicated in the lumbar puncture discussion (p. 651).

After

- Follow the postprocedure guidelines for a lumbar puncture.

TEST RESULTS AND CLINICAL SIGNIFICANCE

▼ Decreased Levels

Alzheimer disease,
Other senile dementia:
> *These patients have low beta amyloid levels in their CSF, possibly because of its deposition in the brain. How these plaques of beta amyloid exert the neurologic damage is unknown.*

RELATED TESTS

Lumbar Puncture (p. 651). This diagnostic procedure is required to obtain the CSF to be studied for beta amyloid proteins.

PET scan (p. 821). PET scanning with amyloid imaging is able to identify plaques within the brain compatible with the changes of Alzheimer's disease.

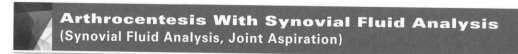

Arthrocentesis With Synovial Fluid Analysis
(Synovial Fluid Analysis, Joint Aspiration)

NORMAL FINDINGS

SYNOVIAL FLUID ANALYSIS

	Normal Findings
Appearance	Clear Straw-Colored
	No Blood
RBC	None
WBC	0-150/mm^3
WBC differential	
Neutrophils	7%
Lymphocytes	24%
Monocytes	48%
Macrophages	10%

Continued

Glucose	Equal to fasting blood glucose
Protein	1-3 dL
LDH	<25 mg/dL
Uric acid	6-8 mg/dL
Gram stain	Negative

INDICATIONS

Arthrocentesis is performed to establish the diagnosis of joint infection, arthritis, crystal-induced arthritis (gout and pseudogout), synovitis, or neoplasms involving the joint. This procedure is also used to identify the cause of joint inflammation or effusion, to monitor chronic arthritic diseases, and to inject antiinflammatory medications (usually corticosteroids) into a joint space.

TEST EXPLANATION

Arthrocentesis is performed by inserting a sterile needle into the joint space of the involved joint to obtain synovial fluid for analysis. Synovial fluid is a liquid found in small amounts within the joints. Aspiration (withdrawal of the fluid) may be performed on any major joint, such as the knee, shoulder, hip, elbow, wrist, or ankle.

The fluid sample is examined microscopically and chemically. A gram stain and culture of the fluid is usually performed. Normal joint fluid is clear, straw colored, and quite viscous because of the hyaluronic acid, which acts as a lubricant. Viscosity is reduced in patients with inflammatory arthritis. Viscosity can be roughly estimated by forcing some synovial fluid from a syringe. Fluid of normal viscosity forms a "string" more than 5 cm long; fluid of low viscosity as seen in inflammation drips in a manner similar to water.

The *mucin clot test* correlates with the viscosity and is an estimation of hyaluronic acid-protein complex integrity. This test is performed by adding acetic acid to joint fluid. The formation of a tight, ropy clot indicates qualitatively good mucin and the presence of adequate molecules of intact hyaluronic acid. Hyaluronic acid can be directly quantified by Enzyme Linked Immunoabsorbent Assay. The mucin clot is poor in quality and quantity in the presence of an inflammatory joint disease, such as rheumatoid arthritis (RA). By itself, synovial fluid should not spontaneously form a fibrin clot (clot without the addition of acetic acid) because normal joint fluid does not contain fibrinogen. If, however, bleeding into the joint (from trauma or injury) has occurred, the synovial fluid will clot.

The synovial fluid glucose value is usually within 10 mL/dL of the fasting serum glucose value. For proper interpretation the synovial fluid glucose and serum glucose samples should be drawn simultaneously after the patient has fasted for 6 hours. The synovial fluid glucose level falls with increasing severity of inflammation. Although lowest in septic arthritis (the synovial fluid glucose value may be less than 50% of the serum glucose value), a low synovial glucose level also may be seen in patients with rheumatoid arthritis. The synovial fluid is also tested for protein, uric acid, and lactate levels. Increased uric acid levels indicate gout. Increased protein and lactate levels indicate bacterial infection or inflammation.

Cell counts are also performed on the synovial fluid. Normally the joint fluid contains less than 200 WBCs/mm^3 and 2000 RBCs/mL. An increased WBC count with a high percentage of neutrophils (over 75%) supports the diagnosis of acute bacterial infectious arthritis. Leukocytes can also occur in other conditions, such as acute gouty arthritis and rheumatoid arthritis. The differential white cell count, however, will indicate monocytosis or lymphocytosis with these later-mentioned diseases.

Bacterial and fungal cultures are usually requested and performed when infection is suspected. The administration of antibiotics prior to arthrocentesis may diminish growth of bacteria from synovial fluid cultures and confound results. Smears for acid-fast stains for tubercle bacilli are also performed on the synovial fluid. Synovial fluid is also examined under polarized light for the presence of crystals, which permits differential diagnosis between gout and pseudogout. (The calcium pyrophosphate dihydrate crystals of pseudogout are birefringent [blue on red background] when examined with a polarized light microscope.)

The synovial fluid is also analyzed for complement levels (p. 172). Complement levels are decreased in patients with systemic lupus erythematosus, rheumatoid arthritis, or other immunologic arthritis. These decreased joint complement levels are caused by consumption of the complement induced by the antigen-antibody immune complexes within the joint cavity.

One of the most important tests routinely performed on synovial fluid is the microscopic examination for crystals. For example, urate crystals indicate gouty arthritis. Calcium pyrophosphate crystals are found in pseudogout. Cholesterol crystals occur in rheumatoid arthritis.

A physician performs this procedure in an office or at the patient's bedside in approximately 10 minutes. The only discomfort associated with this test is from the injection of the local anesthetic. The joint-space pain may worsen after fluid aspiration, especially in patients with acute arthritis. The administration of steroids is also associated with pain for as much as 2 days after the injection.

CONTRAINDICATIONS

- Patients with skin or wound infections in the area of the needle puncture, because of the risk for sepsis

POTENTIAL COMPLICATIONS

- Joint infection
- Hemorrhage in the joint area

PROCEDURE AND PATIENT CARE

Before

- Explain the procedure to the patient.
- Obtain an informed consent if this is the institution's policy.
- Keep the patient on nothing by mouth (NPO) status after midnight on the day of the test. This is done to prevent alterations of the chemical determinations (e.g., glucose) that may be performed with the study. However, this study may be done more conveniently in a physician's office without the patient fasting.

During

- Have the patient lie on his or her back with the joint fully extended.
- Note the following procedural steps:
  1. The skin is locally anesthetized to minimize pain.
  2. The area is aseptically cleansed, and a needle is inserted through the skin and into the joint space.
  3. Fluid is obtained for analysis. The joint area sometimes may be wrapped with an elastic bandage to compress free fluid within a certain area, thereby ensuring maximal collection of fluid.
  4. If a corticosteroid or other medications (e.g., antibiotics) are to be administered, a syringe containing the steroid preparation is attached to the needle and the drug is injected.
  5. The needle is removed, and a pressure dressing may be applied to the site.
  6. Sometimes a peripheral venous blood sample is taken to compare chemical tests on the blood with chemical studies on the synovial fluid.

After

- Assess the joint for any pain, fever, or swelling, which may indicate infection.
- Apply ice to decrease pain and swelling.
- Keep a pressure dressing on the joint to avoid re-collection of joint fluid or development of a hematoma.
- Tell the patient to avoid strenuous use of the joint for the next several days.

TEST RESULTS AND CLINICAL SIGNIFICANCE

Infection,

Septic arthritis:

> *This can be the result of penetrating trauma or blood-borne infection resulting from bacteremia. One would expect to see a red, warm, swollen, and painful joint. The joint fluid would be expected to have a reduced glucose level, increased levels of WBCs, protein, and lactate (because of the lactate produced by the bacteria). Gram stains and cultures (p. 704) may identify the offending organism.*

Degenerative arthritis (osteoarthritis): *Degenerative changes involving the joint space may be caused by excess nongouty crystals within the joint space and cartilage. The course is usually chronic and without acute flare-up. Nonsteroidal antiinflammatory drugs are usually helpful.*

Synovitis: *This can be inflammatory or infectious. The synovial membrane is the tissue surrounding the joint space.*

Neoplasm: *Synovial, cartilaginous, and bony tumors (benign and malignant) can begin in the joint. Protein levels can be expected to be elevated. Microscopy may reveal malignant cells.*

Joint effusion: *Joint effusion (fluid in the joint) causes the joint to be swollen. The fluid is obtained to determine the source of the effusion.*

Systemic lupus erythematosus,

Rheumatoid arthritis:

> *Autoimmune or collagen-vascular diseases can be associated with immunogenic arthritis. One may expect a reduced complement level and increased levels of WBCs and protein.*

Gout,

Pseudogout:

> *Crystal-induced arthritis occurs when urate (gout) or calcium pyrophosphate (pseudogout) is deposited into the joint-surrounding structures and joint surface cartilage. Inflammation follows, and arthritis occurs. In time, cartilage destruction occurs.*

Trauma: *When a joint is injured, a joint effusion may develop. This is usually a transudate. However, if a ligament or cartilage is torn, bleeding may occur within the joint.*

RELATED TEST

Arthroscopy (p. 583). This is an endoscopic procedure designed to directly view the joint space and to provide access to the joint for surgical treatment of disease and injury.

Breast Cyst and Nipple Discharge Fluid Analysis

NORMAL FINDINGS

No evidence of atypical or neoplastic cells

Fluid Analysis Studies

5

INDICATIONS

These two tests are used to attempt to make the diagnosis of cancer within breast cysts or to exclude the diagnosis of breast cancer as a cause of persistent nipple discharge.

TEST EXPLANATION

Fluid from breast cysts or nipple discharge can be examined cytologically for evidence of cancer cells. Most simple cysts (cysts that contain fluid and no tissue—as recognized by ultrasound, p. 871) are benign. The exceptions are if the aspirated fluid is bloody, the cyst repeatedly recurs after aspirations, or if the cyst does not completely collapse after aspiration. The contents of these simple cysts should be sent for cytologic examination. A complex cyst (one that contains some tissue) can be cancerous (cystic adenocarcinoma of the breast) and its contents should also be aspirated and examined microscopically. The cyst aspiration can be directed by palpation of the doctor or by ultrasound.

Cytologic examination of nipple discharge is not terribly reliable in the identification of cancer. Nearly all nonbloody nipple discharge comes from benign pathology. Only 10% to 12% of bloody discharges are related to breast cancer. Of that small percentage, less than half can be detected by a cytologic examination of the nipple discharge. Cellular deterioration can be misinterpreted as atypical or suspicious cytologic changes. This may cause an unnecessary breast biopsy.

POTENTIAL COMPLICATIONS

- Infection in the breast as a result of the needle aspiration
- Pneumothorax as a result of the needle penetrating a thin chest wall in attempting to aspirate a cyst in the posterior portion of the breast
- Hematoma in the breast as a result of intraglandular bleeding from a blood vessel penetrated by the aspirating needle

PROCEDURE AND PATIENT CARE

Before

- Because cyst aspiration may cause intraglandular bleeding that may temporarily distort mammography, a bilateral mammogram may be performed before cyst aspiration.
- Inform the patient of the proposed procedure.
- Allay the patient's concern about anticipated pain related to cyst aspiration. Only a very-small-bore needle is used. If a larger-bore needle is required, local anesthetic is used first.

During

Nipple Discharge

- Note the following procedure:
  1. Express the nipple discharge from the breast.
  2. Smear the discharge onto a clean microscope slide as for a Pap test.
  3. The cells are immediately fixed either by immersing the slide in equal parts of 95% alcohol and ether or by using a commercial spray (e.g., Aqua Net hair spray). The secretions must be fixed before drying because drying will distort the cells and make interpretation difficult. This fixing process kills most infectious organisms so that the specimen is less infectious to the personnel who handle the specimen.
  4. The slide is labeled with the patient's name, date of birth, date of test, and site of the lesion.

Cyst Aspiration

- Note the following procedure:
  1. While the patient is in the supine position, the cyst is identified by palpation or by ultrasound guidance.
  2. The skin overlying the cyst is prepared in a sterile manner.
  3. If a 25-gauge needle is to be used for aspiration, no local anesthetic is required. If, however, the fluid is suspected to be thick, a 20-gauge needle is used. In this circumstance, local anesthetic is infiltrated into the skin.
  4. The needle is inserted through the skin and into the cyst. Fluid is aspirated until the cyst is completely collapsed.
  5. The fluid is injected into a fixative solution (Carbowax) and appropriately labeled as described previously.

After

- Pressure is applied to the aspiration site. An adhesive bandage is applied.
- The patient should be informed that it is not uncommon to develop an ecchymosis in the area of the breast where the aspiration was performed.
- Allay the patient's fears, stating that if clear cyst fluid was obtained, the lesion is most certainly benign.

TEST RESULTS AND CLINICAL SIGNIFICANCE

Cancer,
Benign cyst:
> As indicated previously, cystic adenocarcinoma of the breast is very rare. When clear fluid is obtained and the cyst collapses completely, the cyst is considered to be benign.

Intraductal papilloma: *This is a common cause of breast discharge. Intraductal papillomas are benign, and no treatment is required unless the discharge is copious.*

RELATED TESTS

Ultrasound of the Breast (p. 871). This method of cyst visualization can be used to direct cyst aspiration.
Mammography (p. 1043). Cysts are apparent as soft tissue densities within the breast tissue.

Breast Ductal Lavage

NORMAL FINDINGS

No atypical cells in the effluent

POSSIBLE CRITICAL VALUES

Cancer cells in the effluent

INDICATIONS

This test is performed on women who are at increased risk for developing breast cancer and would make a decision to accept treatment designed to diminish that risk if atypical (premalignant) cells were found in their ducts.

TEST EXPLANATION

The theory behind ductal lavage is that by washing out exfoliated cells from a few breast ducts, the risk of developing breast cancer in the near future can be assessed. If atypical cells are obtained, the risk of developing breast cancer in the next decade may be as high as 4 to 10 times normal. Once that risk is identified, the patient may choose to attempt to alter that risk by using chemopreventive medications (such as selective estrogen receptor modulators) or surgery.

Initially, it was hoped that ductal lavage would identify ductal carcinoma of the breast at its earliest stages. The results of several large studies did not support that fact. Its use has now been limited to women who have been found to be at a statistically higher personal risk for breast cancer by *breast cancer risk models*. These statistical models are based on age of menarche, age of first pregnancy, prior breast surgery, family history, and history of atypical changes in previous breast biopsies. In women found to be at increased risk, many would like more data before they decide to take a medication designed to reduce those risks. If they were found to have atypical cells in the lavage, most would choose to take the medication. If no atypical cells were found, they may choose just close observation.

There are still no data to confirm that the findings do accurately reflect a true risk for breast cancer. Furthermore, there are no data to indicate what a negative lavage means.

CONTRAINDICATIONS

- Patients with prior breast cancer surgery because their risks are known to be high

POTENTIAL COMPLICATIONS

- Infection

PROCEDURE AND PATIENT CARE

Before

- Explain the procedure to the patient. Often these women have already received extensive counseling regarding their risks for breast cancer.
- Be sure the breast examination and mammogram are normal.
- Apply a topical anesthetic to the nipple area for about 30 minutes before the test.

During

- Note the following procedural steps:
  1. Prior to suction, the breast is massaged for a few minutes.
  2. A suction apparatus is applied to the nipple area. Ducts that reveal fluid with the suction are then chosen for cannulation.
  3. A tiny catheter is gently placed into the nipple and the duct is lavage with 5 to 10 mL of saline.
  4. The effluent is then collected in a small tube and sent for cytology.
  5. The procedure is then repeated for other ducts that produced fluid with nipple suction. A separate catheter is used for each duct.
  6. The sites for each cannulated duct are recorded on a grid representing the nipple for future reference.
- This procedure is performed by a surgeon in the office in approximately 30 minutes. There is minimal to moderate discomfort associated with the nipple suction, duct cannulation, and lavage.

TEST RESULTS AND CLINICAL SIGNIFICANCE

Atypical cells: *Atypical cells indicate that the patient is at an increased risk for developing breast cancer and should consider cancer preventive therapy.*

Ductal cancer cells: *Identification of cancer cells presents a very perplexing problem because the location of the cancer often cannot be determined thereby precluding conservative simple excision for treatment. It is prudent to confirm the presence of malignant cells through a second cytopathologic opinion.*

RELATED TESTS

Mammography (p. 1043). This is an x-ray study of the breast that has proved to be a very accurate method of screening and diagnosing breast cancer.

Ductoscopy (p. 603). This test provides an endoscopic view of the breast ducts.

Magnetic Resonance Imaging (MRI) of the Breast (p. 1106). This is a very sensitive method of breast imaging.

 Fetal Fibronectin (fFN)

NORMAL FINDINGS

Negative (≤0.05 mcg/mL)

INDICATIONS

To help predict preterm delivery, some doctors now suggest that women with symptoms of preterm labor be screened for the presence of fetal fibronectin (fFN). The presence of fFN in the cervicovaginal secretions of symptomatic women during weeks 22 through 34 of gestation indicates an increased risk of preterm delivery. However, the absence of fFN is a more reliable predictor that the pregnancy will continue for at least another 2 weeks.

TEST EXPLANATION

Fibronectin may help with implantation of the fertilized egg into the uterine lining. Normally, fibronectin cannot be identified in vaginal secretions after 22 weeks of pregnancy. However, concentrations are very high in the amniotic fluid. If fibronectin is identified in vaginal secretions after 24 weeks, the patient is at high risk for preterm (premature) delivery within the next 2 weeks. Its use is limited to women whose membranes are intact and cervix dilatation of less than 3 cm in women with signs and symptoms of labor.

A negative fFN test result is a highly reliable predictor that delivery will not occur within the next 2 weeks. A positive result is a less reliable predictor of preterm labor: there is still a fair chance that the pregnancy will continue for at least another 2 weeks. The greatest value of the fFN test is the high level of reliability of a negative test result. A negative test result reassures medical providers and expectant parents that the risk of preterm delivery is currently low, and helps reduce the need for medical interventions. A positive fFN result, although less reliable, allows doctors and patients to take preventive measures to delay labor for as long as possible, by hospitalization and/or administering labor-suppressing (tocolytic) medications.

The American College of Obstetricians and Gynecologists (ACOG) currently does not recommend the test for routine screening, as its use has not been shown to be clinically effective in predicting preterm labor in low-risk, asymptomatic pregnancies. This test can be done at the bedside in a few minutes. This quick assay has been shown to be highly concordant with the original enzyme-linked immunosorbent assay (ELISA), which required 48 hours to obtain a result.

Fluid Analysis Studies

5

PROCEDURE AND PATIENT CARE

Before

✗ Explain the procedure to the patient.
✗ Tell the patient that no fasting is required.
- Determine if the patient has had a recent cervical exam. The result may be inaccurate if a cervical exam has been performed within 24 hours.

During

- Note the following procedural steps:
  1. The patient is placed in the lithotomy position.
  2. A vaginal speculum is inserted to expose the cervix.
  3. Vaginal secretions are collected from the posterior vagina and paracervical area with a Dacron swab that comes with the fibronectin laboratory kit.
  4. The slide is labeled with the patient's name, age, estimated date of confinement.
✗ Tell the patient that no discomfort, except for insertion of the speculum, is associated with this procedure.
- Note that this procedure is performed by a physician or other licensed health care provider in several minutes.

After

✗ Inform the patient that usually the result will be available the next day.
✗ Educate the patient of the signs of preterm labor: cramps, vaginal bleeding, uterine contractions, pelvic pressure, or the rupture of membranes.
✗ Encourage the patient to express concerns regarding the plans for preterm delivery.

TEST RESULTS AND CLINICAL SIGNIFICANCE

▲ Increased Levels

High risk for preterm premature delivery: *Fetal fibronectin, a component of the extracellular matrix of fetal membranes, leaks into the cervix when the interaction between the fetal membranes and the uterine wall weakens.*

Human Papillomavirus (HPV Test, HPV DNA Testing)

NORMAL FINDINGS

No HPV present

INDICATIONS

An HPV test is performed to identify genital HPV infection in a woman with an abnormal Pap test.

TEST EXPLANATION

HPV is a small, nonenveloped, double-stranded, circular deoxyribonucleic acid (DNA) tumor virus, classified in the genus *Papillomavirus* of the Papovaviridae family of viruses. More than 100 distinct types of HPV have been identified that infect the genital areas, throat, and mouth of males and females. Approximately 50 of these infect the epithelial membranes of the anogenital tract of women. HPV DNA incorporates itself into the cervical cell genome, promoting its effects through activation of oncogenes and suppression of host cell immune response. HPV protein products prevent DNA repair and programmed cell death, which can lead to instability and unchecked cell growth.

HPV infects the genital epithelium and is spread via skin-to-skin contact. Some strains of HPV cause genital warts, but HPV infections often produce no signs or symptoms. As a result, infected persons are frequently unaware that they are carriers, and transmission occurs unknowingly.

Genital HPV strains are divided into two groups (low and high risk) based on their oncogenic potential and ability to induce viral-associated tumors. Low-risk strains (HPV 6, 11, 42, 43, and 44) are associated with condylomata genital warts and low-grade cervical changes, such as mild dysplasia. Lesions caused by low-risk HPV infection have a high likelihood of regression and little potential for progression, and are considered of no or low oncogenic risk. High-risk strains (HPV 16, 18, 31, 33, 35, 39, 45, 51, 52, 56, 58, 59, 66, and 68) are associated with intraepithelial neoplasia and are more likely to progress to severe lesions and cervical cancer.

A clear causal relationship has been established between HPV infection and cervical cancer (99% of cervical cancers are related particularly to types 6, 11, 16, and 18). HPV is found in almost all cases of cervical malignancies world-wide. Of the high-risk HPV strains, HPV 16 and 18 are the most carcinogenic and most prevalent. HPV 16 is the predominant strain in almost all regions of the world, with the exception of Southeast Asia, where HPV 18 has the highest prevalence. High-grade cervical intraepithelial lesions are most commonly associated with HPV 16 and 18, yet these strains are also frequently found to be the causative factor in minor lesions and mild dysplasia. The latency period between initial HPV exposure and development of cervical cancer may be months or years. Although rapid progression is possible, average time from initial infection to manifestation of invasive cervical cancer is estimated at about 15 years. Women who have normal Pap test results and no HPV infection are at very low risk (0.2%) for developing cervical cancer. Women who have an abnormal Pap test and a positive HPV test are at higher risk (6% to 7% or greater) for developing cervical cancer.

Gardasil is a vaccine that will guard against HPV 6, 11, 16, and 18. The Centers for Disease Control and Prevention (CDC) recommends Gardasil for all girls and boys 11 or 12 years of age. The vaccine is also recommended in young men and women 13 through 26 years of age who have not already received the vaccine or have not completed all booster shots. Gardasil is given as an intramuscular injection in a series of three shots. Second and third boosters are provided at 2 months and 6 months after the first.

The HPV test is now performed routinely on most women but particularly those who have an abnormal Pap test. Pap test results such as "atypical squamous cells of undetermined significance (ASC-US)" or "low-grade squamous intraepithelial lesion" often prompt a routine HPV test. The most commonly used test is the Hybrid Capture II (HC II) DNA assay. It uses ribonucleic acid (RNA) probes in a modified enzyme-linked immunosorbent assay (ELISA) platform to identify the presence or absence of 13 strains of "high-risk" HPV DNA. Another commonly performed method of HPV testing uses nucleic acid probe/polymerase chain reaction.

Numerous sources indicate that more than 60% of women with an abnormal Pap test will test positive for high-risk HPV. If the HPV test is positive, the woman should undergo colposcopy or repeat cytology to look for a more serious cervical lesion such as cancer. It is well known that HPV infection in younger women is more prevalent and will often spontaneously regress, particularly in those under the age of 30. In contrast, persistent high-risk infection peaks in women over 30. As a result, some physicians recommend that HPV testing be reserved for clinical use in the evaluation of women over the age of 30 to 35 or for younger women with ASC-US with a negative Pap test. Most recent studies have suggested that HPV testing is more sensitive than Pap testing in the detection of serious cervical disease.

HPV testing is typically included as a part of regular screening with a Pap test in these women. There is increasing clinical evidence to suggest that HPV DNA screen with cytology triage (Pap/ThinPrep [p. 743], if positive) is more accurate than conventional cervical cancer screening using Pap/ThinPrep alone. Most cervical cancer is associated with HPV 16 and 18, which occur at earlier ages. Once a woman has been vaccinated with Gardasil (which includes HPV 16 and 18 protection), cervical cancer screening may be delayed. (See Table 5-1 for cervical screening.)

TABLE 5-1	American Cancer Society Recommendations for Cervical Screening
Population - by Age	**Recommended Screening**
<21	No screening
21-29	Pap/Thin Prep alone every 3 years
30-65	HPV and Pap/Thin Prep co-testing every 5 years
>65	No screening following adequate negative prior screening
After hysterectomy	No screening
HPV vaccinated	Follow above recommendations (? Delay screening for 3-5 years)

Several clinical professional societies have made recommendations as to the appropriate use of high-risk HPV testing. HPV high risk (oncogenic) testing is suggested for women who are:

- 30 to 65 (without any prior cervical abnormalities). They may extend the interval between screens to 5 years if they use HPV tests in conjunction with the Pap test. The HPV test should not be used in younger women because many of them will have HPV infection that they will naturally clear without treatment.
- 30 years and older with a prior positive test for low-risk HPV
- 30 years and older with atypical cells of undetermined significance (ASC-US)
- Over 21 and have atypical squamous cells of undetermined significance
- Postmenopausal and have ASC-US or a low-grade squamous intraepithelial lesion. Women over 65 should not be screened with Pap or HPV, as long as they have had consistently normal Pap tests and are not at high risk for cervical cancer.
- Any age and have atypical glandular cells or high-grade squamous intraepithelial lesion after colposcopy
- Any age for posttreatment surveillance

HPV cannot be cultured. It cannot be identified easily on routine histology. Molecular testing is the most effective way of identifying HPV. The hybrid capture to test is a liquid/solid phase signal amplification with multiple RNA probes directed against the genomic sequence of 13 high-risk HPV types, including 16 and 18. When combined with the specimen, HPV DNA/RNA hybrids form. Anti-hybrid antibodies can be identified by a particular label.

HPV HR assay is another essay that can be automated but is associated with significant HPV cross-hybridization. Using similar techniques and HPV 16/18 assay is specifically designed for the detection of those particular HPV types. Both use Invader Chemistry Technology. With in situ hybridization procedures the HPV can be directly associated with a particular high-risk histologic cervical lesion. PCR methods allow for target amplification of HPV DNA. Different methods for the detection of the amplified sequence exist.

INTERFERING FACTORS

- HPV testing may be affected by the cellularity of the specimen. Cervical specimens with low cellularity may not provide adequate cells for DNA testing.

PROCEDURE AND PATIENT CARE

Before

Explain the procedure for Pap test (p. 743).

Instruct the patient not to douche or bathe in a tub during the 24 hours before the Pap test. (Some physicians prefer that patients refrain from sexual intercourse for 24 to 48 hours before the test.)

Instruct the patient to empty her bladder before the examination.
 Instruct the patient to reschedule testing if she is menstruating.
 Tell the patient that no fasting or sedation is required.

During

Note the following procedural steps:

1. The patient is placed in the lithotomy position as for a Pap test.
2. With the use of either a cytology brush or a wooden spatula, a cervical mucus specimen is obtained by placing the instrument into the cervical os and rotating 3 to 5 times in clockwise and counterclockwise directions.
3. After specimen collection, rotate the broomlike device or spatula and cytobrush several times in the collection vial to remove the specimen. Firmly cap the vial and discard the collection devices.
4. Affix a patient identification label to the vial.
5. Seal the vial and place in a plastic specimen bag along with a properly completed cytology requisition form, and send to the laboratory.

- Specimens for HPV can be obtained in two ways. Reflex testing uses the residual cell suspension from liquid-based cytology from the original Pap test. A second sample can also be obtained at the time of the original Pap test or during a second procedure. The cervical specimen is then placed into a transport medium in a separate tube for HPV testing.
- Note that a Pap test is obtained by a nurse or a physician in approximately 10 minutes.

 Tell the patient that no discomfort, except for insertion of the speculum, is associated with this procedure.

After

 Inform the patient that usually she will not be notified unless further evaluation is necessary.
 Instruct the patient that HPV is a sexually transmitted disease. All proper precautions should be taken to prevent infecting sexual partners.

TEST RESULTS AND CLINICAL SIGNIFICANCE

HPV infection: *These women should consider more aggressive cervical cancer screening.*

RELATED TEST

Papanicolaou Test (p. 743). This is a commonly performed screening test for cervical/uterine cancer that is performed at the same time the specimen is obtained for HPV testing.

Lumbar Puncture and Cerebrospinal Fluid Examination (LP and CSF Examination, Spinal Tap, Spinal Puncture, Cerebrospinal Fluid Analysis)

NORMAL FINDINGS

Pressure: <20 cm H_2O
Color: clear and colorless
Blood: none

Cells:
  RBC: 0
  WBC
  Total
    Neonate: 0-30 cells/μL
    1-5 years: 0-20 cells/μL
    6-18 years: 0-10 cells/μL
    Adult: 0-5 cells/μL
  Differential
    Neutrophils: 0%-6%
    Lymphocytes: 40%-80%
    Monocytes: 15%-45%
Culture and sensitivity: no organisms present
Protein: 15-45 mg/dl CSF (up to 70 mg/dL in older adults and children)
Protein electrophoresis
  Prealbumin: 2%-7%
  Albumin: 56%-76%
  Alpha$_1$ globulin: 2%-7%
  Alpha$_2$ globulin: 4%-12%
  Beta globulin: 8%-18%
  Gamma globulin: 3%-12%
  Oligoclonal bands: none
  IgG: 0.0-4.5 mg/dL
Glucose: 50-75 mg/dL CSF or 60%-70% of blood glucose level
Chloride: 700-750 mg/dL
Lactic dehydrogenase (LDH): ≤40 units/L for adults, ≤70 units/L for neonates
Lactic acid: 10-25 mg/dL
Cytology: no malignant cells
Serology for syphilis: negative
Glutamine: 6-15 mg/dL

INDICATIONS

This examination may assist in the diagnosis of primary or metastatic brain or spinal cord neoplasm, cerebral hemorrhage, meningitis, encephalitis, degenerative brain disease, autoimmune diseases involving the central nervous system (CNS), neurosyphilis, and demyelinating disorders (e.g., multiple sclerosis, acute demyelinating polyneuropathy).

TEST EXPLANATION

By placing a needle in the subarachnoid space of the spinal column (Figure 5-2), one can measure the pressure of that space and obtain CSF for examination and diagnosis. Lumbar puncture may also be used to inject therapeutic or diagnostic agents and to administer spinal anesthetics. Furthermore, lumbar puncture may be used to reduce intracranial pressure in patients with normal pressure hydrocephalus with pseudotumor cerebri.

CSF is made by selective secretion from the plasma by the choroid plexus (a group of small blood vessels) in the ventricles of the brain. There are three membranes surrounding the brain and spinal cord. From inner to outer, they are the pia mater, arachnoid, and dura mater. The CSF exists within

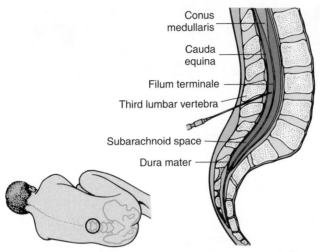

Conus medullaris

Cauda equina

Filum terminale

Third lumbar vertebra

Subarachnoid space

Dura mater

Figure 5-2 Patient position for a lumbar puncture (LP).

the space between the pia mater and the arachnoid (called the subarachnoid space). This fluid (about 150 to 200 mL) bathes and protects the brain and spinal cord. The fluid acts as a shock absorber when head or back trauma or sudden change in position occurs. The CSF transports nutrients and clears metabolic wastes. Because the CSF is made from plasma, its constituents are about the same as plasma. Chloride levels are higher, however. Blood constituents of larger molecular size cannot be secreted by the choroid plexus (blood-brain barrier).

Examination of the CSF includes evaluation for the presence of blood, bacteria, and malignant cells, as well as quantification of the amount of glucose and protein present. Color is noted, and various other tests, such as a serologic test for syphilis (p. 473), are performed.

Occasionally, lumbar puncture is contraindicated because of nearby infection or suspected spinal canal CSF blockage.

Pressure

By attaching a sterile manometer to the needle used for LP, the pressure within the subarachnoid space can be measured. A pressure of 20 cm H_2O or above is considered abnormal and indicative of increased spinal pressure. Because the subarachnoid space surrounding the brain is freely connected to the sub-arachnoid space of the spinal cord, any increase in intracranial pressure will be directly reflected as an increase at the lumbar site. Tumors, infection, hydrocephalus, and intracranial bleeding can cause increased intracranial and spinal pressure. If it is suspected that this normal connection is obstructed by tumor or postinfection scarring, a Queckenstedt-Stookey test is performed (see "Procedure and Patient Care") to document that. Intracranial pressure is related to the volume of CSF fluid, which is determined by the homeostatic balance between production and resorption of CSF. Also, because the cranial venous sinuses are connected to the jugular veins, obstruction of those veins or of the superior vena cava will increase intracranial pressure.

Decreased pressure is noted in hypovolemia (dehydration or shock). A chronic leakage of CSF through a previous LP site, or through a nasal sinus fracture with a dura tear, is associated with reduced pressures.

Pressures are routinely measured at the beginning and the end of an LP. If there is a significant difference in these values, one must suspect a spinal cord obstruction (tumor). In these instances, a small amount of CSF exists below the tumor. Removal of a large percentage of that fluid will drastically reduce

TABLE 5-2	Differential Diagnosis of Causes of Blood in the Cerebrospinal Fluid (CSF)	
	Traumatic Puncture	**Subarachnoid Bleeding**
CSF pressure	Low	High
Duration of bleeding	Decreases when CSF is withdrawn	No change in color when CSF is withdrawn
Clotting	Present	Absent
Repeat lumbar puncture	Not bloody	Bloody
Centrifugation	Clear fluid	Xanthochromia

the pressure. Large differences in opening and closing pressures are also seen in patients with hydrocephalus. If high opening pressures are noted, normal volumes of CSF should not be removed to prevent the risk of cerebellar herniation. One must be aware that a child who is crying and holding the breath may have transient elevations of pressure that reduce as the child relaxes.

Color

Normal CSF is clear and colorless. Xanthochromia (usually refers to a yellow tinge) is commonly used to indicate an abnormal color of CSF. Color differences can occur with hyperbilirubinemia, hypercarotenemia, melanoma, or elevated protein levels.

A cloudy appearance may indicate an increase in the WBC count or protein level. Normally CSF contains no blood. A red tinge to the CSF indicates the presence of blood. Blood may be present because of bleeding into the subarachnoid space or because the needle used in the LP has inadvertently penetrated a blood vessel on the way into the subarachnoid space. These causes of bleeding must be differentiated because it is important to identify and document a subarachnoid bleed (Table 5-2).

With a "traumatic puncture" the blood within the CSF will clot. No clotting occurs in a patient with subarachnoid hemorrhage. Also, with a traumatic tap the fluid clears toward the end of the procedure when successive CSF samples are obtained. This clearing does not occur with a subarachnoid hemorrhage.

Blood

Blood within the CSF indicates cerebral hemorrhage into the subarachnoid space or a "traumatic tap" as just described.

Cells

The number of red blood cells (RBCs) is merely an indication of the amount of blood present within the CSF. Except for a few lymphocytes, the presence of white blood cells (WBCs) in the CSF is abnormal (Table 5-3). The presence of polymorphonuclear leukocytes (neutrophils) is indicative of bacterial meningitis or cerebral abscess. When mononuclear leukocytes are present, viral or tubercular meningitis or encephalitis is suspected. Leukemia or other primary or metastatic malignant tumors may cause elevated WBCs. Pleocytosis is a term used to indicate turbidity of CSF because of an increased number of cells within the fluid. WBCs can be present in the CSF as a result of a "traumatic tap," where the spinal needle hits a blood vessel while the spinal tap is being performed. However, more than 1 WBC per 500 RBCs is considered pathologic and can indicate infection such as meningitis.

TABLE 5-3	Causes of Leukocytes in the Cerebrospinal Fluid	
Cell Type	**Infection**	**Other Diseases**
Neutrophils	Bacterial meningitis	Subarachnoid bleeding
	Tubercular meningitis	Tumor
	Cerebral abscess	
Lymphocytes or plasma cells	Viral, tubercular, fungal, syphilitic meningitis	Multiple sclerosis
		Guillain-Barré syndrome
Eosinophils	Parasitic meningitis	Allergic reaction to radiopaque dyes
Macrophages	Tubercular, fungal meningitis	Hemorrhage, brain infarction

Culture and Sensitivity

Most of the organisms that cause meningitis or brain abscess can be cultured from the CSF. Organisms found also may include atypical bacteria, fungi, or *Mycobacterium tuberculosis*. A Gram stain (p. 704) of the CSF may give the clinician preliminary information about the causative infectious agent. This may allow appropriate antibiotic therapy to be initiated before the 24 to 72 hours necessary to complete the culture and sensitivity report.

There are microorganisms that are viable but cannot be grown in culture. There are also viruses and parasites associated with meningitis and brain abscesses that are not detected by traditional bacterial culture techniques.

The most common causes of meningitis include *Haemophilus influenzae* (in children) and *Neisseria* or *Streptococcus* in adults.

Protein

Normally very little protein is found in CSF because protein is a large molecule that does not cross the blood-brain barrier. The proportion of albumin to globulin is normally higher in CSF than in blood plasma (p. 424) because albumin is smaller than globulin and therefore can pass more easily through the blood-brain barrier. The amount of protein is usually lower in CSF obtained from the cisternal puncture and even lower still with a ventricular puncture, compared with the CSF obtained from an LP. Disease processes, however, can alter the permeability of the blood-brain barrier, allowing protein to leak into the CSF. Examples of diseases that may be associated with a more permeable blood-brain barrier include infectious or inflammatory processes such as meningitis, encephalitis, or myelitis. Furthermore, CNS tumors may produce and secrete protein into the CSF. Obstruction of CSF flow in the spinal canal caused by tumors or a disk is also associated with high protein counts because normal CSF circulation and resorption are impaired by the obstruction.

CSF protein electrophoresis is very important in the diagnosis of CNS diseases. Patients with multiple sclerosis, neurosyphilis, or other immunogenic degenerative central neurologic disease have elevated immunoglobulins in their CSF. Normally, less than 12% of the total protein consists of gamma globulin. An increase in the CSF level of immunoglobulin G (IgG), an increase in the ratio of IgG to other proteins (e.g., albumin), and the detection of oligoclonal gamma globulin bands are highly suggestive of inflammatory and autoimmune diseases of the CNS, especially multiple sclerosis (MS). Myelin basic protein, a component of myelin (the substance that surrounds normal nerve tissue) can be elevated when demyelinating diseases (such as MS or amyotrophic lateral sclerosis) occur. This protein, detected by radioimmunoassay (RIA) of the CSF, can be used to monitor the course of these deteriorating diseases.

Because albumin and prealbumin are not made in the CNS, increased levels of these specific proteins indicate increased permeability of the blood-brain barrier (as discussed previously).

Glucose

The glucose level is decreased when bacteria, inflammatory cells, or tumor cells are present. A blood sample for glucose (p. 253) is usually drawn before the spinal tap is performed. A CSF glucose level less than 60% of the blood glucose level may indicate meningitis or neoplasm.

Chloride

The chloride concentration in CSF may be decreased in patients with meningeal infections, tubercular meningitis, and conditions of low blood chloride levels. An increase in the chloride level in CSF is not neurologically significant; it correlates with the blood levels of chloride (p. 152). CSF is not routinely evaluated for chloride; this test is done only if specifically requested.

Lactic Dehydrogenase

Quantification of lactic dehydrogenase (LDH) (specifically, fractions 4 and 5; p. 329) is helpful in diagnosing bacterial meningitis. The source of LDH is the neutrophils that fight the invading bacteria. When the LDH level is elevated, infection or inflammation is suspected. The elevated WBC count associated with CNS leukemia is also associated with elevated LDH levels. The nerve tissue in the CNS is also high in LDH (isoenzymes 1 and 2). Therefore disease directly affecting the brain or spinal cord (e.g., stroke) is associated with elevated LDH levels.

Lactic Acid

Elevated levels indicate anaerobic metabolism associated with decreased oxygenation of the brain. The CSF lactic acid level is increased in both bacterial and fungal meningitis but not in viral meningitis. The lactic acid level is also increased when the CSF glucose level is very low or the CSF WBC count is elevated. Because lactic acid does not readily pass through the blood-brain barrier, elevated blood lactate levels are not reflected in the CSF. Chronic cerebral hypoxemia or cerebral ischemia (hypoxic encephalopathy) is associated with elevated CSF lactic acid levels. Lactic acid levels can also be increased in patients with some forms of mitochondrial diseases that affect the CNS.

Cytology

Examination of cells found in the CSF can determine if they are malignant. Tumors in the CNS may shed cells from their surface. These cells can float freely in CSF. Their presence suggests neoplasm as the cause of any neurologic symptoms.

Tumor Markers

Increased levels of tumor markers such as carcinoembryonic antigen, alpha-fetoprotein, or human chorionic gonadotropin may indicate metastatic tumor.

Serology for Syphilis

Latent syphilis is diagnosed by performing one of many available serologic tests on CSF. These include the following:
- The Wassermann test
- The Venereal Disease Research Laboratory (VDRL) test (p. 473)
- The fluorescent treponemal antibody (FTA) test (p. 473): The FTA test is considered to be the most sensitive and specific. When test results are positive, the diagnosis of neurosyphilis is made and appropriate antibiotic therapy is initiated.

Glutamine

The CSF can be evaluated for the presence of glutamine. Elevated glutamine levels are helpful in the detection and evaluation of hepatic encephalopathy and hepatic coma. The glutamine is made by increased levels of ammonia, which are commonly associated with liver failure. (See discussion of serum ammonia on p. 59.) Levels of glutamine are also often increased in patients with Reye syndrome.

C-Reactive Protein

As noted on p. 184, C-reactive protein (CRP) is a nonspecific, acute-phase reactant used in the diagnosis of bacterial infections and inflammatory disorders. Elevated CSF levels of CRP have been useful in the diagnosis of bacterial meningitis. Failure to find elevated CSF levels of CRP appears to be strong evidence against bacterial meningitis. Some research studies have shown that CSF levels of CRP have been valuable in distinguishing bacterial meningitis from viral meningitis, tuberculosis meningitis, febrile convulsions, and other central nervous system disorders. Serum levels of CRP (see p. 184) are more frequently used in the diagnosis of bacterial meningitis.

LP is performed by a physician in approximately 20 minutes. This procedure is described as uncomfortable or painful by most patients. Some patients complain of feeling pressure from the needle. Some patients complain of a shooting pain in their legs.

CONTRAINDICATIONS

- Patients with increased intracranial pressure: The LP may induce cerebral or cerebellar herniation through the foramen magnum.
- Patients who have severe degenerative vertebral joint disease: It is very difficult to pass the needle through the degenerated arthritic interspinal space.
- Patients with infection near the LP site: Meningitis can result from contamination of CSF with infected material.
- Patients receiving anticoagulation drugs because of the risk for epidural hematoma.

POTENTIAL COMPLICATIONS

- Persistent CSF leak, causing severe headache
- Introduction of bacteria into CSF, causing suppurative meningitis
- Herniation of the brain through the tentorium cerebelli or herniation of the cerebellum through the foramen magnum: In patients with increased intracranial pressure, the quick reduction of pressure in the spinal column by release through the LP may induce herniation of the brain. This can cause compression of the brainstem, which may result in deterioration of the patient's neurologic status and death. In adults, especially, most clinicians will obtain a computed tomography (CT) scan of the head before performing lumbar puncture to identify intracranial abnormalities and thus avoid the risk of brain herniation.
- Inadvertent puncture of the spinal cord, caused by inappropriately high puncture of the spinal canal
- Puncture of the aorta or vena cava, causing serious retroperitoneal hemorrhage
- Transient back pain and pain or paresthesia in the legs
- Transient postural headache (worse when standing)

PROCEDURE AND PATIENT CARE

Before

- Explain the procedure to the patient. Many patients have misconceptions regarding LP. Allay the patient's fears and allow time to verbalize concerns.

- Obtain informed consent if required by the institution.
- Perform a baseline neurologic assessment of the legs by assessing the patient's strength, sensation, and movement.
- Tell the patient that no fasting or sedation is required.
- Instruct the patient to empty the bladder and bowels before the procedure.
- Explain to the patient that he or she must lie very still throughout this procedure. Movement may cause traumatic injury. Encourage the patient to relax and take deep, slow breaths with the mouth open.

✔ Clinical Priorities

- LP is contraindicated in patients with increased intracranial pressure because the LP may induce cerebral or cerebellar herniation.
- A basic neurologic assessment should be done before this test to especially evaluate the patient's legs for strength, sensation, and movement.
- If a blockage in CSF circulation is suspected in the subarachnoid space, a Queckenstedt-Stookey test may be performed.

During

- Note the following procedural steps:
    1. This study is a sterile procedure that can be easily performed at the bedside. The patient is usually placed in the lateral decubitus (fetal) position (see Figure 5-2).
    2. The patient is instructed to clasp the hands on the knees to maintain this position. Someone usually helps the patient maintain this position. (A sitting position also may be used.)
    3. A local anesthetic is injected into the skin and subcutaneous tissues after the site has been aseptically cleaned.
    4. A spinal needle containing an inner obturator is placed through the skin and into the spinal canal.
    5. The subarachnoid space is entered.
    6. The insert (obturator) is removed, and CSF can be seen slowly dripping from the needle.
    7. The needle is attached to a sterile manometer, and the pressure (opening pressure) is recorded.
    8. Before the pressure reading is taken, the patient is asked to relax and straighten the legs to reduce the intraabdominal pressure, which causes an increase in CSF pressure.
    9. Three sterile test tubes are filled with 5 to 10 mL of CSF. Usually the first tube is sent for chemical and immunologic testing because these results are not affected by any blood if a "traumatic tap" occurs. The second may be sent for culture, and the third is used for microscopic examination.
    10. The pressure (closing pressure) is measured.
- Note that if blockage in CSF circulation in the spinal subarachnoid space is suspected, a *Queckenstedt-Stookey test* may be performed. For this test the jugular vein is occluded either manually by digital pressure or by a medium-sized blood pressure cuff inflated to approximately 20 mm Hg. Within 10 seconds after jugular occlusion, CSF pressure should increase 15 to 40 cm H_2O and then promptly return to normal within 10 seconds after release of the pressure. A sluggish rise or fall of CSF pressure suggests partial blockage of CSF circulation. No rise after 10 seconds suggests a complete obstruction within the spinal canal.

After

- Apply digital pressure and an adhesive dressing to the puncture site.
- Place the patient in the prone position with a pillow under the abdomen to increase the intraabdominal pressure, which will indirectly increase the pressure in the tissues surrounding the spinal cord. This retards continued CSF flow from the spinal canal.

- All testing of the CSF is ordered stat to diminish the false results that may occur because of cellular deterioration, and so on.
- Encourage the patient to drink increased amounts of fluid with a straw to replace the CSF removed during the lumbar puncture. Drinking with a straw will enable the patient to keep the head flat.
- Usually keep the patient in a reclining position for up to 12 hours to avoid the discomfort of potential postpuncture spinal headache. Allow the patient to turn from side to side as long as the head is not raised.
- Label and number the specimen jars appropriately and deliver them to the laboratory immediately after the test. Refrigeration will alter test results. A delay between collection time and testing can invalidate results, especially cell counts.
- Assess the patient for numbness, tingling, and decreased movement of the extremities; pain at the injection site; drainage of blood or CSF at the injection site; and the ability to void. Notify the physician of any unusual findings.

Home Care Responsibilities

- The patient should be kept flat in bed for up to 12 hours to avoid a postprocedure spinal headache.
- Encourage the patient to drink increased amounts of fluid to replace CSF removed during the LP.
- Instruct the patient to report any abnormalities, such as numbness and tingling in the legs, to the physician.

Fluid Analysis Studies

5

TEST RESULTS AND CLINICAL SIGNIFICANCE

Brain neoplasm,

Spinal cord neoplasm,

Metastatic tumor:

> *The CSF can be expected to be turbid, to contain malignant cells, and to have elevated protein and LDH levels.*

Degenerative brain disease,

Autoimmune disorder,

Multiple sclerosis and other demyelinating diseases:

> *The CSF of these patients may be turbid; it may contain increased protein levels (including myelin basic protein) and oligoclonal bands of proteins; and it may be associated with elevated LDH levels.*

Neurosyphilis: *Not only do these patients have elevated protein levels, increased turbidity, and increased LDH levels in their CSF, but immunologic testing is also positive.*

Subarachnoid bleeding,

Cerebral hemorrhage,

Traumatic lumbar puncture:

> *The CSF in these patients has high protein levels, turbid color with xanthochromia, and RBCs.*

Encephalitis,

Myelitis,

Hepatic encephalopathy or coma:

> *Elevated glutamine levels are noted in these patients.*

Meningitis,

Encephalitis,

Cerebral abscess:

> *Elevated WBCs and proteins support the culture findings of infection.*

RELATED TESTS

Glucose (p. 253). This test is concomitantly performed with the LP to assess the CSF glucose level.

Serum Protein (p. 424). Along with the LP, measurement of serum protein levels is helpful in the calculation of many formulas involved in the evaluation of CSF.

Amyloid Beta Protein Precursor (p. 639). This test is performed on CSF to diagnose Alzheimer's disease.

 Pancreatic Enzymes (Pancreatic Secretory Test, Amylase, Lipase, Trypsin, Chymotrypsin)

NORMAL FINDINGS

Volume: 2-4 mL/kg body weight

(HCC^-_3) (Bicarbonate): 90-130 mEq/L

Amylase: 6.6-35.2 units/kg

Trypsin-like immunoreactivity: 10-57 ng/mL

Trypsin: ≥1:96

Chymotrypsin: by report

INDICATIONS

This is a corroborative test used in the evaluation of cystic fibrosis (CF) and pancreatitis (acute and chronic). This test is indicated in children with recurrent respiratory tract infections, malabsorption syndromes, or failure to thrive.

TEST EXPLANATION

CF is an inherited disease characterized by abnormal secretion by exocrine glands within the bronchi, small intestines, pancreatic ducts, bile ducts, and skin (sweat glands). Because of this abnormal exocrine secretion, children with cystic fibrosis develop mucus plugs that obstruct their pancreatic ducts that can lead to significant malabsorption, steatorrhea, and diarrhea. The pancreatic enzymes (e.g., amylase [p. 61], lipase [p. 339], trypsin, and chymotrypsin) cannot be expelled into the duodenum and therefore are either completely absent or present only in diminished quantities within the duodenal aspirate. For the same reasons, bicarbonate and other neutralizing fluids cannot be secreted from the pancreas. In this test, secretin and pancreozymin are used to stimulate pancreatic secretion of these enzymes and bicarbonate into the duodenum. The duodenal contents are then aspirated and examined for pH, bicarbonate, and pancreatic enzyme levels. Amylase is the most frequently measured enzyme. Diminished values are suggestive of cystic fibrosis. Pancreatic enzyme testing is not diagnostic of cystic fibrosis, but is an excellent screening test especially in the newborn with meconium ileus. Genetic testing is required for definitive diagnosis of cystic fibrosis.

Trypsinogen, another pancreatic exocrine enzyme, is measured in the serum as *trypsin-like immunoreactivity*. This test is used to support the diagnosis of chronic pancreatitis. Levels diminish as pancreatic exocrine function becomes increasingly impaired.

When any of these pancreatic enzymes are measured in the serum, they can reflect acute inflammation of the pancreas. Like amylase and lipase, trypsin, chymotrypsin, and trypsin-like immunoreactivity are increased with acute pancreatic inflammation. Likewise, in patients with burned-out chronic pancreatitis, serum measurements of these pancreatic enzymes are low.

Trypsinogen has two isoenzymes that are excreted in the urine. *Trypsinogen-1* is rapidly reabsorbed in the kidneys. *Trypsinogen-2*, however, is not well reabsorbed by the kidneys and concentrations will increase in the urine during acute pancreatitis.

A physician obtains the duodenal contents in approximately 2 hours in the x-ray department. Discomfort and gagging may occur during placement of the Dreiling tube. The pancreatic enzymes are then measured and serially diluted for quantification.

PROCEDURE AND PATIENT CARE

Before

- Explain the procedure to the patient and/or parents.
- Instruct the adult patient to fast for 12 hours before testing.
- Determine pediatric fasting times according to the patient's age.

During

- Note the following procedural steps:
  1. With the use of fluoroscopy, a Dreiling tube is passed through the patient's nose and into the stomach.
  2. The distal lumen of the tube is placed within the duodenum.
  3. The proximal lumen of the tube is placed within the stomach.
  4. Both lumens are aspirated. The gastric lumen is continually aspirated to avoid contamination of the gastric contents in the duodenum aspirate.
  5. A control specimen of the duodenal juices is collected for 20 minutes.
  6. The patient is tested for sensitivity to secretin and pancreozymin by low-dose intradermal injection.
  7. If no sensitivity is present, these hormones are administered intravenously (IV). Secretin can be expected to stimulate pancreatic water and bicarbonate secretion. Pancreozymin can be expected to stimulate pancreatic enzyme (lipase, amylase, trypsin, and chymotrypsin) secretion.
  8. Four duodenal aspirates are collected at 20-minute intervals and placed in the specimen container.
  9. Each specimen is analyzed for pH, volume, bicarbonate, and amylase levels.

After

- Place the aspirated specimens on ice. Send them to the chemistry laboratory as soon as the test is completed.
- Remove the Dreiling tube after completion of the test. Give appropriate nose and mouth care.
- Allow the patient to resume a normal diet.

TEST RESULTS AND CLINICAL SIGNIFICANCE

▲ Increased Levels

Acute pancreatitis: *Damage to pancreatic acinar cells, as in pancreatitis, causes an outpouring of amylase into the intrapancreatic lymph system and the free peritoneum. Blood vessels draining the free peritoneum and absorbing the lymph pick up the excess amylase.*

▼ Decreased Levels

Cystic fibrosis: *These patients do not have adequate levels of exocrine pancreatic enzymes or bicarbonates because of mucus plugging of the small pancreatic duct tributaries.*

Sprue: *The pathophysiology of this observation is not definitely known. It is thought that patients with sprue have a damaged intestinal mucosa. As a result, they do not have a normal stimulatory response to secrete secretin and pancreozymin. Therefore the pancreas is chronically under stimulated. When these hormones are administered, the pancreas can respond to a slight degree, but not as much as normal because of the previous prolonged periods of absence of stimulation.*

Chronic pancreatitis: *These patients do not have adequate levels of exocrinic pancreatic enzymes or bicarbonates because of pancreatic acinar cell destruction.*

RELATED TESTS

Sweat Electrolytes (p. 678). This is the definitive test used in the diagnosis of cystic fibrosis. Skin sweat is analyzed for sodium and chloride content.

Genetic Testing (p. 1093). This is another confirmatory test for cystic fibrosis or hereditary pancreatitis.

Amylase (p. 61), Lipase (p. 339). When measured in the serum, these pancreatic enzymes will be increased in patients with acute pancreatitis.

Paracentesis (Peritoneal Fluid Analysis, Abdominal Paracentesis, Ascitic Fluid Cytology, Peritoneal Tap)

NORMAL FINDINGS

Gross appearance: clear, serous, light yellow, <50 mL
RBCs: none
WBCs: <300/µL
Protein: <4.1 g/dL
Glucose: 70-100 mg/dL
Amylase: 138-404 units/L
Ammonia: <50 µg/dL
Alkaline phosphatase
   Adult male: 90-240 units/L
   Female <45 years: 76-196 units/L
   Female >45 years: 87-250 units/L
Lactic dehydrogenase (LDH): similar to serum LDH
Cytology: no malignant cells
Bacteria: none
Fungi: none
Carcinoembryonic antigen (CEA): <5 ng/mL

INDICATIONS

Paracentesis is performed on patients who have unexplained ascites to determine the cause. It is an important part of evaluating the patient with multiple trauma to rule out abdominal trauma. Paracentesis is also performed to relieve the intraabdominal pressure that accumulates with large-volume ascites.

TEST EXPLANATION

Paracentesis is an invasive procedure entailing the insertion of a needle into the peritoneal cavity for removal of ascitic fluid. The peritoneum is defined as the space between the visceral peritoneum (thin membrane covering all the abdominal organs) and the parietal peritoneum (thin membrane covering the inside of the abdominal wall). Within the peritoneal membrane is an intricate network of capillary

TABLE 5-4   Differentiation Between Transudate and Exudate

	Transudate	Exudate
Total protein fluid/serum ratio	<0.5	>0.5
Total protein level	<3 g/dL	>3 g/dL
LDH fluid/serum ratio	<0.6	>0.6
Albumin gradient	<1.1	>1.1
Serum – Fluid = Albumin gradient		
Specific gravity	>1.015	>1.015
Clotting	None	Present
WBCs	<300/µL	>500/µL
Differential	Mononuclear	Neutrophils
Glucose	Equal to serum	<60 mg/dL
Serum – Fluid = Glucose difference	<30 mg/dL	>30 mg/dL
Appearance	Clear, thin fluid	Cloudy, viscous
Etiology	Cirrhosis, nephrosis, heart failure, low protein	Infection, inflammation, malignancy, collagen-vascular diseases

Fluid Analysis Studies

5

and lymphatic vessels. Fluid is constantly being secreted by the peritoneal membranes and constantly being reabsorbed by those same membranes. If secretion is increased or reabsorption blocked, buildup of peritoneal fluid (ascites) will develop.

Peritoneal fluid is removed for diagnostic and therapeutic purposes. Diagnostically paracentesis is performed to obtain and analyze fluid to determine the cause of the peritoneal effusion. Peritoneal fluid is classified as transudate or exudate (Table 5-4). This is an important differentiation and is very helpful in determining the cause of the effusion. Transudates are most frequently caused by congestive heart failure, cirrhosis, nephrotic syndrome, myxedema, peritoneal dialysis, hypoproteinemia, and acute glomerulonephritis. Exudates are most often found in infectious or neoplastic conditions. However, collagen-vascular disease, pulmonary infarction, gastrointestinal diseases, trauma, and drug hypersensitivity also may cause an exudative effusion.

Therapeutically, this procedure is done to remove large amounts of ascitic fluid from the abdominal cavity. These patients usually experience transient relief of symptoms (shortness of breath, distention, and early satiety) because of the fluid within the abdominal cavity.

The peritoneal fluid is usually evaluated for gross appearance, RBCs, WBCs, protein, glucose, amylase, ammonia, alkaline phosphatase, lactate dehydrogenase (LDH), cytology, bacteria, fungi, and other tests such as CEA levels. Each is discussed separately. Urea and creatinine may be measured if there is a question that the fluid may represent urine from a perforated bladder.

Gross Appearance

Transudative peritoneal fluid may be clear, serous, or light yellow, especially in patients with hepatic cirrhosis. Milk-colored peritoneal fluid may result from the escape of chyle from blocked abdominal or thoracic lymphatic ducts. Conditions that may cause lymphatic blockage include lymphoma, carcinoma, and tuberculosis involving the abdominal or thoracic lymph nodes. The triglyceride value in a chylous effusion exceeds 110 mg/dL.

Cloudy or turbid fluid may result from inflammatory or infectious conditions such as peritonitis, pancreatitis, and appendicitis. Bloody fluid may be the result of a traumatic tap (the aspirating needle penetrates a blood vessel), intraabdominal bleeding, tumor, or hemorrhagic pancreatitis. Bile-stained, green fluid may result from a ruptured gallbladder, acute pancreatitis, or perforated intestines.

Cell Counts

Normally, no RBCs should be present. The presence of RBCs may indicate neoplasms, tuberculosis, or intraabdominal bleeding. Increased WBC counts may be seen with peritonitis, cirrhosis, and tuberculosis.

Protein Count

Total protein levels greater than 3 g/dL are characteristic of exudates, whereas transudates usually have a protein content of less than 3 g/dL. It is now thought that the albumin gradient between serum and ascitic fluid can differentiate better between the transudate and exudate nature of ascites than can the total protein content. This gradient is obtained by subtracting the ascitic albumin value from the serum albumin value. Values of 1.1 g/dL or more suggest a transudate, which is usually caused by portal hypertension due to cirrhosis. Values less than 1.1 g/dL suggest an exudate but will not differentiate the potential cause of the exudate (malignancy from infection or inflammation).

Because there is significant overlap in protein values differentiating transudate from exudate, the total protein ratio (fluid/serum) has been considered to be a more accurate criterion. A total protein ratio of fluid to serum of greater than 0.5 is considered to indicate an exudate.

Glucose

Usually peritoneal glucose levels approximate serum glucose levels. Decreased levels may indicate tuberculous or bacterial peritonitis or peritoneal carcinomatosis.

Amylase

Increased amylase levels may be seen in patients with pancreatic trauma, pancreatic pseudocyst, acute pancreatitis, and intestinal necrosis, perforation, or strangulation. In these diseases, the amylase level is usually less than 1.5 times higher than serum levels.

Ammonia

High ammonia levels occur in ruptured or strangulated intestines and also with a ruptured appendix or ulcer.

Alkaline Phosphatase

Levels of alkaline phosphatase are greatly increased in infarcted or strangulated intestines.

Lactic Dehydrogenase

A peritoneal fluid/serum LDH ratio of greater than 0.6 is typical of an exudate. An exudate is identified with a higher degree of accuracy if the peritoneal fluid/serum protein ratio is greater than 0.5 and the peritoneal fluid/serum LDH ratio is greater than 0.6.

Cytology

A cytologic study is performed to detect tumors. The tumors most often seen are ovarian, pancreatic, colon, and gastric. The interpretation of cytologic changes requires that the pathologist have considerable experience in cytology. It can be difficult to differentiate malignancy from severely inflammatory mesothelial cells. In general, malignant cells tend to clump together and to have a high nucleus/cytoplasm ratio, prominent and multiple nucleoli, and unevenly distributed chromatin.

Cytologic examination of the fluid is improved by spinning down a large volume of fluid and examining the sediment. A large number of cells can be seen and compared with each other.

Bacteria

Usually the fluid is cultured and the antibiotic sensitivities are determined. Gram stains (p. 704) are often performed.

Gram Stain and Bacteriologic Culture

The presence of bacteria may indicate a ruptured intestine, primary peritonitis, or infections such as appendicitis, pancreatitis, or tuberculosis. Culture and gram stains are used to assist in the identification of the organisms that may be involved in the infection. Microbial cultures may provide information concerning possible antibiotic sensitivity or resistance. (See p. 704 for a more thorough discussion of Gram stain, cultures, and sensitivity.) These tests are routinely performed to diagnose bacterial peritonitis. If possible, these tests should be done before initiation of antibiotic therapy.

Fungi

Fungi may indicate histoplasmosis, candidiasis, or coccidioidomycosis.

Carcinoembryonic Antigen

Elevated peritoneal fluid levels for CEA are associated with abdominal malignancy, usually arising from the GI tract.

Paracentesis is performed by a physician at the patient's bedside, in a procedure room, or in the physician's office in less than 30 minutes. Usually the volume removed is limited to about 4 L at any one time to avoid hypovolemia if the fluid is rapidly reaccumulated. Although local anesthetics eliminate pain at the insertion site, the patient may feel a pressure-like pain as the needle is inserted.

CONTRAINDICATIONS

- Patients with coagulation abnormalities or bleeding tendencies
- Patients with only a small amount of fluid and extensive previous abdominal surgery

POTENTIAL COMPLICATIONS

- Hypovolemia if a large volume of peritoneal fluid was removed and the fluid reaccumulates, with the fluid coming from the intravascular volume
- Hepatic coma in a patient with chronic liver disease
- Peritonitis
- Seeding of the needle tract with tumor cells when malignant ascites exists

✓ Clinical Priorities

- The classification of peritoneal fluid as either a transudate or an exudate helps differentiate the cause of the effusion.
- Usually the volume of peritoneal fluid removed is limited to 4 L to avoid hypovolemia if the fluid rapidly reaccumulates.
- The patient should empty the bladder before this test to avoid inadvertent puncture by the aspirating needle during the procedure.
- After this test, the patient should be frequently monitored for hemodynamic changes, especially hypotension, if a large volume of fluid was removed.

PROCEDURE AND PATIENT CARE

Before

- Explain the procedure to the patient.
- Obtain informed consent for this procedure.
- Tell the patient that no fasting or sedation is necessary.
- Have the patient urinate or empty the bladder before the test to avoid inadvertent puncture of the bladder with the aspirating needle.
- Measure abdominal girth.
- Obtain the patient's weight.
- Obtain baseline vital signs.

During

- Note the following procedural steps:
  1. Position the patient in a high-Fowler position in bed.
  2. Paracentesis is performed under strict sterile technique. A paracentesis tray usually contains all necessary supplies.
  3. The needle insertion site is aseptically cleansed and anesthetized locally.
  4. A scalpel may be used to make a stab wound into the peritoneal cavity approximately 1 to 2 inches below the umbilicus.
  5. A trocar, cannula, or needle is threaded through the incision.
  6. A piece of plastic tubing is attached to the cannula. The other end of the tubing is placed in the collection receptacle (usually a container with a pressurized vacuum).

After

- All tests performed on peritoneal fluid should be performed immediately to avoid false results related to chemical or cellular deterioration.
- Place a small bandage over the needle site.
- Label the specimen with the patient's name, date, source of fluid, and diagnosis.
- Send the specimen to the laboratory promptly.
- Observe the puncture site for bleeding, continued drainage, or signs of inflammation.
- Measure the abdominal girth and weight of the patient; compare with baseline values.
- Monitor vital signs frequently for evidence of hemodynamic changes. Watch for signs of hypotension if a large volume of fluid was removed.
- Note any recent antibiotic therapy on the laboratory requisition slip.
- Because of the high protein content of ascitic fluid, albumin infusions may be ordered after paracentesis to compensate for protein loss. Monitor serum protein and electrolyte (especially sodium) levels.
- Occasionally ascitic fluid continues to leak out of the needle track after removal of the needle. A suture can stop that. If this is unsuccessful, a collection bag should be applied to the skin to allow for measurement of the volume of fluid loss.

TEST RESULTS AND CLINICAL SIGNIFICANCE

Exudate

Lymphoma: *These tumors can involve the lymph nodes of the chest and abdomen. Reabsorption of fluid cannot occur, and chylous effusion develops.*

Carcinoma: *When cancer involves the peritoneal membranes, reabsorption of fluid is diminished. Furthermore, the tumors (especially ovarian) can secrete large volumes of fluid. Ascites develops.*

Tuberculosis,

Peritonitis,

Pancreatitis,

Ruptured viscus:

Infections tend to increase peritoneal capillary permeability, and fluid is secreted into the abdominal cavity.

Transudate

Hepatic cirrhosis,

Portal hypertension:

The capillary vessels experience an increased portal venous drainage pressure. Reabsorption is diminished and fluid accumulates.

Nephrotic syndrome,

Hypoproteinemia:

The nephrotic syndrome is characterized by renal albumin wasting. This and other forms of hypoproteinemia are associated with decreased intravascular oncotic pressure. The fluid tends to leak out of the intravascular space into the peritoneum.

Congestive heart failure: *The venous drainage of peritoneum is diminished by the right heart failure that exists and causes increased venous pressures. Peritoneal fluid accumulates.*

Abdominal trauma,

Peritoneal bleeding:

Intraabdominal bleeding or ruptured viscus can be determined by identifying a bloody effusion (hemoperitoneum) or by aspirating bowel contents from the free abdominal cavity.

RELATED TESTS

Glucose, Lactic Dehydrogenase, Protein, and Amylase (pp. 253, 329, 424, and 61, respectively). These blood tests are performed concomitantly to assist in the evaluation of the peritoneal fluid.

Pericardiocentesis

NORMAL FINDINGS

Less than 50 mL of clear, straw-colored fluid without evidence of any bacteria, blood, or malignant cells

INDICATIONS

Pericardiocentesis is performed to determine the cause of an unexplained pericardial effusion. It is also performed to relieve the intrapericardial pressure that accumulates with a large volume of fluid and inhibits diastolic filling.

TEST EXPLANATION

Pericardiocentesis, which involves the aspiration of fluid from the pericardial sac with a needle, may be performed for therapeutic and diagnostic purposes. *Therapeutically* the test is performed to relieve cardiac tamponade by removing blood or fluid to improve diastolic filling. *Diagnostically* pericardiocentesis is performed to remove a sample of pericardial fluid for laboratory examination to determine the cause of the fluid accumulation. This is similar to the evaluation described for pleural fluid on p. 681.

A physician usually performs this procedure in the cardiac catheterization laboratory, operating room, or emergency room in approximately 10 to 20 minutes. This procedure is associated with very little discomfort. Most patients feel pressure when the needle is inserted into the pericardial sac.

CONTRAINDICATIONS

- Patients who are uncooperative, because of the risk of lacerations to the epicardium or coronary artery
- Patients with a bleeding disorder: Inadvertent puncture of the myocardium may create uncontrollable bleeding into the pericardial sac, leading to tamponade.

POTENTIAL COMPLICATIONS

- Laceration of the coronary artery or myocardium
- Needle-induced ventricular arrhythmias (dysrhythmias)
- Myocardial infarction
- Pneumothorax caused by inadvertent puncture of the lung
- Liver laceration caused by inadvertent puncture of that organ
- Pleural or pericardial infection caused by the aspirating needle
- Vasovagal hypotension or arrest

✓ Clinical Priorities

- Therapeutically this test can be performed to relieve cardiac tamponade by removing blood or fluid to improve diastolic filling. Diagnostically it is performed to determine the cause of a fluid accumulation.
- Atropine may be given before the procedure to prevent the vasovagal reflex of bradycardia and hypotension.
- After this test the vital signs are carefully monitored. Pericardial bleeding may be indicated by hypotension and pulsus paradoxus. Temperature elevations may indicate infection.

PROCEDURE AND PATIENT CARE

Before

 Explain the procedure to the patient.
- Obtain informed consent for this procedure.
- Restrict fluid and food intake for at least 4 to 6 hours (if this is an elective procedure).
- Obtain intravenous (IV) access for infusion of fluids and cardiac medications if required.
- Administer pretest medication. Atropine may be given to prevent the vasovagal reflex of bradycardia and hypotension.

During

- Note the following procedural steps:
  1. The patient is placed in the supine position.
  2. An area in the fifth to sixth intercostal space at the left sternal margin (or subxyphoid) is prepared and draped. Alternatively the subxyphoid space is used for access to the pericardium.

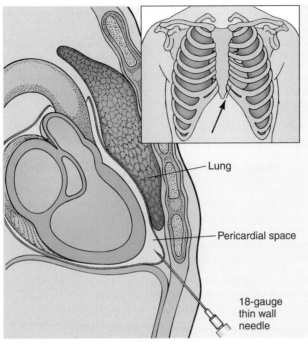

Figure 5-3 Pericardiocentesis using subxiphoid route for aspiration of pericardial fluid. The 18-gauge needle is introduced at 30- to 40-degree angle.

Lung

Pericardial space

18-gauge thin wall needle

3. After a local anesthetic is administered, a pericardiocentesis needle is placed on a 50-mL syringe and introduced into the pericardial sac (Figure 5-3).
4. An electrocardiographic lead is often attached by a clip to the needle to identify any ST-segment elevations, which may indicate penetration into the epicardium. Echocardiography may be used for guidance of the needle.
5. Pericardial fluid is aspirated and placed in multiple specimen containers.
6. Some patients who have recurring cardiac tamponade may require placement of an indwelling pericardial catheter for continuous draining for 1 to 3 days. Occasionally a surgical pericardial window (excision of a small portion of the pericardium) is necessary to prevent recurrent effusions.
7. With certain types of pericarditis, medications (e.g., antibiotics, antineoplastic drugs, corticosteroids) may be instilled during pericardiocentesis to diminish the risk of recurrent effusions.

After

- Closely monitor the patient's vital signs. An increased temperature may indicate infection. Pericardial bleeding would be marked by hypotension or pulsus paradoxus (abnormal decrease in systolic blood pressure during inspiration).
- Label and number the specimen tubes that contain the pericardial fluid and deliver them to the appropriate laboratories for examination. Note the following possibilities:
  1. Usually the fluid is taken to the chemistry laboratory, where the color, turbidity, glucose, albumin, protein, and lactic dehydrogenase levels are obtained. (See the discussion of thoracentesis on p. 681.)

2. A tube of blood often goes to the hematology laboratory, where red and white blood cells are evaluated. (See the discussion of thoracentesis on p. 681.)

3. The bacteriology laboratory performs routine cultures, Gram stains, fungal studies, and acid-fast stains.

4. When malignancy is suspected, the fluid should be sent for cytologic examination.

- All tests performed on pericardial fluid should be performed immediately to avoid false results caused by chemical or cellular deterioration.
- Apply a sterile dressing to the catheter if one has been left for continuing pericardial drainage.
- Establish a closed system if continued pericardial drainage is required. This is usually performed via the straight drainage method.
- Note that to minimize infection, pericardial catheters, if used, are usually removed after 2 days, although there are exceptions. After the sutures are cut and the catheter is removed, apply a sterile dressing to the puncture site.

 Home Care Responsibilities

- Check the dressing frequently for drainage.
- Note that an increased temperature may indicate infection.
- Instruct the patient to report any drop in blood pressure. Hypotension may be a sign of pericardial bleeding.

TEST RESULTS AND CLINICAL SIGNIFICANCE

Pericarditis: *Pericarditis can occur as a sequela to myocardial infarction; myocarditis; viral, bacterial, or tuberculous infections; or collagen-vascular diseases. The fluid is usually an exudate. (See the discussion of thoracentesis on p. 681.)*

Hypoproteinemia,

Nephrotic syndrome:

> *The nephrotic syndrome is characterized by renal albumin wasting. This and other forms of hypoproteinemia are associated with decreased intravascular oncotic pressure. The fluid tends to leak out of the intravascular space into the peritoneum. This fluid is usually a transudate.*

Congestive heart failure: *Normally a small amount of fluid exists within the pericardial space. Fluid is constantly secreted and reabsorbed by the pericardium. If venous pressure of the pericardium is increased as a result of passive congestion of the pericardium associated with congestive heart failure, fluid will accumulate.*

Metastatic cancer: *Neoplasms affecting the pericardium primarily (mesothelioma) or secondarily (breast, lung, ovarian, lymphoma) secrete excess volume of fluid into the pleural space. This fluid is an exudate.*

Blunt or penetrating cardiac trauma,

Rupture of ventricular aneurysm:

> *These events cause sudden accumulation of blood within the closed pericardial space. As a result, diastolic filling is diminished and cardiac output diminishes. Immediate treatment is required if the patient is to survive.*

Collagen-vascular disease: *Patients with these autoimmune diseases can develop an inflammatory pericardial effusion. Usually the effusion develops slowly, allowing enough time for anatomic and functional compensatory changes. Sometimes, however, the effusion is acute enough or large enough to require pericardiocentesis.*

RELATED TESTS

Glucose, Lactic Dehydrogenase (LDH), Protein, and Amylase (p. 253, 329, 424, and 61, respectively). These blood tests are performed concomitantly to assist in the evaluation of the peritoneal fluid.

Chest X-Ray (p. 1014). This is an important part of identifying a pericardial effusion. Furthermore, a chest x-ray should be routinely performed on completion of pericardiocentesis to ensure that a pneumothorax has not iatrogenically occurred.

Electrocardiography (p. 544). This test is simultaneously performed to indicate location of the aspirating needle.

Computed Tomography (CT) of the Chest (p. 1029). This test can accurately assess the volume of fluid in the pericardium.

Semen Analysis (Sperm Count, Sperm Examination, Seminal Cytology, Semen Examination)

NORMAL FINDINGS

Volume: 2-5 mL
Liquefaction time: 20-30 minutes after collection
Appearance: Normal
Motile/mL: $\geq 10 \times 10^6$
Sperm/mL: $\geq 20 \times 10^6$
Viscosity: ≥ 3
Agglutination: ≥ 3
Supravital: $\geq 75\%$ live
Fructose: Positive
pH: 7.12-8
Sperm count (density): ≥ 20 million/mL
Sperm motility: $\geq 50\%$ at 1 hour
Sperm morphology: >30% (Kruger criteria >14%) normally shaped

INDICATIONS

Semen analysis is used to evaluate the quality of sperm, to evaluate an infertile couple, and to document the adequacy of operative vasectomy.

TEST EXPLANATION

Semen production depends on the function of the testicles; semen analysis is a measure of testicular function. Gonadotropin-releasing hormone (Gn-RH) is secreted by the hypothalamus in response to decreased levels of testosterone. Gn-RH stimulates the pituitary to produce follicle-stimulating hormone (FSH) and luteinizing hormone (LH, also called interstitial cell–stimulating hormone). The FSH stimulates the Sertoli cell growth within the seminiferous tubules (location of sperm production). LH stimulates the Leydig cells to produce testosterone, which in turn stimulates the seminiferous tubules to produce sperm. Inadequate sperm production can be the result of primary gonadal failure (because of age, genetic cause [Klinefelter syndrome], infection, radiation, or surgical orchiectomy) or secondary gonadal failure (because of pituitary diseases). These forms of gonadal failure can be differentiated by measuring LH and FSH levels. In primary gonadal failure, LH and FSH levels are increased. In secondary gonadal failure, they are decreased. Stimulation tests using Gn-RH agonists such as leuprolide acetate clomiphene, or human chorionic gonadotropin are also used in the differentiation. Men with *aspermia* (no sperm) or *oligospermia* (<20 million/mL) should be evaluated endocrinologically for pituitary, thyroid, or testicular aberrations.

Semen analysis is one of the most important aspects of the fertility workup because the cause of a couple's inability to conceive often lies with the man. After 2 to 3 days of sexual abstinence, semen is collected and examined for volume, sperm count, motility, and morphology.

The freshly collected semen is first measured for volume. After liquefaction of the white, gelatinous ejaculate, a sperm count is done. Men with very low or very high counts likely are infertile. The motility of the sperm is then evaluated; at least 50% should show progressive motility. Morphology is studied by staining a semen preparation and calculating the number of normal versus abnormal sperm forms. The semen specimen is consideral abnormal if greater than 70% of the sperm have abnormal forms.

More exhaustive semen analysis for male infertility may include a *sperm penetration assay (SPA)*, a multistep laboratory test that offers a biologic assessment of several aspects of human sperm fertilizing ability. *Hyaluronan binding assay (HBA)* is a qualitative assay used to determine the maturity of sperm in a fresh semen sample. The assay is based on the ability of mature, but not immature, sperm to bind to hyaluronan, the main mucopolysaccharide of the egg matrix and a component of human follicular fluid. Hyaluronan-binding capacity is acquired late in the sperm maturation process; immature sperm lack this ability. Therefore a low level of sperm binding to hyaluronan suggests that there is a low proportion of mature sperm in the sample. Similar to the sperm penetration assay, it has been suggested that the HBA assay may be used to determine the need for an intracytoplasmic sperm injection procedure as part of an assisted reproductive technique.

Aside from the conventional parameters of sperm quality such as concentration, motility, and morphology, *sperm DNA integrity* is a potential cause of idiopathic male infertility. Although sperm with fragmented DNA may be able to fertilize oocytes, subsequent embryo and fetal development may be impaired. DNA fragmentation in sperm increases with age. Therefore impaired DNA integrity may be an increasing infertility factor among older couples. Available flow cytometry tests of DNA integrity include the *sperm chromatin structure assay test* and the *sperm DNA fragmentation assay (SDFA) test*. The sperm specimen is considered abnormal if more than 70% of the sperm have abnormal forms.

A single sperm analysis, especially if it indicates infertility, is inconclusive because sperm count varies from day to day. A semen analysis should be done at least twice and possibly a third time, 3 weeks apart. A normal semen analysis alone does not accurately assess the male factor unless the effect of the partner's cervical secretion on sperm survival is also determined. (See the discussion of the Sims-Huhner test on p. 676.) In addition to its value in infertility workups, semen analysis is also helpful in documenting adequate sterilization after a vasectomy. It is usually performed 6 weeks after the surgery. If any sperm are seen, the adequacy of the vasectomy must be suspect.

INTERFERING FACTORS

 Drugs that may cause decreased sperm counts include antineoplastic agents (e.g., methotrexate), cimetidine, estrogens, and methyltestosterone.

✓ Clinical Priorities

- It is best to collect the semen for this test after 2 to 3 days of sexual abstinence.
- For best results the semen specimen should be collected in the physician's office by masturbation.
- A single sperm analysis is inconclusive because the sperm count varies from day to day. A semen analysis should be done two or three times for best results.

PROCEDURE AND PATIENT CARE

Before

- Explain the procedure to the patient.
- Instruct the patient to abstain from sexual activity for 2 to 3 days before collecting the specimen. Prolonged abstinence before the collection should be discouraged, because the quality of the sperm cells, and especially their motility, may diminish.
- Give the patient the proper container for the semen collection.
- Instruct the patient to avoid alcoholic beverages for several days before the collection.
- For evaluation of the adequacy of vasectomy, the patient should ejaculate once or twice before the day of examination to clear the distal portion of the vas deferens.

During

- Note that semen is best collected by ejaculation into a clean container. For best results the specimen should be collected in the physician's office or laboratory by masturbation.
- Note that less satisfactory specimens can be obtained in the patient's home by coitus interruptus or masturbation. Note the following procedural steps:
  1. Instruct the patient to deliver these home specimens to the laboratory within 1 hour after collection.
  2. Tell the patient to avoid excessive heat and cold during transportation of the specimen.

After

- Record the date of the previous semen emission along with the collection time and date of the fresh specimen.
- Tell the patient when and how to obtain the test results. Remember that abnormal results may have a devastating effect on the patient's sexuality.

TEST RESULTS AND CLINICAL SIGNIFICANCE

Infertility: *One of the most common causes of infertility is inadequate sperm production.*

Vasectomy (obstruction of vas deferens): *Semen analysis is necessary before vasectomy can be considered to be adequate.*

Orchitis: *This is usually caused by a virus (varicella) or rarely by a bacterium.*

Testicular failure: *This can be congenital (Klinefelter syndrome) or acquired (e.g., infection). Usually, with acquired forms of testicular failure, sperm are present but in low quantities. With congenital forms of testicular failure, no sperm are seen.*

Hyperpyrexia,

Varicocele:

> *A common finding in sperm analysis is called "stress pattern." This is said to exist when greater than 20% of the sperm have abnormal appearance and sperm counts are low. The stress pattern indicates presence of a varicocele or recent febrile illness.*

Pituitary pathologic condition (adenoma, infarction): *This causes hypospermia because of reduced or absent LH and FSH levels. As a result, spermatogenesis does not occur.*

RELATED TESTS

Antispermatozoal Antibody (p. 96). These antibodies can exist in the blood of males and destroy sperm quality. Furthermore, these antibodies can be produced by women and exist in the cervical mucus, making fertility difficult.

Sims-Huhner (p. 676). The Sims-Huhner test consists of a postcoital examination of the cervical mucus to measure the ability of the sperm to penetrate the mucus and maintain motility. It is used in the diagnostic workup of infertility. This analysis is also helpful in documenting cases of suspected rape by testing the vaginal and cervical secretions for sperm.

Luteinizing Hormone and Follicle-Stimulating Hormone Assay (p. 348). These hormones are useful in determining the pituitary effect on gonadal function and spermatogenesis.

 Sexual Assault Testing

NORMAL FINDINGS

No physical evidence of sexual assault

INDICATIONS

This testing is used to obtain evidence of a recent sexual assault and to obtain specimens to identify sexually transmitted diseases.

TEXT EXPLANATION

The sexual assault victim needs to have psycho-emotional support, treatment of any physical injuries, and accurate and reliable evidentiary testing. Nearly all acute care centers have protocols in place that provide that care to victims of sexual assault. Furthermore, in most circumstances, there are nurses specifically trained in obtaining the appropriate specimens. These nurses know the importance of following the chain of evidence protocols to ensure that evidence is admissible in court.

While being provided with emotional support and assistance, the patient is first interviewed in a nonjudgmental manner. A thorough gynecologic history is obtained. A brief summary of the assault (if there was vaginal, oral, or anal penetration) and timing of the assault is important. After 72 hours, very little evidence persists. It is important to ascertain if the victim changed clothing, showered, or used a douche before coming to the hospital. These will affect the presence of evidence. The general demeanor of the patient, status of the clothing, and physical maturation assessment is documented.

The victim's clothes are removed and separately placed in a paper bag for possible deoxyribonucleic acid (DNA) sources of the victim's or assailant's body parts. Plastic bags are not used because bacteria may grow in them and can destroy DNA. Photographs of all injuries should be obtained, if possible. The victim is then examined for signs of external and internal injuries. A pelvic examination is then performed. A "sexual assault evidence collection kit" is now most commonly used to obtain all the needed specimens. The directions must be carefully followed to ensure that any and all evidence is obtained and is useful toward identification and conviction of any perpetrator (Box 5-1).

Vaginal secretions are obtained for sperm (see p. 671), or other cells from the assailant. Acid phosphatase (see p. 25) or prostate specific antigen (PSA) (see p. 420) are also obtained using this specimen. Cervical secretions are obtained for sexually transmitted disease (STD) (p. 756) testing. These anatomic areas along with the anorectal area are swabbed per directions in the kit. In the male victim, penile and anorectal areas are swabbed. Pubic hair is obtained by combing or plucking. STD testing would include syphilis (p. 473), trichomoniasis (p. 759), gonorrhea (p. 756), and chlamydia (p. 722). Later, blood testing for human immune deficiency virus (HIV) (p. 297) and pregnancy (p. 304) is obtained.

| BOX 5-1 | DNA Evidence Collection: Special Precautions |

To avoid contamination of evidence that may contain DNA, the special sexual assault kit should be used and the following precautions taken:
- Wear gloves and change them often.
- Use disposable instruments or clean them thoroughly before and after handling each sample.
- Avoid touching any area where you believe DNA may be present.
- Avoid talking, sneezing, or coughing over evidence.
- Avoid touching your face, nose, and mouth when collecting and packaging evidence.
- Keep evidence dry and transport it at room temperature.
- Ensure that the chain of custody is maintained at all times.

Next, blood specimens are obtained for DNA testing per the testing kit directions—usually an EDTA containing tube (lavender topped). More blood or urine may also be collected for evidence of mind altering drugs/alcohol or for serologic evidence of STDs. After this testing, a more detailed examination of the vagina, cervix, and rectum are performed using a Wood lamp to more easily identify saliva or sperm from the assailant. These areas are examined for subtle injuries from forced penetration. Two methods used to identify these injuries are the toludine blue dye test and use of a colposcope (see p. 595). The *toludine blue dye test* can also be used to identify recent or healed genital or anorectal injuries. A 1% aqueous solution is applied to the area of concern and washed off with a lubricant (e.g., K-Y Jelly) or a 1% acetic acid solution. Injured mucosa will retain the dye and become more apparent to the naked eye. Finally, the fingernails are scraped underneath because they may potentially contain tissue from the assailant. On completion of the examination, the victim is usually interviewed by the police for further investigation.

Unless medically contraindicated, all victims should be offered antimicrobial therapy to prevent STDs. The following combination of drugs is used in many hospitals: ciprofloxacin 250 mg PO stat dose; doxycycline 100 mg bid for 7 days; and metronidazole 2 g stat. The use of antiretroviral drugs in the prevention of HIV transmission may be recommended and the current guideline for postexposure prophylaxis following needle stick injuries should be used. It may also be advisable to offer victims a hepatitis B vaccination or hepatitis B immunoglobulin as the disease may be fatal. Victims who are at risk for HIV infection should also be given counseling on HIV/acquired immunodeficiency syndrome (AIDS).

A pregnancy test should be done before any treatment or drugs are prescribed. If there is a risk of pregnancy, the victims should be offered postcoital contraception if the rape occurred less than 72 hours before examination by the health worker. If it occurred more than 72 hours but less than 7 days before the examination, an intrauterine contraceptive device may be used to prevent pregnancy. Pregnancy testing may be repeated in the succeeding week after the rape.

CONTRAINDICATIONS

- The patient is emotionally not able to undergo the examination.

INTERFERING FACTORS

- Delays in examination after the alleged attack diminish the possibilities of identifying meaningful evidence.

PROCEDURE AND PATIENT CARE

Before

 Explain the procedure to the patient and provide emotional support.

- Obtain consent to treat the patient or family.
- Notify any family members the patient would like to be present during the examination.
- Assess the patient's emotional condition and determine if the victim is able to undergo sexual assault testing.

During

- Obtain a thorough history as described previously.
- Use the SAPS Sexual Assault Evidence Collection Kit (SAECK) or similar test kit exactly as described to maintain the chain of evidence (see Box 5-1).
- Properly handle the kit specimens to maintain the chain of custody.
- Refrigerate all samples containing biological evidentiary material such as DNA to prevent putrefaction (decomposition).
- It is important to carefully examine all area of the body to help corroborate the victims's version of the alleged events.

After

- Notify police of the alleged assault.
- Assess the patient's need for urgent counseling support and make arrangements, as needed.
- If additional or ongoing counseling is required, the patient should be referred to a trained counselor in victim support.

TEST RESULTS AND CLINICAL SIGNIFICANCE

Rape,
Sexual assault:

> *The psychological effects of a sexual assault in either sex is overwhelming. These patients do best if referred for psychological support. Often the conviction of the offender lessens the fear of the victim. Furthermore, observing just punishment of the offender may hasten healing. It is important to accurately obtain evidence so that all data are admissible and useful to law enforcement agencies.*

Sims-Huhner (Postcoital, Postcoital Cervical Mucus, Cervical Mucus Sperm Penetration)

NORMAL FINDINGS

Cervical mucus adequate for sperm transmission, survival, and penetration; 6 to 20 active sperm per high-power field

INDICATIONS

The Sims-Huhner test consists of a postcoital examination of the cervical mucus to measure the ability of the sperm to penetrate the mucus and maintain motility. It is invaluable in the evaluation of infertility.

TEST EXPLANATION

This study evaluates interaction between the sperm and the cervical mucus. It also measures the quality of the cervical mucus. This test can determine the effect of vaginal and cervical secretions on the activity of the sperm. This procedure is performed only after a previously performed semen analysis has been determined to be normal.

This test is performed during the middle of the ovulatory cycle because at this time the secretions should be optimal for sperm penetration and survival. During ovulation the quantity of cervical mucus is maximal, whereas the viscosity is minimal, thus facilitating sperm penetration. The endocervical mucus sample is examined for color, viscosity, and tenacity (spinnbarkeit). The fresh specimen is then spread on a clean glass slide and examined for the presence of sperm. Estimates of the total number and of the number of motile sperm per high-power field are reported. Normally, 6 to 20 active sperm cells should be seen in each microscopic high-power field; if the sperm are present but not active, the cervical environment is unsuitable (e.g., abnormal pH) for their survival. After the specimen has dried on the glass slide, the mucus can be examined for ferning to demonstrate estrogen effect. The Sims-Huhner study is invaluable in fertility examinations; however, it is not a substitute for the semen analysis. If the results of the Sims-Huhner test are less than optimal, the test is usually repeated during the same or the next ovulatory cycle.

This analysis is also helpful in documenting cases of suspected rape by testing the vaginal and cervical secretions for sperm. This procedure is performed by a physician in approximately 5 minutes. The only discomfort associated with this study is insertion of the speculum.

Fluid Analysis Studies **5**

✓ Clinical Priorities

- This test is performed during the middle of the ovulation cycle, when the secretions should be optimal for sperm penetration and survival.
- Tell the female patient to remain in bed for 10 to 15 minutes after coitus to ensure cervical exposure to the semen. She should then report to the doctor within 2 hours of coitus.

PROCEDURE AND PATIENT CARE

Before

 Explain the procedure to the patient.

Inform the patient that basal body temperature recordings should be used to indicate ovulation.

Tell the patient that no vaginal lubrication, douching, or bathing is permitted until after the vaginal cervical examination, because these factors will alter the cervical mucus.

Inform the patient that this study should be performed after 3 days of male sexual abstinence.

Instruct the patient to remain in bed for 10 to 15 minutes after coitus to ensure cervical exposure to the semen. After this rest period, the patient should report to her physician for examination of her cervical mucus within 2 hours after coitus.

During

- Note that the patient is in the lithotomy position; the cervix is then exposed by an unlubricated speculum. The specimen is aspirated from the endocervix and delivered to the laboratory for analysis.

After

Tell the patient how and when she may obtain the test results.

TEST RESULTS AND CLINICAL SIGNIFICANCE

Infertility: *This test determines the capability of the sperm to function and exist in an environment outside the male urethra. It is the final determinant of the adequacy of sperm. Although semen analysis may indicate an adequate sperm count, etc., if the sperm cannot function within the vaginal or cervical environment, fertility is improbable.*

Suspected rape: *The demonstration of sperm within vaginal secretions indicates that intercourse has occurred.*

RELATED TESTS

Semen Analysis (p. 671). Semen analysis is used to evaluate the quality of sperm, to evaluate an infertile couple, and to document the adequacy of operative vasectomy.

Antispermatozoal Antibody Test (p. 96). These antibodies can exist in the blood of males and destroy sperm quality. Furthermore, these antibodies can be produced by women and exist in the cervical mucus, making fertility difficult.

Luteinizing Hormone and Follicle-Stimulating Hormone Assay (p. 348). These hormones are useful in determining the pituitary effect on gonadal function and spermatogenesis.

 Sweat Electrolytes (Iontophoretic Sweat)

NORMAL FINDINGS

Sodium values in children
    Normal: <70 mEq/L
    Abnormal: >90 mEq/L
    Equivocal: 70-90 mEq/L
Chloride values in children
    Normal: <50 mEq/L
    Abnormal: >60 mEq/L
    Equivocal: 50-60 mEq/L

INDICATIONS

This test is used to diagnose cystic fibrosis. The sweat electrolytes test is indicated in children with recurrent respiratory tract infections, chronic cough, early onset asthma, malabsorption syndromes, late passage of meconium stool, or failure to thrive. This test is also used to screen for the disease in children or siblings of cystic fibrosis (CF) patients.

TEST EXPLANATION

Patients with cystic fibrosis have increased sodium and chloride contents in their sweat. That forms the basis of this test, which is both sensitive and specific for CF. CF is an inherited disease (autosomal recessive) characterized by abnormal secretion by exocrine glands within the bronchi, small intestines, pancreatic ducts, bile ducts, and skin (sweat glands). Sweat, induced by electrical current (pilocarpine iontophoresis), is collected, and its sodium and chloride contents are measured. The degree of abnormality is no indication of the severity of cystic fibrosis; it merely indicates that the patient has the disease.

Patients with CF have a mutation in the CF transmembrane conductance regulator (CFTR) gene. This gene encodes the synthesis of a protein that serves as a channel through which chloride enters and leaves the cells. A mutation in this gene alters the cell's capability to regulate the chloride (and as a result, sodium) transport. Normally, at the base of a sweat gland, sodium and chloride concentrations are very high. As the sweat moves closer to the skin surface, chloride is transported through the lining cells out of the sweat. Sodium follows. By the time the sweat comes to the surface, nearly all of the chloride and sodium has been removed. In patients with CF, the transport of these ions does not occur. The sweat, therefore, has high concentrations of sodium and chloride. Almost all patients with CF have sweat sodium and chloride contents two to five times greater than normal values. In patients with suspicious clinical manifestations, these levels are diagnostic of CF.

Abnormal sweat test results can also occur in patients with glycogen storage diseases, adrenal hypofunction, and G-6-PD deficiency.

The sweat test is not reliable during the first few weeks of life. High serum concentrations of immunoreactive trypsin may be a better test for this age-group. An experienced technologist performs the sweat test in approximately 90 minutes in the laboratory or at the patient's bedside. A small electrical current is experienced during the test, but this is not painful. Generally there is no discomfort or pain associated with this test.

INTERFERING FACTORS

- In a cold room, sweating is inhibited. The room should be warmed or the child covered to maintain body heat.
- Dehydration is associated with reduced volume of sweat and increased concentration of sodium and chloride. The test results are not accurate.
- Values in pubertal adolescents may vary significantly and are not accurate.

PROCEDURE AND PATIENT CARE

Before
⟨✗⟩ Explain the procedure to the patient and/or parents.
⟨✗⟩ Tell the patient and/or parents that no fasting is required.

During
- Note the following procedural steps:
  1. For *iontophoresis,* a low-level electrical current is applied to the test area (the thigh in infants, the forearm in older children) (Figure 5-4).
  2. The positive electrode is covered by gauze and saturated with pilocarpine hydrochloride, a stimulating drug that induces sweating.
  3. The negative electrode is covered by gauze saturated with a bicarbonate solution.
  4. The electrical current is allowed to flow for 5 to 12 minutes.
  5. The electrodes are removed, and the arm is washed with distilled water.
  6. Paper disks are placed over the test site with the use of clean, dry forceps.
  7. These disks are covered with paraffin to obtain an airtight seal, preventing evaporation of sweat.

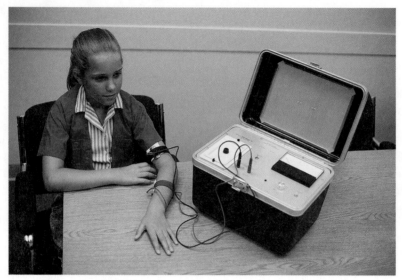

Figure 5-4 Child undergoing sweat test for cystic fibrosis.

8. After 1 hour the paraffin is removed. The paper disks are transferred immediately by forceps to a weighing jar and sent for sodium and chloride analysis.

A *screening test* may be done to detect sweat chloride levels. For screening, a test paper containing silver nitrate is pressed against the child's hand for several seconds. The test is positive when the excess chloride combines with the silver nitrate to form a white powder (silver chloride) on the paper. That is, the child with CF will leave a "heavy" handprint on the paper. A positive screening test is usually validated by iontophoresis.

After

✍ Initiate extensive education, emotional support, and counseling for the patient and/or parents if the results indicate CF.

TEST RESULTS AND CLINICAL SIGNIFICANCE

Cystic fibrosis: *Normally, the sweat produced at the bottom of a sweat duct is rich in chloride and sodium. As the fluid traverses the duct leading to the outer skin level, the chloride (followed by sodium) escapes the lumen through the epithelial cells, leaving only water behind. In patients with CF, the epithelial lining cells of the ducts of sweat glands fail to take up the electrolytes efficiently from the lumen. The sweat at the skin level is therefore high in sodium and chloride.*

RELATED TESTS

Pancreatic Enzymes (p. 660). This is a test whereby pancreatic efflux is measured for amylase and other components. It is a corroborative test for CF.

Genetic Testing (p. 1093). Identification of the cystic fibrosis transmembrane conductance regulator (CFTR) gene is another confirmatory test for the disease. It is more commonly used to identify carriers of the gene that causes CF.

Thoracentesis and Pleural Fluid Analysis
(Pleural Tap)

NORMAL FINDINGS

Gross appearance: clear, serous, light yellow, 50 mL
RBCs: none
WBCs: <300/mL
Protein: <4.1 g/dL
Glucose: 70-100 mg/dL
Amylase: 138-404 units/L
Alkaline phosphatase
    Adult male: 90-240 units/L
    Female <45 years: 76-196 units/L
    Female >45 years: 87-250 units/L
Lactic dehydrogenase (LDH): similar to serum LDH
Cytology: no malignant cells
Bacteria: none
Fungi: none
Carcinoembryonic antigen (CEA): <5 ng/mL

INDICATIONS

Thoracentesis is performed to determine the cause of an unexplained pleural effusion. It is also performed to relieve the intrathoracic pressure that accumulates with a large volume of fluid and inhibits respiration.

TEST EXPLANATION

Thoracentesis is an invasive procedure that entails insertion of a needle into the pleural space for removal of fluid (or rarely, air) (Figure 5-5). The pleural space is defined as the space between the visceral pleura (thin membrane covering the lungs) and the parietal pleura (thin membrane covering the inside of the thoracic cavity). Within the peritoneal membrane is an intricate network of capillary and lymphatic vessels. Fluid is constantly being secreted by the pleural membranes and constantly being reabsorbed by those same membranes. If secretion is increased or reabsorption blocked, pleural fluid will develop.

    Pleural fluid is removed for diagnostic and therapeutic purposes. *Therapeutically,* it is done to relieve pain, dyspnea, and other symptoms of pleural pressure. Removal of this fluid also permits better radiographic visualization of the lung.

    Diagnostically, thoracentesis is performed to obtain and analyze fluid to determine the cause of the pleural effusion. Pleural fluid is classified as transudate or exudate. This is an important distinction and is very helpful in determining the cause of the effusion. See Table 5-4 (p. 663) for differentiation between transudate and exudate. Transudates are most frequently caused by congestive heart failure, cirrhosis, nephrotic syndrome, and hypoproteinemia. *Exudates* are most often found in inflammatory, infectious, or neoplastic conditions. However, collagen-vascular disease, pulmonary infarction, trauma, and drug hypersensitivity also may cause an exudative effusion.

    A decubitus chest x-ray film (p. 1014) is obtained before thoracentesis to ensure that the pleural fluid is mobile and accessible to a needle placed within the pleural space.

5
Fluid Analysis Studies

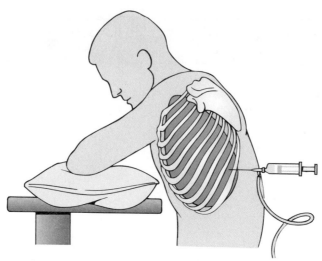

Figure 5-5 Thoracentesis.

Pleural fluid is usually evaluated for gross appearance; cell counts; protein, triglyceride, LDH, glucose, and amylase levels; Gram stain and microbial cultures (for example) *Mycobacterium tuberculosis* and fungi; cytology; CEA levels; and sometimes for other specific tests. Each is discussed separately.

Gross Appearance

The color, optical density, and viscosity are noted as the pleural fluid appears in the aspirating syringe. Transudative pleural fluid may be clear, serous, and light yellow, especially in patients with hepatic cirrhosis. Milk-colored pleural fluid may result from the escape of chyle from blocked thoracic lymphatic ducts. An opalescent, pearly fluid is characteristic of chylothorax (chyle in the pleural cavity). Conditions that may cause lymphatic blockage include lymphoma, carcinoma, and tuberculosis involving the thoracic lymph nodes. The triglyceride value in a chylous effusion exceeds 110 mg/dL.

Cloudy or turbid fluid may result from inflammatory or infectious conditions such as empyema. Empyema is characterized by the presence of a foul odor and thick, pus-like fluid. Bloody fluid may be the result of a traumatic tap (the aspirating needle penetrates a blood vessel), intrathoracic bleeding, or tumor.

Cell Counts

The white blood cells (WBCs) and differential counts are determined. A WBC count exceeding 1000/mL is suggestive of an exudate. The predominance of polymorphonuclear leukocytes usually is an indication of an acute inflammatory condition (e.g., pneumonia, pulmonary infarction, early tuberculosis effusion). When more than 50% of the WBCs are small lymphocytes, the effusion is usually caused by tuberculosis or tumor. Normally, no red blood cells (RBCs) should be present. The presence of RBCs may indicate neoplasms, tuberculosis, or intrathoracic bleeding.

Protein Content

Total protein levels greater than 3 g/dL are characteristic of exudates, whereas transudates usually have a protein content of less than 3 g/dL. It is now thought that the albumin gradient between serum and pleural fluid can differentiate better between the transudate and exudate nature of pleural fluid than can the total protein content. This gradient is obtained by subtracting the pleural albumin value from the serum albumin value. Values of 1.1 g/dL or more suggest a transudate. Values of less than 1.1 g/dL suggest an exudate but will not differentiate the potential cause of the exudate (malignancy from infection or inflammation).

Because there is significant overlap in protein values differentiating transudate from exudate, the total protein ratio (fluid/serum) has been considered to be a more accurate criterion. A total protein ratio of fluid to serum of greater than 0.5 is considered to indicate an exudate.

Lactic Dehydrogenase

A pleural fluid/serum LDH ratio of greater than 0.6 is typical of an exudate. An exudate is identified with a high degree of accuracy if the pleural fluid/serum protein ratio is greater than 0.5 and the pleural fluid/serum LDH ratio is greater than 0.6.

Glucose

Usually pleural glucose levels approximate serum levels. Low values appear to be a combination of glycolysis by the extra cells within an exudate and impairment of glucose diffusion because of damage to the pleural membrane. Values of less than 60 mg/dL also indicate exudate.

Amylase

In a malignant effusion, the amylase concentration is slightly elevated. Amylase levels above the normal range for serum or two times the serum level are seen when the effusion is caused by pancreatitis or rupture of the esophagus associated with leakage of salivary amylase into the chest cavity.

Triglyceride

Measurement of triglyceride levels is an important part of identifying chylous effusions. These effusions are usually produced by obstruction or transection of the lymphatic system caused by lymphoma, neoplasm, trauma, or recent surgery. The triglyceride value in a chylous effusion exceeds 110 mg/dL.

Gram Stain and Bacteriologic Culture

Culture and Gram stains are routinely performed when bacterial pneumonia or empyema is a possible cause of the effusion. These tests identify the organisms involved in the infection and also provide information concerning antibiotic sensitivity. (See p. 704 for a more thorough discussion of Gram stain, cultures, and sensitivity.) If possible, these tests should be done before initiation of antibiotic therapy.

Cultures for *Mycobacterium tuberculosis* and Fungus

Tuberculosis is less often a cause for pleural effusion in the United States today than it was in the past (although its incidence is now on the rise, especially among immuno-suppressed patients). Fungus may be a cause of pulmonary effusion in patients with compromised immunologic defenses. (See p. 768 for more information about tuberculosis culture techniques.)

Cytology

A cytologic study is performed to detect tumors. It is positive in approximately 50% to 60% of patients with malignant effusions. Breast and lung are the two most frequent tumors; lymphoma is the third. The interpretation of cytologic changes requires that the pathologist have considerable experience in cytology. It can be difficult to differentiate malignancy from severe inflammatory mesothelial cells. In general, malignant cells tend to clump together and have a high nucleus/cytoplasm ratio, prominent and multiple nucleoli, and unevenly distributed chromatin.

Cytologic examination of the fluid is improved by spinning down a large volume of fluid and examining the sediment. A large number of cells can be seen and compared with each other. A cytologic study is performed to detect tumor cells.

Carcinoembryonic Antigen

Pleural fluid CEA levels are elevated in various malignant (gastrointestinal [GI], breast) conditions.

Special Tests

The pH of pleural fluid is usually 7.4 or greater. The pH is typically less than 7.2 when empyema is present. The pH may be 7.2 to 7.4 in tuberculosis or malignancy. In some instances the rheumatoid factor (p. 454) and the complement levels (p. 172) are also measured in pleural fluid. Pleural fluid antinuclear antibody (ANA) levels and the pleural fluid/serum ANA ratio are often used to evaluate pleural effusion secondary to systemic lupus erythematosus.

Thoracentesis is performed by a physician at the patient's bedside, in a procedure room, or in the physician's office in less than 30 minutes. Although local anesthetics eliminate pain at the insertion site, the patient may feel a pressure-like pain when the pleura is entered and the fluid is removed.

CONTRAINDICATIONS

- Patients with significant thrombocytopenia, because the aspirating needle may initiate bleeding

POTENTIAL COMPLICATIONS

- Pneumothorax caused by puncture of the lung or entry of air into the pleural space through the aspirating needle
- Intrapleural bleeding because of puncture of a blood vessel
- Hemoptysis caused by needle puncture of a pulmonary vessel
- Reflex bradycardia and hypotension
- Pulmonary edema
- Seeding of the needle track with tumor when malignant pleural effusion exists
- Empyema caused by infection delivered by the aspirating needle

Clinical Priorities

- To prevent needle damage to the lung or pleura, the patient should remain still during this procedure. A cough suppressant may be needed if the patient has a troublesome cough.
- An x-ray film, ultrasound scan, or fluoroscopic view is used to assist in localizing the pleural fluid and in determining the needle insertion site.
- Chest x-ray examinations are done after this procedure to check for pneumothorax. The lungs are carefully assessed for decreased breath sounds, which could be a sign of pneumothorax.

PROCEDURE AND PATIENT CARE

Before

 Explain the procedure to the patient.
- Obtain informed consent for this procedure.
 Tell the patient that no fasting or sedation is necessary.

- ✍ Inform the patient that movement or coughing should be minimized to avoid inadvertent needle damage to the lung or pleura during the procedure.
- Administer a cough suppressant before the procedure if the patient has a troublesome cough.
- Note that an x-ray film or ultrasound scan is often used to assist in location of the fluid. Fluoroscopic examination also may be used.

During

- Note the following procedural steps:
  1. The patient is usually placed in an upright position with the arms and shoulders raised and supported on a padded overhead table. This position spreads the ribs and enlarges the intercostal space for insertion of the needle.
  2. Patients who cannot sit upright are placed in a side-lying position on the unaffected side with the side to be tapped uppermost.
  3. The thoracentesis is performed under strict sterile technique.
  4. The needle insertion site, which is determined by percussion, auscultation, and examination of a chest radiograph film, ultrasound scan, or fluoroscopy, is aseptically cleansed and anesthetized locally.
  5. The needle is positioned in the pleural space, and the fluid is withdrawn with a syringe and a three-way stopcock. Most thoracentesis kits now use a blunt-tip soft catheter over the needle. The needle is withdrawn and the soft Silastic catheter is left in place. The fluid is aspirated. The use of these soft catheters has greatly diminished the incidence of pneumothorax as a complication of this procedure.
  6. Various mechanisms to stabilize the pleural needle or catheter are available to secure the needle depth during the fluid collection.
  7. A short polyethylene catheter may be inserted into the pleural space for fluid aspiration; this decreases the risk of puncturing the visceral pleura and inducing a pneumothorax.
  8. Also, large volumes of fluid may be collected by connecting the catheter to a gravity-drainage system.
- Monitor the patient's pulse for reflex bradycardia and evaluate the patient for diaphoresis and the feeling of faintness during the procedure.

After

- Place a small bandage over the needle site. Usually, turn the patient on the unaffected side for 1 hour to allow the pleural puncture site to heal.
- Label the specimen with the patient's name, date, source of fluid, and diagnosis. Send the specimen promptly to the laboratory.
- All tests done on pleural fluid should be performed immediately to avoid false results caused by chemical or cellular deterioration.
- Obtain a chest x-ray study as indicated to check for pneumothorax.
- Monitor the patient's vital signs.
- Observe the patient for coughing or expectoration of blood (hemoptysis), which may indicate trauma to the lung.
- Evaluate the patient for signs and symptoms of pneumothorax, tension pneumothorax, subcutaneous emphysema, and pyogenic infection (e.g., tachypnea, dyspnea, diminished breath sounds, anxiety, restlessness, fever).
- Assess the patient's lung sounds for diminished breath sounds, which could be a sign of pneumothorax.
- ✍ If the patient has no complaints of dyspnea, normal activity usually can be resumed 1 hour after the procedure.

Fluid Analysis Studies

5

TEST RESULTS AND CLINICAL SIGNIFICANCE

Exudate

Empyema,
Pneumonia:
> *Empyema is most often the result of pneumonia. Occasionally, however, it can follow surgery, pleuritis, or trauma.*

Tuberculosis effusion: *This is usually a bloody effusion that is the result of the primary tuberculous infection of the lung and pleura.*

Pancreatitis: *This pleural effusion is most often a "sympathetic" effusion in response to the inflammatory process below the diaphragm.*

Ruptured esophagus: *The pleural fluid can occur as a result of a free communication of the ruptured esophagus with the pleural cavity. The pleura covering the mediastinum usually prevents this free communication, and the fluid is a "sympathetic" reaction to the mediastinal infection. The fluid, however, subsequently becomes infected and acts as an empyema.*

Tumors: *Neoplasms affecting the pleura primarily (mesothelioma) or secondarily (breast, lung, ovarian) secrete excess volumes of fluid into the pleural space.*

Lymphoma: *The tumor infiltrates the lymph nodes through which the thoracic lymphatic ducts flow. As a result, the lymph fluid is not reabsorbed and collects as a chylous effusion within the pleural space (chylothorax).*

Pulmonary infarction: *This bloody effusion is also a "sympathetic" effusion in response to the necrosis of lung tissue following a pulmonary embolus.*

Collagen-vascular disease: *Rheumatoid arthritis, systemic lupus erythematosus*

Drug hypersensitivity: *An immunogenic pleuritis and subsequent effusion may be the sequelae of autoimmune diseases or drug hypersensitivities as indicated previously.*

Transudate

Cirrhosis,
Congestive heart failure:
> *With increased venous pressure that results from either portal vein hypertension or passive congestion from congestive heart failure, pleural fluid is not absorbed. As a result, pleural fluid accumulates.*

Nephrotic syndrome,
Hypoproteinemia:
> *The nephrotic syndrome is characterized by renal albumin wasting. This and other forms of hypoproteinemia are associated with decreased intravascular oncotic pressure. The fluid tends to leak out of the intravascular space into the pleural space.*

Trauma: *Injury to the thorax, lungs, or great blood vessels can cause bleeding into the pleural space (hemothorax).*

RELATED TESTS

Glucose, Lactic Dehydrogenase (LDH), Protein, and Amylase (pp. 253, 329, 424, and 61, respectively). These blood tests are performed concomitantly to assist in the evaluation of the peritoneal fluid.

Chest X-Ray (p. 1014). This is an important part of identifying a pleural effusion. Furthermore, a chest x-ray should be routinely performed on completion of thoracentesis to ensure that a pneumothorax has not iatrogenically occurred.

Manometric Studies

Overview

Manometric studies evaluate certain areas of the body by using a manometric device to measure and record pressures. These devices can be as familiar to the patient as a blood pressure instrument or as foreign as the one used in oculoplethysmography (OPG) to record eye pressures. Table 6-1 lists the various tests and the areas evaluated.

PROCEDURAL CARE FOR MANOMETRIC STUDIES

Before

- Explain the purpose and procedure to the patient. Patient cooperation is essential in these studies. Many of these studies require informed consent.
- Fasting requirements vary according to the particular study performed. For example, no fasting is required for cystometry. The patient must be fasting for esophageal function studies.

During

- Patient positioning depends on the procedure indicated.
- A particular type of manometer is applied to the patient. For example, blood pressure cuffs are applied to the extremities for arterial plethysmography. A catheter is inserted into the bladder and attached to a pressure monitor for cystometry.
- Patients must remain very still during the procedure. Movement can affect the pressure readings.

TABLE 6-1	Manometric Studies and Areas Evaluated
Test	**Area Evaluated**
Cystometry	Bladder
Esophageal function studies	Esophagus
Oculoplethysmography	Ophthalmic artery
Plethysmography	Arterial pressures
Tilt-table testing	Blood pressure
Urethral pressure profile	Urethra

After

- Aftercare varies with each particular test. For example, some tests (e.g., tourniquet test) require no special aftercare. OPG necessitates some specific eye precautions.

POTENTIAL COMPLICATIONS OF MANOMETRIC STUDIES

There are few complications associated with these tests. The few that do occur vary markedly from test to test. For example, gastric aspiration is a potential complication of esophageal function studies. Conjunctival hemorrhage is a potential complication of OPG.

REPORTING OF RESULTS

Most tests are performed by a technician. The physician reviews the test results and explains them to the patient.

Cystometry (Cystometrogram [CMG])

NORMAL FINDINGS

Normal sensations of fullness and temperature
Normal pressures and volumes
Maximal cystometric capacity
    Male: 350-750 mL
    Female: 250-550 mL
Intravesical pressure when bladder is empty: usually <40 cm H_2O
Detrusor pressure: <10 cm H_2O
Residual urine: <30 mL

Maximal Urethral Pressures in Normal Patients (cm H_2O)

Age (yr)	Male	Female
<25	37-126	55-103
25-44	35-113	31-115
45-64	40-123	40-100
>64	35-105	35-75

INDICATIONS

This test is used to measure pressures within the bladder to identify patients who have bladder dysfunction. It is used in patients with bladder outlet obstruction, urinary incontinence, and questionable neurogenic bladder. It is also used to document progress in treatment of these abnormalities.

TEST EXPLANATION

The purpose of cystometry is to evaluate the motor and sensory function of the bladder when incontinence is present or neurologic bladder dysfunction is suspected. A graphic recording of pressure exerted at varying phases of the filling of the urinary bladder is produced. A pressure/volume relationship of the bladder is determined. This urodynamic study assesses the neuromuscular function of the bladder by measuring the efficiency of the detrusor muscle, intravesical pressure and capacity, and the bladder's response to thermal stimulation.

Cystometry can determine whether a bladder function abnormality is caused by neurologic, infectious, or obstructive diseases. Cystometry is indicated to elucidate the causes of bladder outlet obstruction or frequency and urgency, especially before surgery on the urologic outflow tract. Cystometry is also part of the evaluation for the following: incontinence, persistent residual urine, vesicoureteral reflux, motor and sensory disorders affecting the bladder, and the effect of certain drugs on bladder function.

This test is performed by a urologist in approximately 45 minutes and is often performed at the same time as cystoscopy. The only discomfort is that associated with the urethral catheterization. Nocturnal examinations can be performed to evaluate nocturnal incontinence.

CONTRAINDICATIONS

- Urinary tract infections, because of the possibility of false results and the potential for the spread of infection

Clinical Priorities

- This is an important test for diagnosing bladder dysfunction. It can also document response to therapy.
- Certain medications can be administered during cystometry to distinguish between underactivity of the bladder related to muscle failure and underactivity because of denervation.
- This test can be done at the same time as cystoscopy.
- Patients should be carefully evaluated for infection after this test.

PROCEDURE AND PATIENT CARE

Before

- Explain the purpose and the procedure to the patient.
- Obtain informed consent.
- Tell the patient that no fluid or food restrictions are needed.
- Assure the patient that he or she will be draped to prevent unnecessary exposure.
- Assess the patient for signs and symptoms of urinary tract infection.
- Instruct the patient not to strain while voiding because the results can be skewed.

During

- Note the following procedural steps:
  1. Cystometry, usually performed in a urologist's office or a special procedure room, begins with the patient being asked to void.
  2. The amount of time required to initiate voiding and the size, force, and continuity of the urinary stream are recorded. The amount of urine, the time of voiding, and the presence of any straining, hesitancy, or terminal urine dribbling are also recorded. (See the discussion of urine flow studies, p. 701.)
  3. The patient is placed in a lithotomy or supine position.
  4. A retention catheter is inserted through the urethra and into the bladder.
  5. Residual urine volume is measured and recorded.
  6. Thermal sensation is evaluated by the instillation of approximately 30 mL of room-temperature saline solution into the bladder followed by an equal amount of warm water. The patient reports any sensations.
  7. This fluid is withdrawn from the bladder.
  8. The urethral catheter is connected to a cystometer (a machine used to monitor bladder pressure).
  9. Sterile water, normal saline solution, or carbon dioxide gas is slowly introduced into the bladder at a controlled rate, usually with the patient in a sitting position. While the bladder is slowly filled, pressures are simultaneously recorded. This is called a cystometrogram.
  10. Patients are asked to indicate the first urge to void and then when they have the feeling that they must void. The bladder is full at this point.
  11. The pressures and volumes are plotted on a graph.
  12. The patient is asked to void around the catheter, and the maximal intravesical voiding pressure is recorded.
  13. The bladder is drained for any residual fluid or gas.
  14. If no additional studies are to be done, the urethral catheter is removed.
  15. For urethral pressures, fluid or gas is instilled through the catheter, which is withdrawn while pressures along the urethral wall are obtained. (See the discussion of the urethral pressure profile, p. 700.)
- Throughout the study, ask the patient to report any sensations, such as pain, flushing, sweating, nausea, bladder filling, and an urgency to void.
- Note that certain drugs may be administered during the cystometric examination to distinguish between underactivity of the bladder because of muscle failure and underactivity associated with denervation. Cholinergic drugs (e.g., bethanechol [Urecholine]) may be given to enhance the tone of a flaccid bladder. Anticholinergic drugs (e.g., atropine) may be given to promote relaxation of a hyperactive bladder. If these drugs are to be given, the catheter is left in place.
  After these drugs are given, the examination is repeated 20 to 30 minutes later, using the first test as a control value. The information obtained with the drugs assists in deciding whether drugs will be effective treatment.

After

- Observe the patient for any manifestations of infection (e.g., elevated temperature, chills, or dysuria).
- Examine the urine for hematuria. Notify the physician if the hematuria persists after several voidings.
- Provide a warm sitz bath or tub bath for the patient's comfort if desired.
- Note that pelvic floor sphincter electromyography (p. 576) can be performed to evaluate the urethral sphincter in cases of incontinence.

TEST RESULTS AND CLINICAL SIGNIFICANCE

Neurogenic bladder: *With loss of motor function of the bladder, reduced filling pressures and detrusor pressures are observed. Increased residual volume of urine is also noted. Sensation of fullness and temperature is often diminished or absent. There are several different classifications of neurogenic bladder, some of which are based on the cystometry findings. Spina bifida cord injury, compression, or demyelinating diseases can cause a neurogenic bladder. Diabetic neuropathy, anticholinergics, and alpha-adrenergic antagonists also diminish bladder muscle tone. Extensive pelvic surgery can interrupt the peripheral nerve fibers to the bladder, thereby creating a neurogenic bladder.*

Bladder obstruction: *Bladder outlet obstruction is evidenced by a reduced urine flow, increased intravesicular pressures while voiding, and residual urine volume. Although congenital causes (e.g., urethral valves, phimosis, meatal stenosis) of bladder outlet obstruction can occur, the most common cause of bladder outlet obstruction is a prostatic pathologic condition (cancer or hypertrophy). In women the most common cause of outlet obstruction is a neoplasm (usually of the cervix) or neurogenic bladder (see previous discussion).*

Bladder infection: *Urgency and reduced bladder capacity are noted. Discomfort associated with bladder distention may be enhanced.*

Bladder hypertonicity: *Increased pressures are noted with filling. Capacity is reduced. This occurs with some forms of spastic paralysis. This is most common with upper motor neuron disease or injury.*

Diminished bladder capacity: *This may be the result of post–radiation-therapy fibrosis or an extrinsic tumor compressing the bladder. A fibrotic and inflamed bladder cannot distend adequately. Likewise, when a tumor compresses the bladder, the bladder cannot distend. Capacity is reduced.*

RELATED TESTS

Urine Flow Studies (p. 701). This is a measurement of urine flow per unit of time and is used to diagnose bladder outlet obstruction.

Pelvic Floor Sphincter Electromyography (p. 576). This is a measurement of the electrical activity of the periurethral sphincter function.

Cystography (p. 1036). This is an x-ray contrast study of the bladder. Outlet obstruction is evident on this study.

Esophageal Function Studies (Esophageal Manometry, Esophageal Motility Studies)

NORMAL FINDINGS

Lower esophageal sphincter pressure: 10-20 mm Hg
Swallowing pattern: normal peristaltic waves
Acid reflux: negative
Acid clearing: <10 swallows
Bernstein test: negative

INDICATIONS

This test is used to identify and document the severity of diseases affecting the swallowing function of the esophagus. It is also used to document and quantify gastroesophageal reflux. A wide variety of motor disturbances can be identified. It is commonly used on patients with heartburn, chest pain, or difficulty swallowing.

TEST EXPLANATION

Esophageal function studies include the following:

1. Determination of the lower esophageal sphincter (LES) pressure (manometry)
2. Graphic recording of esophageal swallowing waves, or swallowing pattern (manometry)
3. Detection of reflux of gastric acid back into the esophagus (acid reflux)
4. Detection of the ability of the esophagus to clear acid (acid clearing)
5. An attempt to reproduce symptoms of heartburn (Bernstein test)

Manometric Studies

Two manometric studies are used in assessing esophageal function: (1) measurement of LES pressure and (2) graphic recording of swallowing waves (motility). The LES is a sphincter muscle that acts as a valve to prevent reflux of gastric acid into the esophagus. Free reflux of gastric acid occurs when the sphincter pressures are low. An example of such a disorder in adults is gastroesophageal reflux; in children, it is called chalasia (incompetent or relaxed LES).

With increased sphincter pressure, as found in patients with achalasia (failure of the LES to relax normally with swallowing) and with diffuse esophageal spasms, food cannot pass from the esophagus into the stomach. Increased LES pressures are noted on manometry. In achalasia, few if any swallowing waves are detected. In contrast, diffuse esophageal spasm is characterized by strong, frequent, asynchronous, and nonpropulsive waves.

Acid Reflux With pH Probe

Acid reflux is the primary component of gastroesophageal reflux. Patients with an incompetent LES will regurgitate gastric acid into the esophagus. This will then cause a drop in the esophageal pH during *esophageal pH monitoring*. With the newer and smaller catheters, 24-hour pH monitoring can be performed. Episodes of acid reflux are evident. If they coincide with patient symptoms of chest pain, esophagitis can be incriminated. Transnasal pH catheters can cause discomfort in patients, sometimes resulting in the avoidance of pH testing, which is the "gold standard" for measuring pH levels in the esophagus. This limits the ability to definitively diagnose and ultimately treat gastroesophageal reflux disease (GERD).

With the *wireless pH probes,* patients can eat and drink normally as well as engage in their usual activities while having their pH levels tested. A wireless pH-probe capsule is now being used with increasing frequency. It collects pH data in the esophagus and transmits it via radio frequency telemetry to an external, pager-sized receiver worn by the patient. This allows patients to maintain regular diet and activities during the monitoring period (24 to 48 hours). This small pH capsule is attached to the wall of the esophagus by esophagoscopy (p. 608). Within days, the capsule spontaneously sloughs off the wall of the esophagus and passes through the patient's gastrointestinal tract. After the study is completed, the patient returns the receiver, and the data is downloaded to a computer for analysis.

Acid Clearing

Patients with normal esophageal function can completely clear hydrochloric acid from the esophagus in less than 10 swallows. Patients with decreased esophageal motility (frequently caused by severe esophagitis) require a greater number of swallows to clear the acid.

Bernstein Test (Acid Perfusion)

The Bernstein test is simply an attempt to reproduce the symptoms of gastroesophageal reflux. If the patient suffers pain with the instillation of hydrochloric acid into the esophagus, the test is positive and proves the patient's symptoms are caused by reflux esophagitis. If the patient has no discomfort, a cause other than esophageal reflux must be sought to explain the patient's discomfort.

CONTRAINDICATIONS

- Patients who cannot cooperate
- Patients who are medically unstable

POTENTIAL COMPLICATIONS

- Aspiration of gastric contents

INTERFERING FACTORS

- Eating shortly before the test may affect results.
- Drugs such as sedatives, proton pump inhibitors, histamine α-blockers, and antacids can alter test results.

PROCEDURE AND PATIENT CARE

Before

- Explain the procedure to the patient.
- Obtain informed consent.
- Instruct the patient not to eat or drink anything for at least 8 hours before the test.
- Allay any fears and allow the patient to verbalize concerns. Be sensitive to the patient's fears about choking during the procedure.
- Tell the patient that except for some initial gagging when swallowing the tubes, these tests are not uncomfortable.

During

- Note the following procedural steps:
  1. Esophageal studies are usually performed in the endoscopy laboratory.
  2. The fasting, unsedated patient is asked to swallow two or three very tiny tubes. The tubes are equipped so that pressure measurements can be taken at 5-cm intervals (Figure 6-1).
  3. The outer ends of the tubes are attached to a pressure transducer.
  4. All tubes are passed into the stomach; then three tubes are slowly pulled back into the esophagus. A rapid and extreme increase in the pressure readings indicates the high-pressure zone of the LES.
  5. The LES pressure is recorded.
  6. With all tubes in the esophagus, the patient is asked to swallow. Motility wave patterns are recorded.
  7. The pH indicator probe is placed in the esophagus.
  8. The patient's stomach is filled with approximately 100 mL of 0.1-N hydrochloric acid. A decrease in the pH of the esophageal pH probe indicates gastroesophageal reflux.
  9. Hydrochloric acid is instilled into the esophagus, and the patient is asked to swallow. The number of swallows is counted to determine acid clearing. More than 10 swallows to clear the acid (as determined by the pH probe) indicates decreased esophageal motility.
  10. Finally, 0.1-N hydrochloric acid and saline solution are alternately instilled into the esophagus for the Bernstein test. The patient is not told which solution is being infused. If the patient volunteers symptoms of discomfort while the acid is running, the test is considered positive. If no discomfort is recognized, the test is negative.
- Note that these tests are performed by an esophageal technician in approximately 30 minutes.

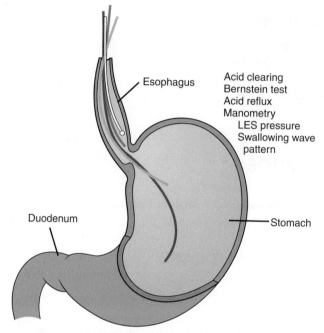

Figure 6-1 Esophageal function studies demonstrating placement of manometry tubes and a pH probe within the esophagus.

Inform the patient that the test results are interpreted by a physician and are available in a few hours.

After

Inform the patient that it is not unusual to have a mild sore throat after placement of the tubes.

TEST RESULTS AND CLINICAL SIGNIFICANCE

Presbyesophagus: *This is a common motility pattern noted among the elderly. It is evident as asynchronous esophageal contractions. As a result, the food is not propelled down the esophagus but, rather, becomes temporarily lodged between the two areas of contraction. This can be quite painful along with causing a functional obstruction to the passage of food.*

Diffuse esophageal spasm: *Spastic synchronously occurring contractions of the esophagus do not allow the food to be propelled down the esophagus but, rather, lodge it temporarily between the two areas of contraction. This, too, can be quite painful along with causing a functional obstruction to the passage of food.*

Chalasia: *Absence of tone in the lower esophageal sphincter allows for free reflux of food and gastric juices into the esophagus. This is a common cause of vomiting in newborns.*

Achalasia: *This is the opposite of chalasia and most commonly occurs in young adults. The tone of the LES is significantly increased. No relaxation of the sphincter occurs. As a result, the LES acts as an obstruction to the passage of food through the esophagus.*

Gastroesophageal reflux,

Reflux esophagitis:

The presence of gastric contents in the esophagus causes esophagitis. The pathophysiology of gastroesophageal reflux is not completely understood. It is known that the LES tone is reduced. This allows acid to reflux into the esophagus. This is evident during pH monitoring. Esophagitis follows, and acid clearing is prolonged because the swallowing function of the inflamed esophagus is reduced.

RELATED TESTS

Esophagoscopy (p. 608). This is an endoscopic test of the esophagus. Reflux esophagitis, esophageal obstruction, achalasia, and other diseases, can be observed.

Barium Swallow (p. 999). This is an x-ray study of the esophagus. Evidence of diseases of the esophagus as listed for esophagoscopy can be visualized.

 Plethysmography, Arterial

NORMAL FINDINGS

<20 mm Hg difference in systolic blood pressure between the lower extremity and the upper extremity

Normal pulse wave amplitude showing a steep upswing; an acute, narrow peak; and a more gentle downslope containing a dicrotic notch (normal arterial pulse wave)

Ankle/brachial ratio: 0.9 to 1.3

INDICATIONS

This is a noninvasive method of identifying and monitoring treatment of arterial occlusive disease.

TEST EXPLANATION

Plethysmography is usually performed to rule out occlusive disease of the lower extremities; however, it also can identify arteriosclerotic disease in the upper extremities. This test does require one normal extremity against which the other extremities may be compared.

Arterial plethysmography is performed by applying three blood pressure cuffs to the proximal, middle, and distal parts of an extremity. Pressure readings are also taken in the upper arm (brachial) artery. These are then attached to a pulse volume recorder (plethysmograph) that enables each pulse wave to be displayed. A reduction in amplitude of a pulse wave in any of the three cuffs indicates arterial occlusion immediately proximal to the area where the decreased amplitude is noted. Also, measurements of arterial pressures are performed at each cuff site. A difference in pressure of greater than 20 mm Hg indicates a degree of arterial occlusion in the extremity. A positive result is reliable evidence of arteriosclerotic peripheral vascular occlusion. However, a negative result does not definitely exclude this diagnosis, because extensive vascular collateralization can compensate for even a complete arterial occlusion.

An *Ankle/Brachial Ratio* of <0.9 indicates peripheral vascular disease in the lower extremity. Arterial plethysmography can also be performed immediately after exercise to determine if symptoms of claudication are caused by peripheral vascular occlusive disease.

Although it is not as accurate as arteriography (see p. 988), plethysmography is performed without serious complications and can be done for extremely ill patients who cannot be transported to the arteriography laboratory.

INTERFERING FACTORS

- Arterial occlusion proximal to the extremity
- Cigarette smoking, because nicotine can cause transient arterial constriction

Clinical Priorities

- A positive result is reliable evidence of arteriosclerotic peripheral vascular occlusion.
- Patients should not smoke for at least 30 minutes before this test because nicotine creates constriction of the peripheral arteries and alters test results.
- This test is usually performed in the noninvasive vascular laboratory or at the bedside by a technologist.

PROCEDURE AND PATIENT CARE
Before

✗ Explain the procedure to the patient.
✗ Inform the patient that this test is painless.
✗ Tell the patient that he or she must lie still during the testing procedure.
- Remove all clothing from the patient's extremities.
✗ Instruct the patient to avoid smoking for at least 30 minutes before the test.
✗ Tell the patient that no fasting is required.

During

- Note the following procedural steps:
  1. The patient is placed in the semirecumbent position.
  2. The cuffs are applied to the extremities and then inflated to 65 mm Hg to increase their sensitivity to pulse waves.
  3. The pulse waves are recorded on the plethysmographic paper.
  4. The amplitudes and form of the pulse wave of each cuff are measured and compared. A marked reduction in wave amplitude indicates arterial occlusive disease.
- Note that this test usually is performed in the noninvasive vascular laboratory or at the patient's bedside by a noninvasive vascular technologist in approximately 30 minutes.
✗ Inform the patient that results are usually interpreted by a physician and are available in a few hours.

After

✗ Encourage the patient to verbalize any concerns regarding the test results.

TEST RESULTS AND CLINICAL SIGNIFICANCE

Arterial atherosclerotic occlusive disease,
Arterial trauma,
Arterial embolization:
   Arterial occlusion is noted by a decreased pressure in the cuff immediately distal to the occlusion.
Small vessel diabetic changes: *Little or no change may be noted in this disease. This type of vascular insufficiency is usually seen in diabetics.*
Vascular diseases (e.g., Raynaud phenomenon): *Arterial occlusion that is episodic is classic for Raynaud phenomenon. This is difficult to identify on plethysmography unless larger vessels of the wrist or hand are involved. Often this diagnosis requires that pressure-sensitive cuffs be placed on the fingers.*

RELATED TESTS

Doppler Arterial Flow Studies (p. 900). This ultrasound examination determines blood flow within the artery suspected to be stenotic. This is a very accurate test of arterial patency.

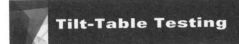

Tilt-Table Testing

NORMAL FINDINGS

<20 mm Hg decrease in systolic blood pressure and <10 mm Hg increase in diastolic blood pressure
Heart rate increase <10 beats/min

INDICATIONS

The tilt-table test is a provocative test used to diagnose vasopressor and vasovagal syncope.

TEST EXPLANATION

Patients with this vasomotor syncope syndrome usually demonstrate symptomatic hypotension and
syncope within a few to 30 minutes of being tilted upright by approximately 60 to 90 degrees. This test
is usually performed with an electrophysiologic study (p. 559). Tilt-table testing is often used to assess
the efficacy of prophylactic pacing in some patients with vasopressor syncope. It is also used to evaluate
the impact of posture on some forms of tachyarrhythmias. Normally a minimal drop in systolic blood
pressure, rise in diastolic blood pressure, and increase in heart rate occur in the tilted position. Patients
with vasopressor or vasovagal syncope demonstrate these changes in an exaggerated fashion and become light-headed and dizzy on assuming the tilted position.

INTERFERING FACTORS

- Patients with dehydration or hypovolemia will demonstrate comparable changes in blood pressure
  and heart rate. This is especially true in elderly patients.
- Patients taking antihypertensive medications or diuretics also may demonstrate similar changes
  when placed in the tilt position.

PROCEDURE AND PATIENT CARE

Before

- Explain the procedure to the patient.
- Obtain informed consent.
- Obtain intravenous (IV) access in the event emergency drugs are required.
- Note that an arterial line can be placed to accurately monitor blood pressure.
- Ask whether the patient has had excessive fluid loss (diarrhea or vomiting) in the previous
  24 hours.
- Record antihypertensive or diuretic medicines that the patient may be taking.

During

- Have the patient lie supine on a horizontal tilt table.
- Obtain the patient's blood pressure and pulse as baseline values before tilting is carried out.
- Note that the table is progressively tilted to 60 to 80 degrees while the patient is being monitored.
  Alternatively, the patient is asked to sit or stand.
- Monitor these vital signs during the procedure.
- Question the patient about the presence of symptoms of dizziness and lightheadedness.

After

- If arterial line was placed, monitor for bleeding after removal of the vascular access.
- Firmly secure a pressure dressing to both sites (arterial and venous).
- Monitor the vital signs as the patient adjusts to positioning changes.

TEST RESULTS AND CLINICAL SIGNIFICANCE

Vasovagal syncope,
Vasomotor syncope: *Tachyarrhythmias, overmedication for hypertension or heart disease, hyperreactive vagal activity, and various forms of vasomotor instability can cause a positive tilt-test result.*

RELATED TEST

Electrophysiologic Study (p. 559). This is a method of studying evoked potentials within the heart. It is used to evaluate patients with syncope, palpitations, or arrhythmias.

Tourniquet Test (Capillary Fragility)

NORMAL FINDINGS

<2 petechiae

INDICATIONS

This test evaluates capillary integrity. It is used to aid in the clinical diagnosis of hemorrhagic fever (Dengue fever).

TEST EXPLANATION

Petechiae occur as a result of increased capillary fragility (microvessels easily rupture and a small amount of bleeding occurs in the skin) or thrombocytopenia (causing spontaneous bleeding in the skin). There are more accurate tests to indicate platelet count (p. 401) and function (p. 404). Petechiae are small, round nonraised red spots in the skin.

Production of petechiae can be induced in patients who have increased capillary fragility or thrombocytopenia. There are two methods of inducing petechiae. The most common is with positive pressure. A blood pressure cuff is applied to an extremity and inflated above venous pressure. The second way is with negative pressure. A suction cup is applied to an area of skin for a particular period of time. Patients with thrombocytopenia, poor platelet function, or purpura will develop more than 10 petechiae per square inch of skin. The number of petechiae can be graded from few to confluent (1 to 4).

INTERFERING FACTORS

- Premenstrual women experience transient episodes of increased capillary fragility.
- Postmenopausal women who do not use hormones experience increased capillary fragility.
- Women, especially those with sun-damaged skin, can have increased capillary fragility.
 Prolonged use of steroids increases capillary fragility.

PROCEDURE AND PATIENT CARE

Before

- Explain the procedure to the patient.
- Obtain an informed consent if required by the institution.
- Tell the patient that no fasting is required.
- Examine the extremity for preexisting petechiae or ecchymoses.

During

Positive Pressure Test

- Place a blood pressure cuff on the upper arm and inflate it to a level above venous pressure (around 70 mm Hg) for 5 minutes.
- Release the cuff pressure.
- Inspect the distal extremity for petechiae.

Negative Pressure Test

- Place a lubricated suction cup (2 cm in diameter) on the upper arm skin.
- Remove the suction after 1 minute.
- Examine the site for petechiae.

After

- Explain the results to the patient.
- If the test is positive, explain to the patient that appropriate precautions should be taken to avoid soft-tissue injury.

TEST RESULTS AND CLINICAL SIGNIFICANCE

Positive: Greater Than 2 Petechiae

Immunologic thrombocytopenia (e.g., idiopathic thrombocytopenic purpura),

Drug-induced thrombocytopenia,

Thromboasthenia (poor platelet function):

Reduced platelets cause spontaneous microbleeding. Nonimmunologic thrombocytopenia is rarely associated with a positive tourniquet test.

Hereditary telangiectasia,

Vascular purpura (autoimmune diseases),

Senile purpura,

Allergic purpura,

Scurvy:

Increased capillary permeability causes petechiae.

Hemophilia: *Spontaneous bleeding causes petechiae.*

RELATED TESTS

Platelet Count (p. 401). This is a direct measurement of platelet number.

Platelet Volume, Mean (p. 407). This is a direct measurement of platelet volume.

Platelet Aggregation (p. 398). This is a direct measurement of platelet function.

Platelet Antibody (p. 399). This test identifies platelet antibodies that destroy the platelet.

Manometric Studies

6

Urethral Pressure Profile (UPP, Urethral Pressure Measurements)

NORMAL FINDINGS

Maximal Urethral Pressures in Normal Patients (cm H_2O)

Age (years)	Male	Female
<25	37-126	55-103
25-44	35-113	31-115
45-64	40-123	40-100
>64	35-105	35-75

INDICATIONS

This test is often a part of cystometry (p. 688). It is used to document reduced urethral pressures in incontinent patients (e.g., females with stress incontinence or males after prostatectomy). It is also used to indicate the degree of compression applied to the urethra from an abnormally enlarged prostate (which will increase UPP value).

TEST EXPLANATION

The UPP indicates the intraluminal pressure along the length of the urethra with the bladder at rest. Indications for this urodynamic investigation include the following:
1. Assessment of prostatic obstruction
2. Assessment of stress incontinence in females
3. Assessment of postprostatectomy sequela of incontinence
4. Assessment of the adequacy of external sphincterotomy
5. Analysis of the effects of drugs on the urethra
6. Analysis of the effects of stimulation on urethral flow
7. Assessment of the adequacy of implanted artificial urethral sphincter devices

This test is usually performed by a urologist in less than 15 minutes. This test is only slightly more uncomfortable than urethral catheterization.

CONTRAINDICATIONS

- Patients with urinary tract infections, because catheterization may induce bacteremia

PROCEDURE AND PATIENT CARE

Before

- Explain the procedure to the patient.
- Obtain informed consent.
- Because many patients are embarrassed by this procedure, assure the patient that he or she will be draped to ensure privacy.
- Tell the patient that no fasting or sedation is required.

During

- Note the following procedural steps:
  1. A catheter is placed into the bladder and attached to a pressure monitor machine.
  2. Fluids (or gas) are instilled through the catheter, which is withdrawn while the pressures along the urethral wall are measured.
  3. A constant infusion of the fluids or gas is maintained by a motorized syringe pump.
  4. The catheter is removed, and the test is completed.

After

- The patient may take a sitz bath, if desired.

TEST RESULTS AND CLINICAL SIGNIFICANCE

Prostatic obstruction secondary to benign prostatic hypertrophy or cancer: *Increased urethral pressures are noted because of the extrinsic compression applied by the enlarged prostate.*

Urinary incontinence: *Reduced urethral pressures are noted because of the reduced tone of the urethral sphincter.*

RELATED TEST

Cystometry (p. 688). This test often includes UPP. This test, which can identify bladder neuromuscular pathologic conditions, is a measure of bladder pressures.

Urine Flow Studies (Uroflowmetry, Urodynamic Studies)

NORMAL FINDINGS

Depend on the patient's age, gender, and volume voided

INDICATIONS

This test is used to evaluate bladder and urethral dysfunction and/or voiding abnormalities. This test is indicated to investigate dysfunctional voiding or suspicious outflow tract obstruction. It is also done before and after any procedure designed to modify the function of the urologic outflow tract.

TEST EXPLANATION

Uroflowmetry is the simplest of the urodynamic techniques, being noninvasive and requiring uncomplicated and relatively inexpensive equipment. This study measures the volume of urine expelled from the bladder per second. If the rate is reduced, outflow obstruction can be documented and measured.

The urine flow depends greatly on the volume of urine voided. Normally, on initiation of urination, flow is slow. However, almost immediately, flow rate rapidly rises until bladder volume quickly decreases. Then the flow decreases rapidly. In patients with outlet obstruction, for example secondary to an enlarged prostate, the flow slowly rises to a level lower than normal. The flow plateaus for a longer time until the bladder volume decreases, and then flow diminishes slowly. The flow rates are highest and most predictable in the urine volume range of 200 to 400 mL. When the bladder contains more

Manometric
Studies

6

than 400 mL of urine, the efficiency of the bladder muscle is greatly decreased. Nomograms of maximal flow versus voided volume may be used for accurate test result interpretation, taking into account the patient's gender and age. If the flow rates are abnormally low, the test should be repeated to check for accuracy.

Modern urine flowmeters provide a permanent graphic recording. If flowmeters are not available, the patient can time the urinary stream with a stopwatch and record the voided volume; from this the average flow is calculated.

In some cases, it is more valuable to analyze several voided volumes and flow rates rather than a single flow rate. If this is to be done, the patient is taught to use a flowmeter. A graph of flow versus volume can be plotted. Together with clinical observation, this provides very valuable information on the severity of outflow obstruction, the likelihood of urinary retention, and the state of compensation or decompensation of the detrusor muscle.

This test is often performed in conjunction with cystometry (p. 688).

PROCEDURE AND PATIENT CARE

Before
- Explain the procedure to the patient.
- Instruct the patient to arrive for the test with a full bladder.
- Instruct the patient how to void into the urine flowmeter.
- Determine the number of flow rates that will be needed.
- Tell the patient that no discomfort is associated with this test.

During
- Note that this test should be performed when the patient has a normal desire to void and in conditions suitable for privacy. The bladder should be adequately full. Essentially all the patient must do is urinate into the flowmeter. Several different types of flowmeters are available.
- Note that the duration of this test is several seconds.

After
- Record the position of the patient, the method of filling the bladder (it should be natural), and whether this study was part of another evaluation.

TEST RESULTS AND CLINICAL SIGNIFICANCE

Dysfunctional voiding: *Flow rates may be normal but intermittent or delayed.*
Outflow tract obstruction: *Flow rates will be diminished significantly, indicating obstruction caused by urethral stricture, prostatic cancer, or hypertrophy. The flow rate curve will plateau at a lower rate and stay there longer than normal.*

RELATED TEST

Cystometry (p. 688). This is a measurement of the pressures within the bladder during filling and micturition. Uroflowmetry may be a part of that study.

Microscopic Studies and Associated Testing

Overview

REASONS FOR PERFORMING MICROSCOPIC STUDIES

Microscopic examinations are essential for the diagnosis and treatment of numerous diseases and infectious processes. Included in this chapter are microbiologic studies and studies that require a microscopic review of tissue. Microbiologic specimens can be collected from many sources, such as tissue and organ biopsies, blood, urine, wound drainage, cervical secretions, and sputum. This testing usually takes place in the microbiology or bacteriology section of the laboratory. Microscopic examination is used in a wide variety of clinical situations, some of which include the following:

1. To evaluate hematologic disorders (bone marrow biopsy, blood smear)
2. To detect sexually transmitted diseases (sexually transmitted disease culture, smear, and wet mount)
3. To evaluate dysfunctional uterine bleeding (endometrial biopsy)
4. To determine liver pathologic conditions (liver biopsy)
5. To detect lung cancer (lung biopsy)
6. To screen for cancer of the vagina, cervix, and uterus (Papanicolaou test)
7. To determine the sensitivity of breast cancer to hormonal therapy (estrogen and progesterone receptor assays)
8. To detect renal disease, such as malignancy, glomerulonephritis, and transplant rejection (renal biopsy)
9. To detect tuberculosis (tuberculosis culture, AFB stain)
10. To evaluate and treat infections (body fluids, wound and soft-tissue culture and sensitivity)
11. To evaluate the urologic tract (see Urinalysis, p. 956)

Microscopic examinations are used to evaluate histologic and cytologic specimens and to identify bacteria (and other infecting organisms). Determination of hormone receptor assay results along with chromatin identification also requires microscopic examination of various types.

Included with microscopic studies are culture and sensitivity testing. Microscopic examination is an important part of identifying an infecting organism. A *Gram stain* is just one of the microscopic examinations performed with microbiology testing. A Gram stain is a method by which all bacteria are classified. All forms of bacteria are grossly classified as gram-positive (blue staining) or gram-negative (red staining). Furthermore, knowledge of the shape of the organism (e.g., spherical, rod shaped) also may be very helpful in the tentative identification of the infecting organism. For example, if the Gram stain indicates gram-negative rods, the infection may be caused by *Escherichia coli*. With knowledge of the Gram stain results, the physician can institute reasonable antibiotic treatment based on past experiences regarding the organism's possible identity and the source of the specimen. The Gram stain can be reported in less than 10 minutes after smearing the specimen on a microscopic slide. Treatment can then be altered based on the final results of culture and sensitivity testing.

The usual culture is obtained from a smear of an infected area (e.g., a wound culture). However, body fluids or tissue can be sent for culture techniques. When plated on the appropriate culture medium, an infecting organism can be expected to grow. Frequently several different kinds of culture media are used in the culture process to maximize the chances of growing the infecting organism. Some bacteria or fungi grow better in one medium than another.

Most of the time the infecting organism is identified from a culture plate on which the organism is growing. In other, rarer situations the infecting organism is found by microscopic review of a tissue specimen. In still other situations the only evidence of infection is derived from serologic testing (e.g., antistreptolysin O titer; see Chapter 2).

Although there are no *potential complications* associated with culture testing, the risks involved in obtaining tissue for microscopic examination may be considerable. They are well outlined in the discussion of each specific study.

PROCEDURAL CARE FOR MICROSCOPIC STUDIES
Before

- Explain the procedure to the patient.
- Inform the patient of any special preprocedure requirements. For example, patients should not douche or tub bathe before cervical cultures for herpes. Men should not void for 1 hour before collection of urethral specimens.

✗ Inform the patient about the collection technique. These techniques vary from being noninvasive (throat culture) to lightly invasive (liver biopsy).

- Invasive studies require an informed consent. Coagulation profiles are often done before invasive studies because of the risk of bleeding.
- If an invasive procedure is to be performed to obtain tissue, the patient should be prepared as if surgery were a possibility because if bleeding or organ injury occurs, the patient must be ready to go to surgery.

During

- Follow universal precautions in handling all specimens because of the risk of transmitting infection or contaminating the specimen.
- Specific protocols for collection are described with each test in this chapter.
- Instruct the patient to remain still during specimen collection. The quality of the specimen depends in part on the cooperation of the patient.

After

- The specimen should be carefully labeled with the patient's name, the source, and any other pertinent information, such as antibiotic therapy.
- The specimen should be promptly transported to the laboratory or pathology department.
- Antibiotic therapy should be initiated after the specimen is collected.
- Vital signs should be carefully evaluated to detect bleeding, infection, or other potential complications of an invasive procedure.
- If the results indicate a sexually transmitted disease (STD), sexual partners should be notified, evaluated, and treated.

LABORATORY HANDLING OF SPECIMENS

The laboratory has protocols to minimize factors that may interfere with testing results. Certain specimens must be processed immediately (such as cerebrospinal fluid [CSF] cultures). Some specimens (such as urine) may be refrigerated if there will be a delay before testing. Stained smears of medically urgent specimens should be evaluated and reported immediately. Cultures should be plated immediately. This is essential to avoid bacterial deterioration. All efforts must be made to avoid the contamination of a culture to decrease the likelihood of incorrect results.

In addition to protocols concerning timeliness in handling of the specimen, the laboratory must also have strict guidelines for rejecting a specimen. An improperly identified specimen is the main reason for rejection. It is obvious that labeling the wrong patient with a diagnosis such as gonorrhea or some other STD can have devastating consequences. Desiccated, poorly preserved specimens, or specimens placed in the wrong container would be considered unsatisfactory.

REPORTING OF RESULTS

Most microbiologic examinations require several days before results are available. The specimens often must go through a staining process that takes at least 24 hours. Some tissue for microscopic examination needs to be sent to reference laboratories for evaluation. Results take much longer to obtain in these cases. Preliminary culture reports and Gram stain results, however, are available much sooner. The quality of microscopic study results depends on the quality of the personnel obtaining, transporting, and handling the specimens. The experience of the physician and technologist reporting the results is also a key component in the process. Microscopic studies are invaluable in making a diagnosis. Not only is communication among the various health care providers imperative, but also reporting must be timely, concise, and accurate.

Acid-Fast Bacilli Smear (AFB Smear)

NORMAL FINDINGS

No bacilli seen

INDICATIONS

This smear (usually of sputum) is used to support the diagnosis of tuberculosis (TB). The diagnosis of TB cannot be made with positive results of an AFB smear by itself. TB cultures are required. AFB smears are also used to monitor treatment of TB. The test is indicated in any patient with a persistent productive cough, night sweats, anorexia, weight loss, fever, hemoptysis, or abnormal chest x-ray. This smear should especially be considered in high-risk patients, such as those who are immunocompromised, are alcoholic, or have had a recent exposure to TB.

TEST EXPLANATION

The most clinically significant AFB is *Mycobacterium tuberculosis*. This is the causative agent in TB. After taking up the fuchsin dye, *M. tuberculosis* is not decolorized by acid alcohol (i.e., it is acid-fast). It is seen under the microscope as a red or pink, rod-shaped organism. If this bacillus is seen, the patient may have active TB. However, other species of microbes such as *Mycobacterium, Nocardia*, and some fungi are also acid-fast. The AFB smear is most commonly performed on sputum. At least 5000 organisms must be present in each milliliter of specimen to be seen on a microscope smear. Other specimens, such as CSF, tissue, and synovial fluid, may be used. Smears may be negative as much as 50% of the time even with positive cultures. One cannot make the diagnosis of TB based only on a positive smear for AFB. Cultures (p. 768) must be positive for a definitive diagnosis. Also, cultures are the only way to determine drug sensitivities for treatment.

AFB is also used to monitor treatment for TB. If after adequate therapy (2 months), the sputum still contains AFB (even though the culture may be negative because of anti-TB drugs), treatment failure should be considered. Cavitary disease may cause this same picture (positive smear, negative cultures).

INTERFERING FACTORS

- False-negative results can occur because of faulty laboratory techniques.
- False-positive results can occur when the water used to suspend the smear on the slide contains a non-TB organism.

Clinical Priorities

- The AFB smear is used to support the diagnosis of TB. A definitive diagnosis requires a sputum culture and sensitivity.
- Inform the patient that sputum must be coughed up from the lungs. The first morning specimen is usually the best.
- Hold antibiotics until after the sputum has been collected.
- If the patient is suspected of having TB, health care professionals should wear an N95 respirator mask when in contact with the patient. Ideally, the patient should be placed on isolation in a negative pressure room.

PROCEDURE AND PATIENT CARE

Before

- Explain the procedure for sputum collection.
- Remind the patient that the sputum must be coughed up from the lungs and that saliva is not sputum. The first morning specimen is usually best.
- Hold antibiotics until after the sputum has been collected.
- Give the patient a sterile sputum container the night before the sputum is to be collected so that the morning specimen may be obtained when the patient awakens.
- Instruct the patient to rinse out his or her mouth with water before the sputum collection to decrease contamination by particles in the oropharynx. Remind the patient not to use antiseptic mouthwash.

During

- For best results, obtain sputum collection when the patient awakens in the morning.
- Collect at least 1 teaspoon of sputum in a sterile sputum container.
- Obtain sputum by having the patient cough after taking several deep breaths.
- If the patient is unable to produce a sputum specimen, stimulate coughing by lowering the head of the patient's bed or by giving the patient an aerosol administration of a warm hypertonic solution.
- Note that other methods to collect sputum, such as endotracheal aspiration, fiberoptic bronchoscopy, and transtracheal aspiration, may be used if necessary.
- For AFB determinations, collect sputum on three separate occasions.

After

- Avoid personal contamination and wear gloves when handling all patient secretions.
- Tell the patient to notify the nurse as soon as the specimen is collected.
- Label the specimen and send it to the laboratory as soon as possible.
- Inform the patient that culture results may take 3 weeks or longer.

TEST RESULTS AND CLINICAL SIGNIFICANCE

Tuberculosis: *Although tuberculosis is highly suspected when AFB is identified on a sputum smear, other organisms can cause positive AFB smears. They may include atypical mycobacteria and some fungi.*

RELATED TESTS

Tuberculin Culture (p. 768). This is the only manner in which the diagnosis of TB can be made with certainty. When TB is grown from the culture of a specimen, the diagnosis of TB can be made and treatment started based on drug sensitivities.

Tuberculin Skin Testing (p. 1126). Purified protein derivative is administered intradermally to test for prior exposure to TB. Skin testing cannot indicate active or dormant TB. Positive results indicate nothing more than previous exposure.

Chest X-Ray (p. 1014). Because TB is usually infective to the lungs from inhalation of airborne infectious material, the chest x-ray examination often demonstrates the results (Ghon complex) of the acute granulomatous infection.

Microscopic Studies

7

Blood Culture and Sensitivity (Blood C&S)

NORMAL FINDINGS

Negative

INDICATIONS

Blood cultures are obtained to detect the presence of bacteria in the blood.

TEST EXPLANATION

Bacteremia (the presence of bacteria in the blood) can be intermittent and transient, except in endocarditis or suppurative thrombophlebitis. The episode of bacteremia is usually accompanied by chills and fever; thus the blood culture should be drawn when the patient manifests these signs to increase the chances of growing bacteria on the cultures. It is important that at least two culture specimens be obtained from two different sites. If one produces bacteria and the other does not, it is safe to assume that the bacteria in the first culture may be a contaminant and not the infecting agent. When both cultures grow the infecting agent, bacteremia exists and is a result of the organism that is growing in the culture. If the patient is receiving antibiotics during the time that the cultures are drawn, the laboratory should be notified. Resin can be added to the culture medium to negate the antibiotic effect in inhibiting growth of the offending bacteria in the culture. If cultures are to be performed while the patient is receiving antibiotics, the blood culture specimen should be taken shortly before the next dose of the antibiotic is administered. All cultures preferably should be performed before antibiotic therapy is initiated.

Culture specimens drawn through an intravenous (IV) catheter are frequently contaminated, and tests using them should not be performed unless catheter sepsis is suspected. In these situations, blood culture specimens drawn through the catheter help to identify the causative agent more accurately than a culture specimen from the catheter tip.

Most organisms require approximately 24 hours to grow in the laboratory, and a preliminary report can be given at that time. Often 48 to 72 hours are required for growth and identification of the organism. Anaerobic organisms may take longer to grow. Cultures may be repeated after antibiotic therapy to assess resolution of the infection. (See Figure 7-1.)

INTERFERING FACTORS

- Contamination of the blood specimen, especially by skin bacteria, may occur.
- Drugs that may alter test results include antibiotics.

PROCEDURE AND PATIENT CARE

Before

- Explain the procedure to the patient.
- Tell the patient that no fasting is required.

During

- Carefully prepare the proposed venipuncture site with an antiseptic solution. Allow the skin to dry.

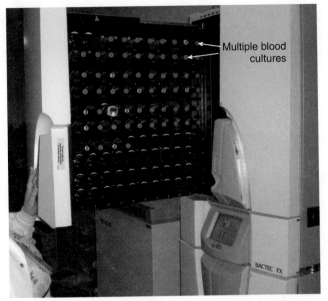

Figure 7-1 Bactec automated blood culture instrument. Note that each blood culture is separately cultured and incubated. CO_2 is monitored in each culture bottle. Positive results are automatically indentified by rising CO_2 levels. If positive, bacteria is isolated and identified, Automated antibiotic sensitivities are then performed.

- Clean the tops of the Vacutainer tubes or culture bottles with an antiseptic solution (such as chlorhexidine, 70% isopropyl alcohol, or Betadine). Allow the area to dry.
- Venous blood by venipuncture from each site is collected into a vacuum blood culture container containing culture media. One is for aerobic, and a second is for anaerobic cultures. A different vacuum container can be used if the amount of blood is less than 3 mL (pediatrics).
- Label the specimen with the patient's name, date, time, and tentative diagnosis.
- Indicate on the laboratory slip the collection site (e.g., left arm or IV line) and any medications that may affect test results.

After

- Transport the culture bottles to the laboratory immediately (within no more than 30 minutes).
- Notify the health care provider as quickly as possible of any positive results so that appropriate antibiotic therapy can be initiated.

TEST RESULTS AND CLINICAL SIGNIFICANCE

Bacteremia: *The bacteria growing in the blood can often be grown in the culture medium within the microbiology laboratory. When bacteremia exists, the patient must be considered gravely ill and antibiotics should be started immediately after blood cultures are obtained.*

Blood Smear (Peripheral Blood Smear, Red Blood Cell Morphology, RBC Smear, WBC Differential)

NORMAL FINDINGS

Normal quantity of red blood cells (RBCs), white blood cells (WBCs), and platelets
Normal size, shape, and color of RBCs
Normal WBC differential count

INDICATIONS

Examination of the peripheral blood smear can provide a significant amount of information concerning drugs and diseases that affect the RBCs, WBCs, or platelets. Furthermore, other congenital and acquired diseases can be diagnosed by an examination of the peripheral blood smear. When special stains are applied to the blood smear, infection, infestation, leukemia, and other diseases can be identified.

TEST EXPLANATION

When adequately prepared and examined microscopically by an experienced technologist or pathologist, a smear of peripheral blood is the most informative of all hematologic tests. All three hematologic cell lines—erythrocytes (RBCs), platelets, and leukocytes (WBCs)—can be examined. In the peripheral blood, five different types of leukocytes can routinely be identified—neutrophils, eosinophils, basophils, lymphocytes, and monocytes. The first three are also referred to as granulocytes. (See discussion of bone marrow biopsy on p. 712 for more information concerning the various elements of blood.)

Microscopic examination of the RBCs can reveal variations in RBC size (anisocytosis), shape (poikilocytosis), color, or intracellular content. Classification of RBCs according to these variables is most helpful in identifying the causes of anemia and the presence of other diseases.

RBC Size Abnormalities

Microcytes (small RBCs)
    Iron deficiency
    Thalassemia
    Hemoglobinopathies
Macrocytes (larger size)
    Vitamin B_{12} or folic acid deficiency
    Reticulocytosis secondary to increased erythropoiesis (RBC production)
    Occasional liver disorder

RBC Shape Abnormalities

Spherocytes (small and round)
    Hereditary spherocytosis
    Acquired immunohemolytic anemia
Elliptocytes (crescent)
    Hereditary elliptocytosis
    Iron deficiency

Codocytes or target cells (thin cells with less hemoglobin)
    Hemoglobinopathies
    Thalassemia
Echinocytes (Burr cells)
    Uremia
    Liver disease

RBC Color Abnormalities

Hypochromic (pale)
    Iron deficiency
    Thalassemia
Hyperchromasia (more colored)
    Concentrated hemoglobin, usually caused by dehydration

RBC Intracellular Structure

Nucleated (normoblasts)
    Mature RBCs are round with a small central pallor without any intracellular structures. They do not
        have a nucleus. Immature RBCs (reticulocytes) do contain intracellular RNA. Immature nucleated
        cells are not normally found in the peripheral blood and indicate increased RBC synthesis.
    Anemia
    Chronic hypoxemia
    "Normal" for an infant
    Marrow-occupying neoplasm or fibrotic tissue
Basophilic stippling (refers to bodies enclosed or included in the cytoplasm of the RBCs)
    Lead poisoning
    Reticulocytosis
Howell-Jolly bodies (small, round remnants of nuclear material remaining within the RBC)
    After a surgical splenectomy
    Hemolytic anemia
    Megaloblastic anemia
    Functional asplenia (after splenic infarction)

WBC Examination

The WBCs are examined for total quantity, percentage of each type of WBC, and degree of maturity. An
increased number of immature WBCs can indicate leukemia or infection. A decreased WBC count indicates a failure of marrow to produce WBCs (drugs, chronic disease, neoplasia, or fibrosis), peripheral
destruction, or sequestration.

Platelet Examination

Finally, an experienced laboratory technologist also can estimate platelet number. Platelets are small
cell fragments that do not contain a nucleus. The contents of the granules in a platelet are released to
promote clotting.

PROCEDURE AND PATIENT CARE

Before

🖉 Explain the procedure to the patient.
🖉 Tell the patient that no fasting is required.

During

- Collect a drop of blood from a finger stick or heel stick (in an infant) and place it on a slide for smearing. The single drop of blood is spread across the slide with a second slide at a 25-degree angle to form a feathered edge.
- If necessary, perform a venipuncture and collect the blood in a lavender-top tube.
- Note that a blood smear is first studied with an automated calculator programmed to recognize abnormal blood cell shapes and other irregularities. A more accurate smear is performed by a technologist. Low counts may be "hand counted" to ensure accuracy. The most accurate smear requires review by a pathologist.

After

- Apply pressure or a pressure dressing to the venipuncture site.
- Assess the venipuncture site for bleeding.

TEST RESULTS AND CLINICAL SIGNIFICANCE

See the list in Test Explanation.

RELATED TESTS

Complete Blood Cell Count and Differential Count (p. 174). This is a battery of tests performed on the peripheral blood to measure the quantity of each blood component.

Bone Marrow Biopsy (see following test). This is a test on the bone marrow, which forms the components of the peripheral blood.

Bone Marrow Biopsy (Bone Marrow Examination, Bone Marrow Aspiration)

NORMAL FINDINGS

Active erythroid cell line, myeloid and lymphoid cell lines, and megakaryocyte (platelet) production:

Cell Type	Range (%)
Neutrophilic Series	49.2-65.0
Myeloblasts	0.2-1.5
Promyelocytes	2.1-4.1
Myelocytes	8.2-15.7
Eosinophilic Series	1.2-5.3
Myelocytes	0.2-1.3
Metamyelocytes	0.4-2.2
Bands	0.2-2.4
Segmented	0-1.3
Basophilic and Mast Cells	0-0.2
Erythrocyte Series	18.4-33.8
Pronormoblasts	0.2-1.3
Basophilic	0.5-2.4
Polychromatophilic	17.9-29.2
Orthochromatic	0.4-4.6

Cell Type	Range (%)
Monocytes	0-0.8
Lymphocytes	11.1-23.2
Plasma Cells	0.4-3.9
Megakaryocytes	0-0.4
Reticulum Cells	0-0.9
Monocyte to Erythrocyte Ratio	1.5 -3.3

Normal iron content demonstrated by staining with Prussian blue

 Critical Values

A physician should be notified when there is a new diagnosis of leukemia, lymphoma, metastatic malignancy, infection, or hemolytic anemia. This notification is usually performed by the interpreting pathologist.

INDICATIONS

Bone marrow examination is an important part of the evaluation of patients with hematologic diseases. Indications for bone marrow examination include the following:
1. To evaluate anemias, leukopenia, or thrombocytopenia
2. To diagnose leukemia, myelodysplastic syndromes, myeloproliferative disorders, and myeloma
3. To assess iron stores and cellularity of the marrow
4. To document bone marrow infiltrative diseases (neoplasm, infection, or fibrosis)
5. To stage lymphomas or other cancers

TEST EXPLANATION

All of the cells circulating through the bloodstream—leukocytes (white blood cells) that fight infections, erythrocytes (red blood cells) that carry oxygen to the tissues, and platelets (clotting cells) that prevent bleeding—are made by precursor cells in a fatty matrix inside the hollow of our bones called bone marrow. At birth there is bone marrow in the hollow space inside all of the bones of the body as well as some bone marrow cells in the liver, spleen, and bloodstream. As the human body grows, the bone marrow cells are confined to the hollow space of the flat bones of the body, specifically, the skull, the sternum, the ribs, or the bones of the pelvis (the iliac bones). When a patient has unexplained abnormal blood counts, has abnormal cells circulating in the blood, or is diagnosed with a disease that can involve the bone marrow (lymphoma) or metastasize to the bone marrow (some carcinomas), a bone marrow biopsy is performed to examine the cells in the marrow space. Because the marrow in adults is in the flat bones, the standard location for sampling bone marrow is the iliac bones of the pelvis. Accepted practice is that the safest location to use for entering the iliac bone to obtain a sample is the posterior superior iliac spine of the pelvis (see Figure 7-2, p. 716). There, the blood-forming cells in the marrow produce the blood cells and release them into the circulation.

By examination of a bone marrow specimen the hematologist can fully evaluate hematopoiesis. Examination of the bone marrow reveals the number, size, and shape of the RBCs, WBCs, and megakaryocytes (platelet precursors) as these cells evolve through their various stages of development in the bone marrow. Samples of the bone marrow can be obtained by either aspiration or bone marrow biopsy.

An aspiration provides a small quantity of different cell types and provides a sample for bone marrow cell morphology immunophenotyping, cytogenetics, or microbiology cultures. An aspiration is usually performed at the same time as the bone marrow biopsy.

Bone marrow biopsy includes estimation of cellularity, determination of the presence of infiltrative diseases (fibrosis or neoplasms, both primary and metastatic), and estimation of iron storage. The bone marrow biopsy is more accurate than the bone marrow aspiration because aspiration removes only a small amount of marrow and may not be truly representative of the entire marrow. Immunophenotyping by flow cytometry is able to identify cell specific antibodies on the surface of the cells examined. Cell percentages are more accurately determined and abnormal cell patterns can be identified. Ploidy status and S-phase analysis are also provided. Florescent hybridization (FISH) analysis is also performed with various DNA probes chosen based on the indication for bone marrow biopsy (e.g., lymphoma). These probes can identify genetic translocations and rearrangements that may impact disease prognosis and treatment.

For the estimation of cellularity, the specimen is examined and the relative quantity of each cell type determined. Leukemias or leukemoid drug reactions are suspected when increased numbers of leukocyte precursors are present. Physiologic marrow leukemoid compensation is also seen with infection. Decreased numbers of marrow leukocyte precursors occur in patients with myelofibrosis, metastatic neoplasia, or agranulocytosis; in elderly patients; and following radiation therapy or chemotherapy. Some drugs can diminish leukocyte production.

Increased numbers of marrow RBC precursors occur with polycythemia vera or as physiologic compensation to blood loss (hemorrhage or hemolysis). Decreased numbers of marrow RBC precursors occur with erythroid hypoplasia following chemotherapy, radiation therapy, administration of other toxic drugs, iron administration, or marrow replacement by fibrotic tissue or neoplasms.

Increased numbers of platelet precursors (megakaryocytes) can be the result of compensation to platelet loss from a recent hemorrhage. They are also seen in some forms of acute and chronic myeloid leukemias. This increase also may be compensatory in patients with platelet sequestration (secondary hypersplenism associated with portal hypertension). Platelet counts decrease, and the marrow compensates by increasing production. Decreased numbers of megakaryocytes occur in patients who have had radiation therapy, chemotherapy, or other drug therapy and in patients with neoplastic or fibrotic marrow infiltrative diseases. Patients with aplastic anemia also have decreased numbers of megakaryocytes.

Increased numbers of lymphocyte precursors occur in chronic, viral, or mycoplasma infections, lymphocytic leukemia, and lymphoma. Plasma cells and lymphocytes are increased in patients with multiple myelomas, lymphomas, hypersensitivity states, rheumatic fever, and other chronic inflammatory diseases.

Estimation of cellularity also can be expressed as a ratio of myeloid (WBC) to erythroid (RBC) cells (M/E ratio). The normal M/E ratio is approximately 3:1. The M/E ratio is greater than normal in those diseases in which leukocyte precursors are increased or erythroid precursors are decreased. The M/E ratio is below normal when either leukocyte precursors are decreased or erythroid precursors are increased.

Drug-induced or idiopathic myelofibrosis can be detected by examination of the bone marrow. Using special stains, one can estimate iron stores with a marrow biopsy.

Bone marrow aspiration/biopsy are performed by a physician. The duration of these procedures is approximately 20 minutes. The patient may have some apprehension when pressure is applied to puncture the outer table of the bone during biopsy-specimen removal or aspiration. The patient probably will feel pain during lidocaine infiltration and pressure when the syringe plunger is withdrawn for aspiration.

CONTRAINDICATIONS

- Patients with acute coagulation disorders, because of the risk of excessive bleeding. A physician must decide whether the procedure is contraindicated for a low platelet count, an elevated INR, or elevated APTT.
- Patients who cannot cooperate and remain still during the procedure
- Patients who cannot comprehend an informed consent.

POTENTIAL COMPLICATIONS

- Hemorrhage. Even in patients with coagulopathy, this is a very rarely occurring event.
- Infection, especially if the patient is leukopenic

Clinical Priorities

- Assess the results of the coagulation studies before bone marrow biopsy. Patients with coagulation disorders usually may not have this procedure because of the risk for excessive bleeding.
- It is essential that patients remain still and cooperate during this invasive procedure.
- During bone marrow aspiration, most patients feel pain during lidocaine infiltration and pressure when the syringe plunger is withdrawn for aspiration.

PROCEDURE AND PATIENT CARE

Before

 Explain the procedure to the patient.
- Obtain a written informed consent for this procedure.

Encourage the patient to verbalize fears because many patients are anxious concerning this study.
- Assess the results of the coagulation studies. Report any evidence of coagulopathy to the physician.
- Obtain an order for sedatives if the patient appears extremely apprehensive.

Remind the patient to remain very still throughout the procedure.

During

- Note the following procedural steps for *bone marrow aspiration*, which is performed on the sternum, iliac crest, anterior or posterior iliac spines, and proximal tibia (in children):
  1. The procedure is usually performed at the patient's bedside using local anesthesia.
  2. A preferred site is the posterior iliac spine, with the patient placed prone or on the side.
  3. The area overlying the bone is prepared with an antiseptic solution and draped in a sterile manner.
  4. The overlying skin and soft tissue, along with the periosteum, is infiltrated with lidocaine.
  5. A small (<1 mm) incision is made in the skin directly over the posterior superior iliac spine.
  6. A large-bore needle containing a stylus is slowly advanced through the soft tissue and into the outer table of the bone (Figure 7-2).
  7. Once inside the marrow, the stylus is removed and a syringe is attached.
  8. A 0.5- to 2-mL sample of bone marrow is aspirated, smeared on slides, and allowed to dry.
- Note the following procedural steps for *bone marrow biopsy*:
  1. The skin and soft tissues overlying the bone are incised.
  2. A core biopsy instrument is "screwed" into the bone.
  3. The biopsy specimen is obtained and sent to the pathology laboratory for analysis.

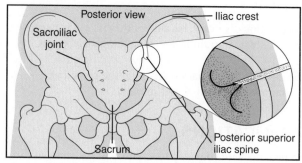

Figure 7-2 Aspiration of bone marrow.

- Note that aspiration is performed by a trained nurse or physician. Bone marrow biopsy is usually performed by a physician. The duration of these studies is approximately 20 minutes.
- Inform the patient that he or she may have some apprehension when pressure is applied to puncture the outer table of the bone during biopsy specimen removal or aspiration.
- Tell the patient that he or she probably will feel pain during lidocaine infiltration and discomfort when the syringe plunger is withdrawn for aspiration.

After

- Apply pressure to the puncture site to arrest minimal bleeding. Apply an adhesive bandage.
- Observe the puncture site for bleeding. Ice packs may be used to help control bleeding.
- Assess for tenderness and erythema, which may indicate infection. Report this to the physician.
- Evaluate the patient for signs of shock (increased pulse rate, decreased blood pressure).
- Normally, place the patient on bed rest for 30 to 60 minutes after the test.
- Note that some patients complain of tenderness at the puncture site for several days after this study. Mild analgesics may be ordered.

🏠 Home Care Responsibilities

- Instruct the patient to observe the puncture site for bleeding.
- Inform the patient that tenderness and erythema may indicate infection. This should be reported to the physician.
- Mild analgesics may be needed for several days after this procedure for tenderness at the puncture site.

TEST RESULTS AND CLINICAL SIGNIFICANCE

Neoplasm,
Myelofibrosis:
> *Infiltrative diseases are evident histologically regarding the specific cause and by demonstrating hypocellularity within the marrow.*

Infection—viral, bacterial, fungal: *Bacterial infection is usually associated with increased neutrophilic elements. However, in overwhelming sepsis, these elements may be depressed. Viral and some fungal infections are characterized by increases in monocytic elements.*

Agranulocytosis: *The marrow has no myeloblast cells.*

Polycythemia vera: *There is an abundance of erythroid cellular elements.*

Multiple myelomas,

Hodgkin disease,

Lymphoma,

Waldenström's macroglobinemia:

These cancers may be associated with overwhelming presence of mononuclear elements within the marrow.

Leukemia: *The myeloid precursor cells are significantly increased and crowd the marrow.*

Hypersensitivity states: *This may be evident as an increase in eosinophilic and basophilic myeloblast elements.*

Acute hemorrhagic marrow hyperplasia: *Following an acute hemorrhage, the erythroid (and to some extent, the myeloid) elements are greatly increased to compensate for the loss of cells in the peripheral blood system.*

Anemia: *If the anemia is because of marrow failure, erythroid precursors will be deficient in number. Specifics about the appearance of the marrow cells (e.g., megaloblasts in B_{12} deficiency) may indicate the cause of the marrow failure. Special stains may reveal deficient iron storage, etc.*

Chronic inflammatory disease,

Rheumatic fever:

Mononuclear precursor elements may be increased.

Acquired immunodeficiency syndrome (AIDS): *Decreased leukocytic elements may be noted, especially as the disease progresses.*

RELATED TEST

Blood Smear (p. 710). These test results are usually reported in the bone marrow biopsy report so as to corroborate the findings and support the indications for the procedure.

Breast Cancer Tumor Analysis (Breast Cancer Predictors, DNA Ploidy Status, S-Phase Fraction, Cathepsin D, HER 2 [c erbB2, neu] Protein, Ki67 Protein, p53 Protein)

NORMAL FINDINGS

DNA Ploidy

Aneuploid is unfavorable

Diploid is favorable

S-phase Fraction

>5.5% is unfavorable

<5.5% is favorable

HER 2 Protein

IHC method: 0 to 1+

FISH method: <2 copies/cell

OncoType Dx method: <10.7 units

Cathepsin D

>10% is unfavorable

<10% is favorable

p53 Protein

>10% is unfavorable

<10% is favorable

Ki67 Protein

>20% is unfavorable

10%-20% is borderline

<20% is favorable

INDICATIONS

This testing is performed on the breast cancer tissue and is used to predict the possibility of breast cancer relapse after curative primary surgery.

TEST EXPLANATION

The most important predictor of recurrent breast cancer is stage of disease, including lymph node status. Patients with positive lymph node metastasis are more likely to develop recurrence. However, nearly 30% of the patients whose tumor has been completely removed and who have no evidence of lymph node metastasis will also develop recurrence. It would be helpful to predict the patients who are destined for recurrence so that they can be selected for systemic therapy, while patients who will not have a recurrence can be spared the morbidity of a treatment that is not needed. Conventional predictors of tumor recurrence such as tumor size, grade, histologic type, and hormone receptors provide some information and are used alongside of the predictors that we mention in this discussion of breast cancer tumor analysis. Although estrogen and progesterone receptors are also breast cancer prognostic indicators, they are discussed separately on pp. 728 and 750. Furthermore, in addition to *HER-2/neu* testing, there are more accurate prognosticators for breast cancer (e.g., breast cancer genomic testing), discussed on p. 1086.

Ploidy (DNA Index) and S-Phase Fraction

Measurement of the rapidity with which the cells in a breast cancer grow includes ploidy status and S-phase analysis. Normally, cells are diploid (one set of paired chromosomes) and have a small number of cells in the S-phase of cell division. During the mitotic phase of cell division, the amount of DNA doubles (two sets of paired chromosomes) in preparation for cell division. Because the more aggressive cancer cells divide more rapidly, many cells are in various stages of the mitotic phase. These cells may have a variable number of chromosome sets (aneuploid).

It has been noted that the more aggressive cancer cells are more often in S-phase (a time of DNA replication in which the amount of DNA in the cell doubles while the ploidy remains the same). This is usually reported as S-phase fraction (SPF), that is, the number of cells in S-phase divided by the total number of cancer cells in the particular specimen. The laboratory methods have been automated by flow cytometry with laser-stimulated DNA fluorescence.

Cathepsin D

This protein catabolic enzyme was found to be absent in resting breast tissue but markedly elevated in malignant tissue. This presence of this protein on the cellular membrane of the malignant cells correlates with higher risk of recurrent breast cancer. The exact cutoff point between favorable prognosis and unfavorable prognosis has yet to be standardized. Like most cell surface protein markers, monoclonal antibody immunohistochemical techniques are used to identify this protein.

HER-2 (c erbB2, neu) Protein

HER-2/neu, which stands for "human epidermal growth factor receptor 2," is a protein associated with a higher aggressiveness in breast cancers. The *HER-2/neu* oncogene encodes a transmembrane tyrosine kinase receptor with extensive similarity to other epidermal growth factor receptors. It is normally involved in the pathways leading to cell growth and survival. Approximately 15% to 20% of breast cancers have an amplification of the *HER-2/neu* gene or overexpression of its protein product. Overexpression of this receptor in breast cancer is associated with increased disease recurrence and worse prognosis.

There are two commonly used methods to measure *HER-2/neu* protein. *Immunohistochemistry (IHC)*, although the easier, can be less accurate. This test measures the production of the HER-2 protein by the tumor. The test results are ranked as 0, 1+, 2+, or 3+. If the results are 3+, the cancer is HER-2–positive. *Fluorescence in situ hybridization (FISH)* has become the "standard criterion" method to measure HER-2/neu protein in tumor tissue. This test method uses fluorescent probes to look at the number of *HER-2* gene copies in a tumor cell. If there are more than two copies of the *HER-2* gene, the cancer is *HER-2* positive. RT-PCR methods are more accurate, but more cumbersome and more costly.

HER-2 testing is also helpful in making treatment decisions. Because tumors that overexpress *HER-2/neu* are more aggressive, more aggressive adjuvant chemotherapy is recommended to women with these tumors. It has been found that the *HER-2* gene can act as a target for an antineoplastic monoclonal antibody drugs (e.g., trastuzumab, Herceptin). Trastuzumab is effective only in breast cancer in which the *HER-2/neu* receptor is overexpressed. One of the mechanisms of trastuzumab after it binds to HER-2 is to halt cell proliferation.

p53 Protein

The *p53* gene is a tumor suppressor gene that is overexpressed in more aggressive breast cancer cells. Mutation of the gene causes overexpression and a buildup of mutant proteins on the surface of the cancer cells. Overexpression of *p53* can be identified by studying the gene or by immunohistochemical staining of paraffin-embedded breast cancer tissue for the mutant proteins.

Ki67 Protein

The *Ki67* gene encodes the synthesis for Ki67 protein that is associated with a more aggressive breast cancer. This protein is identified by immunohistochemical staining of paraffin-embedded breast cancer tissue.

INTERFERING FACTORS

- Delay in tissue fixation may cause deterioration of marker proteins and produce lower values.
- Preoperative use of some chemotherapy agents can decrease levels of some marker proteins.

PROCEDURE AND PATIENT CARE

Before

- Indicate to the patient that an examination for these tumor predictor markers may be performed on their breast cancer tissue.
- Provide psychologic and emotional support to the breast cancer patient.

During

- The surgeon obtains tumor tissue.
- This tissue should be placed on ice or in formalin.
- Part of the tissue is used for routine histology. A portion of the paraffin block is sent to a reference laboratory.

After

Explain to the patient that results are usually available in 1 week.

TEST RESULTS AND CLINICAL SIGNIFICANCE

Unfavorable: *In general, when these prognostic tumor markers are present in high quantities, the cancer acts more aggressively and is associated with a higher risk of recurrence.*

RELATED TESTS

Estrogen Receptor Assay (p. 728) and Progesterone Receptor Assay (p. 750). These are other prognostic markers for breast cancer.

Breast Cancer Genomics (p. 1086). This test is used to predict the possibility of cancer susceptibility to chemotherapy. It is also a powerful indicator of the likelihood of breast cancer recurrence after primary breast cancer surgery.

Cervical Biopsy (Punch Biopsy, Endocervical Biopsy, LEEP Cervical Biopsy, Cone Biopsy, Conization)

NORMAL FINDINGS

Normal squamous cells

! Critical Values

Cancer cells

INDICATIONS

A biopsy of the cervix is performed to more accurately identify and treat premalignant and superficial malignant lesions of the cervix.

TEST EXPLANATION

When a Papanicolaou (Pap) test reveals an "epithelial cell abnormality" or when a pelvic examination reveals a possible neoplastic abnormality in the cervix, a biopsy of that structure is indicated. There are several different methods to perform the biopsy, all of which obtain an increasing amount of tissue. Cervical biopsy procedures include:

- A *simple cervical biopsy*, sometimes called a *punch biopsy*, removes a small piece of tissue from the surface of the cervix. This is often performed during colposcopy, see p. 595.
- An *endocervical biopsy (endocervical curettage)* removes tissue from high in the cervical canal by scraping with a sharp instrument.
- *Loop electrosurgical excision procedure* (LEEP) uses a thin, low-voltage electrified wire loop to cut out abnormal tissue on the cervix and high in the endocervical canal (sometimes called a large loop excision of the transformation zone [LLETZ]).
- A *cone biopsy (conization)* is a more extensive form of a cervical biopsy. It is called a cone biopsy because a cone-shaped wedge of tissue is removed from the cervix. Both normal and abnormal

cervical tissues are removed. This can be performed by LEEP, surgical knife (scalpel), or a carbon dioxide laser.

After colposcopy or a cervical biopsy, LEEP may be used to treat abnormal, precancerous cells found on biopsy. It can also be used to assess the extent and sometimes to treat noninvasive superficial cervical cancers.

CONTRAINDICATIONS

- Patient with active menstrual bleeding
- Pregnant patients

POTENTIAL COMPLICATIONS

- After the surgery, a small number of women (<10%) may have significant bleeding that requires vaginal packing or a blood transfusion.
- Infection of the cervix or uterus may occur. (This is rare.)
- Narrowing of the cervix (cervical stenosis) that can cause infertility. (This is rare.)

PROCEDURE AND PATIENT CARE

Before

- Explain the procedure to the patient.
- Obtain informed consent if required by the institution.
- Instruct the patient to take a non–aspirin-containing analgesic 30 minutes before the procedure.

During

- Note the following procedural steps:
  1. The patient is placed in the lithotomy position, and a vaginal speculum is used to expose the vagina and cervix.
  2. The cervix is cleansed with a 3% acetic acid solution or iodine to remove excess mucus and cellular debris and to accentuate the difference between normal and abnormal epithelial tissues.
  3. Medication may be injected to numb the cervix *(cervical block)*.
  4. With the instrument chosen by the doctor a punch biopsy, endocervical biopsy, LEEP, or cone biopsy is performed.
- Note that a physician performs the procedure in approximately 5 to 10 minutes.
- Although cone biopsy is done in the operating room, the other procedures can be performed in the doctor's office.
- Tell the patient that some women complain of pressure pains from the vaginal speculum and that discomfort may be felt if biopsy specimens are obtained.
- Most women can return to normal activities immediately after a simple cervical biopsy or an endocervical biopsy.
- Most women will be able to return to normal activities within 2 to 4 days after LEEP or cone biopsies. This can vary depending on the amount of tissue removed.

After

- Inform the patient that it is normal to experience the following:
  - Vaginal bleeding if biopsy specimens were taken; suggest that she wear a sanitary pad
  - Mild cramping for several hours after the procedure

- Brownish-black vaginal discharge during the first week
- Vaginal discharge or spotting for about 1 to 3 weeks

 Instruct the patient that sanitary napkins should be used instead of tampons for 1 to 3 weeks.

 Inform the patient when and how to obtain the results of this study.

 Home Care Responsibilities

- Tell the patient that sexual intercourse should be avoided for 3 to 4 weeks.
- Inform the patient that douching should not be done for 3 to 4 weeks.
- Instruct the patient to call the doctor for any of the following symptoms:
  - Fever
  - Spotting or bleeding that lasts longer than 1 week
  - Bleeding that is heavier than a normal menstrual period and contains blood clots
  - Increasing pelvic pain
  - Foul-smelling, yellowish vaginal discharge, which may indicate an infection

TEST RESULTS AND CLINICAL SIGNIFICANCE

Cervical chronic infection,

Cervical intraepithelial neoplasia,

Cervical carcinoma in situ,

Invasive cervical carcinoma,

Endocervical adenocarcinomas:

> *Any of the above lesions can lead to cellular changes on Pap test that could appear to be cancerous and therefore require biopsy. Any visually obvious abnormal lesion on the cervix would also instigate the same.*

RELATED TESTS

Colposcopy (p. 595). Colposcopy is a more thorough evaluation of the cervix and is used to identify malignant and premalignant lesions of the vagina and cervix.

Papanicolaou (Pap) Test (p. 743). Pap tests are the mainstay of screening for cancer of the vagina, cervix, and uterus.

Chlamydia

NORMAL FINDINGS

Negative culture

Antibodies:

Chlamydophila pneumoniae
  IgG: <1:64
  IgM: <1:10
Chlamydophila psittaci
  IgG: <1:64
  IgM: <1:10
Chlamydia trachomatis
  IgG: <1:64
  IgM: <1:10

INDICATIONS

Chlamydia testing is performed on patients with symptoms compatible with the wide variety of diseases this organism can cause. In the United States, its most common form is pelvic inflammatory disease. This form of sexually transmitted disease (STD) commonly presents as pelvic pain and/or vaginal discharge. Cervical cultures or smears are performed on patients who have these complaints. See also Sexually Transmitted Disease Testing (p. 756).

TEST EXPLANATION

There are many *Chlamydia* species that cause various diseases within the human body. *Chlamydia psittaci* causes respiratory tract infections and occurs with close contact with infected birds. *C. pneumoniae,* another species, causes pneumonia. *C. trachomatis* infection is the most frequently occurring STD in developed countries and is also discussed in STD testing (p. 756). Infections of the genitalia are most common, followed by those of the conjunctiva, pharynx, urethra, and rectum. Lymphogranuloma venereum was the first form of venereal disease recognized as a *C. trachomatis* infection; this infection is very common in central Africa. The second serotype of *C. trachomatis* causes the eye disease *trachoma*, which is the most common form of preventable blindness. A third serotype produces genital and urethral infections different from lymphogranuloma. This third type is transmitted by direct contact of the infant with the mother's cervix during vaginal delivery or by direct contact during sexual activity.

Chlamydia infection is thought to be the most widespread STD in the United States. This disease is most prevalent in those younger than 20 years, in nulliparas, and in users of nonbarrier contraceptive methods. Also, in those with multiple or recent, new sexual partners, *Chlamydia* is frequently associated with gonorrhea.

Most women colonized with *Chlamydia* are asymptomatic. *Chlamydia* may be associated with pelvic inflammatory disease, particularly in adolescents.

The *Chlamydia* organism can be detected in many different ways. It seems to be most accurately demonstrated by tissue culture. Although these cultures require a special cell culture line, which takes several days, they are used as the standard criterion against which other methods of detection of *Chlamydia* are measured. It is now possible to detect the *Chlamydia* antigen by utilizing deoxyribonucleic acid (DNA) probes.

With the increasing use of ThinPrep Cervical cytology (see Papanicolaou Test, p. 743), *Chlamydia* infections are being increasingly diagnosed. Transcription mediated amplification can be used to amplify *Chlamydial* ribosomal RNA or using DNA probes on a ThinPrep sample. This same technology can detect *Chlamydia* from a urine specimen.

INTERFERING FACTORS

- Women presently having their routine menses
- Patients undergoing antibiotic therapy

Clinical Priorities

- Because of the rapidly increasing prevalence of *Chlamydia,* screening should take place in all at-risk groups, particularly sexually active adolescents and those with other STDs.
- Females are evaluated for *Chlamydia* by cervical cultures, and males are evaluated by urethral cultures.
- All affected patients should be treated with antibiotics. Sexual partners should be evaluated.

PROCEDURE AND PATIENT CARE

Before

 Explain the procedure to the patient.
- Note that many different methods are used to perform *Chlamydia* tests.
- Tell the patient that minimal discomfort is associated with these procedures.

During

- Collect a venous blood sample in a red-top tube.
- Acute and convalescent serum should be drawn 2 to 3 weeks apart.
- A conjunctival smear is obtained by swabbing the eye lesion with a cotton-tipped applicator or scraping with a sterile ophthalmic spatula and smearing on a clean glass slide.
- Sputum cultures (p. 761) are used to check for C. *psittaci* respiratory infections.
- Refer to p. 757 for cervical culture and p. 758 for urethral cultures.
- Note these procedures are performed by a nurse or physician in several minutes.

After

- Treat patients who have positive smears with antibiotics.
- Tell affected patients to have their sexual partners examined.

TEST RESULTS AND CLINICAL SIGNIFICANCE

Chlamydia infections: *This organism causes many different diseases, as indicated in Test Explanation. In the United States, this is the most significant sexually transmitted infection.*

RELATED TEST

Sexually Transmitted Disease (STD) Testing (p. 756). Discussed here are other STDs and their causative agents.

Colon Cancer Tumor Analysis (Microsatellite Instability [MSI] Testing, DNA Mismatch Repair [MMR] Genetic Testing, BRAF Mutation Analysis, Oncotype DX Colon Cancer Assay)

NORMAL FINDINGS

Recurrence score <10 (on a scale of 0 to 100)
No mismatch repair gene
No microsatellite instability

INDICATIONS

This test is used to indicate the prognosis of a patient recently surgically treated for colon cancer to determine if additional chemotherapy will improve survival. Furthermore this test can be used to indicate the possibility that the colon cancer was hereditary, thereby encouraging other members of the patient's family to undergo testing.

TEST EXPLANATION

Patients with stage 1 colon cancer have a high cure rate with surgery alone. Patients with stage 3 colon cancer benefit from the use of adjuvant chemotherapy. However, patients with stage 2 colon cancer may or may not benefit from adjuvant chemotherapy. Colon cancer tumor analysis can help differentiate stage 2 patients who may benefit from adjuvant chemotherapy. This test is used to indicate the risk of recurrence colon cancer in the years succeeding surgical treatment.

Deficiencies in *DNA mismatch repair (MMR) gene* function, either because of decreased gene expression or mutation, result in the accumulation of DNA alterations that can manifest as abnormal shortening or lengthening of microsatellite DNA sequences in the colon cancer cell. This causes *microsatellite instability (MSI).* Patients with MMR deficient (MMR-D) colon tumors have high MSI and have been shown to have significantly lower colon cancer recurrence risk. Therefore testing the colon tumor for MMR and MSI can assist in determining the likelihood of recurrence after surgery and quantify any benefit from adjuvant chemotherapy.

Furthermore hereditary colon cancers frequently are positive for MSI as compared with sporadic colon cancers. Lynch syndrome (a hereditary form of colon cancer) can be suspected if the tumor is MSI positive. MSI is performed by immunohistochemical identification of specific nucleic acid. MMR genetic testing is most frequently performed by PCR testing.

BRAF is another important gene that is used to indicate the likelihood that a colon tumor is hereditary. BRAF is a kinase-encoding gene in the RAS/RAF/MAPK pathway. The presence of a *BRAF* V600E mutation in a microsatellite unstable tumor indicates that the tumor is probably sporadic and not associated with hereditary non-polyposis colorectal cancer (HNPCC). The lack of this mutation indicates that a tumor may either be sporadic or HNPCC associated.

The *Oncotype DX Colon Cancer Assay* evaluates 12 genes and provides an individualized score reflective of the risk of colon cancer recurrence for individual patients with stage 2 colon cancer. The assay uses a RT-PCR platform to quantitate the level of expression of each of the 12 genes in the panel using the patient's colon tumor. For each patient, the assay produces a recurrence score that is closely associated with the patient's risk of recurrent colon cancer 3 years after surgery (the peak time of recurrence). MMR and MSI testing can complement the information provided by the Oncotype DX Colon Cancer Assay.

PROCEDURE AND PATIENT CARE

Before

🖉 Inform the patient that an examination for these tumor predictor markers may be performed on his or her colon cancer tissue.

🖉 Provide psychological and emotional support to the colon cancer patient.

During

- The surgeon obtains tumor tissue.
- This tissue should be placed on ice or in formalin.
- Part of the tissue is used for routine histology. A portion of the paraffin block is sent to a reference laboratory.

After

🖉 Explain to the patient that results are usually available in 1 week.

TEST RESULTS AND CLINICAL SIGNIFICANCE

Colon cancer with unfavorable prognosis: *This helps determine patients, who by the genomic make up of their colon cancer and other prognostic factors will benefit from the use of adjuvant chemotherapy. Patients whose prognosis is very good by genomic testing will not benefit from the addition of preventive chemotherapy.*

Hereditary colon cancer: *Patients with a BRAF genetic mutation or whose colon cancer has microsatellite instability have an increased risk that their cancer was hereditary. After genetic counseling, other family members may want to consider being tested for genetic predisposition to colon cancer and have early screening testing such as colonoscopy (p. 591) if they are positive.*

RELATED TEST

Genetic Testing (p. 1093). This discussion included genetic testing for other forms of familial colon cancer, including Lynch syndrome and familial polyposis.

Endometrial Biopsy

NORMAL FINDINGS

No pathologic conditions
Presence of a "secretory-type" endometrium 3 to 5 days before normal menses

INDICATIONS

Endometrial biopsy had been used to determine if the patient has adequate ovarian estrogen and progesterone levels. This is indicated in women with suspected ovarian dysfunction (such as women who are nearing menopause, are not menstruating, or are infertile). It is most often used to diagnose and evaluate women who have dysfunctional uterine bleeding and uterine cancer.

TEST EXPLANATION

An endometrial biopsy can determine whether ovulation has occurred. A biopsy specimen taken 3 to 5 days before normal menses should demonstrate a "secretory-type" endometrium on histologic examination if ovulation and corpus luteum formation have occurred. If not, only a preovulatory "proliferative-type" endometrium will be seen. This test can determine if a woman has adequate ovarian estrogen and progesterone levels.

Another major use of endometrial biopsy is to diagnose endometrial cancer, polyps, or inflammatory conditions and to evaluate dysfunctional uterine bleeding.

This procedure is performed by an obstetrician/gynecologist in approximately 10 to 15 minutes. Minor discomfort (menstrual-type cramping) may be felt. It is important to recognize that an endometrial biopsy is not a substitute for a dilation and curettage (D&C). The D&C is much more extensive and tests all surfaces of the endometrium.

CONTRAINDICATIONS

• Patients with infections (e.g., trichomonal, candidal, suspected gonococcal) of the cervix or vagina, because the infection may spread to the uterus

- Patients in whom the cervix cannot be visualized (e.g., because of abnormal position or previous surgery), because the cervix is the access to the uterus
- Patients who are pregnant, because the procedure may induce labor/abortion

POTENTIAL COMPLICATIONS

- Perforation of the uterus
- Uterine bleeding
- Interference with early pregnancy
- Infection

PROCEDURE AND PATIENT CARE

Before

- Explain the procedure to the patient.
- Ensure that written and informed consent for this procedure is obtained from the patient.
- Tell the patient that no fasting or sedation is usually required. Menstrual-type cramping may be experienced.

During

- Note the following procedural steps:
  1. The patient is placed in the lithotomy position, and a pelvic examination is performed to determine the position of the uterus.
  2. The cervix is exposed and cleansed.
  3. A biopsy instrument is inserted into the uterus, and specimens are obtained from the anterior, posterior, and lateral walls. The biopsy can be done with a curette, forceps, or suction device. Suction endometrial biopsy is most commonly performed because it is the least painful and can be performed in the office.
  4. The specimens are placed in a solution containing 10% formalin and sent to the pathologist for histologic or cytologic examination.

After

- Any temperature elevation should be reported to the physician because this procedure may activate pelvic inflammatory disease.
- Advise the patient to wear a pad because some vaginal bleeding is to be expected.
- Instruct the patient to call her physician if excessive bleeding (requiring more than one pad per hour) occurs.
- Inform the patient that douching and intercourse are not permitted for 72 hours after the biopsy.
- Instruct the patient to rest during the next 24 hours and to avoid heavy lifting to prevent increased intraabdominal pressure and uterine hemorrhage.

Home Care Responsibilities

- Instruct the patient to report any temperature elevation to her physician because this procedure may activate pelvic inflammatory disease.
- Advise the patient to wear a sanitary pad after this procedure because some vaginal bleeding is expected. Tell the patient to call her physician for excessive bleeding (more than one pad per hour).
- Tell the patient to avoid heavy lifting after this procedure to prevent increased intraabdominal pressure and possible uterine bleeding.

TEST RESULTS AND CLINICAL SIGNIFICANCE

Anovulation: *Without ovulation the endometrium is persistently in the proliferative stage. No secretory changes are noted.*

Tumor,

Polyps:

  Endometrial adenocarcinoma with or without squamous carcinoma components is the most common uterine cancer. Hyperplastic proliferative polyps are a common cause of dysfunctional uterine bleeding.

Inflammatory condition: *Endometrial infections are rare but do occur. Ascending sexually transmitted diseases (STDs) are the most common type of primary infection not associated with prior surgical instrumentation.*

Estrogen Receptor Assay (ER Assay, ERA, Estradiol Receptor)

NORMAL FINDINGS

Immunohistochemistry

Negative: <5% of the cells stain for receptors
Positive: >5% of the cells stain for receptors

Reverse-Transcriptase Polymerase Chain Reaction (RT-PCR)

Negative: <6.5 units
Positive: >6.5 units

INDICATIONS

Estrogen receptor assay is performed on breast cancer tissue to indicate sensitivity to hormonal manipulative therapy and to indicate prognosis of breast cancer.

TEST EXPLANATION

The ER assay is useful in determining the prognosis and treatment of breast cancer. The assay is used to determine whether a tumor is likely to respond to endocrine therapy. Hormone receptor assays should be performed on all breast cancers. Breast tumors in postmenopausal women tend to be positive more often than in premenopausal women.

Slightly more than half of patients with breast carcinoma who are ER positive respond to endocrine therapy (e.g., tamoxifen, estrogens, aromatase inhibitors, oophorectomy). The response is greater when the progesterone receptors (see p. 750) are also positive. Patients whose breast cancers lack these hormone receptors (i.e., are ER negative) have a much lower chance of tumor response to hormone therapy and may not be candidates for this form of treatment.

Specimens are obtained from surgical specimens by a pathologist. ER assays are performed most commonly using immunohistochemical methods on fixed, paraffin-embedded tissue. Positive reactivity by immunohistochemistry is observed in the nuclei of the tumor cells. This method of measuring ER receptors is considered very accurate. Results are usually available in less than 1 week.

INTERFERING FACTORS

- Delay in tissue fixation or too long in tissue fixative solution may cause deterioration of receptor proteins and may produce lower values.

PROCEDURE AND PATIENT CARE

Before

Explain the biopsy procedure to the patient.

Instruct the patient to discontinue taking hormones before breast biopsy is performed.

- Before biopsy, a gynecologic history is obtained, including menopausal status and exogenous hormone use.

During

- The surgeon obtains tumor tissue.
- This tissue should be placed on ice or in formalin.
- Part of the tissue is used for routine histologic examination. A portion of the paraffin block or a slide containing cancer is used for IHC staining.

After

Explain to the patient that results are usually available in 1 week.

TEST RESULTS AND CLINICAL SIGNIFICANCE

Estrogen receptor positive: *This cancer is more likely to be successfully treated with hormone manipulation in a therapeutic or adjuvant clinical setting. There are other cancers that can have positive hormone receptors (e.g., endometrial/ovarian).*

RELATED TESTS

Progesterone Receptor Assay (p. 750). Like estrogen receptor assay, this test predicts the likelihood of tumor response to endocrine manipulative therapy.

Breast Cancer Genomics (p. 1086). This test is used as a prognosticator indicating the risk of recurrent breast cancer. It is a powerful predictor of benefit from hormone therapy or chemotherapy.

Breast Cancer Tumor Analysis (p. 717). These tests are prognostic as they indicate the risk of tumor recurrence. They also can be predictive of tumor response to some anti–breast cancer therapies.

Fungal Antibody (Antifungal Antibodies; Beta-D-glucan *(1→3)-β-D-glucan, Fungitell)*

NORMAL FINDINGS

No antibodies detected

β-D-glucan:

Negative	Less than 60 pg/mL
Indeterminate	60-79 pg/mL
Positive	≥80 pg/mL

INDICATIONS

This test is used to identify systemic fungal infections.

TEST EXPLANATION

Fungal infections can be superficial, subcutaneous, or systemic (deep). The systemic fungal infections (mycoses) are the most important, for which serologic antibody testing is performed. Generally mycoses are caused by the inhalation of airborne fungal spores. In the United States, the most serious fungal infections are coccidioidomycosis, blastomycosis, histoplasmosis, and paracoccidioidomycosis. These infections start out as primary pulmonary infections. *Aspergillus, Candida,* and *Cryptococcus* systemic infections usually affect only those with compromised immunity (Table 7-1).

Fungal antibody testing is not highly reliable. Antibodies are present in only about 70% to 80% of infected patients. When positive, they merely indicate that the person has an active or has had a recent fungal infection. These antibodies can be identified in the blood or cerebrospinal fluid. In general, more specific antibodies are tested only after screening antibody testing (e.g., complement fixation studies) are performed. Immunodiffusion is most commonly used to detect immunoglobulin (Ig)G antibodies in the blood. IgA and IgM antibodies can also be identified by enzyme immunoassay (EIA). These antibodies can be tested singularly or as a fungal panel. Cross-reactions can occur (e.g., antibodies to blastomycosis can cross-react with histoplasmosis antigens).

(1→3)-β-D-glucan is an enzyme immunoassay used to support the diagnosis of invasive fungal disease (IFD) in at-risk patients. Normally serum contains low levels of (1→3)-β-D-glucan, presumably from yeasts present in the alimentary and gastrointestinal tract. (1→3)-β-D-glucan is produced by most invasive fungal organisms. D-glucan becomes elevated well in advance of conventional clinical signs and symptoms of IFD. As opportunistic infections, IFDs are common among hematologic malignancy and AIDS patients. They account for a growing number of nosocomial infections, particularly among organ transplant recipients and other patients receiving immunosuppressive treatments.

Fungal antigen assays are available to detect a portion of the infecting fungus such as *Aspergillus galactomannan*. This uses ELISA technology. In general, the antigen assays are best used on blood, but CSF may also be studied in some instances. DNA sequencing or PCR can also identify fungal organisms from the specimen or culture tissue. However, negative molecular studies do not rule out infection.

Fungal organisms can be identified by culture growth and macroscopy/microscopy. Fungi components can occasionally be seen on Gram stain. For optimal recovery of organisms, a sufficient specimen

TABLE 7-1 Diseases Resulting from Fungal Infections

FUNGUS	SYSTEMIC DISEASE	ENDEMIC AREA
Candida albicans	Candidiasis, thrush, yeast of mouth/esophagus	Ubiquitous
Cryptococcus neoformans	Infection of the lung, bloodstream; meningitis	Ubiquitous
Histoplasma capsulatum	Pulmonary infection	Caribbean, Central and South America
Coccidioides immitis	Pulmonary infection	Southwestern United States, Mexico, Central America
Aspergillus	Pulmonary infection	Ubiquitous

should be transported within 24 hours of collection. Fungi can be pathogens, colonizers, or contaminants. Correlation of the patient's clinical condition with culture results is necessary. Nucleic Acid Probe/16S rDNA Sequencing/Real-Time Polymerase Chain Reaction is used for the identification of some fungi. Other fungi such as *Coccidioides* are identified by real-time PCR. Fungi can be cultured from blood; body fluids; CSF; fresh tissue; bronchopulmonary secretions; a swab of the ear, nose, and throat; or urine. An accurate fungal culture is labor intensive and requires a highly experience laboratory. Results are not available quickly.

PROCEDURE AND PATIENT CARE

Before
- Explain the procedure to the patient.
- Tell the patient that no fasting or preparation is required.

During
- Collect a venous blood sample in a red-top or any serum separator tube.
- Collect a specimen of other fluids or tissue in a sterile container and immediately transport to the laboratory.
- Indicate on the laboratory slip the particular antibody or panel of antibodies that are to be tested.

After
- Apply pressure or a pressure dressing to the venipuncture site.
- Assess the venipuncture site for bleeding.
- Because some patients with fungal infection may be immunocompromised, instruct the patient to check for signs of infection at the venipuncture site.

TEST RESULTS AND CLINICAL SIGNIFICANCE

▲ Increased Levels

Acute fungal infection: *Fungal antibodies develop only with systemic or deep infections. Negative results do not rule out a fungal disease. Fungal molecular tests are more accurate, but the definitive diagnosis of fungal disease requires a positive culture and identification to be associated with the clinical picture.*

RELATED TESTS

Cultures of the Blood (p. 708), CSF (p. 651), Sputum (p. 761), Throat (p. 765), Urine (p. 973). *When infection is suspected, bacterial infection should be ruled out at the same time appropriate fungal testing is being performed. These cultures predominantly discuss bacterial infection. However, the methodology of specimen accrual is the same.*

Herpes Simplex (Herpesvirus Types 1 and 2, Herpes Simplex Virus Type 1 and 2 [HSV 1 and 2], Herpes Genitalis)

NORMAL FINDINGS

No virus present
No herpes simple virus (HSV) antibodies present

Microscopic Studies

7

INDICATIONS

Herpes testing is performed to diagnose acute initial herpes infections. It is used on patients with suspected initial genital infection. It is also used in immunocompromised patients who have aggressive oral mucosal or genital eruptions compatible with the infection. Furthermore, it is used on patients (especially immunocompromised patients) who have a fever of unknown origin.

Herpes cultures are used to identify active genital herpes infection in women who are expecting to vaginally deliver a baby in the next 6 to 8 weeks.

TEST EXPLANATION

HSV can be classified as either type 1 or type 2. *Type 1* is primarily responsible for oral lesions (blisters on the lips— "cold sores") or even corneal lesions. About half of the patients with HSV 1 develop recurrent infections. HSV 2 is a sexually transmitted viral infection of the urogenital tract. Vesicular lesions may occur on the penis, scrotum, vulva, perineum, perianal region, vagina, or cervix. Initial infections are often associated with generalized symptoms of fever and malaise.

Because most infants become infected if they pass through a birth canal containing HSV, determining its presence at delivery is necessary. Congenital infections may result in problems such as microcephaly, chorioretinitis, and mental retardation in the newborn. Disseminated neonatal herpes virus infections carry a high incidence of infant mortality. A vaginal delivery is possible if no virus is present, but birth by cesarean section is necessary if HSV is present. Viral testing can be performed on males or females to determine the risk for sexual transmission.

Culture is still the standard criterion for HSV detection and can identify HSV in 90% of infected patients. Culture can be performed only during an outbreak. Serologic tests are more easily and conveniently available for detection of HSV 1 and HSV 2 antibodies. *Serologic tests for herpes simplex* are useful to supplement cultures or molecular detection for acute infection. Only about 85% of patients who are culture positive have positive serologies. The advantage of serology tests is that results can be available in a day. Serologic tests for IgG antibodies are available to help differentiate type 1 from type 2 infection. IgG antibodies indicate a previous exposure. IgM antibodies indicate an acute infection, but do not differentiate well between types 1 and 2. Perhaps more than 50% of people in the United States have positive herpes antibodies. Serologic tests for antibodies require repeated blood tests during the acute and convalescent phases of an acute viral outbreak (about 2 weeks apart). A fourfold rise in titer is expected to diagnose acute initial herpes infection. Recurrent infections are far less likely to demonstrate titer elevations.

The antibody tests use immunofluorescent immunoassay or enzyme-linked immunosorbent assay (ELISA) methods. Antibody testing cannot diagnose whether there is active recurrent genital herpes. Culture testing is required.

Fresh tissue is the definitive specimen for detection of HSV, particularly with suspected CNS disease. However, because brain biopsy is an invasive procedure, it is infrequently performed for laboratory diagnosis. Similarly, it is difficult to recover HSV from cerebrospinal fluid (CSF) specimens in culture systems, and the serologic diagnosis of HSV CNS disease has not been informative during early-onset disease. *HSV PCR molecular detection* of HSV DNA from CSF (as well as oral, genital, ocular, and other sites) is a sensitive and specific alternative for detection. PCR is a qualitative assay and results are reported as negative, positive, or indeterminate. The lower limit of detection for PCR is 10 DNA target copies/microliter.

Clinical Priorities

- Neonatal herpes virus infections carry a high incidence of infant mortality. A cesarean delivery may be needed if HSV is present in the pregnant mother.
- Women should refrain from douching and tub bathing for 24 hours before the cervical culture.
- Men should not urinate within 1 hour before a urethral culture because voiding washes secretions out of the urethra.
- If herpes is diagnosed, it should be treated and sexual partners should be evaluated. Although acute outbreaks of herpes genitalis are treatable, this disease is not curable.

PROCEDURE AND PATIENT CARE

Before

- Explain the procedure to the patient.
- Tell the female patient to refrain from douching and tub bathing for 24 hours before the cervical culture is performed.
- Obtain the urethral specimen from the male patient before he voids.
- Note that blood study results can be diagnostic in both males and females.

During

Obtain cultures as follows:

Urethral Culture

1. A culture is taken by inserting a sterile swab gently into the anterior urethra or genital skin lesion of the male patient (see Figure 7-8, p. 758).
2. It is advisable to place the male patient in the supine position to prevent falling if vasovagal syncope occurs during introduction of the cotton swab or wire loop into the urethra.
3. The patient is observed for hypotension, bradycardia, pallor, sweating, nausea, and weakness.

Cervical Culture

1. The female patient is placed in the lithotomy position, and a vaginal speculum is inserted.
2. Cervical mucus is removed with a cotton ball.
3. A sterile cotton-tipped swab is inserted into the endocervical canal and moved from side to side to obtain the culture. If a genital lesion is present, swabs from that area will be more sensitive in indicating infection.

- For *pregnant women with herpes genitalis*, note that the cervix is cultured weekly for the herpes virus beginning 4 to 6 weeks before the due date. Vaginal delivery is possible if the following criteria are met:

1. The two most recent cultures are negative.
2. The woman is not experiencing any symptoms.
3. No lesions are visible on inspection of the vagina and vulva.
4. Throughout pregnancy the woman has not had more than one positive culture, during which she was symptom free.

Blood for Serologic Study

- Obtain a venous blood sample in a red-top tube.

Microscopic Studies

7

Molecular PCR Tissue and Other Fluids
- Obtain CSF (p. 651) or other fluids by sterile technique as described elsewhere in this book.
- Obtain tissue by appropriate biopsy techniques.
- Place specimen in an appropriate container designated by the reference laboratory.

After
- Apply pressure or a pressure dressing to the venipuncture site.
- Observe the venipuncture site for bleeding.
- Inform the patient how to obtain the test results.

TEST RESULTS AND CLINICAL SIGNIFICANCE

Herpes virus infection: *Like other sexually transmitted disease (STDs), this disease can significantly affect patients, their children, and their sexual partners. If herpes or other STDs have been diagnosed, treatment should begin immediately and active sexual partners should be evaluated. Although acute outbreaks of herpes genitalis are treatable, the disease is not curable.*

RELATED TESTS

Sexually Transmitted Disease (STD) Testing (p. 756). Discussed here are other sexually transmitted diseases and their causative agents.
Other STDs are discussed separately:
Chlamydia (p. 722)
Syphilis Detection (p. 473)
Hepatitis Virus Studies (p. 286)
AIDS Serology (p. 297)

Liver Biopsy

NORMAL FINDINGS

Normal liver histology

INDICATIONS

Liver biopsy is a safe, simple, and valuable method of diagnosing pathologic liver conditions.

TEST EXPLANATION

For this study a specially designed needle is inserted through the abdominal wall and into the liver (Figure 7-3). A piece of liver tissue is removed for microscopic examination. Percutaneous liver biopsy is used in the diagnosis of various liver disorders, such as cirrhosis, hepatitis, drug reaction, granuloma, and tumor. Biopsy is indicated for patients with the following conditions that cannot be identified by other tests:
1. Unexplained hepatomegaly
2. Persistently elevated liver enzyme levels
3. Suspected primary or metastatic tumor, as determined by other studies

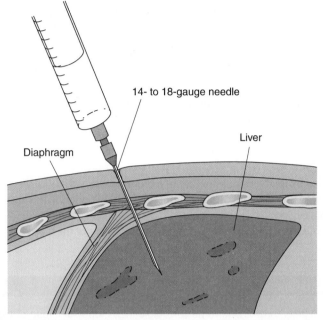

14- to 18-gauge needle

Liver

Diaphragm

Figure 7-3 Liver biopsy. Percutaneous liver biopsy requires the patient's cooperation. The patient must be able to lie quietly and hold his or her breath after exhaling.

4. Unexplained jaundice
5. Suspected hepatitis
6. Suspected infiltrative diseases (e.g., sarcoidosis, amyloidosis)
7. Hemochromatosis and Wilson's disease
8. Diseases in which biopsy is the only way to determine severity of disease

The biopsy may be performed by a "blind" stick or may be directed with the use of a computed tomography (CT) or magnetic resonance imaging (MRI) scan, ultrasound, or laparoscopy. Directed biopsy is used if there is a specific focal area of the liver that is suspect and from which tissue must be obtained (e.g., a metastatic tumor). The "blind" stick is used if the liver is diffusely involved.

This test is performed by a physician in approximately 15 minutes. Minor discomfort may be experienced during injection of the local anesthetic and during needle insertion and biopsy. In the past, blind biopsies were performed with small aspiration or small tissue-sampling needles. With guided biopsies, larger-core needles can obtain a significant amount of tissue for histologic review. This has reduced sampling errors both in placing the needle in the suspicious area and in obtaining enough tissue for histologic study.

CONTRAINDICATIONS

- Uncooperative patients who cannot remain still and hold their breath during sustained exhalation
- Patients with impaired hemostasis
- Patients with anemia who could not tolerate major blood loss associated with inadvertent puncture of an intrahepatic blood vessel

- Patients with infections in the right pleural space or right upper quadrant, because the biopsy may spread the infection
- Patients with obstructive jaundice: In these patients, bile within the ducts is under pressure and may subsequently leak into the abdominal cavity after needle penetration.
- Patients with a hemangioma: This is a very vascular tumor, and bleeding after a biopsy may be severe.
- Patients with ascites, because persistent leak of fluid may occur: Further bile leaks will not seal off.

POTENTIAL COMPLICATIONS

- Hemorrhage caused by inadvertent puncture of a blood vessel within the liver
- Chemical peritonitis caused by inadvertent puncture of a bile duct, with subsequent leakage of bile into the abdominal cavity
- Pneumothorax (collapsed lung) caused by improper placement of the biopsy needle into the adjacent chest cavity

✔ Clinical Priorities

- Assess the coagulation profile before performing a liver biopsy because of the possibility of bleeding.
- After the liver biopsy, instruct the patient to remain on the right side for about 1 to 2 hours. This position decreases the risk of hemorrhage by compressing the liver capsule against the chest wall.
- Carefully evaluate the patient after this test for evidence of hemorrhage (increased pulse rate, decreased blood pressure) and peritonitis (increased temperature).

PROCEDURE AND PATIENT CARE

Before

Explain the procedure to the patient. Many patients are apprehensive about this procedure.
- Obtain a medication history to be certain the patient is not taking medication that could affect coagulation.
- Ensure that all coagulation test results are normal.
- Obtain an informed consent.
Instruct the patient to keep on nothing by mouth (NPO) status after midnight on the day of the test. Surgery may be necessary if a complication occurs. The patient must be prepared for the possibility of surgery.
- Administer any sedative medications as ordered.

During

- Note the following procedural steps:
  1. The patient is placed in the supine or left lateral position.
  2. The skin area used for puncture is locally anesthetized.
  3. The patient is asked to exhale and hold the exhalation. This causes the liver to descend and reduces the possibility of a pneumothorax. Frequently the patient practices exhalation two or three times before insertion of the needle.

4. During the patient's sustained exhalation the physician rapidly introduces the biopsy needle into the liver and obtains liver tissue.
   a. Several types of needles are available.
   b. Often the biopsy needle is inserted under CT guidance. This is especially useful when tissue from a specific area of the liver is needed.
5. The needle is withdrawn from the liver.

- If laparoscopy is used to obtain the biopsy, follow the procedure outlined for laparoscopy (p. 617).

After

- Place the tissue sample into a specimen bottle containing formalin and send it to the pathology department.
- Apply a small dressing over the needle insertion site.
- Place the patient on his or her right side for approximately 1 to 2 hours. In this position the liver capsule is compressed against the chest wall, thereby decreasing the risk for hemorrhage or bile leak.
- Assess the patient's vital signs frequently for evidence of hemorrhage (increased pulse rate, decreased blood pressure) and peritonitis (increased temperature).
- If laparoscopy was performed, provide routine postoperative care.
- Evaluate the rate, rhythm, and depth of respirations. Assess breath sounds. Report chest pain and signs of dyspnea, cyanosis, and restlessness, which may be indicative of pneumothorax.

Clinical Priorities

- Instruct the patient to report signs of bleeding (increased pulse and decreased blood pressure) or peritonitis (increased temperature).
- Tell the patient to avoid coughing and straining that may cause increased intraabdominal pressure. Strenuous activities and heavy lifting should be avoided for 1 to 2 weeks.

TEST RESULTS AND CLINICAL SIGNIFICANCE

Benign tumor (adenoma),
Malignant tumor:
    Primary (hepatoma, cholangiocarcinoma),
    Metastatic (bowel, breast, lung, etc.):
    Biopsies of these focal lesions can be performed and specimens obtained for histologic study. Usually these biopsies are guided by imaging studies.
Abscess,
Cyst:
    These fluid lesions can be aspirated and catheters left for drainage.
Hepatitis,
Infiltrative diseases (e.g., amyloidosis, hemochromatosis, cirrhosis, fat):
    Diffuse liver abnormality is much more easily obtainable by the liver biopsy needle because more tissue contains the pathologic condition.

RELATED TESTS

Computed Tomography (CT) Scan of the Abdomen (p. 1020). This is an x-ray study that provides excellent visualization of the liver for guided biopsy.

Magnetic Resonance Imaging (MRI) Scan of the Liver (p. 1106). This study uses variations in electromagnetic characteristics to provide an accurate image of the liver. Recently technology has advanced to allow the guidance of a biopsy needle to the suspect area within the liver.

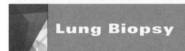

Lung Biopsy

NORMAL FINDINGS

No evidence of pathologic conditions

INDICATIONS

Lung biopsy is indicated to determine the nature of a pulmonary parenchymal nodule that has been identified on plain chest x-ray film or chest computed tomography (CT) scan. Carcinomas, granulomas, infections, and sarcoidosis can be diagnosed with this procedure. This procedure is also useful in detecting environmental exposures, infections, or familial disease, which may lead to better prevention and treatment.

TEST EXPLANATION

This invasive procedure is used to obtain a specimen of pulmonary tissue for a histologic examination by using either an open or a closed technique. The open method involves a limited thoracotomy. The closed technique includes methods such as transbronchial lung biopsy, transbronchial needle aspiration biopsy, transcatheter bronchial brushing, percutaneous needle aspiration biopsy, and video-assisted thoracostomy surgery (VATS).

Note that this procedure is performed by a radiologist, surgeon, or pulmonologist in 30 to 60 minutes. Most patients describe the percutaneous biopsy procedure as painful. Postoperative incisional pain can be expected if the open technique or VATS is used.

CONTRAINDICATIONS

- Patients with bullae or cysts of the lung, because they have a greater risk of pneumothorax with needle lung biopsy
- Patients with suspected vascular anomalies of the lung, because bleeding may occur
- Patients with bleeding abnormalities, because bleeding may occur
- Patients with pulmonary hypertension, because bleeding is more likely to occur
- Patients with respiratory insufficiency, because they are not likely to survive a pneumothorax if it occurs

POTENTIAL COMPLICATIONS

- Pneumothorax
- Pulmonary hemorrhage
- Empyema

Clinical Priorities

- Obtain a medication history to be certain the patient is not taking medication that could affect coagulation.
- Assess the results of the coagulation studies before lung biopsy because postprocedure bleeding can occur.
- The patient is usually kept on nothing by mouth (NPO) status after midnight before this test.
- After this procedure carefully assess the patient for signs of bleeding (increased pulse rate, decreased blood pressure) and shortness of breath.
- A chest x-ray film is usually ordered after the procedure to check for complications (such as pneumothorax).

PROCEDURE AND PATIENT CARE

Before

✍ Explain the procedure to the patient.
- Ensure that informed signed consent is obtained.
✍ Explain to the patient that fasting is usually ordered. The patient may be kept on NPO status after midnight on the day of the test.
- Administer the preprocedural medications 30 to 60 minutes before the test as ordered. Atropine is usually given to decrease bronchial secretions. Meperidine (Demerol) may be used to sedate anxious patients.
✍ Instruct the patient to remain still during the lung biopsy. Any movement or coughing could cause laceration of the lung by the biopsy needle.

During

- Note that the patient's position depends on the method used and that the histologic lung specimen may be obtained by several different methods:

Transbronchial Lung Biopsy
See discussion of bronchoscopy on p. 587.
1. This technique is performed via flexible fiberoptic bronchoscopy using cutting forceps.
2. Fluoroscopy is used to ensure proper opening and positioning of the forceps on the lesions.
3. Fluoroscopy also permits visualization of the "tug" of the lung as the specimen is removed.

Transbronchial Needle Aspiration
See discussion of bronchoscopy on p. 587.
1. The specimen is obtained via a fiberoptic bronchoscope using a needle (Figure 7-4).
2. The bronchoscope is inserted, and the target site is identified using fluoroscopy.
3. The needle is inserted through the bronchoscope and into the tumor or desired area, where aspiration is performed with the attached syringe.
4. The needle is retracted within its sheath, and the entire catheter is withdrawn from the fiberoptic scope.

Transcatheter Bronchial Brushing
1. This is also performed via a fiberoptic bronchoscope (see discussion of bronchoscopy on p. 587).

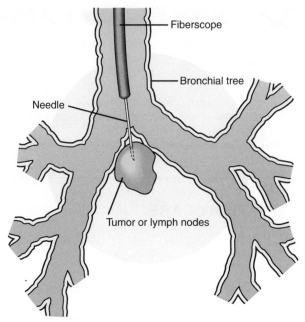

Figure 7-4 Transbronchial needle biopsy. The diagram shows a transbronchial needle penetrating the bronchial wall and entering a mass of subcarinal lymph nodes or tumor.

2. During bronchoscopy a small brush is moved back and forth over the suspicious area in the bronchus or its branches.
3. The cells adhere to the brush, which is then removed and used to make microscopic slides.

Percutaneous Needle Biopsy

1. In this method for obtaining a closed specimen, the biopsy is obtained after using fluoroscopic radiograph or CT scan for localization of the desired site.
2. The procedure is carried out with a cutting needle or by aspiration with a spinal type of needle to obtain a specimen.
3. The main problem with this procedure is potential damage to major blood vessels.
4. During the lung biopsy procedure, assess the patient carefully for signs of respiratory distress (e.g., shortness of breath, rapid pulse rate, cyanosis).

Open Lung Biopsy

1. The patient is taken to the operating room, and general anesthesia is provided.
2. The patient is placed in the supine or lateral position, and an incision is made into the chest wall.
3. After a piece of lung tissue is removed, the lung is sutured.
4. Chest tube drainage is used for approximately 24 hours after an open lung biopsy.
5. This procedure can be performed by thoracoscopy as described in the following section.

Thoracoscopic Biopsy

1. The lung is collapsed with a double-lumen endotracheal tube placed during induction of general anesthesia.

2. With the use of a thoracoscope (similar to a laparoscope [p. 617]), the lung is grasped and a piece is cut off using a cutting/stapling device. Large wedge lung resections can be obtained.
3. The scope and trocars are removed, and a small chest tube is left in place.
4. The tiny incisions are closed, and the procedure is completed.

After

- Place biopsy specimens in appropriate containers for histologic and microbiologic examination.
- Observe the patient's vital signs frequently for signs of bleeding (increased pulse rate, decreased blood pressure) and for shortness of breath.
- Assess the patient's breath sounds and report any decrease on the biopsy side.
- A chest x-ray film is ordered to check for complications (e.g., pneumothorax).
- Observe the patient for signs of pneumothorax (e.g., dyspnea, tachypnea, decrease in breath sounds, anxiety, restlessness).

TEST RESULTS AND CLINICAL SIGNIFICANCE

Carcinoma: *Biopsies of both primary and metastatic lesions can be performed using this technique. The lesion must be peripheral enough to ensure that one of the great vessels will not be punctured.*

Granuloma: *If the lesion is observed to contain calcium, it can be considered to be an old granuloma from previous granulomatous infection. If calcification is not observed, a biopsy of the lesion must be performed to rule out cancer, active fungal infection, or tuberculosis.*

Exposure lung diseases (e.g., black lung, asbestosis): *It is important to recognize and document the presence of exposure lung disease for medical (prognosis and treatment) and legal (workers' compensation or disability) reasons.*

Sarcoidosis: *Sarcoidosis of the lung is an interstitial disease highlighted by chronic inflammation and fibrosis. This is obvious on lung biopsy.*

Infection: *Unusual infections (such as that caused by* Pneumocystis jiroveci*) and unusual fungal diseases require tissue for culture and microscopic identification.*

RELATED TESTS

Bronchoscopy (p. 587). This endoscopic test is the access through which transbronchial biopsy and aspirations are performed.

Computed Tomography (CT) Scan of the Chest (p. 1029). This scan utilizes the method of CT to localize a lung lesion for biopsy.

Pancreatobiliary FISH Testing

NORMAL FINDINGS

No chromosomal ploidy abnormalities

INDICATIONS

This test is used to assist in the diagnosis of pancreatic/biliary cancer.

Microscopic Studies

7

TEST EXPLANATION

It is sometimes difficult to differentiate benign bile duct strictures from early pancreatobiliary cancer. When a stricture is identified on an endoscopic retrograde cholangiopancreatography (ERCP, p. 605), cancer must be considered as a possible cause. If an obvious cancer is not seen at the time of ERCP, a brush is repeatedly swept along the bile duct to obtain duct surface cells for conventional cytology to identify cancer cells. In conventional cytology, the brushing specimens are placed on a slide and stained with a PAP stain. Slides are then interpreted by a cytopathologist to determine whether they show features that are positive for malignancy, suspicious for malignancy, atypical (meaning there are cells that are not normal but cannot be definitely ascribed to a neoplastic process), or negative for malignancy.

With the use of fluorescence in situ hybridization (FISH) testing, three chromosome enumeration probes and a gene-specific probe to P16 tumor suppressor gene are able to determine if more than one pair of chromosomes or P16 genes exists in the cells obtained from the brushings of the bile duct during ERCP. If extra copies of two or more of the chromosomes or P16 genes are evident, the cells are considered to be *polysomic*, which indicates a high chance of malignancy. Based on conventional cytology, FISH testing, and other clinical data, the likelihood of cancer can be calculated.

CONTRAINDICATIONS

- See ERCP.

POTENTIAL COMPLICATIONS

- See ERCP.

INTERFERING FACTORS

- Errors in obtaining a good specimen can influence results.
- Cytologic examination is always affected by physician interpretation.

PROCEDURE AND PATIENT CARE

Before

- Explain the procedure to the patient.
- Obtain informed consent from the patient.
- Keep the patient NPO as of midnight the day of the test.
- Follow the procedure for ERCP (p. 605).

During

- During ERCP, a rounded brush is placed through the accessory lumen of the endoscope and passed repeatedly through the stricture.
- The brush is then swished in a cytology solution for FISH or directly smeared on a slide and preserved for conventional cytology.

After

- Follow the procedure for ERCP.

TEST RESULTS AND CLINICAL SIGNIFICANCE

Sclerosing cholangitis,
Biliary sclerosis,
Strictures of the pancreatobiliary duct:
These benign abnormalities will not be associated with any P16 gene abnormalities.
Pancreatobiliary cancer: *If P16 genetic abnormalities are noted, the likelihood of cancer is very high.*

RELATED TESTS

ERCP (p. 605). With upper GI endoscopic techniques, the pancreatobiliary tree can be accessed for pancreatic biliary FISH testing.

 Papanicolaou Test (Pap Test, Pap Smear, Cytologic Test for Cancer, Liquid-Based Cervical Cytology [LBCC], ThinPrep)

NORMAL FINDINGS

No abnormal or atypical cells

INDICATIONS

Pap test are the mainstay of screening for cancer of the vagina, cervix, and uterus. They are routinely performed on women older than 21 years or on younger women who are sexually active.

TEST EXPLANATION

A Pap test is taken to detect neoplastic cells in cervical and vaginal secretions. This test is based on the fact that normal cells and abnormal cervical and endometrial neoplastic cells are shed into the cervical and vaginal secretions. By examining these secretions microscopically, one can detect early cellular changes associated with infection, premalignant conditions, or an existing malignant condition. The Pap test is 95% accurate in detecting cervical carcinoma; however, its accuracy in the detection of endometrial carcinoma is only approximately 40%.

The Bethesda System for reporting cervical and vaginal cytologic diagnoses was developed and revised by the National Cancer Institute to minimize discrepancy in result reporting and create a standardized framework for reporting results that were clinically useful. A proper patient history is essential to the successful interpretation of cytological specimens and is a regulatory requirement associated with Pap testing. This reporting system was updated in 2001 and includes evaluation of the following five components (Box 7-1):

1. Adequacy of specimen—An indication of the adequacy of the specimen is provided here. The specimen either has enough cells that can be evaluated or does not.
2. General categorization (optional)—This is a quick summary of the cellular findings that allows the clinician to triage results readily.
3. Interpretation/Result—This is a report of the cytopathologist's interpretation of the cells examined. It is not a diagnosis because other diagnostic data may be required to make a diagnosis.
   a. Negative for intraepithelial lesion or malignancy—includes infections such as those caused by *Trichomonas* or *Candida* or reactive changes from an intrauterine device (IUD) or radiation therapy.

Microscopic Studies

7

BOX 7-1	Bethesda System for Reporting Cervical and Vaginal Cytologic Diagnoses

Adequacy of Specimen
- Satisfactory for evaluation
- Unsatisfactory for evaluation
  - Specimen rejected/not processed
  - Specimen processed and examined but unsatisfactory for evaluation

General Categorization
- Negative for intraepithelial lesion or malignancy
- Epithelial cell abnormality
- Other

Specimen Adequacy
- Satisfactory for evaluation
- Unsatisfactory for evaluation
  - Specimen rejected/not processed
  - Specimen processed and examined but unsatisfactory for evaluation

General Categorization
- Negative for intraepithelial lesion for malignancy
- Epithelial cell abnormality
- Other

Interpretation/Results
- Negative for intraepithelial lesion or malignancy
  - Organism causing infection
  - Other nonneoplastic findings
- Epithelial cell abnormalities
- Squamous
  - Atypical squamous cells (ASC)
  - Low-grade squamous intraepithelial lesions (LSIL)
  - High-grade squamous intraepithelial lesions (HSIL)
  - Squamous cell carcinoma
- Glandular cell
  - Atypical glandular cells (AGC)
  - Atypical glandular cells, favor neoplastic (AGC)
  - Endocervical adenocarcinoma in situ
  - Adenocarcinoma

Automated Review and Ancillary Testing

Educational Notes/Suggestions

  b. Epithelial cell abnormalities—These range from atypical to cancer for both the squamous and glandular cancer lines.
4. Automated review and ancillary testing (where appropriate)—This is reported if slides are scanned by automated computer systems (see p. 745). Also the use of any ancillary molecular tests such as human papillomavirus (HPV) (see p. 745) should be specified here.
5. Educational notes (optional)—Here comments are written regarding the significance of the cytology results, or recommendations for further diagnosis are provided.

A more common method of Pap test specimen collection is *liquid-based cervical cytology (LBCC* [more commonly called *ThinPrep*]). With this technique, the specimen obtained from the cervix is placed into a preservative solution instead of smearing it onto a slide as is done during conventional Pap smear testing (CPT). Any blood cells and debris are then isolated by centrifuge, leaving only cervical cells. A thin film of the residuum is then placed on a slide to be evaluated. The specimen can be "split" into two parts. The first is evaluated for cytopathology. In the event that cytologic abnormalities of undetermined significance are found that could be better elucidated with further testing, the cells in the second "split" specimen are used for that testing (to avoid having to obtain another cervical sample). For example, if cellular changes are found that may be related to HPV, the second "split" specimen is tested by real-time PCR for HPV DNA (see p. 648). HPV has been implicated as the cause of more than 95% of cervical cancers.

When compared with CPT, ThinPrep has a significantly greater percentage of satisfactory specimens for Pap testing. A significantly greater percentage of low-grade squamous intraepithelial lesion (LSIL) and high-grade squamous intraepithelial lesion (HSIL) Pap test results were reported using ThinPrep compared with the CPT. The predictive value of a positive ThinPrep test (93.9%) was similar to that for a positive CPT (87.8%) when compared with histology results.

Automated Pap test readings are increasingly being used because the volume of screening Pap tests exceeds the ability of the cytopathologists to spend enough time to accurately interpret the slides. Automation is especially accurate when performed on ThinPrep specimens. The ThinPrep Imaging System, for example, integrates automated imaging with screening by cytotechnologists to identify fields that contain potentially relevant cellular abnormalities. If the cytotechnologist identifies significant abnormalities, the slide is directly examined under a microscope. ThinPrep has replaced Pap testing because with ThinPrep the application of cells to the glass slide is standardized; cells are distributed evenly on the slide; mucus, blood, and inflammatory cells are reduced; fixation is effective and even; higher rates of serious cervical pathology are detected; and the material is less often considered inadequate for interpretation. A slightly different and less expensive technique called the *PapSpin* uses a special brush placed in a collection device and centrifuged to provide a cellular concentrate. The cellular concentrate is then examined microscopically.

Like screening for all cancers, as more studies become available, guidelines change. Furthermore, different medical professional societies may differ on certain aspects of PAP guidelines. Not only has the U.S. Preventive Services Task Force (USPSTF) recommended that the HPV test (p. 648) is appropriate for some women as part of routine cervical cancer screening, but it has also changed its recommendations as follows.

- Women aged 21 to 65 should get Pap tests no more than every 3 years. Previous guidelines, issued in 2003, recommended that women be screened "at least" every 3 years, allowing for annual screens.
- Women aged 30 to 65 may extend the interval between screens to 5 years if they use HPV tests in conjunction with the Pap test. The HPV test should not be used in younger women because many of them will have HPV infection that they will naturally clear without treatment.
- Women under 21 should not be screened for cervical cancer, regardless of sexual history. Previous advice recommended that women begin cervical cancer screening within 3 years of becoming sexually active.
- Women over 65 should not be screened as long as they have had consistently normal Pap tests and are not at high risk for cervical cancer.

The guidelines apply to healthy women who do not have abnormal Pap tests. They do not apply to women who have a history of cervical cancer.

CONTRAINDICATIONS

- Patients menstruating, because this can alter test interpretation
- Patients with known vaginal infections, because the infections can create cellular changes that may be misinterpreted as precancerous

INTERFERING FACTORS

- A delay in fixing a specimen allows the cells to dry, destroys effectiveness of the stain, and makes cytologic interpretation difficult.
- Using lubricating jelly on the speculum can alter the specimen.
- Douching and tub bathing before testing may wash away cellular deposits and interfere with the test results.
- Menstrual flow may alter test results. The best time to perform a Pap test is 2 weeks after the start of the last menses.
- Infections may interfere with hormonal cytology.
- Drugs such as digitalis and tetracycline may alter the test results by affecting the squamous epithelium.

Clinical Priorities

- Pap test should not be collected during menstruation because results may be altered.
- A maturation index can be determined to detect endocrine abnormalities (such as estrogen-progesterone imbalance).

PROCEDURE AND PATIENT CARE

Before

- Explain the procedure to the patient.
- Instruct the patient not to douche or tub bathe during the 24 hours before the Pap test. (Some physicians prefer that the patients refrain from sexual intercourse for 24 to 48 hours before the test.)
- Instruct the patient to empty her bladder before the examination. A full bladder inhibits complete palpation of pelvic structures.
- Tell the patient that no fasting or sedation is required.

During

Note the following procedural steps:

1. The patient is placed in the lithotomy position.
2. A vaginal speculum is inserted to expose the cervix.
3. Material is collected from the cervical canal by rotating a cotton swab moistened with saline or a wooden (plastic for LBCC) spatula within the cervical canal and in the squamocolumnar junction (Figure 7-5). If a maturation index is requested for hormonal information, the smear is taken off the vaginal wall. Care is taken to exclude the cervix.
4. The cells are immediately wiped across a clean glass slide and fixed either by immersing the slide in equal parts of 95% alcohol and ether or by using a commercial spray (e.g., Aqua Net hairspray). The secretions must be fixed before drying, because drying will distort the cells and make interpretation difficult. Furthermore, this fixing process kills any infectious organisms so that the specimen is less infectious to the personnel who handle the specimen.
5. The slide is labeled with the patient's name, age, parity, and date of her last menstrual period. If this is not done, the specimen is considered unsatisfactory for interpretation.

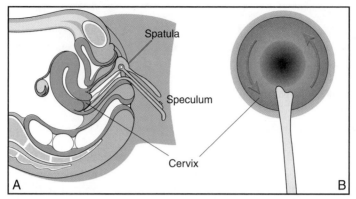

Figure 7-5 Papanicolaou (Pap) test. **A,** Cross-sectional view of the process of obtaining a cervical specimen. **B,** Cervix is scraped with bifid end of a spatula to obtain Pap test.

6. If LBCC is performed, the cervical specimen is placed in the fixative preservative solution. Once placed in this solution, cells can be evaluated anytime within the next 3 weeks (if kept frozen).
7. The patient's medication history (e.g., oral contraceptives) and the reason for the examination should be written on the laboratory request form.

After

- If the Pap test has induced some bleeding, provide the patient with a perineal napkin.
- Note that once in the laboratory, the Pap test slide is stained and reviewed microscopically by the pathologist. Several computer programs are now able to recognize abnormal cells and classify them. These programs are used to assist the pathologist in screening particular cellular smears.
- Inform the patient that usually she will be notified of the test results by her physician only if further evaluation is needed.

TEST RESULTS AND CLINICAL SIGNIFICANCE

Cancer: *The diagnosis of malignancy can be made only on biopsy of the tumor. All patients with suspicious Pap test must be more thoroughly examined with colposcopy, cone biopsy, and/or dilation and curettage.*
Sexually transmitted diseases,
Fungal infection,
Parasite infection,
Herpes infection:
Many of these infectious diseases cause cellular changes on Pap tests. Culture of these organisms, however, is required to make the diagnosis.
Infertility: *Lack of estrogenic effect noted on vaginal Pap tests may indicate ovarian failure in a woman of usual menstrual age.*

RELATED TESTS

Cervical Biopsy (p. 720). A biopsy of the cervix is performed to more accurately identify and treat premalignant and superficial malignant lesions of the cervix.
Colposcopy (p. 595). This is one of the follow-up tests performed for an abnormal Pap test.

Microscopic Studies

7

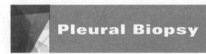

Pleural Biopsy

NORMAL FINDINGS
No evidence of pathologic conditions

INDICATIONS
This test is indicated when the pleural fluid obtained by thoracentesis (p. 681) is exudative fluid, which suggests infection, neoplasm, or tuberculosis. The pleural biopsy is indicated to distinguish among these disease processes. It is also performed when chest imaging indicates a pleural-based tumor, reaction, or thickening.

TEST EXPLANATION
Pleural biopsy is the removal of pleural tissue for histologic examination. Pleural biopsy is usually performed by a percutaneous needle biopsy. It also can be performed via thoracoscopy, which is done by inserting a scope into the pleural space for inspection and biopsy of the pleura (see Thoracoscopy, p. 627). Pleural tissue also may be obtained by an open pleural biopsy, which involves a limited thoracotomy and requires general anesthesia. For this procedure a small intercostal incision is made and the biopsy of the pleura is done under direct observation. The advantage of these open procedures is that a larger piece of pleura can be obtained.

Percutaneous needle biopsies are usually performed by a physician at the patient's bedside, in a special procedure room, or in the physician's office in approximately 30 minutes. Because of the local anesthetic, little discomfort is associated with this procedure. Open biopsies are done in the operating room.

CONTRAINDICATIONS
- Patients with prolonged bleeding or clotting times

POTENTIAL COMPLICATIONS
- Bleeding or injury to the lung
- Pneumothorax

PROCEDURE AND PATIENT CARE
Before
- Explain the procedure to the patient.
- Obtain informed consent for this procedure.
- Tell the patient that no fasting or sedation is required.
- Instruct the patient to remain very still during the procedure. Any movement may cause inadvertent damage by the needle.

During
- Note the following procedural steps for *percutaneous needle biopsy*:
  1. This procedure is usually performed with the patient in a sitting position with his or her shoulders and arms elevated and supported by a padded overhead table.

2. After the presence of the fluid has been determined by the thoracentesis technique, the skin overlying the biopsy site is anesthetized and pierced with a scalpel blade.
3. A needle is inserted with a cannula until fluid is removed. (Some fluid is left in the pleural space after the thoracentesis to make the biopsy easier.)
4. The inner needle is removed, and a blunt-tipped, hooked biopsy trocar, attached to a three-way stopcock, is inserted into the cannula.
5. The patient is instructed to exhale all air and then perform the Valsalva maneuver to prevent air from entering the pleural space.
6. The cannula and biopsy trocar are withdrawn while the hook catches the parietal wall and takes a specimen with its cutting edge.
7. Usually three biopsy specimens are taken from different sites at the same session.
8. The specimens are placed in a fixative solution and sent to the laboratory immediately.
9. After the specimens are taken, additional parietal fluid can be removed.

After

- Apply an adhesive bandage to the biopsy site.
- Note that a chest x-ray film is usually taken to detect the potential complication of pneumothorax.
- Observe the patient for signs of respiratory distress (e.g., shortness of breath, diminished breath sounds) on the side of the biopsy.
- Observe the patient's vital signs frequently for evidence of bleeding (increased pulse rate, decreased blood pressure).
- Ensure that the biopsy specimen is sent to the laboratory immediately.

Home Care Responsibilities

- Instruct the patient to report any signs of shortness of breath.
- Note any signs of bleeding, such as decreasing blood pressure or increasing pulse rate.

TEST RESULTS AND CLINICAL SIGNIFICANCE

Neoplasm: *Pleural tumors can be primary (mesothelioma) or metastatic (breast, lung, ovarian, gastrointestinal, etc.). These tumors are often associated with a pleural effusion.*

Infection: *Lung and pleural space infections can cause thickened pleura and pleural effusions (empyema). Most infections can be identified on Gram stains and cultures of the pleural fluid. However, some infections cannot be identified without tissue for culture or tissue for other forms of identification. This is especially true for the unusual infections occurring in immunocompromised patients* (Pneumocystis jiroveci).

RELATED TESTS

Thoracentesis and Pleural Fluid Analysis (p. 681). This is a procedure whereby pleural fluid is aspirated from the pleural space for analysis.

Chest X-Ray (p. 1014) and Computed Tomography (CT) Scan of the Chest (p. 1029). These x-ray studies visualize most surfaces of the pleura.

Progesterone Receptor Assay (PR Assay, PRA, PgR)

NORMAL FINDINGS

Immunochemistry
Negative: <5% of the cells stain for receptors
Positive: >5% of the cells stain for receptors

Reverse-Transcriptase Polymerase Chain Reaction (RT-PCR)
Negative: <5.5 units
Positive: >5.5 units

INDICATIONS

Progesterone receptor assay is performed on breast cancer tissue to indicate sensitivity to hormone manipulative therapy and to indicate prognosis of breast cancer.

TEST EXPLANATION

The PR assay is used in determining the prognosis and treatment of breast cancer and, to a lesser degree, other cancers. These assays help determine whether a tumor is likely to respond to endocrine therapy. The test is done on breast cancer specimens when a primary or recurrent cancer is identified; it is usually done in conjunction with estrogen receptor (ER) assay (see p. 728) to increase the predictability of a tumor response to hormone therapy. Breast tumors tend to be PR positive in postmenopausal women more often than in premenopausal women. PR-positive tumors are suspected to be associated with a better prognosis than PR-negative tumors. Tumor response rates to hormonal manipulation are found to be potentiated if the ER assay is positive. Response rates are as follows:
    ER positive, PR positive: 75%
    ER negative, PR positive: 60%
    ER positive, PR negative: 35%
    ER negative, PR negative: 25%
The most commonly used laboratory method provides accurate information on paraffin-embedded tissue or fixed slides using immunohistochemical staining for PR proteins. Positive reactivity by immunohistochemistry is observed in the nuclei of the tumor cells. Only a small portion of the tissue is required for testing. Results are usually available in less than 1 week. Only the cancerous tissue is evaluated for PR receptors.

Other tumors (such as ovarian, melanoma, uterine, or pancreatic) are occasionally studied for ER and PR assay. This is mostly done within clinical trials.

INTERFERING FACTORS

⚖ Use of exogenous hormones such as progesterone or estrogen may cause false-negative results.

PROCEDURE AND PATIENT CARE

Before
- Prepare the patient for breast biopsy according to routine protocol.
- Record the menstrual status of the patient.

- Record any exogenous hormone the patient may have used during the last 2 months.
- Instruct the patient to discontinue exogenous hormone therapy before breast biopsy. This is done in consultation with the physician.

During

- The surgeon obtains tissue.
- This tissue should be placed on ice or in formalin.
- Part of the tissue is used for routine histologic examination. A portion of the paraffin block is sent to a reference laboratory.

After

- Provide routine postoperative care.
- Inform the patient that results are usually available in 1 week.

TEST RESULTS AND CLINICAL SIGNIFICANCE

PR positive: *This cancer is more likely to be successfully treated with hormone manipulation in a therapeutic or adjuvant clinical setting.*

RELATED TESTS

Estrogen Receptor Assay (p. 728). Like PR assay, this test predicts the likelihood of tumor response to endocrine manipulative therapy.

Breast Cancer Genomics (p. 1086). This test is used as a prognosticator indicating the risk of recurrent breast cancer. It is also a powerful predictor of benefit from hormone therapy or chemotherapy.

Renal Biopsy (Kidney Biopsy)

NORMAL FINDINGS

No pathologic conditions

INDICATIONS

Renal biopsy is performed for the following purposes:

1. To diagnose the cause of renal disease (e.g., poststreptococcal glomerulonephritis, Goodpasture syndrome, lupus nephritis)
2. To detect primary and metastatic malignancy of the kidney in patients who may not be candidates for surgery
3. To evaluate kidney transplantation rejection, which enables the physician to determine the appropriate dose of immunosuppressive drugs

TEST EXPLANATION

Biopsy of the kidney affords microscopic examination of renal tissue. Renal biopsy is most often obtained percutaneously (Figure 7-6). During this procedure a needle is inserted through the skin and into the kidney to obtain a sample of kidney tissue. The biopsy needle is more accurately placed when guided with CT scan, ultrasonography, or fluoroscopy. These visualization techniques allow more

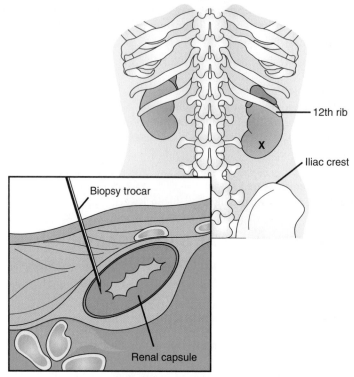

Figure 7-6 Renal biopsy.

precise localization of the desired kidney tissue. This procedure is performed by a physician in approximately 10 to 30 minutes. The biopsy is uncomfortable, but only minimally if enough lidocaine is used.

Occasionally, open renal biopsy is performed. This involves an incision through the flank and dissection to expose the kidney surgically.

CONTRAINDICATIONS

- Patients with coagulation disorders, because of the risk of excessive bleeding
- Patients with operable kidney tumors, because tumor cells may be disseminated during the procedure
- Patients with hydronephrosis, because the enlarged renal pelvis can be easily entered and cause a persistent urine leak requiring surgical repair
- Patients with urinary tract infections, because the needle insertion may disseminate the active infection throughout the retroperitoneum

 Clinical Priorities

- Assess the coagulation profile before performing a kidney biopsy because of the possibility of bleeding. Often hemoglobin and hematocrit values are obtained after the procedure to check for bleeding.
- After a renal biopsy the patient is usually kept in bed on his or her back for about 24 hours.
- After this test, carefully evaluate the vital signs for evidence of bleeding. Inspect the urine for gross hematuria.

POTENTIAL COMPLICATIONS

- Hemorrhage from the highly vascular renal tissue
- Inadvertent puncture of the liver, lung, bowel, aorta, and inferior vena cava
- Infection when an open biopsy is performed

PROCEDURE AND PATIENT CARE

Before

- Explain the procedure to the patient.
- Ensure that written informed consent for this procedure is obtained by the physician.
- Keep the patient on nothing by mouth (NPO) status after midnight on the day of the test in the event that bleeding or inadvertent puncture of an abdominal organ necessitates surgical intervention.
- Assess the patient's coagulation studies (platelet count, prothrombin time, partial thromboplastin time).
- Check the patient's hemoglobin and hematocrit values.
- Note that the patient's blood may need to be typed and crossmatched in case of severe hemorrhage requiring transfusions.
- Tell the patient that no sedative is required.
- Note that the needle biopsy may be done at the bedside.
- If CT scan or ultrasound guidance is to be used, note that the needle biopsy is performed in the radiology or ultrasonography department.

During

- Note the following procedural steps:
  1. The patient is placed in a prone position with a sandbag or pillow under the abdomen to straighten the spine.
  2. Under sterile conditions, the skin overlying the kidney is infiltrated with a local anesthetic (lidocaine).
  3. While the patient holds his or her breath to stop kidney motion, the physician inserts the biopsy needle into the kidney and takes a specimen.
  4. After this procedure is completed, the needle is removed and pressure is applied to the site for approximately 20 minutes.

After

- Apply a pressure dressing.
- Turn the patient on his or her back and have the patient stay in bed for approximately 24 hours.
- Check the patient's vital signs, puncture site, and hematocrit values frequently during the 24-hour period.
- Instruct the patient to avoid any activity that increases abdominal venous pressure (e.g., coughing).
- Assess the patient for signs and symptoms of hemorrhage (e.g., decrease in blood pressure, increase in pulse rate, pallor, backache, flank pain, shoulder pain, light-headedness).
- Evaluate the patient's abdomen for signs of bowel or liver penetration (e.g., abdominal pain and tenderness, abdominal muscle guarding and rigidity, decreased bowel sounds).
- Inspect all urine specimens for gross hematuria. Usually the patient's urine will contain blood initially, but this generally will not continue after the first 24 hours. Urine samples may be placed in consecutive chronologic order to facilitate comparison for evaluation of hematuria. This is referred to as "rack," or serial, urine samples.

Encourage the patient to drink large amounts of fluid to prevent clot formation and urine retention.

• Obtain blood for hemoglobin and hematocrit level determination after the biopsy to assess for active bleeding. One lavender-top tube of blood is needed.

Instruct the patient to avoid strenuous exercise (e.g., heavy lifting, contact sports, horseback riding) or any activity that could cause jolting of the kidney for at least 2 weeks.

Teach the patient the signs and symptoms of renal hemorrhage, and instruct him or her to call the physician if any of these symptoms occur.

Instruct the patient to report burning on urination or any temperature elevations. These could indicate a urinary tract infection.

TEST RESULTS AND CLINICAL SIGNIFICANCE

Renal disease (e.g., poststreptococcal conditions, Goodpasture syndrome, lupus nephritis): *These primary diseases of the kidney have classic histologic appearances. It is important to document the type of renal disease to ensure proper therapy. Immunofluorescent stains are often applied to the tissue to identify renal disease of immunologic origin (e.g., Goodpasture disease).*

Primary and metastatic malignancy of the kidney: *The most common cancers of the kidney are primary renal cell carcinomas. It is dangerous to perform a biopsy of this tumor because it is quite vascular. Furthermore, the biopsy could cause tumor studding along the needle track. However, in cases of metastatic disease, or if medical conditions preclude surgery, tissue can be obtained by kidney biopsy.*

Rejection of kidney transplant: *This is the definitive manner in which rejection is diagnosed. If the problem is caught early enough, the immunosuppressive medication regimen can be altered to stop the rejection process.*

SARS Viral Testing

NORMAL FINDINGS

No SARS virus

INDICATIONS

This test is used to diagnose severe acute respiratory syndrome, or SARS.

TEST EXPLANATION

SARS has now killed more than 100 people and infected some 2600 in 20 countries. A coronavirus causes SARS. China's southern Guangdong province, which includes Hong Kong, is believed to be the source of the virus, which has about an 8- to 10-day incubation period. Symptoms are similar to any pneumonia (fever, chills, and cough). The diagnosis should be suspected in a symptomatic patient who lives in or has traveled to an area where there has been documented transmission of the illness. Routine testing for the SARS virus is not conducted unless a cluster of cases develops and health officials are able to rule out all other infectious agents.

There are three tests that are currently available. These include:

1. *Enzyme-Linked Immunosorbent Assay (ELISA)*—This test detects antibodies to Coronavirus. The test identifies antibodies 20 days after the start of symptoms. That means it cannot be used to detect cases in the early stage of illness.

2. *Immunofluorescence Assay (IFA)*—This method detects SARS antibodies as early as 10 days after infection, but it is a complex and relatively slow test that requires growing the virus in the laboratory.

3. *Reverse-Transcription Polymerase Chain Reaction (RT-PCR)*—This molecular test detects the SARS virus by amplifying ribonucleic acid (RNA) genetic information from a cultured sample by a RT-PCR. It is good at detecting early stages of the infection, and results can be available in 2 days.

The diagnosis can only be made with positive test results in the following situations with:

- One specimen tested on two occasions using the original clinical specimen on each occasion
- Two clinical specimens from different sources (e.g., nasopharyngeal and stool)
- Two clinical specimens collected from the same source on two different days (e.g., two nasopharyngeal aspirates)

Eight of the following types of respiratory specimens may be collected for viral and/or bacterial diagnostics: (1) nasopharyngeal wash/aspirates, (2) nasopharyngeal swabs, (3) oropharyngeal swabs, (4) bronchioalveolar lavage, (5) tracheal aspirate, (6) pleural fluid tap, (7) sputum, and (8) postmortem tissue. Nasopharyngeal wash/aspirates are the specimen of choice for detection of most respiratory viruses.

Serum and blood (plasma) should be collected early in the illness for RT-PCR testing. The reliability of RT-PCR testing performed on blood specimens decreases as the illness progresses. Both acute and convalescent serum specimens should be collected for antibody testing. To confirm or rule out SARS-CoV infection, it is important to collect convalescent serum specimens more than 28 days after the onset of illness.

A virus culture to isolate SARS coronavirus is available but takes a few days for results. The capability to isolate and cultivate the virus is particularly important for epidemiologists and researchers.

PROCEDURE AND PATIENT CARE

Before

✒ Explain the procedure to the patient.
- Observe Standard Precautions and Transmission-Based Precautions.
- Observe strict isolation technique. This disease is contagious.

During

- To obtain a *nasopharyngeal wash/aspirate*, have the patient sit with the head tilted slightly backward. Instill 1 mL to 1.5 mL of nonbacteriostatic saline (pH 7.0) into one nostril. Flush a plastic catheter or tubing with 2 mL to 3 mL of saline. Insert the tubing into the nostril. Aspirate nasopharyngeal secretions. Repeat this procedure for the other nostril. Collect the specimens in sterile vials.
- To obtain a *nasopharyngeal* or *oropharyngeal swabs*, use only sterile Dacron or rayon swabs with plastic shafts. Do not use a cotton swab or swabs with wooden sticks, as they may contain substances that inactivate some viruses and inhibit PCR testing. Insert the swab into the nostril. Leave the swab in place for a few seconds to absorb secretions. Swab both nostrils. (For *oropharyngeal culture*—swab the posterior pharynx and tonsillar areas, avoiding the tongue.)
- To collect *sputum*, educate the patient about the difference between sputum and oral secretions. Have the patient rinse the mouth with water and then expectorate deep cough sputum directly into a sterile screw-cap sputum collection cup or sterile dry container.
- To collect *blood*, collect 5 mL to 10 mL of whole blood in a serum separator tube for serum RT-PCR testing or for ELISA antibody testing. Collect 5 mL to 10 mL of blood in an EDTA (purple-top) tube for plasma testing.

After

- Provide acute care for respiratory illness.
- If shipping the specimen domestically, use cold packs to keep the sample at 4° C. If shipping internationally, pack in dry ice.

TEST RESULTS AND CLINICAL SIGNIFICANCE

SARS: *Initial diagnostic testing for suspected SARS should include chest radiograph, oximetry, blood cultures, sputum for Gram stain and culture, testing for influenza A and B.*

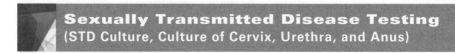

Sexually Transmitted Disease Testing
(STD Culture, Culture of Cervix, Urethra, and Anus)

NORMAL FINDINGS

No evidence of STD (gonorrhea, Chlamydia [p. 722], Trichomonas*)*

INDICATIONS

These cultures and smears are performed for patients who have a vaginal discharge, pelvic pain, urethritis, or penile discharge and are at risk for STDs.

TEST EXPLANATION

In the United States and other countries, some STDs (see Table 7-2, p. 759) have become epidemic, whereas others have become increasingly frequent. In this test discussion, we will concentrate on three common STD organisms: Chlamydia trachomatis (also discussed on p. 722), Neisseria gonorrhoeae, and Trichomonas vaginalis. Whereas *trichomonas* often does not cause any symptoms, these organisms can cause urethritis, vaginitis, endometritis, pelvic inflammatory disease, pharyngitis, proctitis, epididymitis, prostatitis, and salpingitis. Children born of infected mothers may develop conjunctivitis, pneumonia, neonatal blindness, neonatal neurologic injury, and even death.

Specimens for STD infections are obtained on men and women with suggestive symptoms. If the result is positive, sexual partners should be evaluated and treated. Cervical cultures/swabs are usually done for women; urethral swabs and cultures are done for men. Rectal and throat cultures are performed in persons who have engaged in anal and oral intercourse. Because rectal gonorrhea accompanies genital gonorrhea in a high percentage of women, rectal cultures are recommended in all women with suspected gonorrhea. Performing STD testing is also part of the prenatal workup. If the STD culture is positive, treatment during pregnancy can prevent possible fetal complications (e.g., ophthalmia neonatorum) and maternal complications. Rectal and orogastric specimens should be performed on the neonates of infected mothers.

Gram stains of smears or cultures should be taken before a patient begins antibiotic therapy. Cultures for gonorrhea use a special medium such as Thayer-Martin, designed for the cultivation of *Neisseria gonorrhoeae.*

Although cultures are used as the definitive test for documentation of STD infections, nucleic acid (RNA/DNA) probes *(Nucleic Acid Testing, NAT)* are most commonly used for identification of these STD organisms. Each suspected organism must be specifically requested. Some laboratories do routine "genital cultures" that include gonorrhea, beta streptococcus, and *Gardnerella* investigations.

T. vaginalis can be diagnosed via a wet mount, in which "corkscrew" motility is observed. Newer methods, such as rapid antigen testing (similar to Strept Screen, p. 765) and transcription-mediated amplification, have even greater sensitivity, but are not in widespread use. The presence of *T. vaginalis* can also be diagnosed by PCR. Specimens obtained in a Pap test/ThinPrep can also be used for testing.

STD cultures and smears are obtained by a physician or nurse in several minutes. Very little discomfort is associated with these procedures.

INTERFERING FACTORS

- *N. gonorrhoeae* is very sensitive to lubricants and disinfectants.
- Menses may alter test results.
- Female douching within 24 hours before a cervical culture makes fewer organisms available for culture.
- Male voiding within 1 hour before a urethral culture washes secretions out of the urethra.
- Fecal material may contaminate an anal culture.

✓ Clinical Priorities

- If cultures for STDs are positive, sexual partners should be evaluated and treated.
- Women should not douche within 24 hours before cervical cultures because douching may decrease the number of organisms available for culture.
- Men should not urinate within 1 hour before a urethral culture because voiding washes secretions out of the urethra.

PROCEDURE AND PATIENT CARE

Before

 Explain the purpose and procedure to the patient. Use a matter-of-fact, nonjudgmental approach.
Tell the patient that no fasting or sedation is required.

During

Cervical Culture

1. The female patient is told to refrain from douching and tub bathing before the cervical culture.
2. The patient is placed in the lithotomy position, and a moistened, unlubricated vaginal speculum is inserted to expose the cervix (see Figure 7-5, *A,* on p. 747).
3. Excess cervical mucus is removed with a cotton ball held in a ring forceps.
4. A sterile cotton-tipped swab is inserted into the endocervical canal and moved from side to side to obtain the specimen.
5. The swab is placed in sterile saline or a transporting fluid obtained from the laboratory. The specimen should be plated as soon as possible. The specimen should not be refrigerated.

Anal Canal Culture

1. An anal culture of the female or male patient is taken by inserting a sterile, cotton-tipped swab approximately 1 inch into the anal canal (Figure 7-7).
2. If stool contaminates the swab, a repeat swab is taken.

Microscopic Studies

7

Oropharyngeal Culture
1. This culture should be obtained in male and female patients who have engaged in oral intercourse.
2. A throat culture is best obtained by depressing the patient's tongue with a wooden tongue blade and touching the posterior wall of the throat with a sterile cotton-tipped swab.

Urethral Culture
1. The urethral specimen should be obtained from the male patient before he voids. Voiding within 1 hour before collection washes secretions out of the urethra, making fewer organisms available for culture. The best time to obtain the specimen is before the first morning micturition.
2. A culture is taken by inserting a sterile swab gently into the anterior urethra (Figure 7-8).
3. Place the male patient in the supine position to prevent falling if vasovagal syncope occurs during introduction of the cotton swab or wire loop into the urethra.
4. The patient is observed for hypotension, bradycardia, pallor, sweating, nausea, and weakness.
5. In the male, prostatic massage may increase the chances of obtaining positive cultures.

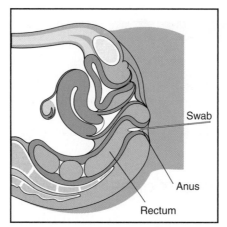

Figure 7-7 Obtaining a specimen of exudate from the rectum.

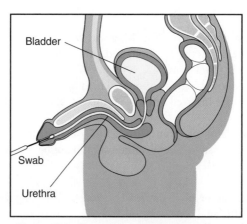

Figure 7-8 Obtaining a urethral specimen.

Urine Culture

Obtain the first voided specimen in the female. (Urine cultures for STD are not helpful in males.) A small quantity of urine is placed in the transporting fluid or sterile empty container obtained from the laboratory.

Pap Test ThinPrep (See p. 743)

After

- Place the swabs for gonorrhea in a Thayer-Martin medium and roll them from side to side.
- Label and send the culture bottle to the microbiology laboratory.
- Transport the specimen to the laboratory as soon as possible.
- Handle all specimens as though they were capable of transmitting disease.
- Do not refrigerate the specimen.
- Mark the laboratory slip with the collection time, date, source of specimen, patient's age, current antibiotic therapy, and clinical diagnosis.
- Advise the patient to avoid intercourse and all sexual contact until test results are available.
- If the culture results are positive, tell the patient to receive treatment and have sexual partners evaluated.
- Note that repeat cultures should be taken after completion of treatment to evaluate therapy.

TEST RESULTS AND CLINICAL SIGNIFICANCE

Gonorrhea,
Chlamydia (p. 722),
Trichomonas:

These and other STDs can be identified by these and other diagnostic tests (Table 7-2).

TABLE 7-2	Sexually Transmitted Diseases (STDs) and Methods of Diagnosis
Disease	**Method of Diagnosis**
Gonorrhea	Cervical, urethral, anal, oropharyngeal cultures
Chlamydia *Lymphogranuloma venereum* *C. trachomatis*	Cervical and urethral cultures, serology, DNA probe testing
Herpes genitalis	Culture from lesion, serology
Syphilis	Serology, fluid cultures (CNS), darkfield slide
Hepatitis	Serology, nucleic acid testing
HIV	Serologic, virologic, nucleic acid testing
Trichomonas vaginalis	Cervical and urethral cultures, urine, ThinPrep PAP, serology, nucleic amplification tests
Candida	Wet mount, fungal culture
Gardnerella vaginalis	Cervical, urethral, anal cultures

Microscopic Studies

7

RELATED TESTS

Tests for the STDs listed in the following are discussed separately:
Chlamydia (p. 722)
Herpes Simplex (p. 731)
Syphilis Detection (p. 473)
Hepatitis Virus Studies (p. 286)
AIDS Serology (p. 297)

Skin Biopsy (Cutaneous Immunofluorescence Biopsy, Skin Biopsy Antibodies, Skin Immunohistopathology, Direct Immunofluorescence Antibody Test)

NORMAL FINDINGS

Normal skin histology
No evidence of IgG, IgA, or IgM antibody, complement C3, or fibrinogen

INDICATIONS

Testing of inflamed skin or mucosa is performed to evaluate and diagnose immunologically mediated dermatitis, such as pemphigoid, pemphigus, bullosa acquisita and bullous lupus erythematosus. It is indicated when an immunologic source for a skin rash is suspected.

TEST EXPLANATION

Autoimmune skin diseases are associated with autoantibodies in the skin and serum. Either can be tested (see Antiscleroderma Antibody, p. 93, and Indirect Immunofluorescence Antibody, p. 197). Direct (testing for antibodies in the *skin*) immunofluorescence antibody (IFA) is most specific and diagnostic. Furthermore, skin/mucosal histology is reported. For this study, a tissue specimen in or around the skin/mucosal lesion is obtained and evaluated by routine histology and by IFA methods. Deposition of human immunoglobulins (IgG, IgA, or IgM), complement C3, or fibrinogen components are determined. This test is also used to confirm the histopathology of skin lesions and monitor the results of treatment. Indirect (testing for IFA detected antibodies in the *serum*) immunofluorescence (IF) testing may be diagnostic when histologic or direct IFA studies are only suggestive, nonspecific, or negative.

PROCEDURE AND PATIENT CARE

Before

Explain the procedure to the patient.
- Obtain an informed consent.

During

- The skin area used for biopsy is anesthetized locally to minimize discomfort. The area chosen for biopsy depends on the disease suspected. For some diseases, the skin lesion is tested. For others, the margin or nearby skin is tested.
- A 4-mm punch biopsy or elliptical tissue excision is obtained.

After

- Apply a dry, sterile dressing over the biopsy site.
- Tell the patient that results may not be available for several days.
- Deliver the specimen (in a container preferred by the reference laboratory) to the local laboratory immediately after the biopsy is taken.

TEST RESULTS AND CLINICAL SIGNIFICANCE

Systemic lupus erythematosus (SLE),
Discoid lupus erythematosus:

> *Lupus erythematosus is associated with acute, subacute, and chronic skin lesions. All are associated with deposits of immunoglobulins and complement in the epidermal basement membrane zone. The acute changes are represented by the butterfly rash of SLE. Subacute changes of SLE are represented by photosensitive ulcers. The chronic changes of discoid lupus are scale-like changes about the neck and face. Once the scale is removed, an ulcer remains until healing and scarring occur.*

Pemphigus,
Bullous pemphigoid:

> *These immunologic dermatitis diseases are highlighted clinically as subepidermal blistering of skin, usually in older adults.*

Dermatitis herpetiformis: *This urticarial immunologic dermatitis is often associated with gluten-sensitive enteropathy.*

RELATED TESTS

Antiscleroderma Antibody (p. 93). This antibody is diagnostic for cutaneous manifestations of scleroderma.
Indirect Immunofluorescence Antibody (p. 197). This test determines the presence of IgG, IgA, and IgM autoantibodies in the serum. This is helpful in the diagnosis of autoimmune skin diseases if the direct IFA skin biopsy is not definitive.

Sputum Culture and Sensitivity (Sputum C&S, Sputum Culture, and Gram stain)

NORMAL FINDINGS

Normal upper respiratory tract

INDICATIONS

Sputum culture is indicated in any patient with a persistent productive cough, fever, hemoptysis, or a chest x-ray picture compatible with a pulmonary infection. This test is used to diagnose pneumonia, bronchiectasis, bronchitis, or pulmonary abscess. Bacterium, fungus, or virus can be cultured.

TEST EXPLANATION

Sputum cultures are obtained to determine the presence of pathogenic bacteria in patients with respiratory infections, such as pneumonia. A *Gram stain* is the first step in the microbiologic analysis of sputum. Through sputum staining, bacteria are classified as gram positive or gram negative. This may be used to guide drug therapy until the C&S report is complete. The sputum sample is then applied to a series of bacterial culture plates. The bacteria that grow on those plates 1 to 3 days later are then identified. Determinations of bacterial sensitivity to various antibiotics (also called *drug sensitivity testing*) are performed to identify the most appropriate antimicrobial drug therapy. This is done by observing a ring of growth inhibition around an antibiotic disk in the culture medium. Sputum for C&S should be collected before antimicrobial therapy is initiated, unless the test is being performed to evaluate the effectiveness of medications already being given. Preliminary reports are usually available in 24 hours. Cultures require at least 48 hours for completion. Sputum cultures for fungus (e.g., *Pneumocystis*) and *Mycobacterium tuberculosis* take 6 to 8 weeks.

PROCEDURE AND PATIENT CARE

Before

𝕏 Explain the procedure for sputum collection to the patient.

𝕏 Remind the patient that sputum must be coughed up from the lungs and that saliva is not sputum (Figure 7-9).

- Hold antibiotics until after the sputum has been collected.
- If an elective specimen is to be obtained, give the patient a sterile sputum container on the night before the sputum is to be collected so that the morning specimen may be obtained on arising.

𝕏 Instruct the patient to rinse out his or her mouth with water before the sputum collection to decrease contamination of the sputum by particles in the oropharynx. Antiseptic mouthwash, however, is to be avoided.

During

- Note that sputum specimens are best taken when the patient awakes in the morning before eating or drinking.
- Collect at least 1 teaspoon of sputum in a sterile sputum container.
- Usually obtain sputum by having the patient cough after taking several deep breaths.

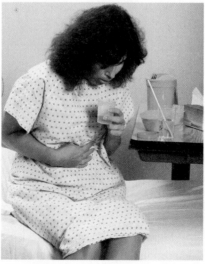

Figure 7-9 Collection of sputum specimen. The specimen should be representative of pulmonary secretions—not saliva.

- If the patient is unable to produce a sputum specimen, stimulate coughing by lowering the head of the patient's bed or giving the patient an aerosol administration of a warm, hypertonic solution.
- Note that other methods to collect sputum include endotracheal aspiration, fiberoptic bronchoscopy, and transtracheal aspiration.

After

✐ Tell the patient to notify the nurse as soon as the sputum is collected.
- Label the sputum and send it to the laboratory as soon as possible.
- Note any current antibiotic therapy on the laboratory slip.

TEST RESULTS AND CLINICAL SIGNIFICANCE

Bacterial infection (e.g., pneumonia),
Viral infection,
Atypical bacterial infection (e.g., tuberculosis),
Fungal infection:
> *Sputum that is obtained for the above-listed types of organisms is plated on several types of culture media to grow the organisms that could grow in the pulmonary tree. Some of these organisms are quite difficult to grow in the laboratory and require great attention to detail to effectively grow these pathogens and demonstrate disease.*

RELATED TEST

Tuberculosis Culture (p. 768). This is the only manner in which the diagnosis of tuberculosis (TB) can be made with certainty. When TB is grown from the culture of a specimen, the diagnosis of TB can be made and treatment based on drug sensitivities can be started.

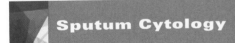

Sputum Cytology

Microscopic Studies

7

NORMAL FINDINGS

Normal epithelial cells

INDICATIONS

Sputum for cytologic examination is indicated for any patient in whom the diagnosis of cancer of the lung is considered. Bronchoscopy and percutaneous lung biopsy have supplanted the need for sputum cytology to a great degree. Now its greatest use is in patients who have abnormal chest x-ray film results, productive cough, and nothing visible on bronchoscopy. It is also used to monitor smokers who have had some atypical changes on prior examination of the lower respiratory tract.

TEST EXPLANATION

Tumors within the pulmonary system frequently slough cells into the sputum. When the sputum is gathered, the cells are examined. If the cytologic examination indicates malignant cells, a lung tumor exists within the mucosa of the trachea, bronchi, and lungs. If only normal epithelial cells are observed, either no malignancy exists or any existing tumor is not shedding cells at that time. Therefore a positive test indicates malignancy; a negative test means nothing. The test is more likely to be positive on smokers who have a chronic productive cough and/or hemoptysis. Furthermore, the more specimens obtained, the greater the accuracy of the test. This test is rarely performed, now that tissue for biopsy can be easily obtained by bronchoscopic biopsy (p. 587).

INTERFERING FACTORS

- False-negative findings can occur as a result of poor cytologic preparation or inadequate specimen acquisition. Interpretation of cytologic changes is difficult, but most pathologists who have had experience with cytology maintain good accuracy. This is usually monitored by quality assurance studies within the pathology department.

PROCEDURE AND PATIENT CARE

Before

- Explain the procedure for sputum collection to the patient.
- Remind the patient that sputum must be coughed up from the lungs and that saliva is not sputum.
- Give the patient a sterile sputum container the night before the sputum is to be collected so that the morning specimen may be obtained on arising.
- Instruct the patient to rinse out her or his mouth with water to decrease contamination of the sputum by particles in the oropharynx.

During

- Note that sputum specimens are best collected when the patient awakes in the morning.
- Collect at least 1 teaspoon of sputum in the sterile sputum container. The container may or may not contain alcohol as an immediate fixative—this varies according to the laboratory. Certainly if a 24-hour specimen is requested, alcohol must be within the container to diminish cellular deterioration during the collection period.
- Usually obtain sputum by having the patient cough after taking several deep breaths.
- If the patient is unable to produce a sputum specimen, stimulate coughing by lowering the head of the patient's bed or with aerosol administration of a warm hypertonic solution.
- Note that other methods to collect sputum include endotracheal aspiration, fiberoptic bronchoscopy, and transtracheal aspiration. Bronchial brushings can obtain excellent specimens for cytologic examination. A brush is placed through the bronchoscope and wiped on the bronchial mucosa. It is then withdrawn back into its sheath and wiped on a dry slide, which is immediately fixed.
- Usually collect sputum for cytologic examination once daily on 3 successive days. The first morning specimen is the best.

After

- Instruct the patient to notify the nurse as soon as the sputum is collected.
- Label the specimen and send it to the laboratory as soon as possible.

TEST RESULTS AND CLINICAL SIGNIFICANCE

Malignancies: *Malignancies of the trachea, bronchus, and lung can be detected. Marked changes in the nuclear/cytoplasmic ratio, size of the cell, and differentiation of the cell indicate suspicious changes. It is now thought that cellular changes progress from benign, normal-looking cells to metaplastic cells, to atypical cells, to frankly cancerous cells. The cytologic report may indicate the cells are somewhere* *within that spectrum. The cells may be labeled benign, abnormal, suspicious, or definitely cancer. The epithelial cells of the lower respiratory system seem to make those progressive changes as the number of years the person smokes increases.*

Benign cellular changes: *This is most commonly related to infection (bronchiectasis), exposure (asbestosis), or viral pneumonitis.*

Asthma: *These patients often have an increased number of eosinophils within their sputum.*

RELATED TEST

Bronchoscopy (p. 587). This is an endoscopic test through which pulmonary lavage can be performed and specimens for cytologic examination can be obtained.

Throat and Nose Cultures

NORMAL FINDINGS

Negative

INDICATIONS

A throat or nose culture is obtained to diagnose bacterial, viral, gonococcal, or candidal pharyngitis. It is indicated on patients who complain of a sore throat, have a fever of unknown cause, or may be chronic carriers of recurrent infection. Nose cultures are used to identify acute nasal and/or sinus infections and to identify carriers of pathogenic bacteria.

TEST EXPLANATION

Because the *throat* is normally colonized by many organisms, culture of this area serves only to isolate and identify a few particular pathogens (e.g., streptococci, meningococci, gonococci, *Bordetella pertussis, Corynebacterium diphtheriae*). Recognition of these organisms requires treatment. Streptococci are most often sought, because a beta-hemolytic streptococcal pharyngitis (Figure 7-10) may be followed by rheumatic fever or glomerulonephritis. This type of streptococcal infection most frequently affects children between the ages of 3 and 15 years. Therefore all children with a sore throat and fever should

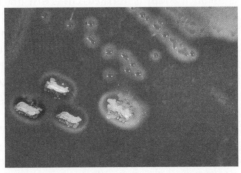

Figure 7-10 Blood agar plate showing beta-hemolytic colonies (clear zone around colony) of group A streptococci, the organism that causes bacterial pharyngitis.

Microscopic Studies

7

have a throat culture done to attempt to identify streptococcal infections. In adults, however, fewer than 5% of patients with pharyngitis have a streptococcal infection. Therefore throat cultures in adults are indicated only when the patient has severe or recurrent sore throat, often associated with fever and palpable lymphadenopathy. These adults often have a history of previous streptococcal infections.

Because Streptococcal pharyngitis remains an important cause of morbidity and is one of the leading reasons for physician visits, it is essential to focus on this organism specifically with throat and nose cultures. Although there are clinical algorithms to assess the probability that pharyngitis is caused by *Streptococcus pyogenes*, the diagnosis of streptococcal pharyngitis cannot be made on clinical grounds alone. Same-day testing by Rapid Antigen Detection Test *(strept screen)* is an important strategy to reduce unnecessary antibiotic use. With these strept screen kits, the streptococcus organism can be identified directly from the swab specimen. The streptococcus is chemically or enzymatically extracted from the swab specimen. It is then tested with the antisera containing the antibodies to group A streptococcus antigen. ELISA (chromatographic immunoassay) are used to detect group A streptococcus. This is a qualitative study with positive and negative results being color coded (in most kits). Obviously some kits perform better than others. False-negative results may occur with any test method if the specimen contains small numbers of streptococci (early in the course of the infection). Therefore a good throat swab is crucial. All antigen-negative swabs should have the negative result confirmed by culture. The rapid serologic tests can be performed in about 15 minutes in any lab or in most physicians' offices that treat children. The final culture report takes at least 2 days.

Infections by group A streptococci are unique because they can be followed by a serious complication (e.g., rheumatic fever, scarlet fever, or glomerulonephritis). Serologic tests (p. 470) are used primarily to determine if a previous group A *Streptococcus* infection (e.g., pharyngitis, pyodermia, pneumonia) has occurred and is the cause of a post-streptococcal disease. These post-streptococcal diseases occur following the infection and after a period of latency during which the patient is asymptomatic. The latency period for glomerulonephritis is approximately 10 days, and for rheumatic fever is about 20 days.

Antibodies (e.g., anti-streptolysin O and antideoxyribonuclease) are directed against streptococcal extracellular products that are primarily enzymatic proteins. Serial rising titers of these antibodies over several weeks, followed by a slow fall in titers, are more supportive than a single titer in the diagnosis of a previous streptococcal infection. The highest incidence of positive results is during the third week after the onset of acute symptoms of the poststreptococcal disease. By 6 months, only about 30% of patients have abnormal titers. By 12 months, levels return to normal.

A routine throat culture uses several different types of culture media (chocolate, streptococcus-specific, and other agar) to grow various bacteria. When a specific streptococcus culture is requested or if the strept screen is negative, the specimen is plated on streptococcus-specific agar only. All cultures should be performed before antibiotic therapy is initiated. Otherwise, the antibiotic may interrupt the growth of the organism in the laboratory. More often than not, however, the physician will want to institute antibiotic therapy before the culture results are reported. In these instances, a Gram stain of the specimen smeared on a slide is most helpful and can be reported in less than 10 minutes. All forms of bacteria are grossly classified as gram-positive (blue staining) or gram-negative (red staining). Knowledge of the shape of the organism (e.g., spherical [coccus], rod-shaped [bacillus]) also can be very helpful in the tentative identification of the infecting organism. With knowledge of the Gram stain results, the physician can institute a reasonable antibiotic regimen based on past experience regarding the organism's possible identity and sensitivity. Most organisms take approximately 24 hours to grow in the laboratory, and a preliminary report can be given at that time. Occasionally, a period of 48 to 72 hours is required for growth and identification of the organism. Cultures may be repeated on completion of appropriate antibiotic therapy to identify resolution of the infection.

Nasal and *pharyngeal* cultures are often done to screen for infections and carrier states caused by various other organisms such as *Staphylococcus aureus*, *Haemophilus influenzae*, *Neisseria meningitidis*, respiratory syncytial virus (RSV), and viruses containing rhinitis. Health care workers in the operating room and newborn nursery may have these cultures performed to screen potential sources of spread once an outbreak occurs in a hospital setting. These cultures are also used to detect infection in elderly and debilitated patients.

INTERFERING FACTORS

Drugs that may affect test results include antibiotics and antiseptic mouthwashes.

PROCEDURE AND PATIENT CARE

Before

Explain the procedure to the patient.

During

- Obtain a *throat culture* by depressing the tongue with a wooden tongue blade and touching the posterior wall of the throat (Figure 7-11) and areas of inflammation, exudation, or ulceration with a sterile cotton swab. Two swabs are preferred. Growth of streptococcus from both swabs is more accurate, and the second swab can also be used in the strept screen. Avoid touching any other part of the mouth. Place the swabs in a sterile container.
- Obtain a *nasal culture* by gently raising the tip of the nose and inserting a flexible swab into the nares. Rotate the swab against the side of the nares. Remove the swab and place it in an appropriate culture tube.
- Obtain a *pharyngeal culture* by gently raising the tip of the nose and inserting a flexible swab along the bottom of the nares. Guide this swab until it reaches the posterior pharynx. Rotate the swab to obtain secretions and then remove it. Place the swab in an appropriate culture tube.
- Wear gloves and handle the specimen as if it were capable of transmitting disease.
- Place the swab in a sterile container and send it to the microbiology laboratory within 30 minutes.
- Note the following *special considerations for specimen collection in young children:*
  1. An adult should hold the child on his or her lap.
  2. The person obtaining the specimen places one hand on the child's forehead to stabilize the head.
  3. The collection is then obtained in a manner similar to that for adults.

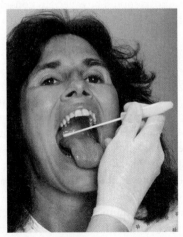

Figure 7-11 Collection of specimen from posterior pharynx.

Microscopic Studies

7

After

- Notify the health care provider of any positive results so that appropriate antibiotic therapy can be initiated.

TEST RESULTS AND CLINICAL SIGNIFICANCE

Acute pharyngitis: *Throat cultures are used to identify pathogenic bacteria such as streptococci,* Coryne-bacterium diphtheriae, *gonococci,* Bordetella pertussis, Neisseria, *and staphylococci.* Candida, *and* Bordetella *infections can also be identified.*

Tonsillar infections: *These infections can be identified and their source determined if the swab is applied adequately to the tonsillar areas.*

Chronic nasal carriers of bacteria: *Some people are chronic carriers of bacterial diseases that can initiate an infection when transferred to others. These people may carry staphylococci, streptococci, influenza, or respiratory syncytial virus.*

RELATED TEST

Streptococcus Serologic Testing (p. 470). This antibody panel is used to identify previous Group A streptococcus infections in a patient who is considered to have a post-streptococcus disease such as rheumatic fever or glomerulonephritis.

Tuberculosis Culture (TB Culture, BACTEC Method, Polymerase Chain Reaction, AFB Smear)

NORMAL FINDINGS

Negative for tuberculosis

INDICATIONS

TB culture is indicated in any patient with a persistent productive cough, night sweats, anorexia, weight loss, fever, and hemoptysis. This diagnosis should be especially considered in high-risk patients, such as those who are immunocompromised, have alcoholism, or have had a recent exposure to TB.

TEST EXPLANATION

The diagnosis of TB can be made only by identification and culture of *Mycobacterium tuberculosis* in the specimen. (See p. 1126 for other TB testing.) Conventional culture techniques for growth, identification, and susceptibility testing of acid-fast mycobacterium take 4 to 6 weeks. Because the patient suspected of having TB cannot be isolated from society for that duration, the disease may spread to many other people while the patient is waiting for the diagnosis. With the resurgence and increasing incidence of TB in the U.S. population (especially among immunocompromised patients with acquired immunodeficiency syndrome [AIDS]), newer, more rapid culture techniques have been identified and are now being utilized.

The BACTEC method is a radiometric culture technique in which the growth medium for culturing mycobacteria is supplanted with a substrate labeled with radioactive carbon (^{14}C). This substrate is used by mycobacteria, and during metabolism, radioactive carbon dioxide ($^{14}CO_2$) is produced from the substrate. The $^{14}CO_2$ is detected quantitatively by counting the radioactivity with the Becton Dickinson Diagnostic Instrument System. The rate and amount of CO_2 produced is directly proportional to the rate and amount of growth occurring on the medium. With this technique, very small quantities of $^{14}CO_2$ can be detected. This permits quick identification of mycobacterial growth. This technique is used not only to isolate mycobacteria from clinical specimens but also to differentiate *M. tuberculosis* complex from other mycobacteria and for antimicrobial susceptibility testing.

Polymerase chain reaction (PCR) genotyping has been developed. With the addition of a deoxyribonucleic acid (DNA) polymerase, genetic chromosomal parts can be multiplied. This allows amplification of genomes, which then can be detected by genetic DNA probes. With genotyping, *M. tuberculosis* can be identified in as little as 36 to 48 hours. With this reduction in diagnostic time, treatment can be started earlier. It is anticipated that the spread of TB therefore will be greatly reduced. The average detection time, however, is longer for extrapulmonary specimens than for sputum specimens. The time for identification is greatly reduced when numerous mycobacteria are present. Generally organisms in specimens from patients already receiving antituberculosis treatment take longer to grow.

After identification and growth of mycobacteria, antibiotic susceptibility testing is performed to identify the most effective antimycobacterial drugs. The culture can be performed on sputum, body fluids, cerebrospinal fluid (CSF), and even biopsy tissue specimens.

When tuberculosis is suspected, a sputum smear for *acid-fast bacillus (AFB)* can be obtained. After taking up a dye, such as fuchsin, *M. tuberculosis* is not decolorized by acid alcohol (i.e., it is acid-fast). It is seen under the microscope as a red, rod-shaped organism. If this bacillus is seen, the patient may have active TB. Other specimens, such as cerebrospinal fluid, tissue, and synovial fluid, may be used. AFB is also used to monitor treatment for TB. If after adequate therapy (2 months) the sputum still contains AFB (even though the culture may be negative because of anti-TB drugs), treatment failure should be considered.

INTERFERING FACTORS

🏺 Antituberculosis drugs that have been started prior to culture could interfere with the growth of TB.

PROCEDURE AND PATIENT CARE

Before

🖎 Explain the procedure to the patient.
🖎 Tell the patient that no fasting is required.

During

- For sputum, obtain an early morning specimen. It is best to induce sputum production with an ultrasonic or nebulizing device.
- Collect three to five early morning specimens. All specimens must contain mycobacteria to make the diagnosis of TB.
- For urine collection, obtain three to five single, clean-voided specimens early in the morning.
- Note that swabs, intestinal washings, and biopsy specimens should be transported to the laboratory immediately for preparation.
- Follow the institution's policy for universal specimen handling. Staff should wear an N95 respirator mask when in contact with the patient. Ideally, the patient should be placed in a negative pressure room.
- Note the following procedural steps:
  1. Once the specimen is received by the laboratory, a decontamination process is applied to it to kill all non-mycobacteria. The specimen is then cultured in the appropriate medium.
  2. With the rapid growth techniques, the specimen is evaluated every 24 hours.

3. When cultural growth is considered adequate, the organisms are stained for acid-fast bacilli and identified (p. 706).

4. With DNA genetic probes, the *Mycobacterium* species is identified.

5. At this point, if *M. tuberculosis* is present, the report will read "culture is positive for mycobacteria." If the species has been identified, this also will be reported.

6. Drug-susceptibility testing then will be carried out and subsequently reported.

After

Instruct the patient in appropriate isolation of sputum and other body fluids to avoid potential spread of suspected TB.

TEST RESULTS AND CLINICAL SIGNIFICANCE

TB

Atypical mycobacterial nontuberculous disease: *These organisms require special medium plates to grow. Any fluid or tissue can be used as a culture specimen. If the lungs are considered to be the sight of infection, sputum or pleural fluid is used. If the kidneys are suspected to be involved, urine should be tested. Others specimens include abdominal fluid, stomach aspirate, and bone tissue.*

RELATED TESTS

Acid-Fast Bacilli Smear (p. 706). This smear is used to support the diagnosis of TB because it cannot, by itself, indicate the diagnosis of TB. The smear (usually of sputum) is also used to monitor treatment for TB.

Tuberculin Skin Testing (p. 1126). Purified protein derivative is administered intradermally to test for prior exposure to TB. Skin testing cannot indicate active or dormant TB. Positive results imply nothing more than previous exposure.

Chest X-Ray (p. 1014). Because TB is usually infective to the lungs due to inhalation of airborne infectious material, the chest x-ray examination often demonstrates the results (Ghon complex) of the acute granulomatous infection.

Interferon Gamma Release Assay (QuantiFERON-TB Gold) (see following test). The IGRA is a whole-blood test for use as an aid in diagnosing *Mycobacterium tuberculosis* infection. It is a measure of the patient's cell–mediated immune response to TB infection.

> **Tuberculosis Testing** (TB Testing, Interferon Gamma Release Assay [IGRA], QuantiFERON-TB Gold [QFT, QFT-G, TB Gold Test, TB Blood Test], Nucleic Acid Amplification for TB [NAAT], TB Antibody)

NORMAL FINDINGS

IGRA Result	Interpretation
Positive	*Mycobacterium tuberculosis* infection likely
Negative	*Mycobacterium tuberculosis* infection unlikely, but cannot be excluded. If TB disease is highly suspected, a negative result does not rule out infection. False-negative results may be seen in immunocompromised patients.

IGRA Result	Interpretation
Indeterminate	Test not interpretable. Collection of a new specimen for testing is recommended if clinically indicated.

INDICATIONS

These tests are used to diagnose active TB infection in patients recently exposed to or suspected to have TB infection.

TEST EXPLANATION

Interferon gamma release assays (IGRA) (e.g., QuantiFERON-TB), NAA tests, and serologic TB testing are used to diagnose active TB infection. The gold standard for making the diagnosis of active TB is the TB culture (p. 768). However, it takes 2 to 6 weeks to obtain results. Identifying acid-fast bacilli in a smear (AFB smear) (p. 706) of the body fluid (usually sputum) is a rapid method of identifying TB in 24 hours. Unfortunately, AFB is not very sensitive or specific. It is often positive in non-tuberculosis mycobacterial diseases. The IGRA is a whole-blood test used in diagnosing *Mycobacterium tuberculosis* infection. The NAAT is a rapid and accurate test of sputum and is used as corroborative information in the diagnosis of TB. Serology testing on blood is also a rapid test used to identify active TB disease infection (Table 7-3).

The value of decreasing the time it takes to make the diagnosis of TB is significant. With an earlier laboratory confirmation of TB disease, treatment can be initiated earlier, patient outcome can be improved, opportunities to interrupt transmission of the disease can be increased, and more effective public health interventions can be instigated. For those reasons, there has been increasing clinical interest in establishing the diagnosis of TB as early as possible. IGRA TB antibody testing and NAA can provide rapid confirmation of TB infection. However, these tests cannot indicate anti-TB drug sensitivities.

The diagnosis of active or latent TB still requires additional testing (including a chest x-ray, sputum smear, and culture). IGRA is a diagnostic aid that measures a component of cell-mediated immune reactivity to *M. tuberculosis*, much like the tuberculin skin testing (TST) (p. 1126). The TST is performed by injecting a small amount of tuberculin purified protein derivative (PPD) into the forearm and examining the injection site at 48 to 72 hours after administration. This skin test assesses an in vivo

Microscopic Studies

7

TABLE 7-3   CDC Recommendations for Initial Sputum Specimens for TB Diagnosis

AFB Smear	NAAT	Diagnosis	Treatment
+	+	TB	Start therapy
−	+	? TB	Await culture results
			Start therapy?
+	−	? TB	Test for PCR inhibitors*
			Repeat NAAT
			Start therapy?
−	−	? TB	Await culture
			Consider other testing

*Inhibitors may include blood, fabrics, tissues, excess salts, ionic detergents, sarkosyl, ethanol, isopropanol, and phenol.

delayed-type hypersensitivity immune response to a polyvalent antigenic mixture in PPD. Unlike TST, however, IGRA can be performed on patients with prior *bacille Calmette-Guérin* (BCG) vaccination without causing a hypersensitivity response. Furthermore, compared with TST, IGRA results are not subject to reader bias and error. Like TST, false negatives can occur in anergic patients.

IGRA cannot differentiate active from latent TB infection. Its use in latent infection is being studied. Because IGRA uses TB-specific antigens as compared with TST that uses nonspecific PPD antigens, IGRA is more accurate and specific. IGRA results are available in 24 hours. Because this is an in vitro test that never exposes the patient to its antigenic proteins, IGRA never generates a "booster" false-positive response. Finally, the elimination of a second patient visit for skin reading makes IGRA an attractive alternative to TST. IGRA can be used for serial surveillance testing up to 12 months after a negative PPD if the initial IGRA is negative.

IGRA and NAAT are used in the same patient population as TST. These include contact investigations, evaluation of recent immigrants, and sequential-testing surveillance programs for infection control, such as those for health care workers.

The IGRA is an ELISA test in which blood samples are mixed with synthetic PPD protein derivative antigens (ESAT-6, TB7.7, and CFP-10). After incubation of the blood with these antigens for 16 to 24 hours, interferon-gamma (IFN-γ) from T-cell lymphocytes is measured. If the patient's T-cell lymphocytes are sensitized to *Mycobacterium tuberculosis* complex organisms (i.e., *Mycobacterium tuberculosis, Mycobacterium bovis, Mycobacterium africanum, Mycobacterium microti,* and *Mycobacterium canetti*), the T-cell lymphocytes in their blood that recognize specific mycobacterial antigens and their lymphocytes will release large quantities of IFN-γ in response to contact with the TB antigens.

The IGRA may be falsely negative in patients with advanced TB because of a suppressed IFN response. The IGRA (unlike some skin tests) does not test for anergy and may be inaccurately negative in immunosuppressed patients. The sensitivity and rate of indeterminate results using IGRA is diminished in immunocompromised persons with HIV infection, AIDS, current treatment with immunosuppressive drugs, selected hematologic disorders, and certain malignancies. These conditions or treatments are known or suspected to decrease responsiveness to the TST, and they might also decrease production of IFN-γ in the IGRA assay. As with a negative TST result, negative IGRA results alone might be insufficient to exclude tuberculosis infection in these persons.

NAAT is designed to identify TB complex DNA in a body fluid (bronchoalveolar lavage, bronchial washing, sputum, stool, pleural/abdominal fluid, tissue, or urine sample). This test provides a rapid result in 24 hours. Like the described rapid tests, NAAT cannot indicate active infection from a previously treated TB infection. NAAT is now standard practice in the United States to aid in the initial diagnosis of patients suspected to have TB. The Centers for Disease Control has indicated that NAAT should be performed on at least one respiratory specimen for each patient with signs and symptoms of pulmonary TB for whom a diagnosis of TB is being considered but is not yet been established and for whom the test results would alter case management.

TB antibody serology is designed to identify IgG antibodies to TB mycobacteria in patients with active TB infections. This blood test can be used in previously vaccinated BCG patients. It is particularly useful in evaluating the effectiveness of anti-TB therapy and documenting a response to therapy. Like IGRA, serology may not be positive in immunocompromised patients, making its use in HIV-infected patients less helpful.

INTERFERING FACTORS

- Heterophile (e.g., human antimouse) antibodies in serum or plasma of certain individuals are known to cause interference with immunoassays. These antibodies from other inflammatory conditions may interfere with specific responses to ESAT-6, CFP-10, or TB7.7 peptides, leading to indeterminate and unreliable results.

- A false-negative interferon gamma release assay (IGRA) result can be caused by the stage of infection (i.e., specimen obtained before the development of cellular immune response), comorbid conditions that affect immune function, or other individual immunologic factors.

PROCEDURE AND PATIENT CARE

Before

⚕ Explain the procedure to the patient or the family.

During

- Collect 1 mL whole blood in each of three lab-specified collection tubes. The accuracy of the IGRA is dependent on the proper collection and incubation of the blood specimen. Blood should fill the tube as close to the 1-mL mark as possible. Underfilling or overfilling the tubes outside the 0.8- to 1.2-mL range may lead to erroneous results.
- Immediately following collection, each specimen tube must be shaken vigorously by shaking the tube up and down 10 times to ensure that the entire inner surface of the tube has been coated with blood. This distributes the stimulating antigens, allowing optimal processing and presentation of the antigens to T cells, which causes release of IFN-γ.
- For NAAT testing, 1 to 3 mL of sputum or body fluid is required. This should be refrigerated in a screw cap sterile container.

After

- Apply pressure or a pressure dressing to the venipuncture site.
- Incubate the blood tubes upright at 37° C for 16 to 24 hours (within 16 hours of collection).

⚕ If the patient's results are positive, educate him or her about the necessary follow-up studies, such as chest radiograph and sputum cultures.

TEST RESULTS AND CLINICAL SIGNIFICANCE

▲ Increased Levels

TB Infection: *Patients with active or dormant TB infections will have elevated levels unless the TB is so advanced as to cause immunodeficiency.*

RELATED TESTS

Tuberculin Skin Testing (p. 1126). This skin test is performed on patients suspected to have TB infection.

Tuberculosis Culture (p. 768). This is the gold standard, most sensitive test for diagnosing mycobacteria.

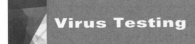
Virus Testing

NORMAL FINDINGS

Negative for viral antibody or antigen
No virus isolated in culture

INDICATIONS

This test is used to diagnose viral diseases and document treatment and immunity.

TEST EXPLANATION

Viral infections are the most common infections affecting children and adults. Viruses are subdivided by the nuclear material they contain (ribonucleic acid [RNA] or deoxyribonucleic acid [DNA]). Infections from viruses are often indistinguishable from bacterial infections. Testing for a virus is indicated when a person with viral symptoms lives or has traveled to an area harboring the virus. Testing is done in the clinical setting when a patient has severe symptoms contributing to significant morbidity. Testing is also performed for epidemiologic reasons to identify a viral outbreak and its extent. Finally, testing can indicate immunity after exposure to the virus or a vaccination.

Viral testing is performed by identifying:

1. Antibodies to a specific antigen in the blood or in other body fluids (e.g., mononucleosis or Epstein-Barr)
2. Antigen parts of the virus by Reverse Transcription Polymerase Chain Reaction (RT-PCR) (e.g., respiratory syncytial or influenza A or B) or Nucleic Acid Amplification Tests (NAAT) (e.g., Dengue)
3. Virus cultured in special media
4. Virus by electron microscopy

Epstein-Barr (p. 217), hepatitis (p. 286), respiratory syncytial, herpes, parainfluenza, HIV (p. 297), Dengue fever, Coxsackie, choriomeningitis, mumps, West Nile (p. 524), arbovirus, equine, cytomegalovirus (p. 200), rubella (p. 457), and influenza A, B are some of the viruses that have highest clinical priorities today.

Most viral infections have common symptoms that are flu-like and include fever, lethargy, headache, and neck/body aches. Certain patients (including infants, the elderly, the immunocompromised, and those with impaired lung function) are at risk for serious complications. Once the diagnosis is confirmed, where possible, aggressive antiviral treatment can be instigated and isolation can be carried out.

Front-line testing measures IgM or IgG antibodies to the virus may or may not be specific to that particular virus. If the front-line testing is positive, confirmatory tests may be carried out. This testing is important for public health officials and researchers. Test results may not correlate with cultures or viral load. Yet for other viral diseases, serology acts as the confirmatory test.

Viral RNA/DNA can be detected by RT-PCR (or in combination with NAAT) in serum (Dengue), or respiratory secretions, including upper and lower respiratory specimens (RSV or influenza). Nasopharyngeal swabs or aspirates are the preferred specimen types. This is particularly useful for suspected infections by influenza A, influenza B, and RSV. Molecular detection of influenza A and B RNA is also available. The sensitivity of the assay is very dependent upon the quality of the specimen submitted. Tracheal aspirates are not acceptable for testing because of the viscous nature of these specimens. Test accuracy depends on viral load in the specimen. Unlike serology, this testing is very specific for the suspected virus. RT PCR viral testing is often performed as panel testing, for example, *respiratory virus panel*. This panel, typically performed on a nasopharyngeal swab or bronchial mucus specimen, is able to detect 12 viruses/viral subtypes (adenovirus, rhinovirus, human meta-pneumovirus, RSV types A/B, parainfluenza types 1 to 3, influenza B, influenza A [with subtypes H1 and H3]). Viral RNA/DNA testing has advantages that make this testing preferable (Box 7-2).

Growth and identification of the virus in culture from a patient specimen provides a definitive diagnosis when positive. The ability to isolate a virus in culture depends on many aspects of the culture process. The first is determining the correct specimen for culture. That depends on the organ involved

BOX 7-2	Advantages of Viral RNA/DNA PCR Testing

- More rapid detection
- Greater recovery of the infecting virus
- Ability to subtype the virus
- Detection of multiple viral infections

TABLE 7-4	Specimen Culture for Common Viruses and Diseases

Common Virus	Specimens	Disease
Adenovirus	Throat culture	Influenza
Influenza	Bronchoscopic aspiration	Pneumonia
Respiratory syncytial	Nose culture	Pharyngitis
Rhinovirus	—	Common cold
Rubella	Throat culture	Skin rash
Rubeola	Skin vesicle	Zoster
Coxsackie	—	Hand, foot, and mouth
Varicella	—	Chickenpox
Arbovirus	Throat culture	Meningitis
Enterovirus	Cerebrospinal fluid (CSF)	Encephalitis
Herpes	Blood	
Cytomegalovirus	Urine, sputum, mouth	CMV infection
Parvovirus	Stool	Skin rash
Adenovirus	Blood	Arthropathy
	Sputum	Upper respiratory infection
Influenza A or B	Throat culture	Flu syndrome
Epstein-Barr	Blood	Mononucleosis
		Epstein-Barr–associated disease

and the type of virus suspected (Table 7-4). Timing is important. Viral load is always greatest in the early stages of the disease. Cultures obtained in the first few days after symptoms begin offer the best chance of identifying the infective culture. Using the correct culture medium is essential. In general, the culture medium used to grow the viral culture is a tissue/cell culture. Different viruses vary greatly in their ability to grow in specific cell cultures. Viral cultures take 3 to 7 days to be reported. Culture results are not an indication of viral load, severity of disease, or disease progression/response to therapy.

INTERFERING FACTORS

- Inadequate specimen, timing, or choice of culture medium will cause false-negative tests.
- The use of a cotton swab or wooden applicator for specimen collection may destroy the virus.

PROCEDURE AND PATIENT CARE

Before

 Explain the procedure to the patient and family.

During

- If blood is the specimen, obtain a venous blood sample in the appropriate tube as determined by the laboratory.
- For other body fluid samples, such as nasopharyngeal or sputum, follow the guidelines below:
    1. Use a closed specimen system to obtain and transport the specimen to the laboratory.
    2. Transport the specimen immediately to the laboratory. Viruses in specimens quickly lose their vitality.
    3. Place samples on ice if delivery to the laboratory is not immediate.
    4. Small volume specimens (e.g., tissue aspirates) are often best transported in a liquid medium. If bacterial cultures are to be performed, use sterile saline solution for transfer.

After

Explain to patient and family that, in most circumstances, testing is carried out at a referral laboratory.

Inform patients that they should observe isolation precautions until results are negative.

Explain that results may not be available for 2 weeks.

TEST RESULTS AND CLINICAL SIGNIFICANCE

Viral Infections (acute and chronic) (see Table 7-4).

RELATED TESTS

Throat and Nose Cultures (p. 765). This test is obtained to diagnose bacterial, viral, gonococcal, or candidal pharyngitis.

Specific discussions are included for each of the following viruses:

Cytomegalovirus (p. 200)
Epstein-Barr (p. 217)
Hepatitis (p. 286)
Herpes (p. 731)
HIV (p. 297)
Rubella (p. 457)
West Nile (p. 524)

Wound and Soft-Tissue Culture and Sensitivity (C&S)

NORMAL FINDINGS

Negative

INDICATIONS

A wound or soft tissue culture is indicated when a wound or soft tissue has signs of infection (redness, warmth, swelling, and pain). In a postoperative patient with a persistent fever of unknown origin, a wound may be probed and cultured even if the signs of infection are not present. Any spontaneous drainage from a wound or soft tissue should be cultured to document infection for treatment and drug sensitivities and to document the appropriateness of skin and wound isolation precautions.

TEST EXPLANATION

Wound cultures are obtained to determine the presence of pathogens in patients with suspected wound infections. Wound infections are most often caused by pus-forming organisms. All cultures should be performed before antibiotic therapy is initiated. Otherwise, the antibiotic may interrupt the growth of the organism in the laboratory. More often than not, however, the physician will want to institute antibiotic therapy after the wound is cultured but before the culture results are reported. In these instances, a *Gram stain* of the specimen smeared on a slide is most helpful and can be reported in less than 10 minutes. All forms of bacteria are grossly classified as gram-positive (blue staining) or gram-negative (red staining). Knowledge of the shape of the organism (e.g., spherical, rod shaped) also may be very helpful in the tentative identification of the infecting organism. With knowledge of the Gram stain results, the physician can institute a reasonable antibiotic regimen based on past experience regarding the organism's possible identity. Most organisms require approximately 24 hours to grow in the laboratory, and a preliminary report can be given at that time. Occasionally 48 to 72 hours are required for growth and identification of the organism. Cultures may be repeated after appropriate antibiotic therapy to assess for complete resolution of the infection.

It is important to recognize that many wound infections contain more than one organism. Multiple organisms may grow on culture. Deep-space wounds, wounds containing necrotic debris or gas, and postoperative wounds commonly contain aerobic and anaerobic bacteria. These different types of organisms require different culture media and conditions for growth.

INTERFERING FACTORS

Drugs that may alter test results include antibiotics.

PROCEDURE AND PATIENT CARE

Before
- Explain the procedure to the patient.
- Assemble all equipment (Figure 7-12).

During
- Aseptically place a sterile cotton swab into the pus of the patient's wound, and then place the swab into a sterile, covered test tube. (Culturing specimens from the skin edge is much less accurate than culturing the suppurative material.)
- If an anaerobic organism is suspected, obtain an anaerobic culture tube from the microbiology laboratory. The specimen is best obtained by aspirating a closed wound and directly transferring the pus to the anaerobic culture tube.
- If wound cultures are to be obtained on a patient requiring wound irrigation, obtain the culture before the wound is irrigated.

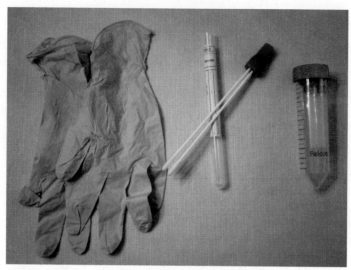

Figure 7-12 Equipment for collection of specimens from an open wound or decubitus ulcer. The specimen obtained with red-tipped applicators is immediately placed into its protective tube. The specimen is adequate for aerobic and anaerobic cultures. Large-volume fluid specimens may be placed in the blue-tipped container. However, this type of container must be transported immediately to the lab if anaerobic cultures are to be added to aerobic cultures.

- If any antibiotic ointment or solution has been previously applied, remove it with sterile water or saline before obtaining the culture several hours later.
- Handle all specimens carefully. These specimens are capable of transmitting disease.
- Indicate on the laboratory slip any medications the patient may be taking that could affect test results.

After

- Transport the specimen to the laboratory immediately after testing (within no more than 30 minutes).
- Notify the physician of any positive results so that appropriate antibiotic therapy can be initiated.
- Note that if pus was observed in the wound or soft tissue, the patient should be immediately placed on skin and wound isolative precautions. The culture report documenting the infection does not need to be received before appropriate protective precautions are instituted.

TEST RESULTS AND CLINICAL SIGNIFICANCE

Wound infection: *The best treatment of a wound infection is incision (widely opening the infection) and providing good drainage. Antibiotics are secondary.*

Nuclear Scanning

Overview

REASONS FOR PERFORMING NUCLEAR MEDICINE STUDIES

With the administration of a radiopharmaceutical and subsequent detection of the photons emitted from a particular organ, anatomic and functional abnormalities of various body areas can be detected. Nuclear medicine studies do not identify the specific cause (disease) of the abnormality. They provide supportive information to be used in conjunction with other diagnostic modalities. There are many indications for nuclear scanning, some of which are listed below:

1. To stage cancer by detecting metastasis (PET scan)—or to test specific organs such as the bone (bone scan), liver (liver scan), or brain (brain scan)
2. To diagnose acute and chronic cholecystitis (gallbladder scan)

3. To detect cerebral pathologic conditions (brain scan)
4. To evaluate gastric emptying (gastric emptying scan)
5. To localize sites of gastrointestinal (GI) bleeding (GI bleeding scan)
6. To diagnose pulmonary embolism (lung scan)
7. To determine perfusion, structure, and function of the kidneys (renal scan) or heart (cardiac scan)
8. To evaluate thyroid nodules (thyroid scan)
9. To evaluate testicular swelling and pain (scrotal scan)
10. To evaluate cardiac function and coronary artery patency

The radionuclides used in diagnostic medicine are artificially produced by either a nuclear reactor or a charged particle accelerator (cyclotron) by irradiating the nuclei and causing them to be unstable. Because of this instability, the nucleus of the radionuclide atom emits radioactive particles (photons in the gamma radiation range). The radionuclides used in nuclear scanning have short half-lives, which refers to the time required for 50% of the radioactive atoms to undergo decay. Technetium-99m (^{99m}Tc) is used extensively in nuclear scanning because its half-life is 6 hours and it emits low levels of gamma rays. Other commonly used radionuclides include gallium, thallium, and iodine.

To get to the desired organ, radionuclides are combined with a transport molecule. This combination of radionuclide and transport molecule is called a *radiopharmaceutical.* A radiopharmaceutical is the compound, labeled with the radionuclide that is administered to the patient and localized in the organ to be studied. For most nuclear scans, radiopharmaceuticals are given intravenously. Less commonly used methods of administration include the oral and inhalation routes. Radiopharmaceuticals concentrate in target organs by various mechanisms. For example, some labeled compounds, such as iodohippurate sodium ^{131}I (Hippuran ^{131}I), are cleared from the blood and excreted by the kidneys. Some phosphate compounds concentrate in the bone and infarcted tissue. Lung function can be studied by imaging the distribution of inhaled gases and aerosols. Other radiopharmaceuticals (such as FDG) are selectively taken up by cancers.

After the radioisotope concentrates in the desired area, it emits gamma rays. The area is scanned with a gamma camera or a scintillation scanner that detects and records the emission of gamma rays. With each gamma ray detected, a light particle is emitted from the scintillation scanner. A computer translates these light readings into a two-dimensional image or scan (scintigram) that is printed in various shades of gray. Using multiple scanners, a three-dimensional image (SPECT) can be obtained. Scintigrams can now be produced in color. The shades of gray or color show the distribution of the radionuclide in the organ. When superimposed on a baseline computerized tomogram (PET/CT), accurate anatomy can be created. Hot spots are areas of increased uptake, and cold spots are areas with decreased uptake of the radionuclide. Normally the uptake of the radionuclide in an organ is diffuse and homogeneous. Hot and cold spots may mean different things on different scans. For example, a cold spot identified in the liver, spleen, or brain would indicate tumor, abscess, or some other space-occupying lesion. A cold spot detected on a thallium scan of the heart would not be suggestive of tumor but rather indicates an area of ischemia or infarction. On bone scan, hot spots may indicate areas of osteoblastic activity surrounding tumor. Arthritis or fracture may also be evident as hot spots. The scanning usually takes place in the nuclear medicine department.

Scanning can be *static,* which means that the patient and the camera are held in one position until an image is completed. Often the patient is rotated into another position for a static image of another view of the same organ. *Dynamic* scanning can also be performed and allows one to evaluate the blood flow to a certain organ, such as the brain or the liver. Single-photon emission computed tomography (SPECT) is a technique in which a gamma camera is serially placed at multiple angles around the entire circumference of the patient. With this method, three-dimensional images can be obtained of the organ to be studied. Increased sensitivity is obtained. Positron emission tomography (PET) scanning can demonstrate anatomic, functional, and biochemical abnormalities in an organ.

Although nuclear scanning includes a risk of radiation for the patient, the risk associated with most radionuclides is much less than that of an x-ray study. The half-lives of the radioisotopes are short, resulting in minimal radiation contamination by way of fecal and urine wastes. Unless the benefit outweighs the risk, nuclear scans are contraindicated in pregnant women and nursing mothers because of the risk of injury to the fetus or infant. To help protect patients and others, patients should take some precautions for 12 hours after injection of radionuclides. Whenever possible, a toilet should be used, rather than a urinal. The toilet should be flushed several times after each use. Spilled urine should be cleaned up completely. After each voiding or fecal elimination, patients should thoroughly wash their hands. All urine- or fecal-soiled clothes should be washed separately.

PROCEDURAL CARE FOR NUCLEAR SCANS

Before

⚡ Explain the procedure to the patient. Assure the patient that radiation exposure is limited and minimal.

- Assess for an allergy to the radiopharmaceutical (especially when iodine is used).
- Note whether the patient has had any recent exposure to radionuclides. The previous study could interfere with the interpretation of the current study.
- Record the patient's age and current weight. This information is sometimes used to calculate the amount of radioactive substance needed.
- Many of the scanning procedures do not require any preparation. However, a few have special requirements. For example, in bone scanning the patient is encouraged to drink several glasses of water between the time of the injection of the isotope and the actual scanning.
- For some studies, blocking agents may need to be given to prevent other organs from taking up the isotope. For example, Lugol iodine solution may be needed to protect the thyroid gland from iodine-tagged radioisotopes. Potassium chloride may be used during a brain scan to prevent an inordinate amount of technetium uptake by the choroid plexus, which would simulate a pathologic condition.

During

- Most radionuclides are injected intravenously. Often the patient is encouraged to drink water between administration of the rad7ioisotope and the scanning. Radionuclides can also be given orally (gastric emptying scan) or by inhalation (ventilation scan).
- The area is scanned at the designated time period. The delay between administration of the radionuclide and scanning depends on the length of time required for the specific organ or tissue to take up the radionuclide and concentrate it. The patient must lie still during the scanning. Scans are usually repeated over a period that may extend from 1 hour to 3 days. The patient returns to the nuclear medicine department for each scanning.

After

⚡ Assure the patient that only tracer doses of radioisotopes have been used and that no precautions against radioactive exposure are necessary.

- Although the amount of radionuclide excreted in the urine is very low, rubber gloves are sometimes recommended if the urine must be handled. Some doctors may advise the patient to flush the toilet several times after voiding.

⚡ Encourage the patient to drink extra fluids to aid in excretion of the isotope from the body.

- If the isotope was injected intravenously, inspect the site for signs of infection, bruising, or hematoma.

REPORTING OF RESULTS

Most tests are performed by a nuclear medicine technologist in the nuclear medicine department. A physician trained in diagnostic nuclear medicine interprets the test results.

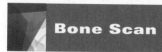

Bone Scan

NORMAL FINDINGS

No evidence of abnormality

INDICATIONS

The bone scan is used to identify metastatic cancer involving the bone. It is often performed on cancer patients as a routine part of staging before and after treatment. To a lesser degree, bone scanning is used to identify pathologic bone conditions that cannot be identified on plain films of the bone (e.g., osteomyelitis, hairline fractures).

TEST EXPLANATION

The bone scan permits examination of the skeleton by a scanning camera after intravenous (IV) injection of a radionuclide material. Usually technetium-99m (^{99m}Tc) is the radionuclide utilized. After injection of the ^{99m}Tc, the radiopharmaceutical is taken up by the bone. Gamma rays are emitted from the ^{99m}Tc through the body and are detected by a scintillation scanner. The scintillation scanner emits light with each photon it receives from the gamma ray. When these light patterns are arranged in a spatial order, a realistic image of the bones is apparent.

The degree of radionuclide uptake is related to the metabolism of the bone. Normally a uniform concentration should be seen throughout the bones of the body. There is symmetric distribution of activity throughout the skeletal system in healthy adults. Urinary bladder activity, faint renal activity, and minimal soft-tissue activity are also normally present. An increased uptake of isotope is abnormal and may represent tumor, arthritis, fracture, degenerative bone and joint changes, osteomyelitis, bone necrosis, osteodystrophy, or Paget disease (Figure 8-1). These areas of concentrated radionuclide uptake are often called hot spots and are detectable months before an ordinary x-ray film can reveal the pathologic condition. Hot spots occur because new bone growth is usually stimulated around areas of abnormality. If a pathologic condition exists and there is no new bone formation around the lesion, the scan will not pick up the abnormality. Increased uptake of radionuclide is also seen in the normal physiologic active epiphyses of children (growth plates).

The major reason a bone scan is performed is to detect metastatic cancer to the bone. All malignancies capable of metastasis may reach the bone, especially those of the prostate, breast, lung, kidney, urinary bladder, and thyroid gland. Bone scans are also useful in staging primary bone tumors such as osteogenic sarcomas and Ewing sarcoma. Bone scans may be serially repeated to monitor tumor response to antineoplastic therapy.

Bone scans also provide valuable information for the evaluation of patients with trauma or unexplained pain. Bone scanning is much more sensitive than routine x-ray films in detecting small and difficult-to-find fractures, especially in the spine, ribs, face, and small bones of the extremities. Bone scans are used to determine the age of a fracture as well. If a fracture line is seen on a plain x-ray film and

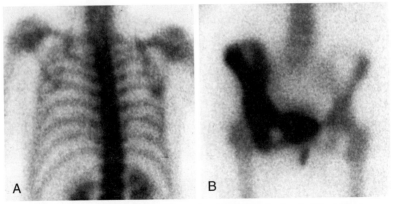

Figure 8-1 Bone scan. **A,** Upper body. **B,** Lower body. There is normal uptake of radionuclide in the bones of the upper body. In the lower body view, the right iliac, ischium, and pubic bones are associated with diffuse increased uptake of radionuclide, consistent with Paget disease.

the uptake around that fracture is not increased on a bone scan, the injury is said to be an "old" fracture, exceeding several months in age.

Although the bone scan is extremely sensitive, unfortunately it is not very specific. Fractures, infections, tumors, and arthritic changes all appear similar in this scan. When plain films fail to identify the classic findings of bone infection (osteomyelitis), bone scans are helpful.

A three-phase bone scan may be performed if inflammation (arthritis) or infection (osteomyelitis, septic arthritis) is suspected. In a three-phase bone scan, imaging is performed at three different times after injection of the radionuclide. Early uptake of the radionuclide would indicate infection or inflammation rather than neoplasm. Uptake of the radionuclide on delayed imaging that had not been present on early imaging would indicate neoplasm.

When the metastasis process is diffuse, virtually all of the radiotracer is concentrated in the skeleton, with little or no activity in the soft tissues or urinary tract. The resulting pattern, which is characterized by excellent bone detail, is frequently referred to as a "superscan." A superscan may also be associated with metabolic bone diseases such as Paget disease, renal osteodystrophy, or osteomalacia. Unlike in metastatic disease, however, the uptake in metabolic bone disease is more uniform in appearance and extends into the distal appendicular skeleton. Intense calvarial uptake disproportionate to that in the remainder of the skeleton is another feature of a metabolic superscan.

The bone scan is performed by a nuclear medicine technologist in 30 to 60 minutes. It is interpreted by a physician trained in nuclear medicine imaging. The injection of the radioisotope causes slight discomfort. There may be some pain caused by lying on the hard scanning table for an hour. In many circumstances, magnetic resonance imaging (MRI) is used in place of bone scans. It is more specific in indicating disease pathology.

CONTRAINDICATIONS

- Patients who are pregnant, unless the benefits outweigh the risk of fetal injury
- Patients who are lactating, because of the risk of contaminating maternal milk

Nuclear Scanning

8

Clinical Priorities

- Bone scans are done mainly to detect metastatic cancer to the bone.
- Bone scans are often repeated to monitor tumor response to antineoplastic therapy.
- Bone scans should not be performed on pregnant or lactating women.

PROCEDURE AND PATIENT CARE

Before

Explain the procedure to the patient.

Assure patients they will not be exposed to large amounts of radioactivity because only tracer doses of the isotope are used.

Tell the patient that no fasting or sedation is required.

Inform the patient that the injection of the radioisotope may cause slight discomfort, nausea, or vomiting.

During

- Note the following procedural steps:
  1. The patient receives an IV injection of an isotope, usually methylene diphosphate (MDP) or hydroxymethylene diphosphate (HDP) in a peripheral vein.
  2. The patient is encouraged to drink several glasses of water between the time of radioisotope injection and the scanning. This facilitates renal clearance of any circulating tracer not picked up by the bone. The waiting period before scanning is approximately 2 to 3 hours.
  3. The patient is instructed to urinate to eliminate any tracer that is in the bladder because it may block the view of the underlying pelvic bones.
  4. The patient is positioned in the supine position on the scanning table in the nuclear medicine department (Figure 8-2).

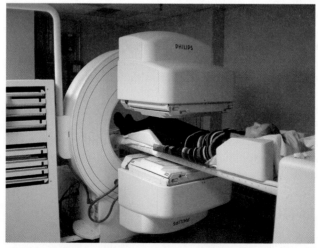

Figure 8-2 Patient undergoing nuclear bone scan. The scintigraphy camera is on the lower part of the body.

5. A scintillation camera is placed over the patient's body and records the radiation emitted by the skeleton.
6. This information is translated into a two- or three-dimensional view of the skeleton, which is then visualized on film.
7. The patient may be repositioned in the prone and lateral positions during the test.

After

- Because only tracer doses of radioisotope are used, remember that no precautions need to be taken to prevent radioactive exposure to other personnel or family present.
- Assure the patient that the radioactive substance is usually excreted from the body within 6 to 24 hours.

Home Care Responsibilities

- Instruct the patient to observe the injection site and to report any redness or swelling.
- Encourage the patient to drink fluids to aid the excretion of the radioactive substance.

TEST RESULTS AND CLINICAL SIGNIFICANCE

Primary or metastatic tumors of the bone: *These can be singular or multiple. It is difficult to specifically diagnose tumor. Serial scans may help.*
Fracture: *Increased uptake in the bone of a patient with anatomic pain is very suggestive of a fracture missed on routine plain films.*
Degenerative arthritis,
Rheumatoid arthritis:
  Increased uptake involving the joints (especially multiple joints) is classic for arthritis.
Osteomyelitis: *Small islands of increased uptake within the bone of a patient with a compatible clinical history indicates infection.*
Bone necrosis: *Decreased uptake (cold spot) may be present if there is not new bone growth surrounding the area of bone necrosis.*
Renal osteodystrophy,
Paget disease:
  These two diseases are usually evident as multiple or diffuse uptake of the tracer in the bones.

RELATED TESTS

Bone (Long) X-Rays (p. 1006). The routine bone x-ray is often used to provide information that is additional or supportive to the bone scan.
Magnetic Resonance Imaging (MRI) (p. 1106). This test is sometimes more reliable in detecting disease or traumatic injury to the bone.

Brain Scan (Cisternogram, Cerebral Blood Flow, DaT Scan)

NORMAL FINDINGS

No areas of altered radionuclide uptake within the brain

Nuclear Scanning

8

INDICATIONS

The usefulness of nuclear brain scan is narrow when compared to CT, MRI, and PET scans of the brain. The cost of these newer scans sometimes precludes their utilization and nuclear brain scanning may be preferably used. This test can be used to identify pathologic conditions (tumor, infarction, infection) involving the cortex. It is used for patients with headaches, epilepsy, and other neurologic symptoms. The nuclear cerebral blood flow brain scan is used to support the diagnosis of cerebral brain death.

TEST EXPLANATION

The brain scan permits examination of the brain by a scanning camera after intravenous (IV) injection of a radionuclide material (Figure 8-3). A technetium-99m (^{99m}Tc) radionuclide, such as hexamethyl-propyleneamine (Tc-HMPAO) or ethyl cysteinate dimer (Tc-ECD), bicisate, or Neurolite, is most commonly used.

Primarily, nuclear brain scan is used to indicate complete and irreversible cessation of brain function (brain death). This determination, when combined with appropriate clinical data, allows for cessation of medical therapy and opportunity for the harvest of potential donor organs. With brain death, there is complete absence of blood perfusion to the brain. In cerebral blood flow scanning, one normally sees an early "arterial visualization phase" followed by a "blood pool phase" in which the venous sinuses but not the brain tissue are seen. In severe brain damage or death, there is usually asymmetric or no blood flow noted on the angiographic phase and an abnormal blood pool phase.

The brain scan can also be used to indicate cerebral vascular occlusion or stenosis. With the use of Diamox (acetazolamide), an accurate assessment of local cerebral blood flow can be determined. Diamox is carbonic anhydrase inhibitor that results in the elevation of Pco_2 in the bloodstream. Normally this causes dilatation of the cerebral blood vessels. If asymmetric blood flow is noted after Diamox injection, cerebral vascular occlusion or stenosis can be suspected.

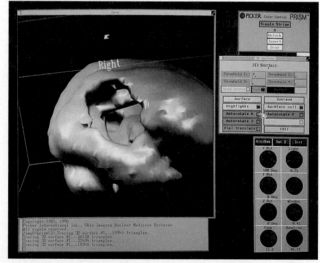

Figure 8-3 Image produced by radionuclide scan. This particular image demonstrates a deficit in cerebral blood flow caused by an arteriovenous malformation.

The brain scan can also document successful therapeutic disruption of the normal blood-brain barrier to inject chemotherapeutic agents into localized brain tumors. Furthermore this scan has been used in the evaluation of patients with seizure disorders, psychiatric disease, and dementia. Although not nearly as accurate as an MRI or PET scan, the nuclear brain scan is able to identify primary brain neoplasms (e.g., gliomas, astrocytomas primary lymphoma) and metastatic tumors. Because sometimes nuclear medicine can indicate tissue viability, nuclear brain scanning is used to differentiate radiation necrosis from recurrent brain viable tumor.

Brain scans are also used to investigate the ventricular system (cisternogram) of the central nervous system. Normal pressure hydrocephalus and ventricular shunt dysfunction can be identified and located. Cisternogram may be performed by injecting radioactive material into the subarachnoid space and then taking serial scans of the head. These scans are useful in evaluating ventricular size and patency of the cerebrospinal fluid (CSF) pathways and reabsorption. Because only a small amount of CSF enters the ventricles, their uptake of radioactive material normally should be minimal. Blocks in the CSF pathways may prevent this reabsorption, however; thus large amounts of isotopes may appear in the ventricles. A cisternogram may also be used to evaluate CSF leakage (e.g., into the nasal sinuses) in patients with recurrent meningitis and to evaluate hydrocephalus.

The technique of single-photon emission computed tomography (SPECT) has significantly improved the quality of brain scanning. With SPECT scanning, the radionuclide is injected and the scintillation cameras are placed to receive images from multiple angles (around the circumference of the head). This technique greatly increases the usefulness of nuclear brain scanning. In general, CT scans, MRI scans, and carotid duplex scans have replaced the brain scan in diagnostic neurology. However, a host of traumatic, inherited, and acquired diseases can be identified with nuclear brain scanning.

A SPECT brain scan using isoflurane I^{123} (also known as phenyltropane) can be helpful in the diagnosis of Parkinson disease. This test is often referred to as a *DaT scan*. Patients with Parkinson's disease experience degeneration of presynaptic dopamine neurotransmitter cells first in the basal ganglia of the brain and then other parts of the brain. Isoflurane tags these neurons with I^{123}. In a healthy brain, isoflurane I^{123} is seen concentrated in the basal ganglia. This is demonstrated as hot spots. In these parts of the brain in which dopamine cells should be remain dark on the brain SPECT scan, Parkinson disease is suspected. These changes may be subtle. There are commonly identified patterns that can separate out Parkinson disease from other forms of brain deterioration or aging.

CONTRAINDICATIONS

- Patients who are pregnant unless the benefits outweigh the risk of fetal damage
- Patients who cannot cooperate during the testing

INTERFERING FACTORS

- Many sedative drugs can affect brain nuclear imaging.
- ACE inhibitors, vasoconstrictors, and vasodilators and can alter blood flow distribution in nuclear brain imaging.

PROCEDURE AND PATIENT CARE

Before

- Explain the procedure to the patient.
- Administer blocking agents as ordered before scanning. For example, potassium chloride prevents an inordinate amount of technetium uptake by the choroid plexus, which would simulate a

pathologic cerebral condition. Similar solutions (e.g., potassium iodine, Lugol iodine solution) may be given orally to block thyroid uptake. Blocking agents are not necessary with the use of ^{99m}Tc diethylenetriamine pentaacetic acid.

- Check for allergy to iodine if an iodinated solution will be used.
- Consider having a sedative ordered for agitated patients.

🖉 Tell the patient that no discomfort is associated with this study other than the peripheral IV puncture required for injection of the radioisotope.

During

- Note the following procedural steps:
  1. After administration of the radioisotope, the patient is placed in the supine, lateral, and prone positions while a counter is placed over the head (Figure 8-4).
  2. The radioisotope counts are anatomically displayed and photographed while the patient remains very still.
  3. When cerebral flow studies are performed, the counter is immediately placed over the head.
  4. The counts are anatomically recorded in timed sequence to follow the isotope during its first flow through the brain.
  5. Another scan is obtained 30 minutes to 2 hours later for identification of pathologic tissues.
- Note that this study is performed by a technologist in the nuclear medicine department in approximately 35 to 45 minutes.

After

🖉 Assure the patient that the radioactive material is usually excreted from the body within 6 to 24 hours.

- Because only tracer doses of radioisotopes are used, remember that no precautions need to be taken to prevent radioactive exposure to other personnel or family present.

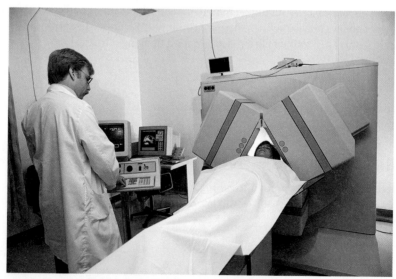

Figure 8-4 Patient positioned for a radionuclide scan of the brain. In this diagnostic study, a small amount of radioactive material crosses the blood-brain barrier to produce an image. This study is known as single-photon emission computed tomography (SPECT).

Encourage the patient to drink fluids to aid in the excretion of the isotope from the body.
• Observe the injection site for redness and swelling.

TEST RESULTS AND CLINICAL SIGNIFICANCE

Cerebral death: *This is noted by asymmetric or absence of cerebral blood flow when associated with other clinical indications of death.*

Cerebral vascular stenosis/occlusion: *Depending on the timing after the incident, affected areas will demonstrate perfusion changes.*

Seizure disorder: *The use of this test for this indication is limited because of the need to withdraw from anti-seizure medication.*

Dementia: *Alzheimer disease can be differentiated from other neurodegenerative diseases using nuclear scanning especially when combined with PET scanning.*

Cerebral neoplasm: *When using radionuclide such as FDG, tumors are obvious by enhancement of radionuclide within the tumor. Primary lymphomas have unique nuclear features that suggest their diagnosis. Metastatic lesions are often multiple and associated with focal increased nuclear activity.*

Brain infection and abscess: *Hypometabolic areas may represent abscess. Increased activity may be noted with acute infection.*

CSF leakage: *The most common site of leakage of CSF is into the nasal cavity. This can be the result of tumor or infection.*

Hydrocephalus: *This is evident on cisternogram. Ventricular shunt dysfunction becomes obvious by lack of nuclear flow.*

RELATED TESTS

Computed Tomography (CT) Scan of the Brain (p. 1026). This test is very accurate in identifying pathologic conditions of the brain. X-rays are directed to the brain from multiple circumferential angles and then gathered to produce multiple images of the brain.

Magnetic Resonance Imaging (MRI) Scan of the Brain (p. 1106). This test does not use x-rays but rather detects electromagnetic differences among the brain tissues. It visualizes the brain from similar angles as the CT scan, producing an accurate image.

PET scan (p. 821). This nuclear spatial scan is particularly useful to identify neoplasm involved in the central nervous system.

Nuclear Scanning

8

> **Breast Scintigraphy** (Breast Scan, Breast-Specific Gamma Imaging [BSGI], Scintimammography, Miraluma Scan, Breast Scintigraphy with Breast-Specific γ-Camera (BSGC)

NORMAL FINDINGS

Negative: Minimal, symmetric, bilateral, and uniform breast uptake equal to soft-tissue uptake

INDICATIONS

This test is used to identify breast cancer, especially in young women with dense breasts in whom the accuracy of mammography is diminished.

TEST EXPLANATION

Nuclear scans of the breast, using technetium (^{99m}Tc)-labeled sestamibi or tetrofosmin as a radiotracer, are used to identify breast cancer in patients whose dense breast tissue precludes accurate evaluation by conventional mammography. To conduct BSGI, patients are given an intravenous injection with a small dose of a tracing agent (Technetium ^{99m}Tc) that emits gamma rays. The radioisotope is transported by passive diffusion into the cell and is sequestered within the mitochondria. Thus cancer cells that usually contain a large number of mitochondria will show an increased uptake of ^{99m}Tc as compared with noncancerous cells. BSGI is a functional scan that indicates physiologic behavior of cells. Cancerous areas show up as "hot spots" on breast specific specialized high-resolution, small field-of-view gamma cameras. The cameras are compact and maneuverable and they can be placed close to the chest to image deep within the breast.

This test has also been used as an adjunct in patients with an indeterminate mammogram abnormality and in women with indeterminate palpable breast masses. However this scan may miss as many as 10% to 15% of cancers, and the false-positive rate is about 15% to 25%. Areas of benign cellular hyperplasia also trap the radiotracer. Because cellular hyperplasia is a common finding in the breast just before menses, imaging at this time in the menstrual cycle should be avoided.

Breast nuclear scans will not replace the role of mammography in breast imaging. Nor will they ever be an effective screening tool for the early detection of breast cancer among large populations. Other technologies currently used for similar post-mammography evaluation include ultrasound (p. 871) and magnetic resonance imaging (MRI) (p. 1106). Each of these technologies has its advantages and limitations. Ultrasound is well tolerated, it does not use ionizing radiation or require intravenous contrast administration, and it is able to identify small lesions in dense breast tissue. MRI of the breast offers accuracy similar to ultrasound and BSGI. However, MRI is not suitable for many patients, such as women with pacemakers, who are claustrophobic, and who cannot lie prone for the required length of the exam. BSGI is not without limitations; it is limited by its inability to reliably image cancers smaller than 1 cm.

CONTRAINDICATIONS

- Patients who are pregnant, unless the benefits outweigh the risk of fetal injury
- Patients who are lactating, because of the risk of contaminating breast milk

PROCEDURE AND PATIENT CARE

Before

- Explain the procedure to the patient. A signed consent form may be required.
- Assure the patient that she will not be exposed to large amounts of radioactivity because only tracer doses of the isotope are used.
- Tell the patient that no fasting or sedation is required.
- Assess the patient for allergies to latex, contrast dyes, or iodine.
- Assess the patient for pregnancy.
- Assess the patient for in situ breast implants.
- Ask the patient to remove all jewelry and clothing above the waist.

During

Note the following procedural steps:

1. The patient may be positioned in the supine, prone, or sitting position.

2. Twenty millicuries of ^{99m}Tc sestamibi is injected intravenously into the arm contralateral to the suspicious breast.
3. Imaging begins a few minutes after injection. A scintillator camera is placed over the breast and records the radiation emitted.
4. This information is translated into a two-dimensional view of the breast, which is then visualized on film.
5. These images are compared with surrounding soft-tissue readings.

After

✗ Tell the patient that because only tracer doses of radioisotope are used, no precautions need to be taken to prevent radioactive exposure to other personnel or family present.

✗ Assure the patient that the radioactive substance is usually excreted from the body within 6 to 24 hours.

✗ Encourage the patient to drink fluids to aid in the excretion of the radioactive substance.

• Observe the injection site for redness or swelling.

TEST RESULTS AND CLINICAL SIGNIFICANCE

Breast cancer,
Hyperplasia of the breast tissue:
>*Rapidly duplicating cells that commonly exist in cancers and in hyperplastic tissue entrap the sestamibi radionuclide. This is demonstrated as a hot region on the breast scan. Not all that lights up is cancer.*

RELATED TESTS

Mammography (p. 1043). This is an x-ray image of the breasts. It is generally the most accurate screening and diagnostic test to identify breast cancer.

Breast Ultrasonography (p. 871). This ultrasound technique is also used to identify and characterize breast pathologic conditions. This test is especially useful to identify breast cysts.

MRI of the Breast (p. 1106). This magnetic resonance imaging of the breast using gadolinium is both an anatomic and functional scan of the breast tissue.

Nuclear Scanning

8

Cardiac Nuclear Scan (Myocardial Perfusion Scan, Myocardial Perfusion Imaging, Myocardial Scan, Cardiac Scan, Heart Scan, Thallium Scan, MUGA Scan, Isonitrile Scan, Sestamibi Cardiac Scan, Cardiac Flow Studies, and Nuclear Stress Test)

NORMAL FINDINGS

Heterogeneous uptake radionuclide throughout the myocardium of the left ventricle
Left ventricular end diastolic volume ≤70 ML
Left ventricular end systolic volume ≤25 ML
Left ventricular ejection fraction >50%
Right ventricular ejection fraction >40%
Normal cardiac wall motion
No muscle wall thickening

TABLE 8-1	Overview of Cardiac Nuclear Scanning			
Scan	**Radionuclide**	**Use**	**Positive Results**	**Comments**
Myocardial perfusion	• ^{99m}Tc Isonitrile (sestamibi) • Tetrofosmin	Identifies ischemic or infarcted heart muscle	Cold spots on stress images are areas of ischemia	Commonly performed with cardiac gating
Myocardial function (MUGA)	• ^{99m}Tc-labeled RBCs	Calculates the cardiac ejection fraction	Reduced cardiac ejection fraction	This is the most accurate method to determine cardiac ejection fraction
Cardiac flow	• ^{99m}Tc alone or ^{99m}Tc-labeled RBCs	Determines the direction of cardiac flow	Abnormal cardiac blood flow patterns	This is most commonly performed in children with suspected cardiac anomalies
Nuclear gated/SPECT ventriculography	• Thallium • ^{99m}Tc	Evaluates muscle wall activity	Poor wall contractility is seen in ischemia or infarction	Commonly done with a perfusion scan
Exercise stress testing	• ^{99m}Tc sestamibi or tetrofosmin	Evaluates muscle wall activity during stress (physical or chemical)	Poor wall contractility is seen in ischemia or infarction	Stress testing commonly includes a perfusion scan and ventriculography

INDICATIONS

This test is used for the evaluation of:
- Coronary vascular disease
- Coronary surgery or angioplasty
- Chest pain
- Shortness of breath
- Elevated cardiac markers (CPK, troponin, or myoglobin)

TEST EXPLANATION

See Table 8-1 for an overview of cardiac nuclear scanning. A cardiac perfusion scan measures the coronary blood flow at rest and during exercise. It is often used to evaluate the cause of chest pain. It may be done after a coronary ischemic event to evaluate coronary patency or heart muscle function.

In this test, radionuclide is injected intravenously into the patient. Myocardial perfusion images are then obtained while the patient is lying down under a single-photon emission computed tomography (SPECT) camera that generates a picture of the radioactivity coming from the heart. This scan can be performed at rest or with exercise such as treadmill or bicycling (*myocardial nuclear stress testing*). Medications may be administered that duplicate exercise stress testing. Vasodilators (dipyridamole, adenosine and Regadenoson) or chronotropic agents (dobutamine) are commonly used. Regadenoson is the most recent A_{2A} adenosine receptor agonist that instigates coronary vasodilatation. It is associated with fewer side effects (e.g., heart block, bronchospasm) and can be injected more quickly.

Although the initial radioisotope used was thallium (thus the name *thallium scan*), technetium agents such as tetrofosmin and sestamibi (isonitrile) are more commonly used today. The uptake of

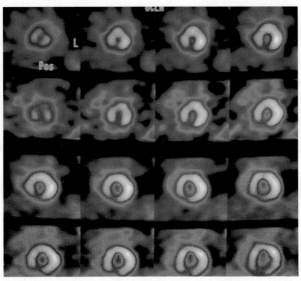

Figure 8-5 Thallium-201 scintigraphy produces a series of images of blood flow and tissue perfusion.

these agents is proportional to the myocardial coronary flow (Figure 8-5). At rest, a coronary stenosis must exceed 90% of the normal diameter before blood flow is impaired enough to see it on the perfusion scan. With exercise stress testing, however, stenosis of 50% becomes obvious. Often stenosis or coronary obstruction is noted by a normal resting perfusion scan followed by stress perfusion scan that demonstrates cold spots compatible with decreased coronary perfusion. Myocardial perfusion scans can be synchronized by gating the images with the cardiac cycle and thereby allowing the visualization and evaluation of cardiac muscle function. The contractility of the muscle wall can be evaluated at the same time. Prior muscle injury is demonstrated by reduced muscle wall motion. Most often, nuclear myocardial scans include both perfusion and gated wall motion images. Cardiac ejection fraction, the end-systolic volume of the left ventricle can be calculated.

Cardiac nuclear stress testing is more accurate than echocardiography stress testing (p. 877) or radiographic stress ventriculography (p. 1008). The nuclear myocardial scan is the best initial imaging study for the detection of myocardial ischemia; however, stress echocardiography is performed more often because it is more readily available and many cardiologists are better trained in echocardiography and are more comfortable with echocardiography. The assessment of myocardial perfusion and function using PET and hybrid positron emission tomography (PET)/CT imaging (p. 822) is becoming more available as the cost of the technology decreases and as positron-emitting radiopharmaceuticals become more available. Myocardial PET scanning provides better cardiac and coronary imaging.

Cardiac nuclear imaging when gated to the cardiac cycle *(Multi Gated Acquisition Scan [MUGA], gated blood pool scan)* can provide an accurate measure of ventricular function through the calculation of the *ventricular ejection fraction* (Figure 8-6). In this scan the patient's red blood cells are tagged with technetium. Red blood cell binding with technetium can be performed in vivo or in vitro. In vivo techniques are more convenient and less time-consuming but in vitro labeling is more efficient, especially in patients who have large indwelling venous access.

Ventricular volumes can be calculated and used to accurately calculate the amount of blood that is ejected from the ventricle with each contraction (ejection fraction). This is used in the initial assessment

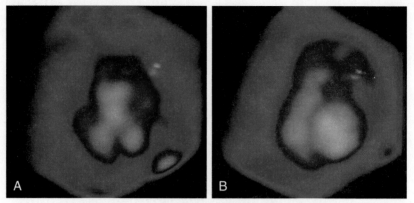

Figure 8-6 Blood pooling imaging. **A,** Systolic frame. **B,** Diastolic frame.

of cardiac function and subsequently to monitor therapy designed to improve cardiac function. Patients with cardiomyopathies (ischemic, infiltrative, inflammatory), cardiac transplant, or drug-induced cardiac muscle toxicity (from doxorubicin or Herceptin) require frequent evaluation of ventricular ejection fraction.

This test is usually performed in a few hours in the nuclear medicine department by a technologist and interpreted by a nuclear medicine physician. Delayed images may be required 24 hours later.

CONTRAINDICATIONS*

- Patients who are uncooperative or medically unstable
- Patients with severe cardiac arrhythmia
- Patients who are pregnant (unless the benefits outweigh the risks) because of fetal exposure to radionuclide material

INTERFERING FACTORS

- Myocardial trauma
- Cardiac flow studies can be altered by excessive alterations in chest pressure (as exists with excessive crying in children).
- Recent nuclear scans (e.g., thyroid or bone scan)
- Drugs, such as long-acting nitrates, may only temporarily improve coronary perfusion and cardiac function.

 Clinical Priorities

- Nuclear scanning is commonly used as the imaging portion of cardiac stress testing to assess myocardial ischemia.
- This test can be used to evaluate myocardial function by measuring the ejection fraction.
- Nuclear scanning is the most accurate method to determine coronary occlusive disease.

---

* See contraindications to cardiac stress testing on p. 540.

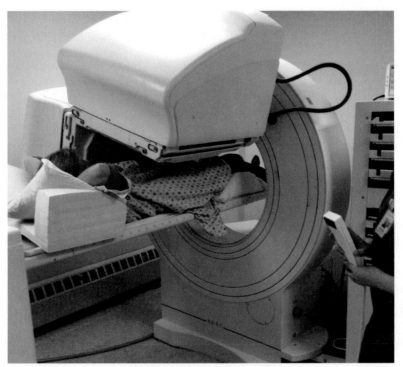

Figure 8-7 Cardiac nuclear scan.

PROCEDURE AND PATIENT CARE

Before

✍Explain the procedure to the patient.

✍Instruct the patient that a short fasting period may be required, especially when using sestamibi or tetrofosmin.

✍Tell the patient that the only discomfort associated with this test is the venipuncture required for injection of the radioisotope.

• Be sure all jewelry is removed from the chest wall.

• Obtain a consent form if stress testing is to be performed.

During

• Take the patient to the nuclear medicine department. Depending on the type of nuclear myocardial scan, each scanning protocol is different.

• Note the following general procedural steps:

1. One or more intravenous (IV) injection of radionuclide material is performed.
2. ECG leads may be applied.
3. Depending on the radionuclide used, scanning is performed 15 minutes to 4 hours later.
4. A SPECT camera is placed at the level of the precordium.
5. If a single gamma camera is used, the patient is placed in a supine position (Figure 8-7), and then may be repositioned to the lateral position and/or in the right and left oblique positions. In some departments, the detector can be rotated around the patient, who remains in the supine position.
6. The gamma ray scanner records the image of the heart, and an image is immediately developed.

7. For an *exercise stress* test, additional radionuclide is injected during exercise when the patient reaches a maximum heart rate. The patient then lies on a table, and scanning is done. A repeat scan may be done 3 to 4 hours later.
8. If an *isonitrile stress test* is needed, the radionuclide material is injected and a scan performed 30 to 60 minutes later for the resting phase. Four hours later, cardiac stress testing is done. After a second injection, scanning is repeated.
- Note that myocardial scans are usually performed in less than 30 minutes by a nuclear medicine technician.
- If nuclear cardiac stress testing is performed, follow routine protocol described on p. 540.

After

Inform the patient that because only tracer doses of radioisotopes are used, no precautions need to be taken against radioactive exposure to personnel or family.

Instruct the patient to drink fluids to aid in the excretion of the radioactive substance.
- Apply pressure or a pressure dressing to the venipuncture site.
- Assess the venipuncture site for bleeding.
- If stress testing was performed, evaluate the patient's vital signs at frequent intervals (as indicated).
- Remove any applied EKG leads.

TEST RESULTS AND CLINICAL SIGNIFICANCE

Coronary artery occlusive disease: *This diagnosis can be made when comparing a resting scan or during a cardiac stress nuclear scan. The manner with which this abnormality becomes evident depends on the radionuclide used.*

Decreased myocardial function associated with ischemia, myocarditis, cardiomyopathy, or congestive heart failure: *These diseases, affecting the myocardium, are evident as hypokinesia of the cardiac wall. Infarcted areas have little or no wall motion. Paradoxical motion may be noted.*

Decreased cardiac output: *Many coronary, myocardial, and valvular diseases are associated with reduced cardiac output. A reduced ejection fraction is an indirect measurement of cardiac output. Often a reduced ejection fraction is the first sign of those diseases.*

RELATED TESTS

Cardiac Stress Testing (p. 540). In this test, stress is provided to maximize the cardiac function. The heart is then often imaged with nuclear scanning to see the effect of the stress.

Cardiac Catheterization (p. 1008). This test provides similar images through the use of radio-opaque dyes injected through catheters placed in and around the heart.

Echocardiography (p. 877). This is an ultrasound directed image of the cardiac muscle and chambers.

> ## Gallbladder Nuclear Scanning (Hepatobiliary Scintigraphy, Hepatobiliary Imaging, Biliary Tract Radionuclide Scan, Cholescintigraphy, DISIDA Scanning, HIDA Scanning, IDA Gallbladder Scanning)

NORMAL FINDINGS

Gallbladder, common bile duct, and duodenum visualize within 60 minutes after radionuclide injection. (This confirms patency of the cystic and common bile ducts.)

INDICATIONS

Cholescintigraphy is valuable in evaluating patients for suspected gallbladder disease. The primary use of this study is to diagnose acute cholecystitis in patients who have acute right upper quadrant abdominal pain. When gallbladder ejection fraction is calculated, chronic cholecystitis can be diagnosed. This study is also used to assist in the diagnosis of extrahepatic biliary obstruction.

TEST EXPLANATION

Through the use of iminodiacetic acid analogues (IDAs) labeled with technetium-99m (^{99m}Tc), the biliary tract can be evaluated in a safe, accurate, and noninvasive manner. These radionuclide compounds are extracted by the liver and excreted into the bile. Gamma rays are emitted from the ^{99m}Tc in the bile through the body and are detected by a scintillation camera. The scintillation camera emits light with each photon it receives from the gamma ray. When these light patterns are arranged in a spatial order, a realistic image of the biliary tree is apparent.

Failure to visualize the gallbladder 60 to 120 minutes after injection of the radionuclide is virtually diagnostic of an obstruction of the cystic duct, which instigates the pathophysiology of acute cholecystitis. Delayed filling of the gallbladder is associated with chronic or acalculous cholecystitis. This procedure is also helpful in diagnosing biliary duct obstructions. The identification of the radionuclide in the biliary tree but not in the bowel is diagnostic of common bile duct obstruction.

This procedure is superior to oral cholecystography, intravenous (IV) cholangiography, ultrasonography, and computed tomography (CT) of the gallbladder in the detection of cholecystitis (Table 8-2). Also, with cholescintigraphy, gallbladder function can be numerically determined by calculating the capability of the gallbladder to eject its contents. It is believed that an ejection fraction below 35% indicates primary gallbladder disease. To a large degree, abdominal ultrasound (p. 866) has replaced this test in the diagnosis of acute cholecystitis.

Occasionally, morphine sulfate is given intravenously during nuclear scanning. The morphine causes increased ampullary contraction. Not only can this reproduce the patient's symptoms of biliary colic, but it also serves to force the bile containing the radionuclide into the gallbladder. If no radionuclide is seen in the gallbladder with the use of morphine within 15 to 60 minutes, the diagnosis of acute cholecystitis is nearly certain. This greatly decreases the scanning time because without morphine it requires 4 hours to obtain a definitive diagnosis of acute cholecystitis.

A nuclear medicine technologist performs this study in 1 to 4 hours in the nuclear medicine department. A physician trained in interpretation of diagnostic nuclear medicine interprets the test in a few minutes. The only discomfort associated with this procedure is the IV injection of radionuclide.

CONTRAINDICATIONS

- Pregnancy, unless the benefits outweigh the risk of fetal injury

INTERFERING FACTORS

- If the patient has not eaten for more than 24 hours, the radionuclide may not fill the gallbladder. This would produce a false-positive result.

PROCEDURE AND PATIENT CARE

Before

Explain the procedure to the patient.

TABLE 8-2	Comparison of Methods of Visualizing the Gallbladder and Biliary System	
Test	**Advantages**	**Disadvantages**
Cholecystography	Easily performed, inexpensive	Will not visualize with acute cholecystitis or if other inflammatory processes are in the abdomen Will not visualize if bilirubin >2 Will not visualize if patient vomits or has diarrhea
IV cholangiography	Easily performed, inexpensive	Will not visualize if bilirubin >2
Endoscopic retrograde cholangiopancreatography (ERCP)	Good visualization of the bile duct Stones can be extracted Stents can be placed to drain bile	Technically difficult May not visualize the gallbladder Invasive procedure
Percutaneous transhepatic cholangiography (PTC)	Good visualization of the biliary tree Stents can be placed to drain bile	Invasive procedure May not visualize the gallbladder
Ultrasound	Easily performed, accurate, inexpensive	May not be accurate for common bile duct pathologic conditions
Scintigraphy (nuclear scanning)	Indicates acute cholecystitis Can visualize the biliary tree even if bilirubin is >2	Not accurate for chronic cholecystitis More complicated to perform Takes several hours to identify pathologic condition May give false-positive results if other inflammatory processes are occurring within the abdomen

Clinical Priorities

- Gallbladder scanning is used primarily to diagnose acute cholecystitis in patients who have acute right upper quadrant pain.
- This procedure is superior to oral cholecystography, IV cholangiography, ultrasonography, and CT of the gallbladder in the diagnosis of cholecystitis.
- This procedure can also determine the ejection fraction of the gallbladder.
- Morphine sulfate can be administered intravenously during scanning to markedly reduce the scanning time from 4 hours to less than 1 hour.

 Assure the patient that he or she will not be exposed to large amounts of radioactivity.

Instruct the patient to fast for 2 to 4 hours before the test.

Avoid morphine or Demerol administration for 4 to 12 hours before the scan.

During

- Note the following procedural steps:
  1. After IV administration of a ^{99m}Tc-labeled IDA (e.g., DISIDA, PIPIDA, HIDA), the right upper quadrant of the abdomen is scanned.
  2. Serial images are obtained over 1 hour.
  3. Subsequent images can be obtained at 15- to 30-minute intervals.
  4. If the gallbladder, common bile duct, or duodenum is not visualized within 60 minutes after injection, delayed images are obtained up to 4 hours later.
  5. Images are recorded on film.
  6. When an *ejection fraction* is to be determined, the patient is given a fatty meal or cholecystokinin is administered to evaluate emptying of the gallbladder. The gallbladder is continually scanned to measure the percentage of isotope ejected.

After

- Obtain a meal for the patient, if indicated.

TEST RESULTS AND CLINICAL SIGNIFICANCE

Acute cholecystitis: *No visualization of the gallbladder will be seen because a gallstone is stuck in the cystic duct, causing acute cholecystitis. The rest of the biliary tree is visualized.*

Chronic cholecystitis,

Acalculous cholecystitis,

Cystic duct syndrome:

Delayed visualization of the gallbladder is seen after several hours. The gallbladder ejection fraction is below 35%. The pathophysiology of cystic duct syndrome is not well known.

Common bile duct obstruction secondary to gallstones, tumor, or stricture: *This is evident when the radionuclide is seen in a large bile duct but not in the bowel. Obstruction of the bile duct must be present.*

RELATED TESTS

See Table 8-2, p. 798.

Ultrasonography of the Gallbladder (p. 866). With the use of ultrasound, gallstones can be identified to be within the gallbladder. The diagnosis of acute cholecystitis cannot be made with the same degree of certainty as it can using biliary scintigraphy.

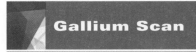

Gallium Scan

NORMAL FINDINGS

Diffuse, low level of gallium uptake, especially in the liver and spleen
No increased gallium uptake within the body

INDICATIONS

Gallium becomes concentrated in areas of the body where white blood cells (WBCs) tend to congregate (areas of tumor, infection, and inflammation). It is used to stage gallium-avid tumors (those that attract high concentrations of gallium; e.g., lymphomas, lung cancer). It is used to locate infection or

Nuclear Scanning

8

inflammation in patients with fever of unknown origin. Finally, it is used to monitor response to treatment of infection, inflammation, or tumor.

TEST EXPLANATION

A gallium scan of the total body is usually performed 24, 48, and 72 hours after an intravenous (IV) injection of radioactive gallium. Most commonly, however, a single scan is performed 2 to 4 days after injection of the gallium. Gallium is a radionuclide that is concentrated in areas of inflammation and infection, by abscesses, and by benign and malignant tumors. Not all types of tumors, however, will concentrate gallium. Lymphomas are particularly gallium avid. Other tumors that can be detected by a gallium scan include sarcomas, hepatomas, and carcinomas of the gastrointestinal (GI) tract, kidney, uterus, stomach, and testicle.

This test is useful in detecting metastatic tumor, especially lymphoma, even when other diagnostic imaging tests are normal. To a large degree, PET scans (p. 821) have replaced the use of gallium scans for the identification of malignancy. The gallium scan also is useful in demonstrating a source of infection in patients with a fever of unknown origin. Gallium can be used to identify noninfectious inflammation within the body in patients who have an elevated sedimentation rate. Unfortunately, this test is not specific enough to differentiate among tumor, infection, inflammation, and abscess. Although a gallium scan is better able to detect sites of chronic inflammation, PET scans are more commonly used to identify areas of acute infection.

Some organs (liver, spleen, bone, colon) normally retain gallium. Therefore a normal total-body gallium scan study would demonstrate some uptake in these organs, but this uptake is much less concentrated than in pathologic areas (e.g., tumor, inflammation).

Another method of scanning is called *SPECT (single-photon emission computed tomography)*. With SPECT scanning, the patient lies supine on the table surrounded by a donut-like gantry. The photon detection camera rotates around the patient to obtain photon counts from 360 degrees. This provides a more detailed image.

A nuclear medicine technologist performs each scan in approximately 30 to 60 minutes. Repeated scanning is required. Repeated injections are not necessary. The test results are interpreted by a physician trained in nuclear medicine and are usually available 72 hours after the injection. No pain or discomfort is associated with this procedure other than the IV injection. However, it occasionally can be uncomfortable to lie still on a hard table for the duration required.

CONTRAINDICATIONS

- Patients who are pregnant, unless the benefits outweigh the risk of fetal injury

INTERFERING FACTORS

- Recent barium studies will interfere with the visualization of the gallium within the abdomen.

Clinical Priorities

- Gallium scanning is useful in detecting metastatic tumor, even when other diagnostic imaging tests are normal.
- Gallium is normally retained in the liver, colon, spleen, and bone. Therefore it is normal to demonstrate small amounts of uptake in these organs during scanning.
- Scanning can be repeated without additional injections of the radionuclide.

PROCEDURE AND PATIENT CARE

Before

Explain the procedure to the patient.
- If ordered, administer a cathartic or enema to minimize increased gallium uptake within the bowel.

During

- Note the following procedural steps:
  1. The unsedated patient is injected with gallium.
  2. A total-body scan may be performed 4 to 6 hours later by slowly passing a scintillation camera over the body.
  3. The images provided by the scintillation camera are recorded on film.
  4. Additional scans are usually taken 24, 48, and 72 hours later.
  5. During the scanning process the patient is positioned in the supine position.

After

Assure the patient that only tracer doses of radioisotopes have been used and that no precautions against radioactive exposure to others are necessary.

TEST RESULTS AND CLINICAL SIGNIFICANCE

Tumor,
Noninfectious inflammation (sarcoidosis, rheumatoid arthritis),
Infection,
Abscess:
  These processes can concentrate gallium, but not with 100% accuracy. These pathologic conditions may exist in patients in whom results of the gallium scan are normal.

Gastric Emptying Scan

NORMAL FINDINGS

Normal values are determined by type and quantity of radiolabeled ingested food.

Time	Lower Normal Limits	Upper Normal Limits
0 minutes		
30 minutes	70%	
1 hour	30%	90%
2 hours		60%
3 hours		30%
4 hours		10%

Values lower than normal represent abnormally fast gastric emptying. Values higher than upper limits represent delayed gastric emptying.

INDICATIONS

This scan is used to determine the rate of gastric emptying. It is used to diagnose gastroparesis or gastric obstruction in patients who have postcibal nausea, vomiting, bloating, early satiety, belching, or abdominal pain.

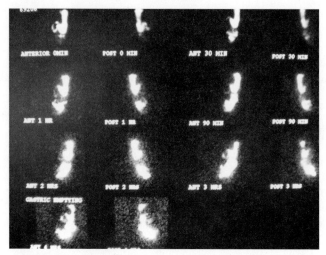

Figure 8-8 Emptying scan. Nuclear content are noted initially in the stomach and duodenum. As time progresses (from 0 minutes on top to 4 hours on bottom), only a portion of the contents within the stomach empty into the small intestine. At 4 hours, 22% of the radionuclide remains in the stomach. Delayed gastric emptying is apparent.

TEST EXPLANATION

In this study the patient ingests a solid or liquid "test meal" containing a radionuclide such as technetium (Tc). The stomach is then scanned until gastric emptying is complete (Figure 8-8). This study is used to assess the stomach's ability to empty solids or liquids and to evaluate disorders that may cause a delay in gastric emptying, such as obstruction (caused by peptic ulcers or gastric malignancies) and gastroparesis. This scan is also useful in determining the patency of a gastrointestinal (GI) surgical anastomosis.

This procedure lasts approximately 4 hours, depending on the gastric emptying time. The test is interpreted by a nuclear medicine physician. Results are available the same day. There is no discomfort associated with the test.

CONTRAINDICATIONS

- Patients who are pregnant or lactating, unless the benefits outweigh the risk of fetal or newborn injury

INTERFERING FACTORS

Drugs that increase gastric emptying time include anticholinergics, opiates, and sedatives/hypnotics. These medications should be withheld for 2 days before testing.

PROCEDURE AND PATIENT CARE

Before

Explain the procedure to the patient.

Assure the patient that no pain is associated with this study.

Inform the patient that only a small dose of nuclear material is ingested. Reassure the patient that this is a safe dose.

Instruct the patient to keep on nothing by mouth (NPO) status after midnight on the day of the test.

Tell the diabetic patient not to take insulin or oral medications before testing because they will be fasting until the next meal.

Tell the patient that smoking is prohibited on the day of examination because exposure to tobacco can inhibit gastric emptying.

During

- Note the following procedural steps:
  1. In the nuclear medicine department the patient is asked to ingest a test meal. In the solid-emptying study the patient eats scrambled egg whites containing Tc.
  In the liquid-emptying study the patient drinks orange juice or water containing technetium-99m diethylenetriamine pentaacetic acid (DTPA) or indium-111 DTPA.
  2. After ingestion of the test meal the patient lies supine under a gamma camera that records gastric images. Images are obtained for 2 minutes every 30 to 60 minutes until gastric emptying is complete. This may take several hours, although each particular timed scan takes only a few minutes.
- With the use of computer calculations of timed images, the rate of gastric emptying can be determined.

After

Assure the patient that he or she has ingested only a small amount of nuclear material. No radiation precautions need to be taken against the patient or his or her body secretions.

TEST RESULTS AND CLINICAL SIGNIFICANCE

Gastric obstruction caused by gastric ulcer or cancer: *Tumors located at the gastric outlet can obstruct or delay gastric emptying. Ulcers, particularly in the duodenum, can cause edema and scarring, which also can cause delay in gastric emptying. The scan, although not specific regarding the cause of the obstruction, will demonstrate prolonged gastric emptying.*

Nonfunctioning GI anastomosis: *Postoperative edema is suspected to be the cause of delayed gastric emptying after gastric surgery. Gastroparesis also may play a role.*

Gastroparesis: *The muscle function required for gastric emptying can be affected by nerve damage caused by diabetes or other neuropathies. There may be endocrine factors (gastrin related) affecting gastric emptying. This process is not uncommon after prolonged periods of gastric obstruction. Here, again, the gastric emptying scan will be prolonged.*

RELATED TEST

Gastroesophageal Reflux Scan (see following test). This is very similarly performed but evaluates the patient for reflux of the gastric contents into the esophagus.

Gastroesophageal Reflux Scan (GE Reflux Scan, Aspiration Scan)

NORMAL FINDINGS

No evidence of gastroesophageal reflux

INDICATIONS

This scan is performed on patients who complain of heartburn, reflux of food, water brash (sour taste in the mouth), aspiration, or paroxysmal nocturnal dyspnea (from nocturnal aspiration). It can detect gastroesophageal reflux and/or aspiration.

TEST EXPLANATION

GE reflux scans are used to evaluate patients with symptoms of heartburn, regurgitation, vomiting, and dysphagia. Also, these scans are used to evaluate the medical or surgical treatment of patients with GE reflux. Finally, aspiration scans may be used to detect aspiration of gastric contents into the lungs and to evaluate swallowing function.

This procedure is performed in the nuclear medicine department in approximately 30 minutes. There is no discomfort associated with this test.

CONTRAINDICATIONS

- Patients who cannot tolerate abdominal compression
- Patients who are pregnant or lactating, unless the benefits outweigh the risk of injury to the fetus or newborn

Age-Related Concerns

- Aspiration scans can be used to evaluate infants for chalasia.
- The tracer is added to the formula or feeding. Films are taken over the next hour, with delayed films taken as needed.

PROCEDURE AND PATIENT CARE

Before

- Explain the procedure to the patient.
- Assure the patient that no pain is associated with this test.
- Instruct the patient to eat a full meal just before the study.

During

- Note the following procedural steps:

GE Reflux Scan

1. The patient is placed in the supine position and asked to swallow 100 to 150 mL of a tracer cocktail (e.g., orange juice, diluted hydrochloric acid, and technetium-99ᵐ–labeled colloid).
2. Images are immediately taken of the patient's esophageal area.
3. The patient is asked to assume other positions to determine whether GE reflux occurs and, if so, in what position.
4. A large abdominal binder that contains an air-inflatable cuff is placed on the patient's abdomen. This is insufflated to increase abdominal pressure.
5. Images are again taken over the esophageal area to determine if any GE reflux occurs.

Aspiration Scan

1. This scan may be performed by adding a radionuclide to the patient's evening meal and keeping the patient in the supine position until the next morning.
2. Images are made over the lung fields to detect esophagotracheal aspiration of the tracer.
3. In *infants* being evaluated for chalasia, the tracer is added to the feeding or formula. Nuclear tracer films are then taken over the next hour, with delayed films as needed.

After

- With the use of computer calculations based on the images of the scans, the severity and percentage of reflux can be calculated.
- Assure the patient that he or she has ingested only a small dose of nuclear material. No radiation precautions need to be taken against the patient or his or her body secretions.

TEST RESULTS AND CLINICAL SIGNIFICANCE

Gastroesophageal reflux: *The radionuclide can be seen to reflux from the stomach into the esophagus. This should diminish or disappear with successful medical or surgical treatment.*

Pulmonary aspiration: *This can be the result of severe gastroesophageal reflux or the result of faulty swallowing function.*

RELATED TEST

Gastric Emptying Scan (p. 801). This is a similarly performed scan designed to identify delayed gastric emptying, which can contribute to gastroesophageal reflux.

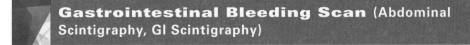

Gastrointestinal Bleeding Scan (Abdominal Scintigraphy, GI Scintigraphy)

NORMAL FINDINGS

No collection of radionuclide in GI tract

INDICATIONS

This study is mainly used to localize sites of GI bleeding.

TEST EXPLANATION

The GI bleeding scan is a test used to localize the site of bleeding in patients who are having active GI hemorrhage. The scan also can be used in patients who have suspected intraabdominal (nongastrointestinal) hemorrhage from an unknown source. Localization of the source of GI or other bleeding can be quite difficult. When surgery is required under these circumstances, it is difficult, cumbersome, and prolonged. The surgeon may have extreme difficulty finding the source of bleeding. The bleeding scan helps localize the bleeding for the surgeon.

Box 8-1 provides an overview of the diagnostic procedures used in evaluating GI bleeding. Many of these studies have limitations that warrant the use of the GI bleeding scan. For example, endoscopy has proved to be extremely useful in determining the source of intestinal bleeding; however, endoscopy is

| BOX 8-1 | Diagnostic Procedures for Gastrointestinal Bleeding |

Upper GI Bleeding (Hematemesis or Blood in the Nasogastric [NG] Tube)
- Esophagogastroduodenoscopy
- Celiac angiography
- Aortography (to rule out aortoduodenal fistula)

Lower GI Bleeding (Hematochezia or Melena)
- Pass NG tube to eliminate upper GI bleeding
- Proctoscopy to eliminate hemorrhoids
- Colonoscopy if patient is stable and bowel is relatively free of stool
- Arteriography if bleeding is fast enough
- GI scintigraphy if bleeding is slow but persistent
- Barium enema if other tests cannot localize bleeding and bleeding is persistent

not helpful if the source is within the small intestine or the colon. Although colonoscopy allows excellent visualization of the colon when it is cleared out, it is extremely difficult to see when acute, active intestinal bleeding is occurring. Arteriography has three limitations in its evaluation of GI bleeding. First, arteriography can determine the site of bleeding, but the rate of bleeding must exceed 0.5 mL/min for detection. Second, if GI bleeding is intermittent, the results of the arteriogram can be falsely negative. Third, arteriography visualizes only the blood vessels to the small bowel, right colon, and transverse colon through a superior mesenteric angiogram. If the left colon and sigmoid vessels are to be visualized (most bleeding comes from these areas), an inferior mesenteric angiogram must be requested. This is more difficult to perform.

The GI bleeding scan has several advantages over arteriography. The GI bleeding scan can detect bleeding if the rate is in excess of 0.05 mL/min. Also, with the use of technetium-labeled RBCs, delayed films (as long as 24 hours) can be obtained to indicate the site of an intermittent or extremely slow intestinal bleed.

A GI scintigram is much more sensitive in locating the site of GI bleeding; however, it is not very specific in pinpointing the site or the cause of bleeding. Usually, when the results of a GI scintigram are positive, the exact source of bleeding cannot be localized any more accurately than indicating the affected quadrant of the abdomen (e.g., right upper, left lower). This test is usually performed by injecting sulfur colloid labeled with technetium-99m (^{99m}Tc) or ^{99m}Tc-labeled red blood cells (RBCs) into the patient. If the patient is bleeding at a rate in excess of 0.05 mL/min, pooling of the radionuclide will ultimately be detected in the abnormal segment of the intestine. Few false-positive results occur. Again, it is important to recognize that the test will only localize the bleeding; it will not indicate the exact pathologic condition causing the bleeding. With this test result, if surgery is required, the surgeon is directed to the abnormal area and hopefully can detect and resect the pathologic bleeding source.

It is important to realize that this test can take at least 1 to 4 hours to obtain useful information. Unstable patients should not leave the intensive care environment for that long. Furthermore, the unstable patient may need to go to surgery in minutes and the surgeon may not have the luxury of taking several hours to determine the region of active bleeding.

CONTRAINDICATIONS

- Patients who are pregnant or lactating unless the benefits outweigh the risk or damage to the fetus or newborn
- Medically unstable patients whose stay in the nuclear medicine department may be risky

INTERFERING FACTORS

- Barium within the GI tract may mask a small source of bleeding.

Clinical Priorities

- GI bleeding scans can localize the bleeding. They cannot indicate the cause of the bleeding.
- Because this test requires several hours, unstable patients may not be candidates for it. They may be unable to leave the intensive care unit for that long.
- Delayed films may be taken up to 24 hours later to detect slow, intermittent, or chronic bleeding.

PROCEDURE AND PATIENT CARE

Before

- Explain the procedure to the patient.
- Assess the patient's vital signs to ensure that they are stable for the patient's transfer to and from the nuclear medicine department.
- Accompany the patient to the nuclear medicine department if vital signs are questionably stable.
- Assure the patient that only a small amount of nuclear material will be administered.
- Instruct the patient to notify the nuclear medicine technologist if he or she has a bowel movement during the test. Blood in the GI tract can act as a cathartic.
- Inform the patient that no pretest preparation is required.
- Instruct the nuclear medicine technologist to notify the nurse of all bloody bowel movements that occur while the patient is in the nuclear medicine department.
- Tell the patient that the only discomfort associated with this study is the injection of the radioisotope.

During

- Note the following procedural steps:
  1. Ten millicuries of freshly prepared ^{99m}Tc-labeled sulfur colloid is administered to the patient intravenously. If ^{99m}Tc-labeled RBCs are to be used, 3 to 5 mL of the patient's own blood is combined with the ^{99m}Tc and reinjected into the patient.
  2. Immediately after administration of the radionuclide, the patient is placed under a scintillation camera.
  3. Multiple images of the abdomen are obtained at short intervals (5 to 15 minutes). Delayed films may be performed as late as 6 to 24 hours later to detect slow, intermittent, or chronic bleeding. The scintigrams are recorded on film.
  4. Detection of radionuclide in the abdomen indicates the site of bleeding. If no bleeding sites are noted in the first hour, the scan may be repeated at hourly intervals for as long as 24 hours.
- Note that areas of the bowel hidden by the liver or spleen may not be adequately evaluated by this procedure. Also, the rectum cannot be easily evaluated because other pelvic structures (e.g., the bladder) obstruct the view. If the initial study is negative and subsequent films give evidence of active bleeding, a repeat scan may be performed.
- Note that this test is usually performed in approximately 20 to 30 minutes if Tc-sulfur colloid is used by a technologist in the nuclear medicine department. The scan may take longer if Tc-labeled red blood cells are used.

After

- Reevaluate the patient's vital signs on return to the nursing unit.
- Assure the patient that only tracer doses of radioisotopes have been used and that no precautions against radioactive exposure to others are necessary.

TEST RESULTS AND CLINICAL SIGNIFICANCE

Ulcers,
Tumors,
Angiodysplasia and other vascular malformations,
Polyps,
Diverticulosis,
Inflammatory bowel disease:
  The mucosa and submucosa in the areas of these diseases are quite friable and can bleed profusely.
Aortoduodenal fistulas: *These usually present as rapid exsanguinating and recurrent upper GI bleeding episodes in a patient who has had prior aortic aneurysm surgery or prior radiation therapy to the area of the midabdomen to upper abdomen.*

RELATED TESTS

Arteriography (p. 988). This is a radiographic study used to evaluate the patient with GI bleeding at a rate greater than 1 mL/min.
Esophagogastroduodenoscopy (p. 608) and Colonoscopy (p. 591). These endoscopic tests can be very helpful in identifying the source of GI blood. In some cases endoscopic therapies can be used to stop the bleeding.

Liver/Spleen Scanning (Liver Scanning)

NORMAL FINDINGS

Normal size, shape, and position of the liver and spleen with no filling defects

INDICATIONS

This test allows for visualization of the liver and spleen. It is indicated in patients with cancer to rule out metastatic tumor to the liver. It is a routine part of tumor staging. It is also indicated in patients with primary tumors (hepatomas) or in patients with cirrhosis who are at high risk for the development of primary hepatomas. Patients with abnormal liver enzymes will also have their liver visualized. Liver scanning is used to monitor liver diseases and response to therapy.

TEST EXPLANATION

This radionuclide procedure is used to outline and detect structural changes of the liver and spleen. A radionuclide, usually technetium-99m (^{99m}Tc)-labeled sulfur colloid, is administered intravenously. Later, a scintillation camera is placed over the right upper and left upper quadrants of the patient's abdomen. This records the distribution of the radioactive particles emitted from the liver and spleen. Images are obtained that are comparable to the gamma ray emission and are recorded digitally or on an analog film.

Because the scan can demonstrate only filling defects greater than 2 cm in diameter, false-negative results may occur in patients with space-occupying lesions (e.g., tumors, cysts, granulomas, abscesses) smaller than 2 cm. The scan may be incorrectly interpreted as positive for filling defects in patients with cirrhosis because of the distortion of the patient's liver parenchyma. The liver scan can detect tumors, cysts, granulomas, abscesses, and diffuse infiltrative processes affecting the liver (e.g., amyloidosis, sarcoidosis).

When a liver filling defect is observed, the most common cause is a benign hemangioma. This can be differentiated from tumor with the use of Tc-labeled red blood cells (RBCs). The patient's own RBCs are labeled with Tc and reinjected into the patient. Immediate uptake of the radionuclide by the filling defect is suggestive of a hemangioma, for which no therapy is usually required.

In general, computed tomography (CT) scans and magnetic resonance imaging (MRI) scans have replaced the liver scan in diagnostics. Single-photon emission computed tomography (SPECT) has significantly improved the quality and accuracy of liver scanning. With SPECT scanning the radionuclide is injected and the scintillation camera is placed to receive images from multiple angles (around the circumference of the liver). This greatly increases the usefulness of nuclear liver scanning. With the use of radioactive carbon, nitrogen, fluorine, or oxygen, anatomic and biochemical changes can be visualized within the liver. This method of liver scanning is called positron emission tomography (PET) scanning (p. 821).

The liver scan can also identify portal hypertension. Normally, most of the radionuclide administered during a liver scan is taken up by the liver. If the liver-to-spleen ratio is reversed (i.e., the spleen takes up more of the radionuclide), reversal of hepatic blood flow exists as a result of portal hypertension.

Splenic hematoma, abscess, cyst, tumor, infarction, and infiltrate processes such as granulomas can be detected. SPECT scanning can also be used to improve visualization of the spleen.

CONTRAINDICATIONS

- Patients who are pregnant or lactating, unless the benefit outweighs the risk of damage to the fetus or infant

INTERFERING FACTORS

- Barium in the gastrointestinal (GI) tract overlying the liver or spleen will produce defects on the scan that may be mistaken for masses.

✓ Clinical Priorities

- This test is a routine part of tumor staging. It is used to rule out metastasis to the liver in cancer patients.
- False-negative results can occur in patients with lesions smaller than 2 cm.
- A combination lung-liver scan can be performed to identify subpulmonic or subdiaphragmatic abscesses.

PROCEDURE AND PATIENT CARE

Before

Explain the procedure to the patient.

Tell the patient that no fasting or premedication is required.

Nuclear Scanning

8

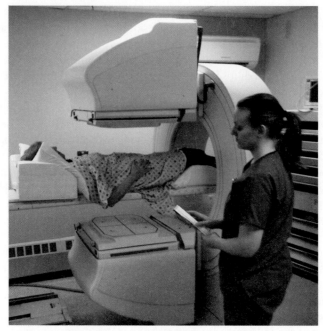

Figure 8-9 Liver/spleen nuclear scan.

🖉 Assure the patient that he or she will not be exposed to large amounts of radiation because only tracer doses of isotopes are used.

🖉 Tell the patient that the only discomfort associated with this procedure is the IV injection of the radionuclide.

During

- Note the following procedural steps:
  1. The patient is taken to the nuclear medicine department, where the radionuclide is administered intravenously. (For inpatients a nuclear medicine technologist may administer the radionuclide at the bedside.)
  2. Thirty minutes after injection, a gamma ray detector is placed over the right upper quadrant of the patient's abdomen.
  3. The patient is placed in supine and prone positions as the camera rotates around the patient (Figure 8-9) so that all surfaces of the liver can be visualized.
  4. The radionuclide image is recorded digitally or on an analog film.
- Note that this procedure is performed by a trained technologist in approximately 1 hour. A physician trained in nuclear medicine interprets the results.

After

🖉 Because only tracer doses of radioisotopes are used, inform the patient that no precautions need to be taken by others against radiation exposure.

TEST RESULTS AND CLINICAL SIGNIFICANCE

Primary or metastatic tumor of the liver or spleen,

Abscess of the liver or spleen,

Hematoma of the liver or spleen,

Hepatic or splenic cyst,

Hemangioma:

These diseases are evident as localized filling defects within the liver/spleen parenchyma.

Lacerations of the liver or spleen: *The organ can be seen to be fractured, with a hematoma within the laceration.*

Infiltrative processes (e.g., sarcoidosis, amyloidosis, tuberculosis, or granuloma of the liver or spleen),

Cirrhosis:

These diseases are apparent as diffuse irregularity in the uptake of the radionuclide within the liver or spleen.

Portal hypertension: *There is reversal of the normal liver/spleen ratio of uptake of the radionuclide. Usually the liver takes up most of the radionuclide. In portal hypertension, with reversal of hepatic portal blood flow, the spleen takes up more of the radionuclide.*

Accessory spleen: *The radionuclide aggregates in extrasplenic sites. This is very helpful to the surgeon who is planning a splenectomy and removal of all spleen tissue for patients with autoimmune thrombocytopenia or hemolytic anemia.*

Splenic infarction: *This is evident as a localized space-filling defect within the spleen in a patient with sudden onset of left upper quadrant pain.*

RELATED TESTS

Computed Tomography (CT) Scan of the Liver and Spleen (p. 1020). This is probably a more accurate test for the evaluation of these organs. However, to make the diagnosis of hemangioma, liver scanning with autologous RBCs labeled with Tc is superior in accuracy to a CT scan.

Magnetic Resonance Imaging (MRI) Scan of the Liver and Spleen (p. 1106). This is considered to be more accurate than the nuclear scans; however, it is more difficult to obtain and more expensive.

Lung Scan (Ventilation/Perfusion Scanning [VPS], V/Q Scan)

NORMAL FINDINGS

Diffuse and homogeneous uptake of nuclear material by the lungs

INDICATIONS

The lung scan is very helpful in making the diagnosis of pulmonary embolism (PE). It is easily and rapidly performed on patients who have sudden onset of noncardiac chest pain or shortness of breath. It is often performed on patients who have unexplained tachycardia or hypoxemia (Box 8-2).

TEST EXPLANATION

This nuclear medicine procedure is used to identify defects in blood perfusion of the lung in patients with suspected PE. Blood flow to the lungs is evaluated using a macroaggregated albumin (MAA) tagged with technetium (Tc), which is injected into the patient's peripheral vein. Because the diameter of the radionuclide aggregates is larger than that of the pulmonary capillaries, the aggregates become temporarily lodged in the pulmonary vasculature. A scintillation camera detects the gamma rays from

Nuclear Scanning

8

BOX 8-2	Diagnosis of Pulmonary Embolism

Symptoms
Chest pain
Shortness of breath
Feelings of impending doom
Pleurodynia (pain with deep inspiration)

Signs
Tachycardia
Hypoxemia
S_4 gallop

Tests	Results
Chest x-ray	Normal, although if the PE progresses to pulmonary infarction, a wedge-shaped abnormality can be identified.
Electrocardiography	Normal, although if the PE is large enough, right heart strain may be evident (i.e., S wave in lead I, Q wave in lead III, and inverted T wave in lead III).
Arterial blood gases	Po_2 is reduced. O_2 saturation is reduced. Pco_2 may be slightly increased.
Lung scan	Poor perfusion to an isolated segment of lung is observed.
V/Q scan	Mismatch of ventilation and perfusion is evident.
Pulmonary angiography	Cutoff of blood flow to one or more segments of the lung and filling defects in the pulmonary arteries or arterioles are observed.
Computerized tomography of the chest	Embolism visible in a branch of the pulmonary artery.

---

within the lung microvasculature. With the use of light conversion a realistic image of the lung is obtained on film.

A homogeneous uptake of particles that fills the entire pulmonary vasculature conclusively rules out PE. If a defect in an otherwise smooth and diffusely homogeneous pattern is seen, a perfusion abnormality exists (Figure 8-10). This can indicate PE. Unfortunately, many other serious pulmonary parenchymal lesions (e.g., pneumonia, pleural fluid, emphysematous bullae) also cause a defect in pulmonary blood perfusion. Therefore, although the scan may be sensitive, it is not specific because many different pathologic conditions can cause the same abnormal results.

The chest x-ray film aids in the interpretation of the perfusion scan because a defect on the perfusion scan seen in the same area as a pulmonary parenchymal abnormality on the chest x-ray film does not indicate PE. Rather, the defect may represent pneumonia, atelectasis, effusion, and so on. When a perfusion defect occurs in an area of the lung that is normal on a chest x-ray study, however, PE is very likely.

Specificity of a perfusion scan also can be enhanced by the concomitant performance of a *ventilation lung scan*, which detects parenchymal abnormalities in ventilation (e.g., pneumonia, pleural fluid, emphysematous bullae). The ventilation scan reflects the patency of the pulmonary airways using xenon gas or technetium (Tc) diethylenetriamine pentaacetic acid (DTPA) as an aerosol. When vascular obstruction (embolism) is present on a perfusion scan, ventilation scans will demonstrate a normal wash-in and a normal wash-out of radioactivity from the embolized lung area. If parenchymal disease (e.g., pneumonia) is responsible for the perfusion abnormality, however, wash-in or wash-out will be

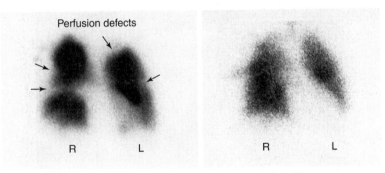

Figure 8-10 Lung scan. **A,** Perfusion. **B,** Ventilation. There are multiple perfusion defects noted on the perfusion lung scan. However, the uptake of radionuclide on the ventilation scan is normal. The combination of findings is because of pulmonary emboli.

abnormal. Therefore the "mismatch" of perfusion and ventilation is characteristic of embolic disorders, whereas the "match" is indicative of parenchymal disease. When ventilation and perfusion scans are performed synchronously, this is called a *ventilation/perfusion (V/Q) scan.*

Most nuclear physicians place the lung scan results in one of several categories: negative for PE, low probability of PE, high probability of PE, or positive for PE.

With the increased availability of rapid access spatial CT scanning of the chest (see p. 1029), the diagnosis of PE is now more easily made with CT scanning of the chest using CT angiography. CT angiography is faster and more accurate than ventilation/perfusion lung scans and is less invasive than pulmonary angiography.

CONTRAINDICATIONS

- Patients who are pregnant unless the benefits outweigh the risk of fetal damage

INTERFERING FACTORS

- Patients with known pulmonary parenchymal or pleural problems (e.g., pneumonia, emphysema, pleural effusion, tumors), which will give the picture of a perfusion defect and simulate PE.

Clinical Priorities

- This nuclear medicine procedure is mainly used to detect PE.
- Because lung scans are sensitive but not specific, several types of pulmonary problems (other than PE) can cause a defect in pulmonary blood perfusion.
- The specificity of a perfusion scan can be improved by the performance of a ventilation scan. When they are performed together, this is called a ventilation/perfusion (V/Q) scan.
- The chest x-ray study aids in the interpretation of the lung scan.

PROCEDURE AND PATIENT CARE

Before

Explain the procedure to the patient.
- Obtain informed consent if required by the institution.

Nuclear Scanning

8

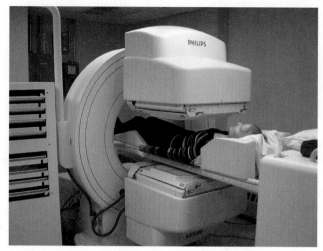

Figure 8-11 Patient positioned for lung scan.

Assure the patient that he or she will not be exposed to large amounts of radioactivity because only tracer doses of isotopes are used.

Tell the patient that no fasting is required.

• Note that a recent (within the last 24 to 48 hours) chest x-ray film should be obtained.

Instruct the patient to remove jewelry around the chest area.

Tell the patient that no discomfort is associated with this test other than the peripheral venipuncture.

During

• The unsedated, nonfasting patient with suspected PE is taken to the nuclear medicine department (Figure 8-11).
• Note the following procedural steps:

Ventilation Scan

1. The patient breathes through a closed-system face mask with a mouthpiece. The radionuclide tracer is then administered into the system.
2. Tc DTPA images are usually obtained before perfusion images and require patient cooperation with deep breathing and appropriate use of breathing equipment to prevent contamination.

Perfusion Scan

1. The patient is given a peripheral intravenous (IV) injection of radionuclide-tagged MAA.
2. While the patient lies in the appropriate position, a gamma ray detector is passed over the patient and records radionuclide uptake.
3. The patient is placed in the supine position with the camera rotating around the patient. This allows for anterior, posterior, and lateral and oblique views, respectively.
4. The results are interpreted by a physician trained in diagnostic nuclear medicine.

• Note that this test is usually performed by a technologist in approximately 30 minutes.

After

Inform the patient that no radiation precautions are necessary.

TEST RESULTS AND CLINICAL SIGNIFICANCE

Pulmonary embolism: *This is evident as a perfusion defect on a perfusion lung scan. It is also apparent as a "mismatch" of ventilation and perfusion on a V/Q scan. Positive results are definitive, but negative results can be false.*

Pneumonia,

Tuberculosis,

Asthma,

Chronic obstructive pulmonary disease,

Tumor,

Atelectasis,

Bronchitis:

    These parenchymal abnormalities can cause perfusion defects. When a defect is apparent on the plain chest x-ray film or a ventilation lung scan, a ventilation/perfusion "match" is identified. Matched defects are not caused by pulmonary emboli, but rather by the above-noted parenchymal disease.

RELATED TESTS

Computed Tomography (CT) Scan of the Lung (p. 1029). This has now become the preferred test to diagnose PE.

Arterial Blood Gases (p. 109). Hypoxemia is the hallmark of PE.

Electrocardiography (p. 544). Although the EKG is usually normal with PE, right heart strain can be identified with large acute PE.

Chest X-Ray (p. 1014). Although PEs are not evident on the plain chest x-ray film, identification of parenchymal abnormalities is important to accurately interpret the perfusion lung scan.

D-dimer (p. 202). This test is used to identify intravascular clotting. It is an excellent screening test for pulmonary embolism.

Meckel Diverticulum Nuclear Scan

NORMAL FINDINGS

No increased uptake of radionuclide in the right lower quadrant of the abdomen

INDICATIONS

This scan is designed to identify a Meckel diverticulum that contains ectopic gastric mucosa. It is indicated in patients who have recurrent lower abdominal pain or in pediatric or young adult patients who have occult gastrointestinal (GI) bleeding.

TEST EXPLANATION

Meckel diverticulum is the most common congenital abnormality of the intestinal tract. It is a persistent remnant of the omphalomesenteric tract. The diverticulum usually occurs in the ileum, approximately 2 feet proximal to the ileocecal valve. Approximately 20% to 25% of Meckel diverticula are lined internally by ectopic gastric mucosa. This gastric mucosa can secrete acid and cause ulceration of the intestinal mucosa nearby. Bleeding, inflammation, and intussusception are other potential complications of this congenital abnormality. The majority of these complications occur by 2 years of age.

Both normal gastric mucosa within the stomach and ectopic gastric mucosa in Meckel diverticulum concentrate technetium-99m pertechnetate. When this radionuclide is injected intravenously, it is concentrated in the ectopic gastric mucosa of Meckel diverticulum. One can then expect to see a hot spot in the right lower quadrant of the abdomen at about the same time as the normal stomach mucosa is visualized. This is a very sensitive and specific test for this congenital abnormality.

It is possible that Meckel diverticulum is present but contains no ectopic gastric mucosa within. Usually this is not symptomatic. No concentration of radionuclide will occur within the diverticulum. This test is not helpful in these cases.

Other conditions can simulate a hot spot compatible with Meckel diverticulum containing ectopic gastric mucosa. Usually these are associated with inflammatory processes within the abdomen (e.g., appendicitis, Crohn disease, or ectopic pregnancy).

PROCEDURE AND PATIENT CARE

Before

- Explain the procedure to the patient.
- Advise the patient to refrain from eating or drinking anything for 6 to 12 hours before the examination.
- A histamine H_2-receptor antagonist is usually given for 1 to 2 days before the scan. This blocks secretion of the radionuclide from the ectopic gastric mucosa and improves visualization of Meckel diverticulum.
- Inform the patient that there is no pain associated with this test.

During

- The patient lies in a supine position, and a large-view nuclear detector camera is placed over the patient's abdomen to identify concentration of nuclear material after intravenous (IV) injection.
- Images are taken at 5-minute intervals for 1 hour.
- Patients may be asked to lie on their left side to minimize the excretion of the radionuclide from the normal stomach because that would flood the intestine with radionuclide and preclude visualization of Meckel diverticulum.
- Occasionally glucagon is provided to prolong intestinal transit time and avoid downstream contamination with the radionuclide.
- Occasionally gastrin is given to increase the uptake of the radionuclide by the ectopic gastric mucosa.

After

- The patient is asked to void, and a repeat image is obtained. This is to ensure that Meckel diverticulum has not been hidden by a distended bladder.
- Inform the patient that no precautions need to be taken by others against radiation because only tracer doses of radioisotopes are used.

TEST RESULTS AND CLINICAL SIGNIFICANCE

Increased uptake in the right lower quadrant: *This is compatible with Meckel diverticula containing ectopic gastric mucosa. As indicated above, if the diverticulum does not contain ectopic gastric mucosa, the test will not be positive. Furthermore, one must be aware that other inflammatory diseases can cause false-positive results.*

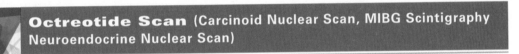

Octreotide Scan (Carcinoid Nuclear Scan, MIBG Scintigraphy Neuroendocrine Nuclear Scan)

NORMAL FINDINGS

No evidence of increased uptake throughout the body

INDICATIONS

Octreotide scans are used to identify and localize neuroendocrine primary and metastatic tumors. This scan is indicated in patients with known neuroendocrine tumors (e.g., carcinoid tumors and gastrinomas). It is used preoperatively to direct the surgeon to primary and metastatic tumors. This scan is also used to monitor therapy of these tumors.

TEST EXPLANATION

Octreotide scan is a specific example of *nuclear peptide scanning* that is increasingly being used to identify neoplasms by their altered state of physiology. Using peptides for which tumors have an increased uptake because of cellular membrane receptors or idiosyncratic physiology (glycolysis, proliferation, angiogenesis, or oxidation) will allow anatomic localization of many previously hidden tumors. These molecular imaging techniques can also provide information regarding the effect of anticancer therapy on tumor growth and survival.

Most neuroendocrine cells have a somatostatin receptor on the cellular membrane. Neuroendocrine tumors retain these receptors. Octreotide is an analogue of somatostatin. When combined with a radiopharmaceutical (such as indium-111 DTPA), the radiolabeled octreotide will attach to the somatostatin receptors of the neuroendocrine tumor cells. With the use of a scintillation camera the uptake can be observed and localized. In pediatrics, metaiodobenzylguanidine (MIBG) is used more frequently than octreotide as the radioisotope for identification of neuroendocrine tumors.

In patients with known neuroendocrine tumors, this test is used to direct the surgeon to the primary and metastatic sites within the body (especially the abdomen). This test is also used in the surveillance of patients who have been or are being treated for these neuroendocrine tumors. When this test is used as a monitor of disease, recurrence or progression can be identified quite easily and accurately. The liver, however, is more difficult to evaluate with octreotide scanning. The use of single-photon emission computed tomography (SPECT) imaging improves the sensitivity of this test. Many different types of hormone-producing tumors can be detected by this scan. Most notable include carcinoid, gastrinoma, insulinoma, glucagonoma, pheochromocytoma, and small cell lung cancer. Other abnormalities can pick up octreotide, including granulomatous infections (such as sarcoidosis or tuberculosis), rheumatoid arthritis, and nonhormonal cancers (breast, lymphoma, and non–small cell lung cancers).

The imaging procedure is performed by a trained technologist in approximately 30 minutes. A physician trained in nuclear medicine interprets the results. The only discomfort associated with this procedure is the intravenous (IV) injection of the radionuclide.

CONTRAINDICATIONS

- Patients who are pregnant or lactating, unless the benefit outweighs the risk of damage to the fetus or infant

Nuclear Scanning

8

INTERFERING FACTORS

- Barium in the gastrointestinal (GI) tract overlying the liver or spleen will produce defects on the scan that may be mistaken for masses.

PROCEDURE AND PATIENT CARE

Before

- Explain the procedure to the patient.
- Tell the patient that no fasting or premedication is required.
- Assure the patient that he or she will not be exposed to large amounts of radiation because only tracer doses of isotopes are used.
- If an iodinated radionuclide is to be used, ensure that the patient does not have an allergy to iodine.
- If an iodinated radionuclide is to be used, administer 5 drops of Lugol iodine solution daily for 3 days. This will block uptake of the radionuclide by the thyroid gland.
- If the patient has been receiving octreotide as a form of antineoplastic treatment, this must be discontinued for 2 weeks before scanning.

During

- Note the following procedural steps:
  1. The patient is taken to the nuclear medicine department, where the radionuclide is administered intravenously. (For inpatients, a nuclear medicine technologist may administer the radionuclide at the bedside.)
  2. One hour after injection, a gamma camera is successively placed over the entire body.
  3. The patient is placed in supine, lateral, and prone positions so that all surfaces can be visualized.
  4. The radionuclide image is recorded on film. SPECT images may also be performed.
  5. After 4 hours the patient is given a strong laxative to clear the octreotide from the bowel.
  6. Repeat scanning is again performed at 2, 4, 24, and 48 hours after administration of the octreotide.

After

- Inform the patient that no precautions need to be taken by others against radiation exposure because only tracer doses of radioisotopes are used.

TEST RESULTS AND CLINICAL SIGNIFICANCE

Carcinoid tumors: *This tumor consists of neuroendocrine argentaffin cells that have somatostatin receptors. They usually arise from the appendix, small bowel, or colon. However, any organ can be the primary site of a carcinoid tumor.*

Neuroendocrine tumors: *Neuroendocrine tumors and other tumors as listed above can take up octreotide.*

Granulomatous infections such as sarcoidosis and tuberculosis: *The pathophysiology of this observation is not well understood.*

Parathyroid Scan (Parathyroid Scintigraphy)

NORMAL FINDINGS

No increased parathyroid uptake

INDICATIONS

This test is used to locate the parathyroid glands before surgery. It also indicates the cause of the hyperparathyroidism.

TEST EXPLANATION

Hypercalcemia can be caused by hyperparathyroidism. Parathyroid hyperplasia, adenoma, or cancer can cause hyperparathyroidism. It is important for the surgeon planning resection of the parathyroid abnormality to know how many parathyroid glands are involved and their locations. Preoperative parathyroid scanning is the most accurate method of providing this information. Parathyroid hyperplasia causes enlargement of all four parathyroid glands. A parathyroid adenoma or cancer, however, causes enlargement of only one parathyroid gland and suppression (decrease in size) of the other three glands. Based on the parathyroid scan, the surgeon will know whether to suspect disease in one or all four of the glands.

Parathyroids are located most commonly on the lateral borders of the thyroid lobes—two on each side. However, parathyroid anatomic location varies considerably, and they may be located anywhere from the upper neck to the lower mediastinum. Parathyroid scanning is also done immediately before surgery to help the surgeon identify the parathyroid glands and particularly the pathologic glands. In this test, the scan is performed on the parathyroid glands as described previously. In the operating room, the surgeon scans the entire anterior neck with a hand-held gamma ray detector. Increased counts are noted in the regions where the parathyroids are located.

Scanning is now done more frequently in newly diagnosed patients. In some centers, scanning is reserved for those patients in whom an initial neck exploration failed to identify all four parathyroid glands and the hypercalcemia persisted after the operation.

There are two methods of parathyroid scanning. The first is the single tracer double phase (STDP) test using technetium-99m (^{99m}Tc) sestamibi or ^{99m}Tc tetrofosmin. With this method, the patient is injected with the sestamibi tracer. Images are obtained at 15 minutes and 3 hours. The tracer initially lights up both the thyroid and the parathyroid glands. At 3 hours, however, the tracer is washed out of all normal endocrine tissue and remains only in the pathologic parathyroid tissue.

The second method is the dual isotope subtraction test in which ^{99m}Tc pertechnetate or iodine 123 (^{123}I) is administered. Only the thyroid gland takes up either of these two later tracers. Scanning is performed. ^{99m}Tc sestamibi is then administered and is taken up by both the thyroid and the parathyroid glands. Scanning is repeated and that first image is then "subtracted" from the second image leaving an image of only the parathyroid glands.

CONTRAINDICATIONS

- Patients who are allergic to iodine if radioactive iodine is to be used
- Patients who are pregnant unless the benefits outweigh the risks

INTERFERING FACTORS

- Patient movement can inhibit the quality of imaging, especially when subtraction scanning is performed.
- Recent administration of x-ray contrast agents can alter test results.
- Iodine-containing foods or drugs (including cough medicines) can affect test results.

Nuclear Scanning

8

PROCEDURE AND PATIENT CARE

Before

🖉 Explain the procedure to the patient.

🖉 Tell the patient that fasting is usually not required. Check with the laboratory.

• Check the patient for allergies to iodine.

🖉 Instruct the patient about medications and food that need to be restricted for weeks before the test (e.g., thyroid drugs, medications or food containing iodine).

• Obtain a history concerning recent contrast x-ray studies, nuclear scanning, or intake of any thyroid-suppressive or antithyroid drugs.

🖉 Tell the patient that no discomfort is associated with this test.

During

There are two methods of parathyroid scanning. Note the following procedural steps:

STDP Method (Single Tracer Double Phase)

1. Technetium-99m sestamibi or tetrofosmin is injected intravenously.
2. At 15 minutes and 3 hours, the patient is placed in a supine position, a detector is passed over the neck and upper chest area, and the radioactive counts are recorded and displayed.
3. Initially the tracer lights up both the thyroid and parathyroid glands. At 3 hours, the tracer remains only in the pathologic parathyroid tissue.

Dual Isotope Subtraction Test

1. Technetium-99m pertechnetate is injected intravenously. Iodine 123 may be administered orally instead.
2. At 15 minutes after IV injection (or 3 to 4 hours after oral administration) the patient is placed in a supine position, a detector is passed over the neck and upper chest area, and the radioactive counts are recorded and displayed. Only the thyroid gland takes up these tracers.
3. Technetium-99m sestamibi is then injected intravenously and imaging is repeated.
4. With the computer, subtraction images are obtained, leaving only the parathyroid gland images.

🖉 Tell the patient that no discomfort is associated with this study.

• A nuclear medicine technologist or a physician in the nuclear medicine department performs this procedure. The duration of the test is approximately 30 minutes. Scanning can be repeated several hours later for the STDP method.

After

🖉 Assure the patient that the dose of radioactive Tc used in this test is minute and therefore harmless. No isolation and no special urine precautions are needed.

TEST RESULTS AND CLINICAL SIGNIFICANCE

Parathyroid adenoma, carcinoma, or hyperplasia: *Adenomas and cancers of the parathyroid gland usually involve only one gland. Hyperplasia of the parathyroids usually involves all four glands. All must be found at the time of surgery. Parathyroid scan provides the location of those glands for the surgeon.*

Aberrantly placed parathyroid tissue in the upper neck, thyroid gland, or mediastinum: *The information provided by this scan can identify abnormally malpositioned parathyroid tissue. This is invaluable to the surgeon when this information is known preoperatively.*

Positron Emission Tomography (PET Scan)

NORMAL FINDINGS

No abnormal areas of increased or decreased uptake

INDICATIONS

PET scanning is used in many areas of medicine, most commonly for evaluation of the heart and brain. It is also commonly used in many aspects of oncology.

TEST EXPLANATION

In PET scanning, radioactive chemicals are administered to the patient. These chemicals are used in the normal metabolic process of the cells of the particular organ being imaged. Positrons emitted from the radioactive chemicals in the organ are sensed by a series of detectors positioned around the patient. Positron counts are received by these detectors and—with the combination of computed tomography—the positron emissions are recorded into a high-resolution three-dimensional image indicating a particular metabolic process in a specific anatomic site (Figure 8-12). Therefore PET provides images representing not only anatomy but also physiology. Like CT scans, MRI merely produces images of the body's anatomy or structure—not its metabolism. In most disease states, physiologic changes precede anatomic changes. Still in other disease states, such as Alzheimer disease, no anatomic changes

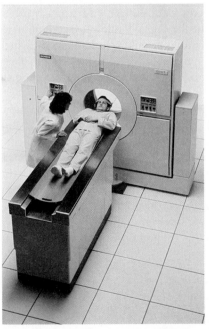

Figure 8-12 Positron emission tomography (PET). Clinical setting for PET. Shown are the Siemens ECAT scanner gantry and patient bed.

TABLE 8-3	Radionuclides Used in PET Scanning
Radionuclide	**Application**
Carbon-11	Cerebral, cardiac, pulmonary perfusion Detection of myocardial infarction Cerebral function
Nitrogen-13	Cerebral and cardiac perfusion Pulmonary inhalation Liver function
Oxygen-15	Cerebral perfusion and oxygen utilization
Fluorine-18	Cerebral function and glucose metabolism
Gallium-68	Cerebral perfusion Lymphoreticular function

occur—yet PET can identify classic physiologic changes that are diagnostic of the disease. Depending on the particular radionuclide used, PET can demonstrate the glucose metabolism, oxygenation, blood flow, and tissue perfusion of any specific area. Pathologic conditions are recognized and diagnosed by alterations in the normal metabolic process.

Certain radioactive chemical compounds provide specific information depending on the information required and the organ being evaluated. A cyclotron is used to create the radioactive chemical. Radioactive oxygen is used to make radioactive water ($H_2^{15}O$). This is used to evaluate blood flow and tissue perfusion of an organ.

Radioactive fluorine is applied to a glucose analog and called fluorodeoxyglucose (FDG). Because most cells use glucose as an energy source, FDG is particularly useful in concentrating in regions of high metabolic activity of a particular organ. Radioactive carbon-labeled glucose is also useful for this purpose. Radioactive nitrogen is used in radioactive ammonia, which can be used in evaluating the liver. Other applications of radionuclides are listed in Table 8-3. PET scanning is becoming more widely applied and commonly used as research continues. Its greatest use thus far has been in the fields of neurology, cardiology, and oncology.

In many centers, PET images can be superimposed with computed tomography (CT) or magnetic resonance imaging (MRI) to produce an anatomically accurate image showing the physiology/metabolism of the organ imaged. With newer units, PET/CT imaging can be performed by the same machine (Figure 8-13). This is called *PET/CT image fusion* or *PET/CT co-registration*. These composite views, which allow the information from two different studies to be digitally correlated and superimposed onto one image, lead to more precise information and accurate diagnoses. The CT images are acquired with the use of iodine contrast. In less than 60 minutes after the FDG is administered, the PET scan is performed in the same unit. The images are imposed on each other. The combined PET/CT scans provide images that pinpoint the location of abnormal metabolic activity within the body.

NEUROLOGY

Most brain imaging is performed with FDG. The brain uses glucose as its sole metabolic fuel. Pathologic areas of the brain that are more metabolically active (such as cancers) more avidly take up FDG than do normal areas. Because of the high physiologic rate at which glucose is metabolized by normal brain

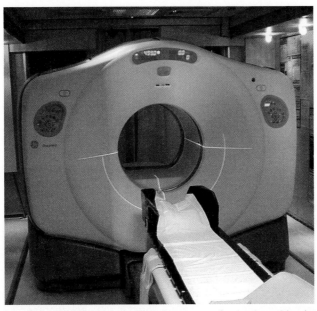

Figure 8-13 PET/CT imaging studies are performed on this uint.

tissue, the detectability of tumors with only modest increases in glucose metabolism, such as low-grade tumors and, in some cases, recurrent tumors, is difficult with FDG. Another radioactive marker that is being used is 3,4-dihydroxy-6-18F-fluoro-L-phenylalanine (18F-FDOPA). This seems to improve visibility of low-grade brain tumors.

Epilepsy, Parkinson disease, and Huntington disease are identified as localized areas of increased metabolic activity indicating rapid nerve firing. Brain trauma resulting in a hematoma or bleeding is evident as decreased metabolic activity in the area of trauma. Stroke can also be identified and its extent determined. With the use of radioactive water ($H_2^{15}O$), brain blood flow can be determined. Areas of decreased blood flow take up less ($H_2^{15}O$) than normal areas and represent areas at risk for stroke.

Alzheimer disease can be recognized by identifying hypometabolism in multiple areas of the brain (temporal and parietal lobe) as scanning is performed during cognitive exercises. PET scanning with amyloid imaging using radioactive markers such as Pittsburgh agent compound B (PiB), flutemetamol, or fluorine-18 has been very helpful in identifying amyloid protein precursors (p. 639) in the brain. These agents bind to the beta-amyloid plaques that are increased in patients with Alzheimer disease. A negative PET scan with amyloid imaging eliminates the possibility of Alzheimer disease in a patient with cognitive impairment. Because other neurologic conditions (especially in elderly people) are also associated with amyloid neuritic plaques, a positive scan does not certainly establish the diagnosis of Alzheimer disease.

Cardiology

PET scans of the heart can show decreased blood flow, indicating coronary artery occlusive disease. PET scans are also used when cardiac muscle function is reduced. A PET scan can indicate whether the dysfunction arises from reversible ischemic muscle that would benefit from revascularization or from muscle tissue that is no longer viable. In the former case, surgical revascularization should be considered. In the latter case, revascularization would not be beneficial.

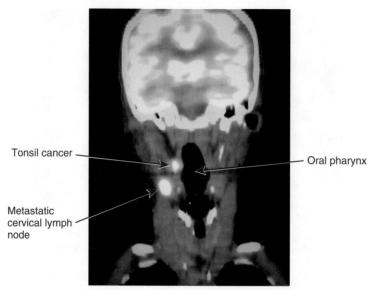

Figure 8-14 PET scan of the head and neck. Avid uptake of normal brain is noted. See two hotspots noted in the neck representing primary tonsil cancer and metastatic cervical lymph node.

Oncology

The most commonly used agent in oncology is FDG because increased glucose metabolism is so prevalent in malignant tumors when compared to normal or benign pathologic tissue. PET can be used to visualize rapidly growing tumors and indicate their anatomic location. It is used to determine tumor response to therapy, identify recurrence of tumor after surgical removal, and differentiate tumor from other pathologic conditions (e.g., infection). PET is particularly helpful in identifying regional and metastatic spread for a particular tumor (Figures 8-14 [head and neck] and 8-15 [chest]). PET is more accurate in oncologic staging than CT scan. Its sensitivity exceeds 95% with a specificity of over 80%. In lung cancer, for example, if the FDG fails to concentrate in any area other than the primary tumor, no spread is suspected and the patient is considered an ideal candidate for surgery. PET has also been particularly useful for identifying metastasis from lung, melanoma, breast, pancreas, colon, lymphoma, and brain cancers.

Rapidly growing tumors are associated with a high metabolic rate and will therefore concentrate FDG particularly well. The amount of uptake of FDG is measured by the Standardized Uptake Value (SUV)—the amount of uptake of FDG in tumor compared to the normal tissue in that same area. SUV helps to distinguish between benign and malignant lesions—the higher the SUV, the more likely the tumor is malignant.

When the SUV is greater than the "cutoff value" (as determined by each institution), cancer rather than a benign pathologic condition is suspected. PET scanning is particularly helpful in the evaluation of solitary pulmonary nodules. CT scans and chest x-rays are inadequate to distinguish benign from malignant lesions. PET scanning can accurately provide that information over 75% of the time.

Bone

A PET/CT scan with a sodium fluoride F18 injection (^{18}F NaF) scans the entire skeletal system and produces high-resolution images of the bones. These images are used to detect areas of abnormal bone growth associated with tumors. This test is more accurate than conventional nuclear bone scans. The

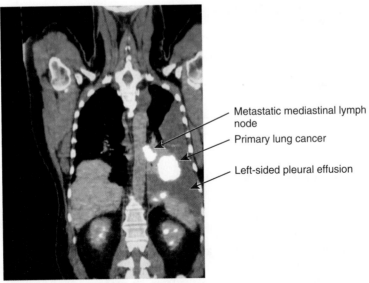

Metastatic mediastinal lymph node

Primary lung cancer

Left-sided pleural effusion

Figure 8-15 PET scan of the chest. Note two hotspots representing a primary lung cancer and multiple mediastinal lymph node metastasis. A large pleural effusion is noted.

PET/CT scan of the bone is particularly helpful for patients with prostate or breast cancer. The uptake of ^{18}F NaF in the skeleton reflects sites of increased blood flow and bone remodeling associated with bone injury or metastatic disease. A bone PET/CT scan's high-resolution images and its ability to scan the entire skeleton make it very helpful in detecting bone disease.

Small parts PET scans are being used with increasing frequency for foot inflammatory pathology. *PET mammography or positron emission mammography (PEM)* is seeing growing use as a tool for diagnostic breast imaging. PEM holds the promise of improving sensitivity and specificity of routine mammography (see p. 1043).

INTERFERING FACTORS

- Recent use (within 24 hours) of caffeine, alcohol, or tobacco may affect test results.
- Ingestion of a small- to moderate-sized meal can cause a marked uptake of FDG in the gut and muscles, thereby leaving little or no radionuclide to be taken up by tumor. This can cause a false-negative result.
- Anxiety can cause increased uptake in multiple areas (e.g., neck, upper mediastinum) of the body. If the patient is anxious, sedatives can be administered 30 minutes before testing. However, these could interfere with PET scanning of the brain if cognitive activities will be used to measure changes in brain activity.
- Mild to moderate exercise can instigate marked uptake of FDG in the muscles thereby leaving little or no radionuclide to be taken up by tumor. This causes a false-negative result.
- The liver and spleen avidly take up FDG. Therefore those organs are difficult to evaluate on PET imaging.
- FDG is excreted by the urinary system. As a result, the bladder may obscure areas of increased uptake in the pelvis.
- Uptake of FDG can occur in the lymph node basin draining the site of the FDG injection. If PET is being done to stage tumors that could metastasize to those lymph nodes, inject the FDG on the contralateral side.

Clinical Priorities

- Test results can be affected by recent use of caffeine, alcohol, or tobacco.
- Tell patients that no sedatives or tranquilizers should be taken, because they may need to perform mental activities during the test.
- After the test, patients should be encouraged to drink fluids and urinate frequently to aid in removal of the radioisotope from the bladder.

PROCEDURE AND PATIENT CARE

Before

- Explain the procedure to the patient.
- Obtain informed consent if required by the institution.
- Inform the patient that he or she may have an intravenous (IV) line inserted.
- Inform the patient that he or she may need to restrict food or fluids for 4 hours on the day of the test. The patient should refrain from alcohol, caffeine, and tobacco for 24 hours.
- Instruct diabetic patients to take their pretest dose of insulin at a meal 3 to 4 hours before the test.
- Tell the patient that no sedatives or tranquilizers should be taken, because he or she may need to perform certain mental activities during the brain PET scan.
- Tell the patient to empty the bladder before the test for comfort. A Foley catheter may be inserted for PET scanning of the pelvic region.
- Tell the patient that the only discomfort associated with this study is insertion of the IV line.
- Depending on the organ being evaluated, specific protocols exist for the examination.

During

- Note the following procedural steps:
  1. The patient is positioned in a comfortable, reclining chair.
  2. The radioactive material can be infused through an IV line or inhaled as a radioactive gas.
  3. The gamma rays that penetrate the tissues are recorded outside the body by a circular array of detectors and are displayed by a computer.
  4. If the brain is being scanned, the patient may be asked to perform different cognitive activities (e.g., reciting the Pledge of Allegiance) to measure changes in brain activity during reasoning or remembering.
  5. Extraneous auditory and visual stimuli are minimized by a blindfold and ear plugs.
  6. If the chest is being scanned, instruct the patient to breathe in a shallow manner until the middle of the chest is reached. Then ask the patient to hold the breath after expiration until the middle of the abdomen is reached. This will improve visibility of the chest anatomy.
- Note that a physician performs this procedure with a trained technologist in approximately 40 to 90 minutes.

After

- Instruct the patient to change position slowly from lying to standing to avoid postural hypotension.
- Encourage the patient to drink fluids and urinate frequently to aid in removal of the radioisotope from the bladder.

TEST RESULTS AND CLINICAL SIGNIFICANCE

Myocardial infarction,
Coronary artery disease:
  *Areas of ischemia or infarction are associated with decreased flow and decreased glucose metabolism.
    This is indicated by hypoconcentration of FDG.*
Cerebrovascular accident (stroke): *These areas are evident as decreased blood flow and metabolism.*
Epilepsy,
Parkinson disease,
Huntington disease:
  Focal areas of increased metabolism are evident during seizure or repetitive activity.
Dementia,
Alzheimer disease:
  *Specific areas of decreased metabolism are noted in classic regions of the brain (temporal and parietal
    lobes).*
Malignant tumor: *Malignancy is associated with increased glucose metabolism in rapidly dividing cells.
  This is indicated by concentration of FDG in levels exceeding SUV cutoff points.*

RELATED TESTS

Computed Tomography (CT) Scanning (p. 1020). This uses a technique that recognizes differences in
  density coefficients to visualize different organs and tissues. Unlike PET, a CT scan cannot provide
  information concerning metabolism or function.
Single-Photon Emission Computed Tomography (SPECT) Scanning (p. 780). This is another form of
  radionuclear imaging that can provide three-dimensional anatomic and perfusion images but lacks
  the capability to indicate metabolism.
Magnetic Resonance Imaging (MRI) (p. 1106). This provides a picture of normal and pathologic anatomy
  by temporarily altering the magnetic field of the cells in the area to be evaluated.

ProstaScint Scan (Radioimmunoscintigraphy [RIS])

NORMAL FINDINGS

No increased uptake outside the prostate gland

INDICATIONS

This test is used to identify and accurately stage prostate cancer.

TEST EXPLANATION

By using a radionuclide that is able to attach to prostate cancer cells only, metastatic prostate cancer
outside the prostate gland can be easily identified. In this scan, mouse monoclonal antibody (capromab)
directed against prostate specific membrane antigen (PSMA) is tagged with indium[111]. PSMA, located
in the cytoplasm of prostate cancer (or transitional cell urogenital cancer), is detected on radionuclide
scan images. Disease outside the prostate (e.g., retroperitoneum, liver, lung, bone) indicates metastatic

Nuclear Scanning

8

prostate cancer. Other radionuclides, such as technetium labeled red blood cells, can be used, but the images provide less accurate results.

This scan is helpful in staging newly diagnosed prostate cancer patients who are at high risk for metastatic disease to the lymph nodes or other organs. This test can also be used to identify recurrent or metastatic disease after curative therapy. This test can document completeness of anti-prostate cancer therapy. Finally this scan helps elucidate abnormalities that may be noted on other diagnostic imaging tests, such as CT scan (especially in patients with prior prostate cancer).

The ProstaScint scan is usually performed in conjunction with other diagnostic testing, such as CT scan, PET scan, or ultrasound. Because of cost and labor intensity, this test is not used routinely for prostate screening.

This test takes about 30 minutes (per day for as many as 5 days) and is performed by a nuclear medicine technologist. It is interpreted by a nuclear medicine physician. There is no discomfort associated with this test other than an intravenous injection.

CONTRAINDICATIONS

- Patients who are allergic to mouse products
- Patients who are unable to be immobile for 1 hour

INTERFERING FACTORS

- Prior bone scans confound image interpretation.
- Areas of inflammation (such as degenerative joint disease, inflammatory bowel disease, or recent trauma) can confound interpretation.

PROCEDURE AND PATIENT CARE

Before

⊠ Explain the procedure to the patient.

⊠ Explain that no fasting is required before the test.

⊠ Instruct the patient to use a mild laxative the evening before imaging. A cleansing enema may be administered 1 hour before imaging. Early in the scanning, radionuclide accumulates in the bowel.

⊠ Tell the patient to void before each image.

During

- After proper identification, the patient is injected with the radiolabeled monoclonal antibody.
- Initial images are obtained 30 minutes after injection. Images are repeated over as many as 5 days.
- The patient is asked to lie on a padded table during imaging.
- A scintigraphy camera is placed over the anterior or posterior surface of the chest, abdomen, and pelvis. Approximately 10 minutes are required for each view.
- The patient may be asked to return the following day or the day after that for repeated images.
- Little or no discomfort is associated with this procedure.
- The procedure takes approximately 1 hour each day over a period of 1 to 5 days.
- This procedure is performed in the nuclear medicine department.

After

Inform the patient that no precautions need to be taken by others against radiation exposure because only tracer doses of radioisotopes are used.

• Encourage the patient to increase oral fluid intake on testing days.

TEST RESULTS AND CLINICAL SIGNIFICANCE

Primary or recurrent prostate cancer: *Prostate cancer cells all have PSMA in the cytoplasm. The monoclonal antibody tagged with nuclear medicine localizes the cancer cells that are seen on nuclear images.*

RELATED TESTS

Prostate Specific Antigen (PSA) (p. 420). This is a screening test for prostate cancer.

CT Scan of the Abdomen and Pelvis (p. 1020). This test is able to identify abnormalities compatible with metastatic prostate cancer. Test results are less specific for prostate cancer.

PET/CT Scan (p. 822). This test is able to identify abnormalities compatible with metastatic prostate cancer. Test results are less specific for prostate cancer.

Renal Scanning (Kidney Scan, Radiorenography, Renography, Radionuclide Renal Imaging, Nuclear Imaging of the Kidney, DSMA Renal Scan, DTPA Renal Scan, Captopril Renal Scan)

NORMAL FINDINGS

Normal size, shape, and function of the kidney

INDICATIONS

Renal scans are used to indicate the perfusion, function, and structure of the kidneys. They are also used to indicate the presence of obstruction or renovascular hypertension. Because this study uses no iodinated dyes, it is safe to use on patients who have iodine allergies or compromised renal function. Renal scans are used to monitor renal function in patients with known renal disease. This scan also plays a large part in the diagnosis of renal transplant rejection.

TEST EXPLANATION

This nuclear medicine procedure provides visualization of the urinary tract after intravenous administration of a radioisotope. The radioactive material is detected by a scintillation camera, which can detect the gamma rays emitted by the radionuclide in the kidney. The scintillation camera information can be translated into light and thereby create a realistic image of the renal structure. That information is collated by a computer, and the amount of gamma ray emission per unit of time can be calculated to determine renal function, vascular insufficiency, or renal obstruction. Scans do not interfere with the normal physiologic process of the kidney. The resultant image (scan) indicates distribution of the radionuclide within the kidney and ureters.

TABLE 8-4	Renal Scanning	
Types	**Purpose**	**Examples of Findings**
Blood flow (perfusion)	Evaluates blood flow to each kidney	Renal artery stenosis, renovascular hypertension, transplant rejection, hypervascular tumors
Structural	Identifies structural abnormalities	Tumor, cyst, abscess, congenital disorders, malposition or absence, horseshoe-shaped kidney
Function (renogram)	Evaluates function by uptake and excretion of radioisotopes	Glomerulonephritis, decreased blood supply, transplant rejection, renal failure
Hypertension	Detects presence and source of renal hypertension	Renal artery stenosis, vascular obstruction
Obstruction	Identifies outflow obstruction	Renal pelvis obstruction, ureter obstruction, bladder outlet obstruction

There are several different types of renal scans, depending on what information is needed (Table 8-4). Different isotopes may be more suitable for different scans, based on the manner in which the kidney handles the radioisotope.

Renal Blood Flow (Perfusion) Scan

This type of renal scan is used to evaluate the blood flow to each kidney. It is used to identify renal artery stenosis, renovascular hypertension, and rejection of renal transplant. Also, it is used to demonstrate hypervascular lesions (renal cell carcinoma) in the kidney.

The basic test is performed by rapid IV injection of the radionuclide (usually technetium-99m diethylenetriamine pentaacetic acid [^{99m}Tc DTPA], ^{99m}Tc disodium monomethane arsenate [DSMA], or iodohippurate sodium ^{131}I) while the patient is positioned under the scintigraphy camera. Computers collate the data obtained by the camera and create a curve of gamma activity per unit of time. Each kidney is compared to the opposite kidney and to the aorta. Decreased gamma activity is noted in the kidney with arterial stenosis or renovascular hypertension. Decreased activity relative to the aorta is noted in a transplanted kidney that is experiencing rejection. Increased gamma activity is noted in the kidney that contains a hypervascular tumor (cancer).

Renal Structural Scan

This type of renal scan is performed to outline the structure of the kidney to identify a pathologic condition that may alter normal anatomic structure (e.g., tumor, cyst, abscess). Congenital disorders (e.g., hypoplasia or aplasia of the kidney, malposition of the kidney) can also be detected. Also, information following renal transplants can be obtained with this scan. A filling defect in the renal parenchyma may indicate a tumor, cyst, abscess, or infarction. Horseshoe-shaped kidney, pelvic kidney, or absence of a kidney may be evident. Anatomic alterations in the parenchymal distribution of tracer may indicate transplant rejection.

^{99m}Tc DTPA or ^{99m}Tc DSMA can be used for this scan. DSMA is particularly good because it is rapidly taken up by the kidney but excreted very slowly, allowing good visualization of the renal structure.

Renal Function Scan (Renogram)

Renal function can be determined by documenting the capability of the kidney to take up a particular radioisotope and excrete it. A well-functioning kidney can be expected to rapidly assimilate the isotope and then excrete the same isotope. A poorly functioning kidney will not be able to take up the isotope rapidly or excrete it in a timely manner. Each radioactive tracer is handled by the kidney in a different manner. Different renal functions can be tested according to which isotope is used:

^{99m}Tc DTPA measures glomerular filtration.

^{99m}Tc DSMA measures tubular cell secretion.

In this study the dose of radionuclide is determined by calculation based on the body weight or surface area. The patient is placed under the scintigraphy camera. The radioisotope is injected, and a computer analyzes the data obtained from the camera. Activity per unit of time equals the function of the kidney, which is plotted on graph paper. This is called a renogram curve (isotope renography). The function tested depends on the radioisotope being used. Disappearance of the isotope is also plotted as part of that same curve and is a measurement of excretory function of the kidney. The curves are plotted, and their shapes can be compared to expected normal values and to the opposite kidney. Furthermore, renal function can be monitored by serially repeating this test and comparing results. Renal function can be noted to be improved or deteriorating, depending on serial comparisons of the curves.

The kidney with diminished renal function (e.g., glomerulonephritis) or decreased blood supply can be expected to not have rapid uptake of activity and rapid disappearance (excretion) of the radionuclide. The curve will be much flatter. This can also be seen in rejection after transplantation. Impending renal failure can be identified with this scan.

Renal Hypertension Scan

This scan is used to determine the presence and the source of renovascular hypertension. This scan usually uses an angiotensin-converting enzyme (ACE) inhibitor (such as captopril).

The captopril scan (captopril renography/scintigraphy) determines the functional significance of a renal artery or arteriole stenosis. After the administration of captopril, the glomerular filtration rate (GFR) in a kidney with a partial vascular obstruction is reduced despite the preservation of renal plasma flow. The GFR in the contralateral kidney is maintained. This would be demonstrated as delayed radioactivity in the affected kidney after injection of a radionuclide. These scans may predict the response of the blood pressure to medical treatment, angioplasty, or surgery.

Renal Obstruction Scan

This scan is performed to identify obstruction of the outflow tract of the kidney because of obstruction of the renal pelvis, ureter, or bladder outlet. In this study the radionuclide is rapidly injected while the patient is under the scintigraphy camera. Activity is measured and plotted per unit of time. After about 10 minutes, a diuretic (Lasix) is administered. The radionuclide in the unobstructed kidney can be seen to rapidly wash out (be excreted) from the kidney. A slow excretion without a wash-out is seen in an obstructed but still functioning kidney. Furthermore, when the collecting system does become visible, it is observed to be dilated.

Often several of these scans are combined to obtain the maximum amount of information about the renal system. A *triple renal study* may use all of these techniques to evaluate renal blood perfusion, structure, and excretion.

Renal scans are superior to other testing in determining renal function, identifying renal infarction, monitoring renovascular hypertension, and identifying primary renal diseases and transplant rejection. This radionuclear scan is also helpful in the evaluation of the following:

Nuclear Scanning

8

- Arterial atherosclerosis or trauma; the renal uptake of the radionucleated material will be delayed or absent on the affected side or sides
- Pathologic renal or ureteral conditions in patients who cannot have IV pyelography (IVP) (p. 1057) because of dye allergies or poor renal function
- Renal tumors, abscesses, or cysts in patients who may have an allergy to iodine; these appear as cold spots because of the nonfunctioning tissue
- Renal or ureteral disease in patients whose renal function is already poor and who would be at risk for further reduction in function if iodinated dye were to be administered

For anatomic abnormalities, tumors, or cysts, ultrasound (p. 866), computed tomography (p. 1020), or MRI (p. 1106) scans are preferable and more accurate.

 Clinical Priorities

- There are several different types of renal scans (such as blood flow, structure, function, obstruction, hypertension) that can be done, depending on what information is needed. Various isotopes are used, depending on how the kidney handles the radioisotopes.
- A renal scan should not be scheduled within 24 hours after an IVP because the iodinated dye may diminish renal function.
- Renal scans can be used to evaluate rejection of a transplant.

CONTRAINDICATIONS

- Patients who are pregnant, unless the benefits outweigh the risk for fetal injury

PROCEDURE AND PATIENT CARE

Before

✗ Explain the procedure to the patient.
- Do not schedule a renal scan within 24 hours after an IVP. The iodinated dye may temporarily diminish renal function.
✗ Assure the patient that he or she will not be exposed to large amounts of radioactivity because only tracer doses of isotopes are used.
✗ Remind the patient to void before the scan.
✗ Tell the patient that no sedation or fasting is required but that good hydration is essential.
✗ Instruct the patient to drink two to three glasses of water before the scan.
✗ Tell the patient that no pain or discomfort is associated with this procedure.
✗ Inform the patient that he or she must lie still during this study.

During

- Note the following procedural steps:
  1. The unsedated, nonfasting patient is taken to the nuclear medicine department.
  2. A peripheral IV injection of radionuclide is given. It takes only minutes for the radioisotopes to be concentrated in the kidneys.
  3. While the patient assumes a prone or sitting position, a gamma ray scintigraphy camera is passed over the kidney area and records the radioactive uptake on film.
  4. For a *Lasix renal scan* or a *diuretic renal scan*, the patient is imaged with DTPA. Images are obtained for 10 to 20 minutes, then Lasix is administered intravenously, and images are obtained for another 20 minutes.

5. For the *captopril renal scan*, the patient is scanned after the administration of an ACE inhibitor, such as captopril.
6. Scans may be repeated at different intervals after the initial isotope injection. For the renal blood flow and the renal function scans, scanning is started immediately after the injection.
7. For *structural renal scans* the patient is asked to lie still for the entire time of the scan (30 minutes).

- Note that the duration of this test varies from 1 to 4 hours, depending on the specific information required. Perfusion scans are done in approximately 20 minutes and functional scans in less than 1 hour. Static structure scans require 20 minutes to 4 hours for completion.
- Note that this study is performed by a nuclear medicine technologist or physician.

After

✗ Inform the patient that because only tracer doses of radioisotopes are used, no precautions need to be taken against radioactive exposure.

✗ Tell the patient that the radioactive substance is usually excreted from the body within 6 to 24 hours. Encourage the patient to drink fluids.

TEST RESULTS AND CLINICAL SIGNIFICANCE

Urinary obstruction: *This is obvious on a renal obstruction scan. After diuresis the obstructed kidney fails to demonstrate excretion (wash-out) of the radionuclide. Prolonged obstruction ultimately leads to total loss of function of the obstructed kidney. That kidney will not light up after injection of a radionuclide.*

Renovascular hypertension: *The renal hypertension scan is performed after administration of captopril. The time for the affected kidney to light up is significantly prolonged.*

Renal infarction: *This can be seen as a wedge-shaped defect on the structural scan and perhaps as decreased blood flow on the perfusion scan.*

Renal arterial atherosclerosis: *This is evident as delayed light-up on the perfusion scan. The plotted curve is flatter than normal.*

Glomerulonephritis,
Pyelonephritis,
Acute tubular necrosis,
Absence of kidney function:
  If significant enough to affect renal function, these diseases are evident on the renal function scans. The affected kidney does not light up as quickly as normal. The plotted curves of function per unit of time are flatter than normal. No uptake is seen with absence of renal function.

Renal tumor,
Renal abscess,
Renal cyst:
  These abnormalities are apparent as filling defects on the renal structural scan.

Congenital abnormalities such as renal aplasia, hypoplasia, and malposition: *These abnormalities are evident on the renal structural scan.*

Renal trauma: *With arterial injury, the renal blood flow scan will demonstrate prolonged or no visualization of the affected kidney. The renal structural scan may demonstrate a laceration of the kidney with extravasation of radionuclide out of the renal capsule.*

Transplant rejection: *This is apparent with many of the scans described in this section. With rejection of a transplanted kidney, one may see reduced blood flow to the transplanted kidney, reduced function of the transplanted kidney, and/or alterations in renal structure of the transplanted kidney.*

RELATED TESTS

Intravenous Pyelography (IVP) (p. 1057). This is an x-ray examination of the kidneys and lower urologic tract. With the use of iodinated IV contrast medium, this test can also provide information about renal function, blood flow, and structure. Renal obstruction can also be demonstrated.

Computed Tomography (CT) (p. 1020). This scan is an x-ray study utilizing the technology of computed tomography. This test can provide information about renal function, blood flow, and structure. Also, renal obstruction can be demonstrated.

Salivary Gland Nuclear Imaging (Parotid Gland Nuclear Imaging)

NORMAL FINDINGS

Normal function of the salivary gland
No tumor or duct obstruction

INDICATIONS

This test is used to evaluate patients with xerostomia (dry mouth), salivary gland pain, tumors, or possible parotid duct obstruction.

TEST EXPLANATION

The ability of the epithelial cells of the salivary glands to transport large pertechnetate from the blood and to secrete it into the saliva provides the principle for imaging the salivary glands. The functional capabilities, structural integrity, and location of the glands can be assessed. Most usually, the parotid gland alone is visualized. Occasionally, the submandibular glands can be seen.

By following the radionuclide immediately after injection, blood flow can be evaluated. Because this blood flow comes from the cerebral arteries, this test is a measure of the patency of those vessels. Tumors have increased blood flow that can be identified during this part of the study. Patients with acute inflammation will also have increase blood flow during the early stages of the test.

In about 10 to 20 minutes after injection, gland function becomes obvious by uptake of the nuclide into the gland. This uptake is usually compared to the thyroid, which is visualized at the same time. Function will be diminished in patients with severe inflammation or autoimmune diseases, such as Sjögren syndrome. Five to 10 minutes later, one should see secretion of nuclear material into the mouth. Salivary calculi will impede excretion and wash-out of the radionuclide because of obstruction of the excretory duct.

Wash-out demonstrates complete salivary gland excretion. Usually the patient is asked to suck on a lemon to encourage rapid wash-out. Static lateral pictures of the salivary glands can demonstrate tumors or cysts. Most commonly the parotid gland is affected by tumors, and usually they are benign. In neoplasm of the salivary glands, wash-out is slow (i.e., the tumor may remain "hot" [retain radionuclide]) for longer periods of time. Nearly 50% of the benign tumors are hot. A cold tumor (does not take up radionuclide as well as "cold" surrounding tissue) is common in malignant tumors.

CONTRAINDICATIONS

- Patients who are pregnant unless the benefits outweigh the risks

INTERFERING FACTORS

- Rinsing mouth before study may reduce excretion.

PROCEDURE AND PATIENT CARE

Before

✗ Explain the procedure to the patient.
✗ Tell the patient that no specific preparation is necessary.
- Make certain that the patient does not receive any thyroid-blocking agents within 48 hours of testing.

During

- Note the following procedure steps:
  1. Tc-99m pertechnetate is injected into the antecubital vein.
  2. Dynamic images are obtained immediately by placing the detector over the facial area. Radioactive counts are recorded and displayed.
  3. Repeat images are obtained every 3 to 5 minutes for total of 15 to 20 minutes.
  4. A salivary gland stimulant is administered following completion of static images. Either lemon juice or a lemon slice should be swished in the mouth and then expectorated.
  5. "Wash-out" images are obtained 5 to 10 minutes after the salivary gland stimulant. The thyroid gland is included for reference/comparison.
- This procedure is performed by a nuclear medicine technologist or a physician in the nuclear medicine department in approximately 35 to 45 minutes.

After

✗ Assure the patient that the dose of radioactive technetium used in this test is minute and therefore harmless. No isolation and no special urine precautions are needed.

TEST RESULTS AND CLINICAL SIGNIFICANCE

See Table 8-5 for Salivary Gland Nuclear Imaging.

TABLE 8-5	Salivary Gland Nuclear Imaging			
	Early Blood Flow	Static Images/Function Phase	Wash-Out	Excretion
Sjögren syndrome	Normal	Poor uptake	Normal	Normal
Benign tumor	Increased or decreased	Local–hot or Local-cold	Poor	Normal
Malignant tumor	Increased	Local–cold	Very slow	Normal
Acute inflammation	Increased	Diffuse–increased early then decreased	Slow	Normal
Chronic inflammation	Normal	Diffuse-decreased	Slow	Normal
Duct obstruction	Decreased	Diffuse-decreased	Slow	Slow or none

Nuclear Scanning

8

Scrotal Nuclear Imaging (Scrotal Scan, Testicular Imaging)

NORMAL FINDINGS

Symmetric and prompt blood flow to both testicles

INDICATIONS

Scrotal imaging is helpful in the diagnosis of patients with a sudden onset of unilateral testicular swelling and pain. Scrotal imaging can differentiate unilateral testicular torsion from other causes of testicular pain (e.g., acute epididymitis, torsion of the testicular appendage, orchitis, strangulated hernia, testicular hemorrhage). This test is not used frequently because scrotal ultrasound can reliably provide the same information more rapidly and more cheaply.

TEST EXPLANATION

Testicular torsion is a surgical emergency requiring prompt surgical exploration to salvage the involved testicle. To provide immediate surgical care, the surgeon must differentiate the condition from other causes of painful testicular swelling that do not require surgery. Use of radionuclide scrotal imaging enables the surgeon to diagnose testicular torsion. This study is usually performed on an emergency basis and in the nuclear medicine department.

The patient is positioned under the gamma camera with the scrotum supported between the abducted thighs. Technetium-99m (^{99m}Tc) pertechnetate is administered, and a dynamic radionuclide nuclear angiogram is obtained. Static images are obtained immediately afterward. An area of decreased perfusion corresponding to the involved testes indicates a high probability of torsion of the testicle. If the clinically involved testis is normally perfused or hypervascular, a disease other than torsion of the testicle (as described earlier) exists.

PROCEDURE AND PATIENT CARE

Before

- Explain the procedure to the patient.
- Tell the patient that no fasting or premedication is required.
- Assure the patient that he will not be exposed to large amounts of radiation because only tracer doses of isotope are used.
- If the patient is a child, encourage the parent(s) to be present.

During

- The patient is placed on a padded table in the supine position.
- The patient's legs are abducted, and the testicles are supported with tape or a lead shield. The penis is taped to the lower abdomen.
- A small intravenous (IV) injection of ^{99m}Tc pertechnetate is administered.
- Radionuclide imaging is then immediately performed over both testicles. Both dynamic and static images are obtained.

After

Inform the patient that because only tracer doses of radioisotopes are used, no precautions need to be taken by others against radiation exposure.

- If the patient is identified as having torsion of the testicle, prepare the patient for surgery.

TEST RESULTS AND CLINICAL SIGNIFICANCE

▲ Increased Testicular Blood Flow

Epididymitis,
Torsion of the testicular appendage,
Orchitis,
Trauma:
   These abnormalities may be associated with increased blood flow to the testicle.

▼ Decreased Testicular Blood Flow

Testicular torsion of the spermatic cord: *Torsion of the testicle inhibits blood flow to the testicle. This will ultimately lead to infarction of the testicle if not treated immediately.*

RELATED TEST

Scrotal Ultrasonography (p. 893). This is now the preferred test to indicate torsion of the testicle. It is more rapidly performed and most accurate.

Sentinel Lymph Node Biopsy (SLNB, Lymphoscintigraphy)

Nuclear Scanning

8

NORMAL FINDINGS

Uptake is noted in one or more lymph nodes. No tumor in the sentinel node.

INDICATIONS

Lymphoscintigraphy is used to identify the "sentinel" lymph node—the one most likely to contain metastasis from a nearby primary tumor. It is used to map the lymphatic drainage of a primary cancer so that surgery can be directed for diagnostic and possibly therapeutic resection of lymph nodes. It is primarily used in breast cancer and melanoma.

TEST EXPLANATION

With this procedure, the first (sentinel) lymph node in line to catch metastatic tumor cells from a primary tumor is identified and biopsied. To stage most breast or melanoma cancers, a lymph node draining the primary site must be evaluated microscopically. With the use of SLNB, the first lymph node in the chain of lymph nodes can be identified and biopsied. If results are negative, as is the case in most patients with small tumors, the rest of the axillary lymph contents can be safely assumed to be free of tumor and are not removed. This saves women from the potential complications associated with a full lymph node dissection including arm swelling, cellulitis, postoperative pain, and reduced range of motion. Furthermore this test can identify unusual locations for lymph node metastasis that would not normally be identified by the surgeon.

To summarize the procedure, a tracer (isosulfan blue dye or technetium [^{99m}Tc] sulfur colloid) is injected into the skin or tissue near the tumor. If technetium is used, a *lymphoscintigraphy scan* is performed about 1 to 2 hours after the injections. There are specific protocols depending on the lymph node basin being studied and on the primary tumor site. Lymph nodes that take up the radionuclide are the sentinel lymph nodes that the surgeon will identify and remove. In the operating room, using a hand-held gamma detector, the surgeon is able to identify the region of maximum radioactivity. These are removed and sent to the pathologists for immediate evaluation. If isosulfan or methylene blue dye is injected, a stained lymphatic vessel is identified by the surgeon in the subcutaneous tissue and followed to the first blue-colored node. The sentinel lymph nodes are the blue, or "hot," nodes closest to the primary tumor.

If the sentinel lymph node is negative on frozen section or imprint cytology (touch prep) pathologic study, the lymph node dissection procedure is not required. If the sentinel lymph node is positive, a full lymph node dissection may be performed. In some instances light microscopy may be negative but subsequent immunohistochemical staining may indicate the presence of cancer in the node. The sentinel lymph node can also be evaluated right in the operating room by using molecular assays for epithelial cell specific components such as cytokeratin or mammaglobin.

This test is quickly becoming an important part of the standard treatment for breast and melanoma cancer surgery. The only discomfort associated with the test is the preoperative injections required around the tumor. The technetium injection and subsequent scanning are usually performed in the nuclear medicine department. When isosulfan blue is used as the lymph node tracer, the injection is administered in the operating room under anesthesia.

Nuclear lymphoscintigraphy is also used to evaluate the lymph node status in patients with Hodgkin disease and other lymphomas. Patients with chronic lymphedema of an extremity may also be evaluated by lymphoscintigraphy.

CONTRAINDICATIONS

- Patients who have a large cancer in which lymph node metastasis is very likely
- Patients in early pregnancy, unless the benefit outweighs the risk of damage to the fetus

POTENTIAL COMPLICATIONS

- Anaphylaxis has been reported with injection of isosulfan blue dye.

PROCEDURE AND PATIENT CARE

Before

🖉 Explain the procedure to the patient.
- Because this is an operative procedure, routine preoperative nursing processes should be carried out, including obtaining operative consent, keeping the patient on nothing by mouth (NPO) status, and surgical site preparation as ordered.

During

Note the following procedural steps:
   Technetium
   1. The patient is taken to the nuclear medicine department, where the radionuclide is injected around the tumor.

2. The site of lymph node drainage is then scanned immediately and 1 to 24 hours later.
3. Lymph node uptake is reported to the surgeon.
4. In the operating room, a handheld gamma detector locates "hot" areas of radionuclide uptake in the lymph node–bearing area. The most proximal "hot" node is excised as the sentinel node.

Isosulfan Blue
1. In the operating room, 4 to 5 mL of isosulfan blue dye is injected around the tumor.
2. After 5 to 9 minutes, a small incision is made overlying the lymph node–bearing area and the proximal blue lymph node is removed as the sentinel lymph node.
- If the sentinel lymph node is negative for tumor, the lymph node dissection procedure is discontinued. If the sentinel lymph node is positive, a complete lymph node dissection may be performed.

After

🖉 Inform the patient that no precautions are required if technetium is used because the radionuclide dose is minimal.
- If isosulfan blue dye is used, the patient's skin may develop a transient blue hue (looking almost like severe cyanosis). This will dissipate over the next 6 hours.

🖉 Warn the patient that the urine will have a blue tinge as a result of the isosulfan blue dye injection.
- Observe the patient for signs of allergy (rare) caused by the blue dye injection.

TEST RESULTS AND CLINICAL SIGNIFICANCE

Metastatic tumor to lymph node,
Normal lymph node:

> *It is important to note that uptake of dye or radionuclide does not indicate whether a lymph node contains metastatic tumor. It only locates the lymph node that is most likely to contain tumor if metastasis occurred.*

Thyroid Scanning (Thyroid Scintiscan)

NORMAL FINDINGS

Normal size, shape, position, and function of the thyroid gland
No areas of decreased or increased uptake

INDICATIONS

This test is used to visualize the thyroid gland when disease of the thyroid is suspected. It is particularly useful in the evaluation of patients with a suspected thyroid nodule. With thyroid nuclear scanning the nodule can be classified and more appropriately treated.

TEST EXPLANATION

Thyroid scanning allows the size, shape, position, and physiologic function of the thyroid gland to be determined with the use of radionuclear scanning. A radioactive substance such as technetium-99m (^{99m}Tc) or Iodine^{131} is given to the patient to visualize the thyroid gland. A scintigraphy camera is passed over the neck area, and an image is recorded (Figure 8-16).

Thyroid nodules are easily detected by this technique. Nodules are classified as functioning *(warm/hot)* or nonfunctioning *(cold)* depending on the amount of radionuclide taken up by the nodule (Figure 8-17). A functioning nodule could represent a benign adenoma or a localized toxic goiter. A nonfunctioning

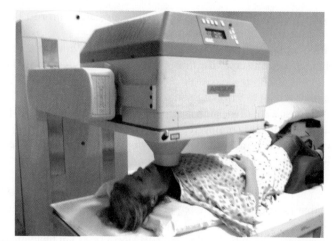

Figure 8-16 Nuclear thyroid scanning technique using cone-down collimator.

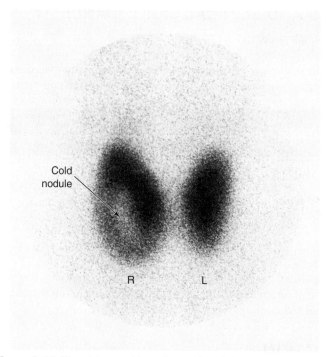

Figure 8-17 Thyroid scan. Note the cold nodule in the right (larger) lobe of the thyroid gland. This finding is consistent with tumor, cyst, or goiter.

nodule may represent a cyst, carcinoma, nonfunctioning adenoma or goiter, lymphoma, or localized area of thyroiditis.

Scanning is useful in patients with the following clinical conditions:

1. Neck or substernal mass.
2. Thyroid nodule. Thyroid cancers are usually nonfunctioning (cold) nodules.
3. Hyperthyroidism. Scanning will assist in differentiating Graves disease (diffusely enlarged hyperfunctioning thyroid gland) from Plummer disease (nodular hyperfunctioning gland).
4. Metastatic tumors without a known primary site. A normal scan excludes the thyroid gland as a possible primary site.
5. Well-differentiated form of thyroid cancer.

Another form of thyroid scan is called the *whole-body thyroid scan*. This scan is performed on patients who have previously had a thyroid cancer treated. Iodine[131] is administered orally, and the entire body is scanned to look for metastatic thyroid tissue. A hot spot would indicate recurrent tumor. Before this test can be performed, all of the thyroid tissue in the neck must be either surgically excised or ablated with radioactive [131]I. If the patient is receiving thyroid replacement therapy, the thyroid medicine must be discontinued at least 6 weeks before testing. This makes any metastatic thyroid tissue, particularly iodine, avid. A high thyroid-stimulating hormone blood level ensures that any thyroid cancer tissue will take up the administered radioactive iodine. This test is performed routinely (every 1 to 2 years) on patients who have had a thyroid cancer larger than 1 cm. Smaller cancers are unlikely to metastasize. Much of the procedure is similar to thyroid scanning.

CONTRAINDICATIONS

- Patients who are allergic to iodine or shellfish, because sometimes iodine is used as the radionuclide
- Patients who are pregnant, unless the benefit outweighs the risk of fetal injury

POTENTIAL COMPLICATIONS

- Radiation-induced oncogenesis: This complication is eliminated if technetium or low-radioactive iodine isomers are used instead of [131]I.

INTERFERING FACTORS

- Iodine-containing foods affect results because the iodine may saturate all of the iodine-binding sites and very little iodine tracer will be taken up by the thyroid. Also, if large quantities of iodine are ingested, the thyroid may shut down and even Tc tracer will not be taken up by the thyroid.
- Recent administration of x-ray contrast agents affects results because these agents contain large quantities of iodine. For the reasons described above, contrast agents should be avoided before thyroid scanning.
- Drugs that may affect test results include cough medicines, multiple vitamins, some oral contraceptives, and thyroid drugs.

✓ Clinical Priorities

- Thyroid nodules are classified as hot or cold, depending on the amount of radionuclide taken up by the nodule.
- The entire body can be scanned to detect metastatic thyroid tissue by the whole-body thyroid scan.
- Iodine in foods or x-ray contrast agents should be avoided before thyroid scanning.

PROCEDURE AND PATIENT CARE

Before

🖎 Explain the procedure to the patient.

• Check the patient for allergies to iodine.

🖎 Instruct the patient about medications that need to be restricted for 6 weeks before the test (e.g., thyroid drugs, medications containing iodine).

• Obtain a history concerning previous contrast x-ray studies, nuclear scanning, or intake of any thyroid-suppressive or antithyroid drugs.

🖎 Tell the patient that fasting is usually not required. Check with the laboratory.

🖎 Tell the patient that no discomfort is associated with this study.

During

• Note the following procedural steps:
  1. A standard dose of radioactive iodine is usually given to the patient by mouth. The capsule is tasteless.
  2. Scanning is usually performed 24 hours later. If intravenous technetium is used, scanning may be performed 2 hours later.
  3. At the designated time, the patient is placed in a supine position and a scintigraphy camera is placed over the thyroid area.
  4. The radioactive counts are recorded and displayed.
• Note that this study is performed by a nuclear medicine technologist in less than 30 minutes.

After

🖎 Assure the patient that the dose of radioactive Tc or iodine used in this test is minute and therefore harmless. No isolation and no special urine precautions are needed.

TEST RESULTS AND CLINICAL SIGNIFICANCE

Adenoma: *This may be evident as a hot nodule if it is functioning or a cold nodule if it is not functioning.*

Toxic and nontoxic goiter: *The toxic goiter will be apparent as a hot nodule. The nontoxic goiter will be a cold nodule.*

Cyst,

Carcinoma,

Lymphoma,

Thyroiditis,

Metastasis:
  These diseases usually appear as cold nodules or filling defects in normal thyroid tissue.

Graves disease: *This disease is evident on thyroid scan as diffuse increased uptake of radionuclide involving the entire thyroid gland.*

Plummer disease: *This disease produces a single or multiple nodular areas of increased uptake.*

Hyperthyroidism,

Hypothyroidism:
  In general, hyperthyroid patients have increased uptake of radionuclide, and hypothyroid patients have reduced uptake.

Hashimoto disease: *This often is apparent as mottled uptake of radionuclide.*

RELATED TESTS

Thyroid Ultrasonography (p. 895). This is an important part of evaluation of the thyroid gland. In general, all solid nodules on ultrasound that are cold on thyroid scan should be considered suggestive of cancer.

Triiodothyronine (T_3), Thyroxine (T_4), Thyroid-Stimulating Hormone (TSH) (pp. 506, 497, and 486, respectively). These tests are the most common methods by which thyroid function is measured. They are more accurate than radioactive iodine uptake and thyroid scanning. No radioactive material needs to be administered to the patient. These tests should be a part of every thyroid evaluation.

Computed Tomography (CT) Scan of the Neck (p. 1029). With CT scan, the thyroid nodule can be more accurately located and its characteristics evaluated for malignancy.

Total Blood Volume (TBV, Red Blood Cell [RBC] Volume)

NORMAL FINDINGS

No deviation from normal

INDICATIONS

Total blood volume measurement may be useful in the following clinical circumstances:

1. Congestive heart failure: The actual amount of fluid overload can be calculated and diuresis can be more appropriately determined.
2. Presurgery: The patient's fluid status can be accurately determined, as can RBC status.
3. Acutely ill patients: There are often large fluid shifts in these patients and TBV may help in guiding IV fluid replacement.
4. Azotemia: Measurement of TBV will indicate if azotemia is prerenal (hypovolemia) or primary renal.
5. Hypertension: TBV may indicate plasma volume overload versus vascular constriction.
6. Anemia: TBV and RBC volumes can indicate accurately the extent of anemia that otherwise could be affected by fluid status, etc.

TEST EXPLANATION

Measurement of total blood volume is an accurate indicator of true plasma (liquid components of blood) measurement. Based on the patient's height, weight, gender, and body composition, a TBV can determine whether the measured volumes are normal, high, or low compared with what would be ideal for the particular patient. The report indicates actual volumes for TBV and RBCs that deviate from normal.

To maintain blood volume within a normal range, the kidneys regulate the amount of water and sodium lost into the urine. For example, if excessive water and sodium are ingested, the kidneys normally respond by excreting more water and sodium into the urine. This auto adjustment is mediated through the renin-angiotensin-aldosterone system. Both angiotensin and aldosterone, although by different mechanisms, stimulate distal tubular sodium reabsorption and decrease sodium and water loss by the kidney and thereby adjust blood volume. Another important hormone in regulating blood volume is vasopressin (antidiuretic hormone [ADH]). This hormone is released by the posterior pituitary. One of its actions is to stimulate water reabsorption in the collecting duct of the kidney, thereby decreasing water loss and increasing blood volume. Blood volume affects cardiac output and blood pressure.

Nuclear Scanning

8

Radioiodine labeled albumin is injected intravenously. Blood is withdrawn every 5 minutes for five samples. The radioactivity is counted and compared with what would be considered normal. A lower amount of the radioactivity in the sample indicates a higher plasma volume. The hematocrit is then used to derive the red cell volume. The total blood volume is obtained by adding the plasma volume and the red cell volume.

Before

Explain the procedure and tell the patient that no fasting is required.

During

- Obtain venous access
- Fifteen minutes after radionuclide injection, the first venous blood specimen is collected in a red-top tube.
- Similar venous blood specimens are obtained every 5 minutes for a total of five samples.

After

- Apply pressure to the intravenous site upon removal after the extracting the last sample.

TEST RESULTS AND CLINICAL SIGNIFICANCE

▲   Increased Levels

Hypervolemia,
Hypertension,
Congestive heart failure,
Primary renal disease,
Polycythemia vera:
  These conditions are associated with increased total blood volume because of too much intravascular fluid or too many RBCs.

▼   Decreased Levels

Dehydration,
Hypovolemia,
Acute bleeding,
Anemia:
  These conditions are associated with decreased total blood volume because of too little intravascular fluid and/or too few RBCs.

RELATED TESTS

Hematocrit (p. 277). *This is a measure of the volume of RBCs in the blood. This measurement is inversely related to the amount of intravascular fluid, given that the RBCs are normal in size.*

WBC Scan (Inflammatory Scan)

NORMAL FINDINGS

No signs of white blood cell (WBC) localization outside the liver or spleen

INDICATIONS

This scan is used to identify and localize occult inflammation or infection. It is used for patients who have a fever of unknown origin, suspected osteomyelitis, or inflammatory bowel disease. It is used to indicate whether or not an abnormal mass (e.g., a pancreatic pseudocyst) is infected.

TEST EXPLANATION

This test is based on the fact that WBCs are attracted to areas of infection or inflammation. When the patient has a suspected infection or inflammation, yet the site cannot be localized, the injection of radiolabeled WBCs may identify and localize that area of inflammation or infection. Appropriate treatment can then be performed. This is especially helpful in patients who have a fever of unknown origin, suspected occult intraabdominal infection, or suspected (yet radiographically unapparent) osteomyelitis. The scan can differentiate infectious from noninfectious processes. Areas of noninfectious inflammation (e.g., inflammatory bowel disease) also take up the radiolabeled WBCs.

This scan requires drawing about 40 to 50 mL of blood from the patient, separating out the WBCs, labeling the WBCs with technetium or indium, and reinjecting them into the patient. Four to 24 hours later, imaging of the whole body may show an area of increased radioactivity suggestive of accumulation of the radiolabeled WBCs in an area of infection or inflammation.

The imaging procedure is performed by a trained technologist in approximately 30 minutes. A physician trained in nuclear medicine interprets the results. The only discomfort associated with this procedure is the intravenous (IV) injection of the radionuclide.

INTERFERING FACTORS

- The reticuloendothelial system (liver, spleen, and bone marrow) tends to accumulate these radiolabeled cells normally.

PROCEDURE AND PATIENT CARE

Before

- Explain the procedure to the patient.
- Assure the patient that he or she will not be exposed to large amounts of radioactivity because only tracer doses of the isotope are used.
- Tell the patient that no preparation or sedation is required.

During

- Note the following procedural steps:
  1. Approximately 40 to 50 mL of blood is withdrawn from the patient, and the WBCs are extracted from the rest of the blood cells. This is usually done by centrifugation. With leukopenia, the WBC count is so low that separating them out from the other blood cellular components would be very difficult. In these instances, donor WBCs are used instead of autologous WBCs. Donor WBCs are also used for human immunodeficiency virus (HIV) positive patients to minimize the risk to laboratory workers.
  2. The WBCs are suspended in saline and tagged with technetium-99m (^{99m}Tc) or indium-111 (^{111}In) lipid-soluble product.
  3. The tagged WBCs are reinjected into the patient.

4. In 4, 24, and 48 hours after injection, a gamma camera is placed over the body.
5. The patient is placed in supine, lateral, and prone positions so that all surfaces of the body can be visualized.
6. The radionuclide image is recorded digitally on a computer monitor and on film.

After

🖎 Inform the patient that because only tracer doses of radioisotopes are used, no precautions need to be taken against radioactive exposure.

TEST RESULTS AND CLINICAL SIGNIFICANCE

Infection (abscess, osteomyelitis, or poststernotomy infections): *The WBCs are localized to the area of infection and show up as increased radionuclear uptake (hot spot).*

Inflammation (e.g., inflammatory bowel disease, arthritis): *Like infection, areas of noninfectious inflammation attract the radiolabeled WBCs.*

Stool Tests

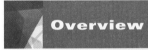

Overview

REASONS FOR PERFORMING STOOL STUDIES

Stool represents the waste products of digested food. It also includes bile, mucus, shed epithelial cells, bacteria, and other inorganic salts. Normally food is passed through the stomach, into the duodenum, and into the small bowel. There, most of the nutrient and electrolyte absorption occurs. The liquid stool is then passed into the colon, where most of the water is reabsorbed.

Stool studies are used to evaluate the function and integrity of the bowel. These studies are performed to evaluate patients with intestinal bleeding, infections, infestations, inflammation, malabsorption, and diarrhea.

In this chapter, we have listed some stool studies that are commonly performed. Other testing can be done on the stool but is more often performed on other specimens. In those situations, the study is listed in the appropriate chapter for the specimen that is more commonly used.

Although these specimens may be unpleasant to obtain, handle, and examine, the information obtained from stool studies is invaluable to proper care of the patient with gastrointestinal (GI) diseases.

PROCEDURAL CARE FOR STOOL STUDIES

Before

Explain the method of stool collection to the patient. Be matter-of-fact to avoid any embarrassment to the patient.

Instruct the patient not to mix urine or toilet paper with the stool specimen.

Instruct the patient to use an appropriate collection container.

- Determine if female patient is menstruating because vaginal blood may contaminate the specimen.
- Observe Standard Precautions when handling stool specimens.

During

- Ask the patient to defecate into a designated container.
- Place a small amount of stool in a sterile collection container.
- If a rectal swab is needed, wear gloves and insert the cotton-tipped swab at least 1 inch into the anal canal. Then rotate the swab for 30 seconds and place it in the clean container.

After

- Handle the stool specimen carefully, as though it were capable of causing infection. Wear gloves when obtaining and handling the specimen.
- Promptly send the stool specimen to the laboratory. Delays in transfer of the specimen may affect test results. If there will be a delay in laboratory handling of the stool specimen, follow laboratory procedures or guidelines concerning storage. Stools for ova and parasites should be kept warm. Stools for enteric pathogens and *Clostridium difficile* should be refrigerated. Another option is to add a preservative to the stool. For example, for stool culture, a buffered glycerol-saline solution may be combined with the stool as a preservative.

REPORTING OF RESULTS

It may take several days or even weeks to obtain results of some stool specimens. However, most stool study results are available within 24 hours.

Apt Test (Downey Test, Qualitative Fetal Hemoglobin Stool Test, Stool for Swallowed Blood)

NORMAL FINDINGS

No newborn blood present
Maternal blood present

INDICATIONS

This is a screening test to indicate if blood present in the stool, emesis, or amniotic fluid of a newborn is fetal blood (possible intestinal bleeding) or swallowed maternal blood.

TEST EXPLANATION

Blood in the stool or emesis of a newborn must be rapidly evaluated. Although an adult can lose hundreds of milliliters of blood, that volume may represent the entire blood volume of a newborn child. Newborns may have a serious disease causing the blood in the intestinal tract or may simply be defecating maternal blood that was swallowed during birth or breastfeeding. It is important to rapidly tell the difference. The Apt test is performed on the stool specimen to differentiate the source of the blood. Fetal hemoglobin is resistant to alkali denaturation; adult hemoglobin (hemoglobin A) is not. When sodium hydroxide is added to the blood, maternal blood will dissolve, leaving only a brown hematin stain. Newborn blood (containing hydroxide-resistant hemoglobin) will not dissolve, and red blood will remain in the specimen. This test can be performed on stool, a stool-stained diaper, amniotic fluid, or vomitus.

PROCEDURE AND PATIENT CARE

Before

- Explain the procedure to the newborn's parents.
- It is important to assess vital signs of a newborn who develops possible intestinal bleeding.

During

- Obtain an adequate stool or vomitus specimen. Only a small amount (several mL) is required.
- In the laboratory, 1% NaOH is added to the specimen. Vomitus is diluted and centrifuged first. Maternal blood turns brown; newborn blood stays red or pink.

After

- If maternal blood is present, reassure the parents and examine the mother for nipple erosion and/or cracking.
- If newborn blood is present, begin close observation and provide support during further diagnostic procedures.

TEST RESULTS

Maternal blood: *A newborn usually defecates maternal blood in the first 3 to 5 days of life. If maternal nipple disease exists, the blood in the stool of a newborn can persist.*

Fetal blood: *This is an indication of disease within the gastrointestinal tract of the newborn and must be evaluated immediately.*

RELATED TEST

Stool for Occult Blood (p. 857). This is a method of identifying occult adult blood or substantiating the presence of adult blood in the stool.

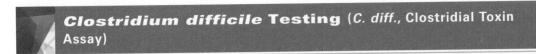

Clostridium difficile **Testing** (*C. diff.*, Clostridial Toxin Assay)

NORMAL FINDINGS

Negative (no *Clostridium* toxin identified)

INDICATIONS

This test is indicated in patients with diarrhea who have been taking antibiotics for more than 5 days. It can also be performed on immunosuppressed patients with diarrhea even though they are not receiving antibiotics.

TEST EXPLANATION

Clostridium difficile–associated diarrhea (CDAD) bacterial infections usually affects the intestine (colitis) and occur in patients who are immunocompromised or taking broad-spectrum antibiotics (e.g., clindamycin, ampicillin, and cephalosporins). The disease severity can range from mild nuisance diarrhea to severe pseudomembranous colitis and bowel perforation. The overwhelming predisposing factor is ongoing antibiotic therapy. Patient age, length of hospital stay, acuity of illness, and comorbidities are risk factors.

The infection possibly results from depression of the normal flora of the bowel caused by the administration of antibiotics. The clostridial bacterium produces two toxins (A and B) that cause inflammation and necrosis of the colonic epithelium. The standard for laboratory detection of *Clostridium difficile* toxins is the cytotoxicity assay in cell cultures. The specificity of the reaction is determined by the neutralization of the toxins with antisera directed to the toxin in the stool. However, the cytotoxin assay is labor intensive and may take up to 48 hours to obtain a result. Toxin detection by EIA is insensitive. *C. difficile* can also be diagnosed by obtaining colonic-rectal tissue for this toxin. Stool cultures (p. 855) for *C. difficile* can be performed but are also labor intensive and take longer to get results.

A PCR assay for the qualitative in vitro rapid detection of *C. difficile* toxin B gene (tcdB) in human liquid or soft stool specimens is available. This method rapidly provides a definitive diagnosis of *C. difficile*. Quickly reaching a definitive diagnosis allows CDAD patients to get the proper treatment without delay and reduce hospital stays for inpatients with CDAD. At the same time they can be placed in isolation sooner to reduce transmission and prevent outbreaks. Definitive results can reduce inappropriate antimicrobial use in negative patients.

A positive PCR result for the presence of the gene-regulating toxin production (tcdC) indicates the presence of *Clostridium difficile* and toxin A and/or B. A negative result indicates the absence of detectable *Clostridium difficile* tcdC DNA in the specimen, but does not rule out *Clostridium difficile* infection. False-negative results may occur because of inhibition of PCR, sequence variability underlying the primers and/or probes, or the presence of *Clostridium difficile* in quantities less than the limit of detection of the assay.

Treatment of CDAD typically involves withdrawal of the associated antimicrobial(s) and, if symptoms persist, orally administered and intraluminally active metronidazole, vancomycin, or fidaxomicin. Intravenous metronidazole may be used if an oral agent cannot be administered. In recent years, a more severe form of CDAD with increased morbidity and mortality has been recognized as being caused by an epidemic toxin-hyperproducing strain of *Clostridium difficile* (NAP1 strain). Many toxin-hyperproducing isolates also contain the binary toxin gene and are resistant quinolones.

PROCEDURE AND PATIENT CARE

Before

🖉 Explain the method of stool collection to the patient. Be matter of fact to avoid embarrassment to the patient.

🖉 Instruct the patient not to mix urine or toilet paper with the stool specimen.

• Handle the specimen carefully, as though it were capable of causing infection. If someone is assisting with the specimen collection, gloves should be worn.

During

🖉 Instruct the patient to defecate into a clean container. A rectal swab cannot be used, because it collects inadequate amounts of stool. The stool cannot be retrieved from the toilet.

• Stool can be obtained from incontinence pads.

- A stool specimen also can be collected by proctoscopy or colonoscopy.
- Place the specimen in a closed container and then transport it to the laboratory to prevent deterioration of the toxin.
- If the specimen cannot be processed immediately, refrigerate it (depending on laboratory protocol).
- Submission of more than one specimen for testing is not recommended.

After

- Maintain enteric isolation precautions on all patients until appropriate therapy is completed.
- Perform hand hygiene.

TEST RESULTS AND CLINICAL SIGNIFICANCE

Antibiotic-related pseudomembranous colitis,
C. difficile colitis:

> *Multiple names exist for the same clinical entity. This infection can progress to toxic megacolon and even death. In the extreme cases of this disease, medical therapy may **not** be adequate, and a total colectomy may be required.*

RELATED TESTS

Sigmoidoscopy (p. 623). This endoscopic test is used to support the diagnosis of pseudomembranous colitis. Also, through this test, good specimens can be obtained for clostridial toxin testing.

Stool Culture (p. 855). This study is performed to identify pathogenic bacteria growing within the bowel.

Fecal Fat (Fat Absorption, Quantitative Stool Fat Determination)

NORMAL FINDINGS

Timed collection:
    ≥18 years: 2-7 g fat/24 hours
    Reference values have not been established for patients who are <18 years of age.
Random collection:
    All ages: 0%-19% fat

INDICATIONS

This test is performed to confirm the diagnosis of steatorrhea. Steatorrhea is suspected when the patient has large, greasy, and foul-smelling stools. Determining an abnormally high fecal fat content confirms the diagnosis.

TEST EXPLANATION

The fecal fat test measures the fat content in the stool. This qualitative or quantitative test is performed to confirm the diagnosis of steatorrhea. Steatorrhea occurs when fat content in the stool is high. Short-gut syndrome and any condition that may cause malabsorption (e.g., sprue, Crohn disease, Whipple disease) or maldigestion (e.g., bile duct obstruction, pancreatic duct obstruction secondary to tumor or gallstones) are also associated with increased fecal fat.

Neutral fats include the monoglycerides, diglycerides, and triglycerides, whereas split fats are the free fatty acids that are liberated from them. Maldigestion (impaired synthesis or secretion of pancreatic enzymes or bile) may cause an increase in neutral fats, whereas an increase in split fats suggests malabsorption.

The total output of fecal fat can be tested on a random stool specimen but is more accurate when total 24-, 48-, or 72-hour collection is carried out. Abnormal results from a random specimen should be confirmed by submission of a timed collection. Test values for random fecal fat collections are reported in terms of percent fat.

INTERFERING FACTORS

▓ Drugs that may *increase* levels of fecal fat include enemas, diaper rash ointments, and laxatives, especially mineral oil.

▓ Drugs that may *decrease* levels of fecal fat include barium and fiber laxatives or supplements.

Age-Related Concerns

- Children with cystic fibrosis have mucous plugs that obstruct the pancreatic ducts. This prevents fat absorption (malabsorption).
- A fat retention coefficient is used in infants and children to determine the difference between ingested fat and fecal fat.
- The fat retention coefficient should be at least 95%. A low value indicates steatorrhea.

PROCEDURE AND PATIENT CARE

Before

✍ Explain the procedure to the patient and/or the parent (if a child).

✍ Instruct the patient to abstain from alcohol ingestion 3 days before testing.

✍ Give the patient instructions regarding the appropriate diet (a diet diary may be requested by the laboratory):

1. For adults, usually 100 g of fat per day is suggested for 3 days before and throughout the collection period.

2. Children, and especially infants, cannot ingest 100 g of fat. Therefore a *fat-retention coefficient* is determined by measuring the difference between ingested fat and fecal fat and then expressing that difference (the amount of fat retained) as a percentage of the ingested fat:

$$(\text{Ingested fat} - \text{Fecal fat}) \div \text{Ingested fat} \times 100\,\% = \text{Fat-retention coefficient}$$

- Note that the normal fat-retention coefficient is 95% or greater. A low value indicates steatorrhea.

✍ Instruct the patient to defecate into a dry, clean container. Occasionally a tongue blade is required to transfer the stool to the specimen container.

✍ Tell the patient not to urinate into the stool container.

✍ Inform the patient that even diarrheal stools should be collected.

✍ Instruct the patient that toilet paper should not be placed in the stool container.

✍ Tell the patient not to take any laxatives or enemas during this test because they will interfere with intestinal motility and alter test results.

During

- Collect each stool specimen and send immediately to the laboratory during the 24- to 72-hour testing period.
- Label each specimen and include the time and date of collection.
- If the specimen is collected at home, give the patient a large stool container to keep in the freezer.

After

Inform the patient that a normal diet can be resumed.

TEST RESULTS AND CLINICAL SIGNIFICANCE

▲ Increased Levels

Cystic fibrosis: *These patients experience maldigestion of fat because their pancreatic function is poor. They cannot absorb fat from the gut. As a result, they have steatorrhea.*

Malabsorption secondary to sprue, celiac disease, Whipple disease, Crohn disease (regional enteritis), or radiation enteritis: *The absorptive capability of the stool is markedly reduced. Transit time is markedly decreased. As a result of these changes, fat is not absorbed. Steatorrhea is the result.*

Maldigestion secondary to obstruction of the pancreatobiliary tree (e.g., cancer, stricture, gallstones): *Exocrine secretion of the pancreatobiliary tree is necessary for digestion of dietary fat. When disease affects these organs, steatorrhea results.*

Short-gut syndrome secondary to surgical resection, surgical bypass, or congenital anomaly: *The transit time in these patients is markedly diminished. The time available for digestion and absorption of fat is inadequate. Steatorrhea results.*

RELATED TEST

D-Xylose Absorption (p. 533). This test is used to evaluate the absorptive capability of the intestines. It is used in the evaluation of patients with suspected malabsorption.

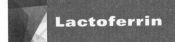

Lactoferrin

NORMAL FINDINGS

None detected

INDICATIONS

Lactoferrin is used to diagnose inflammatory bowel diseases such as ulcerative colitis or Crohn disease. It is also used as a screening test to determine the possibility of bacterial colitis.

TEST EXPLANATION

Lactoferrin is a glycoprotein expressed by activated neutrophils. The detection of lactoferrin in a fecal sample therefore serves as a surrogate marker for inflammatory white blood cells (WBCs) in the intestinal tract. WBCs in the stool are not stable and may be easily destroyed by temperature changes, delays in testing, and toxins within the stool. As a result, WBCs may not be detected by common microscopic methods. Lactoferrin assay has allowed the identification of inflammatory cells in the stool without the use of microscopy.

Detection of fecal lactoferrin allows for the differentiation of inflammatory and noninflammatory intestinal disorders in patients with diarrhea. Usually the test is used as a diagnostic aid to help identify patients with active inflammatory bowel disease (such as Crohn disease or ulcerative colitis) and rule out those with active irritable bowel syndrome, which is noninflammatory. Lactoferrin is also present in patients with bacterial enteritis such as *Shigella, Salmonella, Campylobacter jejuni,* and *Clostridium difficile.* Diarrhea caused by viruses and most parasites is not associated with elevated lactoferrin levels. Lactoferrin testing is often used as a screening test for patients who may have bacterial enteritis. If the stool is negative for lactoferrin, it is unlikely that a stool culture will be positive.

The lactoferrin analyte may be qualitatively detected by two distinct methods: (1) A latex agglutination procedure (the most commonly used) and (2) a microwell enzyme immunoassay procedure. The former method has been used primarily in the evaluation of patients with diagnoses of bacterial infectious gastroenteritis, while the latter method has been developed primarily as a diagnostic aid to distinguish between active inflammatory bowel disease and active noninflammatory irritable bowel syndrome.

INTERFERING FACTORS

- Delays in testing can interfere with test results: The stool specimen should be examined immediately. In some instances a specific stool preservative–enteric transport media (Cary-Blair) can be used.
- Breast feeding can affect test results: Because lactoferrin is a component of human breast milk, the test will be positive in breast-fed children and should not be used to evaluate neonates receiving breast milk. However, the test uses a human lactoferrin–specific antibody that does not cross react with lactoferrin in cow's milk.

PROCEDURE AND PATIENT CARE

Before
🗴 Explain the procedure to the patient.
🗴 Instruct the patient not to mix urine or toilet paper with the specimen.

During
- Stool is collected in a clean bedpan.
- Place at least 5 g of stool in a clean specimen container.

After
- Observe appropriate contamination precautions.
- Transfer the specimen to the laboratory immediately.
🗴 Inform the patient that results are available in less than ½ hour.

TEST RESULTS AND CLINICAL SIGNIFICANCE

Bacterial enteritis,
Acute Crohn disease,
Acute ulcerative colitis:
   Each of these diseases is associated with an inflammatory immune response of WBCs causing positive lactoferrin results.

RELATED TESTS

Stool Culture (p. 855). This test is used to identify the cause of bacterial enteritis.

Colonoscopy (p. 591). This is a commonly performed test to identify inflammatory bowel diseases such as ulcerative colitis and Crohn disease.

Stool Culture (Stool for Culture and Sensitivity [Stool C&S], Stool for Ova and Parasites [O&P])

NORMAL FINDINGS

Normal intestinal flora

No ova or parasite infestation

INDICATIONS

Stool cultures are indicated in patients who have unrelenting diarrhea, fever, and abdominal bloating. One is especially suspicious if the patient has been drinking well water, has been receiving a prolonged course of antibiotics, or has traveled outside of the United States.

TEST EXPLANATION

Normally stool contains many bacteria and fungi. The more common bacteria include *Enterococcus, Escherichia coli, Proteus, Pseudomonas, Staphylococcus aureus, Candida albicans, Bacteroides,* and *Clostridium.* Bacteria are indigenous to the bowel; however, several bacteria act as pathogens within the bowel. These include *Salmonella, Shigella, Campylobacter, Yersinia,* pathogenic *E. coli, Clostridium,* and *Staphylococcus.*

Parasites also may affect the stool. Common parasites are *Ascaris* (hookworm), *Strongyloides* (tapeworm), and *Giardia* (protozoans), and *Cryptosporidium* (especially in acquired immunodeficiency syndrome [AIDS] patients). Identification of any of these pathogens in the stool incriminates that organism as the cause of the infectious enteritis.

Sometimes the normal stool flora can become pathogenic if overgrowth of the bacteria occurs as a result of antibiotics (e.g., *C. difficile*), immunosuppression, or overaggressive catharsis. *Helicobacter pylori* can be found in the stool but indicates an increased risk for peptic ulcer disease and gastritis. Usually, however, this is better cultured from the stomach or determined by a serologic test on the blood.

Infections of the bowel from bacteria, virus, or parasites usually present as acute diarrhea, excessive flatus, abdominal discomfort, and fever. This may progress to toxic megacolon.

INTERFERING FACTORS

- Urine may inhibit the growth of bacteria. Therefore urine should not be mixed with the feces during collection of a stool sample.
- Recent barium studies may obscure the detection of parasites.
- Drugs that may affect test results include antibiotics, bismuth, and mineral oil.

Stool Tests

9

Clinical Priorities

- Stool cultures are usually done on patients with unrelenting diarrhea, fever, and abdominal bloating.
- The normal stool flora can become pathogenic if bacterial overgrowth occurs as a result of antibiotics, immunosuppression, or excessive catharsis.
- Wear gloves when obtaining and handling a stool specimen.

PROCEDURE AND PATIENT CARE

Before

✋ Explain the method of stool collection to the patient. Be matter-of-fact to avoid any embarrassment to the patient.

✋ Instruct the patient not to mix urine or toilet paper with the stool specimen.

✋ Instruct the patient to use an appropriate collection container.

During

✋ Instruct the patient to defecate into a designated clean container.

- Place a small amount of stool in a sterile collection container.
- Send mucus and blood streaks with the specimen.
- If a rectal swab is to be used, wear gloves and insert the cotton-tipped swab at least 1 inch into the anal canal. Then rotate the swab for 30 seconds and place it in the clean container.

Tape Test

- Use this test when pinworms *(Enterobius)* are suspected.
- Place a strip of clear tape in the patient's perianal region. (This is especially helpful in children.)
- Because the female worm lays her eggs at night around the perianal area, apply the tape before bed-time and remove it in the morning before the patient gets out of bed.
- Press the sticky surface of the tape directly to a glass slide and examine microscopically for pin-worm ova.

After

- Handle the stool specimen carefully, as though it were capable of causing infection.
- Promptly send the stool specimen to the laboratory. Delays in transfer of the specimen may affect viability of the organism. If long delays are necessary, obtain a buffered glycerol-saline solution to be combined with the stool and used as a preservative.
- Note that some enteric pathogens may take as long as 6 weeks to isolate.
- When pathogens are detected, maintain isolation of the patient's stool until therapy is completed. Other people who have had close contact with the patient should be tested and treated to prevent spread of the infection.

TEST RESULTS AND CLINICAL SIGNIFICANCE

Bacterial enterocolitis,
Protozoan enterocolitis,
Parasitic enterocolitis:

These organisms can be grown on special culture plates. The parasites can also be detected on smear of the stool. Treatment of these infections must be prompt, especially in children, who can dehydrate rapidly and become septic.

RELATED TEST

Clostridial Toxin Assay (p. 849). This test allows one to make the diagnosis of pseudomembranous colitis based on the presence of the bacterium *C. difficile*.

 Stool for Occult Blood (Stool for OB, Fecal Occult Blood Test [FOBT], Fecal Immunochemical Test [FIT], DNA Stool Sample)

NORMAL FINDINGS

No occult blood within stool

INDICATIONS

This test is used for colorectal cancer screening of asymptomatic individuals. It can also detect occult blood from other causes (e.g., ulcers, hemorrhoids, diverticulosis).

TEST EXPLANATION

Normally only minimal quantities (2 to 2.5 mL) of blood are passed into the gastrointestinal (GI) tract. Usually this bleeding is not significant enough to cause a positive result in the stool for occult blood (OB) testing. This test can detect OB when as little as 5 mL of blood is lost per day.

Tumors of the intestine grow into the lumen and are subjected to repeated trauma by the fecal stream. Eventually the friable neovascular tumor ulcerates and bleeding occurs. Most often, bleeding is so slight that gross blood is not seen in the stool. The blood can be detected by chemical assay or by immunohistochemistry. Guaiac is the most commonly performed chemical assay. The peroxidase-like activity of hemoglobin catalyzes the reaction of peroxide and a chromogen called orthotolidine to form a blue-stained oxidized orthotolidine.

OB can also be detected by immunochemical methods that detect the human globin portion of hemoglobin using monoclonal antibodies. These tests are called *fecal immunochemical test (FIT)* or *immunochemical fecal occult blood test (iFOBT)*. These methods are as sensitive as guaiac testing but are not affected by red meats or plant oxidizers as described below (see Interfering Factors). Immunochemical methods may fail to recognize occult blood from the upper GI tract because the globin is digested by the time it gets in the stool.

The *DNA stool sample test* is more sensitive than guaiac testing in the detection of significant colorectal precancerous, benign, and malignant tumors. Because most precancerous polyps do not bleed, they can be missed by FOBT. In contrast, all precancerous polyps shed cells that contain abnormal DNA. So, a stool-based DNA test designed to detect this DNA promises to be more accurate in the detection of precancerous polyps—which, when detected, can be removed before they turn into cancer.

Benign and malignant GI tumors, ulcers, inflammatory bowel disease, arteriovenous malformations, diverticulosis, and hematobilia (hemobilia) can all cause OB within the stool. Other more common abnormalities (e.g., hemorrhoids, swallowed blood from oral or nasopharyngeal bleeding) may also cause OB within the stool.

When OB testing is properly performed, a positive result obtained on multiple specimens collected on successive days warrants a thorough GI evaluation—usually EGD (see p. 608) and colonoscopy (see p. 591). Regular screening, beginning at age 50, can reduce the number of people who die from colorectal cancer by as much as 60%. There are several tests used for colorectal cancer screening (Table 9-1). Yet despite the availability of such screening tools, more than half of American adults have never undergone

TABLE 9-1 Testing Options for Colorectal Cancer*	
Test	**Frequency**
Fecal occult blood test (FOBT, or FIT)	Every year
Flexible sigmoidoscopy	Every 5 years
Double-contrast barium enema	Every 5 years
Colonoscopy†	Every 10 years
Virtual colonoscopy	Every 10 years

*(See Table 4-3, p. 593, colonoscopy, p. 591). People at higher risk of developing colorectal cancer should begin screening at a younger age, and may need to be tested more frequently.
†Colonoscopy can be used as a follow-up diagnostic tool when the results of another screening test are positive.

colorectal cancer screening. This fact highlights the need for more user friendly testing methods such as stool DNA testing. Several scientific organizations, including the U.S. Preventive Services Task Force (USPSTF) and other federal agencies, recommend regular screening for all adults aged 50 or older.

Reducing or oxidizing agents (such as iron, radish, cantaloupe or cauliflower, and vitamin C) can affect the results of guaiac or fecal immunochemical test (FIT). Furthermore neither FIT nor guaiac testing detects slow upper gastrointestinal (GI) bleeding because globin and heme are degraded during intestinal transit. To evaluate occult GI bleeding in these patients, a fluorometric method that will detect any hemoglobin or heme-derived porphyrins in the stool is very sensitive and provides quantitative results.

INTERFERING FACTORS

- Vigorous exercise.
- Ingestion of red meat within 3 days before testing.
- Bleeding gums following a dental procedure or disease may affect results.
- Ingestion of peroxidase-rich vegetables and fruits (turnips, artichokes, mushrooms, radishes, broccoli, bean sprouts, cauliflower, oranges, bananas, cantaloupes, and grapes) and horseradish may affect results.
- Drugs that may cause GI bleeding include anticoagulants, aspirin, colchicine, iron preparations (large doses), nonsteroidal antiarthritics, and steroids. Although these drugs do not interfere with the performance of the test, they can cause GI bleeding not associated with pathology.
- Drugs that may instigate the peroxidation reaction and cause false-positive results include boric acid, bromides, colchicine, iodine, iron, and rauwolfia derivatives.
- Vitamin C may cause false-negative results by inhibiting the peroxidation reaction.

Clinical Priorities

- This test is part of the routine colorectal cancer screening done on people older than age 50 years.
- Red meats need to be avoided for 3 days before the test. Otherwise, false-positive results could be obtained because red meats contain animal hemoglobin.
- Positive test results for OB indicate the need for a thorough GI evaluation.

PROCEDURE AND PATIENT CARE

Before

🖉 Explain the procedure to the patient.

🖉 Instruct the patient to refrain from eating any red meat for at least 3 days before the test.

🖉 Instruct the patient to refrain from drugs known to interfere with OB testing.

🖉 Instruct the patient in the method of obtaining appropriate stool specimens. Many procedures are available (e.g., specimen cards, tissue wipes, test paper). Tests may be done at home with specimen cards (Hemoccult) and mailed to a local testing laboratory or doctor's office when collected.

🖉 Instruct the patient not to mix urine with the stool specimen.

🖉 Inform the patient about the need for multiple specimens obtained on separate days to increase the test's accuracy.

• Note that in some centers a high-residue diet is recommended to increase the abrasive effect of the stool.

• Be gentle in obtaining stool by digital rectal examination. Traumatic digital examination can cause a false-positive result, especially in patients with prior anorectal disease such as hemorrhoids.

During

Hemoccult Slide Test

1. Place stool samples on one side of guaiac paper. Stool samples should be from two different areas of the specimen.
2. Place two drops of developer on the other side.
3. Note that a bluish discoloration indicates OB in the stool.

Tablet Test

1. Place a stool sample on the test paper.
2. Place a tablet on top of the stool specimen.
3. Put two or three drops of tap water on the tablet and allow to flow onto the paper.
4. Note that a bluish discoloration indicates OB in the stool.

After

🖉 Inform the patient of the results.

🖉 If the tests are positive, inquire whether the patient violated any of the preparation recommendations.

• Refer patient for a thorough GI evaluation if results are positive.

TEST RESULTS AND CLINICAL SIGNIFICANCE

GI tumor (cancers and polyps): *The mucosa overlying neoplasm is friable. Bleeding occurs when stool passes by.*

Peptic diseases (esophagitis, gastritis, and ulceration): *In peptic disease, the mucosa becomes inflamed, thickened, and friable. Bleeding easily occurs. Ulcers can erode into blood vessels within the wall of the gut.*

Varices: *Caused by portal hypertension, these large venous complexes are covered by a thin lining of mucosa. With increased intraabdominal pressure, these can rupture and bleed.*

Inflammatory bowel disease (ulcerative colitis, Crohn disease): *The inflammatory reaction causes a thickened and friable mucosa, which causes bleeding.*

Ischemic bowel disease: *The mucosa of the bowel is the first layer to be affected by diminished blood supply. This mucosa easily sloughs, and minor bleeding can occur.*

Stool Tests

9

GI trauma: *Penetrating or blunt trauma can cause bleeding into the gut.*

Recent GI surgery: *Small amounts of bleeding occur at the new GI anastomosis.*

Hemorrhoids and other anorectal problems: *An anorectal pathologic condition is the most common non-neoplastic cause of blood in the stool.*

RELATED TESTS

Colonoscopy (p. 591). This test allows endoscopic evaluation of the entire colon.

Esophagogastroduodenoscopy (p. 608). This endoscopic procedure visualizes the esophagus, stomach, and duodenum.

Barium Enema (p. 994). This test uses barium to provide x-ray visualization of the colon.

Upper GI Series (p. 1072). This test uses barium to provide x-ray visualization of the upper GI tract.

Small Bowel Series (p. 1064). This test uses barium to provide x-ray visualization of the small intestines.

Septin 9 DNA Methylation Assay (p. 460). This blood test is used to screen asymptomatic patients for colorectal cancer.

Ultrasound Studies

Overview

Ultrasonography is a diagnostic technique in which high-frequency sound waves (ultrasonic waves) are directed at internal body structures, and a record is made of the wave pulses as they are reflected back (echoed) through the tissues. Different acoustic densities differentiate between solid and cystic structures and thereby form an "image" of the organ being studied.

REASONS FOR PERFORMING ULTRASOUND STUDIES

Ultrasonography is performed for any of the following reasons:

1. To determine whether a lump or other abnormality is a fluid-filled cyst or a solid tumor (e.g., kidney, thyroid, breast lesions).
2. To guide needle-directed biopsy of a suspected tumor site to establish a diagnosis (e.g., prostate or breast cancer).
3. To stage a tumor (e.g., esophageal, rectal, or breast cancer).

4. To evaluate pregnancy and placental status.
5. To detect ectopic pregnancy.
6. To determine fetal status, size, and growth.
7. To evaluate disorders of arteries (e.g., aneurysm) and veins (e.g., deep vein thrombosis).

PRINCIPLES OF ULTRASONOGRAPHY

Tissues of different composition reflect sound waves differently, which permits differentiation of normal and diseased tissue. Sound waves are transmitted well through fluid, but not through air, bone, or contrast medium (e.g., barium).

The advantages of ultrasonography are that it is noninvasive and requires no ionizing radiation. Therefore repeated studies can be performed and multiple images obtained with no risk. Because no radiation exposure occurs, ultrasonography can be performed in an office or laboratory or at the bedside. Ultrasonography is less expensive than either computed tomography (CT) or magnetic resonance imaging (MRI).

Ultrasonography is painless. The skin overlying the body area to be evaluated (e.g., heart, gallbladder) is covered with a lubricating gel to provide an air-free barrier between the skin and the ultrasonographic probe, which contains a transducer. The probe is passed over the specific body area, and ultrasonic waves, with frequencies in a range above human hearing, are transmitted through the tissues. The transducer converts the echoes to electric impulses and transforms them into visual images, or sonograms, which can be viewed singly (like a photograph), or in rapid sequence (like a movie), to evaluate the data obtained. Light (hyperechoic) or dark (hypoechoic) areas seen on an ultrasonogram are a result of the manner in which various tissues reflect ultrasonic waves.

In some types of ultrasonography, the probe (transducer) is placed within the body. For example, in transesophageal echocardiography (TEE), the transducer is incorporated in the tip of a fiberoptic endoscope, which is placed in the esophagus, behind the heart; in rectal or prostate ultrasonography, the transducer is introduced through the anus into the rectum; and during surgery, the transducer can be held directly on the organ to be evaluated (e.g., the liver).

Various scans and techniques can be used to display the ultrasonic echoes. Some of these are as follows:

1. *B-scan:* A B-scan image is made up of a series of dots, each indicating a single ultrasonic echo. The position of a dot corresponds to the time elapsed, and the brightness of a dot corresponds to the strength of the echo. Movement of the transducer over the skin yields a two-dimensional cross-sectional image (Figure 10-1).
2. *M-mode scan:* An image obtained with M-mode echocardiography shows the motion (M) of the heart over time.
3. *Real-time imaging:* Multiple transducers are used to display a rapid sequence of data that can be instantaneously converted into accurate anatomic images of the organ being evaluated.
4. *Doppler ultrasound:* As opposed to static ultrasound, in which the sound wave returning to the transducer is the same frequency as that which was emitted, Doppler ultrasound uses a different technique. In Doppler ultrasound of blood vessels, the red blood cells (RBCs) within the vessel distort the frequency of the ultrasound waves. The change in frequency of the ultrasound wave is proportional to the velocity of the RBC. The better the blood flow, the faster the RBCs move by the stationary ultrasound beam, the greater the frequency distortion (or Doppler shift). With this technique, sound waves are transformed into audible sounds or linear graphic recordings. This is important for assessing blood flow through arteries and veins. It is also used with pregnant women to assess the fetal heart rate and with increasing frequency to determine blood flow to organs (e.g., kidney, testicles).

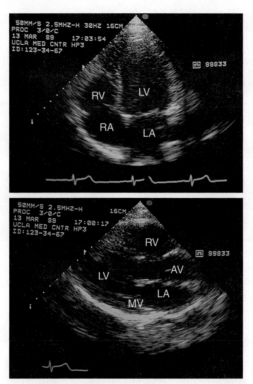

Figure 10-1 Two-dimensional echocardiogram. *RA*, Right atrium; *RV*, right ventricle; *LA*, left atrium; *LV*, left ventricle; *MV*, mitral valve; *AV*, aortic valve.

5. *Color flow Doppler imaging*: This imaging technique is used to determine direction (recorded as colors) and velocity (shades) of blood flow in the chambers of the heart (Figure 10-2). This technique is important in evaluating heart valve regurgitation and blood shunting in patients with heart defects.

6. *Duplex scanning*: Real-time imaging and color flow Doppler imaging combine to demonstrate how the arteries and veins are functioning and velocity and turbulence within the vessels. Duplex scanning is useful to detect plaque within arteries, demonstrate aneurysms, and assess renal or liver transplants for rejection.

7. *Three-dimensional (3D) ultrasound*: This imaging technique is often used during pregnancy to provide 3D images of the fetus. The common obstetric mode is 2D. In 3D fetal scanning, a computer program can construct a 3D image of the fetus that is more realistic than 2D imaging (Figure 10-3). Four-dimensional (4D) shows a 3D picture in real time (e.g., can see fetus moving).

Ultrasonography is often used in conjunction with other diagnostic testing. For example, if a CT scan of the kidney demonstrates a filling defect, an ultrasound scan can indicate whether that defect is a benign fluid-filled cyst or a malignant solid tumor.

PROCEDURAL CARE FOR ULTRASONOGRAPHY

Before

- Most ultrasound procedures require little or no preparation. However, patients undergoing pelvic scanning must have a full bladder, which may become uncomfortable. Patients undergoing

Ultrasound Studies

10

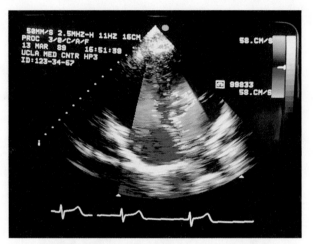

Figure 10-2 Color flow Doppler echocardiography. Flow, or signals, moving toward the transducer are recorded in shades of yellow and red, and those moving away from the transducer are recorded as blue.

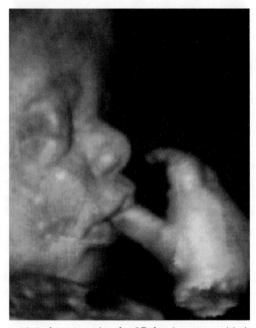

Figure 10-3 An example of a 3D fetal sonographic image.

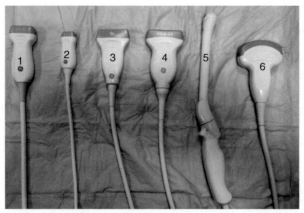

Figure 10-4 US probes (from the left) 1, low frequency sector probe used for abdominal US; 2, high-frequency sector probe used for infant US and intraoperative brain surgery US; 3, linear probe used for vascular US; 4, high-frequency linear probe used for superficial structures such as thyroid, scrotum, or breast; 5, intracavitary probe used for vaginal/rectal US; 6, general low-frequency probe used for abdominal US.

ultrasound examination of the gallbladder should be fasting to avoid gallbladder contraction that usually follows ingestion of a meal. A contracted gallbladder is difficult to identify with ultrasonography.
- Consent is needed if the transducer will be inserted into a body cavity or if an ultrasound-directed biopsy is planned.

During
- Ultrasound examinations are usually performed in an ultrasonography suite but can be performed on the patient unit or in a physician's office.
- A gel lubricant is applied to the tissue overlying the organ to be studied. Air impedes transmission of sound waves, and this lubricant ensures good contact between the skin and the transducer or probe. Different probes are used depending on the area being evaluated (Figure 10-4). Thus sound transmission and reception are enhanced.

After
- Because ultrasonography is noninvasive, no special nursing measures are needed after the study except to help the patient remove the gel.
- Ultrasound examinations can be repeated as often as necessary without harm to the patient. No cumulative effects have been noted.

INTERFERING FACTORS
- Air impedes transmission of ultrasonic waves into the body. The use of a lubricant is essential to ensure good transmission of sound waves to and from the body.
- Barium blocks transmission of ultrasonic waves. For this reason, ultrasonography of the abdomen should be performed before any barium contrast studies.

Ultrasound
Studies

10

- Large amounts of gas in the bowel will distort visualization of abdominal organs, because bowel gas reflects sound. Likewise, ultrasonic evaluation of the lungs yields poor results.
- Obesity may affect the results of the study, because sound waves are altered by fatty tissue. For this reason, it may be difficult to obtain an accurate scan in an obese patient.
- Movement causes artifacts. Some patients may need to be sedated to remain still. Uncooperative patients (especially children) may not be candidates for ultrasonography.
- Because ultrasonography requires direct contact of the transducer and the skin, it may not be possible to perform this study in postoperative patients with dressings.
- The quality of the ultrasound image and the sufficiency of the study depend to a large extent on the abilities of the ultrasound technician performing the study.

POTENTIAL COMPLICATIONS

No potential complications have been directly related to ultrasonography at the intensities used for medical diagnosis. However, in some procedures (e.g., TEE), complications may occur as a result of the invasive method used to place the ultrasound probe inside the body. These complications are described for individual tests.

REPORTING OF RESULTS

The patient can usually observe the scan on a monitor in the room. The technician may point out some findings at that time. Later, the physician will review the scan and explain the results to the patient.

Abdominal Ultrasonography (Abdominal Sonography; Echography; Ultrasonography of the Kidney, Liver, Pancreatobiliary System, Gallbladder, Pancreas, Biliary Tree)

NORMAL FINDINGS

Normal abdominal aorta, liver, gallbladder, bile ducts, pancreas, kidney, and bladder

INDICATIONS

This technique is used to visualize the abdomen and the organs within it. Its uses are many, as described in Table 10-1.

TABLE 10-1	Overview of Abdominal Ultrasonography
Area Visualized	**Possible Findings**
Kidney, bladder	Cysts, tumors, calculi, hydronephrosis, malformations, abscess, transplant rejection
Abdominal aorta	Aneurysm
Liver	Cysts, abscess, dilated hepatic ducts, tumors
Gallbladder, extrahepatic ducts	Gallstones, polyps, dilation secondary to strictures or tumors
Pancreas	Tumors, pseudocysts, inflammation, abscess

TEST EXPLANATION

Through use of reflected sound waves, ultrasonography provides accurate visualization of the abdominal aorta, liver, gallbladder, pancreas, bile ducts, spleen, kidneys, and bladder. The technique of ultrasonography requires the emission of high-frequency sound waves from the transducer to penetrate the organ being studied. The sound waves are bounced back to the transducer and electronically converted to a pictorial image that is recorded on film. Real-time ultrasound provides an accurate picture of the organ being studied. Doppler ultrasound provides information about blood flow to those organs.

The *kidney* (Figure 10-5) is evaluated ultrasonographically for the following reasons:

1. Diagnose and locate renal cysts
2. Differentiate renal cysts from solid renal tumors
3. Demonstrate renal and pelvic calculi
4. Document hydronephrosis
5. Guide a percutaneously inserted needle for cyst aspiration, biopsy, or nephrostomy placement

Ultrasound of the urologic tract is used to detect malformed or ectopic kidneys and perinephric abscesses. Renal transplantation surveillance is possible with ultrasonography. One advantage of kidney sonography over intravenous pyelography (p. 1057) is that it can be performed in patients with impaired renal function, because no intravenous contrast medium is required.

Endourethral urologic ultrasound can also be performed through a stent that has a transducer at its end. The stent probe is placed into the urethra to examine that segment for diverticula. The stent probe can then be advanced into the bladder, where the depth of a tumor into the bladder wall can be measured. With the use of wire lead guidance, the stent probe can be passed into the ureter, where stones (especially those embedded into the submucosa), tumors, or extraurethral compression can be identified and localized. Finally, as the probe is advanced in the proximal ureter, renal tumors or cysts can be better delineated.

The *abdominal aorta* can be assessed for aneurysmal dilation. Sonographic evidence of an aortic aneurysm greater than 5 cm in greatest dimension, or any aneurysm that is documented to be significantly enlarging, is an indication for abdominal aortic aneurysm resection. Ultrasonography is also an ideal way to monitor aneurysms before and after surgery.

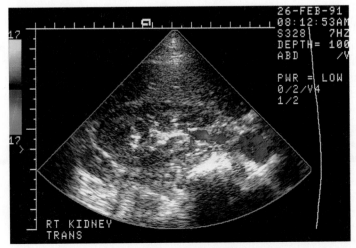

Figure 10-5 Ultrasonogram of the kidney.

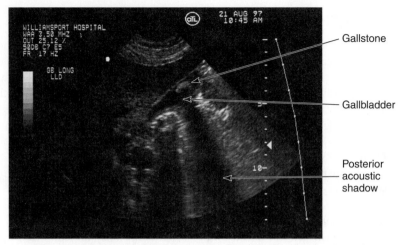

Figure 10-6 Ultrasonogram of the gallbladder. Long-axis view of the gallbladder containing a gallstone. Note the posterior acoustic shadowing, typical for gallstones.

Ultrasonography is used to detect cystic structures of the *liver* (e.g., benign cysts, hepatic abscesses, dilated hepatic ducts) and solid intrahepatic tumors (primary and metastatic). Hepatic ultrasonography can also be performed intraoperatively with a sterile probe. This technique allows accurate location of small, nonpalpable hepatic tumors or abscesses. The *gallbladder* and *extrahepatic ducts* can be visualized for evidence of gallstones (Figure 10-6), polyps, or dilation secondary to obstructive strictures or tumors. The *pancreas* is examined for evidence of tumor, pseudocysts, acute or chronic inflammation, or pancreatic abscess. Repeated ultrasound scans of the pancreas are frequently obtained to document resolution of acute pancreatic inflammatory processes. Often the pancreas is better visualized if the stomach and duodenum are filled with water.

Because ultrasonography requires no contrast material or radiation, it is especially useful in patients who are allergic to contrast media or are pregnant. Fasting is desirable but not mandatory. (See discussion of pelvic ultrasonography [p. 887] for evaluation of pelvic organs.)

INTERFERING FACTORS

- Barium and gas distort the sound waves and alter test results. This test should be performed before any x-ray testing with barium contrast.
- Ultrasound studies are only as good as the skills of the sonographer.
- Obesity may affect the results because sound waves are altered by fatty tissue. It may be difficult to obtain an accurate scan in an obese patient.

✓ Clinical Priorities

- Because this study requires no contrast material and has no associated radiation, it is especially useful in patients allergic to dyes and in pregnant patients.
- The need for preprocedure fasting depends on the organ to be examined.
- Ultrasound of the kidney can be used to evaluate rejection of a kidney transplant.

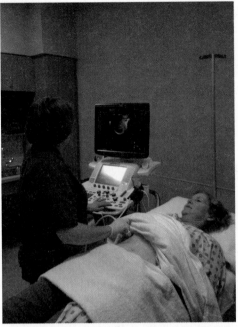

Figure 10-7 Abdominal ultrasound.

PROCEDURE AND PATIENT CARE

Before

☒ Explain the procedure to the patient.

☒ Tell the patient that no discomfort is associated with the procedure.

☒ Tell the patient that fasting may or may not be required, depending on the organ to be examined. No fasting is required for ultrasonography of the abdominal aorta, kidney, liver, spleen, or pancreas, but is preferred before ultrasonography of the gallbladder and biliary tree.

During

- Procedure:
  1. The patient is placed on the ultrasonography table in the prone or supine position, depending on the organ to be examined.
  2. A gel lubricant is applied to the patient's skin to enhance sound wave transmission and reception.
  3. A transducer is placed over the skin (Figure 10-7).
  4. Images are made of the reflections from the organ being studied.
- For water distention of the stomach, the patient is asked to drink 8 to 10 oz of water while standing.
- The test is completed in approximately 20 minutes, usually by an ultrasound technologist, and later is interpreted by a radiologist.

After

- Remove the gel from the patient's skin.
- If a biopsy was performed, refer to the specific organ (e.g., liver biopsy, kidney biopsy) for postprocedure care.

TEST RESULTS AND CLINICAL SIGNIFICANCE
Kidney

Renal cysts and polycystic kidney: *Renal cysts appear as dark (echo free, or hypoechoic) areas with smooth, well-defined walls. In polycystic kidney, these cysts are of various sizes.*

Renal tumor: *Renal tumors appear as white (hyperechoic) areas.*

Renal calculi,

Hydronephrosis,

Ureteral obstruction:
   Obstruction is inferred by identification of dilation of the collecting system.

Perinephric collection (e.g., perirenal abscess, perirenal hematoma): *Perirenal collections of pus or blood appear as a hypoechoic (dark) halo surrounding the kidney.*

Primary renal disease (e.g., glomerulonephritis, pyelonephritis): *Primary renal disease is evidenced by small, isoechoic kidneys, especially at the end stage.*

Pancreas

Tumor: *Pancreatic tumor is evident as an echogenic (solid) mass, usually in the head of the pancreas.*

Cysts or pseudocysts: *These appear as dark (hypoechoic) masses. Neoplastic cysts are difficult to differentiate from pseudocysts. Malignant cystic tumors cannot be differentiated from benign cysts.*

Abscess: *Hypoechoic (dark) areas in an inflamed pancreas could be cysts or abscesses, which cannot be differentiated.*

Inflammation: *Acute inflammation of the pancreas is visualized as an enlarged edematous pancreas. Chronic inflammation is apparent as a small, contracted echogenic (dense) pancreas.*

Gallbladder

Polyps,

Tumor:
   Neoplasms appear as echogenic (solid) masses in the gallbladder that do not move with change in position.

Gallstone: *Ultrasound is accurate for detection of gallstones. An echogenic mass with "shadowing" behind it is the classic appearance of a gallstone.*

Liver

Tumor primary or metastatic: *The ultrasound appearance of liver metastasis is variable. In general, liver neoplasms are echogenic.*

Abscess,

Cysts:
   Liver abscesses and cysts cannot be differentiated with certainty using ultrasonography.

Bile Ducts

Gallstone,

Tumor:
   Tumors and gallstones appear as echogenic masses with posterior acoustic "shadowing" within the bile duct.

Dilation due to stricture, stones, or tumor,

Intrahepatic dilated bile ducts:
   The entire biliary tree is seen as a hypoechoic tube in the portal area or liver.

Abdominal Aorta

Aneurysm: *The aorta appears as a hypoechoic tubular structure in the retroperitoneum. Aortic aneurysm is evident as a saccular dilation.*

Abdominal Cavity

Ascites: *Ultrasound is sensitive for detection of fluid within the abdomen. As little as 10 mL of fluid can be detected.*

Abscess: *Abscesses secondary to appendicitis or diverticulitis are easily demonstrated. Phlegmon (inflammatory involvement of tissue) may surround an abscess.*

RELATED TESTS

Ultrasonography of the Prostate Gland, Testes, Uterus, and Ovaries are discussed separately (pp. 891, 893, and 887, respectively).

Breast Ultrasonography (Ultrasound Mammography Breast Sonogram)

NORMAL FINDINGS

No evidence of cyst or tumor

INDICATIONS

Ultrasound examination of the breast is diagnostically performed to determine if a mammographic abnormality or a palpable lump is a cyst (fluid-filled) or solid tumor (benign or malignant). It is also used in screening for breast cancer for women whose breasts are dense on mammography.

TEST EXPLANATION

In diagnostic real-time ultrasonography, harmless high-frequency sound waves are emitted and penetrate the breast. The sound waves are reflected back to the sensor and arranged in a pictorial image by electronic conversion. Ultrasonography of the breast is useful to:

1. Differentiate cystic from solid breast lesions
2. Identify masses in women with breast tissue too dense for accurate mammography
3. Monitor a cyst to determine whether it enlarges or disappears
4. Measure the size of a tumor
5. Evaluate the axilla in women who are newly diagnosed with breast cancer

Ultrasonography is also useful for examination of symptomatic breasts in women in whom the radiation of mammography is potentially harmful. These include:

1. Pregnant women. Radiation may be harmful to the fetus.
2. Women younger than age 25, who may be at greater oncologic risk from the radiation of mammography.
3. Women who refuse mammography because of unreasonable fear of diagnostic radiation.

With high-quality diagnostic ultrasonography, the characteristics of an abnormality can be evaluated and a reasonable prediction can be made whether it is malignant. Characteristics of malignancy are indicated in Table 10-2. Diagnostic accuracy is improved when breast ultrasonography is combined with mammography

TABLE 10-2	Characteristics of Ultrasound Findings: Benign Versus Malignancy	
Characteristic	**Benign**	**Suspicious for Malignancy**
Contents	Cystic	Solid
Effect on surrounding tissue	No interruption	Invasive
Dimensions	Wider than tall	Taller than wide
Homogeneity of contents	Homogeneous	Heterogeneous
Acoustic effects beyond the lesion	Good sound transmission (acoustic enhancement)	Poor sound transmission (acoustic attenuation)

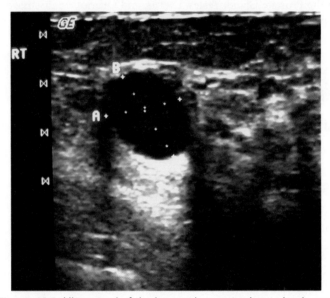

Figure 10-8 Ultrasound of the breast demonstrating a simple cyst of the breast measuring 1.14 by 0.94 cm.

(see p. 1043). Ultrasound is especially useful in patients with an abnormal mass identified on a mammogram, because the nature (cystic or solid) of the mass can be determined. Most cysts are benign. See Figure 10-8.

Ultrasound can be used to locate and accurately direct percutaneous biopsy probes to a nonpalpable breast abnormality for biopsy or aspiration. Ultrasound is painless, harmless, and is without any radiation effects on the breast tissue.

PROCEDURE AND PATIENT CARE

Before

✍ Explain the procedure to the patient and assure the patient that no discomfort is associated with the examination.

✍ Inform the patient that no fasting or sedation is required. Instruct the patient not to apply any lotions or powders to the breasts on the examination day.

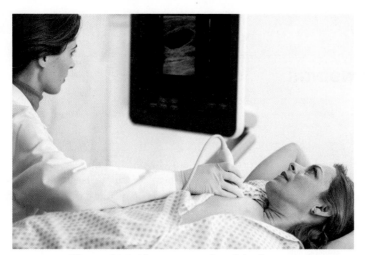

Figure 10-9 Ultrasonography of the breast.

During

- The patient is placed supine, a gel lubricant is applied, and a hand-held transducer is placed directly on the skin overlying the breast (Figure 10-9).
- The test is performed by an ultrasound technician in approximately 15 minutes.

After

- After the test is completed, the gel is removed.

TEST RESULTS AND CLINICAL SIGNIFICANCE

Cyst: *These are apparent as very dark (hypoechoic), well-circumscribed abnormalities with posterior acoustic enhancement. These are benign and no intervention is required unless they are symptomatic.*

Hematoma,

Abscess,

Cancer:
> *These appear as hypoechoic (dark), poorly circumscribed masses with acoustic "shadowing" behind the back wall.*

Fibroadenoma: *These appear as hypoechoic (dark) well-circumscribed lesions within the breast acoustic "enhancement" behind the back wall.*

Fibrocystic disease: *This is evident as diffuse, echogenic, localized tissue within the breast.*

RELATED TESTS

Mammography (p. 1043). This x-ray study of the breast can detect breast abnormalities but cannot differentiate between cystic and solid masses as ultrasonography can.

Magnetic Resonance Imaging (MRI) of the Breast (p. 1106). This test is very sensitive in detecting abnormalities in the breast .

Carotid Artery Duplex Scan (Carotid Ultrasound)

NORMAL FINDINGS

Carotid artery free of plaques and stenosis

INDICATIONS

This Doppler ultrasound test is performed to identify occlusive disease in the carotid artery or its branches. It is recommended in patients with peripheral vascular disease and neurologic symptoms such as transient ischemic attacks (TIAs), hemiparesis, paresthesia, dizziness, syncope, or acute speech or visual deficits. It is also used on patients who are asymptomatic but are found to have a carotid bruit.

TEST EXPLANATION

Carotid duplex scanning is a noninvasive, ultrasound test used to directly detect occlusive disease of the vertebral and extracranial carotid artery. It is called "duplex" because it combines the benefits of two methods of ultrasonography—Doppler and B-mode. With the use of the transducer, a B-mode ultrasound grayscale image of the carotid vessel is obtained. A pulsed Doppler probe within the transducer is used to evaluate blood flow velocity and direction in the artery and to measure the amplitude and waveform of the carotid arterial pulse. A computer combines that information and provides a two-dimensional image of the carotid artery along with an image of blood flow. With this technique, one is able to directly visualize areas of stenotic or occluded arteries and arterial flow disruption. The degree of occlusion is measured in percentage of the entire lumen that is occluded. *Color Doppler Ultrasound (CDU)* can be added to duplex scanning. CDU assigns color for direction of blood flow within the vessel and the intensity of that color is dependent on the mean computed velocity of blood traveling in the vessel. This allows visualization of stenotic areas by seeing slowing or reversal of direction of blood flow at a particular area of the artery. Reversal of blood flow is sometimes associated with contralateral arterial occlusion, which can be easily demonstrated using this technique.

This test is performed by an ultrasound technologist in the ultrasound or radiology department in approximately 15 to 30 minutes. Results are interpreted by a radiologist, usually the same day. No discomfort is associated with the test. The accuracy of this test is limited by the skill of the technologists.

Measurement of the thickness of the wall of the carotid artery (*carotid intima–media thickness [CIMT]*) is used as a measurement of cerebrovascular atherosclerosis specifically and is a predictor of coronary atherosclerosis in general. CIMT is also used to monitor progression of atherosclerosis (particularly in diabetics). It is also used to monitor atherosclerotic regression in patients who are undergoing a treatment for atherosclerosis.

Many studies have documented the relation between the carotid intima–media thickness and the presence and severity of atherosclerosis. Because the carotid artery is elastic, most of its wall represents the intima (innermost part of the arterial wall). The wall of a muscular artery like the femoral artery, on the other hand, is made up mostly of the muscular media. Because atherosclerosis most affects the intima, the carotid artery is best to evaluate. Furthermore, its proximity to the skin in the neck makes it an excellent artery to measure with external ultrasound. The CIMT can also be measured by intravascular ultrasound (see p. 884). Nonatherosclerotic diseases such as intimal hyperplasia and intimal fibrocellular hypertrophy can also cause increased CIMT. More recent research has used the combined carotid artery IMT and femoral artery IMT measurements to more accurately determine the atherosclerotic burden of the coronary arteries.

CIMT measurements above thresholds (0.9 mm) almost certainly indicate atherosclerosis. For every 0.1 mm increase, the risk of a heart attack or stroke increases 15%. CIMT is able to identify and monitor subclinical atherosclerosis. B-mode ultrasound is most commonly used. The intimal-medial thickness is measured and averaged over six sites in each carotid artery. A limitation of carotid artery IMT for the evaluation of coronary artery disease is that it does not accurately assess the total atherosclerotic burden and therefore cannot predict the severity of coronary artery disease or distinguish patients with one-vessel, two-vessel, or more coronary artery disease.

PROCEDURE AND PATIENT CARE

Before

✗ Explain the procedure to the patient.
✗ Tell the patient that no special preparation is required.
✗ Assure the patient that the study is painless.

During

- Place the patient supine with the head supported to prevent lateral motion.
- Note the following procedural steps:
    1. A gel lubricant is used to couple the sound from the transducer to the skin surface.
    2. Images of the carotid artery and pulse waveform are obtained.

After

- Remove the gel from the patient's skin.

TEST RESULTS AND CLINICAL SIGNIFICANCE

Carotid artery occlusive disease: *Narrowing of the lumen of the carotid artery or any of its branches can be accurately determined as a percentage of the vessel occluded (e.g., 90% occlusion). Most often occlusion is a result of atherosclerotic disease.*
Carotid artery aneurysm: *This arterial flow disruption is easily visualized.*

RELATED TEST

Angiography, Carotid (p. 988). This is a more accurate test of the carotid system, and is performed if surgery is contemplated. The angiogram demonstrates where and how extensive occlusive plaques are.

Contraceptive Device Localization (Intrauterine Device [IUD] Localization)

NORMAL FINDINGS

An IUD contraceptive device is located in the endometrial cavity.

INDICATIONS

This ultrasound test is performed to locate an IUD when its string cannot be palpated.

Ultrasound Studies

10

TEST EXPLANATION

When a woman is unable to visualize or palpate the string of an IUD, ultrasonography is indicated to determine whether the IUD has perforated the uterus, been evacuated, or been incorporated with an intrauterine pregnancy. IUDs have a particular type-specific structure and can be easily recognized on a sonogram. If an IUD can be seen on an abdominal x-ray film but cannot be demonstrated in the endometrial cavity on a sonogram, the IUD most likely has perforated the uterus.

IUD localization is performed in approximately 20 minutes. No discomfort is associated with this study other than having a full bladder and the urge to urinate.

INTERFERING FACTORS

- Recent gastrointestinal (GI) contrast studies, because barium severely distorts reflective sound waves
- Air-filled bowel loops, because gas does not transmit sound waves well
- Failure to fill the bladder, which is often used as a reference point for pelvic sonography

PROCEDURE AND PATIENT CARE

Before

- Explain the procedure to the patient.
- Give the patient three to four glasses (200 to 300 mL) of water or other liquid 1 hour before the examination, and instruct her not to void until after the procedure is completed. This will allow the bladder to fill and to be used as a reference point.
- Tell the patient that no fasting or sedation is required.

During

- Note the following procedural steps:
  1. The patient is taken to the ultrasound room and placed supine on the examination table.
  2. The ultrasonographer, usually a radiologist, applies a gel lubricant to the abdomen to enhance sound transmission and reception.
  3. A transducer is passed vertically and horizontally over the skin.
  4. Pictures are taken of the sound waves, and a real-time image is produced.

After

- Remove the lubricant from the patient's skin.
- Provide an opportunity for the patient to void.

TEST RESULTS AND CLINICAL SIGNIFICANCE

Perforation of the uterus: *If an IUD is seen on a plain film of the abdomen but cannot be found in the uterus at ultrasonography, it can be suspected that the IUD has perforated the uterus and is outside it.*

Expulsion of the IUD: *The IUD cannot be located in the uterus or on a plain film of the abdomen.*

Incorporation of the IUD in an intrauterine pregnancy: *The IUD was in place when pregnancy occurred and has become incorporated in the pregnancy.*

Echocardiography (Cardiac Echography, Heart Sonography, Transthoracic Echocardiography [TTE])

NORMAL FINDINGS

Normal position, size, and movement of the cardiac valves and heart muscle wall
Normal directional flow of blood within the heart chambers

INDICATIONS

Echocardiography is performed most commonly to evaluate heart wall motion (a measure of heart wall function) and to detect valvular disease, evaluate the heart during stress testing, and identify and quantify pericardial fluid.

TEST EXPLANATION

Echocardiography is a noninvasive ultrasound procedure used to evaluate the structure and function of the heart. In diagnostic ultrasonography, harmless, high-frequency sound waves emitted from a transducer penetrate the heart and are reflected back to the transducer as a series of echoes (Figure 10-10). These echoes are amplified and displayed on a cathode ray tube. Tracings also can be recorded on moving graph paper or videotape. The study usually includes M-mode recordings, two-dimensional recordings, a Doppler study, and real-time three-dimensional imaging.

M-mode echocardiography produces a one-dimensional recording of the amplitude and rate of motion (M) of the heart structures in real time. This allows the various cardiac structures to be located and studied regarding their movement during a cardiac cycle.

In *two-dimensional echocardiography*, the ultrasonic beam is moved within one sector of the heart. Computer reconstruction produces a two-dimensional image of the spatial relationships within the heart. *Three-dimensional echocardiography* is routinely added to most new cardiac echo procedures. This allows for improved images of the heart wall and valves. The addition of high temporal resolution improves images still further.

Color flow Doppler imaging demonstrates the direction and velocity of blood flow within the heart and great vessels. These variations in blood flow and velocity alter the ultrasound frequency. By assigning computerized weighted numbers to these altered frequencies, origins of velocity change and blood turbulence can be mapped. Altered direction and velocity of blood flow are coded as colors and shades, respectively (e.g., blue and red represent the direction of blood flow; various hues from dull to bright represent blood velocity). The most useful application of the color flow Doppler imaging is to determine the direction and turbulence of blood flow across regurgitant or narrowed valves. Color flow Doppler imaging also may be helpful in assessing proper functioning of prosthetic valves.

Echocardiography is used to diagnose pericardial effusion, valvular heart disease (e.g., mitral valve prolapse, stenosis, regurgitation), subaortic stenosis, myocardial wall abnormalities (e.g., cardiomyopathy), infarction, aneurysm, and cardiac tumors (e.g., myxomas). Atrial and ventricular septal defects and other congenital heart diseases, and postinfarction mural thrombi are also recognized with this testing.

Echocardiography is fast becoming the method of choice for cardiac stress testing. During an exercise or chemical cardiac stress test, ischemic muscle areas are evident as hypokinetic areas within the myocardium. Echocardiography is being used increasingly in emergent evaluation of chest pain. If

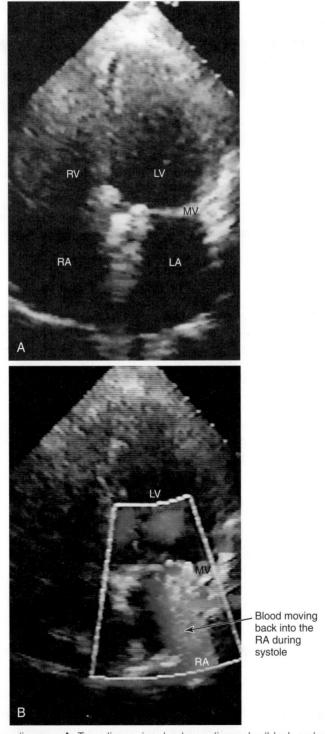

Figure 10-10 Echocardiogram. **A,** Two-dimensional echocardiography (black and white). **B,** Color Doppler echocardiography. The heart is oriented with the ventricles on the upper portion of the picture and the atria on the lower portion. The four chambers of the heart are easily identified. The right side of the heart is seen on the left side of the figure. *RV,* Right ventricle; *LV,* left ventricle; *RA,* right atrium; *LA,* left atrium; *MV,* mitral valve leaflets (white line) closed during systole. On the color Doppler echocardiogram, the blue indicates abnormal reversal of blood flowing from the left ventricle and into the left atrium during systole because of mitral valve regurgitation.

the myocardium is normal and without areas of hypokinesia, no coronary artery occlusive disease is suspected. A hypokinetic or akinetic area, however, indicates ischemia or infarction and that the chest pain is cardiac in origin.

Echocardiography can be performed through the esophagus using a transducer mounted on an endoscope. This procedure is referred to as transesophageal echocardiography (TEE) (p. 897). Fetal echocardiograms enable identification of significant congenital heart disease before birth.

Perflutren (DEFINITY) is an injectable opacifying agent (given by IV bolus or IV infusion) that provides enhancement of the endocardial borders during echocardiography by lowering acoustic impedance and enhancing the intrinsic backscatter of blood in the heart. This improves images of any abnormalities in heart wall activity.

Echocardiography usually takes approximately 45 minutes and is performed by an ultrasound technician in a darkened room in the cardiac laboratory or radiology department. No discomfort is associated with this study other than that the transmission gel is usually cooler than body temperature.

CONTRAINDICATIONS

- Patients who are uncooperative

INTERFERING FACTORS

- Patients with chronic obstructive pulmonary disease (COPD) have a substantial amount of air between the heart and the chest cavity. Air space does not conduct ultrasound waves well.
- In obese patients, the space between the heart and the transducer is greatly enlarged; therefore, accuracy of the test is decreased.

✔ Clinical Priorities

- Echocardiography is rapidly becoming the method of choice of heart imaging for stress testing.
- This test is frequently used in the emergency evaluation of chest pain.
- Because of the large amount of air between the heart and the chest cavity, it is difficult to evaluate patients with COPD using echocardiography. Transesophageal echocardiography is a better test in these patients.

PROCEDURE AND PATIENT CARE

Before

 Assure the patient that the study is painless.
- Include pertinent patient history on the echocardiogram request form.

During

- Note the following procedural steps:
    1. The patient is placed supine.
    2. Electrocardiographic (EKG) leads are placed (p. 544).
    3. A gel, which allows better transmission of sound waves, is placed on the chest wall, over which the transducer is passed.
    4. Ultrasonic waves are directed at the heart, and appropriate tracings are obtained (Figures 10-11 and 10-12).

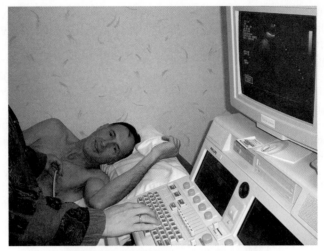

Figure 10-11 Echocardiography laboratory.

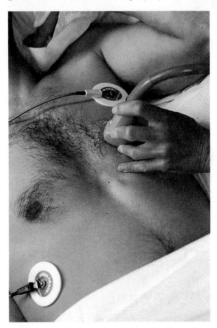

Figure 10-12 Placement of chest leads and transducer on precordium.

After

- Remove gel from the patient's chest wall.
- Inform the patient that the physician must interpret the study and that the results will be available in a few hours.

TEST RESULTS AND CLINICAL SIGNIFICANCE

Valvular heart disease (e.g., stenosis, regurgitation, mitral valve prolapse): *This is readily evident on echocardiograms. All valves can be easily seen with the linear mode. The circulatory effects of valvular disease are apparent on Doppler studies.*

Pericardial effusion: *Fluid around the heart is easily evident. Echocardiography can be used to guide a needle into the pericardial space for aspiration of fluid for analysis and treatment.*

Ventricular or atrial mural thrombi: *When these are evident, anticoagulation therapy is required. These thrombi may be the result of previous myocardial infarction (MI), ventricular aneurysm, congestive heart failure (CHF), or cardiomyopathy.*

Myxomas: *These tumors are often evident as a mass partially attached to the endocardium.*

Poor ventricular muscle motion: *Hypokinesia is evident in a portion of or in the entire myocardial wall in patients with myocardial ischemia, cardiomyopathy, and CHF.*

Ventricular hypertrophy: *This chronic disease is evident as an unusually thickened myocardium.*

Endocarditis: *Vegetations are readily evident on the valves. Aggressive antibiotic or anticoagulation therapy, or both, is needed.*

Septal defects: *Left-to-right shunting is readily evident with color flow Doppler imaging.*

RELATED TEST

Transesophageal Echocardiography (TEE) (p. 897). This test provides information similar to that obtained with transthoracic echocardiography, but TEE allows better visualization of the posterior portion of the heart and thoracic vessels.

Fetal Biophysical Profile (BPP)

NORMAL FINDINGS

Score of 8 to 10 points (if amniotic fluid volume is adequate)

 Critical Values

Score of less than 4 may necessitate immediate delivery.

INDICATIONS

The premise behind the BPP is that assessment of variable factors of fetal biophysical activity are more reliable than examination of a single parameter (e.g., fetal heart rate). Indications for BPP include post-date pregnancy, maternal hypertension, diabetes mellitus, vaginal bleeding, maternal Rh factor sensitization, maternal history of stillbirth, and premature rupture of membranes. The BPP is probably more useful in identifying a fetus that is in jeopardy than in predicting future fetal well-being. Testing usually begins at about 32 weeks, but can be done earlier if maternal complications exist.

TEST EXPLANATION

The BPP is a method of evaluating antepartal fetal status on the basis of five variables: fetal heart rate, fetal breathing movement, gross fetal movement, fetal muscle tone, and amniotic fluid volume. Fetal heart rate reactivity is measured with the nonstress test (p. 569); the other four parameters are measured with ultrasonography. Each variable is scored as either 2 or 0. Therefore 10 is a perfect score, and 0 is the lowest score.

1. *Fetal heart rate reactivity.* Fetal heart rate reactivity is measured and interpreted in the same way as with the nonstress test (p. 569). Fetal heart rate is considered reactive when there are movement-associated fetal heart rate accelerations of at least 15 beats/min above baseline and 15 seconds in

duration, over a 20-minute time period. A score of 2 indicates reactivity; a score of 0 indicates that the fetal heart rate is nonreactive.

2. *Fetal breathing movements.* This variable is assessed on the assumption that fetal breathing movements indicate fetal well-being, and their absence may indicate hypoxemia. Rate and uniformity of fetal breathing become increasingly regular after week 36 of gestation. At least one episode of fetal breathing lasting a minimum of 60 seconds within a 30-minute observation period is scored as 2; absence of this breathing pattern is scored as 0. Several factors can alter fetal breathing movements. For example, fetal breathing movements increase during the second and third hours after maternal meals and also at night. Fetal breathing movements may decrease in conditions such as hypoxemia, hypoglycemia, nicotine use, and alcohol ingestion.

3. *Fetal body movements.* Fetal activity is a reflection of neurologic integrity and function. The presence of at least three discrete episodes of fetal movement within a 30-minute observation period is scored as 2; two or fewer fetal movements in 30 minutes is scored as 0. Fetal activity is greatest 1 to 3 hours after the mother has consumed a meal. For this reason, it is often suggested that this test be scheduled in relation to mealtime.

4. *Fetal muscle tone.* In the uterus, the fetus is normally in a position of flexion, but also stretches, rolls, and moves. The arms, legs, trunk, and head may be flexed and extended. If there is at least one episode of active extension with return to flexion (e.g., opening and closing of a hand), it is scored as 2; slow extension with return to only partial flexion, fetal movement not followed by return to flexion, limbs or spine in extension, and an open fetal hand are scored as 0.

5. *Amniotic fluid volume.* Measurement of amniotic fluid volume is an effective method of predicting fetal distress. Oligohydramnios (too little amniotic fluid) has been associated with fetal anomalies, intrauterine growth restriction, and postterm pregnancy. Immediate delivery is recommended in postterm pregnancy with oligohydramnios because of the high risk of associated problems such as umbilical cord compromise. If there is at least one pocket of amniotic fluid that measures 1 cm in two perpendicular planes, the score is 2; if fluid is absent in most areas of the uterine cavity or else the largest pocket measures 1 cm or less in the vertical axis, the score is 0.

A score of 8 or 10 with an acceptable amount of amniotic fluid is normal. A score of 8 with oligohydramnios or a score of 4 to 6 is equivocal and is interpreted as possibly abnormal. Some clinicians recommend repeating the test within 24 hours; others advocate extending testing after any equivocal test result. A score of 0 or 2 is abnormal and indicates the need for assessment of immediate delivery.

Modifications can be made to the BPP. Some physicians omit the nonstress test if the ultrasound parameters are normal; some include placental grading as a sixth parameter. Information about fetal size, position, and location of the placenta can also be obtained.

Another measure of fetal well-being is the *amniotic fluid index (AFI).* This is determined by using ultrasound to measure the largest collection of amniotic fluid in each of the four quadrants within the uterus. The sum represents a number that is plotted on a graph in which the age of gestation is also taken into account. If the AFI is less than the 2.4 percentile, oligohydramnios is present. If AFI exceeds the 97 percentile, polyhydramnios exists. An abnormal amniotic fluid index observed in antepartum testing is associated with an increased risk of intrauterine growth restriction and overall adverse perinatal outcome. Some suggest that borderline amniotic fluid index be performed twice weekly. Yet other studies have shown AFI to be so weak a predictor for poor neonatal outcome as to be useless. The percentile value seems to be a better indicator than an absolute fluid volume. Oligohydramnios is associated with placental failure or fetal renal problems. Polyhydramnios is associated with maternal diabetes or fetal upper gastrointestinal malformation/obstruction.

Additional information about fetal well-being can be gained from Doppler ultrasound evaluation of the placenta and the *umbilical artery flow velocity.* Changes in umbilical artery flow or direction may indicate fetal stress or illness.

INTERFERING FACTORS

- Maternal hyperglycemia may increase fetal biophysical activity.
- Hypoxemia and trauma may decrease fetal biophysical activity.
- Maternal or fetal infection will affect fetal biophysical activity.
- Occasionally no movement will be noted. If no eye movement or respiratory movement is noted, the fetus may be sleeping.
- Central nervous system stimulants, such as catecholamines, can increase fetal biophysical activity.
- Magnesium sulfate, analgesics, anesthetics, sedatives, and nicotine can depress fetal biophysical activity.

✔ Clinical Priorities

- The BPP is more useful in identifying a fetus in jeopardy than in predicting future fetal well-being.
- The BPP is usually indicated in women with high-risk pregnancies. Testing usually begins around week 32 of gestation, but can be done earlier if there are maternal complications.
- Several BPP variables are affected by the maternal blood glucose level. For this reason, it is often recommended that this test be performed 1 to 3 hours after the mother has eaten.

PROCEDURE AND PATIENT CARE

Before
 Explain the procedure to the patient.
Inform the patient that no fasting is required.
Instruct the patient to eat 2 to 3 hours before the test.

During
- Fetal heart rate reactivity is measured and interpreted from a nonstress test (p. 569).
- Fetal breathing movements, fetal body movements, fetal muscle tone, and amniotic fluid volume are determined by ultrasound imaging (see obstetric ultrasonography, p. 887).

After
If test results are abnormal or equivocal, support the patient in the next phase of the fetal evaluation process.

TEST RESULTS AND CLINICAL SIGNIFICANCE

Fetal asphyxia,
Congenital anomalies,
Oligohydramnios,
Intrauterine growth restriction,
Postterm pregnancy,
Fetal distress or death:
  These situations are easily evaluated with ultrasound.

10 Ultrasound Studies

RELATED TESTS

Fetal Contraction Stress Test (p. 566) and Nonstress Test (p. 569). These tests are performed to monitor fetal heart rate and movement.

Pelvic Ultrasonography (p. 887). This test is used in the obstetric patient to identify a tubal or molar pregnancy, indicate the number of fetuses, and determine fetal age, rate of growth, position, and size.

Intravascular Ultrasound (IVUS)

NORMAL FINDINGS

Normal coronary arteries

INDICATIONS

Intravascular ultrasound (IVUS) is used to determine the presence, progression, and treatment of athlerosclerosis. It can determine the patency of blood vessels, particularly the coronary arteries. IVUS is used to evaluate the need or the effectiveness of coronary artery stents.

TEST EXPLANATION

Percutaneous IVUS imaging requires very small, specially made transducers that are mounted on the tip of an intravascular catheter. The ultrasound catheter tip is slid in over the guidewire and positioned using angiographic techniques, so that the tip is in the blood vessel to be studied. Sound waves are emitted from the catheter tip. The catheter receives and conducts the echo information from the blood vessel out to the external digital ultrasound equipment. The machine then constructs and displays a real-time ultrasound image of a thin section of the blood vessel currently surrounding the catheter tip.

Unlike arteriography, which shows a shadow of the arterial lumen, IVUS shows a tomographic, cross-sectional view of the vessel. This orientation enables direct measurements of lumen dimensions, which are considered to be more accurate than angiographic dimensions. The guide wire is kept stationary and the ultrasound catheter tip is slid backward, usually under motorized control at a pullback speed of 0.5 mm/s. The motorized pullback tends to be smoother than hand movement by the physician. The data obtained can be restructured into a longitudinal image by the ultrasound machine software to create a three-dimensional image of the particular segment of artery that is being studied.

IVUS is an important technology for studying the progression, stabilization, and potential regression of coronary atherosclerosis. IVUS permits imaging of the lumen size, vessel wall structure, and any atheroma that may be present. It allows characterization of atheroma size, plaque distribution, and lesion composition and enables accurate visualization of not only the lumen of the coronary arteries, but also the atheroma that may be "hidden" within the vessel wall. In this way, IVUS has enabled advances in clinical research, providing a more thorough perspective and better understanding of vascular disease. It provides a reproducible, safe, and sensitive method for assessing the development and extent of atherosclerosis, particularly in its earlier, presymptomatic stages. This procedure is predominantly used in the coronary arteries.

Normal coronary arteries usually have a tri-layered appearance on IVUS imaging, which corresponds to the three histologic layers of the arterial wall. The innermost layer is the echogenic (brighter) intima, the middle layer is the echolucent (darker) media, and outermost layer is the echogenic adventitia. The tomographic orientation of IVUS enables visualization of the full 360-degree circumference of the vessel wall, so that lumen dimensions can be directly measured on a cross-sectional image. This allows precise assessment of the extent of disease in vessels that are often difficult to assess with angiography. IVUS also allows excellent resolution of structures within the arterial wall that may represent other atheromatous disease.

IVUS is used in the following clinical situations:

1. Assessment of coronary stent placement and determination of minimum luminal diameter within the stent
2. Determination of the mechanism of stent restenosis (inadequate expansion versus neointimal proliferation) and selection of appropriate therapy (plaque ablation versus repeat balloon expansion)
3. Evaluation of coronary obstruction at a location difficult to image by angiography (such as the left main coronary artery, the ostia of the anterior descending artery, the left circumflex artery, and the right coronary artery)
4. Assessment of a suboptimal angiographic result following stent placement in cases in which the degree of stenosis of a coronary artery is unclear
5. Guidance and assessment for vascular atherectomy
6. Determination of plaque location and circumferential distribution for guidance of directional coronary atherectomy
7. Determination of the extent of atherosclerosis in patients with characteristic anginal symptoms and a positive functional study with no focal stenoses or mild coronary artery disease on angiography. IVUS can directly quantify the percentage of stenosis and give insight into the anatomy of the plaque.
8. Preinterventional assessment of lesion characteristics and vessel dimensions as a means to select an optimal revascularization device
9. Assessment of the changes in plaque volume after lipid-lowering therapy

INTERFERING FACTORS

- The accuracy of ultrasonography depends on the skills of the sonographer (the technician who performs the study).

PROCEDURE AND PATIENT CARE

Before

✋ Explain the procedure to the patient.
- Obtain informed consent.
✋ Tell the patient that fasting is required.

During

- The IVUS probe is placed by coronary angiographic procedures. See p. 988.
- The test is completed in approximately 1 hour, usually by a cardiologist.

After

- See cardiac catheterization (p. 1008) for postprocedure care.

TEST RESULTS AND CLINICAL SIGNIFICANCE

Coronary occlusive disease: *With IVUS the degree of stenosis of a coronary artery can be directly quantified by percentage of stenosis. IVUS can give insight into the anatomy of the plaque when the degree of stenosis of a coronary artery is unclear.*

RELATED TEST

Cardiac Catheterization–Coronary Angiography (p. 988). The anatomy and degree of stenosis of a coronary artery is most commonly determined by this method because it is less technically demanding and provides a better indication of anatomy if heart surgery is required.

Ocular and Orbit Ultrasonography

NORMAL FINDINGS

Normal pattern of orbital and posterior orbital structures

INDICATIONS

Ocular ultrasound is used to examine the eye when the extraocular and intraocular spaces cannot be adequately evaluated by other methods because of disease, scarring, or surgery, and to evaluate the posterior bulbar area for tumors and cysts.

TEST EXPLANATION

Ultrasound of the eye is used to detect intraocular disease such as vitreous hemorrhage, retinal or choroidal detachment, and intraocular foreign bodies. It is also used to identify retro-ocular abnormalities such as tumor (e.g., glioma, meningioma), benign cysts (e.g., dermoid, mucocele), and cavernous hemangioma. Changes in corneal and ocular shape as a result of disease, surgery, or trauma can be identified. Computed tomography (CT) and magnetic resonance imaging (MRI) are also excellent methods to evaluate the ocular and retrobulbar spaces. The orbital fossae and eyes can be evaluated in the fetus by ultrasound if cranial or ocular abnormalities are suspected.

PROCEDURE AND PATIENT CARE

Before

Explain the procedure to the patient.
- Obtain informed consent.
- Topical anesthetic drops are administered to the eyes 5 to 10 minutes before the study.

During

- The ultrasound probe is applied directly to the eye.
- Ultrasound images are obtained.
- Alternatively, ultrasound immersion technique can be performed (i.e., the probe is immersed in a water bath).

After

 Inform the patient that the cornea is still anesthetized and that because no discomfort can be appreciated, it is important to refrain from rubbing or otherwise contacting the eye.

TEST RESULTS AND CLINICAL SIGNIFICANCE

Retinal or choroidal detachment: *This can result from senile deterioration, trauma, or posterior ocular bleeding.*

Thickened orbit: *The most common cause is hyperthyroidism (Graves disease).*

Vitreous opacities: *These "floaters" or dark spots in vision can be caused by foreign bodies, desquamated cells, or hemorrhage.*

Neoplasm: *These include posterior ocular tumors such as melanoma, hemangioma, or metastatic tumors, retrobulbar tumors such as glioma, meningioma, neurofibroma, or metastatic tumor.*

Pelvic Ultrasonography (Obstetric Echography, Pregnant Uterus Ultrasonography, Pelvic Ultrasonography in Pregnancy, Obstetric Ultrasonography, Vaginal Ultrasonography)

NORMAL FINDINGS

Normal fetal and placental size and position
No evidence of pathology in nonpregnant women

INDICATIONS

Pelvic ultrasonography is used in obstetric patients to evaluate the pregnancy and the fetus. It is especially important in high-risk pregnancies. In nonpregnant women, it is used to evaluate the genital tract for disease and to monitor known pelvic disease (e.g., benign ovarian cysts).

See Rectal Sonography (p. 891) for discussion of pelvic ultrasound examination in male patients.

TEST EXPLANATION

Ultrasound examination is a harmless, noninvasive method of evaluating the female genital tract and the fetus. In real-time diagnostic ultrasound, high-frequency sound waves are emitted from the transducer and penetrate the structure to be studied (e.g., uterus, ovaries, parametria, placenta, fetus). These sound waves are reflected back to a sensor within the transducer, and by electronic conversion are arranged into a pictorial image of the studied structure.

Pelvic ultrasonography can be performed with the transducer placed on the anterior abdomen, or in the vagina with a specially designed vaginal probe, which provides the best view of the pelvic organs in a nonpregnant woman. The images obtained with both transducers are complementary. Vaginal ultrasound provides significant accuracy in identifying paracervical, endometrial, and ovarian disease that may not be detected with the anterior abdominal probe. Occasionally abdominal organs fall into the pelvis and preclude good pelvic visualization with the anterior abdominal probe. Vaginal ultrasound provides better visualization under these circumstances. In the obese patient, the thick abdominal wall inhibits good transmission of ultrasonic waves, and vaginal ultrasound is preferred. The anterior abdominal probe, however, provides better visualization of the upper pelvis than does the vaginal probe, especially in pregnant women.

Pelvic ultrasonography may be useful in the *obstetric patient* in the following circumstances:

1. To make an early diagnosis of normal pregnancy or abnormal pregnancy (e.g., tubal pregnancy)
2. To identify multiple pregnancies
3. To differentiate a tumor (e.g., hydatidiform mole) from a normal pregnancy
4. To determine the age of the fetus from the diameter of the head
5. To measure fetal growth rate
6. To identify placental abnormalities such as abruptio placentae and placenta previa
7. To determine the position of the placenta (ultrasound localization of the placenta is done before amniocentesis)
8. To make differential diagnoses of various uterine and ovarian enlargements (e.g., polyhydramnios, neoplasms, cysts, abscesses)
9. To determine fetal position
10. To diagnose ectopic pregnancy
11. To provide a realistic image of the fetus using 3D and 4D imaging (see p. 863) for expectant parents.

Ultrasound is a very accurate and easily performed screening test to recognize risks of fetal abnormalities (see *amniotic fluid index*, p. 882). *Fetal nuchal translucency (FNT)* is an ultrasound measurement of subcutaneous edema in the neck region of the fetus. It is performed at 10 to 14 weeks of gestation. Major heart defects, trisomy 21, and other genetic defects are associated with increased edema in this location at this age of gestation. Screening for chromosomal defects by measurement of FNT identifies 80% of fetuses with trisomy 21 for a false-positive rate of 5%. This is especially helpful for older pregnant women. With FNT, these abnormalities can be identified earlier in the pregnancy when abortion is still possible. Although there may be advantages in early detection of fetal anomalies, there may be a disadvantage that should be considered. Many pregnancies complicated by fetal abnormality, both aneuploidy and other anomalies, will end in an early miscarriage. If these pregnancies are identified early, parents may be asked to make difficult decisions regarding termination of pregnancy. This imposed a potential burden and long-term consequence that may have been avoided had the pregnancy been lost spontaneously.

Pelvic ultrasonography is useful in *nonpregnant women* to monitor the endometrium in patients who take tamoxifen and to aid in the diagnosis of:

1. Ovarian cyst or tumor
2. Tubo-ovarian abscess
3. Uterine fibroids or cancer
4. Pelvic inflammatory disease (PID)
5. Uterine stripe (endometrium)

The procedure is performed in approximately 20 minutes. No discomfort is associated with the study, other than having a full bladder and the urge to void. Some patients may be uncomfortable lying on a hard table.

CONTRAINDICATIONS

- Patients with latex allergy, because vaginal ultrasound requires placement of the probe in a latex condom-like sac

INTERFERING FACTORS

- Patients who have recently undergone barium contrast studies, because barium creates severe distortion of reflective sound waves
- Patients with air-filled bowels, because gas does not transmit sound waves well
- Obesity or failure to fill the bladder, because the image may be uninterpretable

Clinical Priorities

- Pelvic ultrasound can be performed with the transducer placed on the anterior abdomen or in the vagina. Ensure patient privacy.
- Vaginal ultrasound is preferred in the obese patient because a thick abdominal wall inhibits transmission of sound waves.
- A full bladder is essential in patients undergoing transabdominal ultrasonography, to provide a reference point for interpreting pelvic ultrasonograms.
- No discomfort is associated with the study other than having a full bladder and the urge to void.

PROCEDURE AND PATIENT CARE

Before

- Explain the procedure to the patient.
- Assure the patient that the study has no known deleterious effect on maternal or fetal tissues, even if repeated several times.
- Give the patient three to four glasses (200 to 350 mL) of water or other liquid 1 hr before the examination, and instruct her not to void until after the procedure is completed. This will permit visualization of the bladder, which is used as a reference point in pelvic anatomy. The full bladder also displaces the bowel from the pelvis and pushes the uterus and ovaries away from the pubis. The fluid in the bladder acts as a window to the pelvis for transmission of sound waves.
- No water is required for vaginal ultrasonography.
- If a transabdominal ultrasound is required urgently and there is no time to fill the bladder by ingestion or administration of fluids, the bladder can be filled by means of a bladder catheter.
- Tell the patient that no fasting or sedation is required.

During

- Note the following procedural steps:
  1. The patient is taken to the ultrasound room and placed supine on the examining table (Figure 10-13).
  2. The ultrasonographer applies a gel lubricant to the abdomen to enhance sound wave transmission and reception.
  3. A transducer is passed vertically and horizontally over the skin.
  4. If a *vaginal probe* is used, it is inserted in the vagina and angled to identify the various parts of the pelvis.
  5. The sound waves are reflected back by the transducer, and an image appears on the cathode ray tube.
  6. During the examination, fetal structures are usually pointed out to the mother.

After

- Remove the lubricant from the patient's skin.
- Provide an opportunity for the patient to void.

TEST RESULTS AND CLINICAL SIGNIFICANCE

Abdominal or tubal pregnancy: *Extrauterine pregnancy is evident when the placental complex is external to the uterus.*

Ultrasound Studies

10

Hydatidiform mole: *Molar pregnancy can be diagnosed and monitored by ultrasound.*
Intrauterine growth restriction,
Fetal hydrocephalus,
Multiple fetuses,
Fetal death,
Abnormal fetal position (e.g., breech, transverse),
Polyhydramnios:
  Fetal characteristics are easily evaluated with ultrasound (see Fetal Biophysical Profile [p. 881]).
Abnormal position of the placenta (e.g., placenta previa, abruptio placentae): *Placenta position and quality can be evaluated with ultrasonography. Doppler ultrasound can be used to evaluate placental blood flow.*
Neoplasm of the ovaries, uterus, or fallopian tubes: *Ultrasound is sensitive in detection of tumors of the female genital tract. The uterine stripe (endometrial lining of the uterus) is monitored in patients taking medications associated with hyperplasia or cancer (e.g., tamoxifen).*
Cysts: *Ultrasound is the most accurate method to differentiate an ovarian cyst from a solid ovarian tumor. Pure cysts (well-defined hypoechoic mass with clean walls) are more likely to be benign than are complex cysts (containing echogenic material).*
Pelvic inflammatory disease and abscesses: *Abscesses (tubo-ovarian) appear similar to ovarian cysts but can be differentiated by means of their clinical features.*
IUD localization: *This test can locate an IUD.*

RELATED TESTS

Contraceptive Device Localization (p. 875). An IUD can be located with ultrasound when its string cannot be palpated.
Sonography of the Rectum (see following test). This is used in the staging of rectal tumors in men and women.

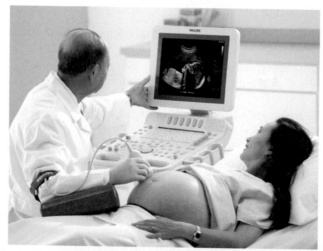

Figure 10-13 Pelvic ultrasonography. Ultrasonography is often used for obtaining diagnostic information on pregnant women.

Prostate and Rectal Sonography

NORMAL FINDINGS

Normal size, contour, and consistency of the prostate gland
Normal mucosa with no polyps, bleeding, cancer, or other perirectal disease

INDICATIONS

Prostate or rectal sonography is helpful in the detection of prostate cancer in patients with an elevated prostate specific antigen (PSA) titer. This study can also be used to stage and monitor rectal cancer and to detect other perirectal diseases.

TEST EXPLANATION

Rectal ultrasound of the prostate is a valuable tool in the early diagnosis of prostate cancer. When combined with rectal digital examination and PSA testing (p. 420), very small prostate cancers can be identified. Rectal prostate sonography is also helpful in evaluating the seminal vessels and other perirectal tissue. Ultrasound is helpful in guiding prostate biopsy (Figure 10-14), and can be helpful in quantifying the volume of prostate cancer. When radiation therapy implantation is required for treatment,

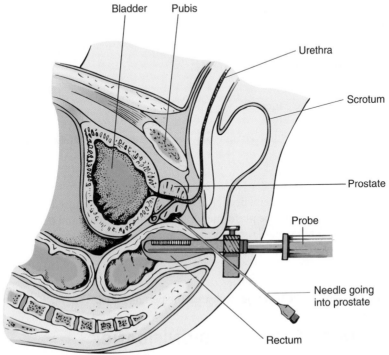

Figure 10-14 Rectal ultrasonography. Diagram demonstrating transrectal biopsy of the prostate.

Ultrasound
Studies

10

ultrasound is used to map the exact location of the prostate cancer. Rectal ultrasound is helpful in staging rectal cancers as well. The depth of transmural involvement and presence of extrarectal extension can be accurately assessed.

Real-time ultrasonography requires the emission of high-frequency sound waves from a special transducer placed in the rectum. The sound waves are reflected back to the transducer and electronically converted into a pictorial image. This test can be performed in the ultrasound section of the radiology department and is now being routinely performed in most urologists' offices. Results are available almost immediately.

CONTRAINDICATIONS

- Patients with latex allergy, because rectal ultrasound requires placement of the probe in a latex condom-like sac

INTERFERING FACTORS

- Stool in the rectum

 Clinical Priorities

- By combining rectal or prostate sonography with a digital rectal examination and PSA test, small prostate cancers can be identified.
- This test can be easily performed in the office of most urologists.
- This test cannot be performed in patients with latex allergy.

PROCEDURE AND PATIENT CARE

Before

- Explain the procedure to the patient.
- Obtained informed consent.
- Tell the patient that a small-volume enema may be required approximately 1 hour before the ultrasound examination.

During

- The patient is placed in the left lateral decubitus position. Privacy is ensured.
- A digital rectal examination may be performed to assess the prostate gland or rectal tumor.
- A draped and lubricated ultrasound probe is placed within the rectum.
- Scans are obtained in various spatial planes.

After

- Provide the patient with tissue material to cleanse the perianal area.

TEST RESULTS AND CLINICAL SIGNIFICANCE

Prostate cancer,
Benign prostatic hypertrophy:
   An enlarged solid prostate mass anterior to the rectum is suggestive of prostate disease.

Prostatitis: *An enlarged bulgy echogenic gland indicates inflammation.*

Seminal vesicle tumor: *An echogenic mass in the region of the seminal vesicle may indicate tumor.*

Prostate abscess,

Perirectal abscess:

    A hypoechoic fluid-filled mass that is well circumscribed indicates abscess, especially if surrounded by a phlegmonous reaction.

Intrarectal or perirectal tumor: *Extent of tumor can be accurately assessed with ultrasound. Lymph node metastasis, if present, is evident.*

RELATED TEST

Pelvic Ultrasonography (p. 887). Discussion of this test describes pelvic ultrasound of the female genital tract and the pregnant uterus.

Scrotal Ultrasonography (Ultrasound of Testes)

NORMAL FINDINGS

Normal size, shape, and configuration of the testicles

INDICATIONS

Ultrasonography of the scrotum allows thorough evaluation of the testes and other scrotal structures for evidence of suspected disease.

TEST EXPLANATION

Scrotal ultrasound is a noninvasive, nonionizing, rapid method for scrotal examination. Through the use of reflected sound waves, ultrasonography provides accurate visualization of the scrotum and its contents. Ultrasonography requires the emission of high-frequency sound waves from the transducer to penetrate the organ being studied. The sound waves are reflected back to the transducer and electronically converted into an accurate digital pictorial image.

    Present uses for scrotal ultrasound include:

1. Evaluation of scrotal masses
2. Measurement of testicular size
3. Evaluation of scrotal trauma
4. Evaluation of scrotal pain and identification of torsion of the testicle
5. Evaluation of occult testicular neoplasm
6. Surveillance in patients with previous primary or metastatic contralateral testicular neoplasms
7. Follow-up of testicular infections
8. Location of undescended testicles
9. Identification of microlithiasis

The scrotum is examined with real-time ultrasound. The testes and extratesticular intrascrotal tissues are examined. The accuracy of scrotal ultrasound is 90% to 95%. Both benign and malignant tumors (primary and metastatic) can be identified with ultrasound. Benign abnormalities (e.g., testicular abscess, orchitis, testicular infarction, testicular torsion) can be identified. Extratesticular lesions such as hydrocele (fluid in the scrotum), hematocele (blood in the scrotum), and pyocele (pus in the scrotum) can be identified. Scrotal and groin ultrasound has been helpful in locating cryptorchid (undescended) testes.

Ultrasound of the scrotum is now the preferred method to identify torsion of the testicle. Ultrasound is a very accurate method of identifying microlithiasis in the testicles. When identified, microcalcifications in the testicle indicate marked increased risk for testicular cancer. Calcifications can also occur following orchitis or trauma. In most cases, both testicles are routinely imaged during the ultrasound exam.

The use of color Doppler is very helpful in determining blood flow to the testicle. With torsion of the testicle, color Doppler will indicate markedly reduced blood flow to the testicle, and immediate surgical exploration is required. Scrotal ultrasound has replaced scrotal nuclear imaging for the diagnosis of testicular torsion because results can be obtained immediately.

Very little discomfort is associated with testicular ultrasound. The study is usually performed by an ultrasound technologist, and the results are interpreted by an ultrasound physician.

PROCEDURE AND PATIENT CARE

Before

✗ Explain the procedure to the patient.
✗ Tell the patient that no fasting is required.

During

- Note the following procedural steps:
  1. Careful examination of the scrotum is performed by the physician. Usually, a short history is obtained. Privacy is ensured.
  2. The scrotum is supported by a towel or cradled by the examiner's gloved hand.
  3. A gel lubricant is applied to the scrotum before scanning. This paste enhances sound wave transmission and reception.
  4. Thorough scanning in the sagittal, transverse, and oblique projections is performed.
- The test takes approximately 20 to 30 minutes.

After

- Remove the gel from the patient's scrotum.

TEST RESULTS AND CLINICAL SIGNIFICANCE

Benign testicular tumor,
Malignant testicular tumor:
   Seminoma of the testicle is evident as a hypoechoic mass in the testicle. Other cancers may appear as hyperechoic dense masses in the testicle.
Testicular infection (e.g., orchitis),
Hydrocele: fluid around the testicle,
Hematocele: blood around the testicle,
Pyocele: pus around the testicle,
Varicocele: venous varicosities in the cord, usually on the left side,
Spermatocele: cystic collection surrounding the cord or epididymis:
   These abnormalities appear as hypoechoic (dark) areas surrounding the testicle or cord.
Epididymitis: *This is apparent as an enlarged epididymis. It is a painful infection involving the epididymis.*

Scrotal hernia: *Bowel contents can be seen in the scrotum and indicate hernia.*

Cryptorchidism: *Cryptorchid (undescended) testes can be located anywhere from the retroperitoneum to the inlet of the scrotum. It is important to locate these organs and evaluate their consistency, because undescended testes are at high risk of becoming malignant.*

Hematoma: *A testicular hematoma from trauma is seen as a hypoechoic mass in the parenchyma of the testicle.*

Testicular torsion: *Inadequate suspension of the testicle in the scrotum results in the testicle twisting around on its blood supply. The testicle appears to have an irregular texture, with echogenic areas that correspond to areas of intratesticular hemorrhage. Doppler ultrasound can indicate reduced blood flow to the testicle.*

Thyroid Ultrasonography (Thyroid Echography, Thyroid Sonography)

NORMAL FINDINGS

Normal size, shape, and position of the thyroid gland

INDICATIONS

The primary purpose of thyroid ultrasound is to indicate whether a thyroid nodule is a fluid-filled cyst (likely benign) or a solid tumor (possibly malignant). Ultrasound is also used to monitor the medical treatment or observation of a thyroid nodule or enlargement and to monitor the contralateral thyroid lobe when one side was surgically removed because of cancer.

TEST EXPLANATION

Ultrasound examination of the thyroid gland is valuable to distinguish cystic from solid thyroid nodules. If the nodule is found to be purely cystic (fluid-filled), the fluid can simply be aspirated (cysts are not cancerous), and surgery is avoided. If the nodule has a mixed or solid appearance, however, a tumor may be present, and surgery may be required for diagnosis and treatment.

This study may be repeated at intervals to determine the response of a thyroid mass to medical therapy. This test is the procedure of choice for studying the thyroid gland in pregnant women, because no radioactive material is used.

An ultrasound technologist usually performs this study in approximately 15 minutes; a radiologist interprets the results. No discomfort is associated with this study.

PROCEDURE AND PATIENT CARE

Before

 Explain the procedure to the patient.

Tell the patient that breathing or swallowing will not be affected by the placement of a transducer on the neck.

Inform the patient that a liberal amount of lubricant will be applied to the neck to ensure effective transmission and reception of sound waves.

Tell the patient that no fasting or sedation is required.

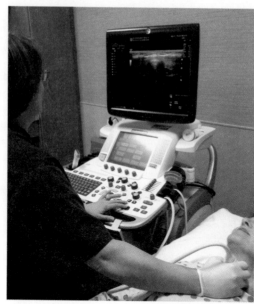

Figure 10-15 Thyroid ultrasound examination.

During

- Note the following procedural steps:
  1. The patient is taken to the ultrasonography department (usually in the radiology department) and placed supine with the neck hyperextended.
  2. Gel is applied to the patient's neck.
  3. A transducer is passed over the gland (Figure 10-15).
  4. Photographs are taken of the image displayed.

After

- Assist the patient in removing the lubricant from the neck.

TEST RESULTS AND CLINICAL SIGNIFICANCE

Cyst: *A thyroid cyst is evident as a hypoechoic, well-circumscribed mass in the thyroid gland.*
Thyroid adenoma,
Thyroid carcinoma,
Goiter:
  These are evident as a solid echogenic mass within the thyroid gland.

RELATED TEST

Thyroid Scanning (p. 839). This nuclear medicine study allows visualization of the thyroid gland after intravenous administration of a radionuclide. Cysts, tumors, and goiters appear as space-occupying filling defects (cold nodule) within the thyroid gland. This study is often performed with ultrasonography of the thyroid. A cold nodule that is solid at ultrasonography is the type of lesion with the greatest chance of being a cancer.

Transesophageal Echocardiography (TEE)

NORMAL FINDINGS

Normal position, size, and movement of the heart muscle, valves, and chambers

INDICATIONS

An ultrasonography probe, placed endoscopically in the distal esophagus or proximal stomach, provides accurate information about the heart muscle, heart valves, heart function, and thoracic aorta. TEE is helpful in evaluation of structures that are inaccessible or poorly visualized by the transthoracic probe approach, especially in patients who are obese or have large lung-air spaces (e.g., chronic obstructive pulmonary disease [COPD]).

TEE is performed for the following reasons:

1. To better visualize the mitral valve
2. To differentiate intracardiac from extracardiac masses and tumors
3. To better visualize the atrial septum (for atrial septal defects)
4. To diagnose thoracic aortic dissection
5. To better detect valvular vegetation indicative of endocarditis
6. To determine cardiac sources of arterial embolism
7. To detect coronary artery disease by identifying areas of muscle wall hypokinesia

TEST EXPLANATION

TEE provides ultrasonic imaging of the heart from a retrocardiac vantage point, avoiding interference by the interposed subcutaneous tissue, bony thorax, and lungs. A high-frequency ultrasound transducer placed in the esophagus at endoscopy provides better resolution than that of images obtained with routine transthoracic echocardiography (p. 877). For TEE, the distal end of the endoscope is advanced into the esophagus. The transducer is positioned behind the heart (Figure 10-16). Controls on the handle of the endoscope permit the transducer to be rotated and flexed in the anteroposterior and right and left lateral planes. TEE images have better resolution than those obtained by routine transthoracic echocardiography because of the higher frequency sound waves and closer proximity of the transducer to the cardiac structures.

TEE can be used intraoperatively to monitor high-risk patients for ischemia. Ischemic muscle movement is much different from normal muscle movement. Because TEE is a sensitive indicator of myocardial ischemia, it can be used to monitor patients undergoing major abdominal, peripheral vascular, and carotid artery procedures who are at high risk for intraoperative ischemia because of coronary artery disease.

Transesophageal echocardiography is more sensitive than electrocardiography (EKG) for detecting ischemia. TEE is also used intraoperatively to evaluate surgical results of valvular or congenital heart disease and to detect air emboli, a serious complication of neurosurgery performed with the patient in the upright position (e.g., cervical laminectomy).

Perflutren (DEFINITY) is an injectable opacifying agent (given by IV bolus or infusion) that provides enhancement of the endocardial borders during echocardiography by lowering acoustic impedance and enhancing the intrinsic backscatter of blood in the heart. This improves images of any abnormalities in the walls of the heart wall activity.

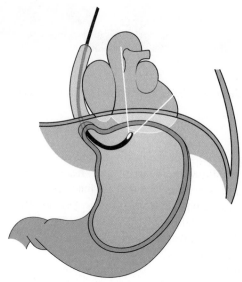

Figure 10-16 Transesophageal echocardiography. Diagram illustrating the location of the transesophageal endoscope in the esophagus.

TEE is performed by a cardiologist or a gastrointestinal endoscopist in approximately 20 minutes in the endoscopy suite or at the bedside. Little discomfort is associated with this test, and light sedation is administered.

CONTRAINDICATIONS

- Patients with known upper esophageal disease
- Patients with known esophageal varices
- Patients with Zenker diverticulum
- Patients with esophageal abnormalities (e.g., stricture diverticula, scleroderma, esophagitis)
- Patients with bleeding disorders
- Patients who have recently undergone esophageal surgery
- Patients who cannot cooperate during the procedure

POTENTIAL COMPLICATIONS

- Esophageal perforation or bleeding
- Cardiac arrhythmias

 Clinical Priorities

- TEE is especially useful in patients who are obese or have COPD.
- TEE can be used intraoperatively to monitor patients at high risk for ischemia.
- TEE is the most sensitive technique for detecting air emboli, a serious complication of neurosurgery performed with the patient in the upright position (e.g., cervical laminectomy).

PROCEDURE AND PATIENT CARE

Before

🖉 Explain the procedure to the patient.
• Obtain informed consent.
🖉 Instruct the patient to fast for 4 to 6 hours before the test.
• Remove all oral prostheses.
• Obtain intravenous access.

During

• Follow the facility's procedural sedation protocols (i.e, sedation, EKG, US, pulse oximetry, etc.).
• Note the following procedural steps:
  1. The pharynx is anesthetized with a locally applied topical agent to depress the gag reflex.
  2. The patient is placed in the left lateral decubitus position.
  3. The endoscope is inserted through the mouth and into the upper esophagus.
  4. The patient is asked to swallow, and the transducer is positioned behind the heart by manipulation through the endoscope.
  5. The room is darkened, and the ultrasound images are displayed on a monitor. Printouts of the ultrasound image can be obtained if desired.

After

• Observe the patient closely for approximately 1 hr after the procedure, until the effects of sedation have worn off.

TEST RESULTS AND CLINICAL SIGNIFICANCE

Myocardial ischemia,
Myocardial infarction (MI):
  These are suspected by presence of abnormal (hypokinetic) wall motion.
Valvular heart disease: *Motion of heart valves is evaluated.*
Intracardiac thrombi: *These can be a cause of arterial emboli. Thrombi usually form in the area of akinetic muscle because of MI or myocardial aneurysm.*
Cardiac valvular vegetation: *This is a result of endocarditis and is a cause of arterial emboli.*
Cardiomyopathy: *Heart muscle is hypokinetic, may or may not be thickened, and may or may not be dilated.*
Marked cardiac chamber dilatation: *This is usually because of chronic congestive heart failure.*
Cardiac tumors: *The most common (although rare) cardiac tumor is a myxoma.*
Thoracic aortic aneurysm: *TEE is considered the standard for diagnosis of dissecting thoracic aortic aneurysm.*
Aortic plaque: *Arterial sclerotic plaques can easily be seen with TEE.*
Pulmonary hypertension: *When pulmonary arterial thrombosis (embolism) is the cause of acute or chronic pulmonary hypertension, TEE can demonstrate that clot.*

RELATED TEST

Echocardiography (p. 877). This test provides the same information as TEE, but the posterior portion of the heart is not as well seen as with TEE.

Ultrasound Studies

10

Vascular Ultrasound Studies (Venous/Arterial Doppler Ultrasound, Venous/Arterial Duplex Scan)

NORMAL FINDINGS

Venous

Normal Doppler venous signal with spontaneous respiration
Normal venous system without evidence of occlusion or thrombus

Arterial

Normal arterial Doppler signal with systolic and diastolic components
No reduction in blood pressure in excess of 20 mm Hg compared with the normal extremity
No evidence of arteriosclerotic stenosis
Normal ankle-to-brachial artery blood pressure index of 0.85 or greater
No evidence of arterial occlusion

INDICATIONS

This ultrasound study provides information about venous or arterial patency without the use of invasive techniques. Venous ultrasound is used to evaluate the patency of the venous system in patients with a swollen painful leg, venous varicosities of the upper or lower extremities, or edematous extremities. Arterial Doppler studies are used in patients with suspected arterial insufficiency (e.g., cerebral vascular symptoms, claudication, poorly healing skin ulcer, cold and pale leg, pulseless extremity, resting pain).

TEST EXPLANATION

Vascular ultrasound studies are used to identify occlusion or thrombosis of the veins. Patency is demonstrated with *Doppler ultrasound* by detecting moving red blood cells (RBCs) within the vein. The Doppler transducer directs an ultrasound beam at the vessel. Moving RBCs scatter the frequency of the beam. The change in frequency of the sound wave reflected back to the transducer is proportional to the velocity of the blood flow. The patency of the venous system can also be identified by evaluating the degree of venous reflux (backward blood flow in the veins of the lower extremities in patients with venous valvular insufficiency). Venous Doppler studies are not accurate for detection of venous occlusive disease of the lower calf.

Vascular duplex scanning is called duplex because it combines the benefits of Doppler with B-mode scanning (see Carotid Ultrasound, p. 874). With the use of the transducer, a B-mode ultrasound gray-scale image of the vessel is obtained. A pulsed Doppler probe within the transducer is used to evaluate blood flow velocity and direction in the artery and to measure the amplitude and waveform of the arterial pulse. A computer combines that information and provides a two-dimensional image of the vessel along with an image of blood flow. With this technique, one is able to directly visualize areas of vascular narrowing or occlusion. The degree of occlusion is measured as a percentage of the entire lumen that is occluded. Also venous thrombosis is suspected when the vein is not easily compressible by the ultrasound probe. Also see Carotid Artery Duplex Scan (p. 874).

Color Doppler ultrasound (CDU) can be added to arterial duplex scanning. CDU assigns color for direction of blood flow within the vessel, and the intensity of that color depends on the mean computed velocity of blood traveling in the vessel. This allows visualization of stenotic areas based on velocity or direction of blood flow in a particular area of the artery. With the use of duplex scanning, an accurate representation of the vessel anatomy and patency can be obtained.

Duplex scanning is routinely used to identify venous thrombosis in patients suspected of having an extremity affected by DVT. It is more rapidly performed and interpreted than venography (p. 1076). In general, venous duplex scanning is less accurate than venography in identifying DVT in the calf or in the iliac veins.

With a single-mode transducer, venous blood flow can be heard audibly and is augmented by an audio speaker as a swishing noise. If the vein is occluded, no swishing sounds are detected. With single-mode arterial Doppler studies, peripheral arteriosclerotic occlusive disease of the extremities can be easily located. By slowly deflating blood pressure cuffs placed on the calf and ankle, systolic pressure in the arteries of the extremities can be accurately measured by detecting the first evidence of blood flow with the Doppler transducer. The extremely sensitive Doppler ultrasound detector can recognize the swishing sound of even the most minimal blood flow. Normally systolic blood pressure is slightly higher in the arteries of the arms than in the legs. If the difference in blood pressure exceeds 20 mm Hg, occlusive disease is believed to exist immediately proximal to the area tested. Lower extremity arterial bypass graft patency can also be assessed with Doppler ultrasound.

INTERFERING FACTORS

- Venous or arterial occlusive disease proximal to the site of testing
- Cigarette smoking, because nicotine can cause constriction of the peripheral arteries and alter the results

Clinical Priorities

- Venous patency is demonstrated with Doppler ultrasound, which detects moving RBCs within a vein.
- Flow velocity and direction within an artery can be evaluated with duplex Doppler scanning.
- Because nicotine can cause vasoconstriction, cigarette smoking is prohibited 30 minutes before and during this test.
- An ankle-to-brachial artery index less than 0.85 indicates significant arterial occlusive disease in the extremity.

PROCEDURE AND PATIENT CARE

Before

- Explain the procedure to the patient.
- Inform the patient that the procedure is painless.
- Remove all clothing from the extremity to be examined.
- Instruct the patient to abstain from cigarette smoking for at least 30 minutes before the test.

During

- Note the following procedural steps:

Venous Doppler Studies
1. A gel lubricant is applied in multiple areas to the skin overlying the venous system of the extremity.
2. In the lower extremity, the deep venous system is usually identified in the ankle, calf, thigh, and groin.

3. The characteristic "swishing" sound indicates a patent venous system. Failure to detect this signal indicates venous occlusion.
4. Usually, both the superficial and deep venous systems are evaluated.

Arterial Doppler Studies

1. Blood pressure cuffs are placed around the thigh, calf, and ankle.
2. A gel lubricant is applied to the skin overlying the artery distal to the cuffs.
3. The proximal cuff is inflated to a level above systolic blood pressure in the normal extremity.
4. The Doppler ultrasound transducer is placed immediately distal to the inflated cuff.
5. The pressure in the cuff is slowly released.
6. The highest pressure at which blood flow is detected by the characteristic swishing Doppler signal is recorded as the blood pressure of that artery.
7. The test is repeated at each successive level.
8. An ankle-to-brachial artery index less than 0.85 indicates significant arterial occlusive disease in the extremity.

• These studies are usually performed in the vascular laboratory or radiology department and take approximately 30 minutes.

After

• Remove the gel from the extremity.
• Inform the patient that the radiologist must interpret the studies and that results will be available in a few hours.

TEST RESULTS AND CLINICAL SIGNIFICANCE

Venous occlusion secondary to thrombosis or thrombophlebitis: *Complete or partial occlusion is apparent at any level above the upper calf. Results are not accurate below the upper calf.*
Venous varicosities: *Doppler ultrasound can recognize flow reversal as a result of incompetent valves of varicose veins.*
Small or large vessel arterial occlusive disease,
Spastic arterial disease (e.g., Raynaud phenomenon),
Small vessel arterial occlusive disease (as in diabetes),
Embolic arterial occlusion,
Arterial aneurysm:

> *These vascular diseases are most evident with duplex Doppler scanning. Color flow Doppler imaging can be done, in which designated colors demonstrate flow velocity and direction. Partial or complete occlusion is readily visualized. Turbulence, as with an aneurysm, is obvious. Reversal of flow that may occur distal to an occluded artery will be evident.*

RELATED TESTS

Venography (p. 1076). This is a radiographic study of the veins of an extremity. It is more accurate for detection of deep venous thrombosis in the lower calf, but no more accurate than Doppler studies in the more proximal extremity. Intravenous iodinated contrast medium used for this test may precipitate an allergic reaction or renal failure.
Arteriography (p. 988). This radiographic study of the arteries of an extremity can more accurately indicate the exact location and anatomy of the arterial occlusion.

Urine Studies

Overview

Urine is derived from filtration of the blood by the nephrons in the kidney. Blood enters the kidney through the renal artery and passes into small capillaries in the glomerulus. There, solute and water are filtered through the capillary and into Bowman capsule. This fluid progressively passes through the capsule and into the renal tubule. More capillaries surround the tubule, and water and other solutes can pass through the tubule into and out of the capillaries according to the body's needs. Within the renal medulla, the collecting system collects all the urine from each nephron and transports it to the renal pelvis. The urine then passes through the ureters and into the bladder. At micturition (voiding), the urine passes through the urethra and out of the body.

Urine is nearly all water, with a small percentage of solutes. All end products of metabolism and all potentially harmful materials are excreted in the urine to maintain normal acid/base balance, fluid and electrolyte balance, and homeostasis.

In general, the urine reflects the blood level for any analyte. If the blood level is elevated and the kidneys are working well, the urine level for that same product can be expected to be high. If the urine level is not high, the kidneys may be diseased, resulting in high levels in the blood. In some instances, certain blood solute products are not filtered from the blood unless "threshold" levels of the solute are exceeded. For example, glucose is not excreted by the kidney unless blood levels exceed approximately 180 mg/dL.

REASONS FOR OBTAINING URINE SPECIMENS

The urine specimen has been referred to as a "fluid biopsy" of the urinary tract. It is usually painlessly obtained, and it provides a great deal of information quickly and economically. Like other specimen tests, urine tests must be carefully performed and properly controlled. Most urine tests are performed for one of the following reasons:

1. To diagnose renal or urinary tract disease (e.g., proteinuria may indicate glomerulonephritis).
2. To monitor renal or urinary tract disease (e.g., urine cultures may be used to monitor the effectiveness of antibiotic therapy for urinary tract infections).
3. To detect metabolic or systemic diseases not directly related to the kidneys (e.g., glucose in the urine may be indicative of diabetes mellitus or Cushing syndrome).

Although blood tests provide valuable information about the body, urinalysis may be preferred for several reasons:

1. Identification of urinary tract infection (UTI) requires a urine specimen.
2. A 24-hour urine collection will reflect homeostasis and disease better than a blood specimen obtained at a random moment of the day.
3. Some products are rapidly cleared by the kidneys and may not be apparent in the blood (e.g., Bence-Jones protein). Results of a blood test may be normal while urinalysis indicates the presence of these products.
4. The serum product being tested may be affected by renal clearance (e.g., sodium). Therefore a urine specimen to measure the sodium concentration will add significant additional information to a serum sodium level.
5. Urine testing is easily performed and does not require an invasive skin puncture.
6. Many urine tests are cheaper than blood tests. The urine test may be less accurate or only qualitative, but that may be all that is needed.

TYPES OF URINE SPECIMENS

The type of urine specimen collected and the collection procedure depend on the test ordered. There are five basic types of urine specimens. In addition, other body fluids can be evaluated to determine whether they contain urine.

First Morning Specimen

To collect a first morning specimen, the patient voids before going to bed. Immediately on rising, the patient collects a urine specimen. The benefits of a first morning specimen are multiple. First, the urine in the bladder overnight represents all of the urine for the previous 6 to 8 hours. Unlike a random spot urine sample, it is a more accurate reflection of the patient's 24-hour urine. Second, postural changes that may affect the urine can be avoided by obtaining the urine specimen immediately on arising. Third, diurnal variations may affect test results. Collecting the first morning specimen allows one to factor in the timing of the testing. Finally, because the urine has been retained in the bladder during a relative overnight fast, it is concentrated, and testing is more likely to detect positive findings. This specimen is ideal for detecting substances such as proteins and nitrates, and is often used to confirm a diagnosis of orthostatic proteinuria.

Although the first morning specimen is frequently the specimen of choice, it is not the most convenient to obtain. It requires that the patient be given instructions and the collection container at least 1 day before the specimen is needed. In addition, the specimen must be preserved if it is not going to be delivered to the laboratory within 2 hours of collection.

Random Urine Specimen

Random urine specimens are usually obtained during daytime hours and without any prior patient preparation. For ease and convenience, routine screening is most often performed on a random specimen. Random testing is usually performed when the substance to be tested does not have significant diurnal variation and its normal concentration is adequate to be detected in a small volume of urine. Random urine is also the specimen of choice for illegal drug screening. This avoids patient tampering with results or changing behavior in anticipation of testing.

Timed Urine Collection

Because substances such as hormones, proteins, and electrolytes are variably excreted over 24 hours, and because of the effects of exercise, posture, hydration, and body metabolism on excretion rates, quantitative urine tests often require a timed collection. These time periods may range anywhere from 2 to 24 hours. Timed collections are of two types. One type includes urine specimens collected at a predetermined time. For example, glucose is often measured 2 hours after a meal (postprandial), because that is when the urine is expected to contain the maximum glucose level. A 2-hour postprandial specimen can be collected after any meal. The second type includes specimens collected at a specific time of day. For example, a specimen for urobilinogen testing is best collected between 2:00 PM and 4:00 PM, when bilinogen is maximally excreted. Depending on the substance being measured and the type of collection, a preservative may be needed to ensure stability throughout the collection period. In addition, certain foods and drugs may need to be avoided during the collection period. Box 11-1 lists some of the more common errors in collecting timed urine specimens.

To collect a timed specimen, the patient is instructed to void and discard the first specimen. This is noted as the start time of the test. All subsequent urine is saved in a special container for the designated period of time. At the end of the specified time period, the patient voids and adds this urine to the specimen container, completing the collection process. (For example, see 24-Hour Urine Collection, p. 906).

BOX 11-1	**Sources of Error in Timed Urine Specimens**

- Loss of specimen
- Inadequate preservative used
- Inclusion of two first morning specimens in a 24-hour collection
- Inaccurate total volume measurement
- Transcription error

Double-Voided Specimen

This collection method is performed to obtain and evaluate fresh urine. To obtain this specimen, the patient first empties the bladder. Shortly thereafter, the patient voids again. The second specimen in the double-voided specimen is the freshest urine and is used for testing. It accurately reflects blood concentrations at that particular time.

Urine Specimen for Culture and Sensitivity

This specimen is collected for examination of bacteria. The specimen must be collected in a sterile container as aseptically as possible. This requires meticulous cleansing of the urinary meatus with an antiseptic preparation to reduce contamination of the specimen by external organisms. A midstream collection technique will cleanse the urethral canal of contaminant bacteria. The specimen should be cultured within 1 hour of collection.

Other Body Fluids

Body fluids can be tested for blood urea nitrogen (BUN) and creatinine to determine whether the fluid is urine. This is done commonly after pelvic surgery. Abdominal fluid serous drainage can look like urine. If the BUN and creatinine concentrations in that fluid are the same as in serum, the fluid is considered to be serous drainage or ascites. If, however, the concentration of BUN and creatinine in the fluid is more than three times that in serum, the fluid is urine. This testing is also helpful in obstetrics to differentiate amniotic fluid from urine.

COLLECTION METHODS

Collection methods vary from those requiring no patient preparation to invasive-type procedures. The reason for the test and the clinical situation determine the appropriate collection method.

Common Collection Methods

Routine Void Specimen. A routine void specimen requires no preparation and is collected by having the patient urinate into an appropriate nonsterile container. Random and first morning specimens are collected in this manner.

Midstream and Clean-Catch Specimens. If a culture and sensitivity study is required or if the specimen is likely to be contaminated by vaginal discharge or bleeding, a clean-catch or midstream specimen is collected. For a clean-catch specimen, meticulous cleansing of the urinary meatus with an antiseptic preparation is necessary to reduce contamination of the specimen by external organisms. In male patients, the foreskin is retracted and the meatus cleansed. Then the cleansing agent must be carefully removed, because it may inhibit growth of any bacteria in the specimen, which would affect the culture and sensitivity determination. For a midstream collection, the patient begins to urinate into a bedpan, urinal, or toilet, then stops. This washes the urine out of the distal urethra. The patient voids 3 to 4 ounces of urine into a sterile container, which is then capped, and the patient is allowed to finish voiding.

24-Hour Urine Collection. The patient is instructed to void and discard the first specimen (e.g., at 8:00 AM on day 1). This is noted as the start time of the 24-hour collection. The patient collects all urine voided up to and including that at 8:00 AM the following morning (day 2). In the laboratory, the total volume of the sample is recorded. After the specimen is thoroughly mixed, a measured sample is withdrawn for analysis. See Box 11-2.

If any urine is removed or discarded during a timed collection, the entire timed collection is invalid. Twenty-four-hour urine collections are more accurate than specimens collected over a shorter time.

BOX 11-2	Guidelines for a 24-Hour Urine Collection

1. Begin the 24-hour collection by discarding the first specimen.
2. Collect all urine voided during the next 24 hours.
3. Show the patient where to store the urine.
4. Keep the urine on ice or refrigerated during the collection period. Foley bags are kept in a basin of ice. Some collections require a preservative. Check with the laboratory.
5. Post the hours for the urine collection in a prominent place to prevent accidentally discarding a specimen.
6. Instruct the patient to void before defecating so that urine in not contaminated by stool.
7. Remind the patient not to put toilet paper in the urine collection container.
8. Collect the last specimen as close as possible to the end of the 24-hour period. Add this urine to the collection.

Some analytes are excreted at different rates throughout the day or night, and random specimens may miss the time of maximal excretion. Also, because greater concentrations of an analyte are present in a 24-hour collection, the chance of a false-negative result is reduced.

Special Collection Methods

Special collection methods are indicated when a specimen cannot be obtained by the more common techniques.

Urethral Catheterization. A urine specimen can be obtained by inserting a sterile catheter through the urethra into the bladder. Although catheterization may cause infection, this collection method is used when patients are unable to void or cannot void when the specimen is required (e.g., during trauma).

In patients with an indwelling urinary catheter in place, a specimen is obtained by attaching a syringe to the catheter at a point distal to the sleeve leading to the balloon. Many tubes have an access (sampling port) area for this type of collection technique. Urine is aspirated and placed in a sterile urine container. (Usually the catheter tubing distal to the puncture site needs to be clamped for 15 to 30 minutes before the aspiration of urine to allow urine to fill the tubing. After the specimen is withdrawn, the clamp is removed.) The urine that accumulates in a plastic reservoir bag should never be used for a urine test.

Suprapubic Aspiration. In suprapubic aspiration, urine is collected directly from the bladder by inserting a needle through the abdominal wall and into the bladder. The urine is aspirated into a syringe and sent for analysis. This method is mainly used to obtain urine for anaerobic culture, when specimen contamination is unavoidable, and in infants and young children. Complications are rare.

Pediatric Collections. Urine specimens from infants and young children are often collected using a pediatric collection bag. This clear, pliable, polyethylene bag has a hypoallergenic skin-adhesive backing around the opening. The perineal skin is cleansed and dried before the specimen bag is applied to the skin. The bag is placed over the penis in male children and around the vagina (excluding the rectum) in female children. Once the bag is in place, the patient is checked every 15 minutes until the urine is collected. The specimen bag should be removed as soon as the urine is collected. Bags may be folded and self-sealed for transportation. If a 24-hour specimen is needed, a tube is attached to the bag and connected to a storage container. This avoids repeated skin preparation and reapplication of adhesive to the child's sensitive skin.

Urine Studies

11

BOX 11-3	Criteria for Rejection of a Urine Sample

- Improper sample identification
- Incorrect urine preservation
- Insufficient urine quantity
- Improper specimen collection
- Missing or incomplete request form
- Visible contamination (e.g., stool)

TRANSPORT, STORAGE, AND PRESERVATION

Disposable plastic containers (100- to 200-mL capacity) with lids are sufficient for most routine urine tests. Screw-top containers are preferred because they are less likely to leak during transportation. Wax-coated cardboard containers should not be used because of the possibility of contaminating the specimen with fatty material. Sterile kits are available for bacterial cultures. Kits usually contain a disposable plastic urine container and cleansing pads.

Rigid, brown, light-resistant plastic containers (approximately 3000-mL capacity) are suitable for most 12- and 24-hour urine collections. These containers have a wide mouth and a leak-proof screw cap. Preservatives may be added to these containers. One-gallon glass jugs may also be used.

Specimen containers must be correctly labeled. Labels should not be placed on the lid, because when the lid is removed the specimen is unlabeled. The patient identification label should be placed directly on the container.

Specimens should be promptly transported to the laboratory. If this is not possible and specimen transportation will be delayed 2 hours or longer, precautions need to be taken to preserve the integrity of the specimen. A variety of changes can occur in an unpreserved specimen. Physical, chemical, and microscopic examinations can all be affected by oxidation, precipitation, and overgrowth of bacteria. Therefore appropriate handling and storage are necessary to ensure that changes do not occur and that accurate results are obtained. Laboratories have written criteria describing when to reject a urine specimen as unsuitable for testing. Box 11-3 lists common criteria for rejecting a urine specimen.

Many analytes require preservatives to maintain viability during the collection period. The proper preservative depends on the type of collection, the delay before testing, and the tests to be performed. No single urine preservative suits all testing requirements. Some analytes require an acidic pH for stability; others are stable in an alkaline pH. For example, acetic acid can be used as a preservative to maintain acidity. Sodium carbonate may be used to maintain alkalinity. Boric acid may be used to inhibit bacterial multiplication. Some analytes are best preserved by refrigeration, which is the easiest means of preserving many urine specimens. If possible, all timed urine specimens should be refrigerated or on ice throughout the collection period. Foley catheter bags can be placed in a basin of ice. Timed specimens may also require the addition of a chemical preservative. For example, sodium fluoride is used to preserve glucose in a 24-hour urine collection. Some analytes need to be protected from light by using a dark collection container or by wrapping the container with foil. Urine for the evaluation of tumor cells may be collected into a container with alcohol. Fixatives (e.g., Saccomanno) also can be used to preserve cytologic specimens.

Collection preservatives may differ among laboratories, depending on (1) testing methods, (2) units of measurement, (3) how often the test is performed, (4) time delays, or (5) transportation to reference laboratories.

URINE REAGENT STRIPS

The urine reagent strip has replaced many complicated individual chemical analyses for determination of various components in the urine. For example, estimation of glucose, albumin, hemoglobin, and bile concentrations, as well as urinary pH, specific gravity, protein, ketone bodies, nitrates, and leukocyte esterase, can be easily determined using a dipstick. Dipsticks are small strips of paper impregnated with a chemical that reacts to products in the urine by changing color. The color correlates with concentrations of the analyte in the urine. Many tests can be performed with one dipstick.

This method of testing involves dipping a "fresh" (not outdated) reagent strip or dipstick into urine and observing the color change on the strip. The color is compared with the color chart on the bottle of reagent strips at the exact time indicated. Dipstick testing is accurate and somewhat quantitative. However, a large number of products in a urine specimen can cause false-positive or false-negative results. Dipstick testing is considered preliminary or for screening. Often more definitive and quantitative studies are necessary to confirm the results.

REPORTING OF RESULTS

Accurate results depend on appropriate collection, transport, storage, and preservation of the urine specimen. To be clinically useful, test results must be promptly reported, because delays can make the data useless. The report must also be delivered to the appropriate medical record keeper and must be presented in a manner that is clear and easily interpreted.

The report should include the test results, reporting units, and reference ranges. Reference ranges vary from institution to institution. Comments may be included to help interpret results. For example, the technologist may note that the urine specific gravity is too low for proper interpretation of results. Proper reporting of "critical" or "panic" values (well outside the usual range of normal) is essential because such results generally require immediate intervention. If these results are called in to a physician or nurse, verification of notification must be properly documented.

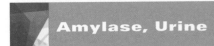

Amylase, Urine

NORMAL FINDINGS

Up to 5000 Somogyi units/24 hours, or 6.5 to 48.1 units/hour
Amylase clearance: <2

INDICATIONS

The urine amylase concentration is used to assist in making the diagnosis of pancreatitis, although other nonpancreatic diseases can also cause elevated urine amylase levels. Urine amylase levels rise later than blood amylase levels. Several days after onset of the disease process, serum amylase levels may be normal while urine levels are significantly elevated. Urine amylase concentration is particularly useful in detecting pancreatitis late in the disease course.

TEST EXPLANATION

Amylase is normally secreted from the pancreatic acinar cells into the pancreatic duct and then into the duodenum. Once in the intestine, it aids catabolism of carbohydrates to their component simple sugars. Destruction of acinar cells (as in pancreatitis) or obstruction to the pancreatic duct flow (as in pancreatic carcinoma) causes outpouring of this enzyme into the bloodstream.

Because the kidneys rapidly clear amylase, disorders that affect the pancreas cause elevated amylase levels in the urine. Serum levels of amylase rise transiently but usually return to normal 1 to 2 days after resolution of the acute phase of disease. Levels of amylase in the urine, however, remain elevated 5 to 7 days after onset of disease. This is an important indicator of pancreatitis in patients who have had symptoms for 3 days or longer.

As with serum amylase (p. 61), urine amylase is sensitive but not specific for pancreatic disorders. Other diseases, such as parotiditis (mumps), cholecystitis, perforated bowel, penetrating peptic ulcer, ectopic pregnancy, and renal infarction, can cause elevated urine levels; however, urine levels are usually highest with pancreatitis. A comparison of the renal clearance ratio of amylase to creatinine provides more specific diagnostic information than either the urine amylase level or the serum amylase level alone. When the *amylase/creatinine clearance ratio* is 5% or more, the diagnosis of pancreatitis can be made with certainty. A ratio less than 5% in a patient with elevated serum and urine amylase levels is indicative of nonpancreatic pathologic conditions (e.g., perforated bowel, macroamylasemia).

INTERFERING FACTORS

- Intravenous dextrose solutions can cause a false-negative result.
- Drugs that may cause *increased* amylase levels include aminosalicylic acid, aspirin, azathioprine, corticosteroids, dexamethasone, ethyl alcohol, glucocorticoids, iodine-containing contrast media, loop diuretics (e.g., furosemide), methyldopa, narcotic analgesics, oral contraceptives, and prednisone.
- Drugs that may cause *decreased* levels include citrates, glucose, and oxalates.

✓ Clinical Priorities

- Urinary levels of amylase remain elevated for 5 to 7 days after disease onset. This is helpful in diagnosing pancreatitis after serum levels have returned to normal.
- When the amylase/creatinine clearance ratio is 5% or higher, the diagnosis of pancreatitis can be made with certainty.

PROCEDURE AND PATIENT CARE

Before

- Explain the procedure to the patient.
- Tell the patient that no fasting is required.
- Record the exact times of urine collection.

During

- See Box 11-2, Guidelines for a 24-Hour Urine Collection, p. 907.
- A 2-hour spot urine specimen can sometimes be used instead of the 24-hour urine collection.
- No preservative is needed.

After

- Send the urine specimen to the laboratory promptly.

TEST RESULTS AND CLINICAL SIGNIFICANCE

▲ Increased Levels

Acute pancreatitis,
Chronic relapsing pancreatitis:

> *Damage to pancreatic acinar cells (as in pancreatitis) causes outpouring of amylase into the intrapancreatic lymph system and the free peritoneum. Blood vessels draining the free peritoneum and absorbing the lymph pick up the excess amylase. The amylase is then cleared by the kidneys, and urine levels rise. Amylase clearance can be expected to be greater than 5.*

Penetrating peptic ulcer into the pancreas,
Gastrointestinal disease:

> *In patients with perforated peptic ulcer, necrotic bowel, perforated bowel, or duodenal obstruction, amylase leaks out of the gut and into the free peritoneal cavity. The amylase is picked up by the blood and lymphatic vessels of the peritoneum. The amylase is cleared by the kidneys, and urine levels rise. Amylase clearance is between 2 and 5.*

Acute cholecystitis,
Parotiditis (mumps),
Ruptured ectopic pregnancy:

> *Amylase is present in the salivary glands, gallbladder, and fallopian tubes. Diseases that affect these organs are associated with elevated urine and blood levels of amylase. Amylase clearance will be between 2 and 5.*

Diabetic ketoacidosis,
Pulmonary infarction,
Osteogenic sarcoma,
Cryoglobulinemia,
Rheumatoid diseases,
Postendoscopic retrograde pancreatography:

> *These clinical situations are sometimes associated with high urine amylase levels.*

RELATED TESTS

Serum Amylase (p. 61). Amylase can be detected in the serum earlier than in the urine. This test is more easily performed and therefore used more frequently to monitor the course of disease.

Lipase (p. 339). Lipase is similar to amylase but is more specific for the pancreas.

Bence-Jones Protein (Free Kappa and Lambda Light Chains)

Urine Studies

11

NORMAL FINDINGS

Kappa total light chain: <0.68 mg/dL
Lambda total light chain: <0.40 mg/dL
Kappa/lambda ratio: 0.7-6.2

INDICATIONS

The detection of Bence-Jones protein in the urine most commonly indicates multiple myeloma (especially when the urine levels are high). The test is used to detect and monitor the treatment and clinical course of multiple myeloma and other similar diseases.

TEST EXPLANATION

Bence-Jones proteins are monoclonal light-chain portions of immunoglobulins found in 75% of the patients with multiple myeloma. These proteins are made most notably by the plasma cells in these patients. They also may be associated with tumor metastases to the bone, chronic lymphocytic leukemias, lymphoma, macroglobulinemia, and amyloidosis.

Immunoglobulin light chains are usually cleared from blood through the renal glomeruli and reabsorbed in the proximal tubules so that urine light-chain concentrations are very low or undetectable. The production of large amounts of monoclonal light chains, however, can overwhelm this reabsorption mechanism. Because the Bence-Jones protein is rapidly cleared from the blood by the kidney, it may be very difficult to detect in the blood; therefore urine is used for this study. Normally urine should contain no Bence-Jones proteins.

Routine urine testing for proteins using reagent strips often does not reflect the type or amount of proteins in the urine. In fact, the strip may show a completely negative result despite large amounts of Bence-Jones globulins in the urine. Proteins in the urine are best identified by *protein electrophoresis* of the urine. With this method, the proteins are separated based on size and electrical charge in an electric field when the urine specimen is applied to a gel plate. Once the various proteins are separated, antisera to specific proteins can be added to the gel and specific precipitin arcs can be identified and quantified (*immunofixation*). Monitoring the urine M-spike is especially useful in patients with light-chain multiple myeloma in whom the serum M-spike may be very small or absent, but in whom the urine M-spike is large.

INTERFERING FACTORS

- Dilute urine may yield a false-*negative* result.
- High doses of penicillin or aspirin can cause false-*positive* results.

PROCEDURE AND PATIENT CARE

Before

- Explain the procedure to the patient.
- Instruct the patient not to contaminate the urine specimen with toilet paper or stool.

During

- Instruct the patient to collect an early morning specimen of at least 50 mL of uncontaminated urine in a container. It may be helpful to know the amount of these proteins excreted over 24 hours. If so, a 24-hour collection may be ordered (see Box 11-2, p. 907).

After

- Immediately transport the specimen to the laboratory. If it cannot be taken to the laboratory immediately, refrigerate it because heat-coagulable proteins can decompose, causing a false-positive test.

TEST RESULTS AND CLINICAL SIGNIFICANCE

▲ Increased Levels

Multiple myeloma (plasmacytoma): *Only about 2% of patients with myeloma do not produce Bence-Jones protein. Detection of Bence-Jones protein at high levels (>60 mg/L) is most common with this malignant disease.*
Chronic lymphocytic leukemia,
Lymphoma,

Metastatic colon, breast, lung, or prostate cancer:
> *Several neoplastic disorders are associated with monoclonal gammaglobulinopathies. Some can produce Bence-Jones protein.*

Amyloidosis: *Primary amyloidosis can produce immunoglobulin light chains similar to those of Bence-Jones protein.*

Waldenström macroglobulinemia: *This malignant lymphoproliferative disease is highlighted by lymphadenopathy, hepatosplenomegaly, anemia, hyperviscosity, and Bence-Jones proteinuria (about 20% of the patients).*

RELATED TEST

Urinalysis (p. 956). Urinalysis includes determination of protein in the urine. If positive, urine electrophoresis (similar to serum protein electrophoresis) can be performed (p. 424).

11 Beta-Prostaglandin F(2) Alpha, Urine

NORMAL FINDINGS

>1000 ng/24 hours

INDICATIONS

Measurement of 11 beta-prostaglandin F(2) alpha in urine is useful in the evaluation of patients suspected of having systemic mastocytosis (systemic mast-cell disease [SMCD]).

TEST EXPLANATION

SMCD is characterized by mast cell infiltration of extracutaneous organs (usually the bone marrow). Focal mast cell lesions in the bone marrow are found in approximately 90% of adult patients with systemic mastocytosis.

Prostaglandin D(2) (PGD2) is generated by human mast cells, activated alveolar macrophages, and platelets. There are a large number of metabolic products of PGD(2), the most abundant is 11 beta-prostaglandin F2 alpha. Although the most definitive test for systemic mast cell disease is bone marrow biopsy (p. 712), measurement of mast cell mediators like beta prostaglandin in urine is advised for the initial evaluation of suspected cases. Elevated levels of 11 beta-prostaglandin F(2) alpha in urine are not specific for systemic mast cell disease and may be found in patients with angioedema, diffuse urticaria, or myeloproliferative diseases in the absence of diffuse mast cell proliferation.

Testing is most commonly performed using a commercially available alpha EIA kit.

PROCEDURE AND PATIENT CARE

Before

 Explain the procedure to the patient.

During

 See Box 11-2, Guidelines for a 24-Hour Urine Collection, p. 907.

 Encourage the patient to drink fluids during the 24 hours unless this is contraindicated for medical purposes.

Urine Studies

11

After

- Send the urine to the chemistry laboratory as soon as the test is completed.

ABNORMAL FINDINGS

▲ Increased Levels

Systemic mast cell disease: *Proliferation of mast cells causes elevation of PGD2 that gets metabolized to 11 beta-prostaglandin F(2) alpha and is then excreted in urine.*

Angioedema,

Diffuse urticaria,

Myeloproliferative diseases:

In the absence of diffuse mast cell proliferation associated with these diseases, PGD2 is abundant from a source other than mast cells, leading to increased 11 beta-prostaglandin F(2) alpha in urine.

Bladder Cancer Markers (Bladder Tumor Antigen [BTA], Nuclear Matrix Protein 22 [NMP22])

NORMAL FINDINGS

BTA: <14 units/mL

NMP22: <10 units/mL

FISH: No chromosomal amplification or deletions noted

INDICATIONS

This test is performed on patients who have had a transurethral resection of a superficial bladder cancer to predict or identify tumor recurrence.

TEST EXPLANATION

The recurrence rate for superficial bladder cancers that have been resected by transurethral cystoscopy is high. Surveillance testing requires frequent urine testing for cytology and frequent cystoscopic evaluations. The use of bladder tumor markers may provide an easier and cheaper method of diagnosing recurrent bladder cancer that also improves accuracy.

Bladder Tumor Antigen (BTA) and Nuclear Matrix Protein 22 (NMP22) are proteins produced by bladder tumor cells and deposited into the urine. Normally, none or very low levels of these proteins are found in the urine. When levels of bladder cancer tumor markers are normal, cystoscopy rarely yields positive results. When these markers are elevated, bladder tumor recurrence is strongly suspected and cystoscopy is indicated to confirm bladder cancer recurrence.

NMP22 may also be a good screening test for patients at increased risk for developing bladder cancer. However, these markers can be elevated in other circumstances (recent urologic surgery, urinary tract infection, or calculi). Cancers involving the ureters and renal pelvis may also be associated with increased BTA and NMP22.

Bladder cancer cells have been found to exhibit aneuploidy (gene amplifications on chromosomes 3, 7, and 17, and the loss of the 9p21 locus on chromosome 9). Using DNA probes, through *fluorescence in situ hybridization (FISH),* these chromosomal abnormalities can be identified with great accuracy. FISH can be performed on cells isolated in a fresh urine specimen or cells available on a ThinPrep slide (similar to Pap tests [see p. 743]). When these chromosomal abnormalities are present, fluorescent staining will be obvious using a fluorescence microscope.

Although not actually a tumor marker, a cytology test is available that can be used in the early detection of bladder cancer recurrence. It is an immunocytofluorescence technique based on a patented cocktail of three monoclonal antibodies labeled with fluorescence markers. These antibodies bind to two antigens: a mucin glycoprotein and a carcinoembryonic antigen (CEA). These antigens are expressed by tumor cells found in bladder cancer patients and exfoliated in the urine.

INTERFERING FACTORS

- These proteins are very unstable. If the urine is not immediately stabilized, false negatives may occur.
- Active infection (including sexually transmitted diseases) of the lower urologic tract can cause false elevations.
- Kidney or bladder calculi can cause false elevations.

PROCEDURE AND PATIENT CARE

Before

✗ Explain the procedure to the patient.
✗ Tell the patient that no fasting is required.

During

- A single voided specimen should be collected before noon.
- The specimen should be transported to the lab immediately to avoid deterioration of the protein.
- If a time delay is required, the specimen should be refrigerated.

After

✗ Explain any other surveillance testing that may be required for bladder cancer follow up.

TEST RESULTS AND CLINICAL SIGNIFICANCE

▲ **Increased Levels**

Bladder cancer: *The rapid cellular synthesis and destruction causes these proteins to be generated and washed into the urine.*

Bone Turnover Markers (BTMs, N-Telopeptide [NTx], Bone Collagen Equivalents [BCEs], Osteocalcin [Bone G1a Protein, BGP, Osteocalc], Pyridinium [PYD] Crosslinks, Bone-Specific Alkaline Phosphatase [BSAP], Amino-Terminal Propeptide of Type 1 Procollagen [P1 NP], C-Telopeptide [CTx])

Urine Studies

11

NORMAL FINDINGS

N-telopeptide
 Urine (nm BCE*/mm creatinine)

---

* BCE = bone collagen equivalents.

Male: 21-83
Female, premenopausal: 17-94
Female, postmenopausal: 26-124
Serum (nm BCE*)
Male: 5.4-24.2
Female: 6.2-19.0
C-telopeptide (ng/mL)
Urine
Adults: 1.03 ± 0.41
Children: 8 ± 3.37
Serum (pg/mL)
Female, premenopausal: 40-465
Female, postmenopausal: 104-1008
Male: 60-700
Amino-terminal propeptide of type I procollagen, serum (mcg/L)
Male: 22-105
Female, Premenopausal: 19-101
Female, Postmenopausal: 16-96
Osteocalcin, serum (ng/mL)
Adult (>22 years)
Male: 5.8-14
Female: 3.1-14
Children and adolescents (male and female)
1 year: not established
1-10 years: 10-50
11-15 years: 10-100
16-22 years: 10-50
Pyridium, urine (nm/mm)
Male: 10.3-33.6
Female: 15.3-33.6
Bone-specific alkaline phosphatase, serum (mcg/L)
Male: 6.5-20.1
Female, premenopausal: 4.5-16.9
Female, postmenopausal: 7-22.4

INDICATIONS

N-telopeptide, bone specific alkaline phosphatase, pyridinium, and osteocalcin are rapid biochemical markers of bone turnover and are used to monitor treatment for osteoporosis.

TEST EXPLANATION

With the increased use of bone density scans (see p. 1002), osteoporosis can now be diagnosed and treated more easily. This has prompted an interest in biochemical markers of bone metabolism. Bone is continuously being turned over—bone resorption by osteoclasts and bone formation by osteoblasts.

---

* BCE = bone collagen equivalents.

Osteoporosis is a common disease of postmenopausal women and is associated with increased bone resorption and decreased bone formation. The result is thin and weak bones that are prone to fracture. The same process is now becoming increasingly recognized in elderly men, as well. Early diagnosis allows therapeutic intervention to prevent bone fracture.

Bone mineral density studies are valuable tools in the identification of osteoporosis; however, they cannot recognize small changes in bone metabolism. Although bone density studies can be used to monitor the effectiveness of therapy, it takes years to detect measurable changes in bone density. Bone turnover markers (BTM), however, can identify significant improvement in a few months after instituting successful therapy. Furthermore, the cost of bone density studies limits the feasibility of performing this test as frequently as may be required to monitor treatment.

Because the levels of BTMs vary according to the time of day and bone volume, these studies are not widely used or helpful in screening for detection of osteoporosis. Their use is in determining the effect of treatment as these markers are compared to pretreatment levels. Levels will decline with the use of antiresorption drugs (such as estrogen, biphosphonates, calcitonin, and raloxifene). BTMs have shown to be accurately predictive of early improvement in bone mineral density and antifracture treatment efficacy. BTMs are also useful in documenting treatment compliance.

"N-" and "C-" telopeptides (NTx) are protein fragments used in type 1 collagen that make up nearly 90% of the bone matrix. The "C" and "N" terminals of these proteins are cross-linked to provide tensile strength to the bone. When bone is broken down, CTx and NTx are released into the bloodstream and excreted in the urine. Serum levels of these fragments have been shown to correlate well with urine measurements normalized to creatinine. Measurements of these fragments show early response to antiresorptive therapy (within 3 to 6 months) and are good indicators of bone resorption. Normal levels can vary with method of testing.

Amino-terminal propeptide of type I procollagen (P1NP), like NTx, is directly proportional to the amount of new collagen produced by osteoblasts. Concentrations are increased in patients with various bone diseases and therapies characterized by increased osteoblastic activity. P1NP is the most effective marker of bone formation and is particularly useful for monitoring bone formation therapies and antiresorptive therapies.

Osteocalcin, or bone Gla protein (BGP), is a noncollagenous protein in the bone and is made by osteoblasts. It enters the circulation during bone resorption as well as bone formation and is a good indicator of bone metabolism. Serum levels of BGP correlate with bone formation and destruction (turnover). Increased levels are associated with increased bone mineral density loss. BGP is a vitamin K–dependent protein. A reduced vitamin K intake is associated with reduced BGP levels. This probably explains the pathophysiology of vitamin K–dependent deficiency osteoporosis.

Pyridinium (PyD) crosslinks are formed during maturation of the type 1 collagen during bone formation. During bone resorption, these pyridinium crosslinks are released into the circulation.

Bone Specific Alkaline Phosphatase (BSAP) is an isoenzyme of alkaline phosphate (p. 47) and is found in the cell membrane of the osteoblast. It is, therefore, an indicator of the metabolic status of osteoblasts and bone formation.

These BTMs cannot indicate the risk for bone fracture nearly as well as a bone density measurement scan. These markers can be used to monitor the activity and treatment of Paget disease, hyperparathyroidism, and bone metastasis.

BTMs are normally high in children because of increased bone resorption associated with growth and remodeling of the ends of the long bones. The levels reach a peak at about age 14, and then gradually decline to adult values. Because estrogen is a strong inhibitor of osteoclastic (bone resorption) activity, loss of bone density begins soon after menopause begins. Marker levels therefore rise after menopause. Most urinary assays are correlated with creatinine excretion for normalization.

INTERFERING FACTORS

- Measurements of these urinary markers can differ by as much as 30% in one person even on the same day. Collecting double-voided specimens in the morning can minimize variability.
- Osteocalcin production is dependent on the availability of vitamins D, C, and K.
- ⚕ Drugs taken for bodybuilding treatments, such as testosterone, can cause *reduced* levels of NTx.

PROCEDURE AND PATIENT CARE

Before

- ✍ Explain the procedure to the patient. Tell the patient to fast 8 hours prior to testing.
- It is important to obtain baseline levels before instituting therapy.
- Note that some laboratories require a 24-hour urine collection.

During

Urine

- Preferably, obtain a double-voided specimen.
  1. Collect the urine specimen 30 to 40 minutes before the time the specimen is needed.
  2. Discard this first specimen.
  3. Give the patient a glass of water to drink.
  4. At the requested time, obtain a second specimen.

Blood

- Collect a venous blood sample in a red-top tube for NTx and/or a lavender- or green-top tube for osteocalcin. Check with laboratory for guidelines with other markers.

After

- Send the specimen to the laboratory for testing.

TEST RESULTS AND CLINICAL SIGNIFICANCE

▲ Increased Levels

Osteoporosis,
Paget disease,
Advanced bone tumors (primary or metastatic),
Acromegaly,
Hyperparathyroidism,
Hyperthyroidism,
Osteodystrophy:
  These diseases are associated with increase activity of osteoblasts and osteoclasts. These bone turnover markers are increased as a result of increased cellular function, increased bone matrix formation, or destruction.

▼ Decreased Levels

Hypoparathyroidism,
Hypothyroidism,
Cortisol therapy,
Effective antiresorptive therapy:
  These situations are associated with decreased activity of osteoblasts and osteoclasts.

RELATED TESTS

Bone Densitometry (p. 1002). This test measures the density of central and peripheral bones. It is a measure of bone mass.

Bone (Long) X-Rays (p. 1006). Plain films can identify advanced bone demineralization and indicate severe osteoporosis.

 Chloride, Urine (Cl)

NORMAL FINDINGS

Adult/elderly: 110-250 mEq/day or 110-250 mmol/day (SI units)
Child: 15-40 mmol/day
Infant: 2-10 mmol/day

INDICATIONS

This test is used with other urinary electrolytes to indicate the state of electrolyte or acid/base imbalance.

TEST EXPLANATION

Chloride is the major extracellular anion. Its main purpose is to maintain electrical neutrality, mostly as a salt with sodium. It follows sodium (cation) losses and accompanies sodium excesses to maintain electrical neutrality. For example, when aldosterone encourages sodium reabsorption, chloride follows to maintain electrical neutrality. Because water moves with sodium and chloride, chloride also affects water balance. Finally, chloride serves as a buffer to assist in acid-base balance. As carbon dioxide (and H cation) increases, bicarbonate must move from the intracellular space to the extracellular space. To maintain electrical neutrality, chloride shifts back into the cell.

A 24-hour urine collection for chloride is useful to evaluate the electrolyte composition of urine and to help determine acid-base imbalances. It is also useful to evaluate the effectiveness of diets with restricted salt (sodium chloride). If sodium and chloride levels are high, the patient is not complying with the diet.

INTERFERING FACTORS

- Urine volume and perspiration can affect chloride levels.
- Dietary salt intake or saline infusion affects urinary levels.
- Drugs that may cause *increased* levels include bromides, diuretics, and steroids.

PROCEDURE AND PATIENT CARE

Before
- Explain the procedure to the patient.
- Tell the patient that no special diet is required.

During
- See Box 11-2, Guidelines for 24-Hour Urine Collection, p. 907.

After

- Transport the urine specimen to the laboratory promptly.

TEST RESULTS AND CLINICAL SIGNIFICANCE

▲ Increased Levels

Dehydration,
Starvation,
Diuretic therapy,
Addison disease:
   Sodium (followed by chloride) reabsorption is decreased.
Increased salt intake,
Intravenous saline infusion:
   Output must equal input to maintain homeostasis. Therefore urinary chloride increases with increased intake.

▼ Decreased Levels

Cushing syndrome,
Conn syndrome,
Steroid therapy,
Congestive heart failure:
   Sodium (followed by chloride) reabsorption is increased.
Malabsorption syndrome,
Prolonged gastric suction or vomiting,
Diarrhea,
Pyloric obstruction,
Diaphoresis,
Reduced salt intake:
   Serum chloride levels are decreased. Therefore urinary chloride is decreased.

RELATED TESTS

Urinary Electrolytes (pp. 942, 946). These are measurements of sodium and potassium electrolytes.
Chloride, Blood (p. 152). This is a measurement of serum chloride level.

Cortisol, Urine (Hydrocortisone, Urine Cortisol, Free Cortisol)

NORMAL FINDINGS

Adult/elderly: <100 mcg/24 hr or <276 nmol/day (SI units)
Adolescent: 5-55 mcg/24 hr
Child: 2-27 mcg/24 hr

INDICATIONS

This test, a measure of urinary cortisol, is performed in patients with suspected hyperfunction or hypofunction of the adrenal gland.

TEST EXPLANATION

An elaborate feedback mechanism for cortisol exists to coordinate the function of the hypothalamus, pituitary gland, and adrenal glands. Corticotropin-releasing hormone (CRH) is made in the hypothalamus. This stimulates adrenocorticotropic hormone (ACTH) production in the anterior pituitary gland. ACTH, in turn, stimulates the adrenal cortex to produce cortisol. The rising levels of cortisol act as a negative feedback and curtail further production of CRH and ACTH. Free or unconjugated cortisol is filtered by the kidneys and excreted in the urine. Elevated urine levels reflect elevated serum cortisol levels.

Cortisol is a potent glucocorticoid released from the adrenal cortex. This hormone affects the metabolism of carbohydrates, proteins, and fats. It has an especially profound effect on glucose serum levels. Cortisol tends to increase glucose by stimulating gluconeogenesis from glucose stores. It also inhibits the effect of insulin and thereby inhibits glucose transport into the cells.

INTERFERING FACTORS

- Pregnancy causes increased cortisol levels.
- Physical and emotional stress can elevate cortisol levels.
- Stress is stimulatory to the pituitary-cortical mechanism, which thereby stimulates cortisol production.
- Drugs that may cause *increased* levels include danazol, hydrocortisone, oral contraceptives, and spironolactone.
- Drugs that may cause *decreased* levels include dexamethasone, ethacrynic acid, ketoconazole, and thiazides.

PROCEDURE AND PATIENT CARE

Before

- Explain the procedure to the patient.
- Assess the patient for signs of physical stress (e.g., infection, acute illness) or emotional stress, and report these to the physician.

During

- See Box 11-2, Guidelines for a 24-Hour Urine Collection, p. 907.

After

- Send the specimen to the laboratory promptly.

TEST RESULTS AND CLINICAL SIGNIFICANCE

▲ Increased Levels

Cushing disease,
Ectopic ACTH-producing tumors,
Stress:
   ACTH is overproduced as a result of neoplastic overproduction of ACTH in the pituitary gland or elsewhere in the body by an ACTH-producing cancer. Stress is a potent stimulus to ACTH production. Cortisol levels rise as a result.
Cushing syndrome (adrenal adenoma or carcinoma): *Neoplasm produces cortisol without regard to the normal feedback mechanism.*

Hyperthyroidism: *Metabolic rate is increased and cortisol levels rise accordingly to maintain elevated glucose needs.*

Obesity: *All sterols are increased in the obese, perhaps because fatty tissue may act as a depository or location of synthesis.*

▼ Decreased Levels

Adrenal hyperplasia: *Congenital absence of important enzymes in the synthesis of cortisol prevents adequate serum levels.*

Addison disease: *As a result of hypofunctioning of the adrenal gland, cortisol levels drop.*

Hypopituitarism: *ACTH is not produced by the pituitary gland destroyed by disease, neoplasm, or ischemia. The adrenal gland is not stimulated to produce cortisol.*

Hypothyroidism: *Normal cortisol levels are not required to maintain the reduced metabolic rate in patients with hypothyroidism.*

RELATED TESTS

Adrenocorticotropic Hormone Stimulation (p. 34). This test is used to evaluate the differential diagnosis of Cushing syndrome or Addison disease.

Adrenocorticotropic Hormone (p. 31). The serum ACTH study is a test of anterior pituitary gland function that affords the greatest insight into the causes of Cushing syndrome (overproduction of cortisol) and Addison disease (underproduction of cortisol).

Cortisol, Blood (p. 179). This is direct measurement of cortisol blood level.

Delta-Aminolevulinic Acid (Aminolevulinic Acid [ALA], δ-ALA)

NORMAL FINDINGS

1.5-7.5 mg/24 hr or 11-57 μmol/24 hr (SI units)

 Critical Values

>20 mg/24 hr

INDICATIONS

This test is used to diagnose porphyria, and in the evaluation of subclinical forms of lead poisoning in children.

TEST EXPLANATION

As the basic precursor for the porphyrins (p. 940), delta-ALA is needed for the normal production of porphobilinogen, which ultimately leads to heme synthesis in erythroid cells. Heme is used in the synthesis of hemoglobin. Genetic disorders (e.g., porphyria) are associated with lack of a particular enzyme vital to heme metabolism. These disorders are characterized by accumulation of porphyrin products in the liver or RBCs. The liver porphyrias are much more common. Symptoms of liver porphyrias include abdominal pain, neuromuscular signs and symptoms, constipation and, occasionally, psychotic behavior. This group of disorders results from enzymatic deficiency in synthesis of heme (a portion of hemoglobin). Acute intermittent porphyria (AIP) is the most common form of liver porphyria and is caused by a deficiency in uroporphyrinogen-1-synthase (also called porphobilinogen deaminase).

Most patients with AIP have no symptoms (latent phase) until the acute phase is precipitated by medication or some other factor (see Box 2-20, p. 517). The acute phase is characterized by abdominal and muscular pain, nausea, vomiting, hypertension, mental symptoms (e.g., anxiety, insomnia, hallucinations, paranoia), sensory loss, and urinary retention. Hemolytic anemia also may develop during the acute phase. These acute symptoms are associated with increased serum and urine levels of porphyrin precursors (aminolevulinic acid, porphyrins, and porphobilinogens).

In lead intoxication, heme synthesis is similarly diminished by the inhibition of ALA dehydrase. This enzyme assists in the conversion of ALA to porphobilinogen. As a result of lead poisoning, ALA accumulates in the blood and urine.

INTERFERING FACTORS

- Drugs that may cause *increased* ALA levels include barbiturates, griseofulvin, and penicillin (see also Box 2-20, p. 517).

PROCEDURE AND PATIENT CARE

Before
- Explain the procedure to the patient.

During
- See Box 11-2, Guidelines for a 24-Hour Urine Collection, p. 907.
- Keep the urine in a light-resistant container with a preservative.
- If the patient has a Foley catheter in place, cover the drainage bag to prevent exposure to light.
- Encourage the patient to drink fluids during the 24 hours unless contraindicated for medical reasons.

After
- Transport the urine specimen promptly to the laboratory.

TEST RESULTS AND CLINICAL SIGNIFICANCE

▲ Increased Levels

Porphyria (acute intermittent, variegate, and coproporphyria): *During the acute phase, porphyrin precursors (including ALA) accumulate in the blood and urine.*

Lead intoxication: *Chronic lead intoxication may be associated with increased ALA, which accumulates in the blood and urine.*

Chronic alcoholic liver disorders,
Diabetic ketoacidosis:
   These diseases are associated with increased ALA. The pathophysiology of these observations is complex and not well defined.

Related Tests

Uroporphyrinogen-1-Synthase (p. 516). This test is used to identify persons at risk for development of porphyria, and to diagnose porphyria in the acute and latent stages.

Porphyrins and Porphobilinogens, (p. 940). This is a quantitative measurement of porphyrins and porphobilinogen in the urine. Helps to define a porphyrin pattern that can classify the type of porphyria.

Glucose, Urine (Urine Sugar)

NORMAL FINDINGS

Random specimen: Negative
24-hour specimen: 50-300 mg/day or 0.3-1.7 mmol/day (SI units)

INDICATIONS

Testing for glucose in the urine is part of routine urinalysis. If present, it reflects the degree of glucose elevation in the blood. Urine glucose tests are also used to monitor the effectiveness of therapy for diabetes mellitus.

TEST EXPLANATION

A qualitative glucose test is part of routine urinalysis. This screening test for the presence of glucose within the urine may indicate the likelihood of diabetes mellitus or other causes of glucose intolerance (see Glucose, p. 253). This diagnosis must be confirmed by other tests (e.g., fasting glucose, glucose tolerance, glycosylated hemoglobin). Urine glucose tests may be used to monitor the effectiveness of diabetes therapy; however, today this is largely supplanted today by fingerstick determinations of blood glucose levels.

In patients with diabetes that is not well controlled with hypoglycemic agents, blood glucose levels can become very high. Normally, glucose is filtered from the blood by the glomeruli of the kidney. In the glomerular filtrate, the glucose concentration is the same as in the blood. Normally, all of the glucose is reabsorbed in the proximal renal tubules. When the blood glucose level exceeds the capability of the renal threshold to reabsorb the glucose (about 180 mg/dL), it begins to spill over into the urine (glycosuria). As the blood glucose level increases, the amount of glucose spilling into the urine also increases.

Glucosuria may occur immediately after eating a high-carbohydrate meal, and in patients with otherwise normal glucose levels or prediabetic patients receiving dextrose-containing intravenous (IV) fluids. Further, glucosuria does not always indicate diabetes but can occur normally or in diseases that affect the renal tubule or in genetic defects in metabolism and excretion of glucose. In these diseases, the renal threshold for glucose is abnormally low. Despite a normal blood glucose concentration, the kidney cannot reabsorb the normal glucose load. As a result, surplus glucose is spilled into the urine. In these patients, results of glucose tolerance tests are normal. Patients with acute severe physical stress or injury can have a transient glucosuria caused by normal compensatory endocrine-mediated responses.

INTERFERING FACTORS

- Any substance that can reduce copper in the Clinitest can produce false-positive results. This may include other sugars (e.g., galactose, fructose, lactose).
- Drugs that may cause *false-positive* results with reagent tablets (e.g., Clinitest) but not with enzyme-impregnated strips (Clinistix, Tes-Tape) include acetylsalicylic acid, aminosalicylic acid, ascorbic acid, cephalothin, chloral hydrate, nitrofurantoin, streptomycin, and sulfonamides.

🏃 Drugs that may cause *false-negative* tests include ascorbic acid (Clinistix, Tes-Tape), levodopa (Clinistix), and phenazopyridine (Clinistix, Tes-Tape).

🏃 Drugs that may *increase* urine glucose levels include aminosalicylic acid, cephalosporins, chloral hydrate, chloramphenicol, dextrothyroxine, diazoxide, diuretics (loop and thiazide), estrogen, glucose infusions, isoniazid, levodopa, lithium, nafcillin, nalidixic acid, and nicotinic acid (large doses).

PROCEDURE AND PATIENT CARE

Before

📖 Explain the procedure to the patient.
- Read the directions on the bottle or container of reagent strips.
- Check the expiration date on the bottle before use.

📖 Inform the patient that urine tests for glucose may be performed at specified times during the day, generally before meals and at bedtime, and that test results may be used to help determine insulin requirements.

During

- Because accuracy is necessary, collect a "fresh" urine specimen. Stagnant urine that has been in the bladder for several hours will not accurately reflect the serum glucose level at testing.
- Preferably, obtain a double-voided specimen by the following method:
  1. Collect a urine specimen 30 to 40 minutes before the time the urine specimen is actually needed.
  2. Discard this first specimen.
  3. Give the patient a glass of water to drink.
  4. At the required time, obtain a second specimen to be tested for glucose.

📖 Inform the patient that testing for glucose can be easily performed using enzyme tests such as Clinistix, Diastix, or Tes-Tape.

- If a 24-hour specimen is required, refrigerate the urine during the collection period. See Box 11-2, Guidelines for a 24-Hour Urine Collection, p. 907.

After

- If bedside or office testing is used, record the urine glucose level on the patient's chart.

TEST RESULTS AND CLINICAL SIGNIFICANCE

▲ Increased Levels

Diabetes mellitus and other causes of hyperglycemia

Pregnancy: *Glycosuria is common in pregnant women. Persistent and significantly high levels may indicate gestational diabetes or other obstetric illness. Also, lactosuria is common in nursing women. Lactose is a reducing substance that may cause false-positive results for glucose, depending on the method of testing.*

Renal glycosuria: *It can occur normally or in patients with diseases that affect the renal tubule. It can also result from genetic defects in the metabolism and excretion of glucose. In these diseases, the renal threshold for glucose is abnormally low. Despite a normal blood glucose level, the kidney cannot reabsorb the glucose it should. As a result, the surplus glucose is spilled into the urine.*

Fanconi syndrome: *Associated with transport defects in the proximal renal tubules, causing glycosuria, this genetic defect can also affect the metabolism and excretion of amino acids and electrolytes.*

Hereditary defects in metabolism of other reducing substances (e.g., galactose, fructose, pentose): *These reducing substances may cause false-positive tests for glucose, depending on the method of testing.*

11   Urine Studies

Increased intracranial pressure (e.g., from tumors, hemorrhage): *The pathophysiology for this observation is not well defined, although many theories exist.*

Nephrotoxic chemicals (e.g., carbon monoxide, mercury, lead): *These chemicals injure the kidney and lower the renal threshold.*

RELATED TESTS

Glucose (p. 253). This is the main screening test for diagnosis of diabetes.

Glycosylated Hemoglobin (p. 266). This is an accurate method for indicating glucose tolerance in the recent past.

Glucose Tolerance (p. 261). This is a test of a patient's capability to handle a glucose load.

Timed Postprandial Glucose (p. 257). This is a timed glucose measurement after a carbohydrate meal.

Glucagon (p. 251). This is a direct measurement of glucagon, which acts to increase glucose in the blood.

Insulin Assay (p. 315). This is a direct measurement of insulin, which acts to decrease glucose in the blood.

17-Hydroxycorticosteroids (17-OCHS)

NORMAL FINDINGS

Adult
    Male: 3-10 mg/24 hr or 8.3-27.6 µmol/day (SI units)
    Female: 2-8 mg/24 hr or 5.2-22.1 µmol/day (SI units)
Elderly: values slightly lower than for adult
Children
    Younger than 8 years: <1.5 mg/24 hr
    8-12 years: <4.5 mg/24 hr

INDICATIONS

This urine study is used to assess adrenocortical function by measuring the cortisol metabolites (17-OCHS) in a 24-hour urine collection.

TEST EXPLANATION

Elevated levels of 17-OCHS are noted in patients with adrenal hyperfunction (Cushing syndrome), whether the condition is caused by a pituitary or adrenal tumor, bilateral adrenal hyperplasia, or ectopic tumors producing adrenocorticotropic hormone (ACTH). Low levels of 17-OCHS are seen in patients with adrenal hypofunction (Addison disease) as a result of destruction of the adrenal glands (by hemorrhage, infarction, metastatic tumor, or autoimmunity), surgical removal of an adrenal gland without appropriate steroid replacement, congenital enzyme deficiency, hypopituitarism, or adrenal suppression after prolonged exogenous steroid ingestion.

Testing the urine for this hormone metabolite is an indirect measure of adrenal function. Urine and plasma levels of cortisol (see p. 920 and p. 179, respectively) provide a much more accurate measurement of adrenal function. Because excretion of cortisol metabolites follows a diurnal variation, 24-hour urine collection is necessary.

INTERFERING FACTORS

- Emotional and physical stress (e.g., infection) and licorice ingestion may cause increased adrenal activity.
- Drugs that may cause *increased* 17-OCHS levels include acetazolamide, chloral hydrate, chlorpromazine, colchicine, erythromycin, meprobamate, paraldehyde, quinidine, quinine, and spironolactone.
- Drugs that may cause *decreased* levels include estrogen, oral contraceptives, phenothiazines, and reserpine.

PROCEDURE AND PATIENT CARE

Before

- Explain the procedure to the patient.
- Note that drugs are usually withheld for several days before urine collection. Check with the physician and laboratory for specific guidelines.
- Assess the patient for signs of stress, and report these to the physician.

During

- Do not administer any drugs that may interfere with test results.
- See Box 11-2, Guidelines for a 24-Hour Urine Collection, p. 907.

After

- Send the urine to the chemistry laboratory as soon as the test is completed.

TEST RESULTS AND CLINICAL SIGNIFICANCE

▲ Increased Levels

Cushing disease,
Ectopic ACTH-producing tumors:
>   *Overproduction of ACTH results from ACTH-producing cancers in the pituitary gland or elsewhere in the body.*

Stress: *Stress is a potent stimulus to ACTH production. Cortisol and 17-OCHS levels rise as a result.*

Cushing syndrome (adrenal adenoma or carcinoma): *The neoplasm produces cortisol without regard to the normal feedback mechanism, and 17-OCHS levels rise.*

Hyperthyroidism: *Metabolic rate is increased, and cortisol and 17-OCHS levels rise accordingly to maintain the elevated glucose needs.*

Obesity: *All sterols are increased in obese patients, perhaps because fatty tissue acts as a depository or location of synthesis.*

▼ Decreased Levels

Adrenal hyperplasia (adrenogenital syndrome): *Congenital absence of important enzymes in the cortisol synthesis process prevents adequate serum and urine levels.*

Addison disease due to adrenal infarction, adrenal hemorrhage, surgical removal of the adrenal glands, congenital enzyme deficiency, or adrenal suppression from steroid therapy: *As a result of hypofunctioning of the adrenal gland, cortisol and 17-OCHS levels are decreased.*

Hypopituitarism: *ACTH is not produced by the pituitary gland destroyed by disease, neoplasm, or ischemia. The adrenal glands are not stimulated to produce cortisol and 17-OCHS.*

Hypothyroidism: *Normal cortisol levels are not required to maintain the reduced metabolic rate in patients with hypothyroidism. Cortisol and 17-OCHS levels are decreased.*

RELATED TEST

Cortisol, Blood (p. 179). This test is a measure of serum cortisol and is performed in patients with suspected adrenal gland hyperfunction or hypofunction.

5-Hydroxindoleacetic Acid (5-HIAA)

NORMAL FINDINGS

2-8 mg/24 hr or 10-40 µmol/day (SI units)
Concentrations in female patients are lower than in male patients.

INDICATIONS

This test is used to identify patients with carcinoid tumor and to monitor their therapy.

TEST EXPLANATION

Quantitative analysis of urine 5-HIAA is performed to detect and monitor the clinical course of carcinoid tumors. Carcinoid tumors are serotonin-secreting tumors that may grow in the appendix, intestine, lung, or any tissue derived from the neuroectoderm. These tumors contain argentaffin-staining (enteroendocrine) cells, which produce serotonin and other powerful neurohormones that are metabolized by the liver to 5-HIAA and excreted in the urine. These powerful neurohormones are responsible for the clinical symptoms (e.g., bronchospasm, flushing, diarrhea) of carcinoid syndrome. This test is used not only to identify carcinoid tumors but also to reevaluate known tumors by means of serial levels of urinary 5-HIAA. Increasing levels of 5-HIAA indicate progression of tumor; decreasing levels indicate a therapeutic response to antineoplastic therapy.

INTERFERING FACTORS

- Bananas, plantain, pineapple, kiwi, walnuts, plums, pecans, and avocados can factitiously elevate 5-HIAA levels.
- Drugs that may cause *increased* 5-HIAA levels include acetanilid, acetophenetidin, glyceryl guaiacolate, methocarbamol, acetaminophen, and reserpine.
- Drugs that may cause *decreased* levels include aspirin, chlorpromazine, ethyl alcohol, heparin, imipramine, isoniazid, levodopa, methenamine, methyldopa, monoamine oxidase (MAO) inhibitors, phenothiazines, promethazine, and tricyclic antidepressants.

PROCEDURE AND PATIENT CARE

Before

- Explain the procedure to the patient.
- Instruct the patient to refrain from eating foods containing serotonin (e.g., plums, pineapples, bananas, eggplant, tomatoes, avocados, walnuts) for several days (usually 3) before and during testing.

During

- See Box 11-2, Guidelines for a 24-Hour Urine Collection, p. 907.
- Keep the specimen on ice or in a refrigerator during the collection period. A preservative is needed to maintain an appropriate pH.

After

- Send the urine specimen to the laboratory promptly.

TEST RESULTS AND CLINICAL SIGNIFICANCE

▲ Increased Levels

Carcinoid tumor of the appendix, bowel, lung, breast, or ovary: *Serotonin is produced by the argentaffin-staining (enteroendocrine) cells within the tumor. The serotonin is metabolized by the liver to 5-HIAA, which is then excreted into the urine.*

Noncarcinoid illness,
Cystic fibrosis,
Intestinal malabsorption:
  These conditions may be associated with elevated 5-HIAA levels. The pathophysiology of these observations is not clear.

▼ Decreased Levels

Depression,
Migraine:
  Serotonin deficit has been noted in these illnesses. The cause is unknown.

17-Ketosteroid (17-KS)

NORMAL FINDINGS

Male: 6-20 mg/24 hr or 20-70 µmol/day (SI units)
Female: 6-17 mg/24 hr or 20-60 µmol/day (SI units)
Elderly: values decrease with age
Child:
  Younger than 12 years: <5 mg/24 hr
  12-15 years: 5-12 mg/24 hr

INDICATIONS

This urine test is performed to assist in evaluation of adrenal cortex function, especially as it relates to androgenic function. It is especially useful for evaluation and monitoring of adrenal hyperplasia (adrenogenital syndrome) and adrenal tumors.

TEST EXPLANATION

This urine test is used to measure adrenocortical function by measuring 17-ketosteroids (17-KSs) in the urine. 17-KSs are metabolites of testosterone and other androgenic sex hormones. The principal 17-KS is dehydroepiandrosterone (DHEA). In men, approximately one third of the hormone metabolites come from testosterone, produced in the testes, and two thirds come from other androgenic hormones, produced in the adrenal cortex. In women and children, almost all 17-KSs are nontestosterone androgenic hormones, produced in the adrenal cortex. Therefore this test is useful in diagnosing adrenocortical dysfunction. It is important to note that 17-KSs are not metabolites of cortisol and do not reflect levels of cortisol production. Elevated 17-KS levels are frequently noted in congenital adrenal hyperplasia and androgenic tumors of the adrenal glands. In these diseases, excess steroid synthesis is of the "noncortisol" androgenic sterols. These diseases frequently cause virilization syndromes. Testicular tumors rarely cause elevated 17-KS levels.

Low levels of 17-KSs have little clinical significance, because of the inaccuracy of determining low levels. The most common cause of low 17-KS levels is stress. During stress, the adrenal glands produce less androgen and more cortisol. In this regard, low 17-KS levels may reflect states of good health.

INTERFERING FACTORS

- Stress may decrease adrenal androgenic activity.
- Drugs that may cause *increased* 17-KS levels include antibiotics, chloramphenicol, chlorpromazine, dexamethasone, meprobamate, phenothiazines, quinidine, secobarbital, and spironolactone.
- Drugs that may cause *decreased* levels include estrogen, oral contraceptives, probenecid, promazine, reserpine, salicylates (prolonged use), and thiazide diuretics.

PROCEDURE AND PATIENT CARE

Before

- Explain the procedure to the patient.
- Withhold all drugs (with physician approval) for several days before the test.
- Assess the patient for signs of stress, and report these to the physician.

During

- See Box 11-2, Guidelines for a 24-Hour Urine Collection, p. 907.
- Encourage the patient to drink fluids during the 24 hours, unless contraindicated for medical reasons.
- This urine collection needs a preservative.
- Keep the collected urine on ice or refrigerated.

After

- Indicate on the laboratory slip the start and end times of the specimen collection.
- Send the specimen to the laboratory as soon as the test is completed.

TEST RESULTS AND CLINICAL SIGNIFICANCE

▲ Increased Levels

Congenital adrenal hyperplasia: *In congenital hyperplasia, an enzyme defect results in underproduction of cortisol. By the normal feedback mechanism, ACTH is maximally produced. The result is maximum noncortisol adrenal (androgenic) sterol production. Levels of 17-KS are therefore elevated. This often causes masculinizing syndrome in female patients and precocious puberty in male patients. Congenital adrenal hyperplasia is the most common cause of elevated 17-KS levels in children.*

Pregnancy: *Pregnancy is associated with slightly higher levels of androgens. 17-KS levels are therefore elevated.*

ACTH administration,

ACTH-secreting ectopic tumors,

Hyperpituitarism:

ACTH stimulates adrenal cortisol and, to a lesser degree, androgenic sterol production. 17-KS levels are therefore elevated in these three clinical situations.

Testosterone-secreting or androgenic-secreting tumors of the adrenal glands, ovaries, or testes: *These tumors are most often associated with elevated 17-KS levels in adults and can produce very high androgen levels. 17-KS levels also can be very high. Adrenal androgenic (mostly DHEA)–producing cancers or adenomas also can produce very high levels of 17-KS.*

Cushing syndrome: *17-KS production varies depending on the cause of adrenal overproduction.*

Stein-Leventhal syndrome: *This masculinizing syndrome is not well understood. Elevated 17-KS levels have been noted.*

▼   Decreased Levels

Severe debilitating disease,

Severe stress or infection,

Chronic disease:

In serious illness, the adrenal glands produce more cortisol and less androgenic hormone. 17-KS levels are therefore low.

Addison disease: *With diminished adrenal function, production of androgenic hormones is reduced. 17-KS levels are therefore low.*

Hypogonadism (Klinefelter syndrome),

Castration:

With reduced testosterone production, 17-KS levels are low.

Hypopituitarism: *Reduced production of ACTH reduces the activity of the adrenal cortex. 17-KS levels are therefore low.*

RELATED TEST

17-Hydroxycorticosteroids (p. 926). This urine test measures the metabolites of cortisol and function of the adrenal cortex.

Microalbumin (MA)

NORMAL FINDINGS

MA: <2 mg/L

MA/creatinine ratio:

    Males: <17 mg/g creatinine

    Females: <25 mg/g creatinine

INDICATION

This test is used as an indicator of complications (kidney, heart, or small vessels) of diabetes. Often it is the first indicator of renal disease.

Urine Studies

11

TEST EXPLANATION

Microalbuminuria refers to an albumin concentration in the urine that is greater than normal, but not detectable with routine protein testing. Normally, only small amounts of albumin are filtered through the renal glomeruli, and that small quantity can be reabsorbed by the renal tubules. However, when the increased glomerular permeability of albumin overcomes tubular reabsorption capability, albumin is spilled in the urine. Preceding this stage of a disease is a period where there is only a very small amount of albumin (microalbuminuria) that would normally go undetected. Therefore MA is an early indication of renal disease.

For the diabetic patient, the amount of albumin in the urine is related to duration of the disease and the degree of glycemic control. MA is the earliest indicator for the development of diabetic complications (nephropathy, cardiovascular disease [CVD], and hypertension). MA can identify diabetic nephropathy 5 years before routine protein urine tests. Diabetics with elevated MA have a 5- to 10-fold increase in the occurrence of CVD mortality, retinopathy, and end-stage kidney disease.

It is recommended that all diabetics older than the age of 12 be screened annually for MA. This can be done on a spot urine specimen using a semiquantitative Micral Urine Test Strip. If MA is present, the test should be repeated two more times. If two of three MA urine tests are positive, a quantitative measurement using a 24-hour urine specimen should be performed.

The presence of MA in nondiabetics is an early indicator of lower life expectancy because of CVD and hypertension. Nondiabetic nephropathies may also be associated with microalbuminuria. Life insurance underwriters are increasingly using MA testing to indicate life expectancy.

Because MA levels may be affected by hydration status, the MA/creatinine ratio can be calculated. This is obtained by determining the ratio of urinary microalbumin to urinary creatinine (an indicator of urine concentration). The ratio is calculated as follows:

$$\frac{\text{Microalbumin (mg/dL)}}{\text{Creatinine (mg/dL)}} \times 1000 \text{ mg/g}$$

INTERFERING FACTORS

- Urinary tract infection, blood, or acid-base abnormalities can cause elevated MA levels and falsely indicate more serious prognosis.
- Vigorous exercise or febrile illnesses may temporarily cause MA in the urine.
- Drugs that may interfere with test results include oxytetracycline.

PROCEDURE AND PATIENT CARE

Before

- Explain the procedure to the patient.
- Ensure that the patient does not have any acute infection or urinary bleeding that could cause a false-positive result.

During

- Collect a fresh urine specimen in a urine container.
- If the urine specimen contains vaginal discharge or bleeding, a clean-catch or midstream specimen will be needed (see p. 906).

- Ensure that the urine sample is at room temperature for testing.
- If using a Micral Urine Test Strip:
  1. Dip the test strip into the urine for 5 seconds.
  2. Allow the strip to dry for 1 minute.
  3. Compare the strip with the color scale on the label. The concentration of the red color is proportional to the amount of MA in the patient's sample.
- For quantification of MA, a 10-mL random sample or a portion of a 24-hour urine specimen is obtained. No preservative is used during the 24-hour collection.

After

- Transport the urine specimen to the laboratory promptly.
- If a 24-hour urine collection is requested, the specimen should be refrigerated. However, it will be warmed to room temperature before testing.

 If the results are positive, inform the patient that the test should be repeated in 1 week.

TEST RESULTS AND CLINICAL SIGNIFICANCE

▲   Increased Levels

Diabetes mellitus,
Myoglobinuria,
Hemoglobinuria,
Bence-Jones proteinuria,
Nephrotoxic drugs,
Nephropathy:
> *These diseases are associated with renal glomerular injury causing the permeability of albumin to exceed the reabsorption in the renal tubule.*

Atherosclerosis,
Lipid abnormalities,
Insulin resistance,
Hypertension,
Myocardial infarction:
> *These diseases also may be associated in some unknown way with increased renal glomerular permeability of albumin.*

Microglobulin (Beta-$_2$ Microglobulin [B$_2$M], Alpha 1 Microglobulin, and Retinol-Binding Protein)

NORMAL FINDINGS

Beta 2 microglobulin:
    Blood: 0.70-1.80 mcg/mL
    Urine: ≤300 mcg/L
    CSF: 0-2.4 mg/L
Alpha 1 microglobulin (urine):
    <50 years: <13 mg/g creatinine
    ≥50 years: <20 mg/g creatinine

Retinol-binding protein (RBP):
    Urine: <163 mcg/24 hours

INDICATIONS

This test is used to evaluate patients with malignancies, chronic infections, inflammatory diseases, and renal diseases.

TEST EXPLANATION

Beta-$_2$ microglobulin (B_2M) is a protein found on the surface of all cells. It is an HLA major histocompatibility antigen that exists in increased numbers on the cell surface and particularly on lymphatic cells. Production of this protein increases with cell turnover. B_2M is increased in patients with malignancies (especially B-cell lymphoma, leukemia, or multiple myeloma), chronic infections, and in patients with chronic severe inflammatory diseases. It is an accurate measurement of myeloma tumor disease activity, stage of disease, and prognosis and, as such, is an important tumor marker. This tumor marker is best determined in the blood.

B_2M, *alpha 1 microglobulin*, and *retinol-binding proteins* pass freely through glomerular membranes and are near completely reabsorbed by renal proximal tubules cells. Because of extensive tubular reabsorption, under normal conditions very little of these proteins appear in the final excreted urine. Therefore an increase in the urinary excretion of these proteins indicates proximal tubule disease or toxicity and/or impaired proximal tubular function. In patients with a urinary tract infection, these proteins indicate pyelonephritis. These proteins are helpful in differentiating glomerular from tubular renal disease. In patients with aminoglycoside toxicity, heavy metal nephrotoxicity, or tubular disease, protein urine levels are elevated. Excretion is increased 100 to 1000 times normal levels in cadmium-exposed workers. This test is used to monitor these workers. Periodic testing is performed on these patients to detect kidney disease at its earliest stage. To date, there are no convincing studies to indicate that one protein has better clinical utility than the other.

B_2M is particularly helpful in the differential diagnosis of renal disease. If blood and urine levels are obtained simultaneously, one can differentiate glomerular from tubular disease. In glomerular disease, because of poor glomerular filtration, blood levels are high and urine levels are low. In tubular disease, because of poor tubular reabsorption, the blood levels are low and urine levels are high. Blood levels increase early in kidney transplant rejection.

Urinary excretion of these proteins can be determined from either a 24-hour collection or from a random urine collection. The 24-hour collection is traditionally considered the gold standard. For random or spot collections, the concentration of alpha-1-microglobulin is divided by the urinary creatinine concentration. This corrected value adjusts alpha-1-microglobulin for variabilities in urine concentration.

Increased CSF levels of B_2M indicate central nervous system involvement with leukemia, lymphoma, HIV, or multiple sclerosis.

Quantitative chemiluminescent immunoassay or nephelometry methods are used to identify these proteins in the urine/serum.

INTERFERING FACTORS

- Results could be affected by recent nuclear imaging when B_2M testing is performed by radioimmunoassay.
- B_2M is unstable in acid urine.

PROCEDURE AND PATIENT CARE

Before

✍ Explain the procedure to the patient to minimize anxiety.

During

Blood

- Collect a venous blood sample in a red-top tube.

Urine

✍ See Box 11-2, Guidelines for a 24-Hour Collection, p. 907.

✍ Encourage the patient to drink fluids during the 24 hours unless this is contraindicated for medical purposes.

- If a single random urine collection is requested, collect specimen for protein and creatinine testing to adjust for urine concentration.

After

- Apply pressure to the venipuncture site.
- Send the urine collection to the laboratory

TEST RESULTS AND CLINICAL IMPLICATIONS

▲ Increased Urine Levels

Renal tubule disease,

Drug-induced renal toxicity,

Heavy metal–induced renal disease:

   In primary renal tubular disease, these proteins cannot be reabsorbed by the renal tubule. Thus they are elevated in excreted urine.

Lymphomas, leukemia, myeloma:

   In patients with advanced disease, glomerular filtration of these proteins exceeds the ability of renal tubules to reabsorb them. Thus they are elevated in excreted urine.

▲ Increased Serum Levels

Lymphomas, leukemia, myeloma,

Glomerular renal disease,

Renal transplant rejection:

   Glomerular filtration of these proteins is diminished and serum levels rise.

Viral infections, especially HIV and cytomegalovirus,

Chronic inflammatory processes:

   Inflammation is associated with increased cell turnover. Thus shedding increases levels of these proteins into the serum.

RELATED TESTS

Microalbumin (p. 931). Like the noted proteins, microalbumin is a marker for renal disease.

BUN (p. 511). This is a measure of renal function.

Creatinine (p. 190). This is a measure of renal function.

Nicotine and Metabolites (Nicotine, Cotinine, 3-Hydroxy-Cotinine, Nornicotine, Anabasine)

NORMAL FINDINGS
Urine

	Unexposed Non-Tobacco User (ng/mL)	Passive Exposure (Non–Tobacco User) (ng/mL)	Abstinent User for >2 Weeks (ng/mL)	Active Tobacco Product User (ng/mL)
Nicotine	<2	<20	<30	1000-5000
Cotinine	<5	<20	<50	1000-8000
3-OH-Cotinine	<50	<50	<120	3000-25,000
Nornicotine	<2	<2	<2	30-900
Anabasine	<3	<3	<3	3-500

Serum

	Unexposed Non-Tobacco User (ng/mL)	Passive Exposure (Non-Tobacco User) (ng/mL)	Abstinent User for >2 Weeks (ng/mL)	Active Tobacco Product User (ng/mL)
Nicotine	<2	<2	<2	30-50
Cotinine	<2	<8	<2	200-800
3-OH-Cotinine	<2	<2	<2	100-500

INDICATIONS

This test is used to document tobacco use. It is used to assess compliance with smoking cessation programs and qualify for surgical procedures. It is also used by insurance companies to determine if the applicant is a smoker.

TEST EXPLANATION

Nicotine is metabolized into cotinine and 3-hydroxy-cotinine which are measurable in urine and serum. The word "cotinine" is actually an anagram of "nicotine"—the eight letters are rearranged. In addition to nicotine and metabolites, tobacco products also contain other alkaloids (anabasine and nornicotine). The purpose of this testing is to differentiate patient tobacco use as the following:

- Active user
- Abstinent >2 weeks
- Passively exposed nonuser
- Unexposed nonuser

Cotinine and 3-hydroxy-cotinine have an in vivo half-life of approximately 20 hours, and are typically detectable from several days to up to 1 week after the use of tobacco. Because the level of these metabolites in the blood is proportionate to the amount of exposure to tobacco smoke, it is a valuable indicator of tobacco smoke exposure. Nicotine and its metabolites can be measured in the serum, urine, or other biofluids (most commonly the saliva). Cotinine is found in urine from 2 to 4 days after tobacco use. Serum/plasma testing is required when a valid urine specimen cannot be obtained (anuretic or dialysis patient) or to detect recent use (within the past 2 weeks). Blood cotinine will increase no matter how the tobacco is used (smoke, chew, dip, or snuff products). Nicotine levels have an in vivo half-life of approximately 2 hours, which is too short to be useful as a marker of smoking status.

Anabasine (only measured in the urine) is present in tobacco products, but not nicotine replacement therapies. Nicotine, cotinine, 3-hydroxy-cotinine, and nornicotine will also be elevated by the use of any of the nicotine replacement gum, patch, or pill products. The presence of anabasine >10 ng/mL or nornicotine >30 ng/mL in urine indicates current tobacco use, irrespective of whether the subject is on nicotine replacement therapy. The presence of nornicotine without anabasine is consistent with use of nicotine replacement products. Heavy tobacco users who abstain from tobacco for 2 weeks exhibit urine nicotine values <30 ng/mL, cotinine <50 ng/mL, anabasine <3 ng/mL, and nornicotine <2 ng/mL. Passive exposure to tobacco smoke can cause accumulation of nicotine metabolites in nontobacco users. Urine cotinine has been observed to accumulate up to 20 ng/mL from passive exposure. Neither anabasine nor nornicotine accumulates from passive exposure.

For smokers, another method of determining tobacco use is expired carbon monoxide. Again, a relatively short half-life (approximately 4 hours) limits the reliability and accuracy. Furthermore, carbon monoxide testing is unable to detect the use of smokeless tobacco.

Urine and salivary cotinine levels are less reliable. Nicotine and metabolite levels will vary by the amount of tobacco used, the use of a filter, the depth of the inhalation, and the size, gender, and weight of the person being tested. Because hydration status and renal function may affect urinary cotinine results, a spot urine cotinine test is always accompanied by a spot urine creatinine.

Quantification of urine nicotine and metabolites while a patient is actively using a tobacco product is useful to define the concentrations that a patient achieves through self-administration of tobacco. The nicotine replacement dose can then be tailored to achieve the same concentrations early in treatment to assure adequate nicotine replacement so the patient may avoid the strong craving he or she may experience early in the withdrawal phase.

Nicotine and metabolites can be accurately quantified with various laboratory methods, including high performance liquid chromatography, gas chromatography/mass spectroscopy, enzyme immunoassay (EIA), and enzyme-linked immunosorbent immunoassay (ELISA). Qualitative assays (including EIA and ELISA) are relatively easy to perform on urine and saliva, but are less accurate than the blood measurement. Absolute laboratory normal values may vary depending on the method of testing.

INTERFERING FACTORS

- Menthol cigarettes may increase cotinine levels because the menthol retains cotinine in the blood for a longer period of time.
- Diluted/adulterated urine may alter results

PROCEDURE AND PATIENT CARE

Before

✍ Explain the procedure to the patient and indicate the type of specimen needed.
- Obtain an accurate history of recent tobacco use.

During

Blood
- Collect venous blood in a red-top, lavender-top (EDTA), or pink-top (K_2 EDTA) tube.

Urine

- Obtain a random spot urine specimen of at least 5 mL.
- Immediately transport the specimen to the laboratory.

Saliva

- Ask the patient to spit at least 1 mL of saliva into a spit container.
- Alternatively, dental gauze rolls can be placed in the mouth for 15 minutes and then placed in a storage container for transport.

After

- Keep the specimens in a cool place if they cannot be transported to the laboratory immediately.

TEST RESULTS AND CLINICAL SIGNIFICANCE

Tobacco exposure: *With even minimal tobacco use, nicotine and metabolite levels will be elevated.*

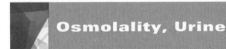

Osmolality, Urine

NORMAL FINDINGS

12- to 14-hour fluid restriction: >850 mOsm/kg H_2O (SI units)
Random specimen: 50-1200 mOsm/kg H_2O or 50-1200 mmol/kg (SI units), depending on fluid intake

INDICATIONS

This test is used to evaluate fluid and electrolyte abnormalities. It is an accurate determination of the kidney's concentrating capabilities. It is also used to investigate antidiuretic hormone (ADH) abnormalities (e.g., diabetes insipidus) and the syndrome of inappropriate ADH (SIADH) secretion.

TEST EXPLANATION

Osmolality is the measurement of the number of dissolved particles in a solution. It is a more exact measurement of urine concentration than specific gravity because specific gravity depends on the number and precise nature of the particles in the urine. Specific gravity also requires correction for the presence of glucose or protein, as well as for temperature; in contrast, osmolality depends only on the number of particles of solute in a unit of solution. Osmolality also can be measured over a wider range than specific gravity and with greater accuracy.

Osmolality is used in the precise evaluation of the concentrating and diluting abilities of the kidney. With normal fluid intake and normal diet, a patient will produce urine of about 500 to 850 mOsm/kg water. The normal kidney can concentrate urine to 800 to 1400 mOsm/kg. With excess fluid intake, a minimal osmolality of 40 to 80 mOsm/kg can be obtained. With dehydration, the urine osmolality should be three to four times the plasma osmolality.

Osmolality is used in the evaluation of kidney function and the ability to excrete ammonium salts. Osmolality may be used as part of the urinalysis when the patient has glycosuria or proteinuria or has had tests that use radiopaque substances. In these situations, the *urine osmolar gap* increases because of other organic osmolar particles. The urine osmolar gap is the sum of all the particles predicted or calculated to be in the urine (electrolytes, urea, and glucose) compared with the actual measurement of the osmolality. The predicted/calculated urine osmolality can then be determined by urine levels of sodium, potassium, glucose, and urea nitrogen:

$$\text{Calculated urine osmolality} = 2 \times ([Na + K]) + [Urea\ nitrogen]/2.8 + [Glucose]/18$$

Normally the osmolar gap is 80 to 100 mOsm/kg of H_2O. The urine osmolality is more easily interpreted when the serum osmolality (see p. 378) is simultaneously performed. More information concerning the state of renal water handling or abnormalities of urine dilution or concentration can be obtained if urinary osmolality is compared with serum osmolality and urine electrolyte studies are performed. Normally the ratio of urine osmolality to serum osmolality is 1.0 to 3.0, reflecting a wide range of urine osmolality.

✔ Clinical Priorities

- This test provides valuable information about fluid and electrolyte abnormalities.
- Urine osmolality is a more exact measure of urine concentration than is specific gravity.
- Urine osmolality is more easily interpreted when the serum osmolality is also measured.

PROCEDURE AND PATIENT CARE

Before

 Explain the procedure to the patient.

🖊 Tell the patient that no special preparation is necessary for a random urine specimen.

🖊 Inform the patient that preparation for a fasting urine specimen may require ingestion of a high-protein diet for 3 days before the test.

🖊 Instruct the patient to eat a dry supper the evening before the test and to drink no fluids until the test is completed the next morning.

During

- Preferably collect a first-voided urine specimen for a random sample.
- Indicate on the laboratory slip the patient's fasting status.

After

- Send the specimen to the laboratory.
- Provide food and fluids for the patient.

TEST RESULTS AND CLINICAL SIGNIFICANCE

▲ Increased Levels

Syndrome of inappropriate antidiuretic hormone (SIADH) secretion: *Several illnesses can produce SIADH secretion. ADH is inappropriately secreted despite factors that normally would inhibit its secretion. As a result, large quantities of water are reabsorbed by the kidney. Less free water is excreted, and the urine osmolality rises.*

Paraneoplastic syndromes associated with carcinoma (e.g., lung, breast, colon): *These cancers act as an autonomous ectopic source for secretion of ADH. The pathophysiology is the same as is described for SIADH.*

Shock: *The normal physiologic response to shock is to minimize the loss of free body water. The kidneys therefore absorb all the free water possible. Urine osmolality rises.*

Hepatic cirrhosis,
Congestive heart failure:
    These illnesses are associated with water retention because of reduced perfusion of the kidneys. Less free body water is excreted, and urine osmolality rises.

▼ Decreased Levels

Diabetes insipidus: *Insufficient secretion of ADH despite physiologic stimulation by increased serum osmolality diminishes the kidneys' capability to concentrate urine. Urine osmolality decreases.*
Excess fluid intake: *Free water overload is excreted into the urine. Urine osmolality decreases.*
Renal tubular necrosis,
Severe pyelonephritis:
    The concentrating capability of the kidneys is reduced. Excess free water is excreted. Urine osmolality decreases.

RELATED TESTS

Serum Osmolality (p. 378). This is a measurement of osmolality of the serum. When combined with urine osmolality, more accurate interpretation of either test is possible.
Antidiuretic Hormone (p. 73). This provides a direct measurement of ADH in the blood.
Antidiuretic Hormone Suppression (p. 76). This test is helpful in evaluation of ADH abnormalities.

Porphyrins and Porphobilinogens (Uroporphyrins, Coproporphyrin, Free Erythrocyte Protoporphyrin [FEP])

NORMAL FINDINGS

Total porphyrins (mcg/24 hr):
    Male: 8-149
    Female: 3-78
Uroporphyrin (mcg/24 hr):
    Male: 4-46
    Female: 3-22
Coproporphyrin (mcg/24 hr):
    Male: <96
    Female: <60
Porphobilinogens: 0-2 mg/24 hr or 0-8.8 μmol/day (SI units)

INDICATIONS

This test is a quantitative measurement of porphyrins and porphobilinogen. It is used along with aminolevulinic acid (ALA) to identify the various forms of porphyria.

TEST EXPLANATION

Porphyria is a group of genetic disorders associated with enzyme deficiencies involved with porphyrin synthesis or metabolism. Porphyrins (e.g., uroporphyrin, coproporphyrin) and porphobilinogens are important building blocks in the synthesis of heme. Heme is incorporated into hemoglobin within the erythroid cells. Porphyrias are classified according to location of the accumulation of the porphyrin precursors. In most forms of porphyria, increased levels of porphyrins and porphobilinogen are found in the urine. Heavy metal (lead) intoxication is also associated with increased porphyrins in the urine.

Variable symptoms are associated with different types of porphyrias. Erythropoietic porphyria is associated with photosensitivity of the eyes and skin. Intermittent porphyria and, less often, variegate and hereditary coproporphyria are associated with abdominal pain and neurologic symptoms. Heavy metal (e.g., lead) intoxication is also associated with increased porphyrins in the urine. Certain drugs can induce porphyria and cause elevated porphyrin levels in the urine (see Box 2-20, p. 517). This test is a quantitative analysis of urinary porphyrins and porphobilinogens. If porphyrins are present, the urine may be colored amber red or burgundy, or even darker after standing in the light.

Urine tests for porphyrins are not as accurate as plasma measurements and pattern identification for the various forms of porphyria. They are accurate, however, in screening for porphyria, especially the intermittent variety. Porphyrin fractionation of erythrocytes and of plasma provides specific assays for primary red blood cell (RBC) porphyrins. These assays are predominantly used to differentiate the various forms of congenital porphyrias. Plasma measurement of *free erythrocyte protoporphyrin (FEP)* is helpful in the diagnosis of iron deficiency anemia or lead intoxication. In these latter diseases, a small amount of excess porphyrin remains in the RBC after heme synthesis. This is measured as FEP.

Although this test can also be done on a fresh stool specimen, random and 24-hour urine collections are more accurate. Colorimetric methods (or spectrophotometry) are used most often. *Porphyrin fractionation* of the various types of porphyrins within the urine allows identification of patterns commonly associated with the various porphyrias. High-performance liquid chromatography is used for that. The diagnosis of porphyria and interpretation of test results are difficult. The American Porphyria Foundation can provide assistance to health care providers in this area.

INTERFERING FACTORS

☖ Drugs that may alter test results include aminosalicylic acid, barbiturates, chloral hydrate, chlorpropamide, ethyl alcohol, griseofulvin, morphine, oral contraceptives, phenazopyridine, procaine, and sulfonamides (see also Box 2-20, p. 517).

PROCEDURE AND PATIENT CARE

Before
✗ Explain the procedure to the patient.
✗ Tell the patient that no fasting is required.

During
Porphobilinogens
- Collect a freshly voided urine specimen.
- Protect the specimen from light.

Porphyrins
- See Box 11-2, Guidelines for a 24-Hour Urine Collection, p. 907.
✗ Instruct the patient to avoid alcohol use during the collection period.
- Keep the specimen on ice or refrigerated during the 24 hours.
- Keep the urine in a light-resistant specimen bottle with a preservative to prevent degradation of the light-sensitive porphyrin.
✗ Encourage the patient to drink fluids during the 24 hours unless contraindicated for medical reasons.

After

- Transport the urine specimen to the laboratory promptly.

TEST RESULTS AND CLINICAL SIGNIFICANCE

▲ Increased Levels

Porphyrias

Acute intermittent porphyria: *Porphobilinogen and to a lesser degree porphyrin levels are elevated during the acute phase. No real increase is noted during the latent phases.*

Congenital erythropoietic porphyria: *Porphobilinogen level is elevated.*

Hereditary coproporphyria: *Coproporphyrin and porphobilinogen levels are elevated.*

Variegate porphyria: *In acute episodes, porphobilinogen and ALA (p. 922) levels are elevated.*

Lead poisoning: *ALA level is most significantly elevated; porphyrin levels are slightly elevated.*

RELATED TESTS

Uroporphyrinogen-1-Synthase (p. 516). Used to identify persons at risk for development of porphyria, and to diagnose porphyria in the acute and latent stages.

Delta-Aminolevulinic Acid (p. 922). Used to diagnose porphyria and in evaluation of children with subclinical forms of lead poisoning.

 Potassium, Urine (K)

NORMAL FINDINGS

25-100 mEq/L/day or 25-100 mmol/day (SI units). Values vary greatly with diet.

INDICATIONS

This test measures the amount of potassium in a spot or 24-hour urine collection to aid in determining electrolyte balance.

TEST EXPLANATION

Potassium is the major cation within the cell. The electrolyte balance of potassium can be measured in a spot or a 24-hour urine collection. A 24-hour collection is essential to evaluate electrolyte (especially hypokalemia) balance, acid-base balance, and renal and adrenal diseases.

The serum potassium concentration depends on many factors. Aldosterone, and to a lesser extent glucocorticosteroids, tends to increase renal losses of potassium. If sodium blood levels are diminished, the renal tubules can reabsorb sodium in exchange for potassium, which is then excreted at increased rates. Acid-base balance depends to a small degree on potassium excretion. In alkalotic states, hydrogen can be reabsorbed in exchange for potassium. The kidneys cannot reabsorb potassium. Therefore potassium intake is balanced by kidney excretion through the urine.

INTERFERING FACTORS

- Dietary intake affects potassium levels.

- Excessive intake of licorice may cause increased levels of potassium in the urine because licorice acts like aldosterone and increases potassium excretion.
- Drugs that may cause increased levels include diuretics, glucocorticoids, and salicylates.

PROCEDURE AND PATIENT CARE

Before

- Explain the procedure to the patient.
- Tell the patient that no special diet is required.

During

- See Box 11-2, Guidelines for a 24-Hour Urine Collection, p. 907.
- Encourage the patient to drink fluids during the 24 hours.

After

- Transport the urine specimen promptly to the laboratory.

TEST RESULTS AND CLINICAL SIGNIFICANCE

▲ Increased Levels

Chronic renal failure: *Sodium loss is increased in some forms of renal failure because of loss of reabsorptive capabilities of the kidneys. Potassium follows sodium loss.*

Renal tubular acidosis: *Reduced excretion of hydrogen increases excretion of potassium.*

Starvation: *To provide energy, protein- and fat-containing tissues are broken down. The cells in those tissues expel potassium into the bloodstream. The potassium is then excreted, at increased levels, into the urine.*

Cushing syndrome,
Hyperaldosteronism:
   Aldosterone increases potassium urinary excretion. Because glucocorticosteroids have an aldosterone-like effect, potassium excretion is also increased in Cushing syndrome.

Excessive intake of licorice: *Licorice has an aldosterone-like effect, as described above.*

Alkalosis: *Hydrogen is reabsorbed in the renal tubules in exchange for potassium excretion.*

Diuretic therapy: *Most diuretics are potassium wasting and increase potassium urinary excretion.*

▼ Decreased Levels

Dehydration: *Decreased renal blood flow associated with dehydration diminishes urinary excretion of potassium.*

Addison disease: *This disease is associated with diminished aldosterone effect on the kidneys. Because aldosterone increases urinary excretion of potassium, reduced levels of aldosterone are associated with reduced urinary potassium levels.*

Malnutrition,
Vomiting,
Diarrhea,
Malabsorption:
   Diminished intake of potassium is matched by diminishing urinary excretion of potassium.

Acute renal failure: *Urinary excretion of potassium is diminished. This is the most common cause of hyperkalemia.*

RELATED TESTS

Sodium, Urine (p. 946). These electrolytes are often measured with potassium. Metabolically, they are intermingled.

Potassium, Urine (p. 942). Direct measurement of potassium in serum.

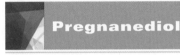
Pregnanediol

NORMAL FINDINGS

Younger than 2 years: <0.1 mg/day
Younger than 9 years: <0.5 mg/day
10-15 years: 0.1-1.2 mg/day
Adult male: 0-1.9 mg/day
Adult female
    Follicular phase: <2.6 mg/day
    Luteal phase: 2.6-10.6 mg/day
    Pregnancy
        First trimester: 10-35 mg/day
        Second trimester: 35-70 mg/day
        Third trimester: 70-100 mg/day

INDICATIONS

This test measures pregnanediol, a metabolite of progesterone. It is used in the evaluation and decision making in women who are having difficulty becoming pregnant or maintaining a pregnancy. It is also used to monitor "high-risk" pregnancies.

TEST EXPLANATION

Urinary pregnanediol is measured to evaluate progesterone production by the ovaries and placenta. The main effect of progesterone is on the endometrium. It initiates the secretory phase of the endometrium in anticipation of implantation of a fertilized ovum. Normally, progesterone is secreted by the ovarian corpus luteum after ovulation. Both serum progesterone levels and urine concentration of progesterone metabolites (pregnanediol and others) are significantly increased during the second half of an ovulatory cycle. Pregnanediol is the most easily measured metabolite of progesterone.

Because pregnanediol levels rise rapidly after ovulation, this study is useful in documenting whether ovulation has occurred and, if so, exactly when. During pregnancy, pregnanediol levels normally rise because of placental production of progesterone. Repeated assays can be used to monitor the status of the placenta in women who have difficulty becoming pregnant or maintaining a pregnancy. Repeated assays can also be used to monitor the status of the placenta in high-risk pregnancy.

Hormone assays for urinary pregnanediol are primarily used to monitor progesterone supplementation in patients with an inadequate luteal phase to maintain an early pregnancy. Urinary assays may be supplemented by plasma assays (progesterone assay, p. 750), which are quicker and more accurate.

INTERFERING FACTORS

▮ Drugs that may cause *increased* levels include adrenocorticotropic hormone (ACTH).
▮ Drugs that may cause *decreased* levels include oral contraceptives and progesterone.

PROCEDURE AND PATIENT CARE

Before

✗ Explain the procedure to the patient.
✗ Tell the patient that usually no special diet is required.
✗ Inform the patient that no sedation or fasting is necessary.

During

- See Box 11-2, Guidelines for a 24-Hour Urine Collection, p. 907.
- Keep the specimen on ice or refrigerated during the 24 hours.
- Check with the laboratory to see if a preservative is needed.

✗ Encourage the patient to drink fluids during the 24 hours.

After

- Record on the laboratory slip the date of the last menstrual period or the week of gestation during pregnancy.

TEST RESULTS AND CLINICAL SIGNIFICANCE

▲ Increased Levels

Ovulation: *Ovulation occurs with development of a corpus luteum, which makes progesterone. Pregnanediol is a metabolite of progesterone.*
Pregnancy: *A healthy placenta produces progesterone. Pregnanediol is a metabolite of progesterone.*
Molar pregnancy: *Hydatidiform mole can produce progesterone, although at lower levels than during pregnancy.*
Luteal cysts of ovary: *The corpus luteum produces progesterone in the nonpregnant woman and in the early stages of pregnancy. Cysts can also produce progesterone for prolonged periods of time. Pregnanediol is a metabolite of progesterone.*
Arrhenoblastoma of ovary: *This tumor can secrete sex hormones or their metabolites (usually testosterone). 17-Hydroxyprogesterone is a precursor of sex hormones. Pregnanediol is a metabolite of progesterone.*
Hyperadrenocorticism,
Adrenocortical hyperplasia:
   Adrenal cortical hormones are secreted at increased rates. 17-Hydroxyprogesterone is a precursor of these cortical hormones. Pregnanediol is a metabolite of progesterone.
Choriocarcinoma of ovary: *This tumor produces progesterone.*

▼ Decreased Levels

Preeclampsia,
Toxemia of pregnancy,
Threatened abortion,
Placental failure,

Fetal death:

> *These obstetrical emergencies are associated with decreased placental viability. Progesterone is made by the placenta during pregnancy. Pregnanediol is a metabolite of progesterone, which is decreased when placental viability is threatened.*

Ovarian neoplasm: *Ovarian epithelial cancers can destroy functional ovarian tissue. Progesterone levels may decrease.*

Amenorrhea,

Ovarian hypofunction:

> *Without ovulation, a corpus luteum will not develop. Progesterone will not be secreted, and progesterone and pregnanediol levels will be lower than expected.*

RELATED TEST

Progesterone Receptor Assay (p. 750). Direct measurements of progesterone in serum.

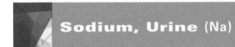

Sodium, Urine (Na)

NORMAL FINDINGS

24-hour collection: 40-220 mEq/day or 40-220 mmol/day (SI units)
Spot urine collection: >20 mEq/L
Fractional excretion (FE_{Na}): 1%-2%

INDICATIONS

This test is used to evaluate fluid and electrolyte abnormalities, especially sodium. It can also be used to monitor therapy for these abnormalities.

TEST EXPLANATION

Many factors regulate sodium balance. Aldosterone causes conservation of sodium by stimulating the kidneys to reabsorb sodium, thus decreasing renal losses. Natriuretic hormone, or third factor, is stimulated by increased sodium levels. This hormone decreases renal absorption and increases renal losses of sodium. Antidiuretic hormone (ADH), which controls the reabsorption of water at the distal tubules of the kidney, affects sodium urine levels by dilution or concentration.

This test evaluates sodium balance in the body by determining the amount of sodium excreted in urine over 24 hours. Sodium is the major cation in the extracellular space. Measuring the amount of sodium in the urine is useful for evaluating patients with volume depletion, acute renal failure, adrenal disturbances, and acid-base imbalances. In the setting of acute renal failure, an increased value will indicate acute tubular necrosis, while a low value would be typical of pre-renal azotemia.

This test is also useful when the serum sodium concentration is low. For example, in patients with hyponatremia caused by inadequate sodium intake, urine sodium will be low. However, in patients with hyponatremia caused by chronic renal failure, urine sodium concentration will be high.

Urine sodium excretions are helpful when the urine output is low (<500 mL/24 hr). However, a more accurate test to determine the cause of reduced urine output is the *fractional excretion of sodium* (FE_{Na}). This is the fraction of sodium actually excreted relative to the amount filtered by the kidney.

FE_{Na} is a calculation based on the concentrations of sodium (Na) and creatinine (Cr) in the plasma and the urine as follows:

$$\text{Fractional excretion of sodium } (FE_{Na}) = \frac{U_{Na} \times P_{Cr}}{P_{Na} \times U_{Cr}} \times 100$$

FE_{Na} is usually greater than 3% with acute tubular necrosis and severe obstruction of the urinary drainage of both kidneys. It is generally less than 1% in patients with acute glomerulonephritis, hepatorenal syndrome, and states of prerenal azotemia (such as congestive heart failure and dehydration). FE_{Na} can also be less than 1% with acute partial urinary tract obstruction.

INTERFERING FACTORS

- Dietary salt intake may increase sodium levels.
- Altered kidney function may affect levels.
- Drugs that may cause *increased* urine sodium levels include antibiotics, diuretics, and prostaglandins.
- Drugs that may cause *decreased* urine levels of sodium includes nonsteroidal antiinflammatory drugs (NSAIDs) and steroids.

PROCEDURE AND PATIENT CARE

Before

- Explain the procedure to the patient.
- Tell the patient that no fasting is required.

During

- See Box 11-2, Guidelines for a 24-Hour Urine Collection, p. 907.
- A spot urine specimen can be obtained and sent to the laboratory if information about urine sodium is needed sooner than 24 hours. In this situation, ask the patient to void in a nonsterile container, and transport the entire volume to the laboratory. The more urine available, the more accurately the spot urine specimen will reflect the 24-hour urine results.
- If FE_{Na} is ordered, venous blood is drawn in a gold-top tube for serum creatinine and sodium measurement.

After

- Transport the urine specimen promptly to the laboratory.

TEST RESULTS AND CLINICAL SIGNIFICANCE

▲ Increased Levels

Dehydration: *Free water is maximally reabsorbed by the kidney, and urine sodium is more concentrated.*

Adrenocortical insufficiency: *Aldosterone and corticosteroids stimulate sodium reabsorption in the distal renal tubules. With inadequate levels of these hormones, sodium will not be reabsorbed, and large amounts are wasted into the urine.*

Diuretic therapy: *Most diuretics work by diminishing sodium reabsorption and increasing sodium loss in the kidney.*

Syndrome of inappropriate antidiuretic hormone secretion (SIADH): *ADH stimulates free water reabsorption in the kidney. With inappropriately high secretion of ADH, free water in the urine is diminished and sodium is more concentrated.*

Diabetic ketoacidosis: *The osmotic diuresis due to hyperglycemia tends to diminish sodium reabsorption in the kidney. Further, sodium salts combine with some ketotic products to further increase sodium losses into the urine.*

Chronic renal failure: *Renal reabsorption of sodium and many other products is diminished in a diseased, nonfunctioning kidney. Urine sodium levels increase.*

▼ Decreased Levels

Congestive heart failure: *Renal blood flow is diminished with reduced cardiac output. The renin-angiotensin system is activated (see pp. 447 to 448), and aldosterone production is stimulated. Aldosterone stimulates renal reabsorption of sodium, and urine levels diminish.*

Malabsorption,

Diarrhea:

   Intestinal absorption of sodium is reduced. The physiologic response is to reduce sodium excretion in the urine.

Cushing disease: *Corticosteroids have an aldosterone-like effect on the kidney, which tends to stimulate renal reabsorption of sodium, and urine levels diminish.*

Aldosteronism: *Aldosterone stimulates renal reabsorption of sodium, and urine levels diminish.*

Inadequate sodium intake: *Intestinal absorption of sodium is very efficient. Therefore it is rare for a nutritional deficiency to occur as sodium insufficiency severe enough to significantly diminish renal excretion. However, with sodium deficit or ongoing sodium losses treated with inadequate sodium replacement, serum sodium levels significantly diminish and the kidneys are maximally stimulated to reabsorb sodium. Urine sodium levels diminish.*

RELATED TESTS

Sodium, Blood (p. 466). This is a direct measurement of sodium levels in blood.

Aldosterone (p. 43). More than any other hormone, aldosterone has a significant effect on blood sodium levels.

Antidiuretic Hormone (p. 73). By affecting free body water excretion, ADH alters sodium levels by virtue of dilution or concentration.

Substance Abuse Testing (Urine Drug Testing, Drug Screening)

NORMAL FINDINGS

Negative

INDICATIONS

Substance abuse testing is used to identify metabolites of illegal drugs used by the person being tested.

TEST EXPLANATION

Drug testing is mostly used by employers and by law enforcement agencies. Employers primarily use drug testing to promote and protect the safety, health, and well-being of their employees. Because many industrial fatalities are attributable to substance abuse, drug-testing programs are common in the workplace. Furthermore, drug use is responsible for decreased productivity and increased absenteeism. Industrial testing is used at the time of preemployment, prepromotion, annual physical, postaccident, or when there is reasonable suspicion. Other times include random testing or for follow-up surveillance of treatment.

Most commonly, a drug screen is performed to detect small amounts of any number of metabolites of commonly used drugs. If the screen result is positive, a more accurate and quantitative test is performed on the same specimen. Drug screens are available for a variety of substances. The most common are amphetamines, barbiturates, benzodiazepines, carisoprodol, cocaine, meprobamate, methamphetamine, opiates (morphine and heroin), cannabinoids (marijuana [tetrahydrocannabinol {THC}]), phencyclidine (PCP), and propoxyphene (Table 11-1). Alcohol testing is most commonly used by law enforcement (see p. 229). Not only is drug testing helpful in identifying users, but it also acts as a deterrent. Athletes are tested for anabolic hormones, stimulants, diuretics, beta blockers, street drugs, anti-estrogens, erythropoietin, and beta-2 agonists that may unfairly improve their performance. Health and life insurance companies routinely test for illicit drugs.

Substance abuse testing, up until recently, has used urine exclusively as the sample of choice. Urine is easily obtained and plentiful, and it contains a large amount of drug and metabolites. More importantly, urine can identify drug usage for several days after the last usage. THC can be identified in the urine for several weeks in chronic users. Blood testing reflects drug usage only during the past few hours. Saliva, breath, hair, and sweat are becoming increasingly important and accurate samples for specific drug testing. These testing methods are very expensive, however. Hair samples detect the presence of drugs used during the past 3 months. In addition, hair and nail samples may be used to detect or document exposure to arsenic and mercury. Nevertheless, urine testing remains the mainstay for drug testing (Figure 11-1).

TABLE 11-1 Typical Multipanel Drug Screen		
Drugs/Drug Classes	**Screen**	**Confirmation***
Marijuana	20 ng/mL	5 ng/mL
Cocaine	150 ng/mL	50 ng/mL
Opiates	300 ng/mL	5 ng/mL
Oxycodone	100 ng/mL	5 ng/mL
Phencyclidine	25 ng/mL	10 ng/mL
Amphetamines	300 ng/mL	200 ng/mL
MDMA (Ecstasy)	500 ng/mL	200 ng/mL
Barbiturates	200 ng/mL	50 ng/mL
Benzodiazepines	200 ng/mL	20 ng/mL
Methadone	150 ng/mL	10 ng/mL
Propoxyphene	300 ng/mL	10 g/mL

*Confirmatory tests are more sensitive and can detect metabolites at lower levels.

Urine Studies

11

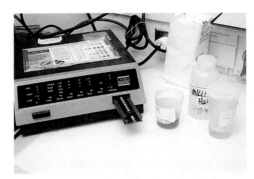

Figure 11-1 Urine sample tested for chemical substance abuse using a chemistry instrument.

The absence of an expected drug(s) and/or drug metabolite(s) may indicate compliance or a difficulty in identifying the substance because of inappropriate timing of specimen collection relative to drug administration, poor drug absorption, diluted/adulterated urine, or limitations of testing. The concentration at which the screening test can detect a drug or metabolite varies within a drug class.

Toxicology screening tests for drug overdose (see Table 2-19 on p. 213) and poisoning (e.g., lead and carbon monoxide, see Table 11-2 on p. 952) are best performed on blood. Results indicate current drug levels, which are used to determine or alter therapy. Toxicology studies are used to incriminate drugs as a cause or factor in the death of a person. They are also used to assess patients when poisoning contributes to an illness.

Substance abuse testing can be ordered as the "drug abuse survey" that is an immunoassay to identify drugs of abuse by class (e.g., amphetamines, barbiturates, benzodiazepines). This testing is directed toward the patient's symptoms or medication history. The results are considered presumptive only. There is high cross-reactivity to over-the-counter medications.

Confirmed drug abuse survey is usually performed by immunoassay as described in the preceding paragraph. However, the results are confirmed by more definitive analytic techniques such as gas chromatography or liquid chromatography/tandem mass spectrometry. This testing method is especially useful for patients who are inclined to deny the results of the drug abuse survey immunoassay. When positive, a specific drug and its quantification are reported.

Because a positive result can have a profound effect on a person's life, job, and accountability, it is not uncommon for a drug abuser to attempt to alter the urine specimen (specimen adulteration). Therefore the urine sample is tested for odor, color, temperature, creatinine, pH, and specific gravity to ensure that it is a proper specimen. If the specimen does not meet these assessment standards, it is rejected and a second specimen is requested.

INTERFERING FACTORS

- Poppy seeds can cause positive opiate results.
- Second-hand marijuana smoke can cause positive results.
- Ibuprofen can cause a *false-positive* THC result in some assay systems.
- Cold remedies can cause *false-positive* amphetamine results in some assay systems, but not with the monoclonal antibody test.
- Antibiotics (e.g., amoxicillin) can cause false-*positive* results for heroin and/or cocaine.
- The aggressive use of diuretics can *decrease* drug levels in the urine.

PROCEDURE AND PATIENT CARE

Before

- Explain the procedure to the patient based on standard guidelines.
- Obtain a list of prescription medicines that the patient is taking that may alter or confuse screening results.
- If the specimen is obtained for medicolegal testing, obtain informed consent.

During

- Collect blood and urine specimens as designated by the laboratory.
- Ensure that patients provide their own urine. Usually, the collection is supervised by a trained health care professional.
- Be sure that the patient does not alter the urine specimen.
- For hair testing, cut 50 strands of hair from the scalp.
- A second confirmatory specimen may be obtained (and is used if the results are positive).

After

- Follow the chain of custody for the specimen as provided by standard guidelines of the institution.
- Place the specimen in the required container for delivery.
- Check the temperature of urine specimens within 3 minutes after voiding. Temperature should be between 97° and 99° F.
- The specimen may be sent to a nationally certified laboratory for federal workers or workplace testing. Local hospital laboratories are often able to test for many drugs.

TEST RESULTS AND CLINICAL SIGNIFICANCE

Positive: *Results above the cutoff level indicate that the person tested may have used illicit drugs in the recent past. More definitive testing is then performed to confirm and quantify the presence of illicit drugs.*

RELATED TEST

Ethanol (p. 229). This is another common form of drug testing used in industry and by law enforcement agencies.

Toxicology

NORMAL FINDINGS

See Tables 11-2 and 11-3 for blood toxicology and urine toxicology, respectively.

INDICATIONS

Toxicology is used to evaluate for drug abuse, overdose, or poisoning.

TEST EXPLANATION

Detection of the most commonly abused nonprescription mood-altering drugs is discussed. These drugs are most commonly used in suicide attempts and chemical poisonings.

TABLE 11-2	Blood Toxicology Screening		
Drug	**Type**	**Therapeutic Level***	**Toxic Level***
Acetaminophen	Analgesic, antipyretic	Depends on use	>250 mcg/mL
Alcohol	—	None	80-200 mg/dL (mild to moderate intoxication) 250-400 mg/dL (marked intoxication) >400 mg/dL (severe intoxication)
Amobarbital	Sedative, hypnotic	0.5-3 mcg/mL	>10 mcg/mL
Butabarbital	Sedative, hypnotic	0.5-3 mcg/mL	>10 mcg/mL
Carboxyhemoglobin (COHb, carbon monoxide)	Gas	None	>30% COHb (beginning of coma)
Glutethimide	Sedative	0.5-3 mcg/mL	>10 mcg/mL
Lead	—	None	>40 mcg/dL
Lithium	Manic episodes of bipolar disorder	0.8-1.2 mEq/L	>2 mEq/L
Meprobamate	Anxiolytic	0.5-3 mcg/mL	>10 mcg/mL
Methyprylon	Hypnotic	0.5-3 mcg/mL	>10 mcg/mL
Phenobarbital	Anticonvulsant	15-30 mcg/mL	>40 mcg/mL
Phenytoin (Dilantin)	Anticonvulsant	10-20 mcg/mL	>20 mcg/mL
Salicylate	Antipyretic, antiinflammatory, analgesic	100-250 mcg/mL	>300 mcg/mL

*Varies according to institution performing the test.

TABLE 11-3	Urine Toxicology Screening for Amphetamines	
Drug	**Therapeutic Level* (mcg/mL)**	**Toxic Level* (mcg/mL)**
Amphetamine	2-3	>3
Dextroamphetamine	0.1-1.5	>15
Methamphetamine	3-5	>40
Phenmetrazine	5-30	>50

*Varies according to institution performing the test.

Testing for drug overdose and poisoning is best performed on blood. Results indicate immediate drug levels, which can indicate or alter therapy. Screening for use or abuse of nonprescription drugs is usually done on urine. Urine specimens are easily obtained without any invasive procedure. Often the specimen is obtained several hours or days after the drug administration. In this case, blood levels are low but urine levels are high. Further, drug metabolic products exist in the urine for longer periods, allowing detection of drug use in the past few hours or days. The disadvantages of urine drug tests are that they cannot indicate with any degree of accuracy when the drug was used and if the drug had any effect on the person's actions at any time. Also, the urine can be altered easily by changing the concentration (by drinking a large volume of water or adding water to the specimen), changing the pH, or adding foreign substances. Urine temperature, specific gravity, and creatinine concentration are often determined in urine specimens to ensure the specimen has not been altered. It is important to define the appropriate chain of transfer of the specimen from the moment it is obtained to the point of testing to prevent tampering.

Because of the impact on a person's life (socially, financially, and legally), positive results must be substantiated by another equally accurate test method. A popular combination is to screen with thin-layer or gas chromatography to separate out the constituents in the specimen, followed by mass spectrometry to identify those constituents.

Toxicology studies are used to incriminate drugs as a cause of or factor in a death. They are also used to assess patients when drug abuse or poisoning is contributing to an illness. Drug abuse is important to recognize in the workplace because of safety issues and in prisons because of disciplinary concerns.

Commonly Abused Drugs

Marijuana (Cannabis). Marijuana is usually detected by identifying one of its metabolites (tetrahydrocannabinol [THC]) in the urine. Most laboratories detect carboxy-THC and use 100 ng/mL as a cutoff. Lower levels from passive inhalation of marijuana may be detected, but are not prosecutable in court. These metabolites can exist in the urine 1 hour after use and for 1 to 3 days afterward.

Cocaine (Including Crack). Benzoylecgonine is a metabolite of cocaine. It is easily detectable in urine 1 to 4 hours after use and for 2 or 3 days. To indicate the timing of cocaine use, serum levels of cocaine must be determined.

Phencyclidine (PCP). PCP or one of its metabolites is detectable in urine about 6 to 18 hours after use and for as long as 3 days.

Amphetamines (Especially Methamphetamine). Amphetamines are identifiable in urine about 3 hours after use and for about 1 or 2 days. One must be careful in assuming abuse with detection of amphetamines, because many over-the-counter (OTC) cold medicines and weight loss medicines contain amphetamine analogs.

Morphine and Other Narcotic Alkaloids. Heroin, morphine, and codeine can be identified in the urine glucuronide conjugated forms 2 hours after use and for 2 to 3 days. Like amphetamines, one must be careful in assuming abuse with detection of codeine, because many OTC pain relievers and cough-suppressive medicines contain codeine.

Barbiturates. Barbiturates can be detected in the blood, urine, or gastric contents by direct immunoassay.

Common Toxins

Lead. See p. 334.

Other Heavy Metals. Heavy metals such as mercury, arsenic, bismuth, and antimony can be identified in the urine.

INTERFERING FACTORS

- Detergents, bicarbonates, salt tablets, or blood can all result in inaccurate drug testing in the urine.

PROCEDURE AND PATIENT CARE

Before

✍ Explain the procedure to the patient or significant others.
- If the specimen is obtained for medicolegal testing, ensure that the patient or family member has signed a consent form.
- Obtain as much information as possible about the drug type, amount, and ingestion time.
- Carefully assess the patient for respiratory distress, a common adverse reaction to drug overdose.

During

- Collect blood or urine specimens as indicated. Urine specimens are collected in the presence of a trained health care professional.
- Collect gastric contents for analysis if indicated.
- Note that hair and nail samples may be used to detect or document exposure to arsenic and mercury.
- Immediately identify the sample and mark the patient's name on the specimen.

After

- Apply pressure or a pressure dressing to the venipuncture site.
- Assess the venipuncture site for bleeding.
- Assess the patient for respiratory distress, a common adverse reaction to drug overdose.
✍ Refer the patient for appropriate drug and psychiatric counseling.
- Follow the predetermined chain of transfer of the specimen to the laboratory for testing. Each person involved in handling the specimen must document his or her place in its handling.
✍ Remind the patient that all positive screening results must be confirmed.

TEST RESULTS AND CLINICAL SIGNIFICANCE

Abuse or use of nonprescription drugs: *Urine is most often used for this testing.*
Heavy metal and lead poisoning: *Blood, urine, cerebrospinal fluid, and tissue specimens may all be used to identify these poisons.*
Suicide attempts: *Determination of toxic levels of drugs is much more accurately determined with blood tests, although urine may also be used.*

RELATED TESTS

Ethanol (p. 229). This is a direct measurement of alcohol level in the blood.
Carboxyhemoglobin (p. 143). This test is used to detect carbon monoxide poisoning.
Delta-Aminolevulinic Acid (p. 922). This test is used to identify lead poisoning.
Drug Monitoring (p. 211). These tests are used to help identify toxic levels of therapeutic drugs such as aspirin and acetaminophen, commonly involved in suicide attempts.
Substance Abuse Testing (p. 948). This test is used to detect illegal drug use.

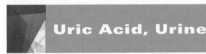

Uric Acid, Urine

NORMAL FINDINGS

250-750 mg/24 hr or 1.48-4.43 mmol/day (SI units)

INDICATIONS

Uric acid levels can be measured in both blood and urine. Urine levels of uric acid are helpful in evaluating uric acid metabolism in gout and for assessing hyperuricosuria in renal calculus formation. This test also helps to identify persons at risk for stone formation.

TEST EXPLANATION

Uric acid is a nitrogenous compound that is the final breakdown product of purine (a deoxyribonucleic acid [DNA] building block) catabolism. (See p. 514 for blood uric acid level.) Seventy-five percent of uric acid is excreted via the kidneys, and 25% by way of the intestinal tract. Elevated uric acid levels (hyperuricemia) may be indicative of gout, a form of arthritis caused by deposition of uric acid crystals in periarticular tissue. An elevated uric acid level in the urine is called uricosuria. Uric acid can become supersaturated in the urine and crystallize to form kidney stones, which can block the renal system.

Uric acid is produced primarily in the liver. Urinary excretion of uric acid depends on uric acid levels in the blood, along with glomerular filtration and tubular secretion of uric acid into the urine. Elevated uric acid levels can cause nephrolithiasis and ureterolithiasis. Uric acid is less well saturated in alkaline urine. As the urine pH rises, more uric acid can exist without crystallization and stone formation. Therefore urine known to have a high uric acid level can be alkalinized by ingestion of a strong base to prevent stone formation.

INTERFERING FACTORS

- Recent use of radiographic contrast agents may increase uric acid levels in the urine.
- Drugs that may interfere with test results include alcohol, antiinflammatory preparations, salicylates, thiazide diuretics, vitamin C, and warfarin.

✔ Clinical Priorities

- This test is helpful in evaluating uric acid metabolism and gout.
- In persons with high uric acid levels, the urine should be kept alkaline to prevent precipitation of kidney stones.

PROCEDURE AND PATIENT CARE

Before

- Explain the procedure to the patient.
- Tell the patient that no special diet is usually required.

During

- See Box 11-2, Guidelines for a 24-Hour Urine Collection, p. 907.
- A preservative may be used. Check with the laboratory.
- Show the patient where to store the urine container.
- Keep the specimen on ice or refrigerated during the entire 24 hours. (Note that some laboratories do not require that the specimen be kept cool.)
- Encourage the patient to drink fluids during the 24 hours.

After

- Transport the urine specimen to the laboratory promptly.

TEST RESULTS AND CLINICAL SIGNIFICANCE

▲ Increased Levels (Uricosuria)

Gout: *Uric acid levels are high in blood. With normal glomerular filtration, levels are high in urine.*
Metastatic cancer,
Multiple myeloma,
Leukemias,
Cancer chemotherapy:
> *Rapid cell destruction associated with rapidly growing cancers (with high cell turnover), and especially after chemotherapy for those rapidly growing tumors, causes the cells to lyse and spill their nucleic acids into the bloodstream. In the liver, these free nucleic acids are converted to uric acid. Blood and urine levels of uric acid increase.*

High-purine diet: *With increased uric acid production caused by a diet high in purines, uric acid levels in the urine will be increased.*
Uricosuric drugs (e.g., ascorbic acid, calcitonin, citrate, dicumarol, estrogens, steroids, iodinated dyes, glyceryl guaiacolate, phenolsulfonphthalein, probenecid, salicylates, and outdated tetracycline): *These drugs increase uric acid excretion into the urine.*
Lead toxicity: *Heavy-metal poisoning is associated with increased uric acid tubular secretion.*

▼ Decreased Levels

Kidney disease: *With decreased glomerular filtration rate and decreased tubular secretion of uric acid, urine levels fall.*
Eclampsia: *The pathophysiology of this observation is not well known.*
Chronic alcohol ingestion: *Chronic acidosis from excessive alcohol ingestion decreases renal tubular secretion of uric acid into the urine.*
Acidosis (ketotic [diabetic or starvation], lactic): *Renal tubular secretion of uric acid into the urine is decreased. Ketoacids, as occur in diabetic or alcoholic ketoacidosis, may compete with uric acid for tubular excretion, which is another cause of decreased uric acid excretion.*

RELATED TEST

Uric Acid, Blood (p. 514). This test is used to diagnose gout.

Urinalysis (UA)

NORMAL FINDINGS

Appearance: clear
Color: amber yellow
Odor: aromatic
pH: 4.6-8.0 (average, 6.0)
Protein
> 0-8 mg/dL
> 50-80 mg/24 hr (at rest)
> <250 mg/24 hr (during exercise)

Specific gravity
> Adult: 1.005-1.030 (usually, 1.010-1.025)

Elderly: values decrease with age
Newborn: 1.001-1.020
Leukocyte esterase: negative
Nitrites: none
Ketones: none
Bilirubin: none
Urobilinogen: 0.01-1 Ehrlich unit/mL
Crystals: none
Casts: none
Glucose (see Urine Glucose, p. 924)
    Fresh specimen: none
    24-hour specimen: 50-300 mg/24 hr or 0.3-1.7 mmol/day (SI units)
White blood cells (WBCs): 0-4 per low-power field
WBC casts: none
Red blood cells (RBCs): ≤2
RBC casts: none

INDICATIONS

Urinalysis (UA) is part of routine diagnostic and screening evaluations. It can reveal a significant amount of preliminary information about the kidneys and other metabolic processes. For example, it can detect urinary tract diseases (e.g., infection, glomerulonephritis, loss of concentrating capacity), and extrarenal disease processes (e.g., glucosuria in diabetes, proteinuria in monoclonal gammopathies, bilirubinuria in liver disease). It is done diagnostically in patients with abdominal or back pain, dysuria, hematuria, or urinary frequency. It is part of routine monitoring in patients with chronic renal disease and some metabolic diseases.

TEST EXPLANATION

Total UA involves multiple routine tests on a urine specimen. This specimen is not necessarily a clean-catch specimen. However, if urinary tract infection (UTI) is suspected, often a midstream, clean-catch specimen is obtained. This urine is then divided into two portions. One is sent for UA, and the other is held in the laboratory refrigerator for culture (see p. 973) if results of UA indicate infection. Routinely, UA includes remarks regarding the color, appearance, and odor; pH; and presence of proteins, glucose, ketones, blood, and leukocyte esterase. In addition, the urine is examined microscopically for RBCs, WBCs, casts, crystals, and bacteria. Because this is a spot urine test, volume is not measured. Volume of urine may be important in many clinical situations; in these cases, a full 24-hour specimen is required. (See Figure 11-2 for automated testing.)

Laboratory Examination

Appearance and Color. Urine appearance and color are noted as part of routine urinalysis. A normal urine specimen should be clear. Cloudy urine may be caused by the presence of pus (necrotic WBCs), RBCs, or bacteria; however, normal urine also may be cloudy because of ingestion of certain foods (e.g., large amounts of fat, urates, phosphates). Urine ranges from pale yellow to amber because of the pigment urochrome (product of bilirubin metabolism). The color indicates the concentration of the urine and varies with specific gravity. Dilute urine is straw colored, and concentrated urine is deep amber.

Abnormally colored urine may result from a pathologic condition or the ingestion of certain foods or medicines. For example, bleeding from the kidney produces dark red urine, whereas bleeding from

11 Urine Studies

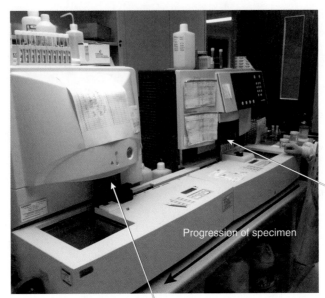

Dipstick auto analysis

Progression of specimen

Microscopic auto analysis

Figure 11-2 Siemens automated urinalysis analyzer. The urine specimen enters the machine on the far right. First, automated dipstick analysis is carried out. The specimen is then transferred to the left of the machine where microscopic automated analysis occurs. The machine will notify the technologist if any significant abnormality is noted. The findings are then individually corroborated. Many specimens can be processed in a short period of time.

the lower urinary tract produces bright red urine. Dark yellow urine may indicate the presence of urobilinogen or bilirubin. Pseudomonas infection may produce green urine. Eating beets may cause red urine, and rhubarb can color the urine brown. Many frequently used drugs also may affect urine color (Table 11-4).

Odor. Determination of urine odor is part of routine urinalysis. The aromatic odor of fresh, normal urine is caused by the presence of volatile acids. Urine of patients with diabetic ketoacidosis has the strong, sweet smell of acetone. In patients with a UTI, the urine may have a very foul odor. Urine with a fecal odor may indicate an enterobladder fistula.

pH. Analysis of the pH of a freshly voided urine specimen indicates the acid-base balance. The urine reflects the work of the kidneys to maintain normal pH homeostasis. Just as the lungs (respiratory component) help compensate for acid-base imbalance, so do the kidneys (metabolic component). The kidneys assist in acid-base balance by reabsorbing sodium and excreting hydrogen.

An alkaline pH is observed in a patient with alkalemia. Also, bacteria, UTI, or a diet high in citrus fruits or vegetables may cause increased urine pH. An alkaline urine is common after eating. Certain medications (e.g., streptomycin, neomycin, kanamycin) are effective in treating UTIs when the urine is alkaline. It is more common for the urine to be acidic. However, acidic urine is also observed in patients with acidemia, which can result from metabolic or respiratory acidosis, starvation, dehydration, or a diet high in meat products or cranberries. In patients with renal tubular acidosis, however, the blood is acidic and the urine is alkaline.

TABLE 11-4   Frequently Used Drugs That May Affect Urine Color

Generic and Brand Names	Drug Class	Urine Color
Cascara sagrada	Stimulant laxative	Red in alkaline urine; yellow-brown in acid urine
Chloroquine (Aralen)	Antimalarial	Rusty yellow or brown
Chlorzoxazone (Paraflex)	Skeletal muscle relaxant	Orange or purple-red
Docusate calcium (Doxidan, Surfak)	Laxative	Pink to red to red-brown
Doxorubicin (Adriamycin)	Antineoplastic	Red-orange
Iron preparations (Ferotran, Imferon)	Hematinic	Dark brown or black on standing
Levodopa	Antiparkinsonian agent	Dark brown on standing
Metronidazole (Flagyl)	Antiinfective	Darkening, reddish-brown
Nitrofurantoin (Macrodantin, Nitrodan)	Antibacterial	Brown-yellow
Phenazopyridine (Pyridium)	Urinary tract analgesic	Orange to red
Phenolphthalein (Ex-Lax)	Contact laxative	Red or purplish pink in alkaline urine
Phenothiazines (e.g., prochlor-perazine [Compazine])	Antipsychotic, neuroleptic, antiemetic	Red-brown
Phenytoin (Dilantin)	Anticonvulsant	Pink, red, red-brown
Riboflavin (vitamin B)	Vitamin	Intense yellow
Rifampin	Antibiotic	Red-orange
Sulfasalazine (Azulfidine)	Antibacterial	Orange-yellow in alkaline urine
Triamterene (Dyrenium)	Diuretic	Pale blue fluorescence

The urine pH is useful in identifying crystals in the urine and determining the predisposition to form a given type of stone. Acidic urine is associated with xanthine, cystine, uric acid, and calcium oxalate stones. To treat or prevent these urinary calculi, urine should be kept alkaline. Alkaline urine is associated with calcium carbonate, calcium phosphate, and magnesium phosphate stones. To treat or prevent these urinary calculi, urine should be kept acidic. See Urinary Stone Analysis, p. 971.

Protein. Protein is a sensitive indicator of kidney function. Normally, protein is not present in the urine because the spaces in the normal glomerular filtrate membrane are too small to allow its passage. If the glomerular membrane is injured, as in glomerulonephritis, the spaces become much larger, and protein (usually albumin, because it is a smaller molecule than the globulins) seeps into the filtrate and then into the urine. If this persists at a significant rate, hypoproteinemia can develop as a result of severe protein loss through the kidneys. This decreases the normal capillary oncotic pressure that holds fluid within the vasculature and causes severe interstitial edema. The combination of proteinuria and edema is known as nephrotic syndrome.

Proteinuria (usually albumin because it is a relatively small protein) is probably the most important indicator of renal disease. The urine of all pregnant women is routinely checked for proteinuria, which can be an indicator of preeclampsia. Urinary protein is used to screen for nephrotic syndrome and for complications of diabetes mellitus, glomerulonephritis, amyloidosis, and multiple myeloma (see test for Bence-Jones protein, p. 911).

If significant protein is noted at urinalysis, a 24-hour urine specimen should be collected so that the quantity of protein can be measured. This test can be repeated as a method of monitoring renal disease and its treatment. Usually, protein loss of more than 3000 mg/24 hr leads to the signs and symptoms of nephrotic syndrome. If proteinuria is identified, a random urine can be analyzed for protein quantification. This estimate of 24-hour protein excretion is usually performed with a urine creatinine, since hydration status and other factors may influence urine concentration. The normal *protein/creatinine ratio* is less than 0.15.

Glucose. See the Blood Glucose testing section on p. 253.

Specific Gravity. Specific gravity is a measure of the concentration of particles (including wastes and electrolytes) in the urine. High specific gravity indicates concentrated urine; low specific gravity indicates dilute urine. Specific gravity refers to the weight of the urine compared with that of distilled water (which has a specific gravity of 1.000). Particles in the urine give it weight, or specific gravity.

Specific gravity is used to evaluate the concentrating and excretory power of the kidneys. Renal disease tends to diminish concentrating capability. As a result, chronic renal diseases are associated with low specific gravity of the urine. Specific gravity must be interpreted in light of the presence or absence of glycosuria and proteinuria. Specific gravity is also a measurement of hydration status. With overhydration, the urine will be more dilute, with lower specific gravity, whereas with dehydration, specific gravity can be expected to be abnormally high. Nephrotoxic diabetes insipidus is associated with very little variation in specific gravity of the urine because the kidney cannot respond to variables such as hydration and solute load.

Measurement of urine specific gravity is easier and more convenient than measurement of osmolality (see p. 938). Specific gravity correlates roughly with osmolality. Knowledge of specific gravity is needed to interpret the results of most parts of the urinalysis. Specific gravity is usually evaluated with a refractometer (which measures the amount of light that can pass through a drop of urine) or a dipstick.

Leukocyte Esterase (WBC Esterase). Leukocyte (WBC) esterase is a screening test used to detect leukocytes in the urine. Positive results indicate UTI. For this examination, chemical testing is performed with a leukocyte esterase dipstick; a shade of purple is considered a positive result. Some laboratories have established screening protocols in which a microscopic examination (see later discussion) is performed only if results of a leukocyte esterase test are positive.

Nitrites. Like the leukocyte esterase screen, the nitrite test is a screening test for identification of UTIs. This test is based on the principle that many (but not all) bacteria produce an enzyme called *reductase*, which can reduce urinary nitrates to nitrites. Chemical testing is done with a dipstick containing a reagent that reacts with nitrites to produce a pink color, thus indirectly suggesting the presence of bacteria. A positive test result indicates the need for a urine culture. Nitrite screening enhances the sensitivity of the leukocyte esterase test to detect UTIs.

Ketones. Normally, no ketones are present in the urine; however, a patient with poorly controlled diabetes and hyperglycemia may have massive fatty acid catabolism. The purpose of this catabolism is to provide an energy source when glucose cannot be transferred into the cell because of insulin insufficiency. Ketones (beta-hydroxybutyric acid, acetoacetic acid, and acetone) are the end products of this fatty acid breakdown. As with glucose, ketones (predominantly acetoacetic acid) spill over into the urine when blood levels in diabetic patients are elevated. Ketonuria is usually associated with poorly controlled diabetes. This test for ketonuria is also important in evaluating ketoacidosis associated with alcoholism, fasting, starvation, high-protein diets, and isopropanol ingestion. Ketonuria may occur with acute febrile illnesses, especially in infants and children.

Bilirubin and Urobilinogen. *Bilirubin* is a major constituent of bile. If bilirubin excretion is inhibited, conjugated (direct) hyperbilirubinemia will result (see p. 121). Obstruction of the bile duct by a gallstone is the classic example of obstructed bilirubin excretion causing conjugated hyperbilirubinemia. Unlike the unconjugated form, conjugated bilirubin is water soluble and can be excreted into the urine. Therefore, bilirubin in urine suggests disease affecting bilirubin metabolism after conjugation or defects in excretion (e.g., gallstones). Unconjugated bilirubin caused by prehepatic jaundice will not be excreted in the urine because it is not water soluble.

Bilirubin is excreted by way of the bile ducts into the bowel. There some of the bilirubin is transformed into *urobilinogen* by the action of bacteria in the bowel. Most of the urobilinogen is excreted from the liver back into the bowel, but some is excreted by the kidneys.

Microscopic Examination of Urine Sediment. Microscopic examination of the sediment from a centrifuged urine specimen provides substantial information about the urinary system. Because many different methods can be used to prepare the sediment for microscopic review, normal values may vary significantly among laboratories. Reference ranges are provided here to recognize marked abnormalities.

Crystals. Crystals found in the urinary sediment on microscopic examination indicate that renal stone formation is imminent, if not already present. By themselves, crystals cause no symptoms until they form stones. Even then, stones produce symptoms only when they obstruct the urinary tract. Uric acid crystals occur in patients with high serum uric acid levels (e.g., gout). Phosphate and calcium oxalate crystals (Figure 11-3) occur in the urine of patients with parathyroid abnormalities or malabsorption states. The type of crystal found varies with the disease and the pH of the urine (see previous discussion on urinary pH). Small amounts of crystalline material and even casts (see next page) can be observed when the specific gravity of the urine is high.

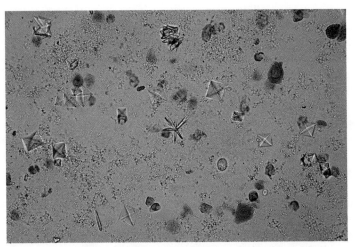

Figure 11-3 Microscopic examination of urine sediment: calcium oxalate crystals. This is the most common crystal structure seen in urine sediment. Note the classic cross-shaped internal configuration.

Casts. Casts are rectangular clumps of materials or cells that form in the renal distal and collecting tubules, where the material is maximally concentrated. These amorphous clumps of material and cells are shaped like tubules, thus the term *cast*. Casts are usually associated with some degree of proteinuria and stasis within the renal tubules. There are two kinds of casts: hyaline and cellular. Casts are best seen on low power of the light microscope. Some casts are nearly clear (hyaline), and the condenser lamp must be dimmed to see them well.

Hyaline Casts. Hyaline casts are conglomerations of protein and are indicative of proteinuria. A few hyaline casts are normally present, especially after strenuous exercise.

Cellular Casts. Cellular casts are conglomerations of degenerated cells. Various types are described in the following paragraphs:

Granular casts. Granular casts result from the disintegration of cellular material into granular particles within a WBC or epithelial cell cast. Granular casts are found after exercise and in various renal diseases.

Fatty casts. In some diseases, the epithelial cells desquamate into the renal tubule. As the cell degenerates, fatty deposits within the cell coalesce and become incorporated with protein into fatty casts. These are associated with glomerular disease or nephrotic syndrome/nephrosis. Free oval fat bodies may also be associated with fatty emboli, which occur in patients with bone fractures.

Waxy casts. Waxy casts may be cell casts, hyaline casts, or renal failure casts. Waxy casts probably represent further degeneration of granular casts. They occur when urine flow through the renal tubule is diminished, giving time for granular casts to degenerate. Waxy casts are associated with chronic renal diseases and chronic renal failure. They also occur in diabetic nephropathy, malignant hypertension, and glomerulonephritis.

Epithelial cells and casts (renal tubular casts). Epithelial cells can enter the urine at any point during the process of urinary excretion. These cells can be shed from the bladder as a result of tumor, infection, or polyps. They can result from cellular contamination of the urine by vaginal or urethral secretions. They can also result from desquamation of renal tubule cells into the lumen of the tubules and collecting system. These cells can form epithelial casts. The material in these cells can disintegrate first into coarse granules and then into fine granules, making granular casts. The presence of occasional epithelial cells is not remarkable; large numbers, however, are abnormal. Tubular (epithelial) casts are most suggestive of renal tubular disease or toxicity.

White blood cells and casts. Normally, few WBCs are found in the urine sediment on microscopic examination. The presence of five or more WBCs in the urine indicates a UTI involving the bladder or kidneys, or both. A clean-catch urine culture should be done for further evaluation. WBC casts are most frequently found in infections of the kidney (e.g., acute pyelonephritis or interstitial nephritis).

Red blood cells and casts. Any disruption in the blood-urine barrier, whether at the glomerular, tubular, or bladder level, will cause RBCs to enter the urine. Hematuria can be microscopic or gross. Patients with more than three RBCs per high-power field in two out of three properly collected urine specimens should be considered to have microhematuria, and hence be evaluated for possible pathologic causes. Bladder, ureteral, and urethral diseases are the most common causes of RBCs in the urine. Pathologic conditions (e.g., tumors, trauma, stones, infection) that involve the mucous membrane in the collecting system can also cause hematuria. RBC casts suggest glomerulonephritis (which may be present in patients with acute bacterial endocarditis, renal infarct, Goodpasture syndrome, vasculitis, sickle cell disease, or malignant hypertension), interstitial nephritis, acute tubular necrosis, pyelonephritis, renal trauma, or renal tumor.

INTERFERING FACTORS

Appearance and Color

- Sperm remaining in the urethra after recent or retrograde ejaculation can cause the urine to appear cloudy.
- Urine that has been refrigerated for longer than 1 hour can become cloudy.
- Certain foods affect urine color. Eating carrots may cause dark yellow urine; beets may cause red urine; rhubarb may cause reddish or brownish urine.
- Urine darkens with prolonged standing because of oxidation of bilirubin metabolites.
- Many drugs, given the right environment, can alter the color of urine. See Table 11-4, p. 959.

Odor

- Some foods (e.g., asparagus) produce a characteristic urine odor.
- When urine stands for a long time and begins to decompose, it has an ammonia-like smell.

pH

- Urine pH becomes alkaline on standing, because of the action of urea-splitting bacteria, which produce ammonia.
- The urine pH of an uncovered specimen will become alkaline because carbon dioxide vaporizes from the urine.
- Dietary factors affect urine pH. Ingestion of large quantities of citrus fruits, dairy products, and vegetables produces alkaline urine, whereas a diet high in meat and certain foods (e.g., cranberries) produces acidic urine.
- Drugs that *increase* urine pH include acetazolamide, bicarbonate antacids, and carbonic anhydrase inhibitors.
- Drugs that *decrease* urine pH include ammonium chloride, chlorothiazide, and mandelic acid.

Protein

- Transient proteinuria may be associated with severe emotional stress, excessive exercise, and cold baths.
- Radiopaque contrast media administered within 3 days may cause false-positive results for proteinuria when turbidity is used as a measure of protein in the urine.
- Urine contaminated with prostate or vaginal secretions commonly causes proteinuria.
- Diets high in protein can cause proteinuria.
- Highly concentrated urine may have a greater concentration of protein than more dilute urine.
- Hemoglobin may cause a positive result with the dipstick method.
- Bence-Jones protein may not appear with the dipstick method.
- Drugs that may cause *increased* protein levels include acetazolamide, aminoglycosides, amphotericin B, cephalosporins, colistin, griseofulvin, lithium, methicillin, nafcillin, nephrotoxic drugs (e.g., arsenicals, gold salts), oxacillin, penicillamine, penicillin G, phenazopyridine, polymyxin B, salicylates, sulfonamides, tolbutamide, and vancomycin.

Specific Gravity

- Recent use of radiographic dyes increases urinary specific gravity.
- Cold temperatures cause falsely high specific gravity.
- Drugs that may cause *increased* specific gravity include dextran, mannitol, and sucrose.

Leukocyte Esterase

- False-positive results may occur in specimens contaminated by vaginal secretions (e.g., heavy menstrual discharge, *Trichomonas* infection, parasites) that contain WBCs.
- False-negative results may occur in specimens containing high levels of protein or ascorbic acid.

Ketones

- Special diets (carbohydrate-free, high-protein, high-fat) may cause ketonuria.
- Drugs that may cause *false-positive* results include bromosulfophthalein, isoniazid, isopropanol, levodopa, paraldehyde, phenazopyridine, and phenolsulfonphthalein.

Bilirubin and Urobilinogen

- Bilirubin is not stable in urine, especially when exposed to light.
- pH can affect urobilinogen levels. Alkaline urine indicates higher levels; acidic urine may show lower levels.
- Phenazopyridine colors the urine orange. This may give the false impression that the patient has jaundice.
- Cholestatic drugs may *reduce* urobilinogen levels.
- Antibiotics reduce intestinal flora, which in turn *decreases* urobilinogen levels.

Crystals

- Radiographic contrast media may cause precipitation of urinary crystals.

WBCs

- Vaginal discharge may contaminate the urine specimen and factitiously cause WBCs in the urine.

RBCs

- Strenuous physical exercise may cause RBC casts.
- Traumatic urethral catheterization may cause RBCs in the urine.
- Overaggressive anticoagulant therapy or bleeding disorders tend to cause RBCs in the urine without concomitant disease.

✔ Clinical Priorities

- A common cause of RBCs in the urine of women is contamination because of menses. Before a more thorough evaluation is begun, determine whether the patient was having a period when the urine specimen was obtained.
- Leukocyte esterase and nitrate tests are screening tests used to detect UTIs. Positive test results indicate the need for urine culture.
- If a UTI is suspected, a midstream, clean-catch specimen is needed.
- If a 24-hour urine collection is needed, it should be refrigerated during the collection period. A preservative may also be necessary.

PROCEDURE AND PATIENT CARE

Before

✍ Explain the procedure to the patient.

During

- Collect a fresh urine specimen in a urine container.
- If the urine specimen contains vaginal discharge or bleeding, a clean-catch or midstream specimen will be needed. This requires meticulous cleaning of the urinary meatus with an antiseptic preparation to reduce contamination of the specimen by external organisms. The cleansing agent must then be completely removed so as not to contaminate the specimen. The *midstream collection* is obtained as follows:
  1. Have the patient begin to urinate into a bedpan, urinal, or toilet, then stop urinating. This washes urine out of the distal part of the urethra.
  2. Correctly position a sterile urine container and have the patient void 3 to 4 ounces of urine.
  3. Cap the container.
  4. Allow the patient to finish voiding.
- Testing for ketones can be performed immediately after urine collection with a dipstick.
- For testing urine specific gravity, a first-voided specimen is best.
- Specific gravity can be measured with a refractometer. Light passes through the specimen, and the refractive index (difference between the velocity of light passing through air and the specimen) is determined.
- An easier method of measuring specific gravity is the dipstick method. A dipstick is placed in the specimen, and the resulting color is compared with a color chart.
- To test for protein, a first-voided specimen is best. Occasionally, however, a 24-hour urine collection is preferred. See Box 11-2, Guidelines for a 24-Hour Urine Collection, p. 907.
- Most laboratories use the dipstick method to determine protein in the urine.
- Nitrite, leukocyte esterase, pH, and ketones are measured with the dipstick method and the results determined by comparison with a color chart.
- Urine sediment is obtained by centrifuging a small volume (10 mL) of urine and discarding the supernatant. The remaining urine is a concentrated sediment that can be microscopically examined.

After

- Transport the urine specimen to the laboratory promptly.
- If the specimen cannot be processed immediately, refrigerate it. If the urine cannot be tested within 2 hours, a preservative may be required.
- If a 24-hour urine collection is requested, the specimen should be refrigerated and may need a preservative during the collection time.
- Casts will break up as urine is allowed to sit. Urine examinations for casts should be performed with fresh specimens.

TEST RESULTS AND CLINICAL SIGNIFICANCE

APPEARANCE AND COLOR

Infection: *Infection may cause turbid, foul-smelling urine. Pseudomonas infection can give a green tint to urine.*
Gross hematuria: *RBCs in the urine cause the urine to be red. This is always a pathologic sign unless the blood is found to be from a source other than the urinary tract. Tumors, trauma, stones, and infection anywhere in the urinary tract can cause RBCs in the urine. Glomerulonephritis, interstitial nephritis, acute necrosis, and pyelonephritis are also associated with hematuria.*

Urine Studies

11

Drug therapy: *See Table 11-4, p. 959.*
Overhydration,
Diabetes insipidus,
Diuretic therapy,
Glycosuria:
   These states produce nearly colorless urine.
Fever,
Excessive sweating,
Dehydration,
Jaundice:
   These states cause dark yellow or orange urine.
Hemoglobinuria,
Myoglobinuria,
Porphyria:
   These illnesses cause wine-colored or even dark brown urine.

ODOR

Ketonuria: *Associated with poor glucose tolerance, ketones in the urine cause a fruity smell.*
Urinary tract infection: *Most infections cause foul smelling urine.*
Enterovesical fistula: *This condition causes urine to smell like stool.*
Maple sugar urine: *This congenital defect in protein metabolism causes the urine to smell like burnt sugar.*
Phenylketonuria: *This disease causes the urine to smell musty.*

pH
▲   Increased Levels

Alkalemia: *The renal component of pH homeostasis causes the excretion of excess base to try to correct acid-base imbalance.*
Urinary tract infections: *Urea-splitting bacteria cause the urine to be alkaline as urea is converted to ammonia.*
Gastric suction,
Vomiting,
Renal tubular acidosis:
   These are all associated with reduced hydrogen ion excretion. Urine pH is increased.

▼   Decreased Levels

Acidemia: *To maintain homeostasis, the kidneys attempt to excrete hydrogen ions, causing the urine pH to be reduced.*
Diabetes mellitus,
Starvation:
   Ketone acids associated with starvation or poor glucose metabolism cause acid urine.
Respiratory acidosis: *Hydrogen ions are excreted and the urine becomes acidotic.*

PROTEIN
▲   Increased Levels

Nephrotic syndrome,
Glomerulonephritis,

Malignant hypertension,

Diabetic glomerulosclerosis,

Polycystic kidney disease,

Lupus erythematosus,

Goodpasture syndrome,

Heavy-metal poisoning,

Bacterial pyelonephritis,

Nephrotoxic drug therapy:
 Renal disease involving the glomeruli is associated with proteinuria.

Trauma: *Protein can spill into the urine as a result of traumatic destruction of the blood-urine barrier.*

Macroglobulinemia: *With increased globulin within the blood, albumin is excreted in an attempt to maintain oncotic homeostasis.*

Multiple myelomas: *Classically, multiple myelomas produce large amounts of proteins (e.g., Bence-Jones protein) in the urine.*

Preeclampsia,

Congestive heart failure (CHF):
 The pathophysiologic factors of these observations are many. Suffice it to say that albumin leaks from the glomeruli, which are temporarily damaged by these illnesses.

Orthostatic proteinuria: *As many as 20% of normal male patients have small amounts of protein in the urine when specimens are obtained from patients in the upright position. The pathophysiology is not known with certainty. It may be associated with passive congestion of the kidney in the upright position. This phenomenon can be diagnosed by obtaining a urine specimen before arising, and another after the patient has been up for 2 hours. The first has no protein, the latter does.*

Severe muscle exertion: *Prolonged muscular exertion can be associated with small amounts of protein in the urine.*

Renal vein thrombosis: *Congestion of the kidney is associated with proteinuria.*

Bladder tumor: *Tumors of the bladder secrete protein into the lumen of the bladder.*

Urethritis or prostatitis: *Inflammation in the periurethral glands or urethra can cause proteinuria.*

Amyloidosis: *Often associated with proteinuria, it may be so severe as to cause nephrotic syndrome. Usually, amyloidosis of the kidney is due to other severe, ongoing disease.*

SPECIFIC GRAVITY

▲ Increased Levels

Dehydration: *The kidneys reabsorb all available free water; thus excreted urine is concentrated.*

Pituitary tumor or trauma: *Syndrome of inappropriate antidiuretic hormone (SIADH) results in excessive water reabsorption and concentrated urine.*

Decreased renal blood flow (as in heart failure, renal artery stenosis, or hypotension): *Urine is concentrated through secretion of antidiuretic hormone (ADH) and the renin-angiotensin system.*

Glycosuria and proteinuria: *These particles of glucose and protein increase specific gravity.*

Water restriction,

Fever,

Excessive sweating,

Vomiting,

Diarrhea:
 The above five clinical situations are associated with diminished blood volume. They cause concentrated urine mediated through secretion of ADH and the renin-angiotensin system.

11 Urine Studies

▼ Decreased Levels

Overhydration: *Excess water is excreted, causing dilute urine with low specific gravity.*

Diabetes insipidus: *Inadequate ADH secretion causes decreased water reabsorption. Excess water is excreted, causing dilute urine with low specific gravity.*

Renal failure: *In chronic renal failure the kidney loses its ability to concentrate urine through water reabsorption. Excess water is excreted, causing dilute urine with low specific gravity.*

Diuresis: *Diuretics tend to cause dilute, voluminous urine flow.*

LEUKOCYTE ESTERASE

Possible UTI: *Detection of leukocyte esterase indicates the presence of WBCs in the urine (pyuria), indicative of urinary tract infection.*

NITRITES

Possible UTI: *Reductase produced by bacteria reduces nitrates to nitrites. The presence of nitrites indicates bacterial infection somewhere in the urinary tract.*

KETONES

Poorly controlled diabetes mellitus,

Starvation,

Alcoholism,

Weight-reduction diets,

Prolonged vomiting,

Anorexia,

Fasting,

High-protein diets,

Glycogen storage diseases:

Impaired glucose metabolism causes catabolism of fat for production of energy. Ketones (betahydroxybutyric acid, acetoacetic acid, and acetone) are formed and spill into the urine.

Febrile illnesses in infants and children,

Hyperthyroidism,

Severe stress or illness:

Hypermetabolic states cause excessive utilization of glucose. Fats are then broken down. Ketones form and spill over into the urine.

Excessive aspirin ingestion: *Aspirin toxicity is associated with reduced glucose production. Ketones form and spill over into the urine.*

Anesthesia: *The pathophysiology of this observation is probably multiple. Drug effect, starvation, and severe illness can all affect ketone formation.*

BILIRUBIN

Gallstones,

Extrahepatic duct obstruction (e.g., tumor, inflammation, gallstone, scarring, or surgical trauma),

Extensive liver metastasis:

Direct physical obstruction of flow of bile from the biliary tree causes elevated serum levels of conjugated (direct) bilirubin, which leads to elevated urine levels of bilirubin.

Cholestasis because of drugs: *Some drugs affect bilirubin metabolism and excretion after glucuronide conjugation. Elevated serum levels of conjugated (direct) bilirubin lead to elevated urine levels of bilirubin.*

Dubin-Johnson syndrome,

Rotor syndrome:

> *These congenital defects in bilirubin metabolism occur after glucuronide conjugation. This causes elevated serum levels of conjugated (direct) bilirubin, which leads to elevated urine levels of bilirubin.*

UROBILINOGEN

▲ Increased Levels

Hemolytic anemia,

Pernicious anemia,

Hemolysis because of drugs:

> *Hemolysis results in increased RBC destruction. This causes more heme to be catabolized into bilirubin. Increased bilirubin is excreted into the bowel. More urobilinogen is made in the bowel. More urobilinogen is reabsorbed from the gut. More urobilinogen is excreted by the kidneys into the urine.*

Hematoma,

Excessive ecchymosis:

> *RBCs in these areas break down, causing large amounts of heme to be catabolized into bilirubin. Increased bilirubin is excreted into the bowel. More urobilinogen is produced in the bowel. More urobilinogen is reabsorbed from the gut. More urobilinogen is excreted by the kidneys into the urine.*

▼ Decreased Levels

Biliary obstruction,

Cholestasis:

> *No bilirubin reaches the bowel for conversion to urobilinogen. Therefore urine levels of urobilinogen are reduced.*

CRYSTALS

Renal stone formation: *Stones form with crystals as a nidus for production. Crystals in small quantities are not pathologic. Crystals do give some insight into metabolic diseases (e.g., gout, hyperparathyroidism) and other congenital defects of protein metabolism.*

Urinary tract infection: *Proteus infection, in particular, is associated with crystal formation, especially if chronic.*

GRANULAR CASTS AND WAXY CASTS

Acute tubular necrosis,

Urinary tract infection,

Glomerulonephritis,

Pyelonephritis,

Nephrosclerosis,

Chronic lead poisoning,

Exercise,

Stress,

Renal transplant rejection:

> *Coarse and fine granular casts represent further degeneration of cellular casts. They appear when urine flow through the collecting system is diminished, allowing time for further degeneration. As a result, nearly any renal disease or toxicity can be associated with granular cast formation. Waxy casts represent further deterioration of granular casts over time.*

Urine Studies

11

FATTY CASTS

Nephrotic syndrome,
Diabetic nephropathy (Kimmelstiel-Wilson syndrome),
Glomerulonephritis associated with streptococcal infection,
Chronic renal disease (glomerulonephritis),
Mercury poisoning:
> *Classically, fatty casts are associated with nephrotic syndrome. Any disease or poison that affects the tubular cells causes them to degenerate and desquamate into the lumen. The fatty deposits within those cells coalesce to mix with protein, to make fatty casts or oval fat bodies.*

Fat embolism: *About 50% of fat embolisms are associated with urinary fat.*

EPITHELIAL CASTS

Glomerulonephritis,
Eclampsia,
Heavy-metal poisoning:
> *Diseases that affect the renal tubule cells and diminish urine flow are associated with epithelial cast formation.*

EPITHELIAL CELLS

Acute renal allograft rejection,
Acute tubular necrosis,
Acute glomerulonephritis because of streptococcal infection:
> *Acute tubule cell injuries cause those cells to be destroyed and desquamate into the lumen of the tubule, to be excreted in the urine.*

HYALINE CASTS

Orthostatic proteinuria,
Fever,
Strenuous exercise,
Stress:
> *These clinical states are often associated with short-term proteinuria and decreased urine flow through the renal collecting system. Proteinaceous (or hyaline) casts develop.*

Glomerulonephritis,
Pyelonephritis,
Congestive heart failure,
Chronic renal failure:
> *These diseases are associated with chronic proteinuria and hyaline cast formation.*

RBCs AND CASTS

▲ Increased RBC Levels

Primary renal diseases (e.g., glomerulonephritis, interstitial nephritis, acute tubular necrosis, pyelonephritis): *These diseases are associated with the deterioration of the blood-urine barrier.*
Renal tumor: *Renal neoplasms are friable and hypervascular. RBCs are common with cancers of the kidney.*
Renal trauma: *Lacerations, contusions, and hematomas ultimately lead to blood in the urine.*
Renal stones,
Cystitis,

Prostatitis,
Tumors of the ureters and bladder,
Traumatic bladder catheterization,
Bladder trauma:
>   *Any mucosal injury or disease will cause bleeding directly into the urine. Hematuria is usually gross (visible to the naked eye).*

▲ Increased RBC Cast Levels

Glomerulonephritis,
Subacute bacterial endocarditis,
Renal infarct,
Goodpasture syndrome,
Vasculitis,
Sickling,
Malignant hypertension,
Systemic lupus erythematosus:
>   *Bleeding from the kidney when associated with reduced urine flow through the kidney can be associated with RBC casts. RBC casts exclude the lower urinary tract as a source of bleeding.*

WBCs AND CASTS

▲ Increased WBC Levels

Bacterial infection in the urinary tract: *WBCs in response to bacterial infections anywhere in the urinary tract can cause leukouria. It may be difficult to differentiate cystitis from urethritis, but it can be done with the two-specimen technique. Ask the patient to void about 20 mL of urine into one container and the rest into another container. More WBCs in the first container indicates urethritis; more in the second container indicates cystitis.*

▲ Increased WBC Cast Levels

Acute pyelonephritis,
Glomerulonephritis,
Lupus nephritis:
>   *Infectious or inflammatory diseases affecting the kidney can be associated with WBC cast formation. The presence of casts excludes the lower urinary tract as a source of the infection or inflammation.*

RELATED TESTS

Glucose, Urine (p. 924). This test is included in routine urinalysis. It warrants separate discussion, however, because of its importance.
Urine Culture and Sensitivity (see p. 973). If urinalysis indicates the possibility of infection, a culture and sensitivity test should be performed.

Urinary Stone Analysis (Renal Calculus Analysis)

NORMAL FINDINGS

All urinary stones are pathologic.

Urine Studies

11

INDICATIONS

Urinary stone analysis is performed to identify the chemicals that make up the kidney stone and to treat any underlying disease that may have caused the stone formation. This information is also used to determine the most effective methods to diminish the chance of another stone.

TEST EXPLANATION

About 5% of American women and 12% of men will develop a kidney stone at some time in their lives. Approximately 80% of stones are composed of calcium oxalate (CaOx) and calcium phosphate (CaP); 10% of struvite (magnesium ammonium phosphate produced during infection with bacteria that possess the enzyme urease); 9% of uric acid (UA); and the remaining 1% are composed of cystine or ammonium acid urate or are diagnosed as drug-related stones. Stones ultimately occur because of a supersaturated phase of these substances from liquid to solid state.

A kidney stone can be as small as a grain of sand or as big as 1 inch (2.5 cm) or larger in diameter. Sometimes a stone can leave the kidney and move down a ureter into the bladder. From the bladder, the stone passes through the urethra and out of the body in urine. Stone passage produces renal colic that usually begins as a mild discomfort and progresses to a plateau of extreme severity over 30 to 60 minutes. If the stone obstructs the ureteropelvic junction, pain localizes to the flank; as the stone moves down the ureter, pain moves downward and anterior. Colic is independent of body position or motion and is described as a boring or burning sensation.

Stones less than 5 mm in diameter have a high chance of passage; those of 5 to 7 mm have a modest chance (50%) of passage, and those greater than 7 mm almost always require urologic intervention. Renal stone burden is best gauged using computed tomography (CT) radiographs (see p. 1020) taken with 5-mm cuts, without infusion of contrast agents. The radiographic appearance and density of stones as measured by CT is a guide to their composition. About 90% of kidney stones can be seen on a KUB abdominal x-ray (see p. 1040).

Analysis is done on a kidney stone to determine its chemical makeup. The test, done on a stone that has been passed in the urine or removed from the urinary tract during surgery, shows the type of stone, which can guide treatment and give information that may prevent more stones from forming. People who have had a kidney stone have a risk for having another one. Therefore prevention measures are important.

Diagnosing a kidney stone includes an initial evaluation based on family history, associated medical conditions, medications, and diet; biochemical blood studies; urinalysis; x-rays; and analysis of the stone itself, if obtained. It also typically includes 24-hour urine collection to analyze volume, pH, calcium, magnesium, phosphate, oxalate, urate, creatinine, sodium, citrate, and cystine. If the stone is caused by a urinary tract infection (struvite or carbonate apatite), treatment of the infection will eliminate recurrence. Treating noninfectious stones will invariably involve some form of dietary manipulation, in particular increasing water intake.

Urinary stones can be partially prevented by altering the composition of the urine. In a simplified format, the following type of stones is often treated as follows:

- Hyperuricuria, predominantly uric acid stones, and cystine stones: Alkalinize urine to increase uric acid solubility with potassium alkali two or three times daily.
- Hypercalciuria and predominantly hydroxyapatite stones: Acidify urine to increase calcium solubility. However, treatment also depends on urine pH and urine phosphate, sulfate, oxalate, and citrate concentrations. Thiazide diuretics reduce urinary calcium and increase urinary volume.
- Hyperoxaluria and calcium oxalate stones: Increase daily fluid intake and consider reduction of daily calcium.
- Magnesium, ammonium, and phosphate stones (struvite): Investigate and treat urinary tract infection.

INTERFERING FACTORS

- Tape used to attach a stone to paper may affect the ability to accurately identify the composition of the stone.

PROCEDURE AND PATIENT CARE

Before

- Explain the procedure to the patient.
- Explain that there are no dietary restrictions for this test.
- Ensure pain relief if the patient is having ureteral colic.
- Obtain a history of any previous urinary stones.
- Provide and explain the use of a strainer into which the patient is to urinate.

During

- See Box 11-2, Guidelines for Collecting a 24-Hour Urine Specimen, p. 907.
- Instruct the patient to urinate into the strainer provided.
- Tell the patient to transfer any particulate matter to a container for laboratory analysis.

After

- Transport the specimen to the laboratory promptly.

TEST RESULTS AND CLINICAL SIGNIFICANCE

Urinary stone: *The composition of the stone will be used to direct further diagnosis and treatment.*

RELATED TESTS

Computed Tomography (CT) Scan (p. 1020). A CT scan of the ureters and kidneys (also called a CT urogram) is the most common way to find kidney stones.

Abdominal Ultrasonography (p. 866). This is a quick method that may also be used to find kidney stones.

Intravenous Pyelogram (IVP) (p. 1057). An IVP can monitor the excretion of dye through the urologic tract. An obstruction could indicate a urinary stone.

Urine Culture and Sensitivity (Urine C&S)

NORMAL FINDINGS

Negative: <10,000 bacteria/mL urine
Positive: >100,000 bacteria/mL urine

INDICATIONS

This test is used to diagnose urinary tract infection (UTI) in patients with dysuria, frequency, or urgency. It is also indicated when patients have fever of unknown origin or when urinalysis (UA) suggests infection.

11 Urine Studies

TEST EXPLANATION

Urine culture and sensitivity tests are performed to determine the presence of pathogenic bacteria in patients with suspected UTIs. Most often, urinary tract infections are limited to the bladder, although the kidneys, ureters, bladder, or urethra can be the source of infection. All cultures should be performed before antibiotic therapy is initiated, because the antibiotic may interrupt the growth of the organism in the laboratory. Most organisms require approximately 24 hours to grow in the laboratory, and a preliminary report can be given at that time. Usually, 48 to 72 hours are required for growth and identification of an organism. Cultures may be repeated after appropriate antibiotic therapy to assess for complete resolution of the infection, especially UTIs.

To save money, a urine sample is collected and divided. Half is sent for urinalysis, and the other half is held in the laboratory refrigerator and cultured only if results of urinalysis indicate a possible infection (e.g., increased number of WBCs, bacteria, high pH, leukocyte esterase).

An important part of any routine culture is assessment of the sensitivity to various antibiotics of any bacteria that are growing in the urine. The health care provider can then prescribe the safest, least expensive, and most effective antibiotic therapy for the specific bacteria.

INTERFERING FACTORS

- Contamination of the urine with stool, vaginal secretions, hands, or clothing will cause false-positive results.
- Drugs that may affect test results include antibiotics.

PROCEDURE AND PATIENT CARE

Before

- Explain to the patient the procedure for collecting a clean-catch (midstream) urine specimen.
- Withhold antibiotics until after the urine specimen has been collected.
- Provide the patient with the necessary supplies for the collection.

During

- Note that a *clean-catch* or *midstream urine collection* is required for culture and sensitivity testing. This requires meticulous cleansing of the urinary meatus with an antiseptic preparation to reduce contamination of the specimen by external organisms. The foreskin must be retracted in male patients. The cleansing agent must be completely removed so it will not contaminate the urine specimen. The midstream collection is obtained as follows:
  1. Have the patient begin to urinate into a bedpan, urinal, or toilet, and then stop urinating. This washes urine from the distal portion of the urethra.
  2. Correctly position a sterile urine container so the patient can void 3 to 4 ounces of urine.
  3. Cap the container.
  4. Allow the patient to finish voiding.
- Note that *urinary catheterization* may be needed for patients unable to void. This procedure is not usually performed, however, because of the risk of introducing organisms into the bladder and because of patient discomfort.
- For inpatients with an *indwelling urinary catheter*, obtain a specimen by attaching a syringe at a built-in sampling port. Aspirate the urine and place it in a sterile urine container. Usually the catheter tubing distal to the puncture site needs to be clamped for 15 to 30 minutes before aspiration of urine to allow urine to fill the tubing. After the specimen is withdrawn, remove the clamp.

- Collect specimens from infants and young children in a disposable pouch called a *U bag*. This bag has adhesive backing around the opening to attach to the child's pubic skin. Clean the urinary meatus before applying the bag.
- Note that *suprapubic aspiration* of urine is a safe method of obtaining urine in neonates and infants. The abdomen is prepared with an antiseptic, and a 25-gauge needle is inserted into the suprapubic area 1 inch above the symphysis pubis. Urine is aspirated into the syringe, then transferred to a sterile urine container.
- Note that in patients with a *urinary diversion* (e.g., ileal conduit), catheterization should be performed through the stoma. Urine should not be collected from the ostomy pouch.
- Urine for culture and sensitivity testing should not be taken from a bedpan or brought from home, because it will be contaminated.

After

- Transport the specimen to the laboratory immediately (within 30 minutes). If this is not possible, the specimen may be refrigerated for up to 2 hours. Urine for cytomegalovirus culture, however, will be rendered useless by refrigeration.
- Notify the health care provider of any positive results so that appropriate antibiotic therapy can be initiated.

TEST RESULTS AND CLINICAL SIGNIFICANCE

Urinary tract infection: *Urine is a good culture medium for bacteria. In case of urinary stasis, obstruction, or incomplete emptying, bacteria infect the urine. UTIs can occur as a result of ascending infections from the urethra, especially in female patients.*

RELATED TEST

Urinalysis (UA) (p. 956). This test is often performed before culture and sensitivity testing. The presence of WBCs, leukocyte esterase, nitrites, or bacteria indicates a UTI.

 Vanillylmandelic Acid (VMA), Homovanillic Acid (HVA), and Catecholamines (Epinephrine, Norepinephrine, Metanephrine, Normetanephrine, Dopamine)

NORMAL FINDINGS
VMA

Adult/elderly: <6.8 mg/24 hr or <35 µmol/24 hr (SI units)
Adolescent: 1-5 mg/24 hr
Child: 1-3 mg/24 hr
Infant: <2 mg/24 hr
Newborn: <1 mg/24 hr

HVA

≥15 years (adults): not applicable
10-14 years: <12 mg/g creatinine
5-9 years: <9 mg/g creatinine

2-4 years: <13.5 mg/g creatinine
1 year: <23 mg/g creatinine
<1 year: <35 mg/g creatinine

Catecholamines

Free Catecholamines
<100 mcg/24 hr or <590 nmol/day (SI units)

Epinephrine
Adult/elderly:
   <20 mcg/24 hr or <109 µmol/day (SI units)
Child:
   0-1 years: 0-2.5 mcg/24 hr
   1-2 years: 0-3.5 mcg/24 hr
   2-4 years: 0-6 mcg/24 hr
   4-7 years: 0.2-10 mcg/24 hr
   7-10 years: 0.5-14 mcg/24 hr

Norepinephrine
Adult/elderly:
   <100 mcg/24 hr or <590 nmol/day (SI units)
Child:
   0-1 years: 0-10 mcg/24 hr
   1-2 years: 0-17 mcg/24 hr
   2-4 years: 4-29 mcg/24 hr
   4-7 years: 8-45 mcg/24 hr
   7-10 years: 13-65 mcg/24 hr

Dopamine
Adult/elderly:
   65-400 mcg/24 hr
Child:
   0-1 year: 0-85 mcg/24 hr
   1-2 years: 10-140 mcg/24 hr
   2-4 years: 40-260 mcg/24 hr
   >4 years: 65-400 mcg/24 hr

Metanephrine
<1.3 mg/24 hr or <7 µmol/day (SI units)

Normetanephrine
15-80 mcg/24 hr or 89-473 nmol/day (SI units)

INDICATIONS

This 24-hour urine test for VMA, HVA, and catecholamines is a screening test for the diagnosis of catecholamine-producing tumors, such as neuroblastoma, pheochromocytoma, and other rare adrenal/neural crest tumors.

TEST EXPLANATION

A pheochromocytoma is a tumor of the chromaffin cells within the adrenal medulla that frequently secretes abnormally high levels of epinephrine and norepinephrine. Likewise, neural crest tumors such as neuroblastoma can also hypersecrete catecholamines. These hormones cause episodic or persistent severe hypertension by producing peripheral arterial vasoconstriction. Dopamine is the precursor of epinephrine and norepinephrine. HVA is a metabolite of dopamine. Metanephrine and normetanephrine are catabolic products of epinephrine and norepinephrine, respectively. VMA (3-methoxy-4-hydroxymandelic acid) is the product of catabolism of both metanephrine and normetanephrine. In pheochromocytoma, one or all of these substances will be present in excessive quantities in a 24-hour urine collection. These hormones may be measured singularly in the urine, but the collective metabolic end products, HVA and VMA, are more easily detected because their concentrations are much higher than any one catecholamine component.

VMA and HVA are primarily used as a screening test for neural crest tumors. These urinary tests can also be used to monitor tumor activity. HVA levels may also be altered in disorders of catecholamine metabolism. For example, monoamine oxidase (MAO) deficiency can cause decreased urinary HVA values, whereas a deficiency of dopamine beta-hydrolase (the enzyme that converts dopamine to norepinephrine) can cause elevated urinary HVA values.

A 24-hour urine test is preferable to a blood test because catecholamine secretion from the tumor may be episodic and could be missed at a random time during the day. A 24-hour urine reflects catecholamine production over an entire day. It is best to perform testing when symptoms (hypertension) of the potential adrenal tumor are significant. At that time, catecholamine production is greatest and can be more assuredly identified. That being said, VMA is not the analyte of choice to rule out a diagnosis of pheochromocytoma. Metanephrines measured in the plasma or urine may be more accurate.

In the past, these urinary tests have been performed by spectrophotometric assays. Now, high-performance liquid chromatography (HPLC)–tandem mass spectrometry has improved the accuracy of this testing. Nevertheless, urine testing is cumbersome and time consuming. With HPLC, measurement of plasma-free metanephrines (see p. 357) has nearly replaced urine testing for pheochromocytoma.

INTERFERING FACTORS

- Increased levels of VMA may be caused by certain foods (e.g., tea, coffee, cocoa, vanilla, chocolate, cider vinegar, soda, licorice).
- Vigorous exercise, stress, and starvation may cause increased VMA levels.
- Falsely decreased levels of VMA may be caused by uremia, alkaline urine, and radiographic iodine contrast agents.
- Drugs that may cause *increased* VMA levels include caffeine, epinephrine, levodopa, lithium, and nitroglycerin. Patients receiving L-dopa should stop taking it for 24 hours before the specimen is obtained.
- Drugs that may cause *decreased* VMA levels include disulfiram (Antabuse), guanethidine, imipramine, monoamine oxidase (MAO) inhibitors, phenothiazines, and reserpine.
- Drugs that may cause *increased* catecholamine levels include alcohol (ethyl), aminophylline, caffeine, chloral hydrate, clonidine (prolonged therapy), contrast media (containing iodine), disulfiram, epinephrine, erythromycin, insulin, methenamine, methyldopa, nicotinic acid (large doses), nitroglycerin, quinidine, riboflavin, and tetracyclines.
- Drugs that may cause *decreased* catecholamine levels include guanethidine, reserpine, and salicylates.

Urine Studies

11

Clinical Priorities

- This test is used primarily to evaluate the hypertensive patient for pheochromocytoma.
- A VMA-restricted diet is essential for 2 to 3 days before and throughout the 24-hour urine collection period.
- This 24-hour urine collection requires a preservative and should be placed on ice or refrigerated.

PROCEDURE AND PATIENT CARE

Before

☒ Explain the dietary restrictions and the 24-hour urine collection procedure to the patient.

☒ For 2 or 3 days before and throughout the 24-hour collection for VMA, place the patient on a VMA-restricted diet. Instruct the patient to avoid coffee, tea, bananas, chocolate, cocoa, licorice, citrus fruit, all foods and fluids containing vanilla, and aspirin. Obtain specific restrictions from the laboratory.

☒ Instruct the patient to avoid taking antihypertensive medications, and sometimes all medications, during this period and possibly longer.

During

- See Box 11-2, Guidelines for a 24-Hour Urine Collection, p. 907.
- Use a preservative. Refrigerate the specimen or keep it on ice over the 24 hours.
- Identify and minimize factors contributing to patient stress and anxiety. Excessive physical exercise and emotion may alter catecholamine test results by causing increased secretion of epinephrine and norepinephrine.

After

- Send the specimen to the laboratory as soon as the test is completed.
- Allow the patient to have foods and drugs that were restricted in preparation for the test.

TEST RESULTS AND CLINICAL SIGNIFICANCE

▲ Increased Levels

Pheochromocytomas,
Neuroblastomas,
Ganglioneuromas,
Ganglioblastomas:
   These tumors can produce catecholamines. HVA/VMA levels will be elevated.
Severe stress,
Strenuous exercise,
Acute anxiety:
   Catecholamines are elevated during physical (serious illness) or emotional stress or after heavy exercise. HVA/VMA levels will be elevated.

RELATED TEST

Pheochromocytoma Suppression and Provocative Testing (p. 389). This is used to identify pheochromocytoma when catecholamine levels are not assuredly diagnostic.

Water Deprivation (Antidiuretic Hormone [ADH] Stimulation)

NORMAL FINDINGS

Neurogenic diabetes insipidus: >9% rise in urine osmolality
Nephrogenic diabetes insipidus: <9% rise in urine osmolality
Psychogenic polydipsia: <9% rise in urine osmolality

INDICATIONS

This test is used to aid in the differential diagnosis of polyuria. Polyuria can occur as a result of neurogenic diabetes insipidus (DI), nephrogenic DI, or psychogenic polydipsia.

TEST EXPLANATION

In this test, the patient is deprived of fluids. Patients who have DI will dehydrate quickly as indicated by a rise in urine and serum osmolality. Patients with primary psychogenic polydipsia take a longer time to dehydrate. Next, ADH is administered. Patients with neurogenic DI have no endogenous ADH but can concentrate their urine and raise urine osmolality if ADH is provided exogenously. Patients with nephrogenic DI have kidneys that are insensitive to ADH. They will experience little or no increase in urine osmolality. Patients who have psychogenic polydipsia will experience a less than 9% increase in urine osmolality.

POTENTIAL COMPLICATIONS

- Severe dehydration may occur in patients with neurogenic DI. If their urine output is high, they should be watched closely during the period of dehydration.

INTERFERING FACTORS

- Diuretics can confuse the results and increase the danger of fluid restriction.

PROCEDURE AND PATIENT CARE

Before

- Explain the procedure to the patient.
- Explain the recommended fluid restriction.
  1. Patients with a urine output of less than 4000/24 hr undergo fluid restriction after midnight before the test.
  2. Patients with a urine output of greater than 4000/24 hr begin fluid restriction at the time the test starts, because they may get dangerously dehydrated if asked to restrict water from midnight.
- The test usually starts at 6 AM and stops at noon.

During

- Obtain and record the patient's body weight hourly for the duration of the procedure.
- Obtain urine osmolality hourly from 6 AM to noon or until three consecutive hourly determinations show a urine osmolality increase of less than 30 mOsm/kg.

- At that point obtain a serum osmolality. It must be greater than 288 mOsm/kg for the patient to be considered adequately dehydrated and water deprived.
- If the body weight drops more than 2 kg, discontinue the test and rehydrate the patient.
- Administer the prescribed dose of vasopressin (or desmopressin, an analog of ADH) subcutaneously.
- Obtain urine osmolality 30 to 60 minutes after the injection.

After

- Rehydrate the patient with oral fluids.
- Record vital signs in both the recumbent and erect position to be sure that no orthostasis exists from inadequate rehydration.
- Observe the venipuncture sites for bleeding.

TEST RESULTS AND CLINICAL SIGNIFICANCE

Rise in Urine Osmolality of More Than 9%

Neurogenic (or central) DI caused by CNS trauma, tumor, or infection. Surgical ablation of pituitary gland: *ADH is not produced in these patients, but the kidneys can respond to exogenously administered ADH by concentrating the urine.*

Little or No Increase in Urine Osmolality During Deprivation Portion of Test or After Injection

Nephrogenic DI caused by primary renal diseases: *Patients with nephrogenic DI because of chronic kidney diseases will experience little or no rise in urine osmolality during the dehydration phase of the test, because the kidney has lost its concentrating abilities. Furthermore, their kidneys are insensitive to the urine-concentrating effect of ADH.*

Hypokalemia: *These patients have the same lack of response as do patients with nephrogenic DI.*

Psychogenic polydipsia: *These patients frequently take longer than usual to dehydrate to a serum osmolality of 288, and the urine osmolality rises less than 9% after vasopressin injection.*

RELATED TESTS

Antidiuretic Hormone (ADH) (p. 73). This is a serum assay for direct measurement of ADH. This test is used in the differential diagnosis of neurogenic DI, nephrogenic DI, or psychogenic polydipsia.

Osmolality, Serum (p. 378). This test is a measurement of solute load in the serum.

Osmolality, Urine (p. 938). This test is a measurement of solute load in the urine.

Sodium, Blood (p. 466). This is a direct measurement of sodium level in the blood.

Sodium, Urine (p. 946). This is a direct measurement of sodium level in the urine.

X-Ray Studies

OVERVIEW

TESTS

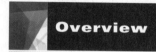

Overview

REASON FOR PERFORMING X-RAY STUDIES

Because x-rays can penetrate human tissue, radiographic studies provide a valuable picture of body structures. These studies can be as simple as routine chest radiography or as complex as dye-enhanced cardiac catheterization. With the increasing concern about radiation exposure, the patient may want to know if the proposed benefit outweighs the risk involved.

X-ray studies are used in a wide variety of clinical conditions, such as the following:

1. To evaluate dye excretion in the urinary system (e.g., intravenous pyelography [IVP], antegrade pyelography, retrograde pyelography).
2. To evaluate arterial occlusive disease (e.g., arteriography of the kidney, adrenal glands, or cerebrum).
3. To evaluate the GI tract with barium contrast medium (e.g., barium enema, upper GI series).
4. To evaluate bone disorders such as fractures, infections, and arthritis (long bone x-ray films).
5. To evaluate the tracheobronchial tree (bronchography).
6. To visualize the heart chambers, arteries, and great vessels (cardiac catheterization).
7. To evaluate the pulmonary and cardiac systems (chest radiography and CT of the chest).
8. To guide needles for biopsy of tumors and aspiration of fluid.
9. To evaluate abdominal organs (computed tomography [CT] of the abdomen).
10. To determine patency of the fallopian tubes (hysterosalpingography).
11. To evaluate abdominal pain or trauma (kidneys, ureter, and bladder [KUB] or obstruction series).
12. To detect breast cancer (mammography).

PRINCIPLES OF RADIOLOGY

X-ray films are radiographs of body structures and look like negatives of photographs. Radiography is based on the ability of x-rays to penetrate tissues and organs differently according to tissue density. X-rays are generated by a machine that passes a high-voltage electrical current through a tungsten filter in a vacuum tube (x-ray tube). As the x-ray passes through body tissues, images are formed on photographic film or digital imaging plate. Images are produced in varying degrees of dark and light, depending on the amount of x-rays that penetrate the tissues. The greater the amount of energy absorbed, the fewer are the x-rays that reach the film and the whiter the image appears on the film. For example, bones appear white (radiopaque) because the x-rays cannot penetrate bone to reach the film. When bones are fractured, the break is visible as a black (radiolucent) line. Because patients with osteoporosis have less calcium in their bones, the bones appear gray and porous on x-ray films. X-rays can easily penetrate air, so areas filled with air or gas (e.g., lungs, bowel) appear black or very dark on x-ray films. Muscles, blood, organs, and other tissues in the body appear as various shades of gray because they are denser than air but not as dense as bone.

By orienting the radiographic machine at different angles in relation to the body or a body part, different views (projections) can be obtained. The two basic views are anteroposterior (AP), in which the x-rays pass through the front of the body (anterior) to the back (posterior), and lateral, in which the x-rays pass through the body from the side. For posteroanterior (PA) views, the x-rays pass through the back of the body to the front. Oblique views are obtained when the x-rays pass through the body at different angles according to how the patient is positioned.

Some of the many types of x-ray procedures include those described in the following sections:

PLAIN RADIOGRAPHY

Plain radiography is performed without contrast material or other augmentation techniques. This procedure is used for routine examination of areas such as the chest, skull, abdomen, and bones.

FLUOROSCOPY

In this radiologic procedure, x-rays pass through the body to a fluorescent viewing screen that is coated with calcium tungstate. The radiologist cannot only view the body organs but can also observe their motion. For example, while a patient swallows barium, its flow through the upper GI tract can be followed, or after administration of a barium enema, the flow of barium through the colon can be observed. Fluoroscopy is used in angiography procedures to guide the catheter to its desired position (e.g., through the heart during cardiac catheterization). Single films (spot films) can be obtained for a permanent record of findings. Videotapes of fluoroscopic procedures (cineradiography) can provide a record of movement for study at a later time. Tapes can be viewed in slow motion to aid in determining abnormal function. The major disadvantage of fluoroscopy is that it exposes the patient to more radiation than standard x-ray procedures do.

TOMOGRAPHY

In CT, computers re-create a three-dimensional, cross-sectional view of body structures after obtaining x-ray information from the entire circumference of the body. The CT scan results from passing x-rays through the body organs at many angles through 360 degrees. The variation in density of each tissue allows for variable penetration of the x-rays. Each degree of density is given a numeric value called a *density coefficient*, which is digitally computed into a shade of gray. An image is then displayed on a cathode ray tube as thousands of dots in various shades of gray. The image can be enhanced by repeating the CT procedure after IV administration of iodine-containing contrast dye. The images can be recorded on film. See Figure 12-11, p. 1020.

CONTRAST STUDIES

In some areas of the body, a contrast agent is necessary to provide better visualization of organs being studied. Contrast material can be administered orally, rectally, intravenously, percutaneously, by inhalation, or through urinary catheterization. For angiography, contrast agent is injected into a blood vessel.

The most commonly used contrast media are barium sulfate for GI studies (Box 12-1); organic iodine for vascular and renal studies; and iodized oils for myelography. These substances are radiopaque (i.e., they block the passage of x-rays) and thus provide excellent contrast to body structures. Air can also be used as a contrast medium, although is much less commonly used lately.

In addition to radiation risks associated with all radiology procedures, contrast studies pose additional potential complications. For example, iodinated dyes may cause a severe allergic reaction, and nephrotoxicity (Box 12-2). Barium sulfate may cause constipation and bowel impaction.

DIGITAL SUBTRACTION ANGIOGRAPHY

Digital subtraction angiography is a type of computerized fluoroscopy in which venous or arterial catheterization is performed to visualize the arteries, especially the carotid and cerebral arteries. The procedure enables small differences in x-ray absorption between an artery and the surrounding tissues to be converted to digital information and stored. It is especially useful when bone blocks visualization

X-Ray Studies

12

| BOX 12-1 | Clinical Responsibilities Associated With Use of Barium Sulfate |

- Barium may interfere with subsequent x-ray studies (e.g., IVP, CT). Tests requiring the use of barium should be performed after other x-ray studies.
- Cathartics are required before tests that require barium, to prevent the possibility of false-positive findings because of food in the bowel.
- Cathartics should always be administered after tests that require barium, to diminish the possibility of barium or fecal impaction.
- The patient should observe the color of stool to ensure that all barium (white) has been eliminated from the intestinal tract.
- Barium should not be administered in patients with acute colitis, especially ulcerative colitis, because it can precipitate development of toxic megacolon.
- Barium should not be administered if GI perforation is suspected. Extravasation of barium from the GI tract may be associated with multiple and recurrent abdominal abscesses.

CT, Computed tomography; *GI*, gastrointestinal; *IVP*, intravenous pyelogram.

| BOX 12-2 | Nephrotoxicity Caused by Contrast Medium |

Definition: Impairment in renal function (increase in serum creatinine by more than 25%) that occurs within 3 days following the intravascular administration of a contrast medium. This occurs in the absence of an alternative etiology.

Risk Factors
- Creatinine >1.5 mg/dL
- Dehydration
- Heart disease (e.g., congestive heart failure)
- Age older than 70 years
- Concurrent administration of nephrotoxic drugs (e.g., nonsteroidal antiinflammatory drugs [NSAIDs])
- Diabetes—especially insulin dependent
- Multiple myeloma
- Heart disease

Clinical Priorities
- Make sure the patient is well hydrated. Depending on the clinical situation, give at least 100 mL oral or intravenous (IV) normal saline (NS) per hour starting 4 hours before to 24 hours after contrast administration. Increase the volume in warm weather.
- Use low- or iso-osmolar nonionic contrast media (e.g., Omniscan Ultravist).
- Stop administration of nephrotoxic drugs for at least 24 hours.
- If possible, use alternate imaging techniques which do not require an iodinated contrast media.
- Do not do any of the following:
  - Give high osmolar contrast media.
  - Administer large doses of contrast media.
  - Administer mannitol and diuretics, particularly loop-diuretics, for 24 hours after contrast.
  - Perform multiple studies with contrast media within a short time period.

of the blood vessel being studied. This study is valuable for preoperative and postoperative evaluation of patients undergoing vascular and tumor surgery.

An image "mask" is made of the area of clinical interest and stored in a computer. After IV injection of contrast material, subsequent images are made. The computer then subtracts the preinjection mask image from the postinjection image. This removes all undesired tissue images (e.g., bone) and leaves an arterial image of high contrast. Venous injection of the dye, rather than arterial injection, averts the complications and risks associated with conventional arteriography. However, arterial injection of contrast material is more often used.

RISKS FOR RADIATION EXPOSURE

All x-ray procedures carry the risk of exposure to radiation. In general, there are three possible types of damage to the body from radiologic procedures.

1. *Somatic effects* ultimately occur in patients exposed to the harmful agent. These may include short-term effects such as blood cell problems or long-term effects such as cancer.
2. *Genetic effects* include damage to future generations as a result of exposure of parent germ cells to a harmful agent. Depending on the type of damage to the germ cell, genetic effects can range from mild to severe (e.g., mental retardation).
3. *Fetal effects* occur as a result of exposure to a harmful agent during the embryonal or fetal stage of development. This type of damage is highly dependent on timing of the exposure with respect to gestational age. Damage can range from mild birth defects to childhood malignancies. The fetus is at greatest risk during early pregnancy, when organs are developing. Radiation exposure during later pregnancy, after development is complete and only growth is occurring, is far less risky to the fetus.

Because of the risks of radiation exposure, x-ray studies should not be performed more often than necessary. For this reason, patients should be adequately prepared for each test, to reduce the need for repeated studies. Patients should be shielded from unnecessary exposure with lead aprons and gloves. During or within 10 to 12 days after normal menses, women can safely undergo diagnostic x-ray studies. Otherwise, no women in the childbearing years should undergo x-ray examination unless a pregnancy test is performed and the results are negative. These restrictions exist to avoid exposure and subsequent injury to a fetus when a woman is unknowingly pregnant.

CONTRAINDICATIONS

Pregnancy is a contraindication for x-ray studies. However, sometimes the benefits of diagnostic x-ray examination outweigh the risks. In those cases, every attempt should be made to minimize exposure of the fetus to x-rays (e.g., use of a lead apron). The contraindications listed below relate to specific types of x-ray studies. Specific details relative to each type of radiographic procedure are discussed later in this chapter.

1. Iodinated dye (e.g., IVP cardiac catheterization)
   - Patients allergic to shellfish or iodinated dye (Table 12-1).
   - Patients with renal disorders, because iodinated contrast is nephrotoxic.
   - Patients who are dehydrated, because they are especially susceptible to dye-induced renal failure.
   - Patients with pheochromocytoma, because a hypertensive crisis may be precipitated by the use of iodine.
2. Arterial or venous puncture (e.g., cardiac catheterization, angiography)
   - Patients with a bleeding disorder, because the arterial or venous puncture site may not stop bleeding.
3. Barium (e.g., upper GI series, barium enema)
   - Patients with suspected perforation of the colon or upper GI tract. In these patients, meglumine diatrizoate (Gastrografin), a water-soluble contrast medium, should be used.

POTENTIAL COMPLICATIONS

- Allergic reaction to iodinated dye: Allergic reactions can include flushing, itching, urticaria, and even severe life-threatening anaphylaxis (evidenced by respiratory distress, decreased blood pressure, or shock). Treatment depends upon the type of reaction. In the unusual event of anaphylaxis,

TABLE 12-1	Signs, Symptoms, and Treatment of Iodine Contrast Allergy		
	Minor Reaction	**Intermediate Reaction**	**Severe or Life-Threatening Reaction**
Incidence	1 of 25	1 of 150	1 of 5000
Signs and symptoms	Nausea, vomiting, mild urticaria	Facial, tongue, or laryngeal edema; bronchospasm; chest pain; chills and fever	Laryngeal and pulmonary edema, hypotension, myocardial depression, cardiac arrhythmias, seizure, ventilatory failure
Treatment	Antihistamines	Antihistamines, possibly steroids, IV fluids, observation, bronchodilators	Antihistamines, steroids, IV fluids, bronchodilators, intubation and ventilation, pressors, antiseizure medications

diphenhydramine (Benadryl), steroids, and epinephrine are included in resuscitative efforts. Oxygen and endotracheal equipment should be on hand for immediate use. To avoid iodine-related allergy, patients with prior allergic reactions should be premedicated before receiving contrast:

Prevention of Allergic Reaction to Iodine

Benadryl 50 mg PO before contrast

Prednisone 50 mg PO the night before testing and Q6 hours times three doses after testing.

Histamine 2 blocker may also be used

Use nonionic contrast

- Catheter-induced embolic stroke (cerebral vascular accident, myocardial infarction).
- Complications associated with the catheter insertion, such as arterial thrombosis, embolism, or pseudoaneurysm.
- Infection at the catheter insertion site.
- Renal failure, especially in elderly patients with chronic dehydration or mild renal failure. Adequate hydration may reduce the likelihood of this complication.
- Lactic acidosis is a rare complication associated with the use of iodinated contrast materials. It is most commonly associated with biguanide oral antihyperglycemic agents (e.g., metformin/Glucophage) used to treat non–insulin-dependent diabetes. This is more common in patients who have impaired renal or hepatic function. These medications should be discontinued for 48 hours before and after a contrast study. Utilization of non-ionic contrast in a well-hydrated patient can minimize the incidence of lactic acidosis.

INTERFERING FACTORS

Factors that can obscure x-ray visualization include:
- Presence of metallic objects (e.g., hemostasis clips, jewelry)
- Barium retained from previous studies
- Large amounts of fecal material or gas in the bowel
- Improper positioning
- Excessive movement

PROCEDURE AND PATIENT CARE

Specific procedures are presented with the discussion of each test.

Before

- Explain the procedure to the patient. Cooperation is necessary, because the patient must lie still during the procedure.
- Obtain informed consent if required by the institution.
- Assess the patient for allergy to iodinated dye. Inform the radiologist if an allergy to iodinated contrast is suspected. The radiologist can prescribe a diphenhydramine and steroid preparation to be administered before testing. Usually, hypoallergenic nonionic contrast material is used for the test.
- Assess the patient for any evidence of dehydration or renal disease. Usually, blood urea nitrogen and creatinine tests are obtained before administration of iodine-containing intravenous contrast. Hydration may be required before the administration of iodine.
- Assess the patient for diabetes. Diabetic patients are particularly susceptible to renal disease caused by the administration of iodine-containing IV contrast. Diabetic patients who take metformin or glyburide are particularly susceptible to lactic acidosis and hypoglycemia. These medications may be discontinued for 1 to 4 days before and 1 to 2 days after the administration of iodine.
- Instruct the patient to remove all jewelry from the area to be imaged.
- Inform the patient of any fasting requirements.
- Depending on the type of test, the patient may be given nothing orally for 2 to 8 hours before testing.
- Mark the site of the patient's peripheral pulses with a pen before arterial catheterization, to permit assessment of the peripheral pulses after the procedure.
- Ensure that the appropriate coagulation studies have been performed and that the results are normal.
- For cerebral angiography, perform a baseline neurologic assessment for comparison with subsequent assessments.
- Administer sedation if indicated.
- Assist the patient with bowel preparation if indicated. For example, a barium contrast study necessitates bowel preparation and, possibly, cleansing enemas.

During

- Instruct the patient to remain motionless throughout the testing. Sometimes patients are asked to hold their breath for periods of time while images are being taken.

After

- If an iodine contrast dye has been used, instruct the patient to drink fluids to avoid dye-induced renal failure and to promote dye excretion.
- If barium contrast was used, laxatives may be indicated to prevent constipation and bowel obstruction.
- Monitor the patient's vital signs. Changes may be noted because of medications used during the tests or from complications such as bleeding.
- Evaluate the patient for delayed reaction to dyes. These may occur within 2 to 6 hours after the test.

REPORTING OF RESULTS

Radiographs are carefully reviewed and the findings reported by the radiologist. Results may be discussed with the patient at the time of testing or within a few days.

X-Ray Studies

12

Arteriography (Angiography; Renal, Mesenteric, Adrenal, Cerebral, and Lower Extremity Arteriography)

NORMAL FINDINGS

Normal arterial vasculature

INDICATIONS

Arteriography of the adrenal glands, kidneys, mesentery, brain, and lower extremity is used to evaluate arterial occlusive disease of these organs and is helpful in evaluation of suspected neoplasms arising from these organs. Arteriography provides the vascular surgeon with an accurate picture of the vascular anatomy of these structures. This is especially important in arterio-occlusive disease involving the arteries to these organs.

TEST EXPLANATION

With the injection of radiopaque contrast material into arteries, blood vessels can be visualized to determine arterial anatomy, vascular disease, or neoplasms. With a catheter usually placed through the femoral or brachial artery and into the desired artery, radiopaque contrast material is rapidly injected while x-ray films are obtained. Blood-flow dynamics, abnormal blood vessels, vascular anomalies, normal and abnormal vascular anatomy, and tumors can be seen. Usually an iodinated contrast agent is used to visualize the arteries.

Digital subtraction angiography (DSA) allows bony structures to be obliterated from the picture. DSA is a sophisticated type of computerized process that, when used with angiography, enables better visualization of the arteries, especially the carotid and cerebral arteries by eliminating bone structures from the image. It is especially useful when adjacent bone inhibits visualization of the blood vessel to be evaluated. For DSA, an image (mask) is made of the area of clinical interest and stored in the computer program. After intraarterial injection of contrast material, subsequent images are made. The computer then subtracts the preinjection mask image from the postinjection image. This removes all the undesired images (e.g., bone) and leaves the arterial image of high contrast and quality.

While nearly all major blood vessels can be visualized through the technique of arteriography, the kidneys, adrenal glands, brain, and abdominal aorta (with lower extremities) are most usually visualized. Coronary arteriography is described under cardiac catheterization (p. 1008).

Renal angiography permits evaluation of blood flow dynamics, demonstration of abnormal blood vessels, and differentiation of a vascular renal cyst from hypervascular renal cancers (Figure 12-1). Arteriosclerotic narrowing (stenosis) of the renal artery is best demonstrated with this study. The angiographic location of the stenotic area is helpful for the vascular surgeon considering repair. Complete transection of the renal artery by blunt or penetrating trauma can also be seen as total vascular obstruction. Highly vascular renal cancers can produce a "blush" of contrast material during angiography.

The adrenal gland and its arterial system can also be visualized by *adrenal arteriography*. Both benign and malignant tumors of the adrenal gland, and bilateral adrenal hyperplasia, can be detected easily with this technique.

Cerebral angiography provides radiographic visualization of the cerebral vascular system with the injection of radiopaque dye into the carotid or vertebral arteries (Figure 12-2). With this procedure, abnormalities of the cerebral circulation (e.g., aneurysms, occlusions, stenosis, arteriovenous

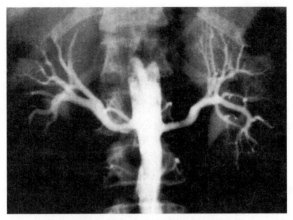

Figure 12-1 Renal arteriogram.

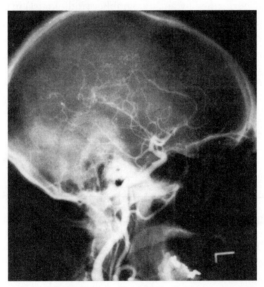

Figure 12-2 Carotid angiogram.

malformations) can be identified. A vascular tumor is seen as a mass containing small, abnormal blood vessels. A nonvascular tumor, abscess, or hematoma appears as a mass that distorts the normal vascular contour.

Lower-extremity arteriography enables accurate identification and location of occlusions within the abdominal aorta and lower-extremity arteries. After the catheter is placed in the aorta or more selectively, into the femoral artery, radiopaque dye is injected. X-ray films are obtained in timed sequence to allow radiographic visualization of the arterial system of the lower extremities. Total or near-total occlusion of the flow of dye is seen in arteriosclerotic vascular occlusive disease. Emboli are seen as total occlusions of the artery. Arterial traumas such as lacerations or intimal tears (laceration of the arterial inner lining) likewise appear as total or near-total obstruction of the flow of dye. Aneurysmal dilation of the aorta or its branches also can be seen. Unusual arterial disorders (e.g., thromboangiitis obliterans [Buerger disease], fibromuscular dysplasia) demonstrate classic arterial "beading," which is pathognomonic.

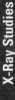

12   X-Ray Studies

Lower-extremity arteriography is usually performed electively in patients with symptoms and signs of peripheral vascular disease. Emergency arteriography, however, is needed when the blood flow to an extremity has ceased suddenly. Immediate surgical therapy is needed and is most effective when the surgeon has knowledge of the cause and location of the sudden occlusion. This knowledge can be obtained only with arteriography.

Arterial vascular balloon dilation and stenting can be performed if a short-segment arterial stenosis is identified. In these instances the wire is placed through the angiocatheter into the area of narrowing. A balloon catheter is inserted over the wire. The dilating balloon is inflated, and the arteriosclerotic plaque is gently and persistently dilated and can then be stented.

With angiography, there is always a concern that the arterial puncture site may not seal, leading to a pseudoaneurysm. More recently, vascular closure products are used to quickly seal femoral artery punctures following catheterization procedures. This allows for early ambulation and hospital discharge. The injection of these materials on the vascular entrance site creates a mechanical seal by sandwiching the arteriotomy between a bioabsorbable anchor and collagen sponge, which dissolve within 60 to 90 days.

This procedure is usually performed by an angiographer (radiologist) in approximately 1 to 2 hours. During the dye injection, remind the patient that an intense, burning flush may be felt throughout the body, but it lasts only a few seconds. The only discomfort is in the area of the groin puncture necessary for arterial access, and discomfort from lying on a hard x-ray table for a long time.

Age-Related Concerns

- The elderly patient with chronic dehydration or who has mildly decreased renal function is at high risk for dye-induced renal failure.
- The postprocedure urinary output in the elderly patient needs to be carefully monitored.

CONTRAINDICATIONS

- Patients allergic to shellfish or iodinated dye
- Patients who are uncooperative or agitated
- Patients who are pregnant, unless the benefits outweigh the risks
- Patients with renal disorders, because iodinated contrast medium is nephrotoxic
- Patients with a propensity for bleeding, because the arterial puncture site may not stop bleeding
- Patients with unstable cardiac disorders
- Patients with dehydration, because they are especially susceptible to dye-induced renal failure

POTENTIAL COMPLICATIONS

- See potential complications associated with iodinated dye on p. 985.
- Hemorrhage from the arterial puncture site used for arterial access
- Arterial embolism or stroke from dislodgement of arteriosclerotic plaque
- Soft-tissue infection around the puncture site
- Renal failure, especially in elderly patients with chronic dehydration or mild renal failure (see Box 12-2, p. 984)
- Dissection of the intimal lining of the artery, causing complete or partial arterial occlusion
- Development of pseudoaneurysm as a result of failure of the puncture site to seal

- Hypertensive crisis: With adrenal angiography, fatal hypertensive crisis may occur in patients with pheochromocytoma. Propranolol (Inderal), a beta-adrenergic blocker, and phenoxybenzamine (Dibenzyline), an alpha-adrenergic blocker, are given for several days before the study to avert precipitation of a malignant hypertensive episode.
- In adrenal angiography, hemorrhage of the adrenal gland, which may lead to adrenal insufficiency
- Lactic acidosis may occur in patients who are taking metformin. On the day of the test, metformin should be held to prevent this complication.

Clinical Priorities

- Assess for allergies to iodinated dye.
- Perform a baseline assessment of the patient's peripheral pulses before arterial catheterization.
- Be certain that coagulation studies (prothrombin time [PT], partial thromboplastin time [PTT], bleeding time) are normal before the test, because of the risk of bleeding.
- After the test, the patient is kept on bed rest for approximately 8 hours to allow complete sealing of the arterial puncture.

PROCEDURE AND PATIENT CARE

Before

- Explain the procedure to the patient. Allay any fears, and allow the patient to verbalize concerns.
- Ensure that written, informed consent for this procedure is in the patient's chart.
- Inform the patient that a warm flush may be felt when the dye is injected.
- See assessment for allergies to iodinated dye on p. 985.
- Determine whether the patient has been taking anticoagulants.
- The patient is allowed nothing orally for 2 to 8 hours before testing.
- Mark the site of the patient's peripheral pulses with a pen before arterial catheterization, to permit assessment of the peripheral pulses after the procedure.
- If the patient does not have peripheral pulses before arteriography, document that fact so that arterial occlusion will not be suspected at the post-angiographic assessment.
- Administer preprocedural medications as ordered.
- If a pheochromocytoma is suspected, administer medications as ordered, to prevent a potentially fatal hypertensive episode.
- Ensure that the appropriate coagulation studies have been performed and that the results are normal.
- For cerebral angiography, perform a baseline neurologic assessment for comparison with subsequent assessment, potentially to diagnose stroke that may be precipitated by the study.
- Remove all valuables and dental prostheses.
- Instruct the patient to void before the study, because iodinated dye can act as an osmotic diuretic.
- Inform the patient that bladder distention may cause some discomfort during the study.

During

- Note the following procedural steps:
  1. The patient may be sedated before being taken to the angiography room, which is usually within the radiology department.
  2. The patient is placed on the x-ray table in supine position (Figure 12-3).
  3. If the femoral artery is to be used, the groin is shaved, prepared, and draped in a sterile manner.

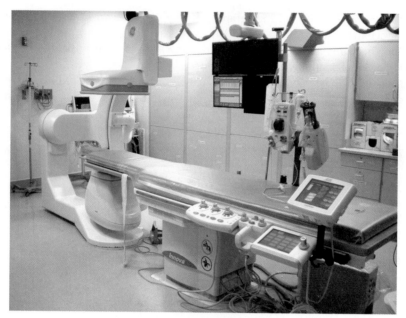

Figure 12-3 Angiography room.

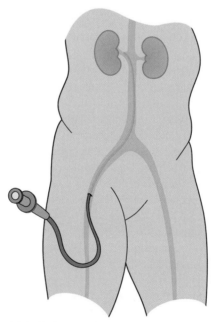

Figure 12-4 Catheter insertion for renal angiography.

4. The femoral artery is cannulated, and a wire is threaded up through the artery and into or near the opening of the artery to be examined (Figure 12-4).
5. A catheter is placed over that wire. The wire and catheter are both visualized fluoroscopically. Because the catheter and wire have curled tips, both can be manipulated directly into the artery to be studied. The wire is removed.

6. Iodinated contrast material is injected through the catheter with an automated injector at a preset, controlled rate, over several seconds.

7. Serial x-rays are obtained in timed sequence to show the arterial injection, and subsequent x-rays are taken to show the venous phase of the injection.

- During adrenal angiography, monitor blood pressure for evidence of malignant hypertensive storm.

After

- After x-ray studies are completed, remove the catheter and apply a pressure dressing to the puncture site.
- Monitor the patient's vital signs for indications of hemorrhage.
- Assess the peripheral arterial pulse in the extremity used for vascular access and compare it with the preprocedural baseline values.
- If cerebral arteriography was performed, perform a neurologic assessment for any signs of catheter-induced embolic stroke syndrome.
- Observe the arterial puncture site frequently for signs of bleeding or hematoma.
- Maintain pressure at the puncture site with a 1- to 2-pound sand bag or intravenous (IV) bag.
- Keep the patient on bed rest for about 8 hours after the procedure to allow complete sealing of the arterial puncture site.
- Assess the patient's extremities for signs of loss of blood supply (e.g., loss of pulses, numbness, pallor, tingling, pain, loss of sensory or motor function).
- Note and compare the color and temperature of the involved extremity with that of the uninvolved extremity.
- Administer mild analgesics for discomfort at the arterial puncture site.
- Notify the physician if the patient has severe, continuous pain.
- Have the patient drink fluids to prevent dehydration caused by the diuretic action of the dye.
- Evaluate the patient for delayed allergic reaction to the dye (dyspnea, rash, tachycardia, hives). This usually occurs within 2 to 6 hours after the test.

Home Care Responsibilities

- Check the arterial puncture site for bleeding and hematoma.
- Monitor the vital signs for evidence of bleeding (increased pulse and decreased blood pressure).
- Instruct the patient to report any signs of numbness, tingling, pain, or loss of function in the involved extremity.
- Encourage the patient to drink fluids to prevent dehydration.

TEST RESULTS AND CLINICAL SIGNIFICANCE

Adrenal Angiography

Pheochromocytoma,
Adrenal adenoma,
Adrenal carcinoma:
>   *These are evident as avascular filling defects within the gland. Pheochromocytomas are epinephrine-producing or norepinephrine-producing tumors that can precipitate a hypertensive crisis during angiography.*

Bilateral adrenal hyperplasia: *Adrenal glands are usually larger and more vascular.*

Arteriography of Lower Extremity

Arteriosclerotic occlusion: *This is evident as a segment of narrowing in an otherwise normal vessel.*

Embolus occlusion: *An embolus may come from the heart or an abdominal aortic aneurysm. Complete interruption in the flow of dye within the blood vessel is seen.*

Primary arterial diseases (e.g., fibromuscular dysplasia, Buerger disease): *Often arteriograms demonstrate findings that are classic for the particular disease.*

Aneurysm: *This is a saccular dilation of a blood vessel. It can rupture or throw off emboli.*

Aberrant arterial anatomy: *Variations in arterial anatomy are well known and usually well delineated by arteriography.*

Tumor neovascularity: *Vascular tumors often have classic findings of arteriovenous shunting, which causes blood to pool in these areas.*

Neoplastic arterial compression: *Nonvascular tumors compress or distort the normal vasculature.*

Brain Arteriography

Vascular aneurysm,

Vascular occlusion or stenosis,

Vascular arteriovenous malformations,

Cerebral vascular thrombosis:
  Arteriographic findings are similar to those described for the lower extremities.

Tumor,

Abscess,

Hematoma:
  These abnormalities distort the normal arterial anatomy.

Kidney Arteriography

Anatomic aberrant blood vessels: *Anatomic abnormalities involving the kidneys are common.*

Renal cyst: *This is an avascular mass in a kidney.*

Renal solid tumor: *Most renal cell carcinomas are very vascular.*

Atherosclerotic narrowing of the renal arteries: *Stenosis or total occlusion of the renal arteries causes decreased blood flow to the kidneys. Vasopressin is stimulated through the angiotensin system (p. 73). Hypertension results.*

Barium Enema (BE, Lower GI Series)

NORMAL FINDINGS

Normal filling, contour, and patency of the colon
Normal filling of the appendix and terminal ileum

INDICATIONS

Lower gastrointestinal (GI) barium contrast study (BE) enables visualization of the colon, distal small bowel, and occasionally the appendix. It is indicated in patients with the following conditions:
- Abdominal pain (but contraindicated in patients with acute abdominal pain)
- Obvious or occult blood in the stools
- Inflammatory bowel disease
- Suspected cancer (bowel or abdominal)

- Abnormal results of an obstruction series (see p. 1051), indicating volvulus or colon obstruction

TEST EXPLANATION

The BE study consists of a series of x-rays that visualize the colon. It is used to demonstrate the presence and location of polyps, tumors, and diverticula. Anatomic abnormalities (e.g., malrotation) also can be detected. Therapeutically, the BE may be used to reduce nonstrangulated ileocolic intussusception in children. Bleeding from diverticula can cease after a BE.

The BE is occasionally used to assess filling of the appendix. When clinical findings suggest possible appendicitis, failure of the appendix to fill with barium may support the diagnosis. Although the colon is the main organ evaluated with a BE, reflux of barium into the terminal ileum also allows adequate visualization of the distal portion of the small intestine. Diseases that affect the terminal ileum, especially Crohn disease (regional enteritis), can be identified. Inflammatory bowel disease and fistulas involving the colon can be demonstrated with BE.

In many cases, air is insufflated into the colon after instillation of barium. This provides air contrast to the barium. With air contrast, the colonic mucosa can be much more accurately visualized. This is called *an air contrast barium enema (ACBE)* or *double-contrast barium enema*, and is used especially when small polyps are suspected. The accuracy of the BE to detect small colonic tumors is approximately 60%, whereas the accuracy of the ACBE to detect small colonic tumors exceeds 85% (Figure 12-5).

This test is usually performed in the radiology department by a radiologist in approximately 45 minutes. Abdominal bloating and rectal pressure occur during instillation of barium.

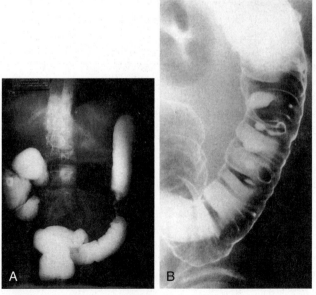

Figure 12-5 A, Single-contrast barium study illustrates obstructing circumferential carcinoma of the sigmoid colon. **B,** Double-contrast barium study shows multiple colonic diverticula. Diverticula on dependent surfaces are barium-filled; diverticula on nondependent surfaces are seen as ring shadows.

CONTRAINDICATIONS

- Patients with suspected perforation of the colon: In these patients, diatrizoate (Gastrografin), a water-soluble contrast medium, is used. No bowel preparation is performed.
- Patients who are unable to cooperate: This test requires the patient to hold the barium in the rectum and colon, which is especially difficult for older adult patients.
- Patients with megacolon: Barium may worsen this condition.

POTENTIAL COMPLICATIONS

- Colonic perforation, especially when the colon is weakened by inflammation, tumor, or infection
- Barium fecal impaction

INTERFERING FACTORS

- Barium in the abdomen from previous barium contrast tests: Barium in the abdomen may interfere with visualization of portions of the colon.
- Significant residual stool in the colon: Stool precludes adequate visualization of the entire bowel wall. Stool may be confused as polyps.
- Spasm of the colon: Spasm can mimic the radiographic signs of a cancer. The use of intravenous (IV) glucagon minimizes spasm.

 Age-Related Concerns: Pediatrics

- Typical preparation in a child may include the following:
  Age ≤2 years:
      Clear-liquid diet for 24 hours before the test
      Nothing by mouth (NPO) for 4 hours before testing
      Pediatric Fleet enema the night before testing, repeated 3 hours before testing
  Age older than 2 years:
      Low-residue diet for 2 days before testing
      Clear-liquid diet (excluding milk) for 24 hours before testing
      PO for 3 hours before testing
      Castor oil the day before testing:
          Age 2-4 years: 1 oz
          Age 5-9 years: 1.5 oz
          Age 10-16 years: 2 oz
      Saline solution enemas the night before testing only if good results were not obtained with castor oil
      Pediatric Fleet enemas until clear, 3 hours before testing
- Be aware of dehydration and electrolyte abnormalities. Instruct the parent to hydrate the child well with electrolyte-containing fluids after the BE.
- The colon in the young child will not tolerate the volume and pressure of instillation of barium that the adult colon can. Both should be reduced.
- A child cannot retain the barium long enough for complete filling of the colon. Thus a rectal tube with a balloon on the end is used. The small balloon is inflated minimally, and the buttocks are taped tightly to prevent premature defecation of the barium.

Age-Related Concerns: Elderly

- Bowel preparation may be difficult for the elderly. Often these patients live alone and cannot administer an enema. Their support system should be evaluated before the day of the BE.
- Older adults become dehydrated easily. Hypovolemia and orthostasis can lead to falling. Further, electrolyte abnormalities may develop, which can alter cardiac rhythm. Bowel preparation may have to be decreased or prolonged over several days to avert these complications. Hydration with electrolyte-containing fluids is vital.
- The elderly have reduced muscle tone, and often cannot retain barium long enough for adequate visualization of the colon. A rectal tube with a balloon at the end is inserted into the rectum, and the balloon is inflated to diminish premature defecation of barium.
- Elimination of residual barium is especially important in chronically constipated older adult patients. Be sure to instruct patients to use a mild cathartic after testing and to continue the cathartic daily until the stool is no longer white.

PROCEDURE AND PATIENT CARE

Before

✍ Explain the procedure to the patient. Encourage the patient to verbalize questions and fears.

✍ Assist the patient with bowel preparation, which varies among institutions. In elderly patients, this preparation can be exhaustive and can cause severe dehydration. Bowel preparation usually includes diet restriction, hydration, orally ingested cathartic, and cleansing enemas. Typical preparation in most adults includes the following:

Day before examination:
1. Give the patient clear liquids (no dairy products) for lunch and supper.
2. Have the patient drink one glass of water or clear fluid every hour for 8 to 10 hours.
3. 2:00 PM: Administer one full bottle (10 ounces) of magnesium citrate or X-Prep (extract of senna fruit).
4. 7:00 PM: Administer three 5-mg bisacodyl (Dulcolax) tablets.
5. Keep the patient NPO after midnight.

Day of examination:
1. Keep the patient NPO.
2. 6:00 AM: Administer a bisacodyl suppository or a cleansing enema, or both.

- Determine whether the bowel is adequately cleansed. When the fecal return is clear, preparation is adequate. If large, solid fecal waste is still being evacuated, preparation is inadequate. Notify the radiologist, who may want to extend the bowel preparation.
- In patients with suspected bowel obstruction, no oral cathartic should be administered. If catharsis is ineffective and enemas are not evacuated, colon obstruction may be present, and the physician should be notified immediately.

✍ Suggest that the patient take reading material to the x-ray department to occupy the time while expelling the barium.

During

- Note the following procedural steps:
1. A balloon rectal catheter is placed.
2. The balloon on the catheter is inflated tightly against the anal sphincter to hold the barium in the colon.
3. The patient is asked to roll in the lateral, supine, and prone positions.

X-Ray Studies

12

4. Barium is dripped into the rectum by gravity.
5. Barium flow is monitored fluoroscopically.
6. The colon is thoroughly examined as the barium progresses through the large colon and into the terminal ileum.
7. The barium is drained out.
8. If an ACBE has been ordered, air is insufflated into the large bowel.
9. The patient is asked to expel the barium, and a postevacuation x-ray film is obtained.
10. The standard procedure for administering barium through a colostomy is to instill the contrast medium through an irrigation cone placed in the stoma. When the x-ray series is completed, the barium is allowed to be expelled from the stoma. A gentle stream of clean water for irrigation is helpful in expelling residual barium. See Box 12-3 for special care of the patient with a colostomy.

After

• Ensure that the patient defecates as much barium as possible.
 Suggest the use of soothing ointments on the anal area to minimize anorectal pain that may result from the aggressive test preparation.
 Encourage ingestion of fluids containing electrolytes to avoid dehydration or electrolyte abnormalities caused by the cathartic agents.
 Encourage rest after the procedure. The cleansing regimen and BE procedure may be exhausting.

Home Care Responsibilities

• Inform the patient that initially stools will be white. Mild cathartics should be given until the stool is no longer white. When all of the barium has been expelled, the stool will return to normal color.
• Note that laxatives may be ordered to facilitate evacuation of the barium.

TEST RESULTS AND CLINICAL SIGNIFICANCE

Malignant tumor: *This is evident as a filling defect in the barium column with an "apple core" appearance.*
Polyps: *These are evident as round filling defects in the barium column. Stool can create this same picture. Persistence in location throughout the study suggests polyps.*
Diverticula: *These are evident as outpouchings of the colon. Diverticulosis refers only to the presence of diverticula. Diverticulitis indicates an infectious inflammation surrounding the diverticula, and is evident as narrowing of the barium column.*

BOX 12-3   Special Care for the Patient With a Colostomy

• Bowel preparation is the same, except enemas are not administered.
• The patient may be asked to irrigate the colostomy with saline solution about 4 hours before the test.
• If a loop colostomy is present (usually in the right upper quadrant of the abdomen), ask the physician which area of the colon is to be studied. If only the distal colon is to be evaluated, oral cathartics will not contribute to the cleansing process. Irrigation and enemas alone are used. If the proximal colon is to be studied, cathartics and proximal irrigation are used.
• Because barium cannot be retained, a balloon catheter is used.
• Elimination of barium is important. Cathartics and irrigation should be administered until the stool is no longer white.

Inflammatory bowel disease (e.g., ulcerative colitis, Crohn disease): *This is evident as narrowing of the barium column as a result of inflammation surrounding the colon. A cobblestone-like pattern is classic for ulcerative colitis. Areas devoid of barium are classic for Crohn disease. The rectum is usually involved in ulcerative colitis, but spared in Crohn disease. Fistulas may be evident in Crohn disease.*

Colonic stenosis secondary to ischemia, infection, or previous surgery: *This is evident as a "non–apple core"–like narrowing of the barium column.*

Perforated colon: *Leakage of contrast is seen with perforation. The most common cause of perforation is cancer or diverticulitis. If perforation is suspected, a water-soluble iodine-containing contrast agent should be used, because it can be absorbed by the body. Barium cannot be absorbed and can cause persistence of infection.*

Colonic fistula: *This is evident as leakage of contrast agent from the colon to another organ (e.g., urinary bladder) or area of the bowel.*

Appendicitis: *Although a diagnosis of appendicitis cannot be made with certainty, it can be supported by lack of barium filling during a BE. The appendix does not fill in 30% to 60% of normal appendixes.*

Extrinsic compression of the colon from extracolonic tumors (e.g., ovarian) or abscess: *This is evident as a convex, rounded distortion of the barium column.*

Malrotation of the gut: *In this congenital abnormality, the cecum, normally in the right lower quadrant of the abdomen, is in the left upper quadrant.*

Colon volvulus: *The cecum or sigmoid portion of the colon can turn on its mesentery and cut off flow of barium to that area of bowel. Sometimes, instillation of barium is therapeutic and can reduce the volvulus.*

Intussusception: *When proximal bowel is invaginated into the distal bowel (intussusception), the flow of barium stops at the tip of the intussusceptum. Sometimes, instillation of barium is therapeutic and can reduce the intussusception. In children the intussusception is usually caused by enlarged lymph nodes in the ileal colic area. In adults, a polypoid tumor usually is the leading cause of the intussusceptum.*

Hernia: *Large groin (usually sliding hernias) or ventral hernias can contain the colon, which is seen outside the abdomen in the hernia sac.*

RELATED TESTS

Colonoscopy (p. 591). Provides direct visualization of the colon mucosa. It is more accurate than BE and enables endoscopic surgery (e.g., biopsy, polypectomy).

Small Bowel Follow-Through (p. 1064). Provides visualization of the small intestine.

Barium Swallow (Esophagogram)

NORMAL FINDINGS

Normal size, contour, filling, patency, and position of the esophagus

INDICATIONS

The barium swallow provides visualization of the lumen of the esophagus. It is indicated in patients with the following symptoms:

- Dysphagia
- Noncardiac chest pain
- Painful swallowing
- Swallowing abnormalities (see swallowing examination [videofluoroscopy], p. 1069)
- Gastroesophageal reflux

TEST EXPLANATION

This barium contrast study is a more thorough examination of the esophagus than that provided by most upper GI series (p. 1072). As in most barium contrast studies, defects in normal filling and narrowing of the barium column indicate tumor, strictures, or extrinsic compression from extraesophageal masses or an abnormally enlarged heart and great vessels. Varices also can be seen as serpiginous linear-filling defects. Anatomic abnormalities such as hiatal hernia, Schatzki rings, and diverticula (Zenker or epiphrenic) can be seen as well.

In patients with esophageal reflux, the radiologist may identify reflux of the barium from the stomach into the esophagus. Muscular abnormalities such as achalasia, and diffuse esophageal spasm, can be easily detected. If perforations or rupture of the esophagus is suspected, it is best to use a water-soluble contrast medium rather than barium. Anatomic abnormalities such as sliding or paraesophageal hiatal hernias can also be detected.

This procedure is usually performed in the radiology department by a radiologist in approximately 15 to 20 minutes. No discomfort is associated with this test.

CONTRAINDICATIONS

- Patients with evidence of bowel obstruction or severe constipation: Barium may create a stonelike impaction.
- Patients with perforated viscus: If barium were to leak, the degree and duration of infection would be much worse. Usually when perforation is suspected, diatrizoate (Gastrografin), a water-soluble iodine-containing contrast medium, is used.
- Patients with unstable vital signs
- Patients who are unable to cooperate during the test

POTENTIAL COMPLICATIONS

- Barium-induced fecal impaction

INTERFERING FACTORS

- Food in the esophagus, which prevents adequate visualization

Clinical Priorities

- This study provides a more thorough examination of the esophagus than is provided by most upper gastrointestinal x-ray studies.
- Barium is not used if perforation or rupture of the esophagus is suspected. In these cases, a water-soluble contrast agent is used.
- After the test, cathartics are recommended to aid in evacuating the barium.

PROCEDURE AND PATIENT CARE

Before

 Explain the procedure to the patient.

Instruct the patient to remain NPO for at least 8 hours before the test. Usually the patient is kept NPO after midnight on the day of the test.

- Assess the patient's ability to swallow. If the patient tends to aspirate, inform the radiologist.

During

- Note the following procedural steps:
  1. The fasting patient is asked to swallow the contrast medium. Usually this is barium sulfate in milkshake-like form; however, if a perforated viscus is possible, diatrizoate (Gastrografin) is used.
  2. As the patient drinks the contrast agent through a straw, the x-ray table is tilted to the near-erect position.
  3. The patient is asked to roll into various positions so that the entire esophagus can be adequately visualized.
  4. With fluoroscopy or videofluoroscopy, the radiologist observes the flow of contrast medium through the entire esophagus.

After

Inform the patient of the need to evacuate all the barium. Cathartics are recommended. Initially, stool will be white, but it will return to normal color with complete evacuation of the barium.

Home Care Responsibilities

- Inform the patient that initially stools will be white. Mild cathartics should be given until the stool is no longer white. When all of the barium has been expelled, the stool will return to normal color.
- Note that laxatives may be ordered to facilitate evacuation of barium.

TEST RESULTS AND CLINICAL SIGNIFICANCE

Total or partial esophageal obstruction: *Usually this is caused by a cancer. However, achalasia or stricture can be so severe that it causes obstruction. Patients complain of dysphagia.*

Cancer: *This is most evident as narrowing in the esophagus or diminished gastroesophageal function.*

Peptic or corrosive (e.g., lye) esophagitis or ulceration: *This can cause bleeding, perforation, scarring, and stricture.*

Scarred strictures: *These are usually a sequela of untreated peptic or corrosive esophagitis.*

Lower esophageal rings: *May be congenital or acquired as a result of long-term reflux.*

Varices: *Submucosal venous varices can result from prolonged portal hypertension.*

Chalasia or achalasia: *Chalasia occurs in infants who have no lower esophageal sphincter function. These children have gastroesophageal reflux. Achalasia is usually acquired, but may be congenital. These patients cannot relax the lower esophageal sphincter, and esophageal obstruction (dysphagia) develops.*

Esophageal motility disorders (e.g., presbyesophagus, scleroderma, diffuse esophageal spasm): *Elderly patients may have asynchronous motility, which prevents swallowed food from progressing through the esophagus.*

Diverticula: *These can be in the upper esophagus (Zenker) and be caused by spasm of the cricopharyngeus muscle (upper esophageal sphincter), or in the lower esophagus (epiphrenic) and be due to paraesophageal infection.*

Extrinsic compression from extraesophageal tumors, cardiomegaly, or aortic aneurysm: *Distorts the normal esophageal anatomy.*

RELATED TEST

Endoscopic Esophagogastroscopy (p. 608). This test enables direct visualization of the esophageal lumen.

Bone Densitometry (Bone Mineral Content [BMC], Bone Absorptiometry, Bone Mineral Density [BMD], DEXA Scan)

NORMAL FINDINGS

Normal: <1 SD below normal (>−1.0)
Osteopenia: 1.0-2.5 SD below normal (−1 to −2.5)
Osteoporosis: >2.5 SD below normal (<−2.5)

INDICATIONS

Bone densitometry systems determine bone mineral content and density to diagnose osteoporosis. They are also used to monitor patients who are undergoing treatment for osteoporosis. Indications include the following:

- Early premenopausal oophorectomy or estrogen-deficiency syndromes (e.g., amenorrhea)
- Plain films indicating osteopenia
- Endocrinopathies known to be associated with osteopenia (e.g., hyperparathyroidism, prolactinoma, Cushing syndrome, male hypogonadism, hyperthyroidism)
- Unexplained or multiple fractures
- Anorexia
- Multiple myeloma
- Prolonged immobility
- Gastrointestinal (GI) malabsorption (proteins and calcium)
- Chronic renal diseases (secondary and tertiary hyperparathyroidism)
- Treatment-related osteopenia (e.g., long-term heparin, breast cancer antihormone therapy, or steroid therapy)
- Monitoring of treatment of osteoporosis (e.g., selective estrogen receptor modulators, bisphosphonates, calcitonins)
- Onset of menopause, to make a better-informed decision regarding the risks and benefits of hormone-replacement therapy (Box 12-4)

TEST EXPLANATION

Osteoporosis and osteopenia, or decreased bone mass, most commonly develop in postmenopausal women. Bones become weak and fracture easily. Diseases associated with osteoporosis include renal failure, hyperparathyroidism, and GI malabsorption syndrome; prolonged steroid therapy and prolonged immobility are predisposing factors. The consequences of osteoporosis are generally vertebral compression fractures and hip fractures. Nationally, these fractures cost billions of health care dollars for medical treatment and long-term custodial care. More important, about 20% of patients older than 45 years will die within 1 year as a consequence of hip/vertebral fracture.

Methods to identify the early stages of osteoporosis are available. The earlier osteoporosis is recognized, the more effective the treatment and the milder the clinical course. If the diagnosis of osteoporosis is delayed until fractures occur or plain film x-rays demonstrate "thin" bones, the success of treatment is less likely.

The diagnosis of osteoporosis should lead to aggressive medical therapy, which can be expensive and is not without risks. Therefore the diagnosis of osteoporosis must be based on accurate data; that is, bone

---

BOX 12-4 | **Patients Recommended for Bone Mineral Density (BMD) Testing**

- Postmenopausal women with at least one additional risk factor (family history, Caucasian descent, thin body habitus)
- All women over 65 years of age
- Women who would consider treatment for osteoporosis or menopause symptoms if BMD would affect the decision
- Women who have received hormone-replacement therapy for prolonged periods
- Men or women who have hyperparathyroidism
- Men or women who are receiving or plan to receive long-term glucocorticoid therapy
- Men or women who are being monitored to assess the efficacy of osteoporosis therapy

---

mineral mass (best measured by bone mineral density [BMD]). Bone densitometry was developed to provide accurate and precise measurement of bone strength based on bone density. Several groups of bones are routinely evaluated because they accurately represent the entire skeleton. The lumbar spine is the best representative of cancellous bone. The radius is the most easily studied cortical bone. The proximal hip (neck of the femur) is the best representative of cancellous and cortical mixed bone. Specific bone sites can be evaluated if they are symptomatic.

There are several methods of measuring BMD. The most commonly used method of determining bone density is *dual-energy densitometry (absorptiometry)*. This method uses a dual-photon source to measure the density of the bone. With dual-energy x-ray absorptiometry *(DEXA)*, x-rays are used to provide two different x-ray energies to produce dual photons in the x-ray spectrum. Because DEXA use two photons, more energy is produced so that bones (spine and hip [femoral neck]) surrounded by more soft tissue can be more easily penetrated. The radius can also be measured with either of these dual-energy techniques.

There are several other methods available to measure BMD. *Quantitative computed tomography (QCT)* uses CT technology to measure central bones, especially the spine. Single x-ray absorptiometry uses a single x-ray beam to measure the density of a peripheral bone (finger, wrist, or heel). *Ultrasound absorption (quantitative ultrasound)* can be used to measure peripheral bones (heel [calcaneus], patella, or midtibia).

Bone mineral density can evaluate the axial skeleton (spine, hips, pelvis) or the peripheral skeleton (forearm, radius, wrist, heal). The former is more accurate. However, when the patient's weight exceeds the weight limit of the study table or severe arthritic changes affect the axial skeleton, only the peripheral skeleton can be tested.

Usually, bone density is reported in terms of standard deviation from mean values. T scores compare the patient's results with those of a group of young, healthy adults. Z scores compare the patient's results with those of a group of age-matched controls. T scores are probably more accurate in predictive value of risk for fracture. The World Health Organization (WHO) has defined osteopenia as bone density value more than 1 standard deviation (SD) below peak bone mass levels in young women, and osteoporosis as a value of more than 2.5 SDs below that same measurement scale.

Based on the BMD of the femoral neck—and other clinical criteria—the risk of a major osteoporotic fracture and the risk of a hip fracture can be calculated (see http://www.shef.ac.uk/FRAX/). This is called *fracture risk assessment*. Furthermore, the identification of vertebral fracture is important in the diagnosis of osteoporosis because the presence of one or more of these fractures is a strong indicator of a patient's future fracture risk at the spine, hip, and other sites. *Vertebral fracture assessment* (VFA) can be performed using the images generated by the DEXA scan. Images of the lower thoracic and lumbar spine are examined. If a vertebral fracture is identified, bone mineral strengthening medications are recommended despite the T score. Presence of a vertebral fracture indicates a substantial risk for a subsequent vertebral or non-vertebral fracture independent of the bone mineral density or other osteoporosis risk factors. VFA is commonly recommended on postmenopausal women with reduced BMD and:

- Age >70
- Height loss >1.6 inches
- Prior vertebral fracture
- Chronic disease with increased risk for vertebral fracture (e.g., COPD, rheumatoid arthritis, or Crohn disease)
- Osteoporosis
- Postmenopausal women chronically receiving glucocorticoid therapy or an aromatase inhibitor

The data are interpreted and reported by a radiologist or a physician trained in nuclear medicine. Bone density studies take about 30 to 45 minutes to perform and are free of any discomfort. Only minimal radiation is used (the total dose of radiation exposure is less than for a chest x-ray study).

Bone mineral density testing is an important part of routine screening testing for postmenopausal women. In general, BMD is recommended every two years to screen for osteoporosis. Women and men with known osteoporotic fractures, hyperparathyroidism, or administration of long-term steroid therapy may benefit from annual BMD testing.

INTERFERING FACTORS

- Barium may falsely increase the density of the lumbar spine. Bone density measurements should not be performed within about 10 days after barium studies.
- Posterior vertebral calcific arthritic sclerosis can falsely increase bone density of the spine.
- Calcified abdominal aortic aneurysm can falsely increase bone density of the spine.
- Internal fixation devices of the hip or radius will falsely increase bone density of those bones.
- Overlying metal jewelry or other objects can falsely increase bone density.
- Previous fractures or severe arthritic changes of the bone to be studied can falsely increase its bone density.
- Metallic clips placed in the plane of the vertebra in patients who have had previous abdominal surgery can falsely increase bone density.
- Previous bone scans can falsely decrease bone density because the photons generated from the bone as a result of the previously administered radionuclide will be detected by the scintillator counter.

Clinical Priorities

- Bone densitometry was developed to provide accurate and precise measurement of bone strength based on bone density.
- According to the WHO, osteopenia is present if the bone density value is >1 SD below peak bone mass levels in young women, and osteoporosis is present if the value is >2.5 SDs below the same level.
- This test should not be performed within 10 days after barium studies, because barium may falsely increase the bone density of the lumbar spine.

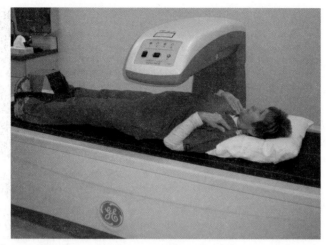

Figure 12-6 Bone densitometry. Note that it is not required that the patient undress. Jewelry, however, must be removed.

PROCEDURE AND PATIENT CARE

Before

✗ Tell the patient that no fasting or sedation is required.

✗ Explain the procedure to the patient.

✗ Ask the patient to remove all metallic objects (e.g., belt buckles, zippers, coins, keys, jewelry) that might be in the scanning path. The patient may stay dressed.

During

- The patient lies supine on an imaging table (Figure 12-6) with the legs supported on a padded box to flatten the pelvis and lumbar spine.
- Under the table, a photon generator is slowly passed under the lumbar spine.
- Above the table, a scintillation (gamma or x-ray) detector camera is passed over the patient parallel to the generator. Images of the lumbar and hip bones are projected on a computer monitor.
- Next, the foot is applied to a brace that internally rotates the nondominant hip, and the procedure is repeated over the hip. A similar procedure is performed to evaluate the radius. When the radius is examined, the nondominant arm is preferred unless there is a history of fracture to that bone.
- Note that there are numerous types of bone densitometry machines. Peripheral units that quickly scan the finger, heel, or forearm are often used to detect patients at risk for osteoporosis. Abnormal results are followed up with the more comprehensive table procedure described above.

After

- On the computer screen, a small window of the lumbar spine, femoral neck, or distal radius is drawn. The computer calculates the number of photons not absorbed by the bone, or bone mineral content (BMC). BMD is computed as follows:

$$BMD = \frac{BMC\ (g/cm^2)}{Surface\ area\ of\ the\ bone}$$

- Findings are compared with data from healthy 25- to 35-year-old women, and the SD above or below the curve is determined. This is the T score. Positive T scores indicate bone stronger than normal;

negative *T* scores indicate bone weaker than normal. *Z* scores are calculated in the same way, but the comparisons are made to those in patients matched for age, sex, race, height, and weight.

TEST RESULTS AND CLINICAL SIGNIFICANCE

Osteopenia (low bone mass),
Osteoporosis:

Osteopenia precedes osteoporosis. The most common cause of osteoporosis is lack of sexual hormones (estrogen in the female, testosterone in the male). Osteopenia may result from primary ovarian failure secondary to menopause or oophorectomy, or pituitary disease. In male patients, osteopenia usually occurs in children with congenital hormone deficiencies.

Hyperparathyroidism: *Excess parathyroid hormone mobilizes calcium from the bone, causing demineralization and bone weakening.*

Chronic renal insufficiency: *Excess phosphates that accumulate as a result of reduced glomerular filtration decrease the calcium in the blood. Parahormone is stimulated to increase calcium levels. Excess parathyroid hormone mobilizes calcium from the bone, causing demineralization and weakening of the bones (secondary hyperparathyroidism). If after persistent parathyroid stimulation the parathyroid glands become autonomous and secrete elevated parahormone despite normal calcium levels, tertiary hyperparathyroidism develops. The bone changes are the same as described above.*

GI malabsorption: *Calcium and protein cannot be absorbed. The bones are depleted of their minerals, and bone density is reduced.*

Cushing syndrome,
Chronic steroid therapy:

Glucocorticosteroids inhibit bone mineralization and decrease bone density.

Chronic heparin therapy: *Heparin binds calcium and other minerals. These minerals are therefore not available for bone growth. Further, these minerals are mobilized from their bone stores. Bone density diminishes.*

Chronic immobility: *The pathophysiology of bone demineralization in the immobilized patient is not clearly understood.*

RELATED TESTS

Bone (Long) X-Rays (see following test). Plain films can identify advanced bone demineralization and indicate severe osteoporosis.

Bone Turnover Biochemical Markers (p. 915). N-telopeptide, bone-specific alkaline phosphatase, pyridinium, and osteocalcin are rapid biochemical markers of bone turnover and are used to monitor treatment for osteoporosis.

Bone (Long) X-Rays

NORMAL FINDINGS

No evidence of fracture, tumor, infection, or congenital abnormalities

INDICATIONS

This x-ray study is performed to evaluate any bone for fracture, infection, arthritis, tendinitis, or bone spurs. Bone age can be determined in children to evaluate growth and development. Primary and metastatic tumors can be identified.

TEST EXPLANATION

X-ray films of the long bones are usually obtained when the patient has complaints about a pertinent body area. Fractures or tumors are readily detected on x-ray studies. Severe or chronic infection involving a bone (osteomyelitis) may be detected. X-ray studies of the long bones also can detect joint destruction and bone spurring as a result of persistent arthritis. Growth patterns can be followed by serial x-ray studies of long bones, usually the wrists and hands. Healing of a fracture can be documented and monitored. X-ray films of the joints reveal the presence of joint effusions and soft-tissue swelling. Calcifications in the soft tissue indicate chronic inflammatory changes of the nearby bursa or tendons. Soft-tissue swelling can also be seen on these similar x-ray films. Because the cartilage and tendons are not directly visualized, cartilage fractures or sprains, and ligamentous injuries cannot be seen.

At least two films obtained at a 90-degree angle are required so that the bone region being studied can be visualized from two different angles (usually anteroposterior and lateral). Some bone studies (e.g., skull, spine, hip) require oblique views to visualize all the parts that need to be seen.

INTERFERING FACTORS

- Jewelry or clothing can obstruct radiographic visualization of part of the bone to be evaluated.
- Previous barium studies can diminish full radiographic visualization of some of the bones surrounding the abdomen (e.g., spine, pelvis).

 Clinical Priorities

- This test can determine bone age to evaluate growth and development. Usually the bones of the wrists and hands are used for this determination.
- When obtaining x-ray films, shield the patient's testes or ovaries, and abdomen if the patient is pregnant, to prevent radiation exposure.

PROCEDURE AND PATIENT CARE

Before

- Explain the procedure to the patient.
- Carefully handle any injured parts of the patient's body.
- Instruct the patient to keep the extremity still while the x-ray film is being obtained. This can sometimes be difficult, especially when the patient has severe pain associated with a recent injury.
- Shield the patient's testes, ovaries, or pregnant abdomen to prevent exposure from scattered radiation.
- Tell the patient that no fasting or sedation is required.

During

- In the radiology department, the patient is asked to place the involved extremity in several positions. An x-ray film is obtained of each position.
- Note that this test is routinely performed by a radiologic technologist within several minutes.
- Tell the patient that no discomfort is associated with this test except perhaps from moving an injured extremity.

After

- Administer an analgesic for relief of pain, if indicated.

TEST RESULTS AND CLINICAL SIGNIFICANCE

Fractures,

Congenital bone disorders (e.g., achondroplasia, dysplasia, dysostosis):
Multiple disorders associated with bone, absence of a bone, or growth and development of bone or bone groups are detected.

Tumors (osteogenic sarcoma, Paget disease, myeloma, metastases): *These can be evident as osteoblastic destruction (radiolucent defects in bone) or osteoclastic reaction (radiopaque areas of bone) to the tumor.*

Infection or osteomyelitis: *These are evident as soft-tissue swelling around the bone infection. Further signs may include periosteal reaction and bony destruction of the affected bone.*

Osteoporosis or osteopenia: *Bone demineralization and thinning indicate osteoporosis. Patients are at increased risk for traumatic and atraumatic fractures.*

Joint destruction (arthritis): *Degenerative and rheumatoid arthritic degenerative changes are seen as narrowing of the joint space because of cartilaginous destruction. Bone spurs and other changes can be noted.*

Bone spurs: *Exophytic growths of bone at pressure points (heels and feet) can cause significant pain.*

Abnormal growth pattern: *Bony development can be evaluated with x-ray films of the wrists, arms, pelvis, and skull. Comparison of findings with those normal for chronologic age provides insight and perspective into possible abnormalities in growth and development.*

Joint effusion: *Swelling and some increased radiodensity of the joint indicate effusion. This may be the result of bleeding, trauma, inflammation, or infection.*

Foreign bodies: *X-ray films of the extremities can demonstrate foreign bodies (usually in the hands and feet).*

Cardiac Catheterization (Coronary Angiography, Angiocardiography, Ventriculography)

NORMAL FINDINGS

Normal heart-muscle motion, normal and patent coronary arteries, normal great vessels, and normal intracardiac pressure and volume

INDICATIONS

Cardiac catheterization is used to visualize the heart chambers, arteries, and great vessels. It is used most often to evaluate chest pain. The study is used to locate the region of coronary occlusion in patients with positive stress test results and to determine the effects of valvular heart disease. Right heart catheterization is the most accurate method to determine cardiac output. It also measures right heart pressures and can be used to identify pulmonary emboli.

TEST EXPLANATION

Cardiac catheterization enables examination of the heart, great blood vessels (aorta, inferior vena cava, pulmonary artery, and pulmonary vein), and coronary arteries. For cardiac catheterization, a catheter is passed into the heart through a peripheral vein (for right-heart catheterization) or artery (for left-heart catheterization). Through the catheter, pressures are recorded and radiographic dyes are injected. With the assistance of computer calculations, cardiac output and other measures of cardiac function can be determined. Cardiac catheterization is indicated for the following reasons:

1. To identify, locate, and quantify the severity of atherosclerotic, occlusive coronary artery disease

2. To evaluate the severity of acquired and congenital cardiac valvular or septal defects
3. To detect congenital cardiac abnormalities, such as transposition of the great vessels, patent ductus arteriosus, and anomalous venous return to the heart
4. To evaluate the success of previous cardiac surgery or balloon angioplasty
5. To evaluate cardiac muscle function
6. To identify and quantify ventricular aneurysms
7. To detect acquired disease of the great vessels, such as atherosclerotic occlusion or aneurysms within the aortic arch
8. To evaluate and treat patients with acute myocardial infarction (MI)
9. To insert a catheter to monitor right-sided heart pressures, such as pulmonary artery and pulmonary wedge pressures, and to measure cardiac output. Cardiac output can be measured only during right heart catheterization. (Table 12-2 provides pressures and volumes used in cardiac monitoring.)
10. To dilate stenotic coronary arteries (angioplasty), to place coronary artery stents, or to perform laser atherectomy

Cardiac catheterization is performed under sterile conditions. In right-heart catheterization, usually the jugular, subclavian, brachial, or femoral vein is used for vascular access (Figure 12-7). In left-heart catheterization, usually the right femoral artery is cannulated, or alternatively, the brachial or radial

TABLE 12-2   Pressures and Volumes Used in Cardiac Monitoring

	Description	Normal Value
Pressures		
Routine blood pressure	Routine brachial artery pressure	90-120/60-80 mm Hg
Systolic left ventricular pressure	Peak pressure in the left ventricle during systole	90-140 mm Hg
End-diastolic left ventricular pressure	Pressure in the left ventricle at the end of diastole	4-12 mm Hg
Central venous pressure	Pressure in the superior cava	2-14 cm H_2O
Pulmonary wedge pressure	Pressure in the pulmonary venules, an indirect measurement of left atrial pressure and left ventricular end-diastolic pressure	Left atrial: 6-15 mm Hg
Pulmonary artery pressure	Pressure in the pulmonary artery	15-28/5-16 mm Hg
Aortic artery pressure	Same as routine blood pressure	
Volumes		
End-diastolic volume (EDV)	Amount of blood present in the left ventricle at the end of diastole	50-90 mL/m^2
End-systolic volume (ESV)	Amount of blood present in the left ventricle at the end of systole	25 mL/m^2
Stroke volume (SV)	Amount of blood ejected from the heart in one contraction (SV = EDV − ESV)	45 ± 12 mL/m^2
Ejection fraction (EF)	Proportion (fraction) of EDV ejected from the left ventricle during systole (EF = SV/EDV)	0.67 ± 0.07
Cardiac output (CO)	Amount of blood ejected by the heart in 1 min	3-6 L/min
Cardiac index (CI)	Amount of blood ejected by the heart in 1 min per square meter of body surface area (CI = CO/body surface area)	2.8-4.2 L/min/m^2 in a patient with 1.5 m^2 of body surface area

X-Ray Studies

12

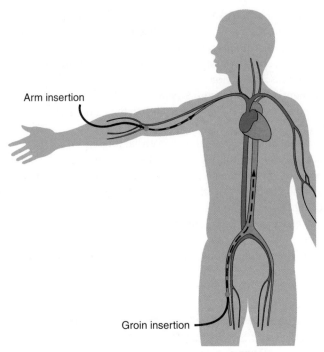

Arm insertion

Groin insertion

Figure 12-7 Insertion sites for cardiac catheterization.

artery. As the catheter is placed into the great vessels of the heart chamber, pressures are monitored and recorded. Blood samples for analysis of oxygen content are also obtained. The catheter is advanced with appropriate guidance into the desired position. After pressures are obtained, angiographic visualization of the heart chambers, valves, and coronary arteries is achieved with the injection of radiographic dye.

Percutaneous transluminal coronary angioplasty and *intracoronary stents* are therapeutic procedures that can be performed during coronary angiography in medical centers where open heart surgery is available. During this procedure, a specially designed balloon catheter is introduced into the coronary arteries and placed across the stenotic area of the coronary artery. This area can then be dilated by controlled inflation of the balloon and subsequently stented. The coronary arteriogram is then repeated to document the effects of the forceful dilation of the stenotic area. Coronary arterial *stents* can be placed at the site of previous stenosis after angioplasty, and maintain patency for longer periods of time.

Atherectomy of coronary arterial plaques can be performed to more permanently open some of the hard, atheromatous plaques. Certain occlusive lesions with characteristics unfavorable for balloon angioplasty appear to be ideally suited for atherectomy. Rotational atherectomy is most commonly used. A tiny rotating knife inside a catheter is moved to the arterial obstruction. A balloon is inflated to position the knife precisely on the fatty deposit. Then the knife shaves the fatty deposit off the wall of the artery. The shavings are collected in the catheter and removed.

Cardiac catheterization is usually performed by a cardiologist in approximately 1 hour. During the dye injection the patient may experience a severe hot flush, which may be uncomfortable but lasts only 10 to 15 seconds. Some patients have a tendency to cough as the catheter is placed in the pulmonary artery. Verbally support the patient as the x-ray films are obtained, because the possibly loud noises may frighten the patient.

Age-Related Concerns

- Elderly patients with chronic dehydration or mild renal failure are at high risk for dye-induced renal failure.
- Urinary output must be carefully monitored after the procedure. Fluid intake needs to be encouraged, because dehydration may be induced by the diuretic action of the dye.

CONTRAINDICATIONS

- Patients who are unable to cooperate during the test
- Patients who would refuse intervention if an amenable lesion were found
- Patients with an iodine dye allergy who have not received preventive medication for allergy
- Patients who are pregnant, unless the benefits outweigh the risk of radiation exposure to the fetus
- Patients with renal disorders, because iodinated contrast material is nephrotoxic
- Patients with a bleeding propensity, because the arterial or venous puncture site may not seal

POTENTIAL COMPLICATIONS

- Cardiac arrhythmias (dysrhythmias)
- Perforation of the heart myocardium
- Renal failure (see Box 12-2, p. 984)
- Catheter-induced embolic cerebrovascular accident (stroke) or MI
- Complications associated with the catheter insertion site, such as arterial thrombosis, embolism, or pseudoaneurysm
- See potential complications to iodinated dye on p. 985.
- Infection at the catheter insertion site
- Pneumothorax after subclavian vein catheterization of the right side of the heart
- Hypoglycemia or acidosis may occur in patients who are taking metformin (Glucophage) and receive iodine dye. The metformin should be held the day of the test to prevent this complication.

 Clinical Priorities

- Assess for allergy to iodinated dye.
- Perform a baseline assessment of the patient's peripheral pulses before catheterization.
- After the test, keep the patient on bed rest for 4 to 8 hours to allow complete sealing of the arterial puncture.
- Assess the puncture site for bleeding, hematoma, and absence of pulse.

PROCEDURE AND PATIENT CARE

Before

- Explain the procedure to the patient.
- Obtain written informed consent.
- Allay the patient's fears and anxieties about the test. Although this test creates tremendous fear in a patient, it is performed often, and complications are rare.
- Instruct the patient to abstain from oral intake for at least 4 to 8 hours before the test.

- Prepare the catheter insertion site as per protocol.
- See assessment for allergy to iodinated dye on p. 985.
- Mark the patient's peripheral pulses with a pen before catheterization. This will facilitate postcatheterization assessment of the pulses in the affected and unaffected extremities.
- Provide appropriate precatheterization sedation as ordered by the physician.
- Instruct the patient to void before going to the catheterization laboratory.
- Remove all valuables and dental prostheses before transporting the patient to the catheterization laboratory.
- Obtain intravenous (IV) access for delivery of fluids and cardiac drugs if necessary.

During

- Take the patient to the cardiac catheterization laboratory (Figure 12-8).
- Note the following procedural steps:
  1. The chosen catheter insertion site is prepared and draped in a sterile manner.
  2. The desired vessel is punctured with a needle.
  3. A wire is placed through the needle and a sheath is placed on the wire and into the vessel.
  4. The angiographic catheter is threaded through the sheath over a guidewire to place the catheter appropriately.
  5. Once the catheter is in the desired location, the appropriate cardiac pressures and volumes are measured.
  6. Cardiac ventriculography is performed with controlled injection of contrast material.
  7. Each coronary artery is catheterized. Cardiac angiography is then carried out with controlled injection of contrast material.
  8. During the injection, x-ray films are rapidly obtained.
  9. The patient's vital signs must be monitored constantly during the procedure.
  10. If *angioplasty* is performed, the following procedural steps are carried out:
      a. The cardiologist appropriately places the catheter and balloon at the stenotic area.
      b. As the electrocardiogram (EKG) tracing is observed, the balloon is inflated and the stenotic areas are forcefully dilated.

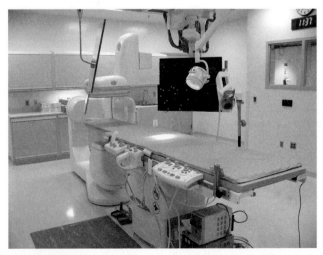

Figure 12-8 Cardiac cathetization lab (Image used with permission, Flagstaff Medical Center, Northen Arizona Healthcare. All rights reserved.)

    c. If signs of myocardial ischemia develop, the balloon is immediately deflated.

    d. Usually, the balloon is inflated for only 10 seconds.

11. After obtaining all required information, the catheter is removed.

12. A chemical vascular closure device designed to seal the arterial puncture site is often placed.

After

- Monitor the patient's vital signs.
- Apply pressure to the site of vascular access.
- Keep the patient on bed rest for 4 to 8 hours to allow complete sealing of the arterial puncture.
- Keep the affected extremity extended and immobilized with sandbags to decrease bleeding.
- Assess the puncture site for signs of bleeding, hematoma, or absence of pulse.
- Assess the patient's pulses in both legs. Compare with preprocedural baseline values.
- Encourage the patient to drink fluids to maintain adequate hydration. Dehydration may be caused by the diuretic action of the dye. Monitor urinary output.
- Evaluate the patient for delayed reaction to the dye (dyspnea, tachycardia, rashes, hives). This usually occurs within the first 2 to 6 hours after the test. Treat with antihistamines or steroids.
- Inform the patient that the angiograms will be reviewed by the cardiologist and that the results will be available in 1 or 2 days.

🏠 Home Care Responsibilities

- Instruct the patient in positioning the extremity to decrease bleeding.
- Check the patient for signs of bleeding (decreased blood pressure and increased pulse).
- Assess the puncture site for bleeding and hematoma.
- Instruct the patient to report any signs of numbness, tingling, pain, or loss of function in the involved extremity.

TEST RESULTS AND CLINICAL SIGNIFICANCE

Coronary artery occlusive disease: *Stenosis in one or more of the coronary arteries (or branches) can be easily identified and located for revascularization with angioplasty or coronary artery bypass grafting.*

Anatomic variation of the cardiac chambers and great vessels: *Ventricular and atrial septal defects, patent ductus arteriosus, and transposition of the great vessels are among many abnormalities that can be identified.*

Ventricular aneurysm: *Aneurysmal dilation of part of the wall muscle because of infarction and weakness is evident at ventriculography.*

Ventricular mural thrombi,

Intracardiac tumor,

Altered blood flow dynamics,

Cardiomyopathy,

Ventricular wall motion deficits,

Acquired or congenital septal defects and valvular abnormalities:

    Ventricular abnormalities are most evident during the ventriculography portion of the study. Some of these abnormalities also cause hemodynamic effects, which are recognized by pressure readings performed during cardiac catheterization.

12 **X-Ray Studies**

Aortic root arteriosclerotic or aneurysmal disease,

Coronary aneurysm,

Coronary fistula,

Anomalies in pulmonary venous return,

Pulmonary emboli:
  Anomalies and diseases of the great vessels are evident following the outflow of dye after ventriculography.

Pulmonary hypertension: *This condition is recognized by pressure readings performed during cardiac catheterization.*

Reduced cardiac output: *Cardiac output is most accurately assessed by right heart catheterization. The right side is catheterized if cardiac output readings are required or valvular diseases of the right side are suspected.*

Arterial oxygen desaturation: *Arterial oxygen saturation may be decreased when mixing of venous and arterial blood occurs. This may be seen with septal defects, transposition of the great vessels, or congenital shunting.*

RELATED TESTS

Cardiac Nuclear Scan (p. 791). This test can provide similar information concerning ventricular wall function and motion. Ejection fraction (a measure of cardiac output) and blood flow dynamics can also be determined. With newer radioisotopes, sites of coronary artery occlusion can be seen.

Computed Tomography (CT) Scan of the Heart (p. 1032). This test is now being applied to the heart and coronary vessels. It holds much promise as a noninvasive substitute for cardiac catheterization.

Chest X-Ray (CXR)

NORMAL FINDINGS

Normal lungs and surrounding structures

INDICATIONS

This is the most commonly obtained x-ray study because it can indicate so much information about the heart, lungs, bony thorax, mediastinum, and great vessels.

TEST EXPLANATION

Chest radiography is important in the complete evaluation of the pulmonary and cardiac systems. This procedure is often part of the general admission screening workup in adult patients. Much information can be provided by the chest x-ray study. Repeated studies enable identification and monitoring of the following conditions:

1. Tumors of the lung (primary and metastatic), heart (myxoma), chest wall (soft-tissue sarcomas), and bony thorax (osteogenic sarcoma)
2. Inflammation of the lung (pneumonia), pleura (pleuritis), and pericardium (pericarditis)
3. Fluid accumulation in the pleura (pleural effusion), pericardium (pericardial effusion), and lung (pulmonary edema)
4. Air accumulation in the lung (chronic obstructive pulmonary disease) and pleura (pneumothorax)
5. Fractures of the bones of the thorax or vertebrae
6. Diaphragmatic hernia
7. Heart size, which may vary depending on cardiac function

8. Calcification, which may indicate large-vessel deterioration or old lung granulomas (from histoplasmosis or some other former infection)
9. Location of centrally placed intravenous access devices
10. Infection in the lung, such as pneumonia or tuberculosis

Most chest x-rays are obtained at a distance of 6 feet, with the patient standing. The sitting or supine position also can be used, but x-ray films obtained with the patient supine will not demonstrate fluid levels or pneumothorax. For a *posteroanterior (PA)* view (projection) the x-rays pass through the back of the body (posterior) to the front (anterior) (Figure 12-9 *A, B*). For an *anteroposterior* view, the x-rays pass through the body from front to back. For a *lateral* view, the x-rays enter from the side (see Figure 12-10 *A, B*). For *oblique* views, x-rays pass through the body at various angles. *Lordotic* views, obtained with the patient recumbent, provide visualization of the apices (rounded upper portions) of the lungs and are usually used to detect tuberculosis. *Decubitus* films are obtained with the patient in the recumbent lateral position, to demonstrate and localize fluid, which becomes dependent in the pleural space (pleural effusion). Table 12-3 (p. 1018) shows the view required for detection of various problems.

Fluoroscopy is an imaging technique that allows real-time moving images (much like a movie) of many different body parts (e.g., barium enema, upper GI, arteriography). When used during the chest x-ray, the lung, diaphragm, and heart motions can be evaluated. This may be helpful in separating a questionable pulmonary nodule from prominent breast nipple. With deep inspiration, a pulmonary nodule will move considerably away from the nipple. Diaphragmatic motion can also be evaluated by fluoroscopy. This is useful in determining diaphragmatic paralysis. Paradoxic diaphragmatic motion associated with prolonged diaphragmatic paralysis motion can be more easily seen with "sniff test." In this test, with chest fluoroscopy, the patient is asked to take a deep sniff through the nose while the diaphragm motion is observed. If the diaphragm rises instead of depresses during the sniff, paradoxic motion is documented (compatible with diaphragmatic paralysis).

Chest x-ray studies are best performed in the radiology department. Studies using a portable x-ray machine may be done at the bedside and are often performed in critically ill patients who cannot leave the nursing unit.

CONTRAINDICATIONS

- Patients who are pregnant, unless the benefits outweigh the risk of radiation exposure to the fetus

INTERFERING FACTORS

- Conditions (e.g., severe pain or shortness of breath because of COPD) that prevent the patient from taking and holding a deep breath
- Scarring from previous lung surgery (makes interpretation difficult)
- Obesity (requires more x-rays to penetrate the body to provide a readable x-ray film)
- Pacemaker, jewelry, body piercing, or undergarments/articles of clothing with metallic components can obstruct identification of radiographic findings.

✓ **Clinical Priorities**

- Chest x-ray studies are best performed in the radiology department but can be performed at the bedside if the patient cannot leave the nursing unit.
- Patient positioning during the test depends on the suspected condition (see Table 12-3, p. 1018).
- To prevent radiation-induced abnormalities, a lead shield is used to cover the testicles in men and the ovaries in women.

X-Ray Studies

12

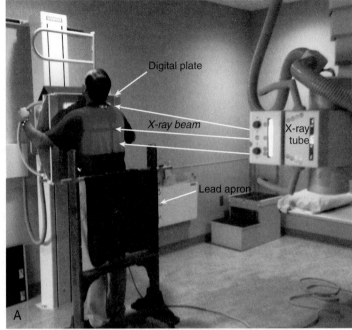

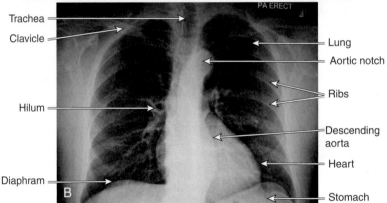

Figure 12-9 **A,** Routine PA view chest x-ray. Note direction of the x-ray beam from the x-ray cathode tube through the patient and to the x-ray digital receptor plate. Also note lead apron for protection from "scatter x-ray". **B,** PA chest radiograph. The diaphragm separates the abdominal contents (including the stomach) from the chest. The heart is situated in the middle of the chest, more toward the left side. The air-filled lungs are represented as dark spaces on either side of the chest. The trachea is seen as a dark shadow in the neck and upper chest. The peak of the descending aorta is the notch. The descending aorta runs vertically in front of the vertebra. The ribs, clavicle, and other bony structures can also be seen as a part of the thoracic cage.

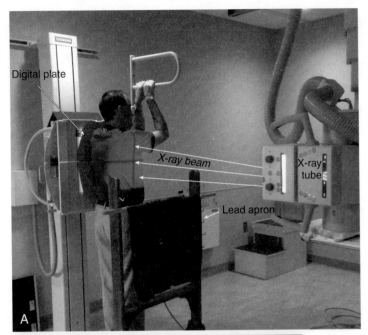

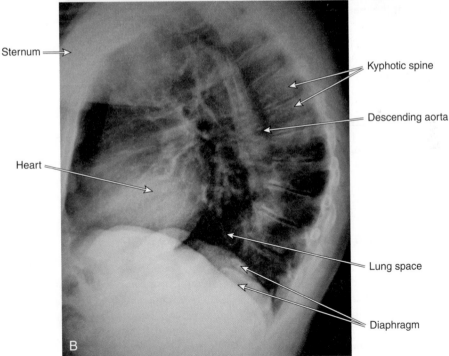

Figure 12-10 **A,** Routine lateral view chest x-ray. Note direction of the x-ray beam from the x-ray cathode tube through the patient and to the x-ray digital receptor plate. Also note lead apron for protection from "scatter x-ray." **B,** Lateral chest radiograph. The heart is situated in anterior chest under the sternum. The air-filled lungs are represented as dark spaces. The descending aorta runs vertically in front of the vertebra. The vertebral bodies are noticed in the posterior chest and are curved due to kyphosis.

X-Ray Studies

12

TABLE 12-3	Patient Position Required to Identify Suspected Problems
Suspected Problem	**Position Required**
Pneumothorax	Erect
Effusion	Lateral decubitus
Widened mediastinum	Erect
Cardiac enlargement	Erect
Fractured rib	Oblique
Tuberculosis	Lordotic

PROCEDURE AND PATIENT CARE

Before

🗶 Explain the procedure to the patient.

🗶 Tell the patient that no fasting is required.

🗶 Instruct the patient to remove clothing to the waist and to put on an x-ray gown.

🗶 Instruct the patient to remove all metal objects (e.g., necklaces, pins) so they do not block visualization of part of the chest.

🗶 Tell the patient that he or she will be asked to take a deep breath and hold it until the images are taken.

• Ensure that the testicles in men and the ovaries in women are covered with a lead shield to prevent radiation-induced abnormalities.

🗶 Inform the patient that no discomfort is associated with chest radiography.

During

🗶 After the patient is correctly positioned, tell him or her to take a deep breath and hold it until the x-ray films are obtained.

• Note that x-ray films are obtained by a radiologic technologist in several minutes.

After

• No special care is required after chest radiography.

TEST RESULTS AND CLINICAL SIGNIFICANCE

Lung

Lung tumors (primary or metastatic): *These are evident as soft-tissue masses in the lung fields.*

Pneumonia: *Increased opacity (lightness) in the lung field indicates pneumonia or atelectatic lung tissue.*

Pulmonary edema: *Increased opacity of the lung is indicative of pulmonary edema, most commonly from congestive heart failure.*

Pleural effusion: *Fluid in the chest wall is evident as increased opacity outside the lung fields, in particular, in the costophrenic margins. A lateral decubitus film will show layering out of free pleural fluid. Entrapped fluid, however, will not layer out.*

Chronic obstructive pulmonary disease: *Increased lung space is classic for COPD.*

Pneumothorax: *Air outside the lung space (pneumothorax) is always abnormal. If large enough, chest tube insertion is required to release the trapped air and re-expand the lung.*

Atelectasis: *Collapse of pulmonary alveoli is evident as white patches or lines in the lung fields.*

Tuberculosis (TB): *Usually in the upper lobes, chronic TB is generally associated with calcification.*

Lung abscess: *Lung abscess is evident as a lung mass with a hollow (radiolucent) center. Sometimes, fungus can grow inside an abscess.*

Congenital lung diseases (hypoplasia): *Congenital aplasia or hypoplasia of the lung tissue is evident by reduced lung tissue on the affected side.*

Pleuritis: *A thickened pleura indicates pleuritis, which is caused by a viral, bacterial, neoplastic, or other cause.*

Foreign body in the chest, bronchus, or esophagus: *Swallowed, aspirated, or penetrating (bullets) foreign bodies can be easily seen.*

Heart

Cardiac enlargement: *When the heart is more than 50% to 60% of the horizontal width of the chest, cardiac enlargement because of congestive heart failure or cardiomyopathy is present.*

Pericarditis,

Pericardial effusion:
  These conditions are evident as an enlarged heart shadow.

Chest Wall

Soft-tissue sarcoma,

Osteogenic sarcoma:
  These primary tumor masses of the bony thorax and chest wall soft tissue are evident as masses arising from those areas.

Fracture of ribs or thoracic spine: *Best seen on lateral or oblique x-ray films, fractures may be displaced or well aligned. They are usually associated with other chest trauma.*

Thoracic scoliosis: *Alterations in thoracic spinal alignment are obvious on chest x-ray films.*

Metastatic tumor to bony thorax: *Osteolytic (dark) or osteoblastic (white) nodules can be seen in the bony thorax. Breast, prostate, kidney, and lung are among the most common cancers to metastasize to the bones in this region.*

Diaphragm

Diaphragmatic or hiatal hernia: *This condition is evident as increased opacity in the posteroinferior mediastinum.*

Mediastinum

Aortic calcinosis: *This is evident as white lines indicating the walls of the calcified aorta.*

Enlarged lymph nodes: *Central masses in the mediastinum indicate enlarged lymph nodes, usually of neoplastic origin.*

Dilated aorta: *This may indicate aneurysm.*

Thymoma,

Lymphoma,

Substernal thyroid:
  These abnormalities often are evident as large soft-tissue masses in the anterosuperior mediastinum.

Widened mediastinum: *Cardiac enlargement, aneurysm, lymph node enlargement, or hematoma may be the cause.*

RELATED TEST

Computed Tomography (CT) of the Chest (p. 1029). This test allows more detailed information concerning pathologic conditions of the chest and its structures.

Computed Tomography, Abdomen and Pelvis
(CAT Scan, Abdomen and Pelvis; CT Scan, Abdomen and Pelvis; Helical/Spiral CT Scan, Abdomen and Pelvis; CT Angiography; CT Colonoscopy; Virtual Colonoscopy)

NORMAL FINDINGS

No evidence of abnormality

INDICATIONS

CT is used in evaluating the abdominal organs and pelvis. CT can be used to guide needles during biopsy of tumor and aspiration of fluid, in staging known neoplasms, and to monitor abdominal disease when serially and repeatedly performed.

TEST EXPLANATION

CT of the abdomen is a noninvasive, yet accurate radiographic procedure used to diagnose pathologic conditions (e.g., tumors, cysts, abscesses, inflammation, perforation of the bowel, intraabdominal bleeding, intestinal or ureteral obstruction, vascular aneurysms, and calculi) in the abdominal and retroperitoneal organs. The CT image results from passing x-rays through the abdominal organs at many angles. The variation in density of each tissue allows variable penetration of the x-rays. Each density is given a numeric value called a density coefficient, which is digitally computed into shades of gray. This is then interpolated to an accurate image on a computer monitor (Figure 12-11). The image can be

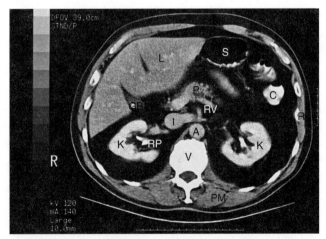

Figure 12-11 CT of the abdomen. Normally many abdominal structures can be seen on a CT scan. *A*, Aorta; *C*, the splenic flexure of the colon (contrast filled); *GB*, gallbladder (containing a gallstone-radiolucent area); *I*, inferior vena cava; *K*, kidney; *L*, liver; *P*, pancreas; *PM*, paraspinal muscles of the back; *R*, bony ribs of the lower chest; *RP*, pelvis of the right renal collecting system; *RV*, left renal vein; *S*, air/contrast filled stomach; *V*, vertebra.

enhanced by repeating the CT scan after intravenous (IV) administration of iodine-containing contrast material. These images can be recorded on x-ray film or captured digitally.

Liver tumors, abscesses, trauma, cysts, and anatomic abnormalities can be seen, and pancreatic tumors, pseudocysts, inflammation, calcification, bleeding, and trauma. The kidneys and urinary outflow tract are well visualized.

Renal tumors and cysts, ureteral obstruction, calculi, and congenital renal and ureteral abnormalities are easily seen with the use of IV contrast material. Calculi can be seen without IV contrast. Extravasation of urine secondary to trauma or obstruction can also be easily demonstrated. Adrenal tumors and hyperplasia are best diagnosed with CT. Some radiology literature indicates that the histology of the tumor can be suggested based on the density coefficients shown on the scan.

Large tumors, perforations of the bowel, and appendicitis can be identified with CT, especially when oral contrast material is ingested (see also virtual colonoscopy below). The spleen can be well visualized for hematoma, laceration, fracture, tumor infiltration, and splenic vein thrombosis with CT. The retroperitoneal lymph nodes can be evaluated. These are usually present, but all nodes with a diameter greater than 2 cm are considered abnormal. The abdominal aorta and its major branches can be evaluated for aneurysmal dilation and intramural thrombi, and the pelvic structures (including the uterus, ovaries, fallopian tubes, prostate gland, and rectum) and musculature can be evaluated for tumors, abscesses, infection, or hypertrophy. Ascites and hemoperitoneum can easily be demonstrated on a CT scan. Tumors, abscesses, or perforation of the pelvis organs can be seen when the CT scan is directed to the pelvis. Perineal CT scanning can demonstrate perianal abscesses or perirectal tumors/infection.

Dynamic CT scanning can be performed during arterial injection of dye to the organ being studied. Dynamic scanning can indicate blood flow and degree of vascularity of an organ or part of an organ in the abdomen.

CT scanning continuously obtains data as the patient is passed through the gantry. With multidetector CT (MDCT) technology, image data can be obtained as the patient is passed through the CT gantry. With the use of multiple collimators (and multiple banks of detectors), large data images can be obtained in a very short period of time. The entire abdomen can be scanned in less than 30 seconds with one breath hold. The "slices" are very thin (1 to 5 mm). With thin slices and rapid accession, breathing and motion distortion are minimized. This produces faster and more accurate images.

With this technique, 200 to 500 individual images can be obtained. Volume imaging with 3D real-time display of the volume of data allows the interpreter to visualize and analyze the data in three dimensions (3-D). Two- and three-dimensional reconstructions of data can provide very accurate images of the intra-abdominal organs and especially the mesenteric vessels in a few seconds. This allows radiologists to see these structures from multiple views and directions.

With the use of *3-D volumetric imaging*, a 3-D perspective can now be added to the abdominal and pelvic organs or tumors that are imaged. This provides data for virtual colonoscope and virtual angiography. *Virtual colonoscopy* uses a CT scanner and computer virtual reality software to look inside the body without needing to insert a colonoscopy (as for conventional colonoscopy, see p. 591). Virtual colonoscopy is an appropriate alternative to screening endoscopic colonoscopy. No sedation is required and no discomfort is experienced. Patients need a cleansing bowel preparation before the test. This procedure takes place in the radiology department. It begins with the insertion of a small flexible rubber tube in the rectum. Air is inserted through this tube to inflate the colon for better visualization. The air acts as a contrast medium. The test is completed in 10 to 20 minutes. Because no sedation is required, patients are free to leave the CT suite without the need for observation and recovery. Patients can resume normal activities after the procedure and can eat, work, or drive without a delay. Unlike with endoscopic colonoscopy, polypectomy and/or biopsy cannot be performed with virtual testing. If abnormalities are found with virtual colonoscopy, conventional colonoscopy is needed.

An increasingly used combination of *fusion CT/PET scans* (see p. 822) is now being used to provide both anatomic and physiologic information that can be fused into one image. This allows the image to locate pathology and indicate whether it is benign or malignant. As directed by the principles described above for colonoscopy, fusion CT/PET scans not only can provide an accurate image of the entire colon, but can also indicate if any abnormality seen is malignant.

Helical *CT arteriography* or *virtual angiography* is done through the use of multichannel helical CT scanning. After IV injection of contrast, CT imaging can demonstrate the arteries in any given organ. 3-D recreations of the aorta and other abdominal vessels are possible. This is particularly helpful in identifying renal artery stenosis and the hepatic vasculature for cancer-related resections. Renal CT arteriography can be used to demonstrate and evaluate each functional phase of urinary excretion. CT angiography is becoming a viable alternative to magnetic resonance imaging (MRI) angiography to assess abdominal aneurysm, iliac vascular occlusion, AV malformations, or vascular tumors.

CT nephrotomography can be done by computerized recreation of a 3-D image of the kidneys, renal pelvis, and ureters. This is particularly helpful in identifying ureteral stone, small tumors of the kidney or collecting system. Utilizing different protocols and radiopaque contrast, kidney function can be evaluated. This does require significant radiation exposure. A different protocol designed to identify ureteral stones can be performed with very little radiation exposure. This is called *CT urogram.*

With the increasing use and development of 3-D volumetric imaging, radiologists have expanded CT scanning to assist pathologists, coroners, and medical examiners to investigate a cadaver for clues as to the cause of death. This is now being termed *"virtual autopsy."* This includes CT or MRI whole-body postmortem imaging. With these techniques, image-directed biopsies can be performed to obtain tissue for the pathologists to review. Postmortem angiograms can be performed to more accurately indicate occlusive disease that may have contributed to death.

CT is usually performed by a radiologist in less than 10 minutes. If dye is used, the procedure time may be doubled, because the abdomen is scanned both before and after administration of the dye. The only discomfort associated with this study is lying still on a hard table and the peripheral venipuncture. Mild nausea is common when contrast dye is used; thus an emesis basin should be readily available. Some patients may experience a salty taste, flushing, and warmth during the dye injection.

CT can be used to aspirate fluid from the abdomen or an abdominal organ, for cultures and other studies; to guide biopsy needles into areas of abdominal tumors to obtain tissue for study; and to guide catheter placement for drainage of intraabdominal abscesses.

CT is an important part of staging and monitoring of many tumors before and after therapy. Treatment of tumors of the colon, rectum, hepatic system, breast, lungs, prostate gland, ovaries, uterus, kidneys, lymph glands, and adrenal gland commonly fails, and recurrence can be detected early with CT.

CONTRAINDICATIONS

- Patients who are allergic to iodinated dye or shellfish
- Patients who are claustrophobic
- Patients who are pregnant, unless the benefits outweigh the risks
- Patients whose vital signs are unstable
- Patients who are profoundly obese (usually over 300 pounds), because the CT table cannot support that much weight

POTENTIAL COMPLICATIONS

- For potential complications of allergy to iodinated dye, see p. 985.
- Acute renal failure from dye infusion: Adequate hydration before the procedure may reduce the likelihood of this complication (see Box 12-2, p. 984).

- Hypoglycemia or acidosis may occur in patients who are taking metformin (Glucophage) and receive iodine dye. The metformin should be held on the day of the test to avoid this complication.

INTERFERING FACTORS

- Presence of metallic objects (e.g., hemostasis clips)
- Retained barium from previous studies
- Large amounts of fecal material or gas in the bowel
- Motion can distort the image: Patients must lie still and hold their breath for several seconds as instructed.

✓ Clinical Priorities

- Check the patient for allergy to iodinated dyes.
- Mild nausea is common when the contrast dye is injected. For this reason, patients are usually kept on nothing by mouth (NPO) status for 4 hours before the test.
- Most patients who are mildly claustrophobic can tolerate this study after appropriate medication with antianxiety drugs.
- Adequate hydration before the test may decrease the possibility of acute renal failure from dye infusion.
- CT can be used to guide needles into abdominal tumors for biopsy or to guide catheters into intraabdominal abscesses for drainage.

PROCEDURE AND PATIENT CARE

Before

Explain the procedure to the patient. Cooperation is necessary, because the patient must lie still during the procedure.
- Obtain informed consent if required by the institution.
- For assessment of allergy to iodinated dye, see p. 985.

Show the patient a picture of the CT machine if the patient has claustrophobia. Most patients who are mildly claustrophobic can be scanned without premedication with antianxiety drugs.
- Keep the patient NPO for at least 4 hours before testing. However, in emergency circumstances, that requirement is not appropriate. Usually, oral contrast is used to separate the gastrointestinal tract from the other abdominal organs. This is usually provided as a water-soluble contrast material that is drunk by the patient several hours before testing. The same contrast can be administered rectally for improved visualization of the rectum and perirectal structures.

During

- Note the following procedural steps:
  1. The patient is taken to the radiology department and placed on the CT table (Figure 12-12).
  2. The patient then is placed in an encircling body scanner (gantry). The x-ray tube travels around the gantry, and images (scans) of the various levels of the abdomen and pelvis are obtained. Any motion will cause blurring and streaking of the final scan. Therefore the patient is asked to remain motionless during x-ray exposure. This problem is eliminated with the use of faster scanning: Data acquisition is so rapid that the entire study can be performed in less than 30 seconds. Motion and breath holding are not a problem. Computer monitoring equipment allows immediate display of the CT image, which is then recorded digitally. In a separate room, the technicians manipulate the

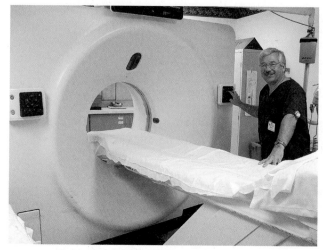

Figure 12-12 CT equipment.

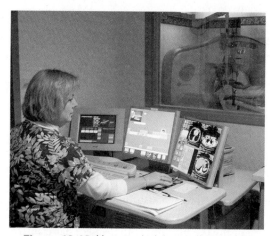

Figure 12-13 X-ray technician performs CT.

CT table and determine the level of the abdomen to be scanned (Figure 12-13). Through audio communication, the patient is instructed to hold his or her breath during x-ray exposure.

3. Better results are obtained with oral or IV administration of iodinated contrast dye. The GI organs can be accurately differentiated from other abdominal organs, and the vessels and ureters are contrasted with the surrounding structures. Contrast agent can sometimes be administered rectally to enable visualization of the pelvic organs. Besides oral contrast, as described above, the blood vessels, kidneys, ureters, and bladder are better visualized with the use of IV iodinated contrast material.

After

✗ Encourage the patient to drink fluids to avoid dye-induced renal failure and to promote dye excretion.

✗ Inform the patient that diarrhea may occur after ingestion of the oral contrast agent.

• Evaluate the patient for delayed reaction to dye (e.g., dyspnea, rash, tachycardia, hives). This may occur 2 to 6 hours after the test. Treat with antihistamines or steroids.

TEST RESULTS AND CLINICAL SIGNIFICANCE

Liver

Tumor, abscess, bile duct dilation: *These are evident as radiolucent (dark) filling defects in the liver parenchyma.*

Pancreas

Tumor, pseudocyst, inflammation, bleeding: *These are evident as solid or cystic masses of the pancreas.*

Spleen

Hematoma, fracture, laceration, tumor, venous thrombosis: *CT of the spleen is the most accurate method of accurately indicating splenic trauma. Tumors, hematomas, and cysts are well demonstrated.*

Gallbladder/Biliary System

Gallstones, tumor, bile duct dilation: *Gallstones are sometimes difficult to see. However, an inflammatory response around the gallbladder is evident. Bile duct dilation is usually evident by demonstration of dilated ducts in the liver parenchyma.*

Kidneys

Tumor, cyst, ureteral obstruction, calculi, congenital abnormalities: *Hydronephrosis is easily evident on a CT scan. Likewise, tumors and cysts can be seen. The density of the renal mass can be computed. If the mass is the same density as water, it can safely be assumed the mass is due to a cyst. The CT scan is not as good as intravenous pyelogram (IVP) in identifying ureteral calculi or ureteral anatomic abnormalities.*

Adrenal gland

Adenoma, cancer, pheochromocytoma, hemorrhage, myelolipoma, hyperplasia: *CT is the most accurate method of evaluating the adrenal glands. It is used not only to diagnose tumors, but also to monitor neoplastic diseases that affect the adrenal glands.*

GI Tract

Perforation, tumor, inflammatory bowel disease, diverticulitis, appendicitis: *Although CT findings are nonspecific as to the cause of an inflammatory mass, CT is sensitive in identification of such a mass. The location and surrounding structures aid in diagnosis of the underlying pathologic process.*

Uterus, Fallopian Tubes, Ovaries

Tumor, abscess, infection, hydrosalpinx, cyst, fibroid: *CT is accurate in evaluation of the pelvis for neoplasms of the ovaries, uterus, or cervix. Likewise, infections and abscess can be identified and drained with CT guidance.*

Prostate

Hypertrophy, tumor: *An enlarged prostate is easily seen on a CT scan. However, benign and malignant disease cannot be differentiated.*

Retroperitoneum

Tumor, lymphadenopathy: *Sarcomas, lymphomas, and inflammation may be evident as masses of increased density in the retroperitoneum.*

Abdominal aneurysm: *The presence of an aortic aneurysm can be determined by CT scanning. Repeated scanning can be performed to see if the aneurysm is expanding. A leak or rupture in the aneurysm can also be identified.*

Peritoneum

Ascites, hemoperitoneum,

Abscess:

Free and localized fluid can be seen on CT scans, especially if GI contrast agent has been used. Sometimes loops of bowel can look like abscess.

RELATED TEST

Magnetic Resonance Imaging (MRI) (p. 1106). This test is less accurate than CT for identification of abdominal disease. However, in certain abdominal areas (e.g., liver and pelvis) it may be better.

Computed Tomography, Brain (CT scan, Brain; Computerized Axial Transverse Tomography [CATT]; Helical/Spiral CT Scan, Brain)

NORMAL FINDINGS

No evidence of disease

INDICATIONS

The first use of CT scanning was in the evaluation of the brain. The brain is well imaged with CT. This test is indicated when CNS disease is suspected. Specifically, CT is useful in the diagnosis of brain tumors, infarction, bleeding, and hematomas. Information about the ventricular system can also be obtained using CT scanning. Multiple sclerosis, Alzheimer and other degenerative abnormalities can be identified.

TEST EXPLANATION

CT of the brain consists of a computerized analysis of multiple tomographic x-ray images taken of the brain tissue at successive layers, providing a three-dimensional (3-D) view of the cranial contents. The CT image provides a view of the head as if one were looking down through its top. The variation in density of each tissue allows for variable penetration of the x-ray beam. An attached computer calculates the amount of x-ray penetration of each tissue and displays this as shades of gray. This is then displayed digitally on a computer monitor as a series of anatomic pictures of coronal and sagittal sections of the brain.

The CT scan is used in the differential diagnosis of intracranial neoplasms, cerebral infarction, ventricular displacement or enlargement, cortical atrophy, cerebral aneurysms, intracranial hemorrhage and hematoma, and arteriovenous (AV) malformation. Magnetic resonance imaging (MRI) of the brain (see p. 1106) is now most commonly used for brain imaging. However, for initial trauma evaluation and for the location and extent of subarachnoid bleeding, CT scan is still preferable.

Visualization of a neoplasm, previous infarction, or any pathologic process that destroys the blood-brain barrier may be enhanced by intravenous (IV) injection of an iodinated contrast dye.

The CT scan continuously obtains images as the patient is passed through the gantry. This produces rapid, accurate images. Because the spiral CT can image the selected area in less than 30 seconds, the entire study can be performed with one breath hold. Therefore breathing and motion misrepresentations are reduced. Images are improved and scan time is reduced. This is particularly helpful in scanning uncooperative adults or children. Through volume averaging, 3-D images can be re-created. Furthermore, when contrast material is used, the entire region can be imaged in just a few seconds after the contrast injection, thereby further improving contrast imaging.

Spiral CT scan is very helpful in re-creation of 3-D images to determine accurate localization of brain tumors. CT arteriography is performed immediately after arterial contrast injection. 3-D re-creations of the carotid artery and its branches are also extremely helpful in the evaluation of cerebral vascular disease.

CONTRAINDICATIONS

- Patients who are allergic to iodinated dye or shellfish
- Patients who are claustrophobic
- Patients who are pregnant, unless the benefits outweigh the risks
- Patients whose vital signs are unstable
- Patients who are very obese (usually over 300 pounds), because the CT table cannot support the weight

POTENTIAL COMPLICATIONS

- For potential complications to iodinated dye, see p. 985.
- Acute renal failure from dye infusion: Adequate hydration before the procedure may reduce the likelihood of this complication (see Box 12-2, p. 984).
- Hypoglycemia or acidosis may occur in patients who are taking metformin (Glucophage) and receive an iodinated dye. Metformin should be held the day of testing to prevent this complication.

PROCEDURE AND PATIENT CARE

Before

- Explain the procedure to the patient. Cooperation is necessary, because the patient must lie still during the procedure.
- Obtain informed consent if required by the institution.
- Keep the patient on nothing by mouth (NPO) status for 4 hours before the study, if oral contrast is to be used.
- Instruct the patient that wigs, hairpins, clips, or partial dentures cannot be worn during the procedure, because they hamper visualization of the brain.
- For assessment of allergy to iodinated dye, see p. 985.
- Tell the patient that he or she may hear a clicking noise as the scanner moves around the head.
- This procedure is performed in the radiology department in less than 1 hour. If dye is administered, the procedure time is doubled.

During

- Note the following procedural steps:
  1. The patient lies supine on an examining table with the head resting on a platform (Figure 12-14).
  2. The scanner passes an x-ray beam through the brain from multiple angles.
- If iodinated contrast will be used, an IV is started and the dye is administered. Scanning is repeated.

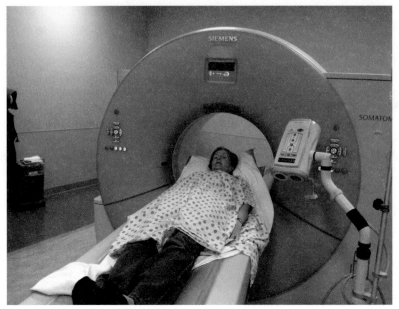

Figure 12-14 CT scan of the brain.

After

✍ Encourage the patient to drink fluids because dye is excreted by the kidneys and causes diuresis.

- Evaluate the patient for delayed reaction to dye (e.g., dyspnea, rash, tachycardia, hives). This usually occurs 2 to 6 hours after the test. Treat with antihistamines or steroids.

TEST RESULTS AND CLINICAL SIGNIFICANCE

Intracranial neoplasm (benign or malignant): *These tumors usually are evident as soft-tissue masses of increased radiolucency (darkness). Adjacent structures are distorted by the tumor's presence. Some benign tumors have calcification within.*

Cerebral infarction: *An infarction can be seen as an area of the brain that is void of contrast material. Reduced cerebral blood flow (CBF) is also noted with xenon scanning.*

Ventricular displacement,

Ventricular enlargement,

Hydrocephalus:

    The fluid-filled ventricles are obvious on CT scans as the least dark areas of the brain. Enlargement may indicate hydrocephalus, with or without increased intracranial pressure. Distortion of the ventricles may be caused by tumor or hemorrhage.

Cortical atrophy: *Brain tissue lucency may change, and the cortical tissue appears thinner.*

Cerebral aneurysm,

AV malformation:

    Aneurysms and AV malformations are seen when intravenous contrast agent is used.

Intracranial hemorrhage,

Hematoma,

Abscess:

    These space-occupying lesions are difficult to differentiate. Serial CT scans may be helpful. In time, hemorrhage will become more diffuse. Hematoma will liquefy and become less radiolucent, and even calcify later. Abscess is often surrounded by edema and will slowly enlarge. Epidural and subdural hematomas are evident as isodense areas of swelling that distort the nearby brain tissue.

Multiple sclerosis: *Classic CT findings with contrast agent can indicate multiple sclerosis with a moderate degree of accuracy. White matter atrophy, periventricular plaques, and spontaneous hypolucent areas in the periventricular area are usually present.*

Brain death: *With xenon scanning, a CBF of zero indicates brain death.*

RELATED TEST

Magnetic Resonance Imaging (MRI), Brain (p. 1106). This test provides an image of the brain that is superior to CT scans. In most institutions, MRI has replaced CT in imaging of the central nervous system.

Computed Tomography, Chest (Chest CT Scan; Helical/Spiral CT Scan, Chest)

NORMAL FINDINGS

No evidence of disease

INDICATIONS

This test is used to more thoroughly evaluate suspected disease in the chest. Questionable or vague abnormalities on the routine chest x-ray can be more thoroughly evaluated with CT scanning of the chest.

TEST EXPLANATION

CT of the chest is a noninvasive yet accurate radiographic procedure for diagnosing and evaluating pathologic conditions such as tumors, nodules, hematomas, parenchymal coin lesions, cysts, abscesses, pleural effusion, and enlarged lymph nodes affecting the lungs and mediastinum. Tumors and cysts of the pleura and fractures of the ribs can also be seen. When an intravenous (IV) contrast material is given, vascular structures can be identified and a diagnosis of aortic or other vascular abnormality can be made. With oral contrast material, the esophagus and upper gastrointestinal (GI) structures can be evaluated for tumor and other conditions. CT provides a cross-sectional view of the chest and is especially useful in detecting small differences in tissue density, demonstrating lesions that cannot be seen with conventional radiography and tomography. The mediastinal structures can be visualized in a manner that cannot be equaled with conventional x-ray films and tomographic scans.

The x-ray image results from using a body scanner (x-ray tube in a circular gantry) to deliver x-rays through the patient's chest at many different angles. The variation in density of each tissue allows for variable penetration of the x-rays. Each density is given a numeric value called a *coefficient*, which is digitally computed into shades of gray. This is then displayed digitally on a computer monitor as a photograph of the anatomic area sectioned by the x-rays.

The CT scan continuously obtains images as the patient is passed through the gantry. With multidetector CT (MDCT) technology, much more image data can be obtained as the patient is passed through the CT gantry. With the use of multiple collimators (and multiple banks of detectors), large data images can be obtained in a very short period of time. The entire chest can be scanned in less than 30 seconds with one breath hold. The "slices" are very thin (1 to 5 mm). With thin slices and rapid accession,

12 X-Ray Studies

breathing and motion distortion are minimized. This produces faster and more accurate images. This is particularly helpful in scanning uncooperative adults and children.

With this CT study 200 to 500 individual images can be obtained. Volume imaging with three-dimensional (3-D) real-time display of the volume of data allows the interpreter to visualize and analyze the data in three dimensions. 2-D and 3-D reconstructions of data can provide very accurate images of the heart (see p. 1032), lungs, chest wall, pleura, esophagus, great vessels, and soft tissue in a few seconds allowing the radiologists to see these structures from multiple views and directions. Utilizing this technology, *virtual bronchoscopy* and *virtual esophagoscopy* will increasingly be used in place of their invasive counterparts.

Spiral CT scan is considered the preferred study to identify pulmonary emboli *(CT pulmonary arteriography)*. It can be performed easily and rapidly. CT scanning of the heart (see p. 1032) is able to identify tiny calcifications in the coronary arteries. This finding is indicative of increased risk for an ischemic event. Pulmonary nodules are particularly well evaluated with this rapid form of CT scanning because breathing misrepresentations are eliminated.

With the use of *3-D volumetric imaging*, a 3-D perspective can now be added to the organs or tumors that are imaged. This provides data for *virtual angiography*.

This procedure is performed by a radiologist in less than 10 minutes. If dye is administered, the procedure time may be doubled because CT scanning is done before and after administration of the contrast dye. The only discomfort associated with this study is from lying still on a hard table and from the peripheral venipuncture. Mild nausea is common when contrast dye is used, and an emesis basin should be readily available. Some patients may experience a salty taste, flushing, and warmth during the dye injection.

CONTRAINDICATIONS

- Patients who are allergic to iodinated dye or shellfish
- Patients who are claustrophobic
- Patients who are pregnant, unless the benefits outweigh the risks
- Patients whose vital signs are unstable
- Patients who are very obese (usually over 300 pounds), because the CT table cannot support the weight

POTENTIAL COMPLICATIONS

- For potential complications for allergies to iodinated dye, see p. 985.
- Acute renal failure from dye infusion: Adequate hydration beforehand may reduce the likelihood of this complication (see Box 12-2, p. 984).
- Hypoglycemia or acidosis may occur in patients who are taking metformin (Glucophage) and receive iodine dye. The metformin should be held on the day of testing to prevent this complication.

Clinical Priorities

- Check the patient for allergy to iodinated dyes.
- Mild nausea is common when the contrast dye is injected. For this reason, patients are usually kept NPO for 4 hours before the test.
- Most patients who are mildly claustrophobic can tolerate this study after appropriate medication with antianxiety drugs.
- Adequate hydration before the test may decrease the possibility of acute renal failure from dye infusion.

PROCEDURE AND PATIENT CARE

Before

🖎 Explain the procedure to the patient. Cooperation is necessary because the patient must lie still during the procedure.

- Obtain informed consent if required by the institution.
- For assessment of allergy to iodinated dye, see p. 985.

🖎 Show the patient a picture of the CT machine and encourage verbalization of concerns about claustrophobia. Most patients who are mildly claustrophobic can tolerate this study after appropriate premedication with antianxiety drugs.

- Keep the patient NPO for 4 hours before the test in the event that contrast dye is administered.

During

- Note the following procedural steps:
  1. The patient is taken to the radiology department and asked to remain motionless in a supine position. Any motion will cause blurring and streaking of the final scan. This problem is eliminated with the use of helical scanning. Data acquisition is so rapid that the entire study can be performed in less than 30 seconds. Motion and breath holding are not a problem.
  2. An encircling x-ray camera (body scanner) takes pictures at varying intervals and levels over the chest area. Monitor equipment allows immediate display, and the image is recorded on x-ray film.
  3. Very often, IV dye is administered to enhance the chest image, and the x-ray studies are repeated.

After

🖎 Encourage patients who received dye injection to increase their fluid intake, because the dye is excreted by the kidneys and causes diuresis.

- Evaluate the patient for delayed reaction to the dye (e.g., dyspnea, rashes, tachycardia, hives). This usually occurs 2 to 6 hours after the test. Treat with antihistamines or steroids.

TEST RESULTS AND CLINICAL SIGNIFICANCE

Lung

Lung tumor (primary or metastatic): *This is evident as soft-tissue masses in the lung fields.*

Pneumonia: *Increased lucency in the lung field indicates pneumonia or atelectatic lung.*

Pleural effusion: *Fluid in the chest wall is evident as increased lucency outside the lung fields, particularly in the costophrenic margins.*

Chronic obstructive pulmonary disease: *Increased lung space is classic for chronic obstructive pulmonary disease (COPD).*

Atelectasis: *Collapse of pulmonary alveoli is evident as white patches or lines in the lung fields.*

Tuberculosis (TB): *Usually in the upper lobes, chronic TB and other granulomatous diseases are usually associated with calcification.*

Lung abscess: *Lung abscess is evident as a lung mass with a hollow (radiolucent) center. Sometimes fungus grows inside the abscess.*

Pleuritis: *A thickened pleura indicates pleuritis, which is from a viral, bacterial, neoplastic, or other cause.*

Heart

Pericarditis,

Pericardial effusion:

These are evident as thickened pericardium with or without fluid around the heart.

12 **X-Ray Studies**

Chest Wall

Soft-tissue sarcoma,

Osteogenic sarcoma:

> *Primary tumor masses of the bony thorax and chest wall soft tissue, they are evident as masses arising from those areas of the chest.*

Fracture (ribs or thoracic spine): *This is usually associated with other chest trauma.*

Metastatic tumor to bony thorax: *Osteolytic (dark) or osteoblastic (white) nodules can be seen in the bony thorax. Breast, prostate, kidneys, and lungs are among the most common cancers to metastasize to the bones in this region.*

Diaphragm

Diaphragmatic or hiatal hernia: *This is evident as increased lucency in the posteroinferior mediastinum.*

Mediastinum

Aortic calcinosis: *Evident as white lines indicating the walls of the calcified aorta.*

Enlarged lymph nodes: *Central-occurring masses in the mediastinum indicate enlarged lymph nodes, usually of a neoplastic etiology.*

Dilated aorta: *This is indicative of aneurysm. Dissection, if present, is obvious on CT scans of the chest.*

Thymoma,

Lymphoma,

Substernal thyroid:

> *These are often evident as large soft-tissue masses in the anterosuperior mediastinum.*

Metastatic tumor to mediastinum: *Esophageal and upper stomach cancers may metastasize to the mediastinal lymph nodes.*

Perforation of esophagus (spontaneous [Boerhaave syndrome] or iatrogenic [following esophageal dilation]): *Meglumine diatrizoate (Gastrografin) that was previously ingested will be seen free in the mediastinum.*

RELATED TEST

Chest X-Ray (p. 1014). This is a routine part of every thorough evaluation of the cardiopulmonary system. Although not so accurate as CT, it provides a tremendous amount of information easily.

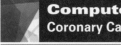

Computed Tomography, Heart (Coronary CT Angiography, Coronary Calcium Score)

NORMAL FINDINGS

No evidence of coronary stenosis; calcium score average for age and gender

INDICATIONS

The exact role of CT of the heart has not been clearly delineated. However, it holds great promise in providing information about the patency of the coronary vessels in patients who have chest pain.

TEST EXPLANATION

With the developments in low-dose x-ray multidetector CT (MDCT) technology, much data can be obtained about the heart and coronary vessels. This test is being used to help stratify patients according to risks of future cardiac events, instigate preventive medicinal interventions (such as statin drugs), monitor progression of coronary vascular disease and effects of statin drugs, evaluate chest pain, and indicate the need for stress testing or coronary angiography.

MDCT produces fast and accurate images of the heart. With the use of multiple collimators (and multiple banks of detectors—usually 4 to 64), large data images can be obtained in a very short period of time. The entire heart can be scanned in 10 seconds with one breath hold. The "slices" are very thin (1 to 5 mm). With thin slices and rapid accession, breathing and motion distortion are minimized.

With advances in software technology, two- and three-dimensional reconstructions of data can provide very accurate images of the heart and coronary vessels in a few seconds, allowing radiologists to see these structures from multiple directions (Figure 12-15). Furthermore, with shorter scanning times, intravenous contrast effect can be greater while using less contrast volume. The newest MDCT scanners allow routine cardiac gating that synchronizes the scanning with each heartbeat, thereby eliminating further motion distortion.

Calcified atheromatous plaques can be seen and quantified (calcium score) with the use of MDCT. The assessment of coronary artery calcification has received considerable attention with respect to its potential role in the early detection of subclinical atherosclerosis and in the diagnostic workup of coronary artery disease. Coronary calcium is a surrogate marker for coronary atherosclerotic plaque. In the coronary arteries, calcifications occur almost exclusively in the context of atherosclerotic changes. Within a coronary vessel or larger segment of the vessel, the amount of coronary calcium correlates moderately closely with the extent of atherosclerotic plaque burden. On the other hand, not every

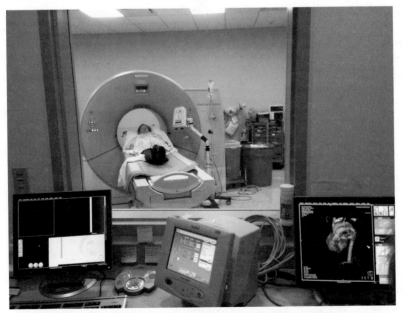

Figure 12-15 CT scan of the heart from the technologist's observer station. Note computer-generated image of heart and great vessels, lower right corner.

TABLE 12-4	Agatston Score Categories			
	Minimal	**Moderate**	**Increased**	**Severe**
Agatston Score	<10	11-99	100-400	>400

serious atherosclerotic coronary plaque is calcified. However, in the vast majority of patients with acute coronary syndromes, coronary calcium can be detected, and the amount of calcium in these patients is substantially greater than in matched control subjects without coronary artery disease.

The *Agatston score* has most frequently been used to quantify the amount of coronary calcium in CT. The distribution of calcification scores in populations of individuals without known heart disease has been studied extensively. From those data we know that the amount of calcification increases with age. Men develop calcifications about 10 to 15 years earlier than women. Furthermore, in the majority of asymptomatic men over 55 years of age and women over 65 years of age, calcification can be detected. These data have been used to create tables that compare the amount of calcium of an individual to a group of people of similar age and gender (percentiles). See Table 12-4 for categorizing absolute Agatston scores.

It is well established that individuals with Agatston scores above 400 have an increased occurrence of coronary procedures (bypass, stent placement, angioplasty) and events (myocardial infarction [MI] and cardiac death) within 2 to 5 years after the test. Individuals with very high Agatston scores (over 1000) have a 20% chance of suffering an MI or cardiac death within a year. Even among elderly patients (over 70 years), who frequently have calcification, an Agatston score above 400 is associated with a higher risk of death.

Variability of the Agatston score can be high for patients with small amounts of calcium but is lower for higher calcium scores. There is a variability of about 20%. Excessively high calcium scores can inhibit the visualization of the coronary arteries. Therefore, when calcium scores are excessively high, injection of radiopaque dye is not performed and coronary CT cannot be carried out.

MDCT can directly and accurately visualize the coronary artery lumen after intravenous injection of a contrast agent *(coronary CT angiography)*. Regular and low heart rates are a prerequisite for reliable visualization of the coronary arteries. Hence, most centers have proposed the administration of a short-acting beta blocker or a calcium-channel blocker before scanning if the heart rate exceeds 60 to 70 beats/min. The use of sublingual nitroglycerin is also recommended to achieve coronary vasodilatation and maximize image quality.

CONTRAINDICATIONS

- Patients who are pregnant
- Patients who are allergic to iodinated dye or shellfish (relative contraindication)
- Patients who are obese, usually more than 300 pounds
- Patients whose vital signs are unstable

POTENTIAL COMPLICATIONS

- Acute renal failure from dye infusion: Adequate hydration beforehand may reduce this likelihood.
- Hypoglycemia or acidosis can occur in patients who are taking metformin (Glucophage) and receive iodine dye. Metformin should be held on the day of testing to prevent this complication.

PROCEDURE AND PATIENT CARE

Before

✗ Explain the procedure to the patient. The patient's cooperation is necessary because he or she must lie still during the procedure.

- Obtain informed consent if required by the institution.
- Assess the patient for allergies to iodinated dye or shellfish.
- Assess the patient's vital signs. If the heart rate exceeds protocol levels, administer a rapid-acting beta blocker or ACE inhibitor per protocol orders.

✗ Show the patient a picture of the CT machine and encourage the patient to verbalize concerns regarding claustrophobia. Most patients who are mildly claustrophobic can tolerate this study after appropriate premedication with antianxiety drugs.

- Keep the patient NPO for 4 hours before the test.

During

- Note the following procedure for the cardiac CT scan:
  1. The patient is taken to the CT department and asked to remain motionless in a supine position because any motion will cause blurring and streaking of the final picture.
  2. EKG leads are applied to synchronize the EKG signal to the image data (gating).
  3. An encircling x-ray camera (body scanner) takes pictures at varying intervals and levels over the heart while the patient holds his or her breath (for about 10 seconds).
  4. A nonenhanced scan is performed first for calcium scoring.
  5. If the calcium scoring is below threshold levels of the protocol, intravenous (IV) dye is rapidly administered through a large-bore IV catheter, and the scan is repeated.
  6. A fast-acting nitrate (usually nitroglycerin) is administered to maximize coronary dilatation.
- Note that a radiologist or cardiologist performs this procedure in about 20 minutes.

✗ Tell the patient that the discomforts associated with this study include lying still on a hard table and peripheral venipuncture.

- Nausea is a common sensation when contrast dye is used. An emesis basin should be readily available.
- Some patients may experience a salty taste, flushing, and warmth during the dye injection.

After

✗ Encourage patients to increase their fluid intake because the dye is excreted by the kidneys and causes diuresis.

- See p. 985 for appropriate interventions concerning the care of patients with iodine allergy.

✗ Tell the patient that a headache from the nitroglycerin is not uncommon.

TEST RESULTS AND CLINICAL SIGNIFICANCE

Coronary vascular disease,
Coronary vascular congenital anomalies:
  The coronary vessels can be visualized completely and any obstruction or anatomic variation is obvious.
Ventricular aneurysm,
Aortic aneurysm or dissection,
Pulmonary emboli,
Cardiac tumors:
  These anatomic abnormalities are obvious even before they become symptomatic.
Myocardial scarring,

X-Ray Studies

12

Cardiac valvular disease:
> *These functional abnormalities are obvious by demonstrating anatomic alterations of the normal heart muscle/valvular motion during a cardiac cycle.*

RELATED TESTS

Cardiac Catheterization (p. 1008). This test is used to visualize the heart chambers, arteries, and great vessels. It is used most often to evaluate chest pain and to locate the region of coronary occlusion in patients with coronary occlusive disease.

Cardiac Nuclear Scan (p. 791). This test is used to detect myocardial ischemia, infarction, cardiac wall dysfunction, and decreased ejection fraction. It is commonly used as the imaging method portion of cardiac stress testing to detect ischemia.

Cystography (Cystourethrography, Voiding, Cystography, Voiding Cystourethrography)

NORMAL FINDINGS

Normal bladder structure and function

INDICATIONS

Cystography enables radiographic visualization of the bladder. It is useful in patients with hematuria, recurrent urinary tract infections (UTIs), and suspected bladder trauma.

TEST EXPLANATION

Filling the bladder with contrast material provides visualization of the bladder for radiographic study. Either fluoroscopic or x-ray films demonstrate bladder filling and collapse after emptying. Filling defects or shadows in the bladder indicate primary bladder tumors. Extrinsic compression or distortion of the bladder is seen with pelvic tumor (e.g., rectal, cervical) or hematoma (secondary to pelvic bone fractures). Extravasation of the dye is seen with traumatic rupture, perforation, and fistula of the bladder. Vesicoureteral reflux (abnormal backflow of urine from bladder to ureters), which can cause persistent or recurrent pyelonephritis, also may be demonstrated during cystography. Although the bladder is visualized during intravenous pyelography (IVP) (p. 1057), primary pathologic bladder conditions are best studied by means of cystography.

A radiologist performs the study in approximately 15 to 30 minutes. This test is moderately uncomfortable if bladder catheterization is required.

CONTRAINDICATIONS

- Urethral or bladder infection or injury: Gram-negative sepsis can occur as a result of catheterization. Existing bladder injury may be made worse by instillation of dye into the bladder.

POTENTIAL COMPLICATIONS

- UTI: May result from catheter placement or instillation of contaminated contrast material.
- Allergic reaction to iodinated dye: Rare, because the dye is not administered intravenously.

Clinical Priorities

- Assess for allergy to iodinated dyes.
- After the test, assess the patient for urinary tract infection, which may result from catheter placement or instillation of contaminated contrast material.
- Encourage the patient to drink fluids to eliminate the dye and to prevent accumulation of bacteria.

PROCEDURE AND PATIENT CARE

Before

- Explain the procedure to the patient.
- Obtain informed consent if required by the institution.
- Give clear liquids for breakfast on the morning of the test.
- Assure the patient that he or she will be draped to prevent unnecessary exposure.
- Insert a Foley catheter if ordered.

During

- Note the following procedural steps:
  1. The patient is taken to the radiology department and placed in a supine or lithotomy position.
  2. Unless a catheter is already present, one is placed.
  3. Approximately 300 mL (much less for children, based on weight) of air or radiopaque dye is injected through the catheter into the bladder, and the catheter is clamped.
  4. X-ray films are taken.
  5. If the patient is able to void, the catheter is removed and the patient is asked to urinate while films are taken of the bladder and urethra (voiding cystourethrogram) (Figure 12-16).

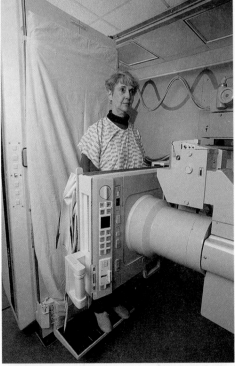

Figure 12-16 Position for voiding cystography.

- Ensure that in male patients a lead shield is placed over the testes to prevent irradiation of the gonads.
- The ovaries in female patients cannot be shielded without blocking bladder visualization. Ensure that female patients are not pregnant.

After
- Assess the patient for signs of UTI.
- Encourage the patient to drink fluids to eliminate the dye and to prevent accumulation of bacteria.

TEST RESULTS AND CLINICAL SIGNIFICANCE

Bladder tumor: *Primary cancers of the bladder are evident as filling defects (radiolucent shadow) in the bladder.*

Pelvic tumor or hematoma: *Any mass that distorts the pelvic anatomy is seen as external compression of the dye-filled bladder.*

Bladder trauma: *Laceration or perforation of the bladder is evident by the finding of dye outside the bladder. This is usually best demonstrated on the postvoid film.*

Vesicoureteral reflux: *Reflux of urine or dye from the bladder into the ureter is obvious with distention of the bladder with dye.*

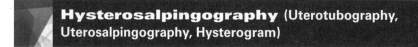

Hysterosalpingography (Uterotubography, Uterosalpingography, Hysterogram)

NORMAL FINDINGS

Patent fallopian tubes
No defects in uterine cavity

INDICATIONS

This test is part of a workup for infertility. The result can indicate patency or obstruction of the fallopian tubes.

TEST EXPLANATION

In hysterosalpingography, the uterine cavity and fallopian tubes are visualized radiographically after the injection of contrast material through the cervix. Uterine tumors, intrauterine adhesions, and developmental anomalies can be seen. Tubal obstruction of the fallopian tubes caused by internal scarring, tumor, infection, or kinking also can be detected. A possible therapeutic effect of this test is that passage of dye through the tubes may clear mucous plugs, straighten kinked tubes, or break up adhesions. This test also may be used to document adequacy of surgical tubal ligation. Its main purpose is in the evaluation of infertility to see if there is any obstruction of the fallopian tubes.

This procedure is performed by a physician in approximately 15 to 30 minutes. The patient may feel occasional, transient menstrual-type cramping and may have shoulder pain caused by subphrenic irritation from the dye as it leaks into the peritoneal cavity.

CONTRAINDICATIONS

- Patients with infections of the vagina, cervix, or fallopian tubes, because of risk of extending the infection
- Patients with uterine bleeding, because contrast material may enter the open blood vessels. Further, clots may be pushed out of the uterus and into the fallopian tubes, causing obstruction.
- Patients who are pregnant, because contrast material may induce abortion

POTENTIAL COMPLICATIONS

- Infection of the endometrium (endometritis)
- Infection of the fallopian tubes (salpingitis)
- Uterine perforation
- Allergic reaction to iodinated dye or shellfish (rare because the dye is not administered intravenously)

INTERFERING FACTORS

- Fecal material or gas in the bowel, which may obscure visualization
- Tubal spasm or excessive traction, which may cause the appearance of a stricture in a normal fallopian tube
- Excessive traction, which may displace adhesions, thereby making tubes appear normal

---

✓ Clinical Priorities

- Check the patient for allergy to iodinated dyes.
- This test is not performed if pregnancy is suspected, because the contrast material might induce abortion.
- After the test, evaluate the patient for signs and symptoms of infection (e.g., fever, increased pulse rate, pain).

PROCEDURE AND PATIENT CARE

Before

 Explain the procedure to the patient. Ask the patient when she had her last menstrual period. If pregnancy is suspected, the test is not performed.
- Obtain informed consent if required by the institution.
- Assess the patient for allergy to iodine dye or shellfish.
- Instruct the patient to take laxatives the night before the test, if ordered.
- Administer enemas or suppositories on the morning of the test, if ordered.
- Administer sedatives (e.g., midazolam [Versed]) or antispasmodics, if ordered, before the test.
- Tell the patient that no food or fluid restrictions are needed.

During

- Note the following procedural steps:
  1. A plain x-ray film of the abdomen is often obtained before the test to ensure that preparation adequately eliminated gastrointestinal gas and feces.

2. After voiding, the patient is placed on the fluoroscopy table in the lithotomy position.
3. A speculum is inserted into the vagina, and the cervix is visualized and cleansed.
4. Contrast material is injected during fluoroscopy, and x-ray films are obtained.
5. More dye is injected so that the entire upper genital tract (uterus and fallopian tubes) can be filled.
6. This test can be considered satisfactorily performed only if the uterus and the tubes are distended to their maximal capacity or fluid flows through the fallopian tubes.

After

🖎 Inform the patient that a vaginal discharge (sometimes bloody) may be present for 1 or 2 days after the test. A perineal pad should be worn.
- Evaluate the patient for delayed reaction to dye (e.g., dyspnea, rash, tachycardia, hives). Treat symptoms with antihistamines or steroids.
🖎 Inform the patient that cramping and dizziness may occur after the study.
🖎 Evaluate the patient for signs and symptoms of infection (e.g., fever, increased pulse rate, pain). Instruct the patient to call her physician and report these symptoms if they occur.

TEST RESULTS AND CLINICAL SIGNIFICANCE

Uterine tumor (e.g., leiomyoma, cancer) or polyps: *Filling defects in the uterus may indicate tumor.*
Developmental anomaly of the uterus (e.g., uterus bicornis): *The anatomy of the uterus can be well visualized and evaluated.*
Intrauterine adhesions: *Usually from previous infection, these adhesions within the uterus can cause infertility.*
Uterine fistula: *Usually traumatic (iatrogenic [e.g., during dilation and curettage]), a fistula is evident as extravasation of dye from the uterus.*
Obstruction, kinking, or twisting of the fallopian tubes secondary to adhesions: *This is indicated by stenosis or complete obstruction. Fertility is unlikely unless tubal patency is reestablished.*
Extrauterine pregnancy: *Early tubal pregnancy can be demonstrated with this study, but there are better and easier ways to determine tubal pregnancy (e.g., CT of the pelvis [p. 1020]).*
Tumor of the fallopian tubes: *Tumors are evident as tubal filling defects.*

Kidney, Ureter, and Bladder X-Ray (KUB, Flat Plate of the Abdomen, Plain Film of the Abdomen, Scout Film)

NORMAL FINDINGS

No evidence of calculi
Normal gastrointestinal (GI) gas pattern

INDICATIONS

This screening x-ray strategy is used to rapidly evaluate the abdomen in patients with abdominal pain or trauma. It can demonstrate pathologic conditions of the urinary or GI system.

TEST EXPLANATION

The KUB is an unenhanced image of the abdomen. It is often referred to as a *plain film or scout film.* The KUB is similar to the supine view on an obstruction series (see p. 1051) and can be performed to

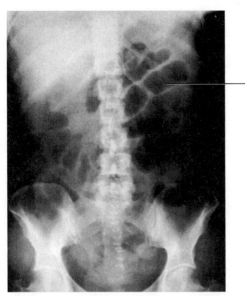

— Dilated loops of small bowel

Figure 12-17 Flat plate of abdomen depicts multiple, somewhat dilated loops of small bowel consistent with postoperative ileus.

demonstrate the size, shape, location, and any malformations of the kidneys and bladder. The KUB can also be used to identify calculi in these organs and in the ureters. This is often one of the first studies done to diagnose other intraabdominal diseases, such as intestinal obstruction, soft-tissue masses, and a ruptured viscus (Figure 12-17). The KUB is useful in detecting abnormal accumulations of gas within the GI tract and identifying ascites. No contrast medium is used for this study.

CONTRAINDICATIONS

- Patients who are pregnant

INTERFERING FACTORS

- Barium retained from previous studies can obscure visualization.

Clinical Priorities

- This test is also called a *plain film* or *scout film* of the abdomen.
- This test involves no contrast dye.
- This is often one of the first tests used in the evaluation of abdominal problems.
- This test should be scheduled before any barium studies.

PROCEDURE AND PATIENT CARE

Before

 Explain the procedure to the patient.

 Tell the patient that no fasting or sedation is required.

- Schedule this study before any barium studies.

- In male patient the testicles should be shielded with a lead apron to prevent their irradiation.
- In female patients, the ovaries cannot be shielded because of their proximity to the kidneys, ureters, and bladder.

✍ Tell the patient that no discomfort is associated with this study.

During

- In the radiology department, the patient is placed in the supine position. X-ray films are obtained of the patient's abdomen (Figure 12-18).
- Note that the KUB is performed by a radiologic technologist in a few minutes, and is interpreted by a radiologist.

After

✍ Tell the patient that results are available in approximately 1 hour.

- If indicated, schedule intravenous pyelography or GI studies after completion of the KUB.

TEST RESULTS AND CLINICAL SIGNIFICANCE

Calculi: *A calcified stone in the area of the KUB where the ureters would be is indicative of a ureteral calculi. Nearly 80% of ureteral stones can be seen on KUB.*

Abnormal accumulation of bowel gas: *Abnormal accumulation of bowel gas can indicate intestinal obstruction or paralytic ileus.*

Ascites: *The classic "ground glass" appearance of the entire abdomen on the KUB films indicates peritoneal effusion.*

Soft-tissue masses: *Large soft-tissue masses can be seen surprisingly well on this plain film without use of any contrast material.*

Ruptured viscus: *Free air (i.e., air outside the bowel but inside the abdomen) is indicative of a perforated viscus.*

Congenital anomalies (e.g., location, size, and number of kidneys): *Because the kidneys can be well visualized with KUB, anomalies are fairly easily detected.*

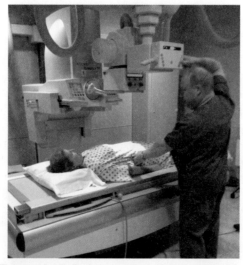

Figure 12-18 Patient positioned for a KUB x-ray.

Organomegaly or bladder distention: *An enlarged liver or spleen is seen as a large soft-tissue mass in the right or left upper quadrant, respectively. A large soft-tissue mass in the midline or pelvis is usually a distended bladder.*

RELATED TEST

Obstruction Series (p. 1051). This study includes a KUB as part of the series of plain film x-rays obtained to evaluate abdominal pain.

Mammography (Mammogram, Digital Mammography)

NORMAL FINDINGS

Breast Imaging Reporting and Database System (BI-RADS®)

Category 1: Negative
Category 2: Benign findings noted
Category 3: Probably benign findings: short-term follow-up is suggested
Category 4: Suspicious findings: further evaluation is indicated
Category 5: Cancer is highly suspected
Category 6: Known breast cancer
Category 0: Abnormality noted for which more imaging is recommended

INDICATIONS

Mammography enables detection of breast cancers, benign tumors, and cysts before they are even palpable. Mammography can be performed for screening (patients without any breast symptom) or diagnostic (patients with breast symptoms, such as a breast lump, pain, nipple discharge, or asymmetry) purposes.

Screening Mammography Guidelines

There are varying guidelines from multiple organizations regarding screening mammography.

National Institute of Health
- Women age 40 and older should have mammograms every 1 to 2 years.
- Women or men who are at higher-than-average risk of breast cancer should talk with their health care providers about whether to have mammograms before age 40 and how often to have them. Those at higher risk would include women with:
  - Personal history of breast cancer
  - Family history—A woman's chance of developing breast cancer increases if her mother, sister, and/or daughter have a history of breast cancer (especially if they were diagnosed before age 50).
  - Certain breast changes on biopsy—A diagnosis of atypical hyperplasia (a non-cancerous condition in which cells have abnormal features and are increased in number) or lobular carcinoma in situ (LCIS) (abnormal cells found in the lobules of the breast) increases a woman's risk of breast cancer. Women who have had two or more breast biopsies for other benign conditions also have an increased chance of developing breast cancer. This increased risk is a result of the condition that led to the biopsy, and not the biopsy itself.

- Genetic alterations (changes)—Specific alterations in *BRCA1, BRCA2* (see p. 1086).
- Radiation therapy ("x-ray therapy")—Women who had radiation therapy to the chest (including the breasts) before age 30 are at an increased risk of developing breast cancer throughout their lives. This includes women treated for Hodgkin lymphoma.

American Cancer Society
- Annual mammograms starting at the age of 40
- Women known to be at increased risk may benefit from earlier initiation of early detection testing and/or the addition of breast ultrasound or magnetic resonance imaging (MRI).

U.S. Preventive Services Task Force
- Screening mammograms before age 50 should not be done routinely and should be based on a woman's values regarding the risks and benefits of mammography.
- Screening mammograms should be done every 2 years beginning at age 50 for women at average risk of breast cancer.

When to Stop Screening

As long as a woman is in reasonably good health and would be a candidate for treatment, she should continue to be screened with mammography. However, if an individual has an estimated life expectancy of less than 5 to 7 years, severe functional limitations, and/or multiple co-morbidities likely to limit life expectancy, it may be appropriate to consider cessation of screening. Chronologic age alone should not be the reason for the cessation of regular screening. That being said, there is insufficient evidence that mammogram screening is effective for women age 75 and older.

Diagnostic Mammography

Women or men older than 25 years should undergo diagnostic mammography if they have breast symptoms, such as a palpable nodule or lump, breast skin thickening or indentation, nipple discharge or retraction, erosive sore of the nipple, or breast pain.

TEST EXPLANATION

Mammography is an x-ray examination of the breast. Careful interpretation of these x-rays can identify cancers (Figure 12-19). In many cases, breast cancers can be detected before they become palpable. It is believed that early detection of breast cancer may improve patient survival. Radiographic signs of breast cancer include fine, stippled, clustered calcifications (white specks on the breast x-ray films); a poorly defined, spiculated mass; asymmetric density; and skin thickening.

Although mammography is not a substitute for breast biopsy, results are reliable and accurate when interpreted by a skilled radiologist. The detection rate for breast cancer with mammography is greater than 85%. This means that less than 15% of breast cancers are missed at mammography. Cancers that are missed are in areas of the breast that are not well imaged by the x-ray (e.g., the high axillary tail of the breast), are in women with very dense breast tissue, or are too small to identify. Nearly 70% of breast cancers are not palpable and are detected only with mammography. Mammography also can detect other diseases of the breast, such as acute suppurative mastitis, abscess, fibrocystic changes, cysts, benign tumors (e.g., fibroadenoma), and intraglandular lymph nodes.

A woman receives minimal radiation exposure during a mammography (about 0.5 rad per view). Females younger than age 25 are most susceptible to the neoplastic effects of ionizing radiation. Therefore, mammography is rarely recommended in young women. Most mammograms include two views of each breast (in the cranial to caudal dimension and in the medial to lateral dimension). It is important to inform the woman

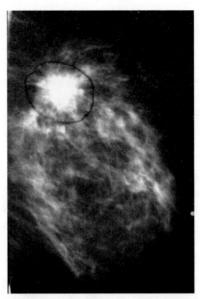

Figure 12-19 Oblique mammogram demonstrating a cancer, encircled in red.

that "callbacks" are not uncommon. If the radiologist sees something that should be more thoroughly evaluated with magnified views, deeper views, or ultrasound, the patient may be "called back" for further testing.

Mammograms can be performed using analog x-rays films or utilizing digital technology *(digital mammography)*. Digital images are viewed on a computer monitor, allowing the radiologist to manipulate the contrast and brightness of the images so as to miss fewer cancers. Portions of the breast image can be magnified. Results of mammography can only suggest a diagnosis of breast cancer. The diagnosis of cancer must be confirmed with microscopic histologic review of a biopsy specimen.

Mammography is performed by a certified radiologic technologist in approximately 10 minutes. The x-ray films are interpreted by an accredited radiologist. Moderate discomfort is associated with mammography. This is caused by the pressure required to compress the breast tissue while the x-ray films are obtained. In patients with tender breasts, this may be painful. The ACR also accredits the mammography machine for quality of picture and accuracy of x-ray dose. The ACR has recommended a standardized method for reporting of mammogram results. This is described under Normal Results.

Mammography can also be used to locate a mammographically identified (i.e., not palpable) lesion for biopsy. One method is *preoperative mammogram localization* of a previously identified abnormality, followed by open biopsy. For this procedure, the patient is taken to the mammography room. A grid printed on transparent adhesive material is attached to the breast containing the abnormality. Craniocaudal and direct lateral views are obtained. With the grid still in place, the radiologist, using the coordinates on the grid, numbs the skin and places a needle into the abnormal area. A wire is then disengaged through the needle into the breast. Repeated mammograms are obtained. The patient is then taken to the operating room. After appropriate anesthesia, an incision is made along the wire, to the abnormal tissue, which is then removed for biopsy. All localizing wire can be placed in a suspicious area of the breast for biopsy by use of stereotactic images (see the following) or by ultrasound (p. 871).

Nonoperative needle biopsy with a *stereotactic biopsy* device is the least invasive manner of obtaining tissue from a nonpalpable mammographic abnormality. For this procedure the patient is placed prone on a specialized table. Through a hole in the table, the breast is placed in a mammography machine under the table. The mammogram is connected to a computer that can identify the exact location of the mammographic abnormality (Figure 12-20). The machine positions the biopsy device in alignment with the lesion. When fired, the biopsy equipment is in the center of the lesion, and specimens are obtained for biopsy. No surgery or sutures are required. Only minimal pain is experienced, because a breast in compression has little skin pain sensation.

Breast tomography (3-D mammography) using multiple mammogram views through different thicknesses of the breast tissue is rapidly becoming a method of interest for the diagnosis of disease of the breast. Unfortunately, these radiographic techniques are too expensive to provide to a large population of non-symptomatic women in screening.

There are multiple other methods of breast imaging. Mammography, however, is the most accurate testing when considering cost-effectiveness and efficiency. MRI of the breast (p. 1106) is more accurate than mammography, but far more expensive and labor intensive. Because of that, it is not applied as a screening modality for most women. However, MRIs are very helpful in the identification of cancer in dense-breasted women. Breast nuclear scintigraphy is also available for breast imaging. Like the MRI, breast scintigraphy is far more expensive and labor intensive than mammography. Radiation exposure with some radionuclides can be quite high. Diagnostic accuracy in comparison with other forms of breast imaging has yet to be determined.

 Clinical Priorities

- The combination of mammography and close physical examination provides the best approach for detecting breast cancer at its earlier stage.
- For mammography, radiation exposure is minimal.
- Some discomfort may be experienced during breast compression. Compression is necessary for visualization of the breast.
- Ten percent of women getting a mammogram may be called back for more directed breast imaging.

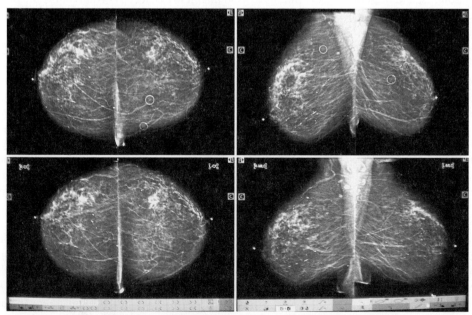

Figure 12-20 The mammography film is placed on the digitizer, and coordinates of the breast lesion are determined and displayed. These coordinates guide the needle to the precise location of the lesion, and the aspirate is drawn for biopsy.

CONTRAINDICATIONS

- Patients who are pregnant, unless the benefits outweigh the risk of fetal damage
- Patients younger than 25 years old

INTERFERING FACTORS

- Talcum powder and antiperspirants give the impression of calcifications within the breast.
- Jewelry worn around the neck can preclude total visualization of the breast.
- Breast augmentation implants can inhibit total visualization of the breast. However, the implants can be displaced so the native breast tissue can be imaged.
- Previous breast surgery can distort mammographic findings.

PROCEDURE AND PATIENT CARE

Before

- Explain the procedure to the patient.
- Inform the patient that some discomfort may be experienced during breast compression. Compression allows better visualization of the breast tissue. Assure the patient that the breast will not be harmed by compression. Premenopausal women with very sensitive breasts can choose to schedule their mammogram 1 to 2 weeks after their menses to reduce any discomfort caused by compression required for the mammogram.
- Tell the patient that no fasting is required.
- Explain to the patient that a minimal radiation dose will be used during the test.
- Instruct the patient to disrobe above the waist and put on an x-ray gown.
- Instruct the patient to report the location of any symptom or lump she may have noted.
- Markers will be placed on any skin bump that may be interpreted to an abnormality on the x-ray image.

During

- Note the following procedural steps:
  1. The patient is taken to the radiology department and stands in front of a mammogram machine.
  2. One breast is placed on the x-ray plate.
  3. The x-ray cone is brought down on top of the breast to compress it gently between the broadened cone and the x-ray plate (Figure 12-21).
  4. The x-ray film is exposed, for a *craniocaudal view.*
  5. The x-ray plate is turned about 45 degrees medially and placed on the inner aspect of the breast.
  6. The broadened cone is brought in medially and again gently compresses the breast. A *mediolateral view* is obtained.
  7. Occasionally *direct lateral* (90-degree) or *magnified spot views* are obtained to more clearly visualize an area of suspicion. Elongated or small cones are applied to the x-ray tube to enhance visualization of a specific area of the breast.

After

- Take the opportunity to instruct the patient in breast self-examination.
- Support the patient in her concerns if additional views are required. It is always frightening if further views are required. Usually these additional views include spot magnified views, which allow the radiologist to better visualize an area of the breast.

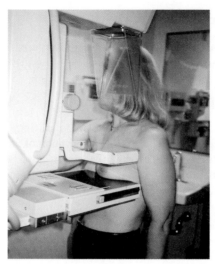

Figure 12-21 Mammography procedure.

TEST RESULTS AND CLINICAL SIGNIFICANCE

Breast cancer: *This can be evident as a radiodense (white) stellate or spiculated mass, a cluster of calcifications, or vague asymmetric radiodensity. When cancer invades the skin, the skin will appear thickened. Also, the nipple can appear inverted if a subareolar cancer exists.*

Benign tumor (e.g., fibroadenoma): *Benign tumors are usually well-rounded masses with discrete borders. Sometimes fibroadenomas can degenerate, and calcifications can develop within. Colloid or medullary cancers can appear similarly well rounded.*

Breast cyst: *Cysts are seen as well-rounded masses with discrete borders. Ultrasound of the breast demonstrates the cysts to be fluid filled.*

Fibrocystic disease: *This is the most common breast finding. Nearly every women has some degree of fibrocystic disease. On mammograms, this is seen as a vague asymmetric radiodensity (white). It can also be evident as calcifications.*

Breast abscess,

Suppurative mastitis:

> *The mammographic findings of infection are increased thickness of the skin, with increased radiodensity of the breast tissue.*

RELATED TESTS

Ultrasound of the Breast (p. 871). An important adjunct to mammography, ultrasound can differentiate between cystic and solid lesions.

Magnetic Resonance Imaging (MRI) of the Breast (p. 1106). Although a more accurate test for breast cancer, its high rate of false positives makes it too expensive for screening.

 Myelography (Myelogram, CT Myelography)

NORMAL FINDINGS

Normal spinal canal

INDICATIONS

Myelography provides radiographic visualization of the subarachnoid space of the spinal canal. The cord, nerve roots, and surrounding meninges can be seen. This test is indicated in patients with severe back pain or localized neurologic signs that suggest narrowing of the spinal canal (e.g., herniated lumbar disk).

TEST EXPLANATION

By placing radiopaque dye into the subarachnoid space of the spinal canal, the contents of the canal can be fluoroscopically outlined. Cord tumors, meningeal tumors, metastatic spinal tumors, herniated intervertebral disks, and arthritic bone spurs can be readily detected with this study. These lesions appear as spinal canal narrowing or as varying degrees of obstruction to the flow of the dye column within the canal. The entire canal (from lumbar to cervical areas) can be examined. Because this test is usually performed with lumbar puncture (LP; see p. 651), all the potential complications of that procedure exist.

Several different contrast materials can be used for myelography. In general, non-ionic low osmolar radiopaque dyes such as iohexol (Omnipaque) or iopamidol (Isovue) are associated with a significantly lower risk of CNS toxicity than some of the oil-based or heavier radiopaque contrast materials. The water-soluble contrast is absorbed by the blood excreted by the kidneys. Oil-based contrast media stays in the subarachnoid space much longer.

After injection of contrast material into the subarachnoid spinal space, images are obtained. These images can be obtained by simple x-ray images of the spine from multiple directions. More commonly additional images are obtained with computed tomography (CT myelography). MRI of the spine (p. 1106) is the preferred modality to image the spine and its contents. Myelography is more time-consuming and invasive than MRI. Plain film or CT myelography is reserved for those patients who do not have access to an MRI or for equivocal cases.

After the procedure, the patient's head and thorax should be elevated 30 to 50 degrees for approximately 6 to 8 hours to reduce upward dispersion of the dye and to prevent contact of the water-soluble agent with the cerebral meninges, which could precipitate a seizure. Bed rest may be ordered for up to 6 hours.

CONTRAINDICATIONS

- Patients with multiple sclerosis, because exacerbation may be precipitated by myelography
- Patients with increased intracranial pressure, because LP may cause herniation of the brain
- Patients with infection near the LP site, because this may precipitate bacterial meningitis
- Patients who are allergic to shellfish or iodinated dye

POTENTIAL COMPLICATIONS

- Headache
- Meningitis
- Herniation of the brain
- Seizures
- Hypoglycemia or acidosis in patients who are taking metformin (Glucophage) and receive iodine dye
- For potential complications to iodinated dye, see p. 985.

Clinical Priorities

- Myelography can be performed with different types of contrast materials. Pantopaque is an oil-based medium; Amipaque and Omnipaque are water-soluble contrast media. Air-contrast myelography can also be performed.
- To avoid herniation of the brain, this test is contraindicated in patients with increased intracranial pressure.

PROCEDURE AND PATIENT CARE

Before

✏ Explain the procedure to the patient.
- Ensure that the physician has obtained written, informed consent for this procedure.
- For assessment of allergy to iodinated dye, see p. 985.

✏ Explain to the patient that he or she must lie very still during the procedure.
- Food and fluid restrictions vary according to the type of dye used. Check with the radiology department for specific restrictions.

✏ Inform the patient that he or she will be tilted into an upside-down position on the table so that the dye can properly fill the spinal canal and provide adequate visualization of the desired area.

During

- Note the following procedural steps:
  1. Lumbar puncture (see p. 651) or cisternal puncture is performed.
  2. A 15-mL sample of CSF is withdrawn, and 15 mL or more of radiopaque dye is injected into the spinal canal.
  3. The patient is placed prone on the tilt table, with the head tilted down.
  4. Representative x-ray images are obtained.
  5. After myelography is performed, the needle is removed and a dressing is applied.

After

- Note that nursing interventions after the procedure depend on the type of contrast agent used.
- See lumbar puncture (p. 651) for appropriate "after" care.

Home Care Responsibilities

- After myelography, safe positioning of the patient's head is determined by the type of dye used in the procedure.
- Encourage the patient to drink fluids to enhance excretion of the dye and to replace CSF.
- Tell the patient to report any signs of meningeal irritation (e.g., fever, stiff neck, occipital headache, photophobia).

TEST RESULTS AND CLINICAL SIGNIFICANCE

Spinal cord tumors (e.g., astrocytoma, neurofibroma, meningioma): *These are seen as radiolucent filling defects in the column of radiopaque dye in the canal.*

Metastatic spinal tumor: *Extrinsic spinal tumors (usually metastatic) are evident as extrinsic radiolucent filling defects in the column of radiopaque dye in the canal.*

Cervical ankylosing spondylosis,

Arthritic lumbar stenosis from arthritic bone spurs:
These bony changes can compress the spinal canal and are evident as distortion of the cord or nerve roots.

Herniated intravertebral disk: *A herniated disk acts as external compression on the spinal cord or the nerve root. The most common areas of disk herniation are L4-L5 and L5-S1.*

Avulsion of nerve roots: *Traumatic avulsion of the nerve root can cause profound neurologic changes.*

Cysts: *Cysts of the cord or meninges surrounding the cord are evident as extrinsic radiolucent filling defects in the column of radiopaque dye in the canal.*

RELATED TEST

Magnetic Resonance Imaging (MRI) (p. 1106). This test is more accurate than myelography for viewing the spinal cord and its surrounding structures.

Obstruction Series

NORMAL FINDINGS

No evidence of bowel obstruction
No abnormal calcifications
No free air

Indications

This x-ray series is used for the evaluation of abdominal pain or suspected obstruction of the intestinal tract.

TEST EXPLANATION

The obstruction series is a group of x-ray images of the abdomen in patients with suspected bowel obstruction, paralytic ileus, perforated viscus, abdominal abscess, kidney stones, appendicitis, or foreign body ingestion. The series of films usually consists of at least two x-ray studies. The first is an *erect abdominal* film, which should include visualization of both diaphragms. The film is examined for evidence of free air under either diaphragm, which is pathognomonic for perforated viscus. This view is also used to detect air-fluid levels within the intestine; the presence of an air-fluid level is compatible with bowel obstruction or paralytic ileus. Occasionally, patients are too ill to stand erect. In this case, an x-ray film can be taken with the patient in the left lateral decubitus position. If free air is present, it will be seen between the liver and the right side of the abdominal wall. Air fluid levels also can be detected.

The second view in the obstruction series is usually a *supine abdominal* x-ray study, similar to the kidney, ureter, and bladder (KUB) study (p. 1040). An abdominal abscess may be seen as a cluster of tiny bubbles within a localized area. A calcification within the ureter could indicate a kidney ureteral stone. A small calcification in the right lower quadrant in a patient with pain in this quadrant may be an appendicolith. A gas-filled, distended bowel is compatible with bowel obstruction or paralytic ileus.

The obstruction series can also be used to monitor the clinical course of gastrointestinal (GI) disease. For example, repeated obstruction series in patients with partial small bowel obstruction or paralytic ileus can indicate clinical worsening or improvement.

Frequently, a *cross-table lateral* view of the abdomen is included in an obstruction series, to detect abdominal aorta calcification, which often occurs in older patients. The calcification represents the anterior wall of the aorta. If an aortic aneurysm exists, this calcification will be seen to protrude from the spine.

The *supine abdominal* x-ray study can be used as a scout image before performing GI or abdominal contrast material-enhanced x-ray studies (e.g., barium enema [p. 994] or intravenous pyelography (IVP) [p. 1057]), to ensure nothing is obstructing adequate visualization of what needs to be studied.

The obstruction series is performed in minutes in the radiology department by a radiologic technologist; however, it can be performed at the bedside with a portable x-ray machine. A radiologist interprets the films. No discomfort is associated with the study.

CONTRAINDICATIONS

• Patients who are pregnant, unless the benefits outweigh the risks

INTERFERING FACTORS

• Previous GI barium contrast study: Although barium within the GI tract can preclude identification of other important calcifications (e.g., kidney stones), it can be helpful in outlining the GI anatomy.

PROCEDURE AND PATIENT CARE

Before

✍ Explain the procedure to the patient.
• Ensure that all radiopaque clothing has been removed.
✍ Remind the patient that no contrast agent will be used.

During

• Although the procedure varies among facilities, usually a supine abdominal x-ray film, erect abdominal film, and perhaps a lower erect chest film are obtained. Often a cross-table lateral x-ray film is also included.

After

• No special care is needed.

TEST RESULTS AND CLINICAL SIGNIFICANCE

Abdominal aortic calcification or abdominal aortic aneurysm: *Abdominal aortic aneurysm is evident by calcification in the anterior wall of the aorta, displaced significantly anterior from the vertebrae.*

Calculi: *A calcified stone in the area where the ureters would be is indicative of ureteral calculi. This finding requires further supportive evidence by means of IVP (p. 1057). Appendicolithiasis (stone in the appendix) is suspected when a patient with right lower quadrant abdominal pain is seen to have a stone in that quadrant.*

Abdominal accumulation of bowel gas: *Abnormal accumulations of bowel gas can indicate intestinal obstruction or paralytic ileus.*

Ascites: *The classic ground-glass appearance of the entire abdomen on the supine abdominal film indicates peritoneal effusion.*

Soft-tissue masses: *Large soft-tissue masses or abscesses can be seen surprisingly well on this plain film x-ray, without contrast material enhancement.*

Ruptured viscus: *Free air (i.e., air outside the bowel but inside the abdomen) is indicative of a perforated viscus.*

Congenital anomalies in the location, size, and number of kidneys: *Because the kidneys are well seen, abnormalities of these features are easily detected.*

Organomegaly or bladder distention: *An enlarged liver or spleen is seen as a large soft-tissue mass in the right or left upper quadrant, respectively. A large soft-tissue mass in the midline or pelvis is usually a distended bladder.*

Foreign body: *A bullet or other solid object is obvious on x-ray films. A surgical sponge or instrument left during surgery is also visible.*

RELATED TEST

Kidney, Ureter, and Bladder (KUB) X-Ray (p. 1040). This is only one component of the obstruction series and therefore does not contribute as much information as does an obstruction series.

Percutaneous Transhepatic Cholangiography (PTC, PTHC)

NORMAL FINDINGS

Normal gallbladder and biliary ducts

INDICATIONS

This procedure allows visualization of the bile ducts and sometimes the pancreatic duct. Patients with jaundice can be evaluated for tumors, gallstones, and other diseases.

TEST EXPLANATION

By passing a needle through the liver and into an intrahepatic bile duct, iodinated dye can be injected directly into the biliary system. The intrahepatic and extrahepatic biliary ducts, and occasionally the gallbladder, can be visualized and studied for partial or total obstruction from gallstones, benign strictures, malignant tumors, congenital cysts, and anatomic variations. This is especially helpful in patients with jaundice. If the jaundice is a result of extrahepatic obstruction, a catheter can be left in the bile duct and used for external drainage of bile. Furthermore, a stent can be placed across a stricture to decompress the biliary system internally.

PTC and endoscopic retrograde cholangiopancreatography (ERCP, p. 605) are the only methods available to visualize the biliary tree in patients with jaundice. ERCP is used more frequently because of its lower complication rate. PTC, however, is the only way to visualize the biliary tree after most gastric surgery. Occasionally (if the pancreatic duct and the common bile duct are from a common channel), part or all of the pancreatic duct can be filled with dye from the same injection. See Table 12-5 for a list of diagnostic tests to visualize the pancreatobiliary system, along with their advantages and disadvantages.

PTC is performed by a radiologist in approximately 1 hour, during which time the patient must lie still. Abdominal pain may be felt for several hours after the test. Occasionally the patient also may have right shoulder-top pain because of diaphragmatic irritation of leaking bile or blood.

CONTRAINDICATIONS

- Patients who are allergic to iodine or shellfish
- Patients with evidence of mild cholangitis: Dye injections increase biliary pressure and cause bacteremia, which may lead to septicemia and shock.

TABLE 12-5	Diagnostic Tests to Visualize the Pancreatobiliary System	
Test	**Advantages**	**Disadvantages**
Intravenous cholangiography	Easy to perform	Poor visualization of ducts
Oral cholecystography	Easy to perform	Visualizes only the gallbladder
ERCP	Good visualization of the pancreas and bile ducts; able to decompress the biliary system	Difficult to perform; complications possible
PTC	Good visualization of the ducts; able to decompress the biliary system	Difficult to perform; complications possible
Nuclear radioscintigraphy	Easy to perform	Poor visualization of the biliary system; not specific as to disease

- Patients who cannot cooperate and remain still
- Patients with prolonged clotting times

POTENTIAL COMPLICATIONS

- For potential complications of iodinated dye, see p. 985.
- Peritonitis caused by bile extravasation from the liver after the needle has been removed
- Bleeding caused by inadvertent puncture of a large hepatic blood vessel
- Sepsis and cholangitis from injection of the dye into an already infected and obstructed bile duct: The pressure of injection pushes the bacteria into the bloodstream, causing bacteremia.

INTERFERING FACTORS

- The presence of barium from a previous upper gastrointestinal (GI) series or barium contrast study may preclude visualization of the biliary tree.

✓ Clinical Priorities

- Check the patient for allergy to iodinated dyes.
- Verify that results of coagulation studies are within the normal range before this test, because bleeding is a potential complication.
- Abdominal pain after the test may be an indication of bleeding or bile extravasation.

PROCEDURE AND PATIENT CARE

Before

Explain the procedure to the patient.
- Obtain informed consent.
- For assessment of allergy to iodinated dye, see p. 985.
- Type and cross-match the patient's blood. The patient may bleed and require a transfusion or surgery.
- Verify that results of coagulation studies are within the normal range.

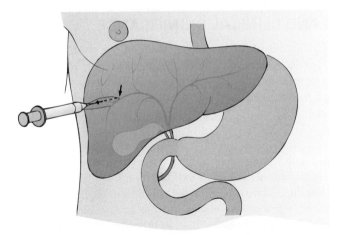

Figure 12-22 Percutaneous transhepatic cholangiography (PTHC).

- Keep the patient on nothing by mouth (NPO) status after midnight on the day of the test. A laxative may be ordered.
- Premedicate the patient as indicated, usually with atropine and meperidine.

During
- Note the following procedural steps:
  1. The patient is placed supine on an x-ray table in the radiology department.
  2. The abdominal wall or lower chest wall (over the liver) is anesthetized with lidocaine (Xylocaine).
  3. With the use of fluoroscopic monitoring, the needle is advanced through the skin and into the liver (Figure 12-22).
  4. When bile flows freely out from the liver through the needle, radiographic dye is injected.
  5. X-ray images are obtained immediately.
  6. If an obstruction is found, a catheter or stent is placed over a guide wire and left temporarily in the biliary tract to establish drainage and decompression of the biliary tract.

After
- Keep the patient on bed rest for several hours.
- Observe the patient for hemorrhage or bile leakage. A small amount of bleeding is normal.
- Keep the patient NPO for a few hours after the test in the event intraabdominal bleeding or bile extravasation develops that requires surgery.
- Repeatedly assess the patient's vital signs for evidence of hemorrhage.
- Assess the patient for signs of bacteremia or sepsis.
- If a catheter is left in the biliary tract, establish a sterile, closed drainage system.
- Withhold high doses of pain medications that may blunt the abdominal signs associated with hemorrhage or bile extravasation.

 Home Care Responsibilities

- Observe the needle insertion site for bleeding and bile leakage.
- Note that fever and chills may indicate bacteremia or sepsis.
- Instruct the patient to report signs of bleeding (increased pulse and decreased blood pressure).

X-Ray Studies

12

TEST RESULTS AND CLINICAL SIGNIFICANCE

Tumors, strictures, or gallstones of the hepatic or common bile duct: *These diseases cause partial or complete obstruction of the biliary tree. Tumors usually cause long strictures. Benign strictures are more likely to cause short segment narrowing. Gallstones usually are evident as rounded radiolucent (dark) filling defects in the bile duct. When they obstruct the bile duct, the obstruction is seen as a soft convex cutoff of the bile duct.*

Sclerosing cholangitis,

Biliary sclerosis:

    These conditions are due to inflammatory or fibrotic changes around the bile ducts; this leads to a long stricture in most of the biliary tree and its radicals.

Cysts of the common bile duct: *These congenital outpouchings of the bile duct may vary in size from tiny and barely noticeable to large and voluminous. The pressure surrounding these cysts can obstruct the normal portion of the bile duct in the closed space of the right upper quadrant of the abdomen.*

Tumors, strictures, inflammation, or true or pseudocysts of the pancreatic duct: *If the pancreatic duct is visualized, these abnormalities can be identified. Pancreatic tumors are evident as long strictures. Postinflammatory strictures are usually short segment narrowing. Neoplastic cysts may be connected to the main pancreatic duct and fill with dye. Pseudocysts, caused by pancreatic duct disruption that follows severe pancreatitis, nearly always connect with the main pancreatic duct and therefore fill with dye.*

Anatomic biliary or pancreatic duct variations: *Duplications, aberrant entry of the pancreatobiliary ducts into the intestine, and other anomalies can be identified.*

RELATED TEST

Endoscopic Retrograde Cholangiopancreatography (ERCP) (p. 605). This is the preferred method of visualizing the pancreatobiliary tree in the patient with jaundice.

Pyelography (Intravenous Pyelography [IVP], Excretory Urography [EUG], Intravenous Urography [IUG, IVU], Retrograde Pyelography, Antegrade Pyelography)

NORMAL FINDINGS

Normal size, shape, and position of the kidneys, renal pelvis, ureters, and bladder

Normal kidney excretory function as evidenced by the length of time for passage of contrast material through the kidneys

INDICATIONS

The test has been mostly replaced by CT scan (p. 1020) because the accuracy of the CT scan is better than IVP. Nevertheless, IVP is still indicated for patients with:

- Pain compatible with urinary stones
- Blood in the urine
- Proposed pelvic surgery to locate the ureters
- Trauma to the urinary system
- Urinary outlet obstruction
- A suspected kidney tumor

TEST EXPLANATION

Pyelography is an x-ray study that uses radiopaque contrast material to visualize the kidneys, renal pelvis, ureters, and bladder. The contrast can be injected intravenously (IVP), through a catheter placed into the ureter (retrograde pyelography), or through a catheter placed into the proximal renal collecting system (antegrade pyelography). IVP testing is not performed as frequently as it was several years ago.

For *IVP*, dye is injected intravenously, filtered out at the kidney by the glomeruli, and then passed through the renal tubules. X-ray films taken at set intervals over the next 30 minutes will show passage of the dye material through the kidneys and ureters and into the bladder. If the artery leading to one of the kidneys is blocked, the dye cannot enter that kidney or part thereof and it will not be visualized. If the artery is partially blocked, the length of time required for the appearance of the contrast material will be prolonged.

With primary glomerular disease (e.g., glomerulonephritis), the glomerular filtrate is reduced, which causes a reduction in the quantity of dye filtered. Therefore it requires more time for kidney visualization. Defects in dye filling of the kidney can indicate renal tumors or cysts.

If the obstruction of the ureter has been of sufficient duration, the collecting system proximal to the obstruction will be dilated (hydronephrosis). Retroperitoneal and pelvic tumors, aneurysms, and enlarged lymph nodes also can produce extrinsic compression and distortions of the opacified collecting system.

IVP can be used to assess the effect of trauma on the urinary system. Renal hematomas distort the renal contour. Renal artery laceration is suggested by non-opacification of one kidney. Laceration of the kidneys, pelvis, ureters, or bladder often causes urine leaks, which are identified by dye extravasation from the urinary system. Furthermore, IVP can assess a patient for congenital absence or malposition of the kidneys. Horseshoe kidneys (connection of the two kidneys), double ureters, and pelvic kidneys are typical congenital abnormalities.

Retrograde pyelography refers to radiographic visualization of the urinary tract through ureteral catheterization and the injection of contrast material. The ureters are catheterized during cystoscopy. A radiopaque material is injected into the ureters, and x-ray films are taken. This test can be performed even if the patient has an allergy to IV contrast dye, because none of the dye injected into the ureters is absorbed.

Retrograde pyelography is helpful in radiographically examining the ureters in patients when visualization with intravenous pyelography is inadequate or contraindicated. When a ureter is obstructed, IVP will visualize only the ureter proximal to the obstruction, if at all. To visualize the distal part of the ureter, retrograde pyelography is necessary. Also, in patients with unilateral renal disease, the involved kidney and collecting system are not visualized because renal function is so poor. As a result, no dye will be filtered into the collecting system (during IVP) by the nonfunctioning kidney. To rule out ureteral obstruction as a cause of the unilateral kidney disease, retrograde pyelography must be done.

Antegrade pyelography provides visualization of the renal pelvis for accurate placement of nephrostomy tubes. This study is used to identify the upper collecting system in an obstructed kidney and used as a map for accurate percutaneous placement of a nephrostomy tube. This is performed on patients who have an obstruction of the ureter and hydronephrosis. With this procedure, the renal pelvis is identified with CT imaging or ultrasound. A needle is placed into the pelvis. Radio-opaque dye is then injected and the entire upper renal collecting system is demonstrated by obtaining x-rays in rapid succession. Proper positioning for the nephrostomy is then decided based on these images.

CONTRAINDICATIONS

- Patients who are allergic to shellfish or iodinated dyes
- Patients who are severely dehydrated, because this can cause renal shutdown and failure (Geriatric patients are particularly vulnerable.)

- Patients with renal insufficiency, as evidenced by a blood urea nitrogen value greater than 40 mg/dL, because the iodinated nephrotoxic dye can worsen kidney function
- Patients with multiple myeloma, because the iodinated nephrotoxic dye can worsen renal function
- Patients who are pregnant, unless the benefits outweigh the risks of radiation exposure to the fetus

POTENTIAL COMPLICATIONS

- Allergy to iodine dye
- Infiltration of contrast dye
- Renal failure. This occurs most often in elderly patients who are chronically dehydrated before the dye injection.
- Hypoglycemia or acidosis may occur in patients who are taking metformin (Glucophage) and receive iodine dye.
- Hemorrhage at the needle puncture site during antegrade pyelography, because the kidney is highly vascular
- Complications associated with *retrograde pyelography* include:
  - Urinary tract infections
  - Sepsis by seeding the bloodstream with bacteria from infected urine
  - Perforation of the bladder or ureter
  - Hematuria
  - Temporary obstruction to ureter caused by ureteral edema

INTERFERING FACTORS

- Fecal material, gas, or barium in the bowel may obscure visualization of the renal system.
- Abnormal renal function studies may prevent adequate visualization of the urinary tract.
- Retained barium from previous studies may obscure visualization. Studies using barium (e.g., barium enema) should be scheduled after an IVP.

PROCEDURE AND PATIENT CARE

Before

- Explain the procedure to the patient. Inform the patient that several x-ray films will be taken over 30 minutes.
- Obtain informed consent if required by the institution.
- Check the patient for allergies to iodinated dye and shellfish.
- Give the patient a laxative (e.g., castor oil) or a cathartic, as ordered, the evening before the test.
- Inform the patient of the required food and fluid restrictions. Some institutions prefer abstinence from solid foods for 8 hours before testing. Some allow a clear-liquid breakfast on the test day.
- Ensure adequate hydration for the patient (IV or oral) before and after the test to avoid dye-induced renal failure.
- Note that pediatric patients will have decreased fasting times, as ordered on an individual basis.
- Note that elderly and debilitated patients should have fasting times indicated specifically for them.
- Note that patients receiving high rates of IV fluids may have infusion rates decreased for several hours before the study to increase the concentration of the dye within the urinary system.
- Assess the patient's blood urea nitrogen and creatinine levels. Abnormal renal function could deteriorate as a result of the dye injection.
- Schedule any barium studies after completion of the IVP.
- Give the patient an enema or suppository on the morning of the study, if ordered.

- If the antegrade or retrograde pyelography will be performed with the patient under general anesthesia, follow routine general anesthesia precautions. Keep the patient NPO after midnight on the day of the test. Fluids may be given intravenously.

During
- Note the following procedural steps:

Intravenous Pyelography
1. The patient is taken to the radiology department and placed in the supine position.
2. A plain film of the abdomen (KUB) is taken to ensure that no residual stool obscures visualization of the renal system. This also screens for calculi in the renal collecting system.
3. Skin testing for iodine allergy is often done.
4. A peripheral IV line is started (if not in place), and a contrast dye (e.g., Hypaque, Renografin) is given.
5. X-ray films are taken at specific times, usually at 1, 5, 10, 15, 20, and 30 minutes and sometimes longer, to follow the course of the dye from the cortex of the kidney to the bladder.
6. The patient is taken to the bathroom and asked to void.
7. A postvoiding film is taken to visualize the empty bladder.

✗ Inform the patient that the dye injection often causes a transitory flushing of the face, a feeling of warmth, a salty taste in the mouth, or even transient nausea. Initial IV needle placement and lying on a hard x-ray table are the only other discomforts associated with IVP.

Retrograde Pyelography
1. The ureteral catheters are passed into the ureters by means of cystoscopy (see p. 598).
2. Radiopaque contrast material (Hypaque or Renografin) is injected into the ureteral catheters, and x-ray films are taken.
3. The entire ureter and renal pelvis are demonstrated.
4. As the catheters are withdrawn, more dye is injected, and more x-ray films are taken to visualize the complete outline of the ureters.
5. A delayed film is often performed to assess the emptying capabilities of the ureter. This is usually done about 5 minutes after the last injection.
6. If obstruction is noted, a stent may be left in the ureter so that the ureter can drain.

✗ Inform the patient that antegrade or retrograde pyelography is uncomfortable. If awake, the patient will feel pressure and an urge to void.

Antegrade Pyelography
1. The renal pelvis is localized by means of ultrasound.
2. Under local anesthesia, a thin-walled needle is advanced into the lumen of the renal pelvis.
3. Contrast material is injected and x-ray films in posteroanterior (PA), oblique, and anteroposterior (AP) views are obtained.
4. The nephrostomy tube is placed over guide wires and its position is affirmed by repeating the x-rays.

After
✗ Maintain on adequate oral or IV hydration for several hours after pyelography to counteract fluid depletion caused by the test preparation. Encourage fluid intake.

✗ Assess the patient's urinary output. A decreased output may be an indication of renal failure. Instruct the patient to report a decreased output.

- Evaluate elderly and debilitated patients for weakness because of the combination of fasting and catharsis necessary for test preparation. Instruct these patients to ambulate only with assistance.

12

X-Ray Studies

- Note the color of the urine; a pink tinge is typically present. Report bright red blood or clots to the physician.
- See p. 985 for appropriate interventions concerning care for patients with iodine allergy.

TEST RESULTS AND CLINICAL SIGNIFICANCE

Pyelonephritis or glomerulonephritis: *Primary renal disease usually is evident as reduced opacification of the kidney with dye. This is because it takes a long time for enough dye to be filtered to the renal system to opacify the kidney.*

Kidney tumor (benign or malignant),

Renal hematoma, laceration,

Cyst or polycystic disease of the kidney:

These are usually evident as a radiolucent (dark) filling defect in the kidney parenchyma. Ultrasound of the kidney (p. 866) is diagnostic for cysts.

Congenital abnormality of the urologic tract: *Congenital anomalies may include absence of a kidney or altered shape, size, or location of a kidney. The collecting system can be duplicated, with more than one ureter per kidney. The bladder can be divided by a congenital septum into two small bladders.*

Renal or ureteral calculi: *Calculi (stones) are evident as radiolucent filling defects that can obstruct the ureters. This is most evident on retrograde pyelography.*

Trauma to the kidneys, ureters, or bladder: *Injury may be evident as leakage of dye from the injured organ. Hematomas are seen as filling defects or radiolucent shadows.*

Tumor of the collecting system: *This can partially or completely obstruct the collecting system.*

Hydronephrosis: *This condition is due to prolonged obstruction of the collecting system distal to the hydronephrotic area. The distal ureter is best evaluated by retrograde pyelography.*

Extrinsic compression of the collecting system (e.g., caused by tumor, aneurysm): *Nonurologic tumors or masses can distort or obstruct the ureters or bladder.*

Bladder tumor: *This is seen as a radiolucent (dark shadow) filling defect in the bladder.*

Prostate enlargement: *This is evident as an extrinsic protrusion into the base of the bladder and inadequate emptying of the bladder because of outlet obstruction.*

RELATED TESTS

Computed Tomography (CT) of the Abdomen (p. 1020). Allows better visualization of the kidneys, ureters, and bladder.

Cystography (p. 1036). Study of the bladder after placement of dye directly into the bladder. With this study, the dye is more concentrated, and more information concerning the bladder can be obtained.

Sialography

NORMAL FINDINGS

No evidence of disease in the salivary ducts and related structures

INDICATIONS

This test is used to identify calculi in the salivary ducts.

TEST EXPLANATION

Sialography is an x-ray procedure used to examine the salivary ducts (parotid, submaxillary, submandibular, sublingual) and related glandular structures after injection of a contrast medium into the desired duct. The procedure is used to detect calculi, strictures, tumors, or inflammatory disease in patients with pain, tenderness, or swelling in these areas. Computed tomography (CT) of the salivary ducts is more reliable for detection of salivary parenchymal tumors or inflammation. Sialography is effective for ductule calculi or strictures.

A radiologist performs this procedure in the radiology department in less than 30 minutes. The patient may feel slight pressure as the contrast medium is injected into the ducts.

CONTRAINDICATIONS

- Patients with mouth infections (e.g., yeast infection), because the infection may be spread to the salivary glands

POTENTIAL COMPLICATIONS

- Allergic reaction to iodinated dye: This is rare, because the dye is not administered intravenously.

PROCEDURE AND PATIENT CARE

Before

- Explain the procedure to the patient. The thought of dye injection in the mouth is frightening to many patients. Provide emotional support.
- Obtain informed consent if required by the institution.
- Instruct the patient to remove jewelry, hairpins, and dentures, which could obscure x-ray visualization.
- Instruct the patient to rinse the mouth with an antiseptic solution to reduce the possibility of introducing bacteria into the ductal structures.

During

- Note the following procedural steps:
  1. X-ray studies are taken before the dye injection to ensure that radiopaque stones are not present, which could prevent the contrast material from entering the ducts.
  2. The patient is placed supine on an x-ray table.
  3. The contrast medium is injected directly into the desired orifice through a cannula or special tiny catheter.
  4. X-ray films are obtained with the patient in various positions.
  5. The patient is given a sour substance (e.g., lemon juice) orally to stimulate salivary excretion of the dye.
  6. Another set of x-ray studies is obtained to evaluate ductal drainage.

After

- Encourage the patient to drink fluids to eliminate the dye.

TEST RESULTS AND CLINICAL SIGNIFICANCE

Calculi,
Strictures:
  These cause obstruction of the duct draining the salivary gland.

X-Ray Studies

12

Tumor: *Most tumors of the salivary glands are benign, and in the parotid gland. These tumors are demonstrated as radiolucent filling defects or distortion of the glandular ductules within the gland.*

Inflammatory disease: *Sialitis (especially parotitis) can result from viral illnesses (e.g., mumps) or bacterial infections.*

Skull X-Ray

NORMAL FINDINGS

Normal skull and surrounding structures

INDICATIONS

This x-ray study is used to evaluate the skull and paranasal sinuses for trauma or disease.

TEST EXPLANATION

An x-ray film of the skull provides visualization of the bones making up the skull, the nasal sinuses, and any central nervous system (CNS) calcification. This study is indicated when a pathologic condition is suspected in any of these structures.

Skull fractures are easily seen as abnormal radiolucent lines in an otherwise radiopaque skull bone (Figure 12-23). Metastatic tumors of the skull can easily be seen as radiolucent spots on an otherwise normal film. Opacification of the nasal sinuses may indicate sinusitis, hemorrhage, or tumor.

Located in the middle of the brain, the pineal gland is thought to regulate biorhythms in mammals. This gland may become calcified after puberty. When calcified, the pineal gland is a useful marker and

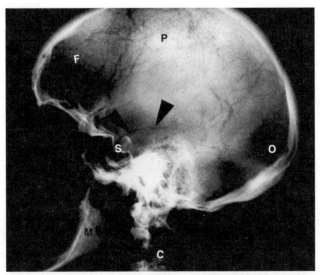

Figure 12-23 Skull x-ray, lateral view. Pointers indicate fracture line in temporal bone. C, Cervical vertabra; *F,* frontal bone; M, mandible; O, occipital bone; *P,* parietal bone; *S,* Sella turcica.

allows the midline of the brain to be easily identified on skull x-ray films. Conditions such as unilateral hematoma or tumor will cause a shift of the midline structures (and the calcified pineal gland) to the side opposite the site of the pathologic condition. Simple skull x-ray films therefore allow easy detection of these unilateral, space-occupying lesions.

The sella turcica is the bony structure surrounding and protecting the pituitary gland. Tumors of the pituitary gland may cause an increase in size or erosion of the sella turcica. These changes can be detected on skull x-ray films.

Most head trauma (or instances where skull injury is suspected) is evaluated with a CT scan of the brain. However, skull x-ray is still the best method of determining skull bone suture lines for the evaluation of children with abnormal head shape/size.

PROCEDURE AND PATIENT CARE

Before

- Explain the procedure to the patient.
- Instruct the patient to remove all objects above the neck, because metal objects and dentures will prevent x-ray visualization of the structures they cover.
- Avoid hyperextension and manipulation of the head if surgical injuries are suspected.
- Tell the patient that no sedation or fasting is required.

During

- The patient is taken to the radiology department and placed on an x-ray table. *Axial* (submentovertical), *half-axial* (Towne), *posteroanterior*, and *lateral* views of the skull are usually obtained (Figure 12-24).
- A radiologic technologist obtains the skull films in a few minutes.
- Tell the patient that the test is painless.

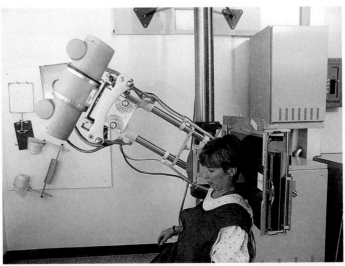

Figure 12-24 Patient positioned for a skull x-ray study (Towne view—anteroposterior projection with posterior view). A lead apron is placed on the patient to prevent unnecessary exposure to radiation.

After

- If a glass eye is present, note this on the x-ray examination request, because it can present a confusing shadow on the x-ray film.

TEST RESULTS AND CLINICAL SIGNIFICANCE

Skull fracture: *This is seen as a radiolucent line in the skull. The normal bone sutures (where the bones have grown together during normal growth and development) can look like fractures to the untrained eye.*

Metastatic tumor: *Breast cancer, Paget disease, myeloma, and many other tumors can metastasize to the skull. Metastatic tumor can be osteolytic (radiolucent) or osteoblastic (radiopaque).*

Sinusitis: *Swelling and mucus in the sinuses are evident as increased density on the x-ray film. Air-fluid levels may be evident also.*

Hemorrhage,

Tumor,

Hematoma:

When unilateral, these abnormalities cause shift of midline structures (including the calcified pineal gland) to the opposite side.

Congenital anomaly: *Many anomalies in the normal growth and development of the skull are obvious.*

RELATED TEST

Computed Tomography (CT) Scan of the Brain (p. 1026). This test can be used to evaluate the skull. Its main purpose is to evaluate the brain.

Small Bowel Follow-Through (SBF, Small Bowel Enema)

NORMAL FINDINGS

Normal positioning, motility, and patency of the small intestine

INDICATIONS

This contrast-enhanced x-ray study of the small intestines is most often used to identify and determine the cause of small bowel obstruction. It is also used to identify tumors, strictures, inflammation, and other congenital or acquired diseases of the small intestine.

TEST EXPLANATION

The SBF study is performed to identify abnormalities in the small bowel. Usually, the patient is asked to drink barium; in patients who cannot drink, barium can be injected through a nasogastric tube. X-ray films are then obtained at timed intervals (usually 30 minutes to 1 hour) to follow the progression of barium through the small bowel. Significant delays in barium transit time may occur as a result of both benign and malignant forms of partial obstruction or diminished intestinal motility (ileus). On the other hand, the flow of barium is faster in patients who have hypermotility of the small bowel (e.g., malabsorption syndromes). Failure of the progression through the small bowel can be seen in patients with complete mechanical small bowel obstruction. Furthermore, SBF series are helpful in identifying and defining the anatomy of small bowel fistulas (abnormal connections between the small bowel and other abdominal organs or skin). Strictures related to Crohn disease or radiation are also evident with SBF.

TABLE 12-6	X-Ray Visualization of the Gastrointestinal (GI) Tract
Study	**Portion of GI Tract Evaluated**
Barium swallow	Esophagus
Upper GI	Lower esophagus, stomach, and upper duodenum
Small bowel series	Duodenum, jejunum, and ileum
Barium enema	Rectum, colon, and distal ileum

A more accurate radiographic evaluation of the small intestine is enabled by the *small bowel enema*. Barium is injected into a tube previously placed in the small bowel. This small bowel enema provides better visualization of the entire small bowel, because the barium is not diluted by gastric and duodenal juices, as when the patient drinks barium. This test is especially useful in the evaluation of partial small bowel obstruction of unknown cause. Tumors, ulcers, and small bowel fistulas are more easily identified and defined with the enema.

Table 12-6 lists x-ray studies used to visualize the gastrointestinal (GI) tract. Note that this procedure is performed by a radiologist in the radiology department in approximately 30 minutes. Inform the patient that this test is not uncomfortable.

CONTRAINDICATIONS

- Patients with a complete small bowel obstruction: The introduction of barium into an obstructed bowel may create a stonelike impaction; however, this is extremely rare.
- Patients with a suspected perforated viscus: Barium should not be used in this situation because it may cause persistent and recurrent infections if it leaks out of the bowel. Meglumine diatrizoate (Gastrografin), a water-soluble contrast medium, can be used if perforation is suspected. However, it becomes diluted rapidly, minimizing the accuracy of the SBF with this contrast medium.
- Patients with unstable vital signs: These patients should be closely supervised during the time required for this study.

POTENTIAL COMPLICATIONS

- Barium-induced small bowel obstruction

INTERFERING FACTORS

- Barium in the intestinal tract from a previous barium x-ray study may obstruct adequate visualization of the area of small bowel to be evaluated.
- Food or fluid within the GI tract may give the false appearance of a filling defect because of a tumor or other mass.
- Morphine can significantly delay small bowel motility.

✓ Clinical Priorities

- More accurate evaluation of the small intestines is provided by the *small bowel enema*, in which barium is injected through a tube placed in the small bowel.
- Barium should not be used in patients with suspected perforated viscus. In these patients, meglumine diatrizoate (Gastrografin), a water-soluble medium, is used.
- Cathartics are recommended after this test to aid in removal of the barium. Stools will return to normal color after evacuation of all the barium.

X-Ray Studies

12

PROCEDURE AND PATIENT CARE

Before

☒ Explain the procedure to the patient.

☒ Instruct the patient not to eat anything for at least 8 hours before the test. Usually, keep the patient NPO after midnight on the day of the test.

☒ Inform the patient that the SBF series may take several hours. Suggest that the patient bring reading material or some paperwork to occupy the time.

• Accompany the patient to the radiology department if vital signs are not stable.

• Arrange for transportation of the hospitalized patient back to the nursing unit between serial films.

During

• Note the following procedural steps:

1. A specially prepared drink containing barium sulfate is mixed as a milkshake, which the patient drinks through a straw.
2. Usually, an upper GI series is performed concomitantly (see p. 1072).
3. Barium flow is followed through the upper GI tract by means of fluoroscopy.
4. At frequent intervals (15 to 60 minutes), repeated x-ray films are obtained to follow the flow of barium through the small intestine until barium is seen flowing into the right colon. This usually takes 60 to 120 minutes, but in patients with delayed progression of the barium, the test may take as long as 24 hours to complete.

Small Bowel Enema

1. Usually performed by placing a long, weighted tube transorally; however, a tube also can be placed into the upper small bowel endoscopically.
2. After the tube is in place, a thickened barium mixture is injected through the tube, and x-ray films are serially obtained as described for SBF.

After

☒ Inform the patient of the need to evacuate all the barium. Cathartics (e.g., magnesium citrate) are recommended. Initially, stools will be white, but should return to normal color with complete evacuation.

TEST RESULTS AND CLINICAL SIGNIFICANCE

Small bowel tumor: *This may be evident as partial or complete small bowel obstruction. Usually, however, tumors are seen as filling defects in the column of barium in the small bowel.*

Small bowel obstruction: *Adhesions are the most common cause of small bowel obstruction, followed by extrinsic tumor, hernia, and stricture from inflammatory bowel disease in adults. Hernias, intussusception, malrotation, bowel atresia, and volvulus are most common in children. Small bowel obstruction can be partial or complete. With complete obstruction, the barium column does not progress past the area of obstruction. With partial obstruction, the barium passes the area of obstruction, but abnormally slowly.*

Inflammatory small bowel disease (e.g., Crohn disease): *Inflammatory bowel disease usually is apparent as a stricture causing partial small bowel obstruction.*

Malabsorption syndromes (e.g., Whipple disease, sprue): *These are usually evident as rapid transit of contrast material through the small bowel.*

Congenital or acquired anatomic anomaly (e.g., malrotation): *Malrotation usually causes the ligament of Treitz (junction of the duodenum and jejunum) to be in the right lower quadrant instead of its normal location in the left upper quadrant. Short bowel syndrome related to surgical small bowel bypass or resection is evident as rapid transit of barium through the small bowel.*

Congenital abnormalities (e.g., small bowel atresia, duplication, Meckel diverticulum): *Bowel atresia or duplication can be noted as bowel obstruction in children. Meckel diverticulum is evident as an out-pouching of the ileum. It may not be apparent until adulthood and may never cause symptoms.*

Small bowel intussusception: *An upper segment of bowel becomes invaginated (swallowed up) into a lower segment. This usually causes bowel obstruction and is most common in children.*

Small bowel perforation: *When contrast leaks out of the intestine, perforation is present.*

Radiation enteritis: *This becomes evident years after radiation therapy. It is demonstrated as a stricture of one or more segments of the small bowel.*

RELATED TEST

Barium Enema (p. 994). This test is contrast material–enhanced x-ray study of the colon. Often the distal small bowel is visualized.

Spinal X-Rays (Cervical, Thoracic, Lumbar, Sacral, or Coccygeal X-Ray Studies)

NORMAL FINDINGS

Normal spinal vertebrae

INDICATIONS

Spinal radiography is used to evaluate back or neck pain.

TEST EXPLANATION

Spinal x-ray studies may be performed to evaluate any area of the spine. They usually include antero-posterior, lateral, and oblique views of these structures. These x-ray films are often obtained to assess back or neck pain, degenerative arthritic changes, traumatic fractures, tumor metastasis, spondylosis (degenerative disease of the spinal structures), and spondylolisthesis (slipping of one vertebral disk over another). Cervical spine x-ray studies are routinely performed in cases of multiple trauma to ensure absence of fracture before the patient is moved or the neck is manipulated. However, CT scanning of the cervical vertebrae is increasingly becoming the standard of practice to ensure that there is no cervical fracture. Spinal radiographs are helpful in evaluating for spinal alignment abnormalities (e.g., kyphosis [Figure 12-25], scoliosis). MRI is another very accurate method of evaluating the spine.

CONTRAINDICATIONS

- Patients who are pregnant, unless the benefits outweigh the risks

PROCEDURE AND PATIENT CARE

Before

 Explain the procedure to the patient.

Instruct the patient to remove any metal objects covering the area to be visualized.

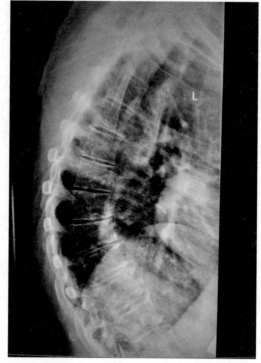

Figure 12-25 Spinal x-ray demonstrating significant thoracic spine kyphosis.

- Immobilize the patient if a spinal fracture is suspected. Apply a neck brace if a cervical spine fracture is suspected.
- Tell the patient that no fasting or sedation is required; however, if a fracture is suspected, the patient may be kept on nothing by mouth (NPO) status.

During

- Note that the patient is placed on an x-ray table. Anterior, posterior, lateral, and oblique x-ray films are obtained of the desired area of the spinal cord. The same views can be obtained with the patient in the standing position.
- A radiologic technologist obtains spinal x-ray films in a few minutes.
- Tell the patient that no discomfort is associated with this study.

After

- Patient positioning and activity depend on test results.

TEST RESULTS AND CLINICAL SIGNIFICANCE

Degenerative arthritis changes: *Bone destruction or spurring is seen in patients with degenerative arthritic changes of the spinal joints.*
Metastatic tumor invasion,

Traumatic or pathologic fracture:

The cervical and lumbar portions of the spine are most frequently injured. Any portion, however, can be affected by metastatic neoplasm (e.g., myeloma, Paget disease, breast or lung cancer). Bone metastasis can lead to fracture without a traumatic event.

Scoliosis,

Spondylosis,

Spondylolisthesis:

These are anatomic alterations of spinal alignment.

Suspected spinal osteomyelitis: *This test is helpful in detecting the infection.*

RELATED TESTS

Computed Tomography (CT) (p. 1029) or Magnetic Resonance Imaging (MRI) (p. 1106) of the Spine. These studies demonstrate spinal anatomy and pathologic conditions better than spinal x-ray studies do. Alignment, however, is best evaluated with plain x-ray studies.

Swallowing Examination (Videofluoroscopy Swallowing Examination)

NORMAL FINDINGS

Normal swallowing function and complete clearing of radiographic material through the upper digestive tract

INDICATIONS

This test is performed to identify the cause of inability to swallow.

TEST EXPLANATION

Problems in swallowing may result from local structural diseases (e.g., tumors, upper esophageal diverticula, inflammation, extrinsic compression of the upper gastrointestinal [GI] tract) or surgery to the oropharyngeal tract. Motility disorders of the upper GI tract (e.g., Zenker diverticulum) and neurologic disorders (e.g., stroke syndrome, Parkinson disease, neuropathies) also may cause difficulty in swallowing. Videofluoroscopy of the swallowing function allows the speech pathologist to delineate more clearly the exact pathologic condition in the swallowing mechanism; this leads to determining the most appropriate treatment and teaching the patient proper swallowing technique.

This test is performed by asking the patient to swallow barium or a barium-containing meal. With videofluoroscopy, the act of swallowing is visualized and documented. Structural abnormalities and functional impairment can be identified easily with the slow-framed progression and reversal possible with videofluoroscopy. This test is similar to barium swallow (p. 999), but finer details of swallowing can be evaluated with videofluoroscopy.

CONTRAINDICATIONS

- Patients who aspirate saliva are not candidates for videofluoroscopy swallowing. Non-swallowing methods of alimentation will be required.

PROCEDURE AND PATIENT CARE

Before

 Explain the procedure to the patient.
Explain to the patient that no preparation is required.

During

- In the radiology department, the patient is asked to swallow a barium-containing meal. The consistency of the meal (e.g., liquid, semi-soft [e.g., applesauce], or solid [e.g., a tea biscuit]) will be determined by the speech therapist and radiologist, to simulate foods to which the patient is to be initially reintroduced. While the patient swallows, videofluoroscopy is recorded in both the lateral and the anterior positions.
- The video is repeatedly examined forward and backward by the radiologist and by the speech pathologist.

After

- No catharsis is required.

TEST RESULTS AND CLINICAL SIGNIFICANCE

Upper GI tract disease,
Neuromuscular disorder,
Achalasia,
Upper GI motility disorder (e.g., stroke syndrome, Parkinson disease, peripheral neuropathy),
Diffuse esophageal spasms,
Zenker diverticulum:

> *These disorders can be associated with swallowing dysfunction at various levels in the swallowing mechanism.*

RELATED TEST

Barium Swallow (p. 999). This test is similar to videofluoroscopy except that multiple still x-ray films are obtained and the entire swallowing mechanism cannot be fully evaluated.

T-Tube and Operative Cholangiography

NORMAL FINDINGS

Normal common bile duct with no dilatation or filling defects
Good runoff of dye through the ampulla of Vater into the duodenum

INDICATIONS

Cholangiography provides visualization of the bile ducts during and after surgery. It is most commonly used to identify common bile duct stones.

TEST EXPLANATION

In *operative cholangiography*, the common bile duct is directly injected with radiopaque material through the cystic duct. This is usually performed during cholecystectomy. Stones appear as radiolucent shadows. Gallstones, tumors, or strictures cause partial or total obstruction of the flow of dye into the duodenum. Visualization of the biliary duct structures enables the surgeon to see the surgical anatomy of the biliary tree. This reduces the possibility of inadvertent common bile duct injury during cholecystectomy. If common duct stones are demonstrated during operative cholangiography, a common duct exploration is performed. Some surgeons perform operative cholangiography in all patients who undergo cholecystectomy. Other surgeons use specific indications for operative cholangiography, including the following:

- Jaundice
- Abnormal liver enzyme levels
- Dilated common bile duct
- Evidence of pancreatitis
- Evidence of small stones in the cystic duct during cholecystectomy

T-*tube cholangiography* is performed postoperatively following T-tube placement during a common duct exploration. Its main purpose is to detect retained common bile duct stones and demonstrate good flow of contrast dye into the duodenum. This test is performed, usually 5 to 10 days after surgery, with use of a T-shaped rubber tube placed in the common bile duct at surgery. If no stones are evident and there is good runoff of bile into the duodenum, the T-tube can be removed. If there are residual stones, the tube tract can be used to extract the stones.

POTENTIAL COMPLICATIONS

- Sepsis caused by increased ductal pressure with dye infusion

INTERFERING FACTORS

- Barium in the abdomen from a previous upper gastrointestinal (GI) series or barium enema x-ray study precludes visualization of the bile duct.

PROCEDURE AND PATIENT CARE

Before

✗ Explain the procedure to the patient when obtaining consent for the main biliary procedure.
✗ Tell the patient that no fasting or sedation is required for T-tube cholangiography. However, routine preoperative nothing by mouth (NPO) status is necessary for operative cholangiography.

During

- Note the following procedural steps:

Operative Cholangiogram
1. Performed through catheterization of the cystic duct during cholecystectomy.
2. Alternatively, a needle or catheter is placed in the common bile duct.
3. The dye is injected directly into the common bile duct.
4. X-ray films are obtained while the patient is on the operating table and are immediately reviewed by the surgeon.

T-Tube Cholangiogram
1. The patient is taken to the radiology department.
2. A sterile dye solution is injected into the T-tube previously placed by the surgeon.
3. X-ray images are obtained of the right upper quadrant of the abdomen with the patient placed in various positions.
- A radiologist or surgeon performs these procedures in approximately 10 minutes.
 Tell the patient that no discomfort is associated with these studies.

After
- Observe for signs of sepsis.
- If a T-tube has been surgically placed, establish a sterile, closed drainage system.

TEST RESULTS AND CLINICAL SIGNIFICANCE

Common bile duct stones: *These appear as radiolucent rounded filling defects in the column of dye within the common bile duct.*
Anatomic variations: *Many types of bile duct congenital anatomic variations can exist and are demonstrated at cholangiography.*
Bile duct cysts: *Though rare, these cysts appear as small to large outpouchings of the bile ducts.*
Stricture or tumor obstructing the common bile duct: *Tumors of the bile duct (cholangiocarcinoma) or extrinsic tumors (e.g., pancreas, colon) can partially or completely obstruct the bile duct. Benign inflammatory or posttraumatic strictures also can cause varying degrees of obstruction.*
Bile duct surgical trauma: *Ligation or laceration of the bile duct is obvious at the time of surgery with the use of cholangiography.*

RELATED TESTS

Endoscopic Retrograde Cholangiopancreatography (ERCP) (p. 605). This is an endoscopic procedure performed to radiographically visualize the bile and pancreatic ducts.
Percutaneous Transhepatic Cholangiography (PTC) (p. 1053). This procedure provides visualization of the bile ducts by percutaneous access to the biliary tree through the liver.

Upper Gastrointestinal Tract X-Ray
(Upper GI Series, UGI)

NORMAL FINDINGS

Normal size, contour, patency, filling, positioning, and transit of barium through the lower esophagus, stomach, and upper duodenum

INDICATIONS

This contrast-enhanced x-ray study provides visualization of the mucosa of the esophageal, gastric, and duodenum lumens. It is indicated in patients with upper abdominal pain, dyspepsia, dysphagia, early satiety, or suspected gastroduodenal obstruction.

TEST EXPLANATION

The upper GI study consists of a series of x-ray images of the lower esophagus, stomach, and duodenum, usually using barium sulfate as the contrast medium. When there is concern for leakage of x-ray contrast through a perforation of the GI tract, however, meglumine diatrizoate (Gastrografin), a water-soluble contrast medium, is used. This test can be performed in conjunction with a barium swallow (p. 999) or small bowel (p. 1064) series, which can precede or succeed the upper GI study, respectively.

The purpose of this examination is to detect ulcerations, tumors, inflammation, or anatomic malposition (e.g., hiatal hernia) of upper GI organs, and obstruction in the upper GI tract. The patient is asked to drink a beverage containing barium. As the contrast agent descends, the lower esophagus is examined for position, patency, and filling defects (e.g., tumors, scarring, varices). As the barium enters the stomach, the gastric wall is examined for benign or malignant ulcerations, filling defects (most often in cancer), and anatomic abnormalities (e.g., hiatal hernia). The patient is placed in a flat or head-down position, and the gastroesophageal area is examined for evidence of gastroesophageal reflux of barium.

As the contrast agent leaves the stomach, patency of the pyloric channel and the duodenum is evaluated. Benign peptic ulceration is the most common pathologic condition affecting these areas. Extrinsic compression caused by tumors, cysts, or enlarged pathologic organs (e.g., liver) near the stomach also can be identified based on anatomic distortion of the outline of the upper GI tract.

A radiologist performs this procedure in approximately 30 minutes. The patient may be uncomfortable lying on the hard x-ray table and may occasionally experience a sensation of bloating or nausea during the test.

CONTRAINDICATIONS

- Patients with complete bowel obstruction
- Patients with suspected upper GI perforation: Water-soluble Gastrografin should be used instead of barium.
- Patients with unstable vital signs: These patients should be supervised during the time required for this test.
- Patients who are uncooperative, because of the necessity of frequent position changes

POTENTIAL COMPLICATIONS

- Aspiration of barium
- Constipation or partial bowel obstruction caused by inspissated barium in the small bowel or colon

INTERFERING FACTORS

- Previously administered barium: This may block visualization of the upper GI tract.
- Poor patient performance
- Incapacitated patient: Such patients cannot assume the multiple positions required for the study.
- Food and fluid in the stomach: They give the false impression of filling defects in the stomach, precluding adequate evaluation of the gastric mucosa.
- Obtundation: These patients cannot safely drink the barium.

X-Ray Studies

12

Clinical Priorities

- When there is a concern for perforation in the GI tract, meglumine diatrizoate (Gastrografin) is used instead of barium. This may cause diarrhea after the procedure.
- For an air-contrast *upper GI study*, the patient swallows a carbonated powder that creates CO_2 in the stomach and aids in visualization of the gastric mucosa.
- After the procedure, a cathartic is necessary to prevent impaction from the barium.

PROCEDURE AND PATIENT CARE

Before

✗ Explain the procedure to the patient. Allow the patient to verbalize concerns.

✗ Instruct the patient to abstain from eating for at least 8 hours before the test. Usually, keep the patient NPO after midnight on the day of the test.

✗ Assure the patient that the test will not cause any discomfort.

During

- Note the following procedural steps:
  1. The patient is asked to drink approximately 16 ounces of barium sulfate. This is a chalky substance usually suspended in milkshake form and drunk through a straw (Figure 12-26). Usually, the drink is flavored to increase palatability.
  2. After drinking the barium, the patient is moved through several position changes (e.g., prone, supine, lateral) to promote filling of the entire upper GI tract.
  3. Films are taken at the discretion of the radiologist as the flow of barium is observed fluoroscopically.

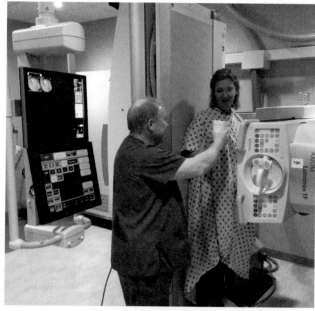

Figure 12-26 Patient receiving barium sulfate drink for upper GI series.

4. The flow of barium is followed through the lower esophagus, stomach, and duodenum.
5. Several x-ray images are obtained throughout the course of the test.
6. For an *air-contrast upper GI study*, the patient is asked to rapidly swallow carbonated powder. This creates CO_2 in the stomach, providing air contrast to the barium within the stomach and increased visualization of the gastric mucosa.

After

📋 Inform the patient that if meglumine diatrizoate (Gastrografin) was used, significant diarrhea may develop. This contrast agent is an osmotic cathartic.

📋 Instruct the patient to use a cathartic (e.g., milk of magnesia) if barium sulfate was used as the contrast medium. Water absorption may cause the barium to harden and create a fecal impaction if catharsis is not carried out.

📋 Instruct the patient to note the stools to ensure that all of the barium has been removed. The stools should return to normal color after the barium is completely expelled, which may take as long as a day and a half.

TEST RESULTS AND CLINICAL SIGNIFICANCE

Esophageal cancer: *Most esophageal cancers occur in the lower esophagus. They are seen as a stricture or complete obstruction of the barium column.*

Esophageal varices: *Serpiginous filling defects indicate esophageal varices.*

Hiatal hernia: *There are two types of hiatal hernias. With a sliding hiatal hernia, the esophagogastric (EG) junction and upper stomach are in the chest. With the rolling type, the EG junction is normal but the fundus of the stomach rolls up into the chest. This latter type can become incarcerated and perforate. Surgical repair is required when this condition is identified.*

Diverticula: *These can be in the upper esophagus (Zenker) and due to spasm of the cricopharyngeus muscle (upper esophageal sphincter), or in the lower esophagus (epiphrenic) and due to paraesophageal infection.*

Gastric cancer: *Cancers can be evident as large polypoid filling defects within the stomach or as ulcerative masses in the wall of the stomach.*

Gastric inflammatory disease (e.g., Ménétrier disease): *Thickened rugae or gastric folds are classic for chronic inflammatory changes of the stomach.*

Benign gastric tumor (e.g., leiomyoma): *Tumors can be small polypoid masses in the stomach or giant tumors that distort the entire upper abdomen.*

Extrinsic compression by pancreatic pseudocyst, cysts, pancreatic tumors, or hepatomegaly: *Masses in the upper abdomen can distort the stomach. Because the stomach is a large sack, it is unusual for that structure to be obstructed by extrinsic compression.*

Perforation of the esophagus, stomach, or duodenum: *Perforation is obvious when contrast material is evident outside the esophagus, stomach, or duodenum.*

Congenital abnormalities (e.g., duodenal web, pancreatic rest, malrotation syndrome): *These are congenital abnormalities that commonly cause duodenal obstruction in infants.*

Gastric ulcer (benign or malignant): *Malignancy can be ulcerative. Benign ulcers (stress or peptic) can also develop.*

Duodenal ulcer: *Most duodenal ulcers are peptic ulcers. They are most commonly seen in the first portion of the duodenum, called the bulb.*

Duodenal cancer: *This is very rare and usually is seen as a filling defect in the column of barium within the duodenum.*

Duodenal diverticulum: *Not uncommon, these outpouchings rarely cause symptoms.*

X-Ray Studies

12

RELATED TEST

Esophagogastroduodenoscopy (EGD) (p. 608). This endoscopic procedure provides better visualization of the upper GI organs. Further, biopsy can be performed with this procedure.

Venography (Phlebography, Venogram)

NORMAL FINDINGS

No evidence of venous thrombosis or obstruction

INDICATIONS

This contrast-enhanced x-ray study of the venous system of the lower or upper extremity is used to identify obstruction or thrombosis of the venous system in patients with a swollen arm or leg.

TEST EXPLANATION

Venography is an x-ray study designed to identify and locate thrombi in the venous system (most commonly in the extremities). Dye is injected into the venous system of the affected extremity. X-ray films are then obtained at timed intervals to visualize the venous system. Obstruction to the flow of dye or a filling defect within the dye-filled vein indicates thrombosis. Positive study results accurately confirm the diagnosis of venous thrombosis; however, negative results—although not so accurate—make the diagnosis of venous thrombosis unlikely. Often both extremities are studied, even when only one leg is suspected to contain deep-vein thrombosis. The normal extremity is used for comparison with the involved extremity. Venography is more accurate than venous Doppler (p. 900) for thrombi in veins below the knee or in the femoral veins. Venography is also performed in the upper extremities to evaluate the more proximal axillary, subclavian, and innominate veins in patients with a swollen arm or hand.

A radiologist performs this study in approximately 30 to 90 minutes. Venous catheterization is only as uncomfortable as a needlestick or a small incision in the foot. The dye may cause the patient to feel a warm flush (although not so severe as with arteriography). Inform the patient that mild degrees of nausea, vomiting, or skin itching also may occasionally occur.

CONTRAINDICATIONS

- Patients with severe edema of the legs, making venous access for dye injection impossible
- Patients who are uncooperative
- Patients who are allergic to iodinated dye or shellfish
- Patients with renal failure, because iodinated dye is nephrotoxic

 Age-Related Concerns

- Elderly persons are particularly vulnerable to renal failure, especially if they are chronically dehydrated (e.g., chronic diarrhea).
- Dehydration after the test can be exacerbated by the diuretic action of the dye.

POTENTIAL COMPLICATIONS

- For potential complications of iodinated dye, see p. 985.
- Renal failure, especially in elderly persons with chronic dehydration or mild renal failure (see Box 12-2, p. 984).
- Subcutaneous infiltration of the dye, causing cellulitis and pain
- Venous thrombophlebitis caused by the dye
- Bacteremia caused by a break in sterile technique
- Venous embolism caused by dislodgement of a deep-vein clot, induced by the dye injection
- Lactic acidosis may occur in patients who are taking metformin (Glucophage) and receive iodine dye. The metformin should be held on the day of the test.

Clinical Priorities

- Check the patient for allergy to iodinated dyes.
- During the dye injection, the patient may feel a warm flush.
- The patient must be encouraged to drink large amounts of fluids after the test to prevent dehydration caused by the diuretic action of the dye.

PROCEDURE AND PATIENT CARE

Before

 Explain the procedure to the patient.

- Obtained informed consent if required for this procedure.
- For assessment of allergy to iodinated dye, see p. 985.
- If needed, provide appropriate pain medication so the patient is able to lie still during the procedure.
- Ensure that the patient is appropriately hydrated before testing. Injection of the iodinated contrast material may cause renal failure, especially in the elderly.

During

- Note the following procedural steps:
  1. The patient is taken to the radiology department and placed supine on the x-ray table.
  2. Catheterization of a superficial vein on the foot is performed. This may require a surgical cutdown.
  3. An iodinated, radiopaque dye is injected into the vein.
  4. X-ray films are obtained to follow the course of the dye up the leg.
  5. Frequently, a tourniquet is placed on the leg to prevent filling of the superficial saphenous vein. All of the dye, therefore, goes to the deep venous system, which contains the most clinically significant thrombosis that can embolize.

After

- Continue appropriate fluid administration to prevent dehydration caused by the diuretic action of the dye.
- Observe the puncture site for infection, cellulitis, or bleeding.
- Assess the patient's vital signs for signs of bacteremia (e.g., fever, tachycardia, chills).
- Evaluate the patient for signs of allergic reaction (e.g., rash, chills, fever, irritability). Treat with antihistamines or steroids.

X-Ray Studies

12

Home Care Responsibilities

- Monitor the puncture site for redness, swelling, or bleeding.
- Note that fever and chills may indicate bacteremia.
- Encourage the patient to drink fluids to prevent dehydration caused by the injected dye.

TEST RESULTS AND CLINICAL SIGNIFICANCE

Obstructed venous system from thrombosis, tumor, or inflammation: *This is evident as complete obstruction of dye flow in the main vein (usually femoral or iliac).*

Acute deep-vein thrombosis: *This is evident as serpiginous filling defects in the column of dye on the wall of the vein.*

RELATED TESTS

Venous Doppler flow studies (p. 900). With the use of ultrasound, blood flow within the vein can be evaluated. Obstruction to flow is easily noted. This test is less invasive, equally accurate (above the knee), and associated with less risk than venography.

Venous Plethysmography. This is a manometric study of the venous system of the extremity. It enables identification of venous occlusion.

Miscellaneous Studies

OVERVIEW

TESTS

Overview

We have tried to organize a multitude of diverse diagnostic tests into groups based on the specimen on which the test was performed and the method of testing. This led to the development of chapters as presented in this text. However, a few tests could not readily be appropriated to any chapter. Therefore this chapter was created to include these important tests. There are no commonalities associated with these tests. All are described separately and in detail.

Allergy Skin Testing

NORMAL FINDINGS

<3 mm wheal diameter
<10 mm flare diameter

INDICATIONS

Skin testing is the most commonly used and easiest method of identifying patients who suffer from allergies. Furthermore, it is a method by which a specific allergen can be determined.

TEST EXPLANATION

When properly performed, skin testing is considered to be the most convenient and least expensive test for detecting allergic reactions. Since the early 1900s, skin testing has been a common practice for establishing a diagnosis of allergy by reexposure of the individual to a specific allergen. Skin testing provides useful confirmatory evidence when a diagnosis of allergy is suspected on clinical grounds. The simplicity, rapidity, low costs, sensitivity, and specificity explain the crucial position skin testing has in allergy testing.

In an allergic patient, an immediate wheal (small swelling, as from an insect bite) and flare (red, inflamed area) reaction follows injection of the specific allergen (that substance to which the person is allergic). This reaction is initiated by immunoglobulin E (IgE) antibodies and is mediated primarily by histamine secreted from mast cells. This usually occurs in about 5 minutes and peaks at 30 minutes. In some patients a "late-phase reaction" occurs; this is highlighted by antibody and cellular infiltration into the area that usually occurs within 1 to 2 hours.

There are three commonly accepted methods of injecting the allergen into the skin. The first method is called the *prick-puncture test* or *scratch test*. In this method, the allergen is injected into the epidermis. Life-threatening anaphylaxis reactions have not been reported with this method. The second method is called the *intradermal test*. Here the allergen is injected into the dermis (creating a skin wheal). Large local reactions and anaphylaxis have been reported with this latter method. For these two tests, the allergen placement part of the test takes about 5 to 10 minutes. The third method is called the *patch test*. This takes much longer because the patient must wear the patch for 48 hours to see if there is a delayed allergic reaction. With this method, needles are not used. Instead, an allergen is applied to a patch that is placed on the skin. It is usually done to detect whether a particular substance (e.g., latex, medications, fragrances, preservatives, hair dyes, metals, resins) is causing an allergic skin irritation, such as contact dermatitis.

Patients with dermographism (nonallergic response of redness and swelling of the skin at the site of any stimulation) develop a skin wheal with any skin irritation, even if nonallergic. In these patients, a false-positive reaction can occur with skin testing. To eliminate these sort of false positives, a "negative control" substance consisting of just the diluent without an allergen is injected at the same time as the other skin tests are performed. Patients who are immunosuppressed because of concurrent disease or medicines may have a blunted skin reaction even in the face of allergy. This would cause false-negative results. To avoid false negatives, a "positive control" substance consisting of a histamine analogue is also injected into the forearm at the time of skin testing. This will cause a wheal and flare response even in the nonallergic patient, unless the patient is immunosuppressed.

For inhalant allergens, skin tests are extremely accurate. However, they are less reliable for food allergies, latex allergies, drug sensitivity, and occupational allergies. Although there is considerable variability in accuracy of skin testing because of poor injection techniques, when performed correctly, skin testing represents one of the major tools in the diagnosis of allergy.

CONTRAINDICATIONS

- Patients with a history of prior anaphylaxis

POTENTIAL COMPLICATIONS

- Anaphylaxis

INTERFERING FACTORS

- False-positive results may occur in patients with dermographism.
- False-positive results may occur if the patient has a reaction to the diluent used to preserve the extract.
- False-negative results may be caused by poor-quality allergen extracts, diseases that attenuate the immune response, or improper technique.
- Infants and the elderly may have decreased skin reactivity.
- Drugs that may *decrease* the immune response (size of wheal and flare) of skin testing include angiotensin-converting enzyme (ACE) inhibitors, beta blockers, corticosteroids, nifedipine, and theophylline.

PROCEDURE AND PATIENT CARE

Before

- Explain the procedure to the patient.
- Observe the following skin-testing precautions:
  1. Be sure that a physician is immediately available.
  2. Evaluate the patient for dermographism.
  3. Have medications and equipment available to handle anaphylaxis.
  4. Proceed with caution in patients with current allergic symptoms.
  5. Pay great attention to the technique chosen for the skin test in order to get accurate results.
  6. Avoid bleeding caused by injection.
  7. Avoid spreading of allergen solutions during the test.
  8. Record the skin reaction at the proper time.
- Obtain a history to evaluate the risk of anaphylaxis.
- Identify any immunosuppressive medications the patient may be taking.
- Evaluate the patient for dermographism by rubbing the skin with a pencil eraser and looking for a wheal at the site of irritation.
- Draw up 0.05 mL of 1:1000 aqueous epinephrine into a syringe before testing in the event of an exaggerated allergic reaction.
- A negative prick-puncture test should be performed before an intradermal test.

During

Prick-Puncture Method (Scratch Test)

- A drop of the allergen solution is placed onto the volar surface of the forearm or back after cleaning the area.
- A 25-gauge needle is passed through the droplet and inserted into the epidermal space at an angle with the bevel facing up.
- The skin is lifted up and the fluid is allowed to seep in. Excess fluid is wiped off after about a minute.

Intradermal Method

- Clean the skin area.
- With a 25-gauge needle, the allergen solution is injected into the dermis by creating a skin wheal. In this method, the bevel of the needle faces downward. A volume of between 0.01 and 0.05 mL is injected.
- In general, the allergen solution is diluted 100- to 1000-fold before injection.

Miscellaneous Studies

13

Patch Method
- Clean the skin area (usually back or arm).
- Apply the patches to the skin (as many as 20-30 can be applied).
- Instruct the patient to wear the patches for 48 hours. Tell the patient to avoid bathing or activities that cause heavy sweating.
- Tell the patient the patches will be removed at the doctor's office. Irritated skin at a patch site may indicate an allergy.

After
- Document allergen solution, location, and patient reaction.
- Evaluate the patient for exaggerated allergic response.
- In the event of a systemic reaction, a tourniquet should be placed above the testing site and epinephrine should be administered subcutaneously.
- With a pen, encircle the area of testing and mark the allergen used.
- Read the skin test at the appropriate time.
- Skin tests are read when the reaction is mature, after about 15 to 20 minutes. Both the largest and smallest diameter of the wheal is determined. The measurements (in millimeters) are averaged.
- The flare is measured in the same manner.
- Observe the patient for 20 to 30 minutes before discharge.

TEST RESULTS AND CLINICAL SIGNIFICANCE

Allergy-Related Diseases
Asthma,
Dermatitis,
Food allergy,
Drug allergy,
Occupational allergy,
Allergic rhinitis,
Angioedema:
> *All of these diseases are immunoreactive (allergic) in their pathophysiology. Specific allergens, when injected or applied to the skin, will cause an allergic reaction of wheal and flare.*

RELATED TEST

Allergy Blood Testing (p. 49). Allergy blood testing is an alternative to allergy skin testing in diagnosing allergy as a cause of a particular symptom complex. It is also useful in identifying the particular allergen affecting a patient. It is particularly helpful when allergy skin testing is contraindicated.

Bioterrorism Infectious Agents Testing
(Botulism, Anthrax, Hemorrhagic Fever, Plague, Smallpox, Tularemia, Brucellosis)

NORMAL FINDINGS
Negative for evidence of infectious agent

INDICATIONS

These tests are indicated if terrorism is suspected because of suspicious illness, or some other type of evidence.

TEST EXPLANATION

Infectious agents used in bioterrorism are many and it would be difficult to discuss each possible agent. This test discusses those agents that humans are most likely to be exposed to in war or in a civilian terrorist attack. Please refer to Table 13-1 for specifics of each agent. All documented cases must be reported to the Department of Public Health.

Botulism Infection

The botulinum toxin produced by *Clostridia botulinum*, a spore-forming anaerobic bacterium, causes the symptoms associated with botulism. The gastrointestinal (GI) tract is the usual port of entry through the ingestion the toxin itself, *C. botulinum* spores, or the actual bacterium. Ingestion of the toxin produces symptoms almost immediately. Symptoms may be delayed if the spores or the bacterium are

TABLE 13-1	Bioterrorism Infectious Agents: Summary Table			
Infection/ Infectious Agent	Site of Entry	Sources	Specimen	Tests
Botulism/ *Clostridium botulinum*	GI mucosal surfaces, lung, wound contamination	Undercooked meats, soil, dust	Blood, stool, vomitus, food	Botulinum toxin, mouse bioassay
Anthrax/*Bacillus anthracis*	Lung, GI	Undercooked meats, inhalation of spores from animal products/skin	Sputum, blood, stool, skin vesicle, food, spores	Culture, Gram stain
Yellow fever/ Hantaan virus, Ebola virus, multiple other viruses	Skin bite	Rodent or mosquito bites	Blood, sputum, tissue	Culture, serology for viral antigens
Plague infections/ *Yersinia pestis*	Skin bite	Infected fleas	Blood, sputum, lymph node aspirate	Culture of organism
Brucellosis/*Brucella abortus, B. canis*, etc.	GI, lung, wound	Infected meats and milk products	Blood, sputum, food	Culture of organism
Smallpox/variola virus	Lungs	Respiratory droplets, direct contact, contaminated clothing	Vesicle	Viral culture or viral identification with electron microscopy
Tularemia/*Francisella tularensis*	Skin, GI tract, lungs	Ingestion of contaminated plants or water	Blood, sputum, stool	Culture of organism

GI, Gastrointestinal.

ingested. Common sources of *C. botulinum* include undercooked meat or sauces exposed to room temperature for prolonged periods. This bacterium can be inhaled by handling the same food or by open wound contamination of soil that contains *C. botulinum*.

The toxin binds irreversibly to the presynaptic nerve terminal at the neuro-muscular junction and prevents the release of acetylcholine necessary for normal muscular function. As a result, one may experience bulbar palsies causing blurred vision, dysphagia, dysarthria and skeletal muscle weakness progressing to flaccid paralysis. Symptoms begin 6 to 12 hours after ingestion of the contaminated food or approximately 1 week after wound contamination. The test used to diagnose this disease involves the identification of the toxin in the blood, stool, or vomitus of the affected individual. The food itself can also be tested. The toxin can be identified by the biologic Mouse Neutralization test. *C. botulinum* can also be cultured in an anaerobic environment from the stool or from contaminated food.

Treatment involves mechanical support of ventilation and nutrition. The use of botulinum antitoxin that can be obtained from the Centers for Disease Control and Prevention (CDC) is the mainstay of treatment. This antitoxin presents a risk of "serum sickness" in nearly one quarter of the patients who receive it.

Anthrax

Anthrax is caused by *Bacillus anthracis*, which is a spore forming gram-positive rod. The organism is widely distributed in the soil and, under natural conditions, grazing animals can become infected and pass it on to those working in close contact with grazing animal products (meat, wool, or hides). It can be contracted by eating undercooked meat or inhaled from animal products (such as wool) or by inhaling the spores. Once inhaled, it is uniformly fatal without treatment. Cutaneous anthrax occurs from contact with contaminated meat, wool, hides, or leather from infected animals.

There are three forms of the disease: cutaneous, gastrointestinal, and pulmonary. Symptoms include fever, malaise, fatigue progressing to cutaneous lesions, or pulmonary failure. Symptoms occur about 2 to 6 days after exposure.

Culturing the organism in sheep blood agar makes the diagnosis. Appropriate specimens for culture would be stool, blood, sputum, or the cutaneous vesicle. Treatment for this disease is early institution of antibiotics and supportive care.

Hemorrhagic Fever (Yellow Fever)

This disease complex has many causative virus families including arenavirus, bunyavirus (including Hantavirus), Filovirus (including Ebola), and flavivirus. Symptoms include fever, thrombocytopenia, shock, multiorgan failure, lung edema, and jaundice. Symptoms develop 4 to 21 days after a mosquito or rodent bite (depending on the disease). This disease is contagious and patients with suspicious symptoms should be quarantined.

The diagnosis is determined by clinical evaluation. However, viral cultures with polymerase chain reaction (PCR) identification, serology, and immunohistochemistry of tissue specimens are possible. There is no specific treatment other than aggressive medical therapy and support of organ failure.

Plague

This disease is caused by the gram-negative coccobacillus *Yersinia pestis*. It is transmitted to humans primarily by the bite of fleas or contact with other human bodily fluids. It has three forms: bubonic (enlarged lymph nodes), septicemic (blood-borne), and pneumonic (aerosol). Pneumonic is, by far, the deadliest form of the infection. Symptoms may include fever, chills, weakness, enlarged lymph nodes, or bacterial pneumonia and respiratory failure.

The diagnosis is made by culture of the blood, sputum, or lymph node aspirate. This disease complex can be treated with antibiotics when started early in the course of the disease. Early testing and diagnosis affects patient outcome. The risk for bioterrorism is weapon attack or spread by aerosol transmission.

Brucellosis

This disease is caused by *Brucella abortus, B. suis, B. melitensis,* or *B. canis*. It is contracted by ingestion of contaminated milk products (especially goat's milk), direct puncture of the skin (by butchers and farmers), or by inhalation. This multisystem disease is characterized by acute or insidious onset of fever, night sweats, undue fatigue, anorexia, weight loss, headache, and arthralgia. Hepatomegaly, splenomegaly, and spondylitis are also common. *Brucella* can be cultured from a blood, sputum, or food specimen. Serology testing is also possible. Diagnosis is confirmed by a fourfold or greater rise in *Brucella* agglutination titer between acute- and convalescent-phase serum specimens obtained greater than or equal to 2 weeks apart and studied at the same laboratory. Demonstration by immunofluorescence of a *Brucella* organism in a clinical specimen is another method of diagnosis. Infections are usually treated with antibiotics.

Smallpox

Smallpox is a serious, contagious, and sometimes fatal infectious disease caused by the variola virus (a deoxyribonucleic acid [DNA] virus). There is no specific treatment for smallpox disease, and the only prevention is vaccination. There are two clinical forms of smallpox. Variola major is the severe and most common form of smallpox, with a more extensive rash and higher fever. Variola minor is a less common presentation of smallpox and a much less severe disease. The disease has been eradicated after a successful worldwide vaccination program. It is very easily spread and is therefore considered a potential bioterrorism weapon. It has the potential to cause widespread disease and death that could devastate a whole city or region.

The first symptoms of smallpox include fever, malaise, head and body aches, and sometimes vomiting. Next a rash occurs in the mouth and then on the skin. This rash proceeds to become pustular. As the pustules dry up and scab, the patient is no longer contagious.

Viral culture, serology, immunohistochemistry, or electron microscopy can make the diagnosis. The best specimen is the vesicular rash. While there is no treatment for the disease, vaccination is available and is offered to all those at risk for bioterrorism.

Tularemia

This disease is caused by a gram-negative bacterium called *Francisella tularensis*. It is contracted by drinking contaminated water or eating vegetation contaminated by infected animals. It can be aerosolized and can contaminate the air or drinking water supplies. When it enters through the skin by an insect bite, tularemia can be recognized by the presence of a lesion and swollen glands. Ingestion of the organism may produce a throat infection, intestinal pain, diarrhea, and vomiting. Symptoms generally appear between 2 and 10 days, but usually 3 days after exposure.

Inhalation of the organism may produce a fever alone or fever combined with a pneumonia-like illness that is difficult to distinguish from influenza or other atypical pneumonias. Diagnosis is made by culture of the blood, sputum, or stool. Although tularemia can be life threatening, most infections can be successfully treated with antibiotics.

PROCEDURE AND PATIENT CARE

Before

- Follow guidelines for safe contact with the patient, who can be highly infectious.
- Maintain strict adherence to all procedures in regard to isolation or contamination of the specimen.
- Biohazard precautions are to be taken with each patient and specimen.
- Laboratory personnel must strictly adhere to all standard precautions and transmission principles.

During

- If an enema is used to obtain a botulinum stool specimen, use sterile water. Saline can negate results.
- Send enough blood for adequate testing. Usually two red-top tubes are adequate. It is best to send the blood specimens on ice.
- If food is sent for testing, it should be sent in its original containers.
- For anthrax or smallpox testing of a cutaneous lesion, soak one or two culture swabs with fluid from a previously unopened lesion.

After

- Identify all potential sources of contamination.
- Isolate individuals who are suspected of having a contagious disease.

TEST RESULTS AND CLINICAL SIGNIFICANCE

See Table 13-1, p. 1083.

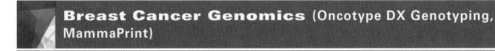

Breast Cancer Genomics (Oncotype DX Genotyping, MammaPrint)

NORMAL FINDINGS

Recurrence score <18 (on scale of 0 to 100)

INDICATIONS

Because molecular genomic studies measure the quantity of specific breast cancer–related genes, they can help predict the possibility of cancer susceptibility to chemotherapy. They also provide a powerful indicator of the likelihood of breast cancer recurrence (local and metastatic) after primary breast cancer surgery.

TEST EXPLANATION

Genomic testing using either Oncotype DX or MammaPrint is a clinically validated, multigene assay that provides a quantitative assessment of the likelihood of distant breast cancer recurrence and also assesses the benefit from certain types of chemotherapy in newly diagnosed breast cancer patients. In early-stage invasive breast cancer, the evaluation of the likelihood of distant recurrence is usually based on multiple pathologic factors, such as nodal status, tumor size and grade, estrogen and progesterone receptors, and *HER-2* status (see p. 717). However, these factors are often inaccurate and cannot quantify the recurrence risk sufficiently to provide significant insight into the risks and benefits of adjuvant chemotherapy. Genomic testing is designed to provide quantitative data to assist in clinical decision making regarding the use of adjuvant systemic therapies.

The Oncotype DX rtPCR assay—performed using formalin-fixed, paraffin-embedded tumor tissue—analyzes the expression of a panel of 21 genes (16 tumor-related genes and 5 reference genes) and provides the results as a recurrence score (0 to 100). The gene panel was selected and the recurrence score calculation derived through extensive laboratory testing followed by appropriate corroboration with multiple clinical studies in which Oncotype's predictability was validated. The MammaPrint, using microarray assay on fresh-frozen breast cancer tissue, analyzes the expression of 70 prognostic genes. A 5-gene IHC assay, the Mammostrat, uses monoclonal antibody biomarkers and a diagnostic algorithm with fresh-frozen cancer tissue. Molecular genomics is sensitive, specific, and highly reproducible and has a wide dynamic range.

Patients whose tumor genomics have low recurrence scores have only a slight chance of recurrence and derive minimal or no benefit from chemotherapy. Patients with tumors that have high recurrence scores have a significant chance of recurrence and can experience considerable benefit from chemotherapy. At present, genomic testing is intended for newly diagnosed patients whose breast cancer is stage I or II, node negative, *HER-2/neu* negative, and estrogen receptor positive. Clinical studies in other populations are currently underway.

CONTRAINDICATIONS

- Patients who would refuse adjuvant therapy because the test is very expensive and results will not affect their treatment

PROCEDURE AND PATIENT CARE

Before

⚕ Explain the significance of the prognostic data available for the patient's tumor.
⚕ Explain the benefits of genomics in helping the physician and the patient make appropriate decisions regarding the use of adjuvant chemotherapy.
- Provide the patient with emotional support through the postoperative period.
- Ensure that the patient's insurance will cover this expensive testing.

During

- After obtaining the specimen, the pathologist will send paraffin-embedded tissue to the centralized laboratory.
- Results will be available in about 2 weeks.

After

⚕ Provide education and support to patients as they evaluate their results.

TEST RESULTS AND CLINICAL SIGNIFICANCES

Breast cancer: *Patients with high recurrence scores are likely to experience early recurrence and will likely benefit from cytotoxic chemotherapy.*

RELATED TESTS

Estrogen/Progesterone Receptor Assay (pp. 728 and 750, respectively). These are also prognostic indicators for breast cancer.
HER-2/neu (p. 717). This is a breast cancer prognosticator and target for monoclonal therapy.

Cell Culture Drug Resistance Testing (CCDRT, Chemosensitivity Assay, Drug Response Assay)

NORMAL FINDINGS

Cells sensitive to planned therapeutic drugs

INDICATIONS

This still-experimental test is performed to evaluate the sensitivity of a patient's cancer cells to anticancer drugs.

TEST EXPLANATION

Cell culture drug resistance testing (CCDRT) refers to testing the reaction of a patient's own cancer cells in the laboratory to drugs that may be used to treat the patient's cancer. The idea is to identify which drugs are more likely to work and which drugs are less likely to work. By avoiding the latter and choosing from among the former, the patient's probability of benefiting from the chemotherapy may be improved. There are multiple tests available for drug sensitivity testing, but all have four common steps. Cancer cells from the patient's tumor must be obtained and isolated. The cells are then isolated with various potentially therapeutic drugs. Assessment of cell survival is then performed and the results are provided. Based on those results, the clinician can recommend more appropriate chemotherapy for a particular cancer. In most cases, this testing is used for patients with refractory or recurrent epithelial tumors (usually breast or ovarian cancer).

PROCEDURE AND PATIENT CARE

Before

Explain the process to the patient. (Tumor cells are usually obtained by a surgical procedure.)

During

- Tumor cells are sent to a reference laboratory. The method of tissue preservation varies among laboratories.

After

- After the results are obtained, appropriate chemotherapy targeted to the patient's tumor cells is administered.

TEST RESULTS AND CLINICAL SIGNIFICANCE

Epithelial cancer: *This testing is still considered experimental because there is no extensive clinical experience to support its accuracy. However, a growing number of studies have shown a superior survival rate for patients treated with drugs targeting their tumor cells.*

Chorionic Villus Sampling (CVS, Chorionic Villus Biopsy [CVB])

NORMAL FINDINGS

No genetic or biochemical disorders

INDICATIONS

CVS is performed in women whose unborn child may be at risk for a life-threatening or life-altering genetic defect. This includes women who (1) are older than 35 years at the time of pregnancy, (2) have had frequent spontaneous abortions, (3) have had previous pregnancies with fetuses or infants with chromosomal or genetic defects (e.g., Down syndrome), (4) have a genetic defect themselves (e.g., hemoglobinopathy), or (5) have increased fetal nuchal transparency or other abnormal ultrasound finding.

TEST EXPLANATION

CVS can be performed at 8 to 12 weeks of gestation for early detection of genetic and biochemical disorders. Because CVS detects congenital defects early, first-trimester therapeutic abortions can be performed if indicated and desired.

A sample of chorionic villi from the chorion frondosum, which is the trophoblastic origin of the placenta, is obtained for analysis. These villi in the chorion frondosum are present from 8 to 12 weeks on and reflect fetal chromosome, enzyme, and deoxyribonucleic acid (DNA) content. This permits much earlier diagnosis of prenatal problems than with amniocentesis, which cannot be done before 14 to 16 weeks. Further, the cells derived by CVS are more easily cultured for karyotyping (determination of chromosomal and genetic abnormalities). Although amniocentesis is the safer procedure, the cells obtained take longer to grow in culture, which further adds to the delay in obtaining results. At this later point, therapeutic abortion for severe genetic defects is more difficult.

POTENTIAL COMPLICATIONS

- Accidental abortion
- Infection
- Bleeding
- Amniotic fluid leakage
- Fetal limb deformities if done before the ninth week of pregnancy
- Rh sensitization

PROCEDURE AND PATIENT CARE

Before

- Explain the procedure to the patient. Encourage patient to have someone accompany her to the appointment for emotional support and to drive home afterward.
- Ensure that signed consent for the procedure has been obtained.
- Tell the patient that no food or fluid restrictions are necessary.
- Encourage the patient to drink at least 1 to 2 glasses of fluid before the test.
- Instruct the patient not to urinate for several hours before the test. A full bladder is an excellent reference point for pelvic ultrasound.
- Assess the vital signs of the mother and fetal heart rate before the test, and again during and on completion of the test.

During

- Note the following procedural steps:
  1. The patient is placed in the lithotomy position, and a sterile speculum is placed into the previously cleansed vagina to visualize the cervix.
  2. A cannula is inserted into the cervix and uterine cavity (Figure 13-1).
  3. Under ultrasound guidance, the cannula is rotated to the site of the developing placenta.
  4. A syringe is attached, and suction is applied to obtain three or more villous samples to ensure sufficient tissue for accurate sampling.

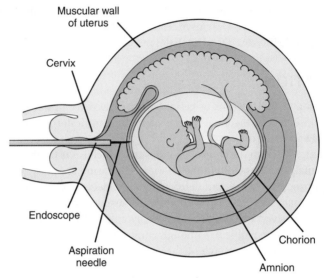

Figure 13-1 Chorionic villus sampling (CVS). Diagram of an 8-week pregnancy showing endoscopic aspiration of extraplacental villi.

5. If ultrasound indicates that the trophoblastic tissue is remote from the cervix, a transabdominal approach similar to that described for amniocentesis (p. 632) may be used.
- This procedure is performed by an obstetrician in approximately 30 minutes.
- Inform the patient that discomfort associated with this test is similar to that of a Papanicolaou test (Pap test).

After

- Some mothers with Rh-negative blood may receive $Rh_o(D)$ immune globulin (RhoGAM) because of the risk for development of maternal antibodies to the fetal blood cells, which could threaten fetal well-being.
- Monitor vital signs, and check the mother for signs of bleeding.
- Schedule an ultrasound in 2 to 4 days to affirm continued viability of the fetus.
- Assess the vaginal area for discharge and drainage; note the color and amount.
- Assess and educate the patient concerning signs of spontaneous abortion (e.g., cramps, bleeding) and endometrial infection (e.g., vaginal discharge, fever, crampy abdominal pain).
- Inform the patient how to obtain the results from the physician. Be sure she understands that the results are usually not available for several weeks (although they may be available much sooner if the test is performed at a major medical center). If results are unclear, amniocentesis may be needed.
- Inform the patient about genetic counseling services if needed to help understand the results or make a decision regarding a problem.

Home Care Responsibilities

- Instruct the mother to immediately report signs of spontaneous abortion (e.g., cramps, bleeding).
- Educate the mother to identify and report signs of endometrial infection (e.g., vaginal discharge, fever, crampy abdominal pain).
- The pregnant mother should be scheduled for an ultrasound 2 to 4 days after CVS to ensure continued viability of the fetus.

TEST RESULTS AND CLINICAL SIGNIFICANCE

Chromosomal, genetic, and biochemical disorders: *Many chromosomal and genetic defects are identified by karyotyping and genetic mapping. Genetic counseling is a vital part of this sort of testing. If therapeutic abortion is an option, the religious, moral, and ethical aspects of this decision need to be considered.*

RELATED TESTS

Obstetric Ultrasonography (p. 887). This test is used to localize trophoblastic tissue.

Amniocentesis (p. 632). Used to indicate fetal well-being and allows tissue sampling for karyotyping and genetic mapping.

Fetoscopy (p. 612). During this test, tissue can be obtained for karyotyping and genetic mapping.

Fetal Nonstress Test (p. 569). This test is used to evaluate the viability of the fetus before, during, and after CVS.

Fluorescein Angiography (FA, Ocular Photography)

NORMAL FINDINGS

Normal retinal/choroidal vasculature

INDICATIONS

This test is performed to diagnose disease affecting the posterior eye including the retina, choroid, and optic nerve. It is also used to monitor disease progression and treatment.

TEST EXPLANATION

With the use of fluorescein angiography, the patency and integrity of the retinal circulation can be determined. It involves injection of sodium fluorescein into the systemic circulation followed by timed-interval photographs performed with a fundus camera. The timed images are then reviewed for specific patterns indicative of disease states. The test is often repeated at intervals to monitor treatment or disease progression.

Fluorescein is a member of the triphenylmethane dyes. When the fluorescein molecules absorb light toward the end of the blue spectrum (465 to 490 nm), the molecules transfer from a basal state to an excited state. In doing so, light of a different wavelength (450 to 465 nm—the yellow-green end of the light spectrum) is emitted. This light emission is then recorded by a specialized camera where very little light outside the blue spectrum is allowed to enter. The camera also has a filter that limits recording of light other than the yellow to green range. With digital technology, color photographs can be obtained at specified times after dye injections. With this technique, baseline photographs are taken prior to fluorescein injection. A 6-second bolus injection of approximately 5 mL of sodium fluorescein is made into a vein in the upper extremity. Photos are taken 10 seconds later and approximately once every second for about 20 seconds, then less often. A delayed image is obtained at 5 and 10 minutes. Some physicians like to see a 15-minute image as well. Normal circulatory filling times are approximate:

0 seconds: Injection of fluorescein
9.5 seconds: Posterior ciliary arteries
10 seconds: Choroidal flush (or pre-arterial phase)

10 to 12 seconds: Retinal arterial stage

13 seconds: Capillary transition stage

14 to 15 seconds: Early venous stage (or lamellar stage, arterial-venous stage)

16 to 17 seconds: Venous stage

18 to 20 seconds: Late venous stage

5 minutes: Late staining

Fluorescein enters the ocular circulation from the internal carotid artery via the ophthalmic artery. The ophthalmic artery supplies the choroid via the short posterior ciliary arteries and the retina via the central retinal artery. However, the route to the choroid is typically less circuitous than the route to the retina. This accounts for the short delay between the "choroidal flush" and retinal filling. Pathologic changes are recognized by the detection of either hyperfluorescence or hypofluorescence. Among the common groups of ophthalmologic disease, fluorescein angiography can detect diabetic retinopathy, vein occlusions, retinal artery occlusions, edema of the optic disc, and tumors.

Fluorescein angiography is often done to follow the course of a disease such as diabetes—a disease that can cause the blood vessels of the retina to leak blood or fluid. Age-related macular degeneration is another disease that can cause the blood vessels of the retina to leak blood or fluid. Both of these abnormalities can be treated with a laser to help prevent loss of vision, and treatment results can be monitored using fluorescein angiography.

The test is performed and interpreted by an ophthalmologist, usually in the office setting. Results are available in less than 30 minutes.

POTENTIAL COMPLICATIONS

Allergic reactions: Allergies to fluorescein dye are rare. If they occur, they may cause a skin rash and
    itching. Severe allergic reactions (anaphylaxis) occur rarely and can be life threatening.

PROCEDURE AND PATIENT CARE

Before

⚕ Explain the procedure to the patient.

- Obtain an informed consent.

⚕ Reinforce the need for the patient to remain still during the few seconds following fluorescein injection.

- Obtain an ocular history of cataracts, prior retinal surgery, or other disease that may inhibit photography.

⚕ Instruct the patient to remove any ocular lenses.

⚕ Inform the patient that there are no dietary restrictions.

- Pupil dilatation can improve access to the posterior eye. If ordered, administer appropriate mydriatic medications. Note, however, that these medications are contraindicated for patients with glaucoma as they may dangerously increase ocular pressures.

During

Note the following procedural steps:

1. The patient is positioned in the fundus camera with the chin on the bar.
2. The patient is told to pick a spot in the far distance and concentrate on that spot during the examination.
3. Intravenous access is obtained.
4. Fluorescein dye is injected with the assistance of an autoinjector.
5. Photographs are taken by the ophthalmologist at timed intervals.

- This test is performed and interpreted by an ophthalmologist, usually in the office setting. Results are available in less than 30 minutes.

After

- Remove the intravenous access device and apply pressure to the venipuncture site.
- Inform the patient that fluorescein dye is excreted by the kidneys and to expect very yellow urine for the next 24 hours.
- Document the procedure and the patient's response.

TEST RESULTS AND CLINICAL SIGNIFICANCE

▲ Increased Levels

Tumor,
Detached retina,
Trauma,
Inflammation,
Retinitis pigmentosa,
Papilledema:
  Hyperfluorescence is caused by neovascularity that occurs with neoplasm or inflammation. It is also seen with destruction of vascular integrity associated with these ocular diseases.
Diabetic retinopathy: *Capillary microaneurysms in the retina are often the earliest signs of diabetic retinopathy.*

▼ Decreased Levels

Diabetes,
Vascular disease,
Radiation to the eye,
Hemorrhage,
Edema,
Prior photocoagulation therapy:
  These diseases will cause hypofluorescence because the arterial flow is interrupted by these diseases.

Genetic Testing (Breast Cancer [BRCA] and Ovarian Cancer, Colon Cancer, Cardiovascular Disease, Tay-Sachs Disease, Cystic Fibrosis, Melanoma, Hemochromatosis, Thyroid Cancer, Paternity [Parentage Analysis] and Forensic Genetic Testing)

NORMAL FINDINGS

No genetic mutation

INDICATIONS

Genetic testing is used to identify a predisposition to disease, establish the presence of a disease, establish or refute paternity, or to provide forensic evidence used in criminal investigations.

TEST EXPLANATION

As research progresses and the Human Genome Project provides more information, precise and accurate methods of identification of normal and mutated genes are becoming more common. The use of gene amplification methods has contributed to the explosion of genetic information in regard to disease

| BOX 13-1 | Breast Cancer Screening in Women With *BRCA* Mutations |

- Monthly breast self-examination starting at age 18
- Semiannual clinical breast examination starting at age 25
- Yearly mammogram starting at age 25
- Semiannual breast MRI (p. 1106)

propensity. These exquisite and sensitive laboratory methods are revolutionizing medicine and the courtrooms. Tests for defective genes known to be associated with certain diseases are now commonly used in screening populations of people who have certain phenotypes and family history compatible with a genetic mutation. Genetic testing is done in addition to a family history (pedigree). Whereas a family history is not always reliable, accurate, or available, genetic testing is very accurate in its determination of risks. Preventive medicine or surgery can be provided to eliminate disease development. Reproductive counseling and pregnancy prevention can preclude the conception of children who are likely to suffer the consequence of disease. Paternity and forensic genetic testing can accurately place responsibility, guilt, and innocence.

The ethics and disadvantages to this genetic testing are presently being discussed. Patients may face financial discrimination for health or life insurance or employment if the results are positive. The Health Insurance Portability and Accountability Act (HIPAA) protects patients from discrimination based on genetic information. This testing may be expensive and not covered by insurance. The information obtained by testing may cause great emotional turmoil in affected individuals or their family. The information obtained by medical genetic testing should be shared with the patient only. If the patient chooses to allow others to know the information, the patient must direct that release of information. Voluntary genetic testing should always be associated with aggressive counseling and support. Because of the potential changes in life for other family members, each person receiving the genetic information must be counseled separately.

Breast Cancer and Ovarian Cancer Genetic Testing

Inherited mutations in *BRCA* (BReast CAncer) genes indicate an increased susceptibility for development of breast cancer. The two genes in which mutations are most commonly seen are *BRCA1* and *BRCA2*. The *BRCA1* gene exists on chromosome 17. *BRCA 2* is on chromosome 13. These genes encode tumor suppressor proteins. More than half of the women who inherit mutations will develop breast cancer by the age of 50 compared with less than 2% of women without the genetic defect. See Box 13-1 for screening recommendations for those with *BRCA* mutations.

The *BRCA* genes also confer an increased susceptibility for ovarian cancer. In the normal population, less than 2% of women develop ovarian cancer by age 70. Of women with mutations of the *BRCA1* gene, 44% develop ovarian cancer by that age. Ovarian cancer is less commonly associated with the *BRCA2* gene (20%). Furthermore, a woman who has already had breast cancer and who has a *BRCA* mutation has a 65% chance of developing a contralateral breast cancer in her lifetime (compared with less than 15% of women without the genetic defect). The woman with breast cancer and a *BRCA* genetic defect has a 10 times greater risk of developing ovarian cancer as a second primary cancer when compared with similar women without the mutated form of the gene. See Box 13-2 for ovarian cancer screening for those with *BRCA* mutations.

These mutations have an autosomal dominant inheritance pattern, indicating that women who inherit just one genetic defect can develop the phenotypic cancers. Men with *BRCA* genetic mutations (most commonly *BRCA2*) are at an increased risk for the development of breast, prostate, and colon cancer. In addition, they can pass the mutation to their daughters. Because *BRCA* is an autosomal dominant gene, 50% of the children are at risk. See Table 13-2 for determining who should be tested for *BRCA* mutations.

| BOX 13-2 | Ovarian Cancer Screening in Women With *BRCA* mutations |

- Transvaginal ultrasound every 6 to 12 months
- CA-125 blood test every 6 to 12 months

Start at age 25 or 10 years before the youngest age at which ovarian cancer was diagnosed in the family.

| TABLE 13-2 | Who Should Be Tested for *BRCA* Mutations? |

Patient With Breast Cancer	Family History (With at Least One Characteristic)
Diagnosed <40 years of age.	No other family history
Diagnosed around 50 years of age with two primary breast cancers	One relative around 50 years of age with breast cancer One relative with ovarian cancer
Diagnosed at any age	Two relatives with ovarian cancer Two relatives with breast cancer Male with breast cancer Personal history of ovarian cancer Ashkenazi Jewish heritage First- or second-degree relative with *BRCA* mutation
Male breast cancer at any age	One relative with breast cancer or ovarian cancer Ashkenazi Jewish heritage First- or second-degree relative with *BRCA* mutation

The value of testing a select group of women who may be at high risk for *BRCA* genetic mutations includes:

1. Identification of those who are at high risk for developing breast or ovarian cancer
2. Consideration of interventions for those who test positive for *BRCA* mutations (e.g., prophylactic mastectomy and/or oophorectomy, or chemoprevention with tamoxifen)
3. Adoption of aggressive screening surveillance testing, which includes the following:
   - Breast: Physical examination, mammography (see p. 1043) starting at age 25, and semiannual breast MRI imaging
   - Ovary: Transvaginal ultrasound (see p. 887) starting at age 25
   - Semiannual CA-125 (see p. 134) testing starting at age 25
4. Estimation of potential for passing the mutated *BRCA* gene to offspring

The method of testing includes obtaining a blood sample from a patient who has breast or ovarian cancer. Through reverse-transcriptase polymerase chain reaction (RT-PCR) amplification, the deoxyribonucleic acid (DNA) is sequenced and amplified for quantitation. If results are positive, blood samples of other family members are specifically tested for that particular genetic mutation only. Therefore, testing is expensive for the first person examined because the search is for any number of potential genetic mutations. However, for the other family members, it is much less expensive because the search has been narrowed to only a single genetic mutation.

Colon Cancer Genetic Testing

Two common forms of colon cancer are associated with a strong familial link. The first is familial adenomatous polyposis (FAP). These patients present with hundreds of polyps in their colon—one or two of which degenerate into cancer. The second type is hereditary nonpolyposis colorectal cancer (HNPCC).

TABLE 13-3	Risk for Hereditary Nonpolyposis Colorectal Cancer–Related Cancers	
Cancer Type	**Hereditary Nonpolyposis Colorectal Cancer (%)**	**General Population (%)**
Colorectal	80	2
Endometrial	60	1.5
Ovarian	12	1
Gastric	13	<1

HNPCC is also known as the Lynch syndrome. These patients are more difficult to recognize because they do not have polyps; colon cancers develop de novo.

FAP is caused by a genetic mutation in the *5 q 21-22 (APC)* gene on chromosome 5. Like *BRCA* genes, these genes are responsible for the synthesis of tumor-suppressor proteins. HNPCC is associated most often with mutations (defective DNA mismatch repair) of *MLH 1, MLH 2,* and *MLH 6* genes. These genes are on chromosome 5 and are important for genome stability (prevention of chromosomal breakage and exchange). HNPCC is associated with several other cancers (Table 13-3), especially endometrial cancer.

These genetic defects are autosomal dominant, indicating that a person with just one defective gene can develop any of the phenotypic cancers. Furthermore, their children have a 50% chance of receiving the genetic mutation with its inherent cancer risks from the affected parent. Characteristics of FAP or HNPCC include:

1. Early-onset colorectal cancer (usually before the age of 50)
2. Polyps in large numbers (FAP only)
3. Cancer in the proximal colon
4. Cancers that tend to be more aggressive
5. Cancers that are found at a later stage
6. Often associated with other cancers

A family member meeting the following criteria should consider genetic testing:

1. A family must have three (two first-degree) relatives with colorectal cancer
2. At least two generations of the family must be affected
3. Colorectal cancer must be found in at least one individual under the age of 50

The value of testing a family who may be at high risk for a genetic mutations includes:

1. Identification of those who are at high risk for developing colorectal or other cancers
2. Consideration of interventions for those who test positive for *APC* or *MLH* mutations (e.g., prophylactic proctocolectomy and/or hysterectomy, or chemoprevention with nonsteroidal antiinflammatory drugs [NSAIDs], which have been shown to reduce the incidence of colon polyps and cancers)
3. Adoption of aggressive screening surveillance testing, which includes:
   - Colon: Annual colonoscopy (p. 591) starting at age of 25
   - Uterus: Transvaginal ultrasound (see p. 887) and endometrial biopsy starting at age 25
4. Estimation of potential for passing the mutated *APC* or *MLH* gene to offspring

The laboratory methods of genetic testing are similar to those described for *BRCA* testing discussed previously.

Cardiovascular Disease Genetic Testing

Because half of all patients with cardiovascular disease (CVD) do not have the traditional risk factors (cholesterol, obesity, diabetes, and high blood pressure), these factors alone may fall short in the identification of patients at high risk for cardiac disease. Although a family history is helpful in identifying families at risk for CVD, genetic testing is more accurate and—if confirmed—more predictive among individuals in such a family. The angiotensinogen *(AGT)* gene demonstrates the strongest and most consistent associations with CVD. This gene is on chromosome 1. This is an autosomal recessive gene. When a patient has just one *AGT* mutation, the risk for CVD is moderately elevated. When an individual has two *AGT* genetic mutations, the risk for CVD is nearly triple that of the general population. These patients have early age onset of hypertension, myocardial infarction (MI), and hypertrophic cardiomyopathy. With genetic testing of individuals in families in which CVD is predominant, early therapeutic interventions (e.g., aggressive lipid-lowering agents and aggressive use of antihypertensives) may preclude disease.

Mutations in sarcomeric genes cause early-onset cardiac channelopathies and cardiomyopathies. These are rare but potentially lethal heart conditions that include long QT syndrome (LQTS), catecholaminergic polymorphic ventricular tachycardia (CPVT), hypertrophic cardiomyopathy (HCM), arrhythmogenic right ventricular cardiomyopathy, and dilated cardiomyopathy (DCM). Patients with a sarcomeric gene mutation are nearly three times more likely to suffer an adverse cardiac outcome (cardiovascular death, nonfatal ischemic stroke, or progression to severe heart failure). Identifying patients with these genetic mutations can help diagnose a patient's disease, guide treatment options, and determine whether family members are at risk.

Tay-Sachs Disease Genetic Testing

Tay-Sachs disease is characterized by the onset of severe mental and developmental retardation in the first few months of life. Affected children become totally debilitated by 2 to 5 years of age and die by age 5 to 8. Another form of the same disease is "late-onset Tay-Sachs" or chronic GM2, also known as gangliosidosis. The basic defect in affected children is a mutation in the hexosaminidase gene, which is on chromosome 15. This gene is responsible for the synthesis of hexosaminidase [HEX] (p. 290), an enzyme that normally breaks down a fatty substance called GM2 gangliosides. When this enzyme is not present in sufficient quantities, gangliosides build up in the nervous system and cause the debilitation characteristic of this disease. Ashkenazi (Eastern European) Jews and non-Jewish French Canadians, particularly those in the Cajun population in Louisiana, are affected most. This gene is an autosomal recessive gene. Carriers have one defective gene. Affected individuals have both genes defective. A "carrier couple" has a 25% chance of having a child affected with the disease.

At present, there is no treatment for the disease. It is important to identify carriers so that reproductive counseling can be provided. Hexosaminidase protein testing (p. 290) has been extremely effective for identification of carriers and affected individuals. However, sometimes the results of HEX protein tests are inconclusive or uncertain. Furthermore, genetic testing is used to diagnose "late-onset" Tay-Sachs. Both the test for the protein and that for the gene mutation are performed on a blood sample or on chorionic villus samples obtained during amniocentesis (p. 632). Genetic testing is performed using amino acid sequencing and comparison.

Cystic Fibrosis Genetic Testing

Cystic fibrosis (CF) is caused by a mutation in the cystic fibrosis transmembrane conductance regulator *(CFTR)* gene. This gene encodes the synthesis of a protein that serves as a channel through which chloride enters and leaves cells. A mutation in this gene alters the cell's capability to regulate the chloride (and therefore sodium) transport. As a result, the lungs and digestive tract of CF patients fill with thick mucus. As bacteria invade their mucus-filled lungs, CF patients experience frequent lung infection. As mucus blocks the pancreas, inefficient digestion results.

There are thousands of potential mutations that are fatally deleterious to the *CFTR* gene. However, the most common mutation that accounts for 70% of the CF cases is known as the Delta AF508. Currently more than 30 genetic mutations can be recognized to cause CF, and these account for 90% of the cases.

The *CFTR* gene is an autosomal recessive gene located on chromosome 7. A carrier has one mutated gene. The person affected by CF has both defective genes. Genetic testing is now used to identify carriers of CF and identify neonates with the disease, and detecting fetal disease during pregnancy. The sweat chloride test (p. 678) is a more easily performed and cheaper way to diagnose the disease in affected children. Therefore the use of genetic testing for CF is often limited to those with a family history of CF, partners of patients with CF, and pregnant couples with a family history of CF. The main purpose of CF genetic testing is to identify carriers who could conceive a child with CF.

It is important to recognize that not all patients who have the CF genetic mutation will develop the disease. Further, because only a few mutations that may cause CF can be detected, a negative test does not necessarily eliminate the possibility of being affected by the diseases.

Genetic testing can be performed on blood samples or on samples taken during chorionic villus sampling (CVS) (p. 1088) or during amniocentesis (p. 632). Polymerase chain reaction (PCR) is used to amplify the locus for the *CTFR* gene. Amplification products are then hybridized to probes for the 36 most common *CFTR*-related mutations, using a line probe assay. Several laboratory methods are used to separate out the sequences for study.

Melanoma Genetic Testing

Recent progress in the genetics of cutaneous melanoma has led to the identification of two melanoma susceptibility genes: the tumor suppressor gene *CDKN2A* encoding the p16 protein on chromosome 9p21 and the *CDK4* gene, on chromosome 12q13. The *p16* genetic mutation is by far the most common form of hereditary melanoma. Characteristics of familial melanoma include frequent multiple primary melanomas, early age of onset of first melanoma, and frequently the presence of atypical or dysplastic nevi (moles). Family members with the following characteristics may consider testing for *p16* genetic mutations:

- Multiple diagnoses of primary melanoma
- Two or more family members with melanoma
- Melanoma and pancreatic cancer
- Melanoma and a personal/family history of multiple atypical nevi
- Relatives of a patient with a confirmed *p16* genetic mutation

Approximately 20% to 40% of families with three or more affected first-degree relatives show inheritance of mutations in the *p16* gene. Fifteen percent of patients with multiple melanoma will have a *p16* mutation. The average age at diagnosis is 35 years for those with a mutation in *p16* versus 57 years in the general population. Carriers of the *p16* gene mutation also have an increased risk for pancreatic cancer.

Once a *p16* mutation is identified, education of all family members about the need for sun protection is essential. Commencing at the age of 10 years, family members should have a baseline skin examination with characterization of moles. It is recommended that an appropriately trained health care provider carry out skin examinations every 6 to 12 months. A monthly self-examination or examination by parent, partner, or family member should also be performed. Individuals should be taught about routine self-examination in the hope that this will prompt earlier diagnosis and removal of melanomas. The significance of change in shape and size of pigmented lesions should be understood, and the rules regarding asymmetry, border, color, and diameter (i.e., the ABCD rules) are often helpful in this regard.

Hemochromatosis Genetic Testing

The diagnosis of hemochromatosis is traditionally made by using serum iron studies. When hereditary hemochromatosis is suspected, mutation analysis of the *hemochromatosis-associated HFE genes* (*C282Y* and *H63D*) is done. Hereditary hemochromatosis (HH), an iron overload disorder considered to be the most common inherited disease in Caucasians, affects 1 in 500 individuals. Increased intestinal iron absorption and intracellular iron accumulation lead to progressive damage of the liver, heart, pancreas, joints, reproductive organs, and endocrine glands. Without therapy, males may develop symptoms between 40 and 60 years of age and women after menopause.

A large, but as yet undefined, fraction of homozygotes for this disease do not develop clinical symptoms (i.e., penetrance is low). Patients with symptoms and early biochemical signs of iron overload consistent with hereditary hemochromatosis should be tested. Relatives of individuals with hereditary hemochromatosis should also be studied. HFE genotyping could improve disease outcomes of the disease. Serum iron markers are monitored at more frequent intervals if an HFE mutation is detected and phlebotomy therapy is initiated earlier. Early initiation of phlebotomy therapy reduces the frequency or severity of hemochromatosis-related symptoms and organ damage.

Thyroid Cancer Genetic Testing

The *RET* proto-oncogene, located on chromosome subband 10 q11.2, encodes a receptor tyrosine kinase expressed in tissues and tumors derived from neural crest. Genetic testing for *RET* germline mutation has shown 100% sensitivity and specificity for identifying those at risk for developing inherited medullary thyroid cancer (multiple endocrine neoplasia [MEN] 2A, MEN 2B, or familial medullary thyroid carcinoma [FMTC]).

Use of the genetic assay allows earlier and more definitive identification and clinical management of those with a familial risk for medullary thyroid cancer. Medullary thyroid carcinoma is surgically curable if detected before it has spread to regional lymph nodes. However, lymph node involvement at diagnosis may be found in up to 75% of patients for whom a thyroid nodule is the first sign of disease. Thus there is an emphasis on early detection and intervention in families, which are affected by the familial cancer syndromes of MEN types 2A and 2B and FMTC, which account for one fourth of medullary thyroid cancer.

After genetic counseling, most family members who test positive undergo surgery to remove the thyroid gland. First-degree relatives of those with medullary thyroid carcinoma that appears to be sporadic in origin also undergo testing to verify that the patient's tumor is not caused by an inheritable form of this disease. RET testing is considered the standard of care in MEN 2 families because clinical decisions are made based on the results of such gene testing.

Paternity Genetic Testing (Parentage Analysis)

Deoxyribonucleic acid (DNA) testing is the most accurate form of testing to prove or exclude paternity when the identity of the biologic father of a child is in doubt. By comparing DNA characteristic of the mother and child, it is possible to determine characteristics that the child inherited from the biologic mother. Thus any remaining DNA must have come from the biologic father. If the DNA from the tested man is found to contain these paternal characteristics, then the probability of paternity can be determined. Testing is 99% accurate. However, in cases when the suspected fathers are close siblings, differentiation cannot be as certain.

Several particular regions (short tandem repeats [STRs]) of several chromosomes are copied by PCR. Frequency of repeated sequencing is then measured, usually by electrophoresis. The number of repeat sequences on the STR varies by individual. Testing is so reliable that it is admissible in court. Testing can be done on a mouth swab, blood, or CVS sample. Results are usually available in 1 to 3 weeks.

Many parents are given misinformation at the time of twin births regarding whether the twins are identical or fraternal. DNA samples from siblings can be analyzed in a manner described to indicate twinship. Again, these tests are 99% accurate.

Unfortunately, prenatal testing of the fetal components for paternity testing requires invasive testing such as chorionic villus sampling or amniocentesis. There are times, particularly in circumstances of rape, when early pregnancy paternity identification is desired. *Noninvasive prenatal paternity testing* can now be performed accurately by extracting and amplifying fetal chromosome alleles from maternal

Miscellaneous Studies

13

blood. This is a difficult process because "cell-free maternal DNA" quickly degrades fetal DNA. Now with the addition of cell stabilizers to maternal blood, cell-free maternal DNA is minimized and fetal DNA can be obtained. By using single nucleotide polymorphisms to distinguish fetal DNA from maternal DNA, an accurate prediction of paternity can be made.

Forensic Genetic Testing

Forensic DNA testing is used with increasing frequency in today's courtrooms because of its accuracy. In a courtroom, the reliability of the evidence can protect the individual and society as a whole. Further, DNA testing can be so conclusive that it often motivates plea bargaining and thereby reduces court time. It can quickly establish guilt or innocence beyond a reasonable doubt. Like paternity testing, forensic DNA testing is based on the fact that each individual is genetically different (except for twins). Through the use of PMR chemical probes, or through restriction length polymorphism methods, the DNA content of a person can be determined from nearly any body part. Furthermore, because DNA does not change or deteriorate even after death, testing can be performed on any body part, cadaver, or live person. Specimens considered adequate for DNA testing include blood, teeth, semen, saliva, bone, nails, skin scrapings, and hair. Forensic testing is also used for body identification. In time, central Federal Bureau of Investigation (FBI) data recording methods may allow for the collation of DNA data similar to the database of hundreds of millions of fingerprints on file.

CONTRAINDICATIONS

- Patients who are not emotionally able to deal with the results: The wishes of family members who do not want to know the results should be respected.

PROCEDURE AND PATIENT CARE

Before

- Explain the procedure to the patient.
- Tell the patient that no fasting is required.
- It is recommended that all patients who undergo testing should receive genetic counseling.
- Tell the patient the time it will take to have the results back.
- Inform the patient of the high costs of genetic testing and that it may not be covered by all medical insurance plans.

During

- Obtain the specimen in a manner provided by the specialized testing laboratory.
  Blood is collected in a lavender-top tube. Cord blood can be used for infants.
  Buccal swab: A cotton swab is placed between the lower cheek and gums. It is twisted and then placed on a special paper or in a special container. Usually two to four swabs are requested.
  Amniotic fluid: At least 20 mL of fluid is preferred.
  Chorionic villus sampling: 10 mg of cleaned villi are sent as prescribed by the testing laboratory.
  Product of conception: 10 mg of placental tissue is preserved in a sterile medium.
  Other body parts: As much tissue as is available is sent for testing.

After

- Document the procedure and the patient's response.
- Apply pressure or a pressure dressing to the venipuncture site.

Be sure that the patient has an appointment scheduled for obtaining the results. It is very upsetting for a patient and family to wait for the results.

 Arrangements should be made to ensure genetic and emotional counseling after abnormal results are obtained.

TEST RESULTS AND CLINICAL SIGNIFICANCE

Genetic carrier state: *These people carry one autosomal genetic recessive gene mutation. They themselves rarely have any abnormal phenotype (disease characteristics). However, if a child is conceived with a similar carrier, the child has a 25% chance of having the disease.*

Affected state: *These individuals have the phenotype demonstrating the genetic defect. This can occur if the person has either one autosomal dominant gene or two autosomal recessive genes. These people may not live long enough to have children of their own.*

RELATED TESTS

Sweat Electrolytes (p. 678). This is the definitive test to diagnose CF.

Hexosaminidase A (p. 290). This is the definitive test to diagnose Tay-Sachs disease.

Mammography (p. 1043). This is the most commonly used test to screen for breast cancer.

CA-125 Tumor Marker (p. 134). This is a commonly used test to screen high-risk patients for ovarian cancer.

Helicobacter pylori Testing (*Campylobacter pylori*, Anti–*Helicobacter pylori* Immunoglobulin G [IgG] Antibody, *Campylobacter*-Like Organism [CLO] Test, Rapid Urease Test, *H. pylori* Antigen Stool Test, Urea Breath Test [UBT, *H. pylori* breath test])

NORMAL FINDINGS

Serology

IgM
≤30 U/mL (negative)
30.01-39.99 U/mL (equivocal)
≥40 U/mL (positive)

IgG
<0.75 (negative)
0.75-0.99 (equivocal)
≥1 (positive)

Breath Test

No evidence of *H. pylori*

Stool Test

No evidence of *H. pylori*

INDICATIONS

This test is used to detect *Helicobacter pylori* infections. It is indicated in patients who are suspected of having peptic ulcers (active or past history), gastric MALT lymphoma, melena, hematemesis, weight loss, persistent vomiting, dysphagia, or anemia.

TEST EXPLANATION

H. pylori, a bacterium is a gram-negative (p. 704) bacillus that infects the mucus overlying the gastric mucosa and the mucosa cells that line the stomach. It is a major risk factor for gastric and duodenal ulcers, chronic gastritis, or even ulcerative esophagitis. It is also a class I gastric carcinogen. Gastric colonization by this organism has been reported in about 90% to 95% of patients with a duodenal ulcer, 60% to 70% of patients with a gastric ulcer, and about 20% to 25% of patients with gastric cancer. Although some infected patients are asymptomatic, most individuals develop peptic symptoms within 2 weeks of exposure.

Approximately 10% of healthy persons younger than 30 years of age have *H. pylori* without disease or symptoms. Gastric "colonization" increases with age, with people older than age 60 years having rates at a percentage similar to their age. Testing should only be performed on symptomatic patients because a large percentage of *Helicobacter pylori*–colonized individuals would have positive results. All patients who test positive for *H. pylori* should be treated with aggressive antibiotics.

There are several methods of detecting the presence of this organism (Table 13-4). A single gold standard test does not exist. The organism can be cultured from a specimen of mucus obtained through a gastroscope (see p. 608). The specimen is plated on an enriched medium (such as chocolate or Skirrow's medium) and incubated for 5 to 7 days at 37° C. Although the delay in diagnosis is not preferred, culture can provide sensitivities for antibiotic therapy choices.

The organism can also be detected on histology of a gastric mucosal biopsy (from the antrum and greater curvature of the corpus) using Gram, silver, Giemsa, or acridine orange stains or by immunofluorescence or immunoperoxidase methods. It may be several weeks before the results are available from cultures or extensive histology. It is preferable to start treatment before that time on a patient with symptomatic or active ulcer disease. For that reason, *rapid urease testing* for *H. pylori* is available. *H. pylori* is capable of breaking down high quantities of urea because of its capability to produce great amounts of an enzyme called urease, which can be found in the lining of the stomach of infected patients. In the rapid urease test, a small piece of gastric mucosa (obtained through gastroscopy) is placed onto a specialized testing gel/agar containing a pH indicator. If *H. pylori* organisms are present in the gastric mucosa, the urease (made by the *H. pylori*) will change the pH and the color of the test material. Results are available in 3 hours.

A *breath test* is also available for the detection of *H. pylori*. It is may be used as first-line testing in symptomatic patients. In the breath test, radioactive carbon urea (^{13}C urea) is administered orally. The

TABLE 13-4	Tests Commonly Used to Detect *Helicobacter pylori* Infection
Test	**Advantages**
Invasive (Specimen Obtained by Endoscopy)	
Culture	Can determine antibody sensitivity
Urease	Quick and simple
Noninvasive	
Serology	Convenient and inexpensive
C^{13} urea breath	Safer and less expensive than endoscopy

urea is absorbed through the gastric mucosa, where, if *H. pylori* is present, the ^{13}C urea is converted to ammonia and $^{13}CO_2$. The $^{13}CO_2$ is then taken up by the capillaries in the stomach wall and delivered to the lungs. There the $^{13}CO_2$ is exhaled and will be detected in the exhaled breath. The breath test is very reliable but is expensive and labor laden.

Although *H. pylori* does not survive in the stool, an enzyme-linked immunosorbent assay (EIA) using a polyclonal anti–*H. pylori* capture antibody can detect the presence of *H. pylori* antigen in a fresh stool specimen. Stool testing is very accurate. Stool tests are mostly used in monitoring the eradication of *Helicobacter pylori* after therapy.

Serologic testing is an inexpensive and noninvasive method of diagnosis of *H. pylori* infection. It is also used as a supportive diagnostic in which no preparation or abstinence from antacids is required. It is the least sensitive of the *H. pylori* tests. The IgG anti–*H. pylori* antibody is most commonly used. It becomes elevated 2 months after infection and stays elevated for more than a year after treatment. The IgA anti–*H. pylori* antibody, like IgG, becomes elevated 2 months after infection but decreases 3 to 4 weeks after treatment. The IgM anti–*H. pylori* antibody is the first to become elevated (about 3 to 4 weeks after infection) and is not detected 2 to 3 months after treatment. These antibody titers are fast becoming the gold standard for *H. pylori* detection. These antibodies can be detected with use of a small amount of blood obtained by fingerstick. Serologic testing is often used several months after treatment to document eradication of *H. pylori* infection. Serologic testing is also used to corroborate the findings of other *H. pylori* testing methods. Because serology may lack specificity, nonserologic tests described in the preceding paragraphs can be used to confirm *Helicobacter pylori* infection.

INTERFERING FACTORS

- *H. pylori* can be transmitted by contaminated endoscopic equipment during endoscopic procedures.
- Sensitivity can be reduced in patients who are actively bleeding from ulcers.
- Rapid urease tests can *be falsely negative* if the patient uses antacid therapy within the week before testing.
- Bismuth (Pepto Bismol) or sucralfate (Carafate) will suppress mucosal uptake of the urea and interfere with test results.
- The concomitant use of a proton pump inhibitor, such as Prilosec, Nexium, Prevacid, or Protonix, will also inhibit urea absorption and diminish the sensitivity of all testing methods.

PROCEDURE AND PATIENT CARE

Before
- Explain the procedure to the patient.
- Tell the patient that no fasting is required for the blood test.
- If a biopsy or culture will be obtained by endoscopy, see discussion of esophagogastroduodenoscopy (EGD) on p. 608.
- If culture is to be performed, be sure the patient has not had any antibiotic, antacid, or bismuth treatment for 5 to 14 days before the endoscopy.

During
- Collect a *venous blood* sample according to the protocol of the laboratory performing the test.
- A *gastric* or *duodenal biopsy* or *specimen of mucus* can be obtained by endoscopy. Keep the specimen moist by the addition of 2 to 5 mL of sterile saline solution or other wetting agent as required by the laboratory. Place in a sterile container. Minimize transport time for cultures.
- Follow the following steps for the *Breath Test*:
  1. Verify that female patients are not pregnant.

2. Give a dose of radioactive ^{14}C or nonradioactive ^{13}C urea by mouth. Follow the guidelines of the laboratory.
3. Follow all the testing precautions for handling radioactive pharmaceuticals.
4. Several minutes after the patient has swallowed the carbon dose, provide the patient with 2 oz of water.
5. Breath samples are collected in any one of a number of gas collection devices depending on how and when the sample will be analyzed.

After

- Apply pressure or a pressure dressing to the venipuncture site.
- Assess the venipuncture site for bleeding.
- If endoscopy was used to obtain a culture, see procedure for esophagogastroduodenoscopy on p. 608. The specimen should be transported to the laboratory within 30 minutes after collection.

TEST RESULTS AND CLINICAL SIGNIFICANCE

▲ Increased Levels

Acute and chronic gastritis,
Recurrent duodenal ulcer,
Gastric ulcer,
Gastric carcinoma:

> The above-noted illnesses are associated with the presence of H. pylori. Whether the infection is causative or contributive is not well known.

RELATED TESTS

Gastrin (p. 248). This test is a measure of serum gastrin. This hormone stimulates gastric acid secretion. Oversecretion can cause recurrent peptic ulcers. The initial symptoms may be similar to those of chronic *H. pylori* infection.

Esophagogastroduodenoscopy (p. 608). This endoscopic procedure is used to directly biopsy the gastric mucosa for definitive *H. pylori* identification.

Laboratory Genetics

NORMAL FINDINGS

No genetic/chromosomal abnormalities

INDICATIONS

Laboratory genetics is used to identify a broad range of diseases and predisposition to diseases. Its use is extensive and growing daily in the field of laboratory medicine.

TEST EXPLANATION

Genetic laboratory testing has become a vital part of identifying diseases of inborn errors in metabolism, such as phenylketonuria (PKU). These genetic laboratory tests have also proved to be helpful in the identification, classification, and prognostication of many oncologic diseases, such as leukemias. The heredity of diseases can be more accurately traced with the use of laboratory genetics.

There are many different laboratory methods used in genetic testing and each is particularly helpful for study of a particular disease. It is not the intent of this manual to explain the details of commonly used genetic laboratory methods. However, it is important to be aware of the availability and ability of genetic laboratory testing in clinical medicine.

Molecular genetics is used to detect mutation carriers, diagnose genetic disorders, test at-risk fetuses, and identify patients at high risk of developing adult-onset conditions (such as Huntington disease or familial cancers). In addition, full-gene analysis is available for diseases such as cystic fibrosis, beta globin, and hereditary hemorrhagic telangiectasia. Once a mutation is identified in a family, a family-specific mutation micro array testing can be performed.

Biochemical genetics is frequently used to diagnose one of many metabolic disorders that affect the body's ability to produce or break down amino acids, organic acids, and fatty acids. Early identification of such a metabolic disorder may prevent serious health problems, as well as death. Biochemical genetic testing can be used as a supplemental newborn screening for inborn errors of metabolism (e.g., PKU, creatine, tyrosine disorders). Biochemical genetics is also helpful in the evaluation of malabsorption syndromes. For some of these disorders, more precise DNA testing for causative mutations is also available. Biochemical testing can differentiate heterozygous carriers from non-carriers of genes by metabolite and enzymatic analysis of physiologic fluids and tissues.

Cytogenetics is used to identify chromosome disorders that cause spontaneous abortions, congenital malformations, mental retardation, or infertility. It is used to evaluate women with gonadal dysgenesis and couples with repeated spontaneous miscarriages. Additionally, the field of cytogenetics is very important in the diagnosis and classification of leukemias, lymphomas, myeloma, and myeloproliferative diseases. This laboratory method also helps with decisions about treatment and monitoring disease status and recovery.

Fluorescence in situ hybridization (FISH) testing uses genomic microarray probes to identify well-characterized hereditary genetic microdeletion, microduplication, or rearrangement inherited disorders (such as DiGeorge syndrome). It is also helpful in the evaluation of oncology specimens (see Breast Cancer Tumor Analysis, p. 717). Many disease-specific FISH panels target subtelomeric and pericentromeric sites and locations of known microdeletion syndromes. FISH testing can assist in the diagnosis and monitoring of patients with cancer (such as breast, leukemia, and lymphomas). It can help determine the specific type of cancer present, predict disease course, and determine a course of treatment.

Microarray genetic testing can identify diseases associated with oligonucleotide and SNP-based genetic diseases. Single nucleotide polymorphisms (SNP, snips, or snippets) are variations in the genetic code at a specific point on the DNA. Like cytogenetic techniques, microarray analysis identifies unbalanced chromosomal abnormalities (loss and/or gain of DNA) in patients with unexplained abnormal phenotypes. Examples include persons with mental retardation, developmental delay, dysmorphic features, congenital anomalies, and autism. In addition, the SNP-based array will also identify long contiguous stretches of homozygosity, which may suggest an increased likelihood for a recessive condition or uniparental disomy.

Microarray FISH testing is also used to determine the presence of a genetic deletion/duplication in a family with a known inheritable disease. FISH testing is used to determine ploidy status of newborns or of cancers. FISH techniques are often used in the evaluation of amniotic fluid, products of conception, and chorionic villi.

CONTRAINDICATIONS

- Individuals/families not prepared to deal with the social and medical issues of inherited disease.

PROCEDURE AND PATIENT CARE

Before

Explain the procedure to the patient

- When testing for inheritable diseases, obtain the services of a licensed genetic counselor to inform the patient and family of the testing methods and potential results. The counselor will also provide the patient and family with potential actions that may need to be taken if the results are positive.

During

- Provide appropriate specimen to the laboratory.
- For blood, collect venous blood in a green-top (sodium heparin) tube.
- Testing is performed in a central reference laboratory and special specimen preparation may be required.

After

- If testing for inheritable diseases, ensure that arrangements have been made with the genetics counselor to provide the results to the patient and family members.

TEST RESULTS AND CLINICAL SIGNIFICANCE

Genetic errors in metabolism,

Inheritable chromosomal abnormalities,

Cancer,

Autism,

Mental retardation,

Spontaneous abortion:

The preceding list mentions just a few of the abnormalities in which laboratory genetics has had some clinical impact. This is a rapidly growing field of laboratory medicine that changes daily.

RELATED TESTS

Genetic Testing (p. 1093). These tests are used to identify disease, determine paternity, and provide forensic evidence in criminal investigations.

Breast Cancer Tumor Analysis (p. 717). These tests use many of the laboratory genetic methods described in this section.

Magnetic Resonance Imaging (MRI, Nuclear Magnetic Resonance Imaging [NMRI])

NORMAL FINDINGS

No evidence of pathology or injury

INDICATIONS

The indications for MRI change constantly as new uses for this technique are discovered. Its most important indications include evaluation of the central nervous system (CNS), neck and back, bones and joints, heart, and the breasts.

TEST EXPLANATION

MRI is a noninvasive diagnostic scanning technique that provides valuable information about the body's anatomy by placing the patient in a magnetic field. MRI is based on how hydrogen atoms behave when they are placed in a magnetic field and then disturbed by radiofrequency signals. The unique feature about MRI is that it does not require exposure to ionizing radiation. MRI has several advantages over computed tomography (CT) scanning, including the following:

- MRI provides better contrast between normal tissue and pathologic tissue.
- Obscuring bone artifacts that occur in CT scanning do not occur in MRI scanning.
- Because rapidly flowing blood appears dark, which results from its quick motion, many blood vessels appear as dark lumens. This provides a natural contrast between the blood vessels and other tissues when using MRI.
- Because spatial information depends only on how the magnetic fields are varied in space, it is possible to image the transverse, sagittal, and coronal planes directly with MRI.

MRI is useful in the evaluation of the following areas:

- Head and surrounding structures (see Figure 13-2)
- Spinal cord and surrounding structures (see Figure 13-3)
- Face and surrounding structures
- Neck
- Mediastinum
- Heart and great vessels
- Liver and biliary tree
- Kidney
- Prostate
- Bones and joints
- Breast
- Extremities and soft tissues
- Pancreas

An important advantage of MRI is that serial studies can be performed on the patient without any health risk. This is useful in assessing the response of cancer to radiotherapy and chemotherapy. A major disadvantage of MRI is that patient eligibility is reduced in comparison to CT scanning. For example, examination of patients requiring cardiac monitoring or having metal implants, metal joint replacements, pins for open reduction of fractures, pacemakers, or cerebral aneurysm clips will result in image degradation and may endanger the patient.

An *MRI of the brain* (Figure 13-2) *and meninges* is particularly accurate in identifying benign and malignant neoplasms. It is able to identify and quantify brain edema, ventricular compression, hydrocephalus, and brain herniation. Intracranial hemorrhage can also be seen on MRI. *Magnetic resonance spectroscopy (MRS)* is a noninvasive procedure that generates high-resolution clinical images based on the distribution of chemicals in the body. This is particularly useful in the brain, where certain chemical metabolites will enhance the image of a high-grade malignancy. MR spectroscopy has also been used to assess chemical abnormalities in the brain associated with HIV infection without having to perform a brain biopsy. This procedure has been used in a wide variety of disorders, including stroke, head injury, coma, Alzheimer disease, and multiple sclerosis.

MRI has revolutionized the practice of orthopedic surgery. It is particularly helpful in the determination of anatomic changes in muscle and joints (particularly knee and shoulder).

Magnetic resonance angiography (MRA) is a noninvasive procedure for viewing possible blockages in arteries. MRA has been useful in evaluation of the extracranial carotid artery and large-caliber intracranial arterial and venous structures. Cardiac abnormalities, aortic aneurysm, and anatomic variants can be identified. This procedure also has proved useful in the noninvasive detection of intracranial

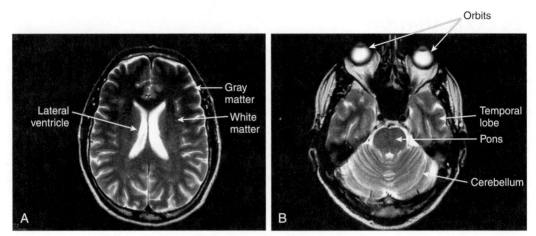

Figure 13-2 **A** and **B,** Normal MRI of the upper and lower brain levels. Note that gray matter is portrayed light and white matter is portrayed dark.

aneurysms and vascular malformations, and especially in renal artery stenosis. Coronary angiography with the resolution of most magnets is sufficient for the detection of stenosis in the large coronary arteries or venous bypass grafts but is inadequate for the detection of stenosis in smaller branches of the coronary tree.

MRI of the breast has expanded significantly over the past few years. With examiner experience, this procedure is more sensitive and specific than mammography or ultrasonography of the breast. Furthermore, lesions that previously were difficult to visualize (e.g., those close to the chest wall) are easily seen with this technique. MRI is fast becoming a reliable technique for breast imaging. MRI of the breast is used for accurate localized staging of breast cancer by demonstrating an excellent three-dimensional image of a cancer and high sensitivity for other smaller synchronously occurring breast cancers that are missed on mammography. MRI of the breast is helpful for preoperative surgical staging and the identification of postoperative positive margins. MRI of the breast can demonstrate response of a primary breast cancer to chemohormonal therapy. This study is particularly helpful in differentiating postoperative scar tissue from breast cancer recurrence. MRI of the breast is the most accurate method of determining fracture of a breast implant. Most breast protocols use a dynamic contrast enhancement pattern on fat suppressed images. Most protocols use gadolinium contrast agents. Cancers tend to enhance more rapidly than benign lesions. The washout of the contrast agent is slower than benign tumors. Interpretive radiologists use both the anatomic changes of breast tumors and gadolinium enhancement washout curves to differentiate benign from malignant tumors.

With the addition of a needle-guiding system to the MRI, breast tumors can be non-operatively and accurately localized and also biopsied. MRI of the breast is expensive and labor intensive. For that reason, it is not an effective screening tool, except for women who are at extremely high risk for the development of breast cancer.

Significant improvement in *MRI of the heart* and great vessels has moved this noninvasive diagnostic procedure into the mainstream of clinical cardiology. Cardiac MRI already is considered the procedure of choice in the evaluation of pericardial disease and intracardiac and pericardiac masses; for imaging the right ventricle and pulmonary vessels; and for assessing many forms of congenital heart disease, especially after corrective surgery. There is increasing support for the use of MRI in the assessment of ischemic heart disease. The ventricle size, shape, and blood volumes can be evaluated. Cardiac valvular abnormalities, cardiac septal defects, and suspected intracardiac or pericardiac masses or thrombi can be identified. Pericardial disease (e.g., pericarditis or effusion) is easily identified. Ventricular muscle changes from ischemia or infarction can be determined. Finally advanced MRI techniques are able to evaluate the coronary vessels directly.

Phase-contrast magnetic resonance imaging (PC-MRI) of the heart quantifies velocity and blood flow in the great arteries. Measurements of blood flow in the aorta and pulmonary trunk produce a wealth of information, including cardiac outputs of the left and right ventricles, regurgitant volumes and fraction of the aortic and pulmonary valves, and shunt ratio. Regurgitant fraction is a particularly important parameter that determines the need for valvular repair or replacement. Shunt ratio is an important parameter for evaluating the need for closing shunt lesions caused by atrial septal defects and ventricular septal defects. Velocity of moving blood is related to the pressure gradients. This relationship is used to estimate pressure gradient across stenotic cardiovascular lesions.

A combined diagnostic session of cine MRI for morphology and function, first past perfusion MRI, and late enhancement MRI to assess the heart viability is feasible in less than an hour and answers most of the relevant questions clinicians have regarding heart function and coronary patency. Stress cardiac MRI can be performed using nitrates, dobutamine, and adenosine. When beta blockers are added to EKG gating, cardiac volumes and images can be better portrayed.

Magnetic resonance cholangiopancreatography (MRCP) allows noninvasive imaging of the biliary tree, gallbladder, pancreas, and pancreatic duct. It is used to:

- Identify pancreatobiliary tumors, stones, inflammation or infection.
- Evaluate patients with pancreatitis to detect the underlying cause.
- Help in the diagnosis of unexplained abdominal pain.
- Provide a less invasive alternative to endoscopic retrograde cholangiopancreatography (ERCP).

Unlike ERCP, MRCP is not a therapeutic procedure in which papillotomy or sphincterotomy can be performed in the event that these ducts are obstructed. Indications for the use of MRCP include unsuccessful or contraindicated ERCP; patient preference for noninvasive imaging; patients considered to be at low risk of having pancreatic or biliary disease; patients in which the need for therapeutic ERCP is considered unlikely; and those with a suspected neoplastic cause for pancreatic or biliary obstruction. Complication rates are much lower for MRCP than ERCP.

MRI of the liver has improved significantly with the use of gadolinium-like contrast agent called gadoxetate (Eovist). Imaging with this agent provides extremely sharp imaging where liver and biliary tumors smaller than a centimeter can be identified. Contrast between tissues can be created by the development of the magnetic fields. However, there are multiple gadolinium-based contrast agents available to enhance MRI imaging/contrast.

Magnetic resonance enterography (MRE) is used to identify inflammatory bowel disease. It is also helpful in determining extra luminal bowel pathology. MRI is an effective tool in liver imaging and in the staging of known prostate cancers.

One of the most common uses is *MRI of the cervical or lumbar spine* (Figure 13-3). The main purpose of this test is to determine the cause of neck or back pain, respectively. The MRI is the most accurate test to identify herniated disk disease. Using different MRI protocols, an *MRI myelogram* can be performed where the spinal fluid appears white and the solid tissue (disks/nerves) appears dark. Herniated disks are easily seen and graded as to their compression on the nerves. Furthermore, MRI of the spine is able to identify subtle changes associated with early infiltrating diseases such as metastatic cancer. An *upright MRI* can scan patients in any position. The upright MRI can scan patients in their positions of symptoms (such as pain or numbness) including weight-bearing positions, such as sitting, standing, or bending. The upright MRI can provide diagnostic images of the cervical spine, lumbar spine, and the joints over their full range of motion (such as cervical flexion/extension). The front-open and top-open design of the upright MRI nearly eliminates possible claustrophobia and accommodates larger patients.

Miscellaneous Studies

13

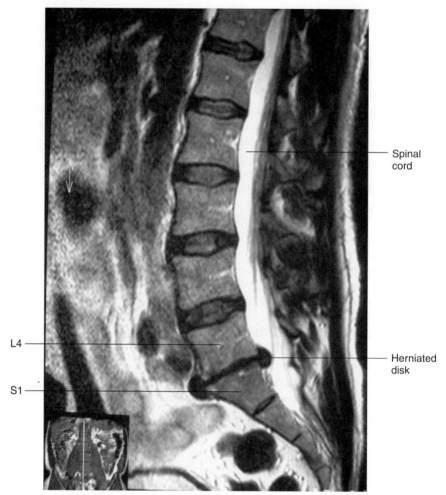

Spinal cord

L4

S1

Herniated disk

Figure 13-3 MRI of the spine demonstrating a herniated disk between lumbar vertebrae 4 and sacral vertebrae 1 compressing the spinal cord.

POTENTIAL COMPLICATIONS

- Gadolinium-based contrast agents (gadopentetate dimeglumine [Magnevist], gadobenate dimeglumine [MultiHance], gadodiamide [Omniscan], gadoversetamide [OptiMARK], gadoteridol [ProHance]) have been linked to the development of nephrogenic systemic fibrosis (NSF) or nephrogenic fibrosing dermopathy (NFD). A creatinine, BUN, and/or estimated GFR (p. 193) may be obtained, especially in adults over the age of 60.

CONTRAINDICATIONS

- Patients who are extremely obese, usually more than 300 lb
- Patients who are confused or agitated

- Patients who are claustrophobic, if an enclosed scanner is used. This can be overcome with the administration of anti-anxiety medication.
- Patients who are unstable and require continuous life support equipment, because most monitoring equipment cannot be used inside the scanner room. Magnet-adaptive equipment is becoming available for use in the MRI scanner room.
- Patients with implantable metal objects (e.g., pacemakers, cardioverter defibrillators, extensive cardiac stents, infusion pumps, aneurysm clips, inner ear implants, metal fragments in one or both eyes), because the magnet may move the object in the body and injure the patient. Piercings, braces, and retainers need to be removed.

INTERFERING FACTORS

- Movement during the scan may cause artifacts on MRI.
- Permanent retainers will cause an artifact on the scan.

✅ Clinical Priorities

- The patient must remain motionless for long intervals during MRI because movement can distort the images.
- Many patients experience a sense of claustrophobia during this test. Sedation may be necessary. This problem is decreased with an open MRI machine.
- This test cannot be performed in patients with any implanted metal objects (e.g., pacemakers). The magnet may move the object within the body and cause injury to the patient.

PROCEDURE AND PATIENT CARE

Before

 Explain the procedure to the patient.

 Inform the patient that there is no exposure to radiation.

- Obtain informed consent if required by the institution.

 Tell the patient that he or she can drive without assistance after the procedure unless anti-anxiety medications are administered to treat claustrophobia.

 Tell parents of young patients that they may read or talk to a child in the scanning room during the procedure. There is no risk of radiation from the procedure.

- Assess the patient for any contraindications for testing (e.g., aneurysm clips).

 If available, show the patient a picture of the scanning machine (Figure 13-4) and encourage verbalization of anxieties. Some patients may experience claustrophobia. Anti-anxiety medications may be helpful for those with mild claustrophobia. If possible, an open MRI system can be used for these patients.

 Tell patients that a microphone within the MRI tube allows them to communicate with personnel performing the study (Figure 13-5).

 Instruct the patient to remove all metal objects (e.g., dental bridges, jewelry, hair clips, belts), because they will create artifacts on the scan. The magnetic field can damage watches and credit cards. Also, movement of metal objects within the magnetic field can be detrimental to patients or staff within the field.

 Tell the patient wearing a nicotine patch (or any other patch with a metallic foil backing) to remove it. These patches can become intensely hot during the MRI and can cause burns.

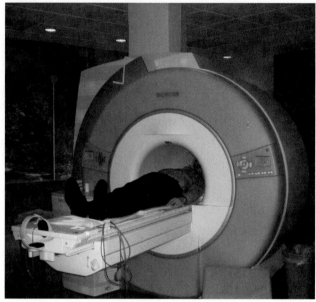

Figure 13-4 Siemens MRI. Note spacious short tube combining high-quality imaging without concerns for claustrophibia.

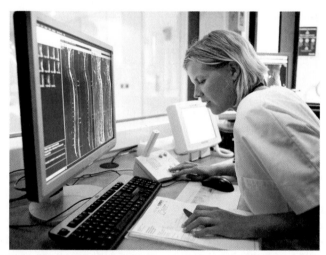

Figure 13-5 Technologist performs magnetic resonance imaging.

🖉 Inform the patient that he or she will be required to remain motionless during this study. Any movement can cause artifacts on the scan.

🖉 Tell the patient that during the procedure he or she may hear a thumping sound. Earplugs are available if the patient wishes to use them.

🖉 Inform the patient that fluid or food restrictions may be required before abdominal MRI.

🖉 For comfort, instruct the patient to empty the bladder before the test.

During

- Note the following procedural steps:
  1. The patient lies on a platform that slides into a tube containing the cylinder-shaped tubular magnet.
  2. For cardiac MRI, EKG leads are applied (p. 544).
  3. The patient is instructed to lie very still during the procedure. The patient may be asked to stop breathing for short periods of time.
  4. During the scan, the patient can talk to and hear the staff via microphone or earphones placed in the scanner.
  5. A contrast medium called gadolinium is a paramagnetic enhancement agent that crosses the blood-brain barrier. It is especially useful for distinguishing hypermetabolic abnormalities like tumors. If this is to be administered, approximately 10 to 15 mL is injected in a vein. Imaging can begin shortly after the injection. No dietary restrictions are necessary before using this agent.
- Note that a qualified radiologic technologist performs this procedure in approximately 30 minutes to several hours.
- ✒ Tell the patient that the only discomfort associated with this procedure may be lying still on a hard surface and a possible tingling sensation in teeth containing metal fillings. Also, an injection may be needed for administration of the contrast medium.

After

✒ Inform the patient that no special postprocedural care is needed.

TEST RESULTS AND CLINICAL SIGNIFICANCE

Brain

Cerebral tumor: *Natural contrast can be accentuated by varying the MRI coil. Brain tumors can be specifically diagnosed. On T1-weighted images, tumors are radiolucent (dark), whereas on T2-weighted images they are radiopaque (white). MRI is particularly useful in evaluating the pituitary gland. With gadolinium, primary brain tumors light up quickly.*

Aneurysm: *This condition is evident as compression of normal brain tissue by an enlarged vascular abnormality that is made more apparent with gadolinium. Bleeding or edema may be present with aneurysmal leak.*

Arteriovenous (AV) malformation: *MRA is useful in this problem. Large AV malformations can be seen with regular MRI as large radiolucent masses in the brain tissue.*

Hemorrhage,
Atrophy of the brain,
Subdural hematoma,
Abscess:
  MRI can demonstrate intracranial hemorrhage, abscess, or atrophy.

Degenerating diseases (e.g., multiple sclerosis, hypoxic encephalopathy, encephalomyelitis): *Specific characteristics of these diseases can be detected with MRI.*

Hydrocephalus: *This condition is evident as tremendous enlargement of the ventricular system of the brain.*

Heart

Coronary occlusive disease: *With the addition of gadolinium, stenosis in large coronary vessels can be detected. With the use of "chemical stress" testing, stenosis in smaller coronary vessels can be identified.*

Valvular heart disease: *With the use of PC-MRI, cardiac valve function can be assessed.*

Intracardiac and pericardiac masses: *Tumors and clots can easily be seen.*

Ventricular dilatation and hypertrophy: *From these images, ventricular volumes can be calculated.*

Breast

Cancer: *For high-risk patients, MRI of the breast is useful for asymptomatic women. MRI of the breast is helpful in identifying second synchronously occurring breast cancers. Images obtained from the MRI can help the surgeon plan local excision of the cancer. The extent of the ductal carcinoma in situ (DCIS) can be well demonstrated with MRI.*

Implant disruption: *MRI is the most accurate test to indicate disruption of a foreign breast implant.*

Benign tumors: *With a fairly high degree of specificity, MRI may be able to separate benign from malignant tumors. However, biopsy is always required.*

Gastrointestinal

Pancreatic cancer: *With the use of MRCP, pancreatic biliary tumors can be identified and localized. This is an alternative to ERCP.*

Inflammatory bowel disease: *With the use of oral contrast, intestinal diseases are being increasingly studied with MRI.*

Other

Herniated lumbar and cervical disks: *MRI is very sensitive for detection of these abnormalities. It is the diagnostic test of choice. MRI not only can determine disk herniation, but also demonstrate consequential nerve compression.*

Tumor (primary or metastatic): *MRI is especially useful for detection of liver, lung, and soft-tissue lesions.*

Joint disorders: *MRI is especially useful for evaluation of knee and shoulder injuries.*

Destructive lesion of bone: *With multiple-weighted images, tumors, osteomyelitis, and other destructive diseases of bone, and especially the spine, can be well demonstrated.*

Vascular disease: *Occlusive disease can be identified in the vessels of brain, chest, abdomen, and extremities.*

RELATED TEST

Computed Tomography (CT) (p. 1020). MRI and CT are not mutually exclusive. However, there are several instances in which CT scan is preferable to MRI. In most institutions, CT scanning is more readily available, especially for the patient requiring emergency imaging.

 Oximetry (Pulse Oximetry, Ear Oximetry, Oxygen Saturation)

NORMAL FINDINGS

≥95%

 Critical Values

≤75%

INDICATIONS

Oximetry is used to monitor arterial O_2 saturation levels (SaO_2) in patients at risk for hypoxemia. This includes patients who are undergoing surgery, cardiac stress testing, mechanical ventilation, heavy sedation, or lung function testing, or who have multiple trauma. It is also used as an indicator of partial pressure of oxygen (Po$_2$) in patients who may experience hypoventilation, sleep apnea, or dyspnea. This test is commonly used to titrate O$_2$ levels in hospitalized patients.

TEST EXPLANATION

Oximetry is a noninvasive method of monitoring Sao$_2$ (i.e., ratio of oxygenated hemoglobin to total hemoglobin). Sao$_2$ is expressed as a percentage; for example, Sao$_2$ of 95% indicates that 95% of the total hemoglobin attachments for O$_2$ have O$_2$ attached to them. Sao$_2$ is an accurate approximation of O$_2$ saturation obtained from arterial blood gas study (see p. 109). By correlating Sao$_2$ with the patient's physiologic status, a close estimate of Po$_2$ can be obtained.

Oximetry is typically used to monitor oxygenation status during the perioperative period and in patients receiving heavy sedation or mechanical ventilation. This test is also used in clinical situations such as pulmonary rehabilitation programs, stress testing, and sleep laboratories. Oximetry can be used to monitor response to drug therapy (e.g., theophylline). Pulse oximetry is constantly monitored during the perioperative period, and the results are one of the discharge criteria used in the postanesthesia unit.

Fetal oxygen saturation monitoring (FSpo$_2$) is very useful in the monitoring of fetal well-being during delivery. When the fetal heart rate becomes significantly abnormal (nonreassuring), C-section is often performed because of concern for fetal well-being. However, with FSpo$_2$, an accurate measure of fetal O$_2$ saturation can be determined and, if normal, C-section can be avoided. The technology is based on the same principle as adult pulse oximetry except that the machine is far more sensitive to accurately read saturations of less than 70%. After membranes are ruptured, and if the baby is in vertex position with good cervical dilatation, a specialized probe can be placed on the temple or cheek of the fetus for FSpo$_2$ monitoring. Expertise is required for appropriate placement of the sensor. The O$_2$ saturation is displayed on a monitor screen as a percentage. The normal O$_2$ saturation for a baby in the womb, receiving oxygenated blood from the placenta, is usually between 30% and 70%. When FSpo$_2$ is less than 30% for several minutes, there is marked and progressive deterioration in fetal well-being as hypoxia and acidemia progress.

O$_2$ levels can also be measured in various body tissues. For example, monitors that continuously measure tissue O$_2$ partial pressures are attached to a small catheter placed in the brain, heart, or peripheral muscle. *Brain tissue oxygen testing* and monitoring is the most common use of this technology. Used to monitor the condition of the brain following severe head trauma, it is a measure of cerebral blood flow and pulmonary oxygenation. It is more accurate than intracranial pressure in indicating brain injury.

INTERFERING FACTORS

- Extreme vasoconstriction diminishes blood flow to the peripheral vessels, which decreases the accuracy of oximetry.
- Extreme alteration in temperature may diminish the accuracy of oximetry.
- Oximetry cannot differentiate carboxyhemoglobin saturation from O$_2$ saturation. Therefore, in cases of suspected smoke or carbon monoxide (CO) inhalation, oximetry should not be used to monitor oxygenation. The levels will be falsely elevated.
- Digital motion can alter accurate readings.
- Severe anemia affects the accuracy of comparison of oximetry and Po$_2$ levels.
- Fingernail polish and fake nails will interrupt digital readings. The earlobe can be used as an alternative.
- Skin with dark pigmentation can impair digital readings.

Clinical Priorities

- Oximetry is typically used to monitor O_2 status during the perioperative period, and in patients receiving conscious sedation. It is invaluable for titrating O_2 levels.
- Oximetry cannot differentiate carboxyhemoglobin from O_2 saturation. The level could be falsely elevated in patients with smoke or CO inhalation.
- The oximetry probe cannot be used on fingertips with nail polish. In such cases, the earlobe can be used.

PROCEDURE AND PATIENT CARE

Before

✍ Explain the procedure to the patient.
✍ Tell the patient that no fasting is required.

During

- Rub the patient's fingertip or, if the ear will be used, earlobe or pinna (upper portion of the ear) to increase blood flow.
- Clip the monitoring probe or sensor to the finger or ear. A beam of light passes through the tissue, and the sensor measures the amount of light the tissue absorbs (Figure 13-6).
- This study is usually performed by a nurse's aide or nurse at the patient's bedside in a few seconds.
✍ Tell the patient that no discomfort is associated with this study.

After

- No special aftercare is needed.

TEST RESULTS AND CLINICAL SIGNIFICANCE

▲ Increased Levels

Increased fraction of inspired oxygen (Fio_2),
Hyperventilation:
   With increased alveolar O_2 caused by breathing more rapidly or increasing the O_2 in inspired air, Po_2 and O_2 can be expected to increase.

▼ Decreased Levels

Hypoventilation,
Inadequate O_2 in inspired air (suffocation):
   When ventilation is reduced enough to affect Po_2, oximetry values diminish.
Atelectasis, mucus plug, bronchospasm, pneumothorax, pulmonary edema, acute respiratory distress syndrome, restrictive lung disease: *Non-aerated portions of the lung are still perfused with unoxygenated blood. This blood returns to the heart with little or no oxygen. The O_2 content is diluted, and oximetry values diminish.*
Atrial or ventricular cardiac septal defects: *Unoxygenated blood gains access to oxygenated blood by direct shunting. By dilution, the O_2 content of the mixed blood returning to the heart is lowered, as is that of arterial blood.*
Severe hypoventilation states (e.g., oversedation, neurologic somnolence): *Without air exchange, Po_2 levels decrease.*
Pulmonary emboli: *When ventilation is reduced, oximetry values diminish.*

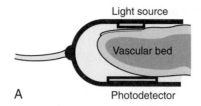

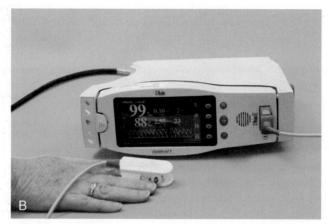

Figure 13-6 Oximetry. **A,** The pulse oximeter passes a beam of light from a light-emitting diode through a vascular bed to a photodetector. The amount of light absorbed by the oxygen-saturated hemoglobin is measured by the sensor to determine the oxygen saturation level. **B,** Pulse oximeter displays oxygen saturation and pulse rate.

RELATED TESTS

O_2 Saturation (p. 109). This is an indication of the percentage of hemoglobin saturated with O_2. This is part of arterial blood gas measurements.

Po_2 (p. 109). This is a measure of the tension (pressure [P]) of oxygen dissolved in the plasma. This pressure determines the force of O_2 to diffuse across the alveolocapillary membrane. This is part of arterial blood gas measurements.

O_2 Content (p. 109). This is a calculated number that represents the amount of O_2 in the blood.

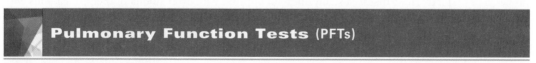

Pulmonary Function Tests (PFTs)

NORMAL FINDINGS

Vary with patient age, sex, height, and weight

INDICATIONS

The primary reasons for performing pulmonary function studies include the following:

1. *Preoperative evaluation of the lungs and pulmonary reserve.* When planned thoracic surgery will result in loss of functional pulmonary tissue, as in lobectomy (removal of part of a lung)

13 Miscellaneous Studies

or pneumonectomy (removal of an entire lung), a significant risk of pulmonary failure exists if the preoperative pulmonary function is already severely compromised by other diseases, such as chronic obstructive pulmonary disease (COPD).

2. *Evaluation of response to bronchodilator therapy.* In some patients with a spastic component to COPD, long-term use of bronchodilators may be useful. Pulmonary function studies performed before and after the use of bronchodilators will identify this group of patients.

3. *Differentiation between restrictive and obstructive forms of chronic pulmonary disease.* Restrictive defects (e.g., pulmonary fibrosis, tumors, chest wall trauma) occur when ventilation is disturbed by limitation of chest expansion. Inspiration is primarily affected. Obstructive defects (e.g., emphysema, bronchitis, asthma) occur when ventilation is disturbed by increased airway resistance. Expiration is primarily affected.

4. *Determination of the diffusing capacity of the lungs (D_L).* Rates are based on the difference in concentration of gases in inspired and expired air.

5. *Performance of inhalation tests in patients with inhalation allergies.*

TEST EXPLANATION

Pulmonary function tests are performed to detect abnormalities in respiratory function and to determine the extent of pulmonary abnormality. Pulmonary function tests routinely include spirometry, measurement of airflow rates, and calculation of lung volumes and capacities. Gas diffusion and inhalation tests (bronchial provocation) are also performed when requested, but not routinely. Exercise pulmonary stress testing can also be performed to provide data concerning pulmonary reserve. During this staged test, the patient performs an aerobic function such as stationary biking or walking on a treadmill.

Spirometry is performed first. A spirometer is a machine that can measure air volumes. When a time element is added to the tracing, airflow rates can be determined. Based on age, height, weight, race, and sex, normal values for volumes and flow rates can be predicted. Values greater than 80% of predicted values are considered normal. Spirometry provides information about obstruction or restriction of airflow. Spirometry supports the diagnosis of COPD and chronic restrictive pulmonary disease (CRPD).

Measurement of airflow rates provides information about airway obstruction. This portion of the study adds a time element to spirometry. When flow is plotted on the Y axis and volume is plotted on the X axis, flow/volume curves (isoflow loops) can be drawn when the patient is asked to maximally inhale, then forcefully exhale while being timed. The shape of the curve can be interpreted to identify and quantify airway obstruction. If airflow rates are significantly diminished (<60% of normal) or if requested by the physician, the test can be repeated after bronchodilators are administered by nebulizer. If the airflow rates improve by 20%, use of bronchodilators may be recommended for the patient. Emphysema or restrictive lung disease usually does not improve with bronchodilator therapy. Patients with an asthmatic component to COPD will benefit from bronchodilators.

Measurement of lung capacity (combination of two or more measurements of lung volume) can be performed using nitrogen or helium washout techniques. This provides further information about air trapping within the lung.

Gas exchange studies measure the diffusing capacity of the lung (D_L), that is, the amount of gas exchanged across the alveolar-capillary membrane per minute. Most laboratories use carbon monoxide (CO) to measure D_L, because CO has a great affinity for hemoglobin and only a small concentration is needed. Because of this affinity of hemoglobin for CO, the only limiting factor to the transfer of the gas is its rate of diffusion across the alveolar-capillary membrane (which is what is measured). Gas exchange is abnormal in congestive heart failure, pneumonia, and other diseases that fill the alveoli with fluid or exudate. Any disease that causes deposition of material in the interstitium of the lung (e.g., acute respiratory distress syndrome [ARDS], collagen-vascular disease, Goodpasture syndrome, pulmonary fibrosis) will decrease gas exchange.

Pulmonary function tests routinely include the following:

Forced vital capacity (FVC): Amount of air that can be forcefully expelled from a maximally inflated lung position. Less than expected values occur in obstructive and restrictive pulmonary diseases.

Forced expiratory volume in 1 second (FEV$_1$): Volume of air expelled during the first second of FVC. In obstructive pulmonary disease, airways are narrowed and resistance to flow is high. Therefore not so much air can be expelled in 1 second, and FEV$_1$ is less than the predicted value. In restrictive lung disease, FEV$_1$ is decreased because the amount of air originally inhaled is low, not because of airway resistance. Therefore the FEV$_1$/FVC ratio should be measured. In restrictive lung disease a normal value is 80%, and in obstructive lung disease this ratio is considerably less. The FEV$_1$ value will reliably improve with bronchodilator therapy if a spastic component to obstructive pulmonary disease exists.

Maximal midexpiratory flow (MMEF) or forced midexpiratory flow: Maximal rate of airflow through the pulmonary tree during forced expiration. This test is independent of the patient's effort or cooperation. MMEF volumes are lower than expected in obstructive pulmonary diseases and normal in restrictive pulmonary diseases.

Maximal volume ventilation (MVV) (formerly, maximal breathing capacity): Maximal volume of air that a patient can breathe in and out during 1 minute. It is less than the expected value in both restrictive and obstructive pulmonary disease.

A comprehensive pulmonary function study also may include evaluation of the following lung volumes and lung capacities (Figure 13-7):

Tidal volume (TV or V$_T$): Volume of air inspired and expired with each normal respiration.

Inspiratory reserve volume (IRV): Maximal volume of air that can be inspired from end of normal inspiration. It represents forced inspiration over and beyond V$_T$.

Expiratory reserve volume (ERV): Maximal volume of air that can be exhaled after normal expiration.

Residual volume (RV): Volume of air remaining in the lungs following forced expiration.

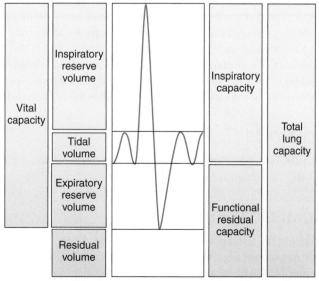

Figure 13-7 Relationship of lung volumes and capacities.

Inspiratory capacity (IC): Maximal amount of air that can be inspired after normal expiration.

$$IC = TV + IRV$$

Functional residual capacity (FRC): Amount of air left in the lungs after normal expiration.

$$FRC = ERV + RV$$

Vital capacity (VC): Maximal amount of air that can be expired after maximal inspiration.

$$VC = TV + IRV + ERV$$

Total lung capacity (TLC): Volume to which the lungs can be expanded with greatest inspiratory effort.

$$TLC = TV + IRV + ERV + RV$$

Minute volume (MV), or minute ventilation: Volume of air inhaled and exhaled per minute.

Dead space: Part of VT that does not participate in alveolar gas exchange. Includes air within the trachea.

Forced expiratory flow (FEF): Portion of airflow curve most affected by airway obstruction.

   $FEF_{200-1200}$: Rate of expired air between 200 mL and 1200 mL during FVC.

   FEF_{25-75}: Rate of expired air between 25% and 75% of flow during FVC.

Peak inspiratory flow rate (PIFR): Flow rate of inspired air during maximum inspiration. It indicates large (trachea and bronchi) airway disease.

Peak expiratory flow rate (PEFR): Maximum airflow rate during forced expiration.

Spirometry is the standard method for measuring most relative lung volumes; however, it is incapable of providing information about absolute volumes of air in the lung. Thus a different approach is required to measure residual volume, functional residual capacity, and total lung capacity. Two of the most common methods of obtaining information about these volumes are *body plethysmography* and *gas dilution tests.*

In *body plethysmography,* the patient sits inside an airtight box, inhales or exhales to a particular volume (usually functional residual capacity, FRC), and then a shutter drops across the breathing tube. The subject makes respiratory efforts against the closed shutter. Changes in total lung volumes can be easily measured instead of calculated. From those values, assuming pressures in the box are stable, airway resistance and lung compliance can be measured. Body plethysmography is particularly appropriate for patients who have airspaces within the lung that do not communicate with the bronchial tree.

Gas dilution or gas exchange studies measure the diffusing capacity of the lung (D_L) (i.e., the amount of gas exchanged across the alveolar-capillary membrane per minute). Gases like helium have densities lower than air. These gases are not affected by turbulent airflow. As a result, the use of helium provides an extremely accurate method of measuring even the most minimal airway resistance existing in small airways. This is used to test *volume of isoflow (VisoV)* that is helpful in identifying early obstructive changes.

CONTRAINDICATIONS

- Patients who are in pain, because of the inability for deep inspiration and expiration
- Patients who are unable to cooperate because of age or mental incapability

POTENTIAL COMPLICATIONS

- Light-headedness during the test, because of relative hyperventilation
- Fainting during FVC maneuver, because of Valsalva effect
- Asthmatic episode, precipitated by inhalation studies; bronchodilators may be necessary for immediate treatment

Clinical Priorities

- Patient cooperation is essential for PFTs. These tests cannot be performed in patients with pain (e.g., from surgery, fractured ribs) or any problem (e.g., mental instability) that precludes cooperation.
- Because inhalation studies can precipitate an asthmatic episode, bronchodilators may be needed for immediate treatment.

PROCEDURE AND PATIENT CARE

Before

- Explain the test to the patient.
- Inform the patient that cooperation is necessary for accurate results.
- Instruct the patient not to use any bronchodilators (if requested by health care provider) or to smoke for 6 hours before this test.
- The use of small-dose meter inhalers and aerosol therapy may be withheld before this study. Verify with the health care provider.
- Measure and record the patient's height and weight before this study to determine predicted values.
- List on the laboratory slip any medications the patient is taking.

During

- Note the following procedural steps:

Spirometry and Airflow Rates

1. The unsedated patient is taken to the pulmonary function laboratory.
2. The patient breathes through a sterile mouthpiece into a spirometer, which measures and records the values.
3. The patient is asked to inhale as deeply as possible and then forcibly exhale as much air as possible. This is repeated several (usually two to three) times. The two best values are used for calculations. This test may be repeated with bronchodilators if values are deficient.
4. The machine computes FVC, FEV_1, FEV_1/FVC, PIFR, PEFR, and MMEF.
5. The patient is asked to breathe in and out as deeply and frequently as possible for 15 seconds. The total volume breathed is recorded and multiplied by 4 to obtain MVV.
6. The patient is asked to breathe in and out normally into the spirometer and then exhale forcibly from the end-tidal volume expiration point, to measure ERV.
7. The patient is asked to breathe in and out normally into the spirometer and then inhale forcibly from the end-tidal volume expiration point, to measure IC.
8. The patient is asked to breathe in and out maximally (but not forced), to measure VC and calculated TLC.

Gas Exchange: Diffusing Capacity of Lung (D_L).

1. The D_L for any gas can be measured as part of pulmonary function studies.
2. The D_L of CO is usually measured by having the patient inhale a CO mixture.
3. $D_L co$ is calculated by analysis of the amount of CO exhaled compared with the amount inhaled.

Inhalation Tests (Bronchial Provocation Studies)

1. These tests may be performed during pulmonary function studies to establish a cause-and-effect relationship in some patients with inhalant allergies.

2. The *Provocholine challenge* test is typically used to detect the presence of hyperactive airway disease. This test is not indicated in patients with asthma.
3. Care is taken during this challenge test to reverse any severe bronchospasm with prompt administration of an inhalant bronchodilator (e.g., isoproterenol).

After

- Patients with severe respiratory problems occasionally are exhausted after PFTs, and will need rest.
- Document the procedure and the patient's response.

TEST RESULTS AND CLINICAL SIGNIFICANCE

Pulmonary fibrosis,

Interstitial lung diseases:

Interstitial lung diseases are highlighted by perialveolar inflammation followed by fibrosis. Asbestosis, ARDS, radiation fibrosis, collagen-vascular diseases, Goodpasture disease, amyloidosis, sarcoidosis, and end-stage hypersensitivity pneumonitis are some of the more common etiologic factors. Usually the FEV_1/FVC ratio is normal. Lung volumes and capacities are reduced. Hypoxemia is common. Diffusing capacity is markedly reduced.

Tumor: *Cancers of the peripheral small bronchi may not cause any changes in pulmonary function studies. Tumors of the trachea (rare) and large bronchi (common) cause a reduction in PIFR.*

Chest wall trauma: *Fractured ribs or recent surgery inhibits a patient's ability to fully cooperate with pulmonary requirements. As a result, most lung volumes and capacities will be reduced.*

Emphysema,

Chronic bronchitis,

Asthma:

Patients with COPD can be expected to have reduced airflow rates (FEV_1, FEF_{25-75}, $FEF_{200-1200}$) and abnormal airflow curves (loops). RV and ERV are increased. VC is reduced. In patients with asthma, this is reversible to a large degree with the use of bronchodilators.

Inhalant pneumonitis (e.g., farmer's lung, miner's lung): *These patients have reduced lung volumes, impaired diffusing capacity, and exercise-induced hypoxemia. There is little airflow rate abnormality.*

Post-pneumonectomy: *As expected, lung volumes and capacities are reduced. With no preexisting obstructive disease, no changes in airflow rates would be expected.*

Bronchiectasis: *These patients, with chronic and recurrent bronchiole infection pockets, have reduced airflow rates (FEV_1, FEF_{25-75}, $FEF_{200-1200}$) and abnormal airflow curves (loops), which may be reversible. They also may have some reaction to methacholine challenge.*

Airway infection: *Patients with acute bronchitis may experience transient airflow obstruction, as determined by reduced airflow rates (FEV_1, FEF_{25-75}, $FEF_{200-1200}$) and abnormal airflow curves (loops), which return to normal when the infection has resolved.*

Pneumonia: *These patients may have reduced lung volumes and capacities. Without other concurrent lung disease, there is no airflow obstruction. Diffusing capacity is impaired.*

Neuromuscular disease: *Patients with impaired muscle strength because of neuromuscular diseases (e.g., multiple sclerosis, myasthenia gravis) have reduced lung volumes and capacities.*

Hypersensitivity bronchospasm: *These patients have reversible airway obstruction (FEV_1, FEF_{25-75}, $FEF_{200-1200}$) and abnormal airflow curves (loops) when induced by methacholine challenge. Airflow rates are reduced. Lung volumes may also be affected.*

RELATED TESTS

Arterial Blood Gases (p. 109). Measurements of arterial blood O_2 and CO_2 pressure and content are useful in determining pulmonary function and calculating lung volumes and capacities.

Chest X-Ray (p. 1014). Pulmonary function can, to a small degree, be assessed with x-ray films of the chest. Hyperexpanded lungs are evidence of chronic obstructive airway disease. Pulmonary fibrosis, pneumonia, and bronchiectasis may also be evident.

Sleep Studies (Polysomnography [PSG], Multiple Sleep Latency Tests [MSLT], Multiple Wake Test [MWT])

NORMAL FINDINGS

Respiratory disturbance index (RDI): fewer than five episodes of apnea per hour
Normal progress through sleep stages
No interruption in nasal or oral airflow
End tidal CO_2: 30-45 mm Hg
Oximetry: ≥90%; no oxygen desaturation of >5%
Minimal snoring sounds
EKG: no disturbances in rate or rhythm
No evidence of restlessness
No apnea
MSLT: onset of sleep >9 minutes

INDICATIONS

Sleep studies are indicated in any person who snores excessively; experiences narcolepsy, excessive daytime sleeping, or insomnia; or has motor spasms while sleeping; and in patients with documented cardiac rhythm disturbances limited to sleep time.

TEST EXPLANATION

There are many types of sleep disorders. Most, however, are associated with impaired nighttime sleep and excessive daytime drowsiness. Sleep disorders can be caused by alterations in sleep times (e.g., night-shift workers), medications (stimulants), or psychiatric problems (e.g., depression, mania). In general, sleep disorders can be categorized as follows:

- *Dyssomnia:* Includes insomnia, sleep apnea, narcolepsy, and restless leg syndrome
- *Parasomnia:* Includes sleep walking, sleep talking, sleep terrors, and rapid eye movement disorders

Sleep studies can identify the cause of the sleep disorders and indicate appropriate treatment. Sleep studies include polysomnography (PSG) and testing for wakefulness and sleepiness. A full PSG would include:

- *Electroencephalography:* Limited to two or more channels (see p. 549)
- *Electrooculography:* Documents eye movements (see Electronystagmography, p. 557)
- *Electromyography:* Demonstrates muscle movement, usually of the chin and legs (see p. 554)
- *Electrocardiography:* EKG (see p. 544)
- *Chest impedance:* Monitors chest wall movement and respirations
- *Airflow monitors:* Measures amount of airflow in and out of the mouth and nose

- *CO_2 monitor:* Measures expiratory CO_2 levels
- *Pulse oximetry:* Monitors tissue oxygen levels (see p. 1114)
- *Sound sensors:* Used to document snoring sounds
- *Audio/video recordings:* Used to document restless motions and fitfulness
- *Esophageal pH probe:* Used only if gastroesophageal reflux is considered to be a cause of paroxysmal nocturnal dyspnea and coughing (see p. 691)

On occasions when sleep apnea alone is suspected, a four-channel PSG is performed. This more simplified test includes the electrocardiogram (EKG), chest impedance, airflow monitor, and O_2 oximetry. Video and/or audio recordings are performed also. Often a *sleep-screening study* is performed to see if full sleep studies are indicated. This is done by using pulse oximetry during sleep. If no hypoxia occurs, significant sleep apnea would be rare and full studies are not indicated.

Sleep apnea can be obstructive or central. Obstructive apnea is by far the most common and is caused by muscle relaxation of the posterior pharyngeal muscles. Breathing stops for 10 to 40 seconds. Central sleep apnea is highlighted by simple cessation of breathing rather than obstructed airway. Primary cardiac events that lead to significant and transient reduction in cardiac output can also cause apnea. Apnea from either cause is associated with increase in heart rate, decreased O_2 levels, change in brain waves, and increased expiratory CO_2. Obstructive apnea is also associated with progressively diminished airflow.

Narcolepsy is a frequent and irresistible need for sleep during daytime hours. Sleepiness can occur even during conversation or driving. Sleep studies can diagnose narcolepsy.

The restless leg syndrome is associated with an acute sensation of discomfort during periods of inactivity. It is difficult for affected patients to fall asleep and to stay asleep. Video monitoring identifies periodic limb movement—jerking of the legs associated with electroencephalogram (EEG) evidence of sleep interruption.

Parasomnias include sleepwalking and sleep-talking. Sleep terrors, associated with sudden awakening with screaming or fighting to escape a terrifying dream that the patient cannot recall, is another example of this sleep disorder.

Another sleep disorder is called rapid eye movement (REM) disorder. Normally during REM sleep, one experiences varying degrees of muscle paralysis. However, patients with REM disorders do not. They may act out their dreams in a way that varies from calling out to violent behavior. These patients can vividly recall their dreams.

Insomnia is an inability to sleep. Although it is the most common form of sleep disorder, it is usually acute and short-lived. However, when it is persistent, a sleep study is indicated. Often the pretest questionnaire can pinpoint stress or restless leg syndrome.

During a sleep study, electrodes for the EKG, EEG, electrooculography, and electromyography are applied. The chest impedance belt monitors are also placed. Under audiovisual monitoring the patient is placed in a comfortable room and sleeps. During sleep, information is synchronously gathered. The various stages of sleep architecture are determined by the EEG, and the physiologic changes during each stage are documented. By the use of the EEG, five stages of sleep can be identified (Table 13-5). The sleep study will be repeated after the patient has been using CPAP or a dental fixture for therapy. On therapy, no sleep apnea should be noted. If the sleep apnea is significant on the first night of study, a "split study" can be performed where the sleep is interrupted after 4 hours and a CPAP machine is provided for the next 4 hours. During that time, appropriate CPAP settings are calibrated to reduce apneic episodes and, at the same time, minimize uncomfortable side effects.

Testing for obstructive sleep apnea is performed in a specially constructed sleep laboratory. This is a well-insulated room in which external sounds are blocked and room temperature is easily controlled. It is performed by a certified sleep technologist and interpreted by a physician trained in sleep disorders. The study is usually completed in one night, although occasionally two nights are required. A second day is often required to administer the *multiple sleep latency test (MSLT)* or the *multiple wake test (MWT)*. The MSLT is a measure of the patient's ability to sleep during a series of structured naps. The MWT is a measure of the patient's ability to not fall asleep during a period of what should

TABLE 13-5	Stages of Sleep by EEG Changes		
Stage	Timing	EEG Changes	Time Normally Spent per Stage (%)
I	Onset of sleep	Low voltage theta/alpha waves	3-9
II	Light sleep	Sleep spindles and K complexes	47-67
III	Deeper sleep	Delta waves	3-21
IV	Deep sleep/dream sleep	High-amplitude, slow delta waves	20-29
REM	Rapid eye movement	Low-voltage, frequent nonalpha waves	20-29

be wakefulness. These tests are used to diagnose narcolepsy that follows a night of inadequate sleep. These tests can also be used to determine the success of therapy for sleep disorders.

These tests can also be used to determine the success of therapy for sleep disorders. The sleep study can be repeated after the patient has started using CPAP or a dental fixture for therapy. While on therapy, no sleep apnea should be noted. Because of the expense and the psycho-emotional difficulties associated with testing in a sleep laboratory, there has been significant growth in unattended *home sleep studies*. The patient is attached to a multichannel monitor by a sleep technician as previously described. The technician does not remain in attendance. The monitoring device records key data so that a sleep disorder can be identified.

Actigraphy can be used to determine sleep patterns and circadian rhythms. A sleep actigraph is a simple device that is worn like a wrist watch. It can be used during normal activities (except swimming or bathing) for several days and nights. It does not require an overnight stay at a sleep center. Doctors can use actigraphy to help diagnose sleep disorders, including circadian rhythm disorders, such as jet lag and shift work disorders. This test can also detect how well sleep treatments are working. Actigraphy can be used with PSG or alone. In some cases, it can replace the need for PSG.

INTERFERING FACTORS

- Psychologic insomnia associated with being in a sleep center
- Environmental noises, temperature changes, or other sensations
- Times for sleep testing different from usual times may affect sleep patterns and should be avoided

PROCEDURE AND PATIENT CARE

Before

- Explain the procedure to the patient.
- Tell the patient that caffeine products should be avoided for several days before testing as they may delay onset of sleep.
- Sedatives are prohibited as they will alter usual sleep patterns.
- Reassure the patient that monitoring equipment will not interrupt the sleeping pattern.
- Allow the patient to express concerns about videotaping and other forms of monitoring.
- Several sleep rating questionnaires are completed by both the patient and his or her sleeping partner.
- Age, weight, and medial history are recorded.

During

- Electrodes for EKG, EEG, electrooculography, and electromyography are applied. Excessive hair may need to be shaved in male patients.

- Airflow, oximetry, and impedance monitors are applied.
- Once the patient is comfortable, he or she is allowed to sleep.
- The lights are turned off and monitoring begins before the patient is asleep.
- For PSG, the patient is asked to sleep per usual process.

Multiple Sleep Latency Testing
- The test is typically done in the morning.
- The patient is asked to nap about every 2 hours throughout the testing period.
- The nap is terminated after 20 minutes.
- Between naps the patient must stay awake.

Multiple Wake Testing
- The patient is asked to stay awake and not nap.
- Monitoring is similar to that described for PSG except for impedance, sound, and airflow monitors.

After
- On completion of the sleep cycle, the monitors and electrodes are removed.
- Test results take several days to collate and interpret.

TEST RESULTS AND CLINICAL SIGNIFICANCE

Obstructive sleep apnea: *Patients experience apneic episodes for 10 seconds or more. They experience synchronous periods of O_2 desaturation and experience sleep disturbances on EEG, increase in cardiac rate, and decreased airflow.*

Central sleep apnea: *Patients do not have the stimulus to breathe during the apneic episode. Otherwise, the findings are nearly the same as for obstructive sleep apnea. Snoring and chest impedance extremes are absent. Cardiac arrhythmia may be observed.*

Insomnia: *These patients demonstrate a delay in falling asleep. They may also show evidence of restless leg syndrome.*

Narcolepsy: *These patients will demonstrate EEG changes compatible with sleep rather than napping. The time in which they fall asleep is less than 5 minutes on repeated napping.*

Restless leg syndrome: *These patients will experience excessive extremity motion before and after sleep.*

Parasomnia: *These patients may demonstrate sleepwalking or phonating.*

REM disorder: *These patients may sleep restlessly and move about as if fighting or escaping terror.*

Tuberculin Skin Testing (TST, Tuberculin Test, Mantoux Test, PPD Test)

NORMAL FINDINGS

Negative, reaction <5 mm

INDICATIONS

Tuberculin testing is performed for persons who are:
1. Suspected of having active TB (e.g., patients with suspicious chest x-ray findings, productive cough with negative routine cultures, hemoptysis, or undetermined weight loss)

2. At increased risk for progression to active TB
3. At increased risk for latent TB infection (LTBI) (e.g., health care workers, recent transplant organ recipients, HIV patients, recent immigrants, IV drug abusers, or those in close contact with someone known to have TB)
4. At low risk for LTBI, but are tested for other reasons (e.g., entrance to college)

TEST EXPLANATION

Purified protein derivative (PPD) of the tubercle bacillus is injected intradermally. If the patient is infected with or has been exposed to TB (whether active or dormant), lymphocytes will recognize the PPD antigen and cause a local inflammatory reaction (Boxes 13-3 and 13-4). Although this test is used to detect TB infection, results do not indicate whether the infection is active or dormant. If test results are negative but the physician strongly suspects TB, testing with "second-strength" PPD can be performed. If these test results are negative, the patient has not been exposed to TB (see p. 768 for tuberculosis culture). Results of PPD skin testing usually become positive 6 weeks after infection. Once positive, the reaction usually persists for life. Box 13-5 lists patients in whom test results may revert to negative or fail to become positive.

The PPD test also can be used as part of a series of skin tests performed to assess the immune system. If the immune system is nonfunctioning because of poor nutrition or chronic illness (e.g., neoplasia, infection, AIDS), PPD test results will be negative despite active or dormant TB infection. Other pathogens used in skin tests to test immune function include *Candida*, mumps virus, and *Trichophyton*, organisms most people in the United States have been exposed to. It has been well established that any surgery is associated with greater mortality in patients with negative skin tests than in patients who react to these common pathogen skin tests. Box 13-6 lists skin tests for other diseases.

There is now an alternative to skin testing. For example, the *QuantiFERON-TB Gold Test (QFT)* is a blood test used as an aid in diagnosing *Mycobacterium tuberculosis* infection (see Tuberculosis Testing, p. 770).

Laboratory testing for TB is usually performed as part of routine prenatal evaluation in pregnant women. Often this may be the mother's first contact with the health care system in several years.

BOX 13-3	Criteria for Positive PPD Test Results in Patients With No Previous PPD Results

Diameter of Induration 48-72 Hours After PPD Injection

≥5 mm (high risk)
- Human immunodeficiency virus (HIV) infection
- Close recent contact with a person with active TB
- Patients with chest x-ray findings consistent with old, healed TB granulomatous infection

≥10 mm (moderate risk)
- Foreigners from continents with high TB rate (e.g., Asia, Africa, South America)
- Intravenous drug abusers
- Economically poor in the United States
- Nursing home residents
- Medical conditions associated with high risk for TB (e.g., malnutrition, post-gastrectomy, steroid use, cancer, diabetes)
- Worker in a long-term care facility

≥15 mm
- Persons who do not fulfill above criteria

BOX 13-4	Criteria for Positive PPD Conversion in Patients With Previously Documented Negative PPD

- Younger than 35 years old: Increase in PPD-induced induration of ≥10 mm within 2 years of last PPD test
- Older than 35 years old: Increase in PPD induration of ≥15 mm within 2 years of last PPD test

BOX 13-5	Conditions in Which PPD Test Results May Demonstrate No Reaction Despite Patient Exposure or Will Revert to Negative

- Fully cured TB
- Malnutrition
- Immunocompromised (e.g., from acquired immunodeficiency syndrome [AIDS], cancer therapy, advanced cancers [e.g., leukemia, lymphoma])
- Overwhelming infection (e.g., bacterial, viral, or miliary TB)
- Steroid therapy
- Sarcoidosis

BOX 13-6	Skin Tests for Other Diseases

- Schick test: Shows previous exposure to diphtheria
- Dick test: Demonstrates antibody development to group A streptococci (scarlet fever)
- Allergy skin testing: Evaluates molds, dust, pollen, other allergens (see p. 1079)

PPD testing is associated with no complications, except in patients known to have active TB or who have been vaccinated against TB. In these patients, local reaction may be so severe as to cause complete skin slough, requiring surgical care. PPD testing will not cause active TB because the test solution contains no live organisms.

CONTRAINDICATIONS

- Patients with active TB
- Patients who have received the immunization against PPD with *bacille Calmette-Guérin (BCG)* because these patients will demonstrate a positive reaction to PPD vaccine even if they have never had TB infection
- Patients who have a skin rash that would make it hard to read the skin test.

INTERFERING FACTORS

- Subcutaneous injection of PPD may cause a negative reaction. The injection must be intradermal for induration to occur.
- Immunocompromised patients will not react to PPD despite exposure to TB.
- Improper storage of PPD can cause false-negative results.
- Improper dosage of PPD can cause false-negative results.

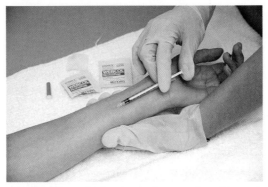

Figure 13-8 Intradermal injection in forearm for skin testing.

 Clinical Priorities

- Positive PPD test results indicate previous exposure, not necessarily active infection. Active infection should be ruled out with appropriate cultures and other diagnostic tests.
- PPD testing should not be performed in patients with active TB or patients who have received BCG vaccine, because local skin reaction may cause complete skin slough requiring surgery.
- If the immune system is nonfunctioning because of poor nutrition or chronic illness, PPD test results may be negative even if the patient has active or dormant TB infection.
- If the immune system is nonfunctioning because of poor nutrition or chronic illness, PPD test results may be negative even if the patient has active or dormant TB infection.

PROCEDURE AND PATIENT CARE

Before
✍ Explain the procedure to the patient.
✍ Assure the patient that TB will not develop from this test.
- Assess the patient for previous history of TB. Report a positive history to the physician.
- Evaluate the patient's history for previous PPD results and BCG immunization.

During
- Prepare the volar (inner) forearm with alcohol, and allow it to dry.
- Intradermally inject PPD (Figure 13-8). A skin wheal (nearly 1 cm) should develop.
- Circle the area with indelible ink. Do not cover with a Band-Aid.
- Record the time when the PPD was injected.

After
- Have a health care professional read the results in 48 to 72 hours.
- Examine the test site for induration (hardening), and encircle the area of induration. Measure the area of induration (not redness) in millimeters.
- If the test results are positive, ensure that the physician is notified and the patient is given appropriate treatment.
- If the test results are positive, check the patient's arm 4 to 5 days after the test to be certain that a severe skin reaction has not occurred.

TEST RESULTS AND CLINICAL SIGNIFICANCE
Positive Results
TB infection,

Nontuberculous *Mycobacteria* infection:

> *Positive results indicate previous exposure, not necessarily active infection. Active infection should be ruled out with appropriate cultures and other diagnostic tests.*

Negative Results
Possible immunoincompetence in chronically ill patients: *Immunocompromised patients and patients who have not been exposed to TB will not react to PPD. In other patients, positive results can revert to negative (see Box 13-5). Immunocompromised patients will not respond to other common pathogens.*

RELATED TESTS
Acid-Fast Bacilli Smear (p. 706). This smear (usually sputum) is used to support the diagnosis of TB. By itself it cannot confirm a diagnosis of TB. This smear test is also used to monitor treatment for TB.

Chest X-Ray (p. 1014). Because TB is most usually infective to the lungs, as a result of inhalation of airborne infectious material, the chest x-ray film often demonstrates the results (Ghon complex) of acute granulomatous infection.

Tuberculosis Culture (p. 768). This is the only way to confirm a diagnosis of TB. When TB is grown from culture of a specimen, the diagnosis of TB can be made and treatment based on drug sensitivities can be started.

Tuberculosis Testing (p. 770). This is a blood test that can identify active and latent TB infection.

 Urea Breath Test (UBT, *H. pylori* breath test)

NORMAL FINDINGS
<50 dpm (if ^{14}C is used)

<3% (if ^{13}C is used)

INDICATIONS
This test is used to detect *Helicobacter pylori (H. pylori)* infections. It is indicated in patients who have recurrent or chronic gastric or duodenal ulceration or inflammation. When the *H. pylori* infection is successfully treated, the ulcer or inflammation will usually heal.

TEST EXPLANATION
H. pylori is a bacterium that can be found in the mucus overlying the gastric mucosa and in the mucosa (cells that line the stomach). It is a risk factor for gastric and duodenal ulcers, chronic gastritis, or even ulcerative esophagitis. This gram-negative bacillus is also a class I gastric carcinogen. Gastric colonization by this organism has been reported in about 90% to 95% of patients with a duodenal ulcer; in 60% to 70% of patients with a gastric ulcer; and in about 20% to 25% of patients with gastric cancer. There are several serologic and microscopic methods of detecting *H. pylori* (see *Helicobacter pylori* Testing, p. 1101).

The UBT is the noninvasive test of choice for diagnosis of *H. pylori* infection. It is based on the capability of *H. pylori* to metabolize urea to CO_2 because of the organism's capability to produce a large amount of urease. In the breath test, carbon (^{13}C) labeled urea is administered orally. The urea is then absorbed through the gastric mucosa. If *H. pylori* is present, the urea will be converted to $^{13}CO_2$. The $^{13}CO_2$ is then taken up by the capillaries in the stomach wall and delivered to the lungs where it is exhaled. The labeled carbon can be measured by gas chromatography or a mass spectrometer.

This test has been simplified to the point that two breath samples collected before and 30 minutes after the ingestion of urea in a liquid form suffice to provide reliable diagnostic information. Labeling urea with ^{13}C is becoming increasingly popular because it is a nonradioactive isotope of ^{14}C and is innocuous. It can be safely used in children and women of childbearing age.

INTERFERING FACTORS

- Dietary constituents with a natural abundance of ^{13}C, such as maize, cane, and corn flour, can cause increased levels.
- Bismuth (Pepto Bismol) or sucralfate (Carafate) will suppress mucosal uptake of the urea and interfere with test results.
- The concomitant use of a proton pump inhibitor, such as Prilosec, Nexium, Prevacid, or Protonix, will also inhibit urea absorption.

PROCEDURE AND PATIENT CARE

Before

- Explain the procedure to the patient.
- Instruct the patient to abstain from oral intake for 6 hours before testing.
- If radioactive carbon (rare) is being used, be sure that female patients are not pregnant.
- When providing the isotopic urea to the patient, instruct the patient as to proper administration (per local laboratory routine).

During

- Several minutes after the patient has swallowed the carbon dose, provide the patient with 2 oz of water.
- Breath samples are collected in any one of a number of gas collection devices depending on how and when the sample will be analyzed.

After

- Instruct the patient to resume medications and normal diet
- If radioactive carbon was used, instruct the patient to drink plenty of fluids to facilitate excretion of the radioisotope.

TEST RESULTS AND CLINICAL SIGNIFICANCE

H. pylori infection: *This bacterium is detected in infected patients.*

RELATED TESTS

Helicobacter pylori Testing (p. 1101). This is the main serologic method of detecting *H. pylori* infection.
Esophagogastroduodenoscopy (p. 608). This endoscopic procedure is used to directly biopsy the gastric mucosa for definitive *H. pylori* identification.

BIBLIOGRAPHY

Bain LJ, Barker W, Loewenstein CA, Duara R: Towards an earlier diagnosis of Alzheimer disease (Proceedings of the 5th MCI Symposium, 2007), *Alzheimer Dis Assoc Disord* 22:99–110, 2008.

Ball EM, et al: Diagnosis and treatment of sleep apnea within the community: the Walla Walla project, *Arch Intern Med* 157(4):419–424, 1997.

Bird TD, Miller BL: Dementia. In Fauci AS et al, editors: *Harrison's principles of internal medicine,* ed 17, New York, 2008.

Brenner H, et al: Protection from colorectal cancer after colonoscopy, *Ann Int Med* 154:22–30, 2011.

Castle PE, et al: Five year experience of human papilloma virus DNA and Papanicolaou test co-testing, *Obstet Gynecol* 113:595–600, 2009.

Catalona WJ, et al: Use of the percentage of free prostate-specific antigen to enhance differentiation of prostate cancer from benign prostatic disease, *JAMA* 279(19):1542, 1998.

Catto AJ, et al: Plasminogen activator inhibitor-1 (PAI-1) 4G/5G promoter polymorphism and levels in subjects with cerebrovascular disease, *Thromb Haemost* 77(4):730–740, 1997.

Cavert W, Balfour HH: Detection of antiretroviral resistance in HIV-1, *Clin Lab Med* 23:915–928, 2003.

Centers for Disease Control and Prevention: Seasonal influenza: http://www.cdc.gov/flu/.

Christenson RH, et al: Multi-center determination of galectin-3 assay performance characteristics: anatomy of a novel assay for use in heart failure, *Clin Biochem* 43:683–690, 2010.

Collinson PO: The need for point of care testing: an evidence-based appraisal, *Scand J Clin Lab Invest Suppl (UCR)* 230:67–73, 1999.

Cooper D, et al: Maraviroc versus efavirenz, both in combination with zidovudine-lamivudine, for the treatment of antiretroviral-naive subjects with CCR5-tropic HIV-1 infection, *J Infect Dis* 201:803–813, 2010.

Danesh J, et al: C-reactive protein and other circulation markers of inflammation in the prediction of coronary heart disease, *N Engl J Med* 350(14):1387–1397, 2004.

de Boer RA, et al: Predictive value of plasma galectin-3 levels in heart failure with reduced and preserved ejection fraction, *Ann Med* 43:60–68, 2011.

DeLuca HF: Overview of general physiologic features and functions of vitamin D, *Am J Clin Nutr* 80(suppl 6): 1689S–1696S, 2004.

Dirkmann D, Hanke AA, Görlinger K, Peters J: Hypothermia and acidosis synergistically impair coagulation in human whole blood, *Anesth Analg* 106:1627–1632, 2008.

Etzioni R, et al: Is prostate-specific antigen velocity useful in early detection of prostate cancer? A critical appraisal of the evidence, *J Natl Cancer Inst* 99:1510–1514, 2007.

Felker GMFiuzat MShaw LK, et al: Galectin-3 in ambulatory patients with heart failure: results from the HF-ACTION Study, *Circ Heart Fail* 5(1):72–78, 2012.

Ferlay J, et al: Estimates of worldwide burden of cancer in 2008, *Int J Cancer* 127:2893–2917, 2010.

Foster G, Stocks C, Borofsky S: Emergency department visits and hospital admissions for kidney stone disease, 2009. Healthcare costs and utilization project statistics, *AHRQ* 139, July 2012.

Giannitsis E, Katus HA: Strategies for clinical assessment of patients with suspected acute coronary syndromes, *Scand J Clin Lab Invest Suppl (UCR)* 230:36–42, 1999.

Gray W, et al: The future of cytopathology in Europe. Will the wider use of HPV testing have an impact on the provision of cervical screening? *Cytopathology* 18:278–282, 2007 (review).

Grundy SM, et al: Implications of recent clinical trials for the National Cholesterol Education Program Adult Treatment Panel III Guidelines, *Circulation* 110(2):227–239, 2004.

Hackam DG, Anand SS: Emerging risk factors for atherosclerotic vascular disease, *JAMA* 290(7):932–940, 2003.

Hancock RD: Venipuncture vs. arterial catheter activated partial thromboplastin times in heparinized patients, *Dimens Crit Care Nurs* 12(5):238–245, 1993.

Hasbun R, et al: Computed tomography of the head before lumbar puncture in adults with suspected meningitis, *N Engl J Med* 345(24):1727–1733, 2001.

Hirsch MS, et al: Antiretroviral drug resistance testing in adult HIV-1 infection: 2008 recommendations of an International AIDS Society-USA Panel, *Clin Infect Dis* 47:266–285, 2008.

Hirsch R, et al: NGAL is an early predictive biomarker of contrast-induced nephropathy in children, *Pediatr Nephrol* 22(12):2089–2095, 2007.

Ho GY, et al: Natural history of cervicovaginal papillomavirus infection in young women, *N Engl J Med* 338(7):423–428, 1998.

Holick MF: Vitamin D deficiency, *N Engl J Med* 357:266–281, 2007.

Kägi G, Bhatia KP, Tolosa E: The role of DAT-SPECT in movement disorders, *J Neurol Neurosurg Psychiatry* 81(1):5–12, 2010.

Kitchener HC, et al: Comparison of HPV DNA testing and liquid base cytology, *Eur J Cancer* 47:864–871, 2011.

Knight EL, et al: Atrial natriuretic peptide and the development of congestive heart failure in the oldest old: a seven-year prospective study, *J Am Geriatr Soc* 47:407–411, 1999.

Kohler HP, Grant PJ: Plasminogen-activator inhibitor type I and coronary disease, *N Engl J Med* 342(24):1792–1801, 2000.

Lensing AW, et al: A comparison of compression ultrasound with color Doppler ultrasound for diagnosis of symptomless postoperative deep vein thrombosis, *Arch Intern Med* 157(7):758–762, 1997.

Levin B, et al: Screening and surveillance for the early detection of colorectal cancer and adenomatous polyps, *CA Cancer J Clin* 58(3):130–160, 2008.

Li N, et al: HPV distribution in 30,848 invasive cervical cancers worldwide, *Int J Cancer* 128:927–935, 2011.

Lok DJ, et al: Prognostic value of galectin-3, a novel marker of fibrosis, in patients with chronic heart failure: data from the DEAL-HF study, *Clin Res Cardiol* 99:323–328, 2010.

Lorenz MW, et al: Prediction of clinical cardiovascular events with carotid intima-media thickness: a systematic review and meta-analysis, *Circulation* 115(4):459–467, 2007.

Mayrand M, et al: Human papillomavirus DNA versus Papanicolaou screening tests for cervical cancer, *N Engl J Med* 357(16):1579–1588, 2007.

Meerhoff TJ, et al: Detection of multiple respiratory pathogens during primary respiratory infection: nasal swab versus nasopharyngeal aspirate using real-time polymerase chain reaction, *Eur J Clin Microbiol Infect Dis* 29:365–371, 2010.

Mullins MD, et al: The role of spiral volumetric computed tomography in the diagnosis of pulmonary embolism, *Arch Intern Med* 160(3):293–298, 2000.

Murphy MJ, Berding CB: Use of measurements of myoglobin and cardiac troponins in the diagnosis of acute myocardial infarction, *Crit Care Nurs* 19(1):58–66, 1999.

Mussolino ME, et al: Phalangeal bone density and hip fracture risk, *Arch Intern Med* 157(4):433–438, 1997.

Nordberg A: Amyloid plaque imaging in vivo: current achievement and future prospects, *Eur J Nucl Med Mol Imaging* 35(suppl 1):S46–S50, 2008.

Novel H1N1 Flu (swine flu): Available from http://www.cdc.gov.

O'Brien JT: Role of imaging techniques in the diagnosis of dementia, *Br J Radiol* 80(2):S71–S77, 2007.

O'Brien JT, et al: Progressive brain atrophy on serial MRI in dementia with Lewy bodies, AD, and vascular dementia, *Neurology* 56:828–834, 2001.

Olaison L, et al: Fever, C-reactive protein, and other acute-phase reactants during treatment of infective endocarditis, *Arch Intern Med* 157(8):885–892, 1997.

O'Shaughnessy JA: Recent advances in the treatment of metastatic breast cancer, *Clin Oncol Updates* 5(2):1–20, 2002.

Pagana KD, Pagana TJ: *Mosby's diagnostic and laboratory test references*, ed 11, St Louis, 2011, Mosby.

Parente DB, et al: Potential role of diffusion tensor MRI in the differential diagnosis of mild cognitive impairment and Alzheimer's disease, *Am J Roentgenol* 190:1369–1374, 2008.

Pearson TA, et al: Markers of inflammation and cardiovascular disease, *Circulation* 107:499–511, 2003.

Pickhardt PJ, et al: Computed tomographic virtual colonoscopy to screen for colorectal neoplasia in asymptomatic adults, *N Engl J Med* 349(23):2191–2200, 2005.

Plebani M, Zaninotto M: Cardiac marker: present and future, *Int J Clin Lab Res* 29(2):56–63, 1999.

Polascik TJ, Oesterling JE, Partin AW: Prostate-specific antigen: a decade of discovery—what we have learned and where we are going, *J Urol* 162:293–306, 1999.

Potter SR, Reckwitz T, Partin AW: The use of percent free PSA for early detection of prostate cancer, *J Androl* 20(4):449–453, 1999.

Preisman S, Kogan A, Itzkovsky K, Leikin G, et al: Modified TEG evaluation of platelet dysfunction patients undergoing coronary artery surgery, *Eur J Cardiothorac Surg* 37:1367–1374, 2010.

Quintero E, et al: Colonoscopy versus fecal immunochemical testing in colorectal cancer screening, *J Med* 336:697–706, 2012.

Rao JK, et al: The role of antineutrophil cytoplasmic antibody (c-ANCA) testing in the diagnosis of Wegener granulomatosis, *Ann Intern Med* 123(2):925–932, 1995.

Rice MS, MacDonald DC: Appropriate roles of cardiac troponins in evaluating patients with chest pain, *J Am Board Fam Pract* 12(3):214–218, 1999.

Ridker PM: Evaluating novel cardiovascular risk factors: can we better predict heart attacks? *Ann Intern Med* 130(11):933–937, 1999.

Ridker PM, et al: C-reactive protein, the metabolic syndrome, and risk of incident cardiovascular events, *Circulation* 107:391–397, 2003.

Ronco G, et al: Human papillomavirus testing and liquid-based cytology in primary screening of women younger than 35 years: results at recruitment for a randomised controlled trial, *Lancet Oncol* 7(7):547–555, 2006.

Rosen CJ, Tenenhouse A: Biochemical markers of bone turnover, *Postgrad Med* 104(4):101–114, 1998.

Ross R: Atherosclerosis—an inflammatory disease, *N Engl J Med* 340:115–126, 1999.

Rypins E, et al: Scintigraphic determination of equivocal appendicitis, *Am Surg* 66(9):891–895, 2000.

Saraiya M, et al: Cervical cancer screening, *Int Med* 170:977–985, 2010.

Saslow D, et al: American Cancer Society guidelines for the early detection of cervical neoplasia and cancer, *CA Cancer J Clin* 52:342–362, 2002.

Savarino V, Vigneri S, Celle G: The 13C urea breath test in the diagnosis of *Helicobacter pylori* infection, *Gut* 45(suppl 1):I18–I22, 1999.

Shariat SF, et al: Urine detection of survivin is a sensitive marker for the noninvasive diagnosis of bladder cancer, *J Urol* 171:626–630, 2004.

Smith RA, Cokkinides V, Brawley OW: Cancer screening in the United States, 2008: a review of current American Cancer Society guidelines and cancer screening issues, *CA Cancer J Clin* 58(3):161–179, 2008.

Smith RA, et al: American Cancer Society guidelines for breast cancer screening: update 2003, *CA Cancer J Clin* 53:141–169, 2003.

Solomon PR, Murphy CA: Early diagnosis and treatment of Alzheimer's disease, *Expert Rev Neurother* 8:769–780, 2008.

Stevens LA, et al: Estimating GFR using serum cystatin C alone and in combination with serum creatinine: a pooled analysis of 3418 individuals with CKD, *Am J Kidney Dis* 51(3):395–406, 2008.

Stolzenber-Solomon RZ, et al: A prospective nested case-control study of vitamin D status and pancreatic cancer risk in male smokers, *Cancer Res* 66:10213–10219, 2006.

Sutinen J: Etiology of central nervous system infections in the Philippines and the role of serum C-reactive protein in excluding acute bacterial meningitis, *Int J Infect Dis* 3(2):88–93, 1998.

Swenson L, et al: Deep sequencing to infer HIV-1 co-receptor usage: application to three clinical trials of maraviroc in treatment-experienced patients, *J Infect Dis* 203:237–245, 2011.

Swenson L, et al: Deep V3 sequencing for HIV type 1 tropism in treatment-naive patients: a reanalysis of the MERIT trial of maraviroc, *Clin Infect Dis* 53:732–742, 2011.

Thompson MA, et al: Antiretroviral treatment of adult HIV infection: 2010 recommendations of the International AIDS Society-USA Panel, *JAMA* 304:321–333, 2010.

VanMeurs JB, et al: Homocysteine levels and the risk of osteoporotic fracture, *N Engl J Med* 350(20):2033–2041, 2004.

Vogester M, Jacob K: B-type natriuretic peptide (BNP): validation of an immediate response assay, *Clin Lab* 47:29–33, 2001.

Wagner J, et al: Noninvasive prenatal paternity testing from maternal blood, *Int J Legal Med* 123:75–79, 2009.

Walsh PC, et al: Chemoprevention of prostate cancer, *J Med* 362:1237–1238, 2010.

Weintraub NL, et al: Acute heart failure syndromes: emergency department presentation, treatment, and disposition: current approaches and future aims: a scientific statement from the American Heart Association, *Circulation* 122:1975–1996, 2010.

Yeh ET, Willerson JT: Coming of age of C-reactive protein, *Circulation* 107:370–372, 2003.

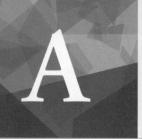

D

E

List of Tests by Body System

Tests in this list are grouped by the following body systems: cancer, cardiovascular, endocrine, gastrointestinal, hematologic, hepatobiliary, immunologic, miscellaneous, nervous system, pulmonary, reproductive system, skeletal system, and urologic system.

Cancer Studies

Acid phosphatase, 25
Bence-Jones protein, 911
Beta$_2$ microglobulin (B$_2$M), 360
Bladder cancer markers, 914
Bladder tumor antigen (BTA), 914
Bone scan, 782
Breast cancer genetic screening, 1093
Breast cancer genomics, 1086
Breast cancer tumor analysis, 717
Breast ductal lavage, 645
Breast scintigraphy, 789
CA 15-3 and CA 27-29 tumor markers, 130
CA 19-9 tumor marker, 132
CA-125 tumor marker, 135
Carcinoembryonic antigen (CEA), 145
Cell culture drug resistance testing, 1087
Ductoscopy, 603
Estrogen receptor assay, 728
Gallium scan, 799
Lymphoscintigraphy, 837
Mammography, 1043
Melanoma genetic testing, 1093
Microglobulin, 933
Neuron-specific enolase, 369
Nuclear matrix protein 22 (NMP22), 914
Octreotide scan, 817
Ovarian cancer genetic screening, 1093
Papanicolaou test, 743
Parotid gland scan, 834
Progesterone receptor assay, 750
ProstaScinct Scan, 827
Prostate specific antigen (PSA), 420

Salivary gland nuclear scan, 834
Sentinel lymph node biopsy, 837
Serotonin and chromogranin A, 462
Sputum cytology, 763
Squamous cell carcinoma antigen, 469
Thyroglobulin (Tg), 484

Cardiovascular Studies

Adenosine stress, 540
Aldosterone, blood, 43
Antimyocardial antibody, 86
Antistreptolysin O titer, 470
Apolipoprotein, 106
Arteriography (renal, adrenal, cerebral, lower extremity), 988
Aspartate aminotransferase (AST), 119
Atrial natriuretic peptide (ANP), 367
Brain natriuretic peptide (BNP), 367
CHF peptides, 367
Cardiac catheterization, 1008
Cardiac nuclear scan, 791
Cardiac stress testing, 540
Cardiovascular genetic screening, 1093
Catecholamines, 975
Cholesterol, 154
Computed tomography (CT), heart, 1032
Creatine kinase (CK), 186
Creatine phosphokinase, 186
C-type natriuretic peptide (CNP), 367
Digital subtraction angiography, 988
2,3-Diphosphoglycerate, 208
Dipyridamole thallium scan, 540
Dobutamine stress, 540
Doppler studies (venous and arterial), 900
Echocardiography, 877
Electrocardiography (ECG, EKG), 544
Electrophysiologic study (EPS), 559
Galectin-3, 245
Holter monitoring, 571

Endocrine Studies

Hepatobiliary Studies

Immunologic Studies

Miscellaneous Studies

Nervous System Studies

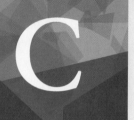

Panel Testing

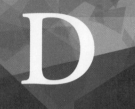

Abbreviations for Diagnostic and Laboratory Tests

A

AAT	Alpha$_1$-antitrypsin
ABEP	Auditory brainstem evoked potential
ABGs	Arterial blood gases
ACE	Angiotensin-converting enzyme
ACT	Activated clotting time
ACTH	Adrenocorticotropic hormone
ADH	Antidiuretic hormone
AFB	Acid-fast bacilli
AFP	Alpha-fetoprotein
A/G ratio	Albumin/globulin ratio
AIT	Agglutination inhibition test
ALA	Aminolevulinic acid
ALP	Alkaline phosphatase
ALT	Alanine aminotransferase
AMA	Antimitochondrial antibody
ANA	Antinuclear antibody
ANC	Absolute neutrophil count
ANCA	Antineutrophil cytoplasmic antibody
ANP	Atrial natriuretic peptide
APCA	Anti–parietal cell antibody
APTT	Activated partial thromboplastin time
ASMA	Anti–smooth muscle antibody
ASO	Antistreptolysin O titer
AST	Aspartate aminotransferase

B

B$_2$M	Beta$_2$ microglobulin
BE	Barium enema
BMC	Bone mineral count
BMD	Bone mineral density
BPP	Biophysical profile
BRCA	Breast cancer
BTA	Bladder tumor antigen
BSAP	Bone specific alkaline phosphatase
BNP	Brain natriuretic peptide
BUN	Blood urea nitrogen

C

Ca	Calcium
CAT	Computerized axial tomography
CBC	Complete blood cell count
CrCl	Creatinine clearance
CEA	Carcinoembryonic antigen
CK	Creatine kinase
Cl	Chloride
CLO	*Campylobacter*-like organism
CMG	Cystometrogram
CMV	Cytomegalovirus
CNP	C-type natriuretic peptide
CO	Carbon monoxide
CO$_2$	Carbon dioxide
COHb	Carboxyhemoglobin test
CP, CPK	Creatine phosphokinase
CRP	C-reactive protein
C&S	Culture and sensitivity
CSF	Cerebrospinal fluid
CST	Contraction stress test
CT	Computed tomography
cTnI	Cardiac troponin I
cTnT	Cardiac troponin T
CVB	Chorionic villi biopsy
CVS	Chorionic villi sampling
CXR	Chest x-ray

D

D&C	Dilation and curettage
DEXA	Dual-energy x-ray absorptiometry
DHEA	Dehydroepiandrosterone
DIC	Disseminated intravascular coagulation
DSMA	Disodium monomethane arsonate renal scan
DPA	Dual-photon absorptiometry
DSA	Digital subtraction angiography
DST	Dexamethasone suppression test

E

EBV	Epstein-Barr virus
ECG, EKG	Electrocardiogram
ECHO	Echocardiography
EEG	Electroencephalogram
EFS	Esophageal function studies
EGD	Esophagogastroduodenoscopy
EIA	Enzyme immunoassay
ELISA	Enzyme-linked immunosorbent assay
EMA	Endomysial antibody
EMG	Electromyography
ENG	Electroneurography
EP	Evoked potential
EPO	Erythropoietin
EPS	Electrophysiologic study
ER	Estrogen receptor
ERCP	Endoscopic retrograde cholangiopancreatography
ESR	Erythrocyte sedimentation rate
EUG	Excretory urography

F

FBS	Fasting blood sugar
FDPs	Fibrin degradation products
Fe	Iron
fFN	Fetal fibronectin
FIT	Fecal immunochemical test
%FPSA	Percent free prostate-specific antigen
FSH	Follicle-stimulating hormone
FSPs	Fibrin split products
FTA-ABS	Fluorescent treponemal antibody absorption test
FTI	Free thyroxine index
FUT	Fibrinogen uptake test
FVL	Factor V-Leiden

G

G-6-PD	Glucose-6-phosphate dehydrogenase
GAD ab	Glutamic acid decarboxylase antibody
GB series	Gallbladder series
GE reflux	Gastroesophageal reflux
GER scan	Gastroesophageal reflux scan
GGT	γ-Glutamyl transferase
GGTP	γ-Glutamyl transpeptidase
GH	Growth hormone
GHb, GHB	Glycosylated hemoglobin
GI series	Gastrointestinal series
GTT	Glucose tolerance test

H

HAA	Hepatitis-associated antigen
HAI	Hemagglutination inhibition
HAV	Hepatitis A virus
Hb, Hgb	Hemoglobin
HBcAb	Hepatitis B core antibody
HBcAg	Hepatitis B core antigen
HBV	Hepatitis B virus
HCG	Human chorionic gonadotropin
HCO_3	Bicarbonate
HCS	Human chorionic somatomammotropin
Hct	Hematocrit
Hcy	Homocysteine
HDL	High-density lipoprotein
5-HIAA	5-Hydroxyindoleacetic acid
HIDA	Hepatic iminodiacetic acid
HIV	Human immunodeficiency virus
HLA	Human lymphocyte antigen
HPL	Human placental lactogen
HPV	Human papillomavirus
HSV-2	Herpes simplex virus, type 2
HTLV	Human T-cell lymphotrophic virus

I

Ig	Immunoglobulin
IAA	Insulin autoantibody
ICA	Islet cell antibody
IFE	Immunofixation electrophoresis
IGF	Insulin-like growth factor
INR	International normalization ratio
ITT	Insulin tolerance test
IVC	Intravenous cholangiography
IV-GTT	Intravenous glucose tolerance test
IVP	Intravenous pyelography
IVU, IUG	Intravenous urography

K

K	Potassium
KS	Ketosteroid
KUB	Kidney, ureter, and bladder x-ray study

L

LAP	Leucine aminopeptidase
LATS	Long-acting thyroid-stimulator
LDH	Lactic dehydrogenase
LDL	Low-density lipoprotein
LE	Lupus erythematosus
LES	Lower esophageal sphincter
LFTs	Liver function tests
LH	Luteinizing hormone

LP	Lumbar puncture
Lp(a)	Lp(a) lipoprotein
L/S ratio	Lecithin/sphingomyelin ratio
LS spine	Lumbosacral spine

M

MCH	Mean corpuscular hemoglobin
MCHC	Mean corpuscular hemoglobin concentration
MCV	Mean corpuscular volume
M/E ratio	Myeloid/erythroid ratio
Mg	Magnesium
MPG	Mean plasma glucose
MPV	Mean platelet volume
MRA	Magnetic resonance angiography
MRI	Magnetic resonance imaging
MUGA	Multigated acquisition cardiac scan

N

Na	Sodium
NMR	Nuclear magnetic resonance
NMP22	Nuclear matrix protein 22
NST	Nonstress test
NTx	N-Telopeptide

O

OB	Occult blood
OCT	Oxytocin challenge test
OGTT	Oral glucose tolerance test
17-OHCS	17-Hydroxycorticosteroids
O&P	Ova and parasites
OPG	Oculoplethysmography

P

P	Phosphorus
PAB	Prealbumin
PAI-1	Plasminogen activator inhibitor-1
PAP	Prostatic acid phosphatase
PAPP	Pregnancy-associated plasma protein
Pb	Lead
Pco_2	Partial pressure of carbon dioxide
PET	Positron-emission tomography
PFTs	Pulmonary function tests
pH	Hydrogen ion concentration
PKU	Phenylketonuria
PMN	Polymorphonuclear (type of WBC)
PNH	Paroxysmal nocturnal hemoglobinuria
Po_2	Partial pressure of oxygen
PO_4	Phosphate
PPBS	Postprandial blood sugar
PPD	Purified protein derivative

PPG	Postprandial glucose
PR	Progesterone receptor
PRA	Plasma renin assay
PSA	Prostate-specific antigen
PSG	Polysomnography
PT	Prothrombin time
PTH	Parathormone, parathyroid hormone
PTC, PTCH	Percutaneous transhepatic cholangiography
PTT	Partial thromboplastin time
PYD	Pyridium

R

RAIU	Radioactive iodine uptake
RAST	Radioallergosorbent test
RBC	Red blood cell
RDW	Red cell distribution width
RF	Rheumatoid factor
RIA	Radioimmunoassay
RPR	Rapid plasma reagin test
RRA	Radioreceptor assay

S

S&A	Sugar and acetone
SACE	Serum angiotensin-converting enzyme
SARS	Severe acute respiratory syndrome
SBF	Small bowel follow-through
SER	Somatosensory evoked responses
SGOT	Serum glutamic oxaloacetic transaminase
SGPT	Serum glutamic pyruvic transaminase
SLE	Systemic lupus erythematosus
SPECT	Single-photon emission computed tomography
STS	Serologic test for syphilis

T

T_3	Triiodothyronine
T_4	Thyroxine
TBG	Thyroxine-binding globulin
TBII	Thyroid binding inhibitory immunoglobulin
TBPA	Thyroxine-binding prealbumin
TDM	Therapeutic drug monitoring
TEE	Transesophageal echocardiography
TGs	Triglycerides
TIBC	Total iron-binding capacity
TPI	Treponema pallidum immobilization
TRAP	Tartrate-resistant acid phosphatase
TRF	Thyrotropin releasing factor
TRH	Thyrotropin releasing hormone

T&S	Type and screen
TSH	Thyroid-stimulating hormone
TSI	Thyroid-stimulating immunoglobulin
TTE	Transthoracic echocardiography

U

UA	Urinalysis
UGI series	Upper gastrointestinal series
UPP	Urethral pressure profile
US	Ultrasound

V

VDRL	Venereal Disease Research Laboratory
VER	Visual evoked response
VLDL	Very-low-density lipoprotein
VMA	Vanillylmandelic acid
VPS	Ventilation/perfusion scanning

W

| WBC | White blood cell |
| WNL | Within normal limits |

Appendix D

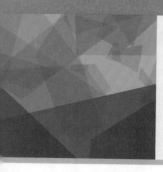

Index

Page numbers followed by *b* indicates boxes; *f* indicates illustrations, and *t* indicates tables.

H

T